a LANGE medical book

Pathophysiology of Disease:
An Introduction to Clinical Medicine

Eighth Edition

Edited by

Gary D. Hammer, MD, PhD
Millie Schembechler Professor of Adrenal Cancer
Director, Endocrine Oncology Program
Rogel Cancer Center
University of Michigan
Ann Arbor, Michigan

Stephen J. McPhee, MD
Professor of Medicine, Emeritus
Division of General Internal Medicine
Department of Medicine
University of California, San Francisco
San Francisco, California

New York   Chicago   San Francisco   Athens   London   Madrid
Mexico City   Milan   New Delhi   Singapore   Sydney   Toronto

1 2 3 4 5 6 7 8 9   DSS   23 22 21 20 19 18

ISBN 978-1-260-02650-4
MHID 1-260-02650-7
ISSN 1079-6185

Notice

Medicine is an ever-changing science. As new research and clinical experience broaden our knowledge, changes in treatment and drug therapy are required. The authors and the publisher of this work have checked with sources believed to be reliable in their efforts to provide information that is complete and generally in accord with the standards accepted at the time of publication. However, in view of the possibility of human error or changes in medical sciences, neither the authors nor the publisher nor any other party who has been involved in the preparation or publication of this work warrants that the information contained herein is in every respect accurate or complete, and they disclaim all responsibility for any errors or omissions or for the results obtained from use of the information contained in this work. Readers are encouraged to confirm the information contained herein with other sources. For example and in particular, readers are advised to check the product information sheet included in the package of each drug they plan to administer to be certain that the information contained in this work is accurate and that changes have not been made in the recommended dose or in the contraindications for administration. This recommendation is of particular importance in connection with new or infrequently used drugs.

This book was set in Minion Pro by Cenveo® Publisher Services.
The editors were Amanda Fielding and Harriet Lebowitz.
The production supervisor was Richard Ruzycka.
Project management was provided by Radhika Jolly.
Cover images:
Central nervous system (Shutterstock)
Legionella pneumophila (iStock)
Small intestine (iStock)
Tumor cells (iStock)

McGraw-Hill Education books are available at special quantity discounts to use as premiums and sales promotions or for use in corporate training programs. To contact a representative, please visit the Contact Us pages at www.mhprofessional.com.

Contents

Authors

Weiyun Z. Ai, PhD, MD
Assistant Clinical Professor of Medicine
Division of Hematology/Oncology
Helen Diller Family Comprehensive Cancer Center
University of California, San Francisco School of Medicine
San Francisco, California
weiyun.ai@ucsf.edu
Neoplasia

Gregory Barsh, MD, PhD
Professor of Genetics and Pediatrics, Emeritus
Stanford University School of Medicine
Stanford, California
gbarsh@stanford.edu
Genetic Disease

Karen C. Bloch, MD, MPH
Associate Professor of Medicine and Health Policy
Division of Infectious Diseases
Department of Medicine
Vanderbilt University School of Medicine
Nashville, Tennessee
karen.bloch@vanderbilt.edu
Infectious Diseases

Jennifer J. Chang, MD, AAHIVS
Fellow in HIV Medicine
David Geffen School of Medicine
at the University of California, Los Angeles
Los Angeles, California
jenniferjwchang@gmail.com
Disorders of the Immune System

Mark S. Chesnutt, MD
Professor of Medicine
Pulmonary & Critical Care Medicine
Department of Medicine and Dotter
Department of Interventional Radiology
Oregon Health & Science University
Director, Critical Care
VA Portland Health Care System
Portland, Oregon
chesnutm@ohsu.edu
Pulmonary Disease

Matthew A. Ciorba, MD
Associate Professor of Medicine
Director, Inflammatory Bowel Disease Program
Division of Biology & Biomedical Sciences
Division of Gastroenterology
Washington University School of Medicine
St. Louis, Missouri
mciorba@wustl.edu
Gastrointestinal Disease

Dru Claar, MD
House Officer, Internal Medicine (Pulmonary)
Pulmonary & Critical Care Medicine
University of Michigan Hospitals
Ann Arbor, Michigan
dclaar@umich.edu
Pulmonary Disease

Erika Darrah, PhD
Assistant Professor of Medicine
Division of Rheumatology
Department of Medicine
Johns Hopkins University School of Medicine
Baltimore, Maryland
edarrah1@jhmi.edu
Inflammatory Rheumatic Diseases

J. Ben Davoren, MD, PhD
Clinical Professor of Medicine
Associate Chief of Staff, Clinical Informatics
San Francisco Veterans Affairs Medical Center
Division of Hematology/Oncology
Department of Medicine
University of California, San Francisco School
of Medicine
San Francisco, California
ben.davoren@va.gov
Blood Disorders

Suzanne M. Donovan, MD, MPH
Clinical Professor of Medicine
Division of Infectious Diseases
Department of Medicine
David Geffen School of Medicine
at the University of California, Los Angeles
sdonovanmd@gmail.com
Disorders of the Immune System

Tobias Else, MD
Assistant Professor of Internal Medicine
Division of Metabolism, Endocrinology & Diabetes
Department of Internal Medicine
University of Michigan Medical School
Ann Arbor, Michigan
telse@umich.edu
*Disorders of the Adrenal Medulla, Disorders of the
Hypothalamus & Pituitary Gland, Disorders of the
Adrenal Cortex*

Nazanene H. Esfandiari, MD
Associate Professor of Internal Medicine
Division of Metabolism, Endocrinology & Diabetes
Department of Internal Medicine
University of Michigan Medical School
Ann Arbor, Michigan
nazanene@umich.edu
Thyroid Disease

Lauren Fishbein, MD, PhD
Assistant Professor of Medicine
Division of Endocrinology, Metabolism and Diabetes
University of Colorado School of Medicine
Aurora, Colorado
lauren.fishbein@ucdenver.edu
Disorders of the Adrenal Medulla

Christina T. Fiske, MD, MPH
Assistant Professor of Medicine
Division of Infectious Diseases
Department of Medicine
Vanderbilt University School of Medicine
Nashville, Tennessee
christina.fiske@vanderbilt.edu
Infectious Diseases

Mikkel Fode, MD, PhD
Department of Urology
Herlev & Gentofte Hospital
University of Copenhagen
Herlev, Denmark
mikkelfode@gmail.com
Disorders of the Male Reproductive Tract

Timothy L. Frankel, MD
Assistant Professor of Surgery
Department of Surgery
University of Michigan Medical School
Ann Arbor, Michigan
timofran@med.umich.edu
Disorders of the Exocrine Pancreas

Janet L. Funk, MD
Professor of Medicine
Division of Endocrinology
University of Arizona School of Medicine
Tucson, Arizona
jfunk@email.arizona.edu
Disorders of the Endocrine Pancreas

Allan C. Gelber, MD, MPH, PhD
Professor of Medicine
Division of Rheumatology
Department of Medicine
Johns Hopkins University School of Medicine
Baltimore, Maryland
agelber@jhmi.edu
Inflammatory Rheumatic Diseases

Gary D. Hammer, MD, PhD
Millie Schembechler Professor of Adrenal Cancer
Director, Endocrine Oncology Program
Rogel Cancer Center
University of Michigan
Ann Arbor, Michigan
ghammer@umich.edu
*Introduction, Disorders of the Hypothalamus & Pituitary
Gland, Disorders of the Adrenal Cortex*

Michael Heung, MD, MS
Associate Professor of Internal Medicine
Division of Nephrology
Department of Internal Medicine
University of Michigan Medical School
Ann Arbor, Michigan
mheung@umich.edu
Renal Disease

Gerald Hsu, MD, PhD
Assistant Clinical Professor of Medicine
Division of Hematology/Oncology
Department of Medicine
San Francisco Veterans Affairs Medical Center
University of California, San Francisco School
of Medicine
San Francisco, California
gerald.hsu@ucsf.edu
Blood Disorders

Erika B. Johnston-MacAnanny, MD
Attending Physician
Shady Grove Fertility Center
Women's Hospital 1602
Richmond, VA
Erika_Johnston2002@yahoo.com
Disorders of the Female Reproductive Tract

Mandana Khalili, MD, MAS
Professor of Medicine
Director of Clinical Hepatology
Zuckerberg San Francisco General Hospital
Department of Medicine
University of California San Francisco School of Medicine
San Francisco, California
mandana.khalili@ucsf.edu
Liver Disease

Jeffrey L. Kishiyama, MD
Associate Clinical Professor
Division of Allergy and Immunology
Department of Medicine
University of California, San Francisco School of Medicine
San Francisco, California
Disorders of the Immune System

Fred M. Kusumoto, MD, FACC
Professor of Medicine
Division of Cardiovascular Diseases
Department of Medicine
Mayo Clinic Jacksonville
Jacksonville, Florida
kusumoto.fred@mayo.edu
Cardiovascular Disorders: Heart Disease

Yeong S. Kwok, MD
Clinical Assistant Professor
Division of General Internal Medicine
Department of Internal Medicine
University of Michigan Medical School
Ann Arbor, Michigan
ykwok@med.umich.edu
Case Studies, Case Study Answers

Stuart M. Levine, MD, FACP
President & Chief Medical Officer
MedStar Harbor Hospital
Senior Vice President
MedStar Health
Baltimore, Maryland
stuart.m.levine@medstar.net
Inflammatory Rheumatic Diseases

Catherine Lomen-Hoerth, MD, PhD
Professor of Neurology
ALS Research Center at UCSF
Department of Neurology
University of California, San Francisco School of Medicine
San Francisco, California
catherine.lomen-hoerth@ucsf.edu
Nervous System Disorders

Timothy H. McCalmont, MD
Professor of Pathology, Dermatology, and Oral Medicine
Departments of Pathology and Dermatology
University of California, San Francisco
San Francisco, California
tim.mccalmont@ucsf.edu
Diseases of the Skin

Stephen J. McPhee, MD
Professor of Medicine, Emeritus
Division of General Internal Medicine
Department of Medicine
University of California, San Francisco School of Medicine
San Francisco, California
stephen.mcphee@ucsf.edu
Introduction, Thyroid Disease

Jason C. Mills, MD, PhD, AGAF
Professor of Medicine
Division of Gastroenterology
Departments of Medicine, Pathology & Immunology, Developmental Biology
Washington University School of Medicine
St. Louis, Missouri
jmills@wustl.edu
Gastrointestinal Disease

Igor Mitrovic, MD
Jack and DeLoris Lange Endowed Chair in Systems Physiology I
Professor of Physiology
Department of Physiology
University of California, San Francisco School of Medicine
San Francisco, California
igor.mitrovic@ucsf.edu
Cardiovascular Disorders: Vascular Disease

Mark M. Moasser, MD
Professor of Medicine
Division of Hematology/Oncology
Department of Medicine
Helen Diller Family Comprehensive Cancer Center
University of California, San Francisco School of Medicine
San Francisco, California
mark.moasser@ucsf.edu
Neoplasia

Nizar A. Mukhtar, MD
Transplant Hepatologist
Director, Liver Tumor Board
Liver Center and Organ Transplant Program
Swedish Medical Center
Seattle, Washington
nizar.mukhtar@swedish.org
Liver Disease

Dana A. Ohl, MD
Professor of Urology
Chief, Division of Andrology and Urologic Health
Department of Urology
University of Michigan Medical School
Ann Arbor, Michigan
daohl@umich.edu
Disorders of the Male Reproductive Tract

Bansari G. Patel, MD
Assistant Professor of Obstetrics and Gynecology–
    Reproductive Medicine
Department of Obstetrics and Gynecology–Reproductive
    Medicine
Wake Forest Baptist Medical Center
Wake Forest University School of Medicine
Winston-Salem, North Carolina
bgpatel@wakehealth.edu
Disorders of the Female Reproductive Tract

Rachel L. Perlman, MD
Associate Professor of Internal Medicine
Division of Nephrology
Department of Internal Medicine
University of Michigan Medical School
Ann Arbor, Michigan
rperlman@umich.edu
Renal Disease

Laura B. Pincus, MD
Associate Professor of Dermatology
Departments of Dermatopathology and Oral Pathology
University of California, San Francisco School
    of Medicine
San Francisco, California
laura.pincus@ucsf.edu
Diseases of the Skin

Thomas J. Prendergast, MD
Professor of Medicine
Section Chief, Pulmonary & Critical Care Medicine
Portland Veterans Affairs Medical Center
Oregon Health & Science University
Portland, Oregon
thomas.prendergast@va.gov
Pulmonary Disease

Shane C. Quinonez, MD
Clinical Assistant Professor of Pediatrics and Medical
    Genetics
Co-Director, Biochemical Laboratory, Michigan Medical
    Genetics Laboratory
University of Michigan Medical School
Ann Arbor, Michigan
squinon@med.umich.edu
Genetic Disease

Vikram G. Shakkottai, MD, PhD
Associate Professor of Neurology and Molecular &
    Integrative Physiology
University of Michigan Medical School
Ann Arbor, Michigan
vikramsh@umich.edu
Nervous System Disorders

Dolores M. Shoback, MD
Professor of Medicine
Endocrine Research Unit
San Francisco Veterans Affairs Medical Center
Department of Medicine
University of California, San Francisco School
    of Medicine
San Francisco, California
dolores.shoback@ucsf.edu
*Disorders of the Parathyroids & Calcium and
    Phosphorus Metabolism*

Thomas H. Sisson, MD
Professor of Pulmonary & Critical Care Medicine
Department of Internal Medicine
University of Michigan Medical School
Ann Arbor, Michigan
tsisson@med.umich.edu
Pulmonary Disease

Jens Sønksen, MD, PhD
Professor of Urology
Department of Urology
Herlev & Gentofte Hospital
University of Copenhagen
Herlev, Denmark
jens@sonksen.dk
Disorders of the Male Reproductive Tract

Christopher J. Sonnenday, MD, MHS
Associate Professor of Surgery
Department of Surgery
University of Michigan Medical School
Ann Arbor, Michigan
csonnend@umich.edu
Disorders of the Exocrine Pancreas

Robert N. Taylor, MD, PhD
Professor, Reproductive Endocrinology & Infertility
Department of Obstetrics & Gynecology
University of Utah School of Medicine
Salt Lake City, Utah
rob.taylor@hsc.utah.edu
Disorders of the Female Reproductive Tract

Sunny Wang, MD
Assistant Clinical Professor of Medicine
Division of Hematology/Oncology
University of California
San Francisco VA Medical Center
San Francisco, California
sunny.wang@ucsf.edu
Blood Disorders

Preface

Goal and Audience

The goal of *Pathophysiology of Disease: An Introduction to Clinical Medicine*, as outlined in the introductory chapter (Chapter 1), is to introduce students to clinical medicine by reviewing the pathophysiologic basis of the symptoms and signs of various common diseases.

The book has proved useful as a text for both Pathophysiology and Introduction to Clinical Medicine courses in medical schools, and it has been popular in similar courses in nursing schools, physician assistants' training programs, and other allied health programs. It is valuable to students early in their medical school years by highlighting the clinical relevance of their basic science courses, and in preparation for their USMLE Step 1 examinations. The book is also helpful to students engaged in their internal medicine and surgery clerkships, and to house officers as an up-to-date summary of relevant physiology and a source of key references. Practitioners (both general internists and specialists who provide generalist care) will find it beneficial as a refresher text, designed to update their knowledge of the mechanisms underlying 132 commonly encountered diseases and disorders. Nurses, nurse-practitioners, physician assistants, and other allied health practitioners have found that its concise format and broad scope facilitate their understanding of these basic disease entities.

Pathophysiology of Disease has been widely adopted in the United States, Canada, and the United Kingdom, and it has been translated into Spanish, Italian, Chinese, Japanese, Greek, and Turkish. Both the text and its Case Study Questions and Answers are also available online at accessmedicine.mhmedical.com, the online version of McGraw-Hill's many medical textbooks (search under "Books, Library, Basic Science" for "Pathophysiology," listed alphabetically).

New Features for This Edition

In preparation for this eighth edition, the editors and authors reviewed the entire book. There have been many text revisions aimed at updating information, improving clarity, and eliminating minor errors. With emphasis on recent pertinent reviews, references have been entirely updated, as have figures and tables. "Checkpoints," collections of review questions, continue to appear throughout the chapters and have been revised.

Examples of Substantive New Content Found in This Eighth Edition

- Update on components and physiology of normal immunity
- Most recent surveillance case definition for HIV infection
- Explication of the concepts of innate immunity and pathogen-associated molecular patterns
- Totally revised chapter on neoplasia, including 19 new figures and 4 new tables
- New figure illustrating iron transport and regulation in the duodenal enterocyte
- New chapter section on urticaria (perivascular dermatitis)
- New chapter section on various forms of spinocerebellar ataxia
- Clarification in text and figures of regional alterations in the overall distribution of ventilation and perfusion referred to as $\dot{V}/\dot{Q}$ mismatch, including concepts of anatomic versus alveolar (wasted ventilation) dead space and right-to-left shunt
- Update on genetic factors implicated in asthma risk, as well as allergic versus nonallergic asthma
- Newly rewritten section on idiopathic pulmonary fibrosis as a prototypic restrictive (interstitial) lung disease
- Extensive revision of sections on pulmonary edema, adult respiratory distress syndrome (ARDS), and pulmonary venous thromboembolism
- Expanded material on paragangliomas
- New figures on mechanisms leading to nonalcoholic fatty liver disease and to hepatic steatosis
- New table summarizing adverse prognostic signs in acute pancreatitis derived from the Acute Pancreatitis Classification Working Group's 2012 classification, a revision of the Atlanta international consensus classification and definitions of acute pancreatitis
- New table summarizing genetic syndromes associated with pancreatic cancer

- New table summarizing the prevalence of various causes of end-stage renal disease for U.S. Medicare recipients in the 2016 U.S. Renal Data System
- Revised flowchart summarizing the pathogenesis of bone diseases in chronic kidney disease
- Updated information on familial hypocalcuric hypercalcemia, malignant hypercalcemia, autosomal dominant hypocalcemia, and the autoimmune polyendocrine failure syndromes
- The American Diabetes Association's new diagnosis and etiologic classification of diabetes mellitus
- New figure illustrating the amino acid sequence and covalent structure of human proinsulin
- New schematic diagram of glucose-stimulated insulin release from the pancreatic β cell
- New figure showing how pancreatic islet cell secretions of glucagon (from α cells) and insulin (from β cells), which are reciprocally regulated by glucose, play key roles in maintaining glucose homeostasis
- Diagram demonstrating stages in the development of type 1 diabetes mellitus with the appearance of β-cell autoantibodies, followed by dysglycemia, insulinopenia, and then frank hyperglycemia
- Review of mechanisms of the newest classes of pharmacologic agents approved for type 2 diabetes mellitus
- New figure illustrating modifiable cardiovascular risk factors in individuals with diabetes
- New figure illustrating the control of energy homeostasis by arcuate nucleus neurons, both stimulatory and inhibitory neurons with regard to food intake
- Updated information on fine-needle aspiration biopsy of thyroid nodules
- Update on thyroid disorders in pregnancy
- New schematic drawing of the sequence of changes that occur in the alveolar secretory units and duct system of the female breast before, during, and after pregnancy and lactation
- Update of indicators of mild to moderate versus severe preeclampsia-eclampsia
- Incorporation of new International Federation of Gynecology and Obstetrics classification system for pathogenesis of abnormal uterine bleeding
- Update to pathogenesis and pathophysiology of inflammatory myopathies and rheumatoid arthritis
- New chapter section on spondyloarthropathies, including ankylosing spondylitis, reactive arthritis, inflammatory bowel disease–associated arthritis, and psoriatic arthritis
- Updated references throughout the text, including articles mainly from 2015, 2016, and 2017
- Revised and updated figure citations throughout the text

Case Study Questions and Answers

Each chapter ends with a collection of Case Studies. These clinical problems give readers an opportunity to test their understanding of the pathophysiology of each clinical entity discussed and to apply their knowledge to exemplar clinical situations. In this eighth edition, Yeong S. Kwok, MD, of the University of Michigan, has added an additional 12 Case Studies with questions, bringing the total number to 132, or one for each of the clinical entities discussed in the book's 24 chapters. New Case Study topics include:

- Down syndrome as a result of a balanced robertsonian translocation
- Chronic granulomatous disease
- Malignant hypercalcemia
- Cerebellar ataxia
- Urticaria
- Ulcerative colitis
- Type 1 diabetes mellitus
- Subclinical hypothyroidism
- Subclinical hyperthyroidism
- Amenorrhea caused by polycystic ovary syndrome
- Abnormal vaginal bleeding as a result of endometrial cancer
- Spondyloarthropathy as a result of ankylosing spondylitis

As before, detailed analyses of the Cases appear in Chapter 25: Case Study Answers. There, Dr. Kwok has updated the Answers to the existing 120 Case Study Questions to reflect the changes made by chapter authors in their revisions, and he has added Answers to the Questions for the 12 new Case Studies.

Changes in Authors

With this eighth edition, the authorship of many chapters has evolved and transitioned—this should not be surprising given the book's multiple editions since it was first published in 1992 and given the transition in location of the book's lead editor from the University of California, San Francisco (Stephen J. McPhee, MD), to the University of Michigan (Gary Hammer, MD, PhD). The editors wish to welcome aboard the following new contributors who are joining the book's authors and to thank the following past contributors who are now departing the book:

- Shane C. Quinonez, MD, of the University of Michigan, has taken over the current revision of Chapter 2, *Genetic Disease*, from Greg Barsh, MD, PhD, of Stanford University; Dr. Barsh, who has been this chapter's author since the book's first edition, will continue as a coauthor for this eighth edition only
- Jennifer J. Chang, MD, and Suzanne M. Donovan, MD, MPH, joined Jeffrey L. Kishiyama, MD, in revising Chapter 3, *Disorders of the Immune System*. Sadly, Dr. Kishiyama died during the final production process for this edition; please see the **In Memoriam** below
- Christina T. Fiske, MD, MPH, of Vanderbilt University, has joined Karen C. Bloch, MD, MPH, in revising Chapter 4, *Infectious Diseases*
- Weiyun Z. Ai, PhD, MD, of UCSF, has assisted chapter author Mark M. Moasser, MD, by revising the hematologic disorders section of Chapter 5, *Neoplasia*

- J. Ben Davoren, MD, PhD, of UCSF, has replaced Sunny Wang, MD, with Gerald Hsu, MD, PhD, as coauthor of Chapter 6, *Blood Disorders*; we would like to thank Dr. Wang for her revisions for the sixth and seventh editions
- Vikram G. Shakkottai, MD, PhD, of the University of Michigan, has taken over the current revision of Chapter 7, *Nervous System Disorders*, from Catherine Lomen-Hoerth, MD, PhD, of UCSF; Dr. Lomen-Hoerth will continue only once more as coauthor for this eighth edition
- Laura B. Pincus, MD, of UCSF, has replaced Melissa M. Meier, MD, as the coauthor, with Timothy H. McCalmont, MD, of Chapter 8, *Diseases of the Skin*; we would like to thank Dr. Meier for her revisions for the seventh edition
- Thomas H. Sisson, MD, and Dru Claar, MD, of the University of Michigan, have taken over the current revision of Chapter 9, *Pulmonary Disease*, from Mark S. Chesnutt, MD, and Thomas J. Prendergast, MD, of Oregon Health and Sciences University; Drs. Chesnutt and Prendergast will continue as coauthors for this eighth edition only. We would like to acknowledge Dr. Prendergast for his role in coauthoring the original chapter in the book's first edition and for his revisions for the next seven editions, and Dr. Chesnutt for his assistance with the seventh and eighth editions
- Lauren Fishbein, MD, PhD, of the University of Colorado, is now coauthor of Chapter 12, *Disorders of the Adrenal Medulla*, with Tobias Else, MD, of the University of Michigan; after the sixth and seventh editions, Gary Hammer, MD, PhD, has now "retired" from coauthorship of this chapter
- Matthew A. Ciorba, MD, of the Washington University at St. Louis, has now joined his colleague Jason C. Mills, MD, PhD, as coauthor of Chapter 13, *Gastrointestinal Disease*; we are thankful for the past contributions of Thaddeus S. Stappenbeck, MD, PhD, to its revision for the sixth and seventh editions
- Mandana Khalili, MD, MAS, of UCSF, is now working with Nizar A. Mukhtar, MD, of Seattle's Swedish Medical Center in producing the current revision of Chapter 14, *Liver Disease*; we are grateful to Blaire Burman, MD, of UCSF for assistance with the seventh edition revision
- Timothy L. Frankel, MD, has now joined his University of Michigan colleague Christopher J. Sonnenday, MD, MHS, in producing the current revision of Chapter 15, *Disorders of the Exocrine Pancreas*
- Joachim H. Ix, MD, has now "retired" from coauthorship of Chapter 16, *Renal Disease*, which is now coauthored by Rachel Leah Pearlman, MD, and Michael Heung, MD, MS; we thank Dr. Ix for his revisions in the fifth, sixth, and seventh editions
- Deborah E. Sellmeyer, MD, has now "retired" from coauthorship with Dolores M. Shoback, MD, of Chapter 17, *Disorders of the Parathyroids & Calcium and Phosphorus Metabolism*; we thank Dr. Sellmeyer for her contributions to the fifth, sixth, and seventh editions

- Nazanene H. Esfandiari, MD, of the University of Michigan, has replaced Douglas C. Bauer, MD, of UCSF, as the coauthor, with Stephen J. McPhee, MD, of Chapter 20, *Thyroid Disease*; we thank Dr. Bauer for his revisions for the second through seventh editions and note that Dr. McPhee, who has been this chapter's author or coauthor for the prior seven editions, will continue as coauthor for this eighth edition only
- Bansari G. Patel, MD, at Wake Forest University, now joins Erika B. Johnston-MacAnanny, MD, now in Richmond, VA, and Robert N. Taylor, MD, PhD, now at the University of Utah, as a coauthor of Chapter 22: *Disorders of the Female Reproductive Tract*
- Mikkel Fode, MD, PhD, and Jens Sønksen, MD, PhD, of Herlev & Gentofte Hospital of the University of Copenhagen in Herlev, Denmark, and Dana A. Ohl, MD, of the University of Michigan, have assumed authorship of Chapter 23, *Disorders of the Male Reproductive Tract*; after seven editions, Stephen J. McPhee, MD, has now "retired" from authorship or coauthorship of this chapter
- Allan C. Gelber, MD, MPH, PhD, and Stuart M. Levine, MD, have been joined by a new coauthor, Erika Darrah, PhD, of Johns Hopkins University, for Chapter 24, *Inflammatory Rheumatic Diseases*; the chapter authors and textbook editors gratefully acknowledge the intellectual contributions of Antony Rosen, MB, ChB, BSc (Hons), to the content of this chapter in the book's third through seventh editions

With these transitions, the content of more than two-thirds of this eighth edition has greatly benefited from the new contributors' viewpoints and inputs (for instance, by including 36 new illustrations in the book's attractive four-color design and layout).

In Memoriam: Jeffrey L. Kishiyama, MD

We are saddened to report that, following submission of the revision of Chapter 3, *Disorders of the Immune System*, for the eighth edition of *Pathophysiology of Disease*, its lead author, Jeffrey L. Kishiyama, MD, died.

A graduate of Stanford University with a degree in biology and economics, Dr. Kishiyama received his MD from Creighton University School of Medicine. He did his internal medicine residency at Northwestern University, after which he completed a fellowship in allergy and immunology at the University of California, San Francisco (UCSF). Thereafter, Dr. Kishiyama spent many years on the faculties of both UCSF and Stanford University, where he served in a variety of positions, including director of the UCSF Clinical Immunology Laboratory and director of the UCSF Stanford Allergy and Immunology training program. In addition to his academic positions, Dr. Kishiyama maintained an active clinical practice, treating patients at Allergy Asthma Associates of Northern California.

Jeff first joined the authors of *Pathophysiology of Disease* as a coauthor with Richard Shames, MD, for its third and fourth editions, published in 2000 and 2003. Thereafter, Jeff continued as a solo author for the fifth edition in 2006, the sixth edition in 2010, and the seventh edition in 2014. For the eighth edition, he recruited coauthors Jennifer J. Chang, MD, Fellow in HIV Medicine, and Suzanne M. Donovan, MD, MPH, Clinical Professor of Medicine, Division of Infectious Diseases, of the UCLA School of Medicine.

Jeff was a superb contributor to *Pathophysiology*, helping to make understandable the increasingly complex field of immunology. Through the years, our readers, particularly our student readers, have been most grateful for his gift in this regard. As one small example, Jeff more than tripled the size of the introductory table of acronyms and abbreviations used throughout both Chapter 3 and the entire book.

We will greatly miss having Jeff as an outstanding (and timely!) contributor to our wonderful book.

With the publication of this eighth edition, the editors want to extend special thanks, not only to the contributors old and new, but also to the students and colleagues who have offered helpful comments and criticisms for each of the previous editions. The authors and editors continue to welcome comments and recommendations for future editions, in writing or via email. The editors' and authors' institutional and email addresses are given in the Authors section.

Gary D. Hammer, MD, PhD
Ann Arbor, Michigan

Stephen J. McPhee, MD
San Francisco, California

Introduction

Gary D. Hammer, MD, PhD, &
Stephen J. McPhee, MD

A man cannot become a competent surgeon without the full knowledge of human anatomy and physiology, and the physician without physiology and chemistry flounders along in an aimless fashion, never able to gain any accurate conception of disease, practicing a sort of popgun pharmacy, hitting now the malady and again the patient, he himself not knowing which.

Sir William Osler (1849–1919)

Osler expresses particularly well the relationship between the basic sciences and clinical medicine in the aphorism cited above. Indeed, ever since the Middle Ages, wise physicians and others concerned with the sick and their care have realized that most human disease may be understood in a real sense as disordered physiology (pathophysiology). Something (eg, a mutation [pathogenic variant] in a gene or invasion by a bacterial organism) triggers an illness, and the body reacts with molecular, cellular, and systemic responses that are the symptoms and signs of the disease. Therefore, with proper knowledge of the body's normal structure and function, and the ways in which these can become disordered, comes the ability to understand disease and to design rational and effective treatment. In addition, of course, the relationship between pathophysiology and disease is a two-way street. Diseases may be viewed as "experiments of nature" that may uncover previously unknown or unappreciated physiologic mechanisms, and the investigation of these physiologic mechanisms in normal individuals advances our fundamental biomedical knowledge. Therefore, it is important that students understand normal structure and function, and how they can become disordered, and apply this knowledge to disease.

The aim of this book is to provide students with an introduction to clinical medicine through the study of diseases as manifestations of pathophysiology. The authors (all experts in their respective fields) have provided a brief review of the relevant normal structure and function of each system in the body, followed by a description of the underlying pathophysiologic mechanisms that underlie several common diseases related to that system. With this approach comes an explication of the symptoms and signs of each disease state and an essential framework for the student's later mastery of treatment strategies. Several subject areas that are not restricted to a single body system are also covered (eg, neoplasia and infectious disease), but the same approach is used in these instances as well. For the most part, diagnosis and treatment are not covered here but are left for later, more detailed study and textbooks such as the annually updated *Current Medical Diagnosis & Treatment.* No attempt is made here to be comprehensive or complete; the pathophysiology section of each chapter discusses one to five relevant clinical entities, based either on their frequency (eg, coronary artery disease and hypertension) or on their importance to understanding how physiologic systems may become disordered (eg, fragile X mental retardation or pheochromocytoma). The aim is to introduce students to diseases as manifestations of disordered function and to start them thinking about the related symptoms and signs in terms of their pathophysiologic basis.

This is the eighth edition of this basic science textbook, first published in 1992. It has grown from 20 to 25 chapters, with the number of clinical entities discussed increasing and the number of case study problems increasing gradually from 38 when debuted in the third edition, to 89 in the fourth and fifth editions, to 111 in the sixth, to 120 in the seventh, and now to 132 in this eighth edition. In addition, the authorship of chapters has gradually transitioned, with 18 new authors or co-authors in this eighth edition alone (compared to the seventh edition). Finally, with the rapid expansion in our understanding of the genetic and genomic origin of many pathophysiologic entities, the amount of content devoted to this particular disease mechanism has greatly increased. In this new edition, for example, a revised Table 15–9 gives a much longer listing of the genetic syndromes associated with pancreatic cancer. And a newly rewritten Chapter 5 provides a detailed explanation of the genetic and genomic origins of neoplastic disorders—including several types of epithelial neoplasms (carcinomas); mesenchymal, neuroendocrine, and germ cell neoplasms (neuroendocrine tumors, testicular germ cell cancers, and sarcomas); and hematologic neoplasms (lymphomas and acute and chronic leukemias).

Genetic Disease

Shane C. Quinonez, MD, &
Gregory Barsh, MD, PhD

Mechanisms of cellular and tissue dysfunction in genetic diseases are as varied as the organs they affect. To some extent, these mechanisms are similar to those that occur in non-heritable disorders. For example, a fracture resulting from decreased bone density in osteoporosis heals in much the same way as one caused by a defective collagen gene in osteogenesis imperfecta, and the response to coronary atherosclerosis in most individuals does not depend on whether they have inherited a defective low-density lipoprotein (LDL) receptor. Thus, the pathophysiologic principles that distinguish genetic disease focus not so much on the affected organ system as on the mechanisms of genetic and genomic changes, inheritance, and molecular pathways from genotype to phenotype.

This chapter begins with a discussion of the terminology used to describe inherited conditions, the prevalence of genetic disease, and some major principles and considerations in medical genetics. Important terms and key words used throughout the chapter are defined in Table 2–1.

Next, a group of disorders caused by pathogenic variants (formerly termed "mutations") in collagen genes is discussed (ie, **osteogenesis imperfecta**). Although osteogenesis imperfecta is often considered a single entity, different pathogenic variants and different genes subject to alteration lead to a wide spectrum of clinical phenotypes. The different types of osteogenesis imperfecta exhibit typical patterns of autosomal dominant or autosomal recessive inheritance and are, therefore, examples of so-called **mendelian conditions**. To show how environmental factors can influence the relationship between genotype and phenotype, another mendelian condition, **phenylketonuria**, is discussed. This serves as a paradigm for newborn screening

programs and for treatment of genetic disease. Several genetic conditions have been found to depend not only on the gene being inherited but also on the phenotype or the sex of the parent. As an example of a condition that exhibits non-autosomal inheritance, **fragile X–associated mental retardation syndrome** is discussed. This syndrome not only is the most common inherited cause of mental retardation but also illustrates how different types of pathogenic variants can explain the perplexing phenomenon of **genetic anticipation**, in which the severity of a mendelian syndrome appears to progress with every generation of inheritance. Another group of disorders that depend on the phenotype and sex of the parent consists of those that affect the mitochondrial genome. As examples, **Leber hereditary optic neuropathy (LHON)** and **myoclonic epilepsy with ragged red fibers (MERRF)** are considered. These illustrate the principles of mitochondrial inheritance and its pathophysiology. **Aneuploidy** is discussed as one of the most common causes of human genetic disorders that does not affect DNA structure but instead alters the normal chromosome content per cell. The example that is considered, **Down syndrome**, has had a major impact on reproductive medicine and reproductive decision making and serves to illustrate general principles that apply to many aneuploid conditions. Finally, this chapter considers how genome sequences and sequencing are improving our understanding of pathophysiology for many diseases. With the completion of the annotation of the human genome and technological advances that allow individual genomes to be sequenced rapidly and inexpensively, prospects are at hand to identify genetic components of any human phenotype and to provide medical care that is truly personalized.

UNIQUE PATHOPHYSIOLOGIC ASPECTS OF GENETIC DISEASES

Although the phenotypes of genetic diseases are diverse, their causes are not. The primary cause of any genetic disease is a change in the sequence or cellular content of DNA that

ultimately deranges gene expression. Most genetic diseases are caused by an alteration in DNA sequence that alters the synthesis of a single gene product. However, some genetic

TABLE 2–1   Glossary of terms and keywords.

Term	Definition
Acrocentric	Refers to the terminal location of the centromere on chromosomes 13, 14, 15, 21, and 22.
Allelic heterogeneity	The situation in which multiple alleles at a single locus can produce one or more disease phenotypes.
Amorphic	Refers to pathogenic variants that cause a complete loss of function for the respective gene and therefore yield the same phenotype as a complete gene deletion.
Aneuploidy	A general term used to denote any unbalanced chromosome complement.
Antimorphic	Refers to pathogenic variants that, when present in heterozygous form opposite a nonmutant allele, will result in a phenotype similar to homozygosity for loss-of-function alleles.
Ascertainment bias	The situation in which individuals or families in a genetic study are not representative of the general population because of the way in which they are identified.
Autosomal	Located on chromosomes 1–22 rather than X or Y.
CpG island	A segment of DNA that contains a relatively high density of 5′-CG-3′ dinucleotides. Such segments are frequently unmethylated and located close to ubiquitously expressed genes.
Dictyotene	The end of prophase during female meiosis I in which fetal oocytes are arrested prior to ovulation.
Dominant	A pattern of inheritance or mechanism of gene action in which the effects of a variant allele can be observed in the presence of a nonmutant allele.
Dominant negative	A type of pathophysiologic mechanism that occurs when a mutant allele interferes with the normal function of the nonmutant gene product.
Dosage compensation	Mechanism by which a difference in gene dosage between two cells is equalized. For XX cells in mammals, decreased expression from one of the two X chromosomes results in a concentration of gene product similar to an XY cell.
End-product deficiency	A pathologic mechanism in which absence or reduction in the product of a particular enzymatic reaction leads to disease.
Epigenetic	Refers to a phenotypic effect that is heritable, through somatic cell division and/or across organismal generations, but that does not depend on variation in DNA sequence. Instead, epigenetic inheritance is associated with alterations in chromatin structure such as DNA methylation or histone modification that can be transmitted during cell division.
Expressivity	The extent to which a variant genotype affects phenotype, including the tissues that are affected, and the severity of those effects.
Fitness	The effect of a variant allele on an individual's ability to produce offspring.
Founder effect	One of several possible explanations for an unexpectedly high frequency of a deleterious gene in a population. If the population was founded by a small ancestral group, it may have, by chance, contained a large number of carriers for the deleterious gene.
Gamete	The egg or sperm cell that represents a potential reproductive contribution to the next generation. Gametes have undergone meiosis and so contain half the normal number of chromosomes found in zygotic cells.
Gene dosage	The principle that the amount of product expressed for a particular gene is proportionate to the number of gene copies present per cell.
Genetic anticipation	A clinical phenomenon in which the phenotype observed in individuals carrying a deleterious gene appears more severe in successive generations. Possible explanations include ascertainment bias or a multistep mutational mechanism such as expansion of triplet repeats.
Haplotype	A set of closely linked DNA sequence variants on a single chromosome.
Hemizygous	A term referring to the presence of only one allele at a locus, either because the other allele is deleted or because it is normally not present; eg, X-linked genes in males.
Heterochromatin	One of two alternative forms of chromosomal material (the other is euchromatin) in which chromosomal DNA is highly condensed and, usually, devoid of genes that are actively transcribed.
Heteroplasmy	The mixture of abnormal and normal mitochondrial DNA molecules in a single cell.

(continued)

TABLE 2–1   Glossary of terms and keywords. (continued)

Term	Definition
Heterozygote advantage	One way to explain an unexpectedly high frequency of a recessively inherited pathogenic variant in a particular population. During recent evolution, carriers (ie, heterozygotes) are postulated to have had a higher fitness than homozygous wild-type individuals.
Heterozygous	Having two alleles at the same locus that are different.
Homozygous	Having two alleles at the same locus that are the same.
Hypermorphic	Refers to a variant that has an effect similar to increasing the number of normal gene copies per cell.
Hypomorphic	Refers to a variant that reduces but does not eliminate the activity of a particular gene product.
Imprinting	Most commonly, the process whereby expression of a gene depends on whether it was inherited from the mother or the father.
Linkage disequilibrium	A condition in which certain combinations of closely linked alleles, or haplotypes, are present in a population at frequencies not predicted by their individual allele frequencies.
Locus heterogeneity	A situation in which pathogenic variants of different genes produce similar or identical phenotypes. Also referred to as genetic heterogeneity.
Mendelian	A form of inheritance that obeys the "laws" or principles of heredity postulated by Gregor Mendel, ie, segregation, independent assortment and dominance; clinically, these are commonly expressed as autosomal dominant, autosomal recessive, X-linked dominant, or X-linked recessive.
Monosomy	A reduction in zygotic cells from two to one in the number of copies for a particular chromosomal segment or chromosome.
Mosaicism	A situation in which a genetic alteration is present in some but not all of the cells of a single individual. In germline or gonadal mosaicism, the alteration is present in germ cells but not somatic cells. In somatic mosaicism, the genetic alteration is present in some but not all of the somatic cells (and is generally not present in the germ cells).
Neomorphic	Refers to a variant that imparts a novel function to its gene product and consequently results in a phenotype distinct from an alteration in gene dosage.
Nondisjunction	Failure of two homologous chromosomes to separate, or disjoin, at metaphase of meiosis I, or the failure of two sister chromatids to disjoin at metaphase of meiosis II or mitosis.
Penetrance	In a single individual of a variant genotype, penetrance refers to whether the variant genotype can be inferred based on defined phenotypic criteria. In a population, reduced penetrance refers to the rate at which individuals of a variant genotype cannot be recognized according to specific phenotypic criteria.
Phenotypic heterogeneity	The situation that occurs when pathogenic variants of a single gene produce multiple different phenotypes.
Postzygotic	A mutational event that occurs after fertilization and that commonly gives rise to mosaicism.
Premutation	A genetic change that does not result in a phenotype itself but has a high probability of developing a second alteration—a fully pathogenic variant/full mutation—that does cause a phenotype.
Primordial germ cell	The group of cells set aside early in development that go on to give rise to gametes.
Recessive	A pattern of inheritance or mechanism of gene action in which a particular mutant allele harboring a pathogenic variant causes a phenotype only in the absence of a normal allele. Thus, for autosomal conditions, the variant or disease phenotype is manifest when two copies of the allele harboring a pathogenic variant are present. For X-linked conditions, the variant or disease phenotype is manifest in cells, tissues, or individuals in which the normal allele is either inactivated (a heterozygous female) or not present (a hemizygous male).
Robertsonian translocation	A type of translocation in which two acrocentric chromosomes are fused together with a single functional centromere. A carrier of a robertsonian translocation with 45 chromosomes has a normal amount of chromosomal material and is said to be euploid.
SNP	Single nucleotide polymorphism—one of the most common types of genetic variation. There are approximately 1 million common SNPs in the human genome (those that exist at a frequency >1%), and billions of rare single-nucleotide variants (at a frequency >0.001%). Most do not affect protein structure, but the common SNPs may serve as valuable markers for determining the effect of genetic variation on complex and common diseases and disorders such as diabetes, heart disease, hypertension, and obesity.
Structural variant	A deletion, insertion, or more complex rearrangement, usually caused by recombination between repetitive elements. Also referred to as "copy number variant" (CNV) and the most common type of genomic variation. Most structural variants involve deletions or insertions that are relatively small (<10 kb) and do not cause any clinical phenotype. Larger structural variants (>100 kb) are increasingly likely to have clinical effects.

(continued)

TABLE 2–1   Glossary of terms and keywords. (continued)

Term	Definition
Substrate accumulation	A pathogenetic mechanism in which deficiency of a particular enzyme causes disease because the substrate of that enzyme accumulates in tissue or blood.
Triplet repeat	A three-nucleotide sequence that is tandemly repeated many times; ie, $(XYZ)_n$. Alterations in length of such simple types of repeats (dinucleotide and tetranucleotide as well) occur much more frequently than most other kinds of pathogenic variants; in addition, alteration in the length of trinucleotide repeats is the molecular basis for several heritable disorders.
Trisomy	An abnormal situation in which there are three, instead of two, copies of a chromosomal segment or chromosome per cell.
Variant	A genetic sequence alteration. A variant can be classified further using modifiers such as "pathogenic," "likely pathogenic," "uncertain significance," "likely benign," and "benign." Use of this nomenclature has replaced the previously used terms "polymorphism" and "mutation."

diseases are caused by (1) structural rearrangements that result in deletion or duplication of a group of closely linked genes or (2) abnormalities during mitosis or meiosis that result in an abnormal number of chromosomes per cell. In most genetic diseases, every cell in an affected individual carries the mutated gene or genes as a consequence of its inheritance via a mutant egg or sperm cell (**gamete**). However, mutation of the gametic cell may have arisen during its development, in which case somatic cells of the parent do not carry the variant, and the affected individual is said to have a "de novo variant." In addition, some variants may arise during early embryogenesis, in which case tissues of the affected individual contain a mixture, or **mosaic**, of abnormal and normal cells. Depending on the time of embryogenesis and cell type in which a new variant arises, an individual may carry the alteration in some but not all of their germ cells (**germline mosaicism**), some but not all of their somatic cells (**somatic mosaicism**), or both.

It is helpful to begin with a brief review of terms that are commonly used in discussing genetic disease with patients and their families. Although genes were recognized and studied long before the structure of DNA was known, it has become common to regard a **gene** as a short stretch of DNA, usually but not always <100,000 base pairs (bp) in length, that encodes a product (usually protein) responsible for a function within the cell. DNA length is typically measured in base pairs, kilobase pairs (kb), or megabase pairs (Mb); chromosomes vary in length from about 46 Mb to 245 Mb. The **locus** is where a particular gene lies on its chromosome. A gene's DNA sequence nearly always has slight differences when compared across many unrelated individuals within a population. These variant versions of a gene are referred to as different **alleles** of that gene. A genetic variant arises via a biochemical event such as a nucleotide change, deletion, or insertion that has produced a new allele. The historic terms "polymorphism" and "mutation" are rarely used in current scientific and clinic discourse. A "polymorphism" was defined as a benign variant when it exhibited a population frequency greater than 1% in DNA sequence and did not contribute to disease manifestation. A "mutation" was defined as a pathogenic change in DNA sequence that did contribute to disease manifestation.

The term "variant" is now the recommended term to define a change in DNA sequence from the population norm and is used with the following modifiers: "pathogenic," "likely pathogenic," "uncertain significance," "likely benign," and "benign." Many changes in the DNA sequence of a gene, such as those within introns or at the third "wobble" position of codons for particular amino acids, do not affect the structure or expression of the gene product; therefore, although all variants result in a biochemical or molecular biologic phenotype (ie, a change in DNA), only some of them result in a clinically abnormal phenotype.

At the molecular level, variant sequences are usually detected through laboratory evaluation (DNA sequencing) and are referred to as a single nucleotide variant (SNV) if a single base pair change has occurred. At the clinical level, variant alleles are recognized by their effect on a phenotype such as human leukocyte antigen (HLA) type or hair color. Two copies or alleles of each autosomal gene (ie, genes on chromosomes 1–22) are present per cell. Individuals carrying identical copies are **homozygous**, whereas individuals whose two copies differ from each other are **heterozygous**. These terms—"homozygous" and "heterozygous"—can apply to the DNA sequence, the protein product, or the clinical phenotype. In other words, an individual may be heterozygous for a single nucleotide polymorphism (SNP) that does not alter the protein product, heterozygous for a deletion that causes a genetic disease, or heterozygous for a DNA sequence alteration that causes a change in protein structure but does not cause disease.

This discussion helps to illustrate the use of the word **phenotype**, which refers simply to any characteristic that can be measured, with the type of measurement depending on the characteristic. Hair color and height are phenotypes readily apparent to a casual observer that are not obviously associated with disease; diabetes and coronary artery disease are disease phenotypes that typically require clinical investigation to be recognized; and restriction fragment length polymorphisms (RFLPs), simple sequence length polymorphisms (SSLPs), and SNPs are molecular biologic phenotypes that can be detected only with a laboratory test.

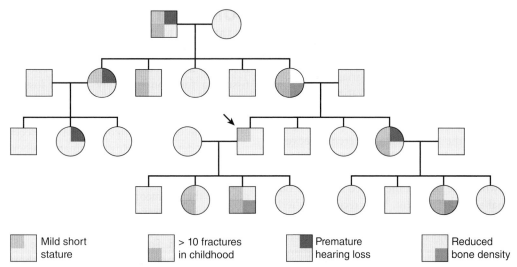

| | Mild short stature | | > 10 fractures in childhood | | Premature hearing loss | | Reduced bone density |

FIGURE 2–1 Penetrance and expressivity in type I osteogenesis imperfecta. In this schematic pedigree of the autosomal dominant condition of type I osteogenesis imperfecta, nearly all affected individuals exhibit different phenotypic features that vary in severity (variable expressivity). As is shown, type I osteogenesis imperfecta is fully penetrant, because every individual who transmits the pathogenic variant is phenotypically affected to some degree. However, if mild short stature in the individual indicated with the arrow had been considered to be a normal variant, then the condition would have been nonpenetrant in this individual. Thus, in this example, judgments about penetrance or nonpenetrance depend on the criteria for normal and abnormal stature.

PENETRANCE & EXPRESSIVITY

One of the most important principles of human genetics is that two individuals with the same mutated gene may have different phenotypes. For example, in the genetic condition of type I osteogenesis imperfecta, pedigrees may occur in which there are both a phenotypically affected grandparent and an affected grandchild even though the obligate carrier parent of the grandchild with the identical genetic variant is asymptomatic (Figure 2–1). Given a set of defined criteria, phenotypic expression of the condition in individuals known to carry the pathogenic variant gene is described as **penetrance**. In other words, if 7 of 10 individuals older than 40 with the type I osteogenesis imperfecta mutation have an abnormal bone density scan, the condition is said to be 70% penetrant by that criterion. Penetrance may vary both with age and according to the set of criteria being used; for example, type I osteogenesis imperfecta may be 90% penetrant at age 40 when the conclusion is based on a bone density scan in conjunction with laboratory tests for abnormal collagen synthesis. **Reduced penetrance**, or **age-dependent penetrance**, is a common feature of dominantly inherited

conditions (see below) that often have a relatively high **fitness** (the extent to which individuals carrying an altered allele produce offspring relative to individuals who carry a normal allele); Huntington disease and polycystic kidney disease are examples of disorders with low **fitness**. Genetic conditions that result in a high degree of embryonic lethality have low **fitness**.

The same altered gene giving rise to a spectrum of different phenotypes is referred to as **variable expressivity**. For example, blue scleras and short stature may be the only manifestations of type I osteogenesis imperfecta in a particular individual, whereas a sibling who carries the identical mutation may be confined to a wheelchair as a result of multiple fractures and deformities. The pathogenic variant is penetrant in both individuals, but its expression is variable. Both reduced penetrance and variable expressivity may occur in individuals who carry the same altered allele; therefore, phenotypic differences between these individuals must be due to the effects of other "modifier" genes, to environmental interactions, or to chance.

MECHANISMS OF MUTATION & INHERITANCE PATTERNS

Genetic variants can be characterized both by their molecular nature—nucleotide deletion, insertion, substitution—and by their effects on gene activity (ie, no effect [neutral or silent],

complete loss of function [amorphic variant], partial loss of function [hypomorphic variant], gain of function [hypermorphic variant], or acquisition of a new property [neomorphic variant]). Geneticists who study experimental organisms frequently use specific deletions to ensure that an altered allele causes a loss of function, but human geneticists rely on biochemical or cell culture studies to assess both losses and gains of function. Amorphic and hypomorphic variants are probably the most frequent types of pathogenic variant in human genetic disease because there are many ways to interfere with a protein's function.

For autosomal genes, the fundamental difference between dominant and recessive inheritance is that, with dominant inheritance, the disease state or phenotypic trait being measured is apparent when one copy of the altered allele and one copy of the normal allele are present. With recessive inheritance, two copies of the altered allele must be present for the disease state or trait to be apparent. However, for genes that lie on the X chromosome, the situation is slightly different because females have two X chromosomes and males have only one. X-linked dominant inheritance occurs when one copy of an abnormal gene causes the disease phenotype (in males and females); X-linked recessive inheritance occurs when two copies of an abnormal gene cause the disease phenotype (in females). Because most pathogenic variants are amorphic or hypomorphic, however, one copy of an X-linked abnormal allele in males is not "balanced" with a normal allele, as it would be in females; therefore, in X-linked recessive inheritance, one copy of an abnormal allele is sufficient to produce a disease phenotype in males, a situation referred to as **hemizygosity**.

RECESSIVE INHERITANCE & LOSS-OF-FUNCTION PATHOGENIC VARIANTS

Most recessive pathogenic variants are due to loss of function of the gene product, which can occur from a variety of causes, including failure of the gene to be transcribed or translated and failure of the translated gene product to function correctly. There are two general principles to keep in mind when considering loss-of-function variants. First, because expression from the normal allele usually does not change (ie, there is no **dosage compensation**), gene expression in a heterozygous carrier of a loss-of-function allele is reduced to 50% of normal. Second, for most biochemical pathways, a 50% reduction in enzyme concentration is not sufficient to produce a disease state. Thus, most diseases resulting from enzyme deficiencies such as phenylketonuria (Table 2–2) are inherited in a recessive fashion.

DOMINANT INHERITANCE & LOSS-OF-FUNCTION PATHOGENIC VARIANTS

If 50% of a particular product is not enough for the cell or tissue to function normally, then a loss-of-function variant in this gene produces a dominantly inherited phenotype. Such pathogenic variants often occur in structural proteins; an example is type I osteogenesis imperfecta, which is considered in detail later. Most dominantly inherited phenotypes are actually **semidominant**, which means that an individual who carries two copies of the abnormal allele is affected more severely than someone who carries one abnormal and one normal copy. However, for most dominantly inherited conditions, individuals homozygous for two pathogenic variants are rarely observed. For example, inheritance of achondroplasia, the most common genetic cause of very short stature, is usually described as autosomal dominant. However, rare matings between two affected individuals have a 25% probability of producing offspring with two copies of the abnormal gene. This results in homozygous achondroplasia, a condition that is very severe and usually fatal in the perinatal period; thus, achondroplasia exhibits semidominant inheritance. Huntington disease, a dominantly inherited neurologic disease, is the only known human condition in which the homozygous abnormal phenotype is identical to the heterozygous abnormal phenotype (sometimes referred to as a "true dominant").

DOMINANT NEGATIVE GENE ACTION

A special kind of pathophysiologic mechanism, referred to as dominant negative, occurs frequently in human genetic diseases that involve proteins that form oligomeric or polymeric complexes. In these disorders, the abnormal allele gives rise to a structurally abnormal protein that interferes with the function of the normal allele. Note that any molecular lesion (ie, deletion, nonsense, missense, or splicing) can produce a loss-of-function allele. However, only molecular lesions that yield a protein product (ie, splicing, missense, or nonsense variants) can result in a dominant negative allele. Type II osteogenesis imperfecta, described later, is an example of a dominant negative pathogenic variant.

Although the terms "dominant" and "recessive" are occasionally used to describe specific pathogenic variants, a DNA sequence alteration itself cannot, strictly speaking, be dominant or recessive. The terms are instead appropriate to the effect of a pathogenic variant on a particular trait. Therefore, in characterizing a particular pathogenic variant as "recessive," one is referring to the effect of the variant on the trait being studied.

MUTATION RATE & THE PREVALENCE OF GENETIC DISEASE

At the level of DNA sequence, nucleotide variants (substitutions, small insertions, or small deletions) in humans occur at a rate of approximately 2×10^{-8} per nucleotide per human generation, or 150 new variants per diploid genome. However, only about 5% of the human genome is protein coding, so most new variants have no effect. Still, with approximately 23,000

TABLE 2-2   Phenotype, inheritance, and prevalence of selected genetic disorders.

Disorder	Phenotype	Genetic Mechanism	Incidence
Down syndrome	Intellectual disability and growth deficiencies, dysmorphic features, internal organ anomalies	Chromosomal imbalance; caused by trisomy 21	≈1:700; increased risk with advanced maternal age
Fragile X–associated mental retardation syndrome	Intellectual disability, characteristic facial features, large testes	X-linked; progressive expansion of unstable DNA causes failure to express gene encoding RNA-binding protein	≈1:1500 males; can be manifested in females; multistep mechanism
Sickle cell anemia	Recurrent painful crises, increased susceptibility to infections	Autosomal recessive; caused by a single missense mutation in beta-globin	≈1:400 blacks
Cystic fibrosis	Recurrent pulmonary infections, exocrine pancreatic insufficiency, infertility	Autosomal recessive; caused by multiple loss-of-function mutations in a chloride channel	≈1:2000 whites; very rare in Asians
Leber hereditary optic neuropathy	Acute or subacute blindness, occasional myopathy or neurodegeneration	Pathogenic variant of electron transport chain encoded by mtDNA	≈1:50,000–1:10,000
Myoclonic epilepsy with ragged red fibers	Uncontrolled periodic jerking, muscle weakness	Pathogenic variant of mitochondrial tRNA in mtDNA	≈1:100,000–1:50,000
Neurofibromatosis	Multiple café-au-lait spots, neurofibromas, increased tumor susceptibility	Autosomal dominant; caused by multiple loss-of-function variants in a signaling molecule	≈1:3000; ≈50% are new mutations
Duchenne muscular dystrophy	Muscular weakness and degeneration	X-linked recessive; caused by multiple loss-of-function variants in muscle protein	≈1:3000 males; ≈33% are new mutations
Osteogenesis imperfecta	Increased susceptibility to fractures, connective tissue fragility, blue scleras	Phenotypically and genetically heterogeneous	≈1:10,000
Phenylketonuria	Intellectual disability and growth deficiencies	Autosomal recessive; caused by multiple loss-of-function variants in phenylalanine hydroxylase	≈1:10,000

genes in the human genome and an estimated deleterious "per locus" mutation rate of 10^{-5} per generation, the chance of a new deleterious variant occurring in any one individual is about 20%. Furthermore, assuming 10 billion new births in the last millennium, every gene in the human genome has probably been mutated (in a deleterious manner) about 100,000 different times. However, from a clinical perspective, only about 6000 single-gene disorders have been recognized to cause a human disease. In considering possible explanations for this disparity, it seems likely that deleterious variants of many single genes are lethal very early in development and thus not clinically apparent, whereas deleterious variants in other genes do not cause an easily recognizable phenotype. The overall frequency of disease attributable to defects in single genes (ie, mendelian disorders) is approximately 1% of the general population.

Table 2–2 lists the major symptoms and signs (phenotypes), genetic mechanisms, and prevalence of the diseases considered in this chapter as well as of several others. The most common conditions, such as neurofibromatosis, cystic fibrosis, and fragile X–associated mental retardation syndrome, will be encountered at some time by most health care professionals regardless of their field of interest. Other conditions, such as Huntington disease and adenosine deaminase deficiency, although of academic and pathophysiologic interest, are not likely to be seen by most practitioners.

Many common conditions such as atherosclerosis and breast cancer, while in a minority of cases are caused by a single-gene disorder, usually do not show strictly mendelian inheritance patterns but have some genetic component evident from familial aggregation or twin studies. These conditions are usually described as **multifactorial**, which means that the effects of one or more mutated genes and environmental differences all contribute to the likelihood that a given individual will manifest the phenotype.

ISSUES IN CLINICAL GENETICS

Most patients with genetic disease present during early childhood with symptoms that ultimately give rise to a diagnosis such as fragile X–associated mental retardation or Down syndrome. The major clinical issues at presentation are arriving at the correct diagnosis and counseling the patient and family regarding the natural history and prognosis of the condition. It is important to assess the likelihood that the same condition will occur again in the family and determine whether it can be diagnosed prenatally. These issues are the subject matter of genetic counseling by medical geneticists and genetic counselors.

Understanding the pathophysiology of genetic diseases that interfere with specific metabolic pathways—so-called inborn errors of metabolism—has led to effective treatments for selected conditions such as phenylketonuria, maple syrup urine disease, and homocystinuria. Many of these diseases are rare, but efforts are underway to develop treatments for common single-gene disorders such as Duchenne muscular dystrophy, cystic fibrosis, and hemophilia. Some forms of therapy are directed at replacing the mutant protein, whereas others are directed at ameliorating its effects.

CHECKPOINT

1. Define gene, locus, allele, variant, heterozygosity, hemizygosity, and phenotype.
2. How is it possible for two individuals with the same pathogenic variant to experience differences in the severity of an abnormal phenotype?
3. Explain the pathophysiologic difference between variants that act via loss of function and those that act via dominant negative gene action.

PATHOPHYSIOLOGY OF SELECTED GENETIC DISEASES

OSTEOGENESIS IMPERFECTA

Osteogenesis imperfecta is a condition inherited in mendelian fashion that illustrates many principles of human genetics. It is a heterogeneous and pleiotropic group of disorders characterized by a tendency toward bone fragility. Advances in the last two decades demonstrate two genetically different groups: the "classical" group, in which more than 90% of cases are caused by pathogenic variants of the *COL1A1* or *COL1A2* genes, which encode the subunits of type I collagen, proα1(I) and proα2(I), respectively, and a newer group, caused by loss-of-function pathogenic variants in other proteins required for proper folding, processing, and collagen secretion. More than 100 different abnormal alleles have been described for osteogenesis imperfecta; the relationships between different DNA sequence alterations and the type of disease (genotype–phenotype correlations) illustrate several pathophysiologic principles in human genetics.

Clinical Manifestations

The clinical and genetic characteristics of osteogenesis imperfecta are summarized in Table 2–3, in which the timing and severity of fractures, radiologic findings, and presence of additional clinical features help to distinguish four different subtypes. This classification was presented more than 30 years ago. Over the past decade, it has become clear that there are more than a dozen different genes in which pathogenic variants can cause osteogenesis imperfecta, and that the utility of alternative or more extended nosologic approaches depends on whether the condition is being considered from the perspective of patients, caregivers, or molecular geneticists.

All forms of osteogenesis imperfecta are characterized by increased susceptibility to fractures ("brittle bones"), but there is considerable phenotypic heterogeneity, even within individual subtypes. Individuals with type I or type IV osteogenesis imperfecta present in early childhood with one or a few fractures of long bones in response to minimal or no trauma; x-ray films may reveal mild osteopenia, little or no bony deformity, and often evidence of earlier subclinical fractures. However, most individuals with type I or type IV osteogenesis imperfecta do not have fractures in utero. Type I and type IV osteogenesis imperfecta are distinguished by the severity (less in type I than in type IV) and by scleral hue, which indicates the thickness of this tissue and the deposition of type I collagen. Individuals with type I osteogenesis imperfecta typically have blue scleras, whereas the scleras of those with type IV are normal or slightly gray. In type I, the typical number of fractures during childhood is 10–20; fracture incidence decreases after puberty, and the main features in adult life are mild short stature, a tendency toward conductive hearing loss, and occasionally dentinogenesis imperfecta. Individuals with type IV osteogenesis imperfecta generally experience more fractures than those with type I and have significant short stature caused by a combination of long bone and spinal deformities, but they often are able to walk independently. Approximately 60% of the cases of type I and type IV osteogenesis imperfecta represent de novo previously undescribed pathogenic variants; in the remainder, the history and examination of other family members reveal findings consistent with autosomal dominant inheritance. In most cases, identified pathogenic variants are unique to an individual or family.

Type II osteogenesis imperfecta presents at or before birth (diagnosed by prenatal imaging) with multiple fractures, bony

TABLE 2-3   Subtypes of dominant osteogenesis imperfecta.

Type	Phenotype	Genetics	Molecular Pathophysiology
Type I	**Mild:** Short stature, postnatal fractures, little or no deformity, blue scleras, premature hearing loss	Autosomal dominant	Loss-of-function variant in proα1(I) chain resulting in decreased amount of mRNA; quality of collagen is normal; quantity is reduced twofold
Type II	**Perinatal lethal:** Severe prenatal fractures, abnormal bone formation, severe deformities, blue scleras, connective tissue fragility	Sporadic (autosomal dominant)	Structural variant in proα1(I) or proα2(I) chain that has mild effect on heterotrimer assembly; quality of collagen is severely abnormal; quantity also often reduced
Type III	**Progressive deforming:** Prenatal fractures, deformities usually present at birth, very short stature, usually nonambulatory, blue scleras, hearing loss	Autosomal dominant[1]	Structural variant in proα1(I) or proα2(I) chain that has mild effect on heterotrimer assembly; quality of collagen is severely abnormal; quantity can be normal
Type IV	**Deforming with normal scleras:** Postnatal fractures, mild to moderate deformities, premature hearing loss, normal or gray scleras, dental abnormalities	Autosomal dominant	Structural variant in the proα2(I), or, less frequently, proα1(I) chain that has little or no effect on heterotrimer assembly; quality of collagen is usually abnormal; quantity can be normal

[1]Autosomal recessive in rare cases.

deformities, increased fragility of nonbony connective tissue, and blue scleras, and usually results in death in infancy. Two typical radiologic findings are the presence of isolated "islands" of mineralization in the skull (wormian bones) and a beaded appearance to the ribs. Nearly all cases of type II osteogenesis imperfecta represent a new dominant pathogenic variant, and there is no family history. Death usually results from respiratory difficulties.

Type III osteogenesis imperfecta presents at birth or in infancy with progressive bony deformities, multiple fractures, and blue scleras. It is intermediate in severity between types II and IV; most affected individuals will require multiple corrective surgeries and lose the ability to ambulate by early adulthood. Unlike other forms of osteogenesis imperfecta, which are nearly always due to variants that act dominantly, type III may be inherited, very rarely, in a recessive manner.

Although different subtypes of osteogenesis imperfecta can often be distinguished biochemically, the classification presented in Table 2–3 is primarily clinical rather than molecular, and the disease phenotypes for each subtype show a spectrum of severities that overlap one another. For example, a few individuals diagnosed with type II osteogenesis imperfecta based on the presence of severe bony deformities in utero will survive for many years and thus overlap the type III subtype. Similarly, some individuals with type IV osteogenesis imperfecta have fractures in utero and develop deformities that lead to loss of ambulation. Distinguishing this presentation from type III osteogenesis imperfecta may be possible only if other affected family members exhibit a milder course.

Additional subtypes of osteogenesis imperfecta have been suggested for individuals that do not match types I–IV, and there are additional disorders associated with congenital fractures that are usually not considered to be "classic" osteogenesis imperfecta. In particular, work over the past several years has identified 11 additional genes in which pathogenic variants can cause autosomal recessive osteogenesis imperfecta and has provided additional insight into the genetic pathophysiology. In general, recessively inherited osteogenesis imperfecta is caused by loss-of-function variants in genes whose protein product is required for proper protein folding, intracellular processing, and trafficking of type I collagen.

Pathophysiology

Osteogenesis imperfecta is a disease of type I collagen, which constitutes the major extracellular protein in the body. It is the major collagen in the dermis, the connective tissue capsules of most organs, and the vascular and gastrointestinal (GI) adventitia and is the only collagen in bone. A mature type I collagen fibril is a rigid structure that contains multiple type I collagen molecules packed in a staggered array and stabilized by intermolecular covalent cross-links. Each mature type I collagen molecule contains two α1 chains and one α2 chain, encoded by the *COL1A1* and *COL1A2* genes, respectively (Figure 2–2). The α1 and α2 chains are synthesized as larger precursors with amino and carboxyl terminal "propeptide" extensions, assemble with each other inside the cell, and are ultimately secreted as a heterotrimeric type I procollagen molecule. During intracellular assembly, the three chains wind around each other in a triple helix that is stabilized by interchain interactions between hydroxylated proline and adjacent carbonyl residues. There is a dynamic relationship between the post-translational action of prolyl hydroxylase and assembly of the triple helix, which begins at the carboxyl terminal end of the molecule. Increased levels of hydroxylation result in a more stable helix, but helix formation prevents further prolyl hydroxylation. The nature of the triple helix causes the side chain of every third amino acid to point inward, and steric constraints allow only a proton

FIGURE 2–2 Molecular assembly of type I procollagen. Type I procollagen is assembled in the endoplasmic reticulum from three proα chains that associate with each other beginning at their carboxyl terminals. An important requirement for proper assembly of the triple helix is the presence of a glycine residue at every third position in each of the proα chains. After secretion, the amino and carboxyl terminal propeptides are proteolytically cleaved, leaving a rigid triple helical collagen molecule with very short non–triple-helical domains at both ends. (Modified and reproduced, with permission, from Alberts BA. *Molecular Biology of the Cell*, 4th ed. Garland Science, 2002. [Fig. 19-47].)

in this position. Thus, the amino acid sequence of virtually all collagen chains in the triple-helical portion is $(Gly-X-Y)_n$, where Y is proline about one-third of the time.

The fundamental defect in most individuals with type I osteogenesis imperfecta is reduced synthesis of type I collagen resulting from loss-of-function variants in *COL1A1*. In most cases, the abnormal *COL1A1* allele gives rise to greatly reduced (partial loss-of-function) or no (complete loss-of-function) mRNA. Because the normal *COL1A1* allele continues to produce mRNA at a normal rate (ie, there is no dosage compensation), heterozygosity for a complete loss-of-function variant results in a 50% reduction in the total rate of proα1(I) mRNA synthesis, whereas heterozygosity for a partial loss-of-function variant results in a less severe reduction. A reduced concentration of proα1(I) chains limits the production of type I procollagen, leading to (1) a reduced amount of structurally normal type I collagen and (2) an excess of unassembled proα2(I) chains, which are degraded inside the cell (Figure 2–3).

There are several potential molecular defects responsible for *COL1A1* pathogenic variants in type I osteogenesis imperfecta, including alterations in a regulatory region leading to reduced transcription, splicing abnormalities leading to

reduced steady-state levels of RNA, and deletion of the entire *COL1A1* gene. However, in many cases, the underlying defect is a single base pair change that creates a premature stop codon (also known as a **"nonsense mutation"**) in an internal exon. In a process referred to as nonsense-mediated decay, partially synthesized mRNA precursors that carry the nonsense codon are recognized and degraded by the cell. With collagen and many other genes, production of a truncated protein (as might be predicted from a nonsense mutation) would be more damaging to the cell than production of no protein at all. Thus, nonsense-mediated decay, which has been observed to occur for mutations in many different multiexon genes, serves as a protective phenomenon and is an important component of the genetic pathophysiology.

An example of these principles is apparent from considering type II osteogenesis imperfecta, which is caused by structurally abnormal forms of type I collagen and is more severe than type I osteogenesis imperfecta. Pathogenic variants in type II osteogenesis imperfecta can be caused by defects in either *COL1A1* or *COL1A2* and usually are missense alterations of a glycine residue that allow the abnormal peptide chain to bind to normal chains in the initial steps of trimer assembly (see Figure 2–3). However, triple-helix formation is ineffective, often because amino acids with large side chains are substituted for glycine. Ineffective triple-helix formation leads to increased post-translational modification by prolyl hydroxylase, a reduced rate of secretion, and activation of the unfolded protein stress response. These appear to be critical events in the cellular pathogenesis of type II osteogenesis imperfecta, because glycine substitutions toward the carboxyl terminal end of the molecule are generally more severe than those at the amino terminal end.

These considerations help to explain why type II osteogenesis imperfecta is more severe than type I and exemplify the principle of dominant negative gene action. The effects of an amino acid substitution in a proα1(I) peptide chain are amplified at the levels of both triple-helix assembly and fibril formation. Because every type I procollagen molecule has two proα1(I) chains, only 25% of type I procollagen molecules will contain two normal proα1(I) chains, even though only one of the two *COL1A1* alleles is mutated. Furthermore, activation of the unfolded protein stress response appears to be a key event in the pathophysiology of the disease, as discussed further below. Finally, because each molecule in a fibril interacts with several others, incorporation of an abnormal molecule can have disproportionately large effects on fibril structure and integrity.

Collagen pathogenic variants that cause type III and type IV osteogenesis imperfecta are diverse and include glycine substitutions in the amino terminal portion of the collagen triple helix, a few internal deletions of *COL1A1* and *COL1A2* that do not significantly disturb triple helix formation, and some unusual alterations in the non–triple-helical extensions at the amino and carboxyl terminals of proα chains.

Recessively inherited osteogenesis imperfect can be caused by loss of function for a key prolyl hydroxylase encoded by

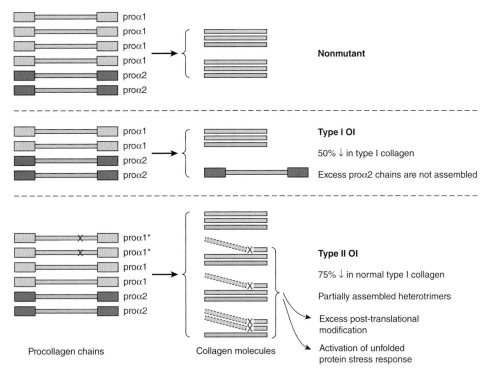

FIGURE 2–3 Molecular pathogenesis of type I and type II osteogenesis imperfecta (OI). The *COL1A1* gene normally produces twice as many proα chains as the *COL1A2* gene. Therefore, in normal cells, the ratio of proα1 to proα2 chains is 2:1, which corresponds to the ratio of α1 and α2 chains in intact collagen molecules. In type I osteogenesis imperfecta, a variant (X) in one of the *COL1A1* alleles (*) results in failure to produce proα1 chains, leading to a 50% reduction in the total number of proα1 chains, a 50% reduction in the production of intact type I collagen molecules, and an excess of unassembled proα2 chains, which are degraded inside the cell. In type II osteogenesis imperfecta, a pathogenic variant in one of the *COL1A1* alleles results in a structural alteration that blocks triple-helix formation and secretion of partially assembled collagen molecules containing the abnormal chain. (Adapted from Nussbaum RL et al. *Thompson & Thompson Genetics in Medicine*, 7th ed. Saunders Elsevier, 2007.)

the *PLOD2* gene, one of three genes—*CRTAP*, *LEPRE1*, and *PPIB*—that encode members of a protein complex that resides within the rough endoplasmic reticulum and facilitates the folding and processing of type I collagen, as well as several additional genes whose protein products are required for intracellular trafficking and secretion of type I collagen. A common pathway for all types of osteogenesis imperfecta involves a combination of reduced production of type I collagen in the extracellular matrix and/or dysfunctional intracellular collagen processing and maturation.

Genetic Principles

As already described, most cases of type I osteogenesis imperfecta are caused by partial or complete loss-of-function variants in *COL1A1*. Moreover, in approximately 60% of affected individuals, the disease is caused by a de novo previously unidentified pathogenic variant. In addition, there are many ways in which DNA sequence alterations can reduce gene expression. Consequently, there is a wide range of abnormal alleles (ie, **allelic heterogeneity**), which represents a challenge for the development of molecular diagnostic tests. Using current sequencing strategies, the pathogenic variant is identifiable in almost all patients affected with types I–IV osteogenesis imperfecta. Identifying the pathogenic variant or variants in a

patient and their family allows for precise recurrence risk estimates and for prenatal testing, if desired.

For types III and IV osteogenesis imperfecta, pathogenic variants can occur in *COL1A1* or *COL1A2* (ie, **locus heterogeneity**), and in this situation, linkage analysis is more difficult because one cannot be sure which locus is abnormal.

For both type I and type IV osteogenesis imperfecta, the most important question in the clinical setting often relates to the natural history of the illness. For example, reproductive decision making in families at risk for osteogenesis imperfecta is influenced greatly by the relative likelihood of producing a child who will never walk and will require multiple orthopedic operations versus a child whose major problems will be a few long bone fractures and an increased risk of mixed sensorineural and conductive hearing loss in childhood and adulthood. As evident from the prior discussion, different abnormal genes and different abnormal alleles, as well as other genes that modify the osteogenesis imperfecta phenotype, can contribute to this **phenotypic heterogeneity**.

In type II osteogenesis imperfecta, a single copy of the abnormal allele causes the abnormal phenotype and, therefore, has a dominant mechanism of action. Although the type II phenotype itself is never inherited, there are rare situations in which a phenotypically normal individual harbors a *COL1A1* pathogenic variant allele among their germ cells. These individuals with

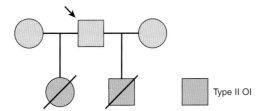

Type II OI

FIGURE 2–4 Gonadal mosaicism for type II osteogenesis imperfecta. In this idealized pedigree, the phenotypically normal father (indicated with the arrow) has had two children by different mates, each of whom is affected with autosomal dominant type II osteogenesis imperfecta (OI). Analysis of the father showed that some of his spermatozoa carried a *COL1A1* pathogenic variant, indicating that the explanation for this unusual pedigree is germline mosaicism. (Adapted from Cohn DH et al. Recurrence of lethal osteogenesis imperfecta due to parental mosaicism for a dominant mutation in a human type I collagen gene [*COL1A1*]. Am J Hum Genet. 1990;46:591.)

so-called **gonadal mosaicism** can produce multiple offspring with type II osteogenesis imperfecta (Figure 2–4), a pattern of segregation that can be confused with recessive inheritance. In fact, many other pathogenic variants, including Duchenne muscular dystrophy, which is X linked, and type 1 neurofibromatosis, which is autosomal dominant, also occasionally show unusual inheritance patterns explained by gonadal mosaicism.

CHECKPOINT

4. When and how does type II osteogenesis imperfecta present? To what do these individuals succumb?
5. What are two typical radiologic findings in type II osteogenesis imperfecta?
6. Explain how nonsense-mediated decay can help protect individuals affected by a genetic disease.

PHENYLKETONURIA

Phenylketonuria represents one of the most dramatic examples of how the relationship between genotype and phenotype can depend on environmental variables. Phenylketonuria was first recognized as an inherited cause of intellectual disability in 1934, and systematic attempts to treat the condition were initiated in the 1950s. The term "phenylketonuria" denotes elevated levels of urinary phenylpyruvate and phenylacetate, which occur when circulating phenylalanine levels, normally between 0.06 and 0.1 mmol/L, rise above 1.2 mmol/L. Thus, the primary defect in phenylketonuria is **hyperphenylalaninemia**, which itself has a number of distinct genetic causes.

The pathophysiology of phenylketonuria illustrates several important principles in human genetics. Hyperphenylalaninemia itself is caused by **substrate accumulation**, which occurs when a normal intermediary metabolite fails to be eliminated properly and its concentrations become elevated to toxic levels.

The most common cause of hyperphenylalaninemia is deficiency of the enzyme phenylalanine hydroxylase, which catalyzes the conversion of phenylalanine to tyrosine. Individuals with pathogenic variants in phenylalanine hydroxylase usually do not suffer from the absence of tyrosine because this amino acid can be supplied to the body by mechanisms independent of phenylalanine hydroxylase. In other forms of phenylketonuria, however, additional disease manifestations occur as a result of **end-product deficiency**, which occurs when the downstream product of a particular enzyme is required for a key physiologic process.

A discussion of phenylketonuria also helps to illustrate the rationale for, and application of, population-based screening programs for genetic disease. More than 10 million newborn infants per year are tested for phenylketonuria, and the focus today in treatment has shifted in several respects. First, "successful" treatment of phenylketonuria by dietary restriction of phenylalanine is, in general, accompanied by subtle neuropsychologic defects that have been recognized only in the last decade. Thus, current investigations focus on alternative treatment strategies such as somatic gene therapy, as well as on the social and psychologic factors that affect compliance with dietary management. Second, a generation of females treated for phenylketonuria are now bearing children, and the phenomenon of **maternal phenylketonuria** has been recognized in which in utero exposure to maternal hyperphenylalaninemia results in congenital abnormalities regardless of fetal genotype. The number of pregnancies at risk has risen in proportion to the successful treatment of phenylketonuria and represents a challenge to public health officials, physicians, dieticians, and geneticists in the future.

Clinical Manifestations

The incidence of hyperphenylalaninemia varies among populations. In African Americans, it is about 1:50,000; in Yemenite Jews, about 1:5000; and in most Northern European populations, about 1:10,000. Post-natal growth restriction, moderate-to-severe intellectual disability, recurrent seizures, hypopigmentation, and eczematous skin rashes constitute the major phenotypic features of untreated phenylketonuria. However, with the advent of widespread newborn screening programs for hyperphenylalaninemia, the major phenotypic manifestations of phenylketonuria today occur when treatment is partial or when it is terminated prematurely during late childhood or adolescence. In these cases, there is a variety of neurocognitive deficits and psychiatric problems that can develop, including deficits in executive functioning and anxiety, depression, and phobias.

Newborn screening for phenylketonuria is performed on a small amount of dried blood obtained at 24–72 hours of age. From the initial screen, there is about a 1% incidence of positive or indeterminate screening results, and in such cases, a more quantitative measurement of plasma phenylalanine is then performed, ideally before 2 weeks of age. In neonates who undergo this confirmatory testing, the diagnosis of phenylketonuria is ultimately validated in about 1%, providing an estimated phenylketonuria prevalence of 1:10,000, although there is great geographic and ethnic variation (see prior discussion).

Infants in whom a diagnosis of phenylketonuria is confirmed are usually placed on a dietary regimen in which a semisynthetic formula low in phenylalanine can be combined with regular breast feeding. This regimen is adjusted empirically to maintain a plasma phenylalanine concentration at or below 1 mmol/L, which is still several times greater than normal but similar to levels observed in so-called **benign hyperphenylalaninemia** (see later discussion), a biochemical diagnosis which is not associated with phenylketonuria and has no clinical consequences. Phenylalanine is an essential amino acid, and even individuals with phenylketonuria must consume small amounts to avoid protein starvation and a catabolic state. Most children require between 25–50 mg/kg/d of phenylalanine, and these requirements are met by combining natural foods with commercial products designed for phenylketonuria treatment. When dietary treatment programs were first implemented, it was hoped that the risk of neurologic damage from the hyperphenylalaninemia of phenylketonuria would have a limited window and that treatment could be stopped after childhood. However, it now appears that even mild hyperphenylalaninemia in adults (>1.2 mmol/L) is associated with neuropsychologic and cognitive deficits; therefore, dietary treatment of phenylketonuria should probably be continued indefinitely.

As an increasing number of treated females with phenylketonuria reach childbearing age, a new problem—fetal hyperphenylalaninemia via intrauterine exposure—has become apparent. Newborn infants in such cases exhibit microcephaly and growth restriction of prenatal onset, congenital heart disease, and severe developmental delay regardless of fetal genotype. Rigorous control of maternal phenylalanine concentrations from before conception until birth reduces the incidence of fetal abnormalities in maternal phenylketonuria, but the level of plasma phenylalanine that is "safe" for a developing fetus is 0.12–0.36 mmol/L—significantly lower than what is considered acceptable for phenylketonuria-affected children or adults on phenylalanine-restricted diets.

Pathophysiology

The normal metabolic fate of free phenylalanine is incorporation into protein or hydroxylation by phenylalanine hydroxylase to form tyrosine (Figure 2–5). Because tyrosine, but not phenylalanine, can be metabolized to produce fumarate and acetoacetate, hydroxylation of phenylalanine can be viewed both as a means of making tyrosine a nonessential amino acid and as a mechanism for providing energy via gluconeogenesis during states of protein starvation. In individuals with pathogenic variants in phenylalanine hydroxylase, tyrosine becomes an essential amino acid. However, the clinical manifestations of the disease are caused not by absence of tyrosine (most

FIGURE 2–5 Metabolic fates of phenylalanine. Because catabolism of phenylalanine must proceed via tyrosine, the absence of phenylalanine hydroxylase leads to accumulation of phenylalanine. Tyrosine is also a biosynthetic precursor for melanin and certain neurotransmitters, and the absence of phenylalanine hydroxylase causes tyrosine to become an essential amino acid.

people get enough tyrosine in the diet in any case) but by accumulation of phenylalanine. Transamination of phenylalanine to form phenylpyruvate normally does not occur unless circulating concentrations exceed 1.2 mmol/L, but the pathogenesis of central nervous system (CNS) abnormalities in phenylketonuria, while still being elucidated, is currently felt to be related more to phenylalanine itself than to its metabolites. In addition to a direct effect of elevated phenylalanine levels on energy production, protein synthesis, and neurotransmitter homeostasis in the developing brain, phenylalanine can also inhibit the transport of neutral amino acids across the blood–brain barrier, leading to a selective amino acid deficiency in the cerebrospinal fluid. Thus, the neurologic manifestations of phenylketonuria are felt to be due to a general effect of substrate accumulation on cerebral metabolism. The pathophysiology of the eczema seen in untreated or partially treated phenylketonuria is not well understood, but eczema is a common feature of other inborn errors of metabolism in which plasma concentrations of branched-chain amino acids are elevated. Hypopigmentation in phenylketonuria is probably caused by an inhibitory effect of excess phenylalanine on the production of dopaquinone in melanocytes, which is the rate-limiting step in melanin synthesis.

Approximately 90% of infants with persistent hyperphenylalaninemia detected by newborn screening have typical phenylketonuria caused by a defect in phenylalanine hydroxylase (see later discussion). Of the remainder, most have benign hyperphenylalaninemia, in which circulating levels of phenylalanine are between 0.1 mmol/L and 1 mmol/L. However, approximately 1% of infants with persistent hyperphenylalaninemia have defects in the metabolism of tetrahydrobiopterin (BH_4), which is a stoichiometric cofactor for the hydroxylation reaction (Figure 2–6). Importantly, BH_4 is required not only for phenylalanine hydroxylase but also for tyrosine hydroxylase and tryptophan hydroxylase. The products of these latter two enzymes are catecholaminergic and serotonergic neurotransmitters; thus, individuals with defects in BH_4 metabolism suffer not only from phenylketonuria (substrate accumulation) but also from absence of important neurotransmitters (end-product deficiency). Affected individuals develop a severe neurologic disorder in early childhood

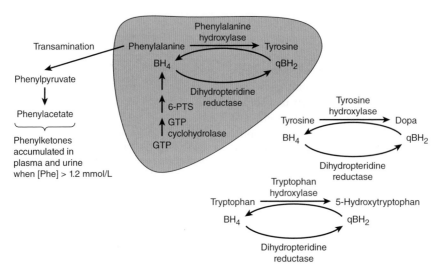

FIGURE 2–6 Normal and abnormal phenylalanine metabolism. Tetrahydrobiopterin (BH$_4$) is a cofactor for phenylalanine hydroxylase, tyrosine hydroxylase, and tryptophan hydroxylase. Consequently, defects in the biosynthesis of BH$_4$ or its metabolism result in a failure of all three hydroxylation reactions. The absence of phenylalanine hydroxylation has phenotypic effects because of substrate accumulation, but the absence of tyrosine or tryptophan hydroxylation has phenotypic effects as a result of end-product deficiency. (6-PTS, 6-pyruvoyltetrahydrobiopterin synthetase; qBH$_2$, quinonoid dihydrobiopterin.)

manifested by hypotonia, inactivity, and developmental regression and are treated not only with dietary restriction of phenylalanine but also with dietary supplementation with BH$_4$, dopa, and 5-hydroxytryptophan.

Genetic Principles

Phenylketonuria is one of several mendelian conditions that have a relatively high incidence, others being cystic fibrosis, Duchenne muscular dystrophy, neurofibromatosis type I, and sickle cell anemia (see Table 2–2). These conditions share no single feature: Some are recessive, some dominant, some autosomal, some X-linked; some are lethal in early childhood, but others have very little effect on reproduction (and transmission to subsequent generations). In fact, the incidence of a mendelian condition is determined by a balance of factors, including the rate at which new variants occur and the likelihood that an individual carrying a pathogenic variant will transmit it to their offspring. As mentioned earlier, the latter characteristic—the probability, compared with the general population, of transmitting one's genes to the next generation—is called **fitness**. Reduced fitness exhibited by many genetic conditions such as Duchenne muscular dystrophy or type 1 neurofibromatosis is balanced by an appreciable **new mutation rate**, so that the incidence of the condition remains constant in successive generations.

For recessive conditions like phenylketonuria or sickle cell anemia (or X-linked recessive conditions such as Duchenne muscular dystrophy), another factor that can influence disease incidence is whether heterozygous carriers experience a selective advantage or disadvantage for survival to reproductive age compared with homozygous normal individuals. For example,

the relatively high incidence of sickle cell anemia in individuals of West African ancestry is due in part to **heterozygote advantage**, conferring resistance to malaria. Because the detrimental effects of homozygosity for the hemoglobin B sickle allele (*HBB*^{S}) are balanced by the beneficial effects of heterozygosity, the overall frequency of the *HBB*^{S} allele has increased over time in populations in which malaria is endemic.

A final factor that may contribute to the high incidence of a mendelian disease is **genetic drift**, which refers to the fluctuation of gene frequencies due to random sampling over many generations. The extent of fluctuation is greatest in very small populations. A related phenomenon is the **founder effect**, which occurs when a population founded by a small number of ancestors has, by chance, a high frequency of a deleterious gene. A founder effect and genetic drift can operate together to produce large changes in the incidence of mendelian diseases, especially in small populations founded by a small number of ancestors. In the case of phenylketonuria, the fitness of affected individuals has until recently been very low, and de novo variants are exceedingly rare; however, population genetic studies provide evidence for both a founder effect and heterozygote advantage.

Phenylketonuria is also representative of a class of mendelian conditions for which efforts are under way to develop gene therapy, such as hemophilia and ornithine transcarbamylase deficiency. A thorough understanding of the pathophysiology of these conditions is an important prerequisite to developing treatments. Each of these conditions is caused by loss of function for an enzyme expressed specifically in the liver; therefore, attempts to deliver a normal gene to affected individuals have focused on strategies to express the gene in hepatocytes. However, as is the case for benign hyperphenylalaninemia, individuals with very low levels of enzymatic activity are clinically normal, and successful gene therapy might, therefore, be accomplished by expressing the target gene in only a small proportion of hepatic cells.

FRAGILE X–ASSOCIATED MENTAL RETARDATION SYNDROME

Fragile X–associated mental retardation syndrome produces a combination of phenotypic features that affect the CNS, the testes, and the cranial skeleton. These features were recognized as a distinct clinical entity more than 50 years ago. A laboratory test for the syndrome was developed during the 1970s, when it was recognized that most affected individuals exhibit a cytogenetic abnormality of the X chromosome:

failure of the region between bands Xq27 and Xq28 to condense at metaphase. Instead, this appears in the microscope as a thin constriction that is subject to breakage during preparation, which accounts for the designation "fragile X." Advances in the last decade have helped to explain both the presence of the fragile site and the unique pattern of inheritance exhibited by the syndrome. In some respects, fragile X–associated mental retardation syndrome is similar to other genetic conditions caused by X-linked pathogenic variants: Affected males are impaired more severely than affected females, and the condition is never transmitted from father to son. However, the syndrome appears to break the rules of mendelian transmission in that at least 20% of carrier males manifest no signs of it when family pedigrees are analyzed. Daughters of these nonpenetrant but "transmitting males" are themselves nonpenetrant but produce affected offspring, male and female, with frequencies close to mendelian expectations (Figure 2–7). About half of carrier females (those with one normal and one abnormal X chromosome) exhibit a significant degree of intellectual disability. These unusual features of the syndrome were explained when the subchromosomal region spanning the fragile site was isolated and shown to contain a segment in which the triplet sequence CGG was repeated many times: $(CGG)_n$. The number of triplet repeats is very polymorphic but normally less than 60. A repeat size between 60 and 200 does not cause a clinical phenotype or a cytogenetic fragile site but is unstable and subject to additional amplification, leading to typical features of the syndrome (Figures 2–8 and 2–9).

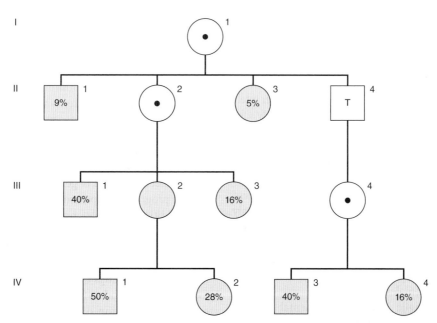

FIGURE 2–7 Likelihood of fragile X–associated mental retardation syndrome in an artificial pedigree. The percentages shown indicate the likelihood of clinical manifestation according to position in the pedigree. Because individuals carrying the abnormal X chromosome have a 50% chance of passing it to their offspring, penetrance is twice that of the values depicted. Penetrance increases with each successive generation owing to the progressive expansion of a triplet repeat element (see text). Expansion is dependent on maternal inheritance of the abnormal allele; thus, daughters of normal transmitting males (indicated with a T in II-4) are nonpenetrant. Obligate carrier females are indicated with a central dot. (Reproduced, with permission, from Nussbaum RL, Ledbetter DH. Fragile X syndrome: a unique mutation in man. Annu Rev Genet. 1986;20:109. Permission conveyed through Copyright Clearance Center.)

Genotype	CpG island	...(CGG)$_n$...	FMR-1 mRNA
Nonmutant (active X)	Unmethylated	$n = 30 \pm 25$	Expressed
Nonmutant (inactive X)	Methylated	$n = 30 \pm 25$	Not expressed
Premutation	Unmethylated	$55 \leq n \leq 200$	Expressed
Full mutation	Methylated	$n \geq 200$	Not expressed

FIGURE 2–8 Molecular genetics of fragile X–associated mental retardation syndrome. The cytogenetic fragile site at Xq27.3 is located close to a small region of DNA that contains a CpG island (see text) and the *FMR1* gene. Within the 5′ untranslated region of the *FMR1* gene lies an unstable segment of repetitive DNA 5′–(CGG)$_n$–3′. The table shows the methylation status of the CpG island, the size of the triplet repeat, and whether the *FMR1* mRNA is expressed depending on the genotype of the X chromosome. Note that the inactive X chromosome in normal females has a methylated CpG island and does not express the *FMR1* mRNA. The methylation and expression status of *FMR1* in premutation and full-mutation alleles applies to males and to the active X chromosome of females; premutation and full-mutation alleles on the inactive X chromosome of females exhibit methylation of the CpG island and fail to express the *FMR1* mRNA.

Clinical Manifestations

Fragile X–associated mental retardation syndrome is usually recognized in affected boys because of developmental delay apparent by 1–2 years of age, small joint hyperextensibility, mild hypotonia, and a family history of intellectual disability in maternally related males. Affected females generally have either milder intellectual disability (when compared to affected males) or only subtle impairments of visuospatial ability, and the condition may not be evident or diagnosed until it is suspected after identification of an affected male relative. In late childhood or early adolescence, affected males begin to exhibit large testes and characteristic facial features, including mild coarsening, large ears, a prominent forehead and mandible, a long face, and relative macrocephaly (considered in relation to height). The syndrome is extremely common and affects about 1:1500–1:1000 males. Virtually all affected males are born to females who are either affected or carry the premutation, and there are no well-recognized cases of new premutations in males or females.

The inheritance of fragile X–associated mental retardation syndrome exhibits several unusual features and is often described in terms of empiric risk figures (see Figure 2–7). In particular, the likelihood that an individual carrying an abnormal chromosome will manifest clinical features depends on the number of generations through which the abnormal chromosome has been transmitted and the sex of the transmitting parent. For example, nonpenetrant transmitting males tend to

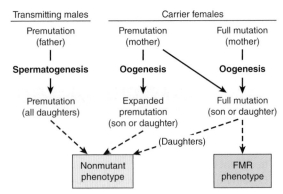

FIGURE 2–9 Transmission and amplification of the fragile X–associated mental retardation syndrome triplet repeat. The heavy arrows show expansion of the triplet repeat, which is thought to occur postzygotically after the premutation or full mutation is transmitted through the female germline. The dashed arrows represent potential phenotypic consequences. Daughters with the full mutation may not express the fragile X–associated mental retardation phenotype, depending on the proportion of cells in which the mutant allele happens to lie on the inactive X chromosome. (Adapted from Tarleton JC et al. Molecular genetic advances in fragile X syndrome. J Pediatr. 1993;122:169.)

occur in the same sibship with each other and with nonpenetrant carrier females. This is reflected in low risk figures for brothers and sisters of transmitting males: 9% and 5%, respectively, compared with 40% and 16% for their maternal grandsons and granddaughters. This latter observation, in which the penetrance or expressivity (or both) of a genetic disease seems to increase in successive generations, is sometimes referred to more generally as **genetic anticipation**.

Genetic anticipation in fragile X–associated mental retardation syndrome is caused by progressive expansion of the triplet repeat. A similar phenomenon occurs in several neurodegenerative disorders such as Huntington disease and spinocerebellar ataxia (ie, grandchildren are affected more severely than grandparents). The neurodegenerative disorders are caused by production of abnormal proteins; fragile X–associated mental retardation is caused by failure to produce a normal protein. Although the biochemical mechanisms are different, the underlying molecular causes of genetic anticipation are identical and involve progressive expansion of an unstable triplet repeat.

In addition to triplet repeat expansion, genetic anticipation can be caused by **bias of ascertainment**, which occurs when a mild or variably expressed condition first diagnosed in grandchildren from a three-generation pedigree is then easily recognized in siblings of the grandchildren who are available for examination and testing. In contrast to genetic anticipation caused by expansion of a triplet repeat, anticipation caused by bias of ascertainment affects the *apparent*, rather than the actual, penetrance.

Pathophysiology

Amplification of the (CGG)$_n$ repeat at the fraXq27.3 site affects both methylation and expression of the *FMR1* gene.

This gene and the unstable DNA responsible for the expansion were isolated on the basis of their proximity to the cytogenetic fragile site in Xq27.3. *FMR1* encodes an RNA-binding protein that regulates translation of mRNA molecules carrying a characteristic sequence in which four guanine residues can form intramolecular bonds, a so-called G quartet structure.

The $(CGG)_n$ repeat is located in the 5′ untranslated region of the *FMR1* gene (see Figure 2–8). This segment is highly variable in length; the number of repeats, n, is equal to about 30 ± 25 in individuals who are neither affected with nor carriers for fragile X–associated mental retardation syndrome. In transmitting males and in unaffected carrier females, the number of repeats is usually between 70 and 100. Remarkably, alleles with fewer than 50 repeats are very stable and almost always transmitted without a change in repeat number. However, alleles with 55 or more repeats are unstable and often exhibit expansion after maternal transmission; these individuals are said to carry a **premutation**. Although premutation carriers do not develop a typical fragile X–associated mental retardation syndrome, studies indicate that female premutation carriers exhibit a 20% and 15% incidence of premature ovarian failure and fragile X–associated tremor/ataxia syndrome (FXTAS), respectively. Male premutation carriers are at an increased risk for FXTAS compared to female carriers, with an overall incidence of 45% in individuals older than 50 years. In both cases, the mechanism is likely to be explained by somatic expansion of the premutation (see later discussion). The degree of expansion is related to the number of repeats; premutation alleles with a repeat number less than 60 rarely are amplified to a full mutation, but premutation alleles with a repeat number greater than 90 are usually amplified to a full mutation. The number of repeats in the full mutation—observed both in affected males and in affected females—is always greater than 200 but is generally heterogeneous, suggesting that once this threshold is reached, additional amplification occurs frequently in somatic cells.

Expansion from a premutation to a full mutation has two important effects: *FMR1* gene transcription is shut off, and DNA surrounding the transcriptional start site of the *FMR1* gene becomes methylated. The clinical phenotype is caused by failure to produce *FMR1*; in addition, methylation of surrounding DNA has important implications for molecular diagnosis. Methylation occurs in a so-called **CpG island**, a several-hundred-base-pair segment just upstream of the *FMR1* transcriptional start site that contains a high frequency of 5′-CG-3′ dinucleotides compared with the rest of the genome. Methylation of the CpG island and expansion of the triplet repeat can be easily detected with molecular biologic techniques, which are the basis of the common diagnostic tests for individuals at risk.

Genetic Principles

In addition to the tendency of $(CGG)_n$ premutation alleles to undergo further amplifications in length, the molecular genetics of fragile X–associated mental retardation syndrome exhibit several unusual features. As described previously, each phenotypically affected individual carries a full mutation defined by a repeat number greater than 200, but the exact repeat number exhibits considerable heterogeneity in different cells and tissues.

Diagnostic testing for the number of CGG repeats is usually performed on lymphocytes taken from a small amount of peripheral blood. In individuals who carry a repeat number less than 50, each cell has the same number of repeats. However, in phenotypically affected males or females (ie, those with a repeat number greater than 200), many of the cells may have a different number of repeats. This situation, often referred to as **somatic mosaicism**, indicates that at least some of the amplification is **postzygotic**, meaning that it occurs in cells of the developing embryo after fertilization. In addition to the DNA methylation associated with an abnormal *FMR1* gene, methylation of many genes is a normal process during development and differentiation that helps to regulate gene expression. Cells in which a particular gene should not be expressed frequently shut off that gene's expression by alterations to chromatin structure that include DNA modification by methylation and histone modification by methylation and/ or acetylation. For example, globin should be expressed only in reticulocytes; albumin should be expressed only in hepatocytes; and insulin should be expressed only by pancreatic β cells. During gametogenesis and immediately after fertilization, specific patterns of chromatin modification characteristic of differentiated cells are erased, only to be reestablished in fetal development. In this way, DNA methylation and other chromatin modifications provide a reversible change in gene structure that can be inherited during mitosis of differentiated cells yet erased during meiosis and early development. This type of alteration—a heritable phenotypic change that is not determined by DNA sequence—is broadly referred to as **epigenetic**.

Analysis of fragile X–associated mental retardation syndrome pedigrees reveals that one of the most important factors influencing whether a premutation allele is subject to postzygotic expansion is the sex of the parent who transmits the premutation allele (see Figures 2–7 and 2–9). As discussed, a premutation allele transmitted by a female expands to a full mutation with a likelihood proportionate to the length of the premutation. Premutation alleles with a repeat number between 52 and 60 rarely expand to a full mutation, and those with a repeat number greater than 90 nearly always expand. In contrast, a premutation allele transmitted by a male rarely if ever expands to a full mutation regardless of the length of the repeat number.

The notion that alleles of the same DNA sequence can behave very differently depending on the sex of the parent who transmitted them is closely related to the concept of **gametic imprinting**, which describes the situation that occurs when expression of a particular gene depends on the sex of the parent who transmitted it. Gametic imprinting affects a handful of genes involved in fetal or placental growth, including insulin-like growth factor 2 (*IGF2*) and the type 2 IGF receptor (*IGF2R*); for example, the *IGF2* gene is expressed only on the paternally derived chromosome, whereas in some individuals, the *IGF2R* gene is expressed only on the maternally derived chromosome. The mechanisms responsible for gametic imprinting depend on biochemical modifications to the chromosome that occur during gametogenesis; these modifications do not affect the actual DNA sequence but are stably transmitted for a certain number of cell divisions (ie, they are epigenetic and contribute to the pathogenesis of certain types of cancer).

CHECKPOINT

11. Explain why fragile X–associated mental retardation syndrome exhibits an unusual pattern of inheritance.
12. What is genetic anticipation? What are two explanations for it?
13. What is an epigenetic change?

LEBER HEREDITARY OPTIC NEUROPATHY, MYOCLONIC EPILEPSY WITH RAGGED RED FIBERS & OTHER MITOCHONDRIAL DISEASES

In nearly every cell in the body, the indispensable job of turning nutrients into energy takes place in mitochondria, ubiquitous subcellular organelles with their own genomes and unique rules of gene expression. Over the past decade, defects in mitochondrial function have become increasingly recognized as important human causes of diseases, from rare conditions whose study has led to a deeper understanding of pathophysiologic mechanisms to common conditions such as diabetes and deafness. On one level, the consequences of defective mitochondrial function are predictable and nonspecific: Inability to generate sufficient adenosine triphosphate (ATP) leads to accumulation of lactic acid, weakness, and, eventually, cell death. However, every mitochondrion contains multiple mitochondrial genomes; every cell contains multiple mitochondria; the requirements for energy production vary from one tissue to another; and, most importantly, pathogenic variants in mitochondrial DNA affect only a fraction of mitochondrial genomes within a given individual. Because of these characteristics, defects in mitochondrial function present clinically with symptoms and signs that are both specific and protean. In addition, mitochondrial DNA is transmitted by eggs but not by sperm, leading to a unique and characteristic pattern of inheritance.

Clinical Manifestations

First described by a German physician in 1871, Leber hereditary optic neuropathy (LHON) presents as painless bilateral loss of vision that occurs in young adults, more commonly in males. Loss of vision can be sudden and complete or subacute and progressive, proceeding from central scotomas to blindness over 1–2 years and usually affecting both eyes within 1–2 months. The condition is occasionally associated with neurologic findings, including ataxia, dysarthria, or symptoms of demyelinating disease, and may be associated also with cardiac conduction abnormalities. Ophthalmologic examination shows peripapillary telangiectasia, microangiopathy, and vascular tortuosity; in patients with neurologic findings (and some without), CNS imaging studies may reveal abnormalities of the basal ganglia and corpus striatum.

By contrast to LHON, myoclonic epilepsy with ragged red fibers (MERRF) was recognized as a distinct clinical entity relatively recently. The usual presenting symptoms are episodic epilepsy, periodic muscle jerking (myoclonus), and progressive skeletal weakness, but the onset and severity of the symptoms are variable. The term "ragged red fibers" refers to the histologic appearance of muscle from affected individuals, in which abnormal mitochondria accumulate and aggregate in individual muscle fibers. Other symptoms may include sensorineural hearing loss, ataxia, cardiomyopathy, and dementia.

Pathophysiology

The central energy-producing machinery of the mitochondria, complexes I–V of the electron transport chain, contains approximately 90 proteins. The majority are encoded by the nuclear genome and, like proteins required for replication, transcription, and translation of the mitochondrial genome, are imported into the mitochondria after translation. The mitochondrial genome itself (mtDNA) is 16,569 bp in length and encodes 13 proteins that are transcribed and translated in mitochondria; mtDNA also encodes mitochondrial ribosomal RNA and 22 mitochondrial tRNA species. Complexes I, III, IV, and V of the electron transport chain contain subunits encoded by both mtDNA and the nuclear genome, whereas the proteins that form complex II are encoded entirely in the nuclear genome.

LHON and MERRF are both caused by pathogenic variants in mtDNA; LHON is caused by pathogenic variants in a component of the electron transport chain, whereas MERRF is caused by pathogenic variants of mitochondrial tRNA, usually tRNA^{Lys}. Thus, from a biochemical perspective, LHON is caused by a specific inability to generate ATP, whereas MERRF is caused by a general defect in mitochondrial protein synthesis. However, the pathophysiologic mechanisms that lead from defective mitochondrial function to specific organ abnormalities are not completely understood. In general, organ systems affected by mitochondrial diseases are those in which ATP production plays a critical role, such as skeletal muscle and the CNS. In addition, defects in electron transport can cause excessive production of toxic free radicals, leading to oxidative damage and cell death, and may contribute to age-related dementia. Finally, several proteins that normally reside within mitochondria play key roles in the control of apoptosis; thus, primary abnormalities in mitochondrial integrity can contribute to disease both by decreasing energy production and by increasing programmed cell death.

Genetic Principles

For mitochondrial proteins encoded by the nuclear genome and imported into mitochondria after translation, defects that cause disease are inherited in a typical mendelian fashion. mtDNA, however, is transmitted by the egg and not the sperm, in part because the egg contains more than 1000 times more mtDNA molecules than the sperm. Therefore, for diseases like LHON and MERRF caused by defects in mtDNA, the conditions show a characteristic pattern of maternal inheritance (Figure 2–10) in which all offspring of an affected female are at risk but affected males never transmit the condition.

A second unique feature of diseases caused by mutations in mtDNA is the mosaic nature of the pathogenic variants within individual cells. Typically, a single cell contains 10–100 separate mtDNA molecules; in the case of an mtDNA pathogenic variant, usually only a fraction of the molecules carry the variant, a situation referred to as **heteroplasmy**. The levels of heteroplasmy may vary considerably among different individuals and among different tissues; furthermore, a female primordial germ cell with a mixture of normal and abnormal mtDNA molecules can transmit different proportions to daughter eggs (Figure 2–11). An mtDNA pathogenic variant present in all molecules is said to be homoplasmic. For both LHON and MERRF, levels of abnormal mtDNA may vary from about 50% to about 90%; in general, the severity of the condition correlates with the extent of heteroplasmy.

A final principle that is apparent from the pathophysiology of mitochondrial diseases is genetic interaction between the nuclear and mitochondrial genomes. One of the best examples is the sex difference in LHON, which affects four to five times as many males as females. This observation suggests that there may be a gene on the X chromosome that modifies the severity of a mitochondrial tRNA^{Lys} pathogenic variant and underscores the observation that, even though mtDNA itself encodes for a set of key mitochondrial components, most mitochondrial proteins are encoded by the nuclear genome.

DOWN SYNDROME

The clinical features of Down syndrome were described over a century ago. Although the underlying cause—an extra copy of chromosome 21—has been known for more than four decades, the nearly complete DNA sequence of chromosome 21—some 33,546,361 base pairs—has only recently been determined, and the relationship of genotype to phenotype is just beginning to be understood. Down syndrome is broadly representative of **aneuploid** conditions, those caused by a deviation from the normal chromosome complement (**euploidy**). Chromosome 21, which contains a little less than 2% of the total genome, is one of the **acrocentric** autosomes (the others are 13, 14, 15, and 22), one in which nearly all the DNA lies on one side of the centromere. In general, aneuploidy may involve part or all of an autosome or sex chromosome. Most individuals with Down syndrome have 47 chromosomes (ie, one extra chromosome 21, or **trisomy 21**) and are born to parents with normal karyotypes. This type of aneuploidy is usually caused by **nondisjunction** during meiotic segregation: the failure of two homologous chromosomes to separate (disjoin) from each other at anaphase. In contrast, aneuploid conditions that affect part of an autosome or sex chromosome must at some point involve DNA breakage and reunion. DNA rearrangements are an infrequent but important cause of Down syndrome and are usually evident as a karyotype with 46 chromosomes in which one chromosome 21 is fused via its centromere to another acrocentric chromosome. This abnormal chromosome is described as a **robertsonian translocation** and can sometimes be inherited from a carrier parent (Figure 2–12). Thus, Down syndrome may be caused by a variety of different karyotypic abnormalities, which have in common a 50% increase in **gene dosage** for nearly all of the genes on chromosome 21.

Clinical Manifestations

Down syndrome is the most common identifiable cause of intellectual disability, occurring in approximately once in every 700 live births and accounting for 15–20% of the intellectually disabled population. The likelihood of conceiving a child with Down syndrome is related exponentially to increasing maternal age. Historically, because screening programs were offered to pregnant women older than 35 years (Figure 2–13), most children with Down syndrome have been born to women younger than 35 years. Updated recommendations, though, recommend that screening be offered to all pregnant women, regardless of age. When not identified prenatally, Down syndrome is usually suspected shortly after birth from the

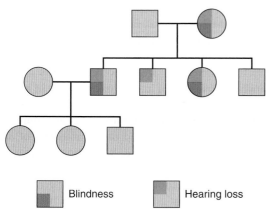

Blindness   Hearing loss

FIGURE 2–10 Maternal inheritance. An idealized pedigree illustrating maternal inheritance, which occurs in disease caused by pathogenic variants in mitochondrial DNA. Mothers transmit the variant mtDNA to all of their offspring, but fathers do not. Variable expressivity and reduced penetrance are a consequence of different levels of heteroplasmy.

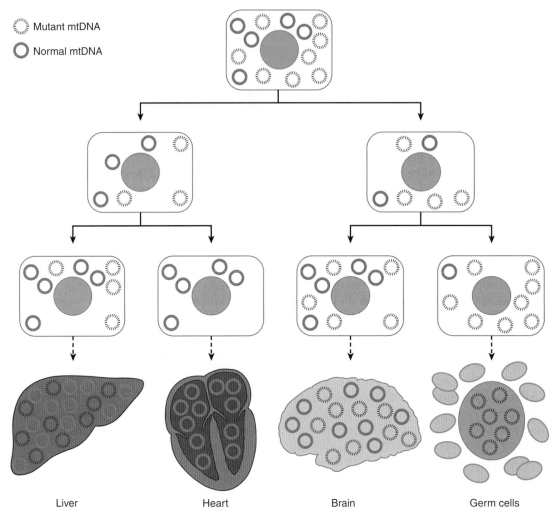

FIGURE 2–11 Heteroplasmy and variable expressivity. The fraction of variant mtDNA molecules within a cell is determined by a combination of random chance and selection at the cellular level during embryonic development. Adult tissues are mosaic for cells with different fractions of variant mtDNA molecules, which helps to explain why mitochondrial dysfunction can produce different phenotypes and different levels of severity.

presence of characteristic facial and dysmorphic features such as brachycephaly, epicanthal folds, small ears, transverse palmar creases, and hypotonia (Table 2–4). Approximately 50% of affected children have congenital heart defects that come to medical attention in the immediate perinatal period because of cardiorespiratory problems. Strong suspicion of the condition on clinical grounds is usually confirmed by molecular testing within 2–3 days.

A great many minor and major anomalies occur with increased frequency in Down syndrome, yet two affected individuals rarely have the same set of anomalies, and many single anomalies can be seen in unaffected individuals. For example, the incidence of a transverse palmar crease in Down syndrome is about 50%, ten times that of the general population, yet most individuals in whom transverse palmar creases are the only unusual feature do not have Down syndrome or any other genetic disease.

The natural history of Down syndrome in childhood is characterized mainly by developmental delay, growth restriction, and immunodeficiency. Developmental delay is usually apparent by 3–6 months of age as failure to attain age-appropriate developmental milestones and affects all aspects of motor and cognitive function. The mean IQ is between 30 and 70 and declines with increasing age. However, there is a considerable range in the degree of intellectual disability in adults with Down syndrome, and many affected individuals can live semi-independently. In general, cognitive skills are more limited than affective performance, and only a minority of affected individuals are severely impaired. Restriction of linear growth is moderate, and most adults with Down syndrome have statures 2–3 standard deviations below that of the general population. In contrast, weight growth in Down syndrome exhibits a mild proportionate increase compared with that of the general population, and most adults with Down syndrome are overweight. Although increased susceptibility to infections is a common clinical feature at all ages, the nature of the underlying abnormality is not well understood, and laboratory abnormalities can be detected in both humoral and cellular immunity.

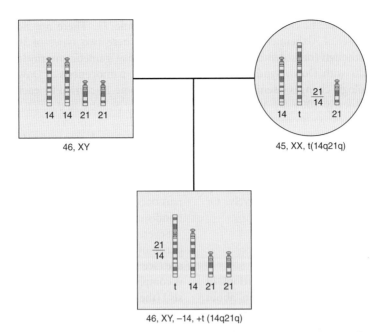

FIGURE 2-12 Mechanisms leading to Down syndrome: a pedigree in which the mother is phenotypically normal yet is a balanced carrier for a 14;21 robertsonian translocation. She transmits both the translocation chromosome and a normal chromosome 21 to her son, who also inherits a normal chromosome 21 from his father. Three copies of chromosome 21 in the son cause Down syndrome. (Adapted from Nussbaum RL et al. *Thompson & Thompson Genetics in Medicine,* 7th ed. Saunders Elsevier, 2007.)

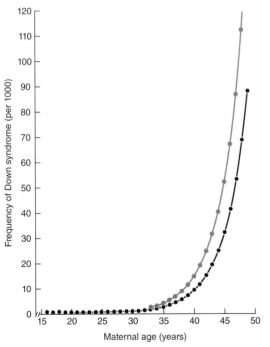

FIGURE 2-13 Relationship of Down syndrome to maternal age. The frequency of Down syndrome rises exponentially with increasing maternal age. The frequency at amniocentesis (blue symbols) is slightly higher than in live-born infants (black symbols) because miscarriages are more likely in fetuses with Down syndrome. (Data from Scriver CR et al, eds. *The Metabolic and Molecular Bases of Inherited Disease,* 8th ed. McGraw-Hill, 2001.)

TABLE 2-4 **Phenotypic features of trisomy 21.**

Feature	Frequency
Upslanting palpebral fissures	82%
Excess skin on back of neck	81%
Brachycephaly	75%
Hyperextensible joints	75%
Flat nasal bridge	68%
Wide gap between first and second toes	68%
Short, broad hands	64%
Epicanthal folds	59%
Short fifth finger	58%
Incurved fifth finger	57%
Brushfield spots (iris hypoplasia)	56%
Transverse palmar crease	53%
Folded or dysplastic ear	50%
Protruding tongue	47%

Data from Scriver CR et al, eds. *The Metabolic and Molecular Bases of Inherited Disease,* 7th ed. McGraw-Hill, 1995.

One of the most prevalent and dramatic clinical features of Down syndrome—premature onset of Alzheimer disease—is not evident until adulthood. Although frank dementia is not clinically detectable in all adults with Down syndrome, the incidence of typical neuropathologic changes—senile plaques and neurofibrillary tangles—is nearly 100% by age 35. The major causes of morbidity in Down syndrome are congenital heart disease, infections, and leukemia. Life expectancy depends to a large extent on the presence of congenital heart disease; survival to ages 10 and 30 years is approximately 60% and 50%, respectively, for individuals with congenital heart disease and approximately 85% and 80%, respectively, for individuals without congenital heart disease.

Pathophysiology

The advent of molecular markers for different portions of chromosome 21 provided considerable information about when and how the extra chromosomal material arises in Down syndrome, and the Human Genome Project has provided a list of the approximately 230 genes found on chromosome 21. In contrast, much less is known about why increased gene dosage for chromosome 21 should produce the clinical features of Down syndrome.

For trisomy 21 (47,XX+21 or 47,XY+21), cytogenetic or molecular markers that distinguish between the maternal and paternal copies of chromosome 21 can be used to determine whether the egg or the sperm contributed the extra copy of chromosome 21. There are no obvious clinical differences between these two types of trisomy 21 individuals, which suggests that gametic imprinting does not play a significant role in the pathogenesis of Down syndrome. If both copies of chromosome 21 carried by each parent can be distinguished, it is usually possible to determine whether the nondisjunction event leading to an abnormal gamete occurred during anaphase of meiosis I or meiosis II (Figure 2–14). Studies such as these show that approximately 75% of cases of trisomy 21 are caused by an extra maternal chromosome, that approximately 75% of the nondisjunction events (both maternal and paternal) occur in meiosis I, and that both maternal and paternal nondisjunction events increase with advanced maternal age.

Several theories have been proposed to explain why the incidence of Down syndrome increases with advanced maternal age (see Figure 2–13). Most germ cell development in females is completed before birth; oocytes arrest at prophase of meiosis I (the **dictyotene** stage) during the second trimester of gestation. One proposal suggests that biochemical abnormalities that affect the ability of paired chromosomes to disjoin normally accumulate in these cells over time and that, without a renewable source of fresh eggs, the proportion of eggs undergoing nondisjunction increases with maternal age. However, this hypothesis does not explain why the relationship between the incidence of trisomy 21 and advanced maternal age holds for paternal as well as maternal nondisjunction events.

Another hypothesis proposes that structural, hormonal, and immunologic changes that occur in the uterus with advanced

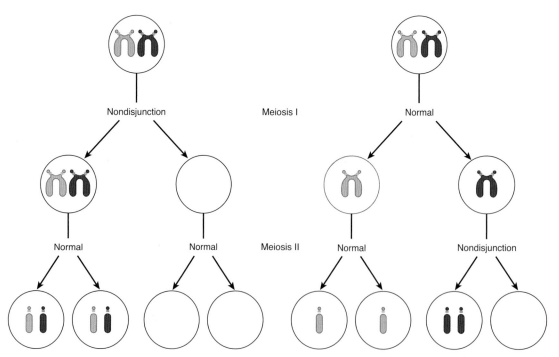

FIGURE 2–14 Nondisjunction has different consequences depending on whether it occurs at meiosis I or meiosis II. The abnormal gamete has two copies of a particular chromosome. When nondisjunction occurs at meiosis I, each of the copies originates from a different chromosome; however, when nondisjunction occurs at meiosis II, each of the copies originates from the same chromosome. Both cytogenetic and molecular polymorphisms can be used to determine the stage and the parent in which nondisjunction occurred. (Adapted, with permission, from Thompson MW et al. *Genetics in Medicine*, 5th ed. Saunders, 1991. Copyright © Elsevier.)

age produce an environment less able to reject a developmentally abnormal embryo. Thus, an older uterus would be more likely to support a trisomy 21 conceptus to term regardless of which parent contributed the extra chromosome. This hypothesis can explain why paternal nondisjunction errors increase with advanced maternal age. However, it does not explain why the incidence of Down syndrome resulting from chromosomal rearrangements (see later discussion) does not increase with maternal age.

These and other hypotheses are not mutually exclusive, and it is possible that a combination of factors is responsible for the relationship between the incidence of trisomy 21 and advanced maternal age. A number of environmental and genetic factors have been considered as possible causes of Down syndrome, including exposure to caffeine, alcohol, tobacco, or radiation, and the likelihood of carrying one or more genes that would predispose to nondisjunction. Although it is difficult to exclude all of these possibilities from consideration as minor factors, there is no evidence that any of these factors plays a role in Down syndrome.

The recurrence risk for trisomy 21 is not altered significantly by previously having affected children. However, approximately 5% of Down syndrome karyotypes have 46 rather than 47 chromosomes as a result of robertsonian translocations that usually involve chromosomes 14 or 22. As described, this type of abnormality is not associated with increased maternal age; however, in about 30% of such individuals, cytogenetic evaluation of the parents reveals a so-called balanced rearrangement such as 45,XX,+t(14q;21q). Because the robertsonian translocation chromosome can pair with both of its component single acrocentric chromosomes at meiosis, the likelihood of segregation leading to unbalanced gametes is significant (Figure 2–15), and the recurrence risk to the parent with the abnormal karyotype is much higher than for trisomy 21 (Table 2–5). Approximately 1% of Down syndrome karyotypes show mosaicism in which some cells are normal and

TABLE 2–5 Risk for Down syndrome depending on parental sex and karyotype.

Karyotype of Parent	Risk of Abnormal Live-Born Progeny	
	Female Carrier	**Male Carrier**
46,XX or 46,XY	0.5% (at age 20) to 30% (at age 30)	<0.5%
Rb(Dq;21q) (mostly 14)	10%	<2%
Rb(21q;22q)	14%	<2%
Rb(21q;21q)	100%	100%

Data from Scriver CR et al, eds. *The Metabolic and Molecular Bases of Inherited Disease,* 7th ed. McGraw-Hill, 1995.

some abnormal. Somatic mosaicism for trisomy 21 or other aneuploid conditions may initially arise either prezygotically or postzygotically, corresponding to nondisjunction in meiosis or mitosis, respectively. In the former case (in which a zygote is conceived from an aneuploid gamete), the extra chromosome is presumably lost mitotically in a clone of cells during early embryogenesis. The range of phenotypes seen in mosaic trisomy 21 is great, ranging from mild intellectual disability with subtle dysmorphic features to "typical" Down syndrome, and does not correlate with the proportion of abnormal cells detected in lymphocytes or fibroblasts. Nonetheless, on average, intellectual disability in mosaic trisomy 21 is generally milder than in nonmosaic trisomy 21.

Genetic Principles

A fundamental question in understanding the relationship between an extra chromosome 21 and the clinical features of Down syndrome is whether the phenotype is caused by

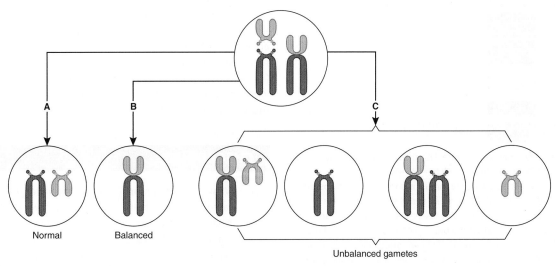

FIGURE 2–15 Types of gametes produced at meiosis by a carrier of a robertsonian translocation. In a balanced carrier for a robertsonian translocation, different types of segregation at meiosis lead to several different types of gametes, including ones that are completely normal (A), ones that would give rise to other balanced translocation carriers (B), and ones that would give rise to aneuploid progeny (C).

abnormal gene expression or an abnormal chromosomal constitution. An important principle derived from studies directed at this question is that of **gene dosage**, which states that the amount of a gene product produced per cell is proportionate to the number of copies of that gene present. In other words, the amount of protein produced by all or nearly all genes that lie on chromosome 21 is 150% of normal in trisomy 21 cells and 50% of normal in monosomy 21 cells. Thus, unlike the X chromosome, there is no mechanism for dosage compensation that operates on autosomal genes.

Experimental evidence generally supports the view that the Down syndrome phenotype is caused by increased expression of specific genes and not by a nonspecific detrimental effect of cellular aneuploidy. Rarely, karyotypic analysis of an individual with Down syndrome reveals a chromosomal rearrangement (usually an unbalanced reciprocal translocation) in which only a very small portion of chromosome 21 is present in three copies per cell (Figure 2–16). These observations suggest that there may be a critical region of chromosome 21, which, when present in triplicate, is both sufficient and necessary to produce Down syndrome.

The concept that altered gene dosage of a group of closely linked genes can produce a distinct clinical phenotype is also supported by the observation that an increasing number of congenital anomaly syndromes have been found to be caused by so-called **copy number** or **structural variants**, often mediated by homologous segments of DNA that lie at both ends of deletion and/or insertion breakpoints. Such structural

TABLE 2–6   Phenotype and karyotype of some contiguous gene syndromes.

Syndrome	Phenotype	Deletion
Langer–Gideon	Intellectual disability, microcephaly, bony exostoses, redundant skin	8q24.11–q24.3
WAGR	Wilms tumor, aniridia, gonadoblastoma, intellectual disability	11p13
Prader–Willi	Intellectual disability, growth deficiencies, hypotonia, obesity, hypopigmentation	15q11–q13
Miller–Dieker	Severe intellectual disability, absence of cortical gyri (lissencephaly) and corpus callosum	17p13.3

variants, which can be easily detected with molecular genetic techniques, result in an increase and/or decrease in gene copy number for one or more genes. **Contiguous gene syndromes**, described in Table 2–6, are generally rare, but they have played important roles in expanding our understanding of the pathophysiology of aneuploid conditions.

Carriers for robertsonian translocations that involve chromosome 21 can produce several different types of unbalanced gametes (see Figure 2–15). However, the empiric risk for such a carrier bearing an infant with Down syndrome is higher than for other aneuploid conditions, in part because embryos with other types of aneuploidies are likely to result in miscarriages early in development. Thus, the consequences of trisomy for embryonic and fetal development are proportionate to the number of genes expressed to 150% of their normal levels. Because monosomy for chromosome 21 (and other autosomes) is virtually never seen in live-born infants, a similar line of reasoning suggests that a 50% reduction in gene expression is more severe than a 50% increase. Finally, female robertsonian translocation carriers exhibit much higher empiric recurrence risks than male carriers, which suggests that (1) selective responses against aneuploidy can operate on gametic as well as somatic cells and (2) spermatogenesis is more sensitive to aneuploidy than oogenesis.

FIGURE 2–16 Down syndrome (DS) critical region. Rarely, individuals with Down syndrome will have chromosomal rearrangements that cause trisomy for just a portion of chromosome 21. The *APP*, *SOD1*, *ETS2*, *CRYA1*, and *CBS* genes encode proteins (amyloid precursor, superoxide dismutase, the Ets2 transcription factor, crystallin, and cystathionine beta-synthase, respectively) that may play a role in the pathogenesis of Down syndrome. Analysis of two sets of individuals (indicated by the two vertical lines) suggests that the genes responsible for Down syndrome lie in the region of overlap. (Reproduced, with permission, from Thompson MW et al. *Genetics in Medicine*, 5th ed. Saunders, 1991.)

CHECKPOINT

14. What are the common features of the variety of different karyotypic abnormalities resulting in Down syndrome?
15. What are the major categories of anomalies in Down syndrome, and what is their natural history?
16. Explain why trisomy 21 is associated with such a wide range of phenotypes from mild intellectual disability to that of "typical" Down syndrome.

IMPACT OF THE HUMAN GENOME PROJECT AND GENOME SEQUENCING ON PATHOPHYSIOLOGY

The major goal of the Human Genome Project has been to determine the identity and gain an understanding of all the genes of human beings and to apply this information to the diagnosis and treatment of human disease. An international collaboration, in which U.S. efforts were coordinated by the National Human Genome Research Institute, achieved a primary milestone in 2003 when the approximately 3 billion–nucleotide human genome DNA sequence was determined.

Understanding the function of all human genes has been facilitated by determining genome sequences for other living organisms. Some are closely related to humans on an evolutionary time scale, such as the chimpanzee, whose genome is approximately 98% the same as humans and whose last common ancestor with humans lived approximately 6 million years ago. Others are more distantly related, such as the laboratory mouse, the fruit fly, or baker's yeast, but nonetheless serve as valuable model organisms for experimental biologists. Even the laboratory mouse, whose last common ancestor with humans lived approximately 100 million years ago, shares more than 95% of its genes with the human genome. These considerations underscore the important genetic principle that the processes of evolution have left valuable molecular footprints that can be used to learn more about human biology.

One important advance of the Human Genome Project in the last decade has been a catalog of common human genetic variation, usually referred to as the HapMap (for "Haplotype Map"), in which millions of SNPs have been genotyped among individuals of diverse genetic ancestry, including populations from Asia, Africa, the Americas, and Europe. Because common genetic differences are a major determinant of susceptibility to conditions such as diabetes mellitus, hypertension, obesity, and schizophrenia, a principal goal of the HapMap is to develop a molecular understanding of those determinants. Importantly, the HapMap catalog of common human genetic variation makes it possible to predict DNA sequence variation for specific segments of the genome, even when that sequence has not been measured directly. The underlying reason is that, in most cases, closely linked SNPs are not independently distributed among humans but are nonrandomly associated in clusters known as haplotype blocks. For example, if two closely linked SNPs are each found at a frequency of 30%, chromosomes that carry both SNPs may exist at a frequency considerably different from 9%, which would be the prediction if the two SNPs were completely independent. This phenomenon, referred to as **allelic association** or **linkage disequilibrium**, is a result of human evolutionary and population history; the extent to which new SNPs (that arise by mutation) become separated from closely adjacent SNPs (by recombination) depends on the distance between adjacent SNPs and the effects of population history on the chances for recombination.

The idea that measuring human genetic variation on a genome-wide scale could provide insight into common diseases such as hypertension, schizophrenia, and cancer underscores the perspective that there is a spectrum of genetic disease from rare conditions inherited in a mendelian fashion (which have been the major subject of this chapter) to so-called complex genetic or multifactorial conditions, for which the incidence of the disease is influenced by a combination of genes, environment, and chance. Identifying genetic components of multifactorial conditions is an important goal of the field of genetic epidemiology, in which epidemiology-based study designs are applied to populations whose familial structure is uncertain or unknown, and SNP measurements in candidate genes are treated as hypothetical risk factors. For example, the epsilon 4 allele of the apolipoprotein E gene (*APOE4*) is found in approximately 15% of the population and increases the risk of both atherosclerosis and late-onset Alzheimer disease. However, *APOE4* is just one of many genes that influence susceptibility to these important conditions, and a major goal of the HapMap is to identify and characterize those genes, both to develop new treatments and to provide as much information as possible to physicians and their patients regarding disease susceptibility as a function of genetics.

Indeed, there is much excitement today about the potential of personalized genetic medicine, in part due to recent advances in several different areas. First, technological advances now make it possible to efficiently measure variation at millions of SNPs in individual patient samples as a routine laboratory test. These kinds of tests have been applied to thousands of individuals in so-called case–control studies to identify particular SNPs that occur more or less frequently in cases versus controls. Second, advances in the design and analysis of this type of approach, known as a **genome-wide association study** (GWAS), have been very successful in identifying new genetic determinants for obesity, diabetes, inflammatory bowel disease, coronary artery disease, and other common conditions.

A second important advance in the Human Genome Project has been the drive to develop new technological approaches for efficient and inexpensive DNA sequencing. So-called **next-generation sequencing** instruments use an innovative combination of molecular biologic, computational, and optical principles and have revolutionized our approach to biomedical research and medical care. The scale of technological advance is staggering: Sequencing the first human genome cost several billion dollars and required the effort of several thousand scientists over a decade; today, a single laboratory technician can sequence a genome on a benchtop instrument for a thousand dollars. This advanced sequencing technology has resulted in the generation of vast amounts of sequence data, which requires equally advanced bioinformatic technologies for analysis and interpretation.

The availability and low cost of genome sequencing are having an enormous impact on our approach to the diagnosis and pathophysiologic understanding of genetic disease. For example, the ability to compare entire genome sequences (or partial sequences of the protein-coding regions, or **exomes**) of individuals affected with rare syndromes is rapidly leading to the identification of pathogenic variants that cause thousands of different conditions, including recessively inherited forms of osteogenesis imperfecta, many unexplained syndromes that involve intellectual disability, and neuropsychiatric conditions such as autism. In addition, the ability to compare genome sequences of different tissues or biopsy samples from the same individual allows unprecedented insight into the pathophysiology of many cancers, identifying, for example, a catalog of DNA sequence alterations that have occurred and, in some cases, have helped to drive the progression of blood cancers, brain tumors, breast cancer, prostate cancer, and melanoma.

The future of genetic medicine will be greatly informed by these advances; many scientists envision that powerful but inexpensive laboratory tests that measure genetic variation across the entire genome will soon be used routinely to predict individual susceptibility to common and rare diseases and take appropriate steps to intervene and/or modify the course of those conditions. For example, individuals at high risk for certain types of cancer may benefit from aggressive screening programs.

Genetic differences may also help identify subgroups of patients whose course is likely to be more or less severe and who may respond to a particular treatment. The latter approach is part of the larger field of pharmacogenomics, in which sequence variation in the hundreds of genes that influence drug absorption, metabolism, and excretion is a major determinant of the balance between pharmacologic efficacy and toxicity. One might imagine, for example, that tests for specific nucleotide differences in a set of genes unique to a particular situation might be used to help predict the pathophysiologic response to alcoholic liver damage, type of regimen used to treat leukemia, and course of infectious diseases like tuberculosis or HIV infection.

CASE STUDIES

Yeong Kwok, MD

(See Chapter 25, p. 741–44 for answers)

CASE 1

A 4-year-old boy is brought in with pain and swelling of the right thigh after a fall in the home. An x-ray film reveals an acute fracture of the right femur. Questioning of the mother reveals that the boy has had two other known fractures—left humerus and left tibia—both with minimal trauma. The family history is notable for a bone problem during childhood in the boy's father that got better as he grew into adulthood. A diagnosis of osteogenesis imperfecta is entertained.

Questions

A. What are the four types of osteogenesis imperfecta? How are they genetically transmitted?
B. Which two types are most likely in this patient? How might they be distinguished clinically?
C. Further workup results in a diagnosis of type I osteogenesis imperfecta. What clinical features may the boy expect in adult life?
D. What is the pathogenesis of this patient's disease?

CASE 2

A newborn girl tests positive for phenylketonuria (PKU) on a newborn screening examination. The results of a confirmatory serum test done at 2 weeks of age are also positive, establishing the diagnosis of PKU.

Questions

A. What are the metabolic defects in persons with PKU?
B. How do these defects lead to clinical disease in persons not treated with dietary restrictions appropriate for PKU?
C. What is the genetic pattern of inheritance? What are some possible explanations for why the gene for the condition has persisted in the gene pool despite the obvious disadvantages for affected individuals?

CASE 3

A young woman is referred for genetic counseling. She has a 3-year-old boy with developmental delay and small joint hyperextensibility. The pediatrician has diagnosed fragile X–associated mental retardation. She is currently pregnant with her second child at 14 weeks of gestation. The family history is unremarkable.

Questions

A. What is the genetic mutation responsible for fragile X–associated mental retardation? How does it cause the clinical syndrome of developmental delay, joint hyperextensibility, large testes, and facial abnormalities?

B. Which parent is the probable carrier of the genetic mutation? Explain why this parent and the grandparents are phenotypically unaffected.

C. What is the likelihood that the unborn child will be affected?

CASE 4

A 16-year-old boy presents with worsening vision for the past 2 months. He first noticed that he was having trouble with central vision in his right eye, seeing a dark spot in the center of his visual field. The dark spot had gotten larger over time, and he had also developed a central loss of vision in his left eye. Two of his maternal uncles had loss of vision, but his mother and another maternal uncle and two maternal aunts had no visual difficulties. No one on his father's side was affected. Physical examination reveals microangiopathy and vascular tortuosity of the retina. Genetic testing confirms the diagnosis of Leber hereditary optic neuropathy.

Questions

A. What is the central defect in Leber hereditary optic neuropathy (LHON)?

B. How is this disorder inherited, and what is the principle of heteroplasmy?

C. What explains the fact that males are much more likely to be affected than females?

CASE 5

A 40-year-old woman, recently married and pregnant for the first time, comes to the clinic with a question about the chances of having "a Down syndrome baby."

Questions

A. What is the rate of occurrence of Down syndrome in the general population? What are some of the common clinical features?

B. What major genetic abnormalities are associated with Down syndrome? How might these abnormalities lead to the clinical features of the syndrome?

C. How might this woman's age contribute to her risk of having a child with Down syndrome?

CASE 6

A 25-year-old woman recently gave birth to a baby diagnosed with Down syndrome. Neither she nor the baby's father have a personal or family history of Down syndrome. Karyotyping of the parents shows that the mother has a balanced robertsonian translocation: 45,XX,+t(14q;21q).

Questions

A. What are common phenotypic features of babies with Down syndrome?

B. What is the chance that this couple would have a subsequent child with Down syndrome?

C. Why does the extra genetic material of chromosome 21 lead to Down syndrome?

REFERENCES

Osteogenesis Imperfecta

Forlino A et al. Osteogenesis imperfecta. Lancet. 2016 Apr 16;387(10028):1657–71. [PMID: 26542481]

Marom R et al. Pharmacological and biological therapeutic strategies for osteogenesis imperfecta. Am J Med Genet C Semin Med Genet. 2016 Dec;172(4):367–83. [PMID: 27813341]

Van Dijk FS et al. Osteogenesis imperfecta: clinical diagnosis, nomenclature and severity assessment. Am J Med Genet A. 2014 Jun;164A (6):1470–81. [PMID: 24715559]

Phenylketonuria

Blau N. Genetics of phenylketonuria: then and now. Hum Mutat. 2016 Jun;37(6):508–15. [PMID: 26919687]

Hood A et al. Variability in phenylalanine control predicts IQ and executive abilities in children with phenylketonuria. Mol Genet Metab. 2014 Apr;111(4):445–51. [PMID: 24568837]

Thomas J et al; PRISM investigators. Pegvaliase for the treatment of phenylketonuria: results of a long-term phase 3 clinical trial program (PRISM). Mol Genet Metab. 2018 May;124(1):27–38. [PMID: 29653686]

Singh RH et al. Recommendations for the nutrition management of phenylalanine hydroxylase deficiency. Genet Med. 2014 Feb;16(2):121–31. [PMID: 24385075]

Vockley J et al. Phenylalanine hydroxylase deficiency: diagnosis and management guideline. Genet Med. 2014 Feb;16(2):188–200. [PMID: 24385074]

Fragile X–Associated Mental Retardation Syndrome

Grigsby J. The fragile X mental retardation 1 gene (FMR1): historical perspective, phenotypes, mechanism, pathology, and epidemiology. Clin Neuropsychol. 2016 Aug;30(6):815–33. [PMID: 27356167]

Kidd SA et al. Fragile X syndrome: a review of associated medical problems. Pediatrics. 2014 Nov;134(5):995–1005. [PMID: 25287458]

Tassone F. Advanced technologies for the molecular diagnosis of fragile X syndrome. Expert Rev Mol Diagn. 2015;15(11):1465–73. [PMID: 26489042]

LHON, MERFF & Other Mitochondrial Diseases

Gorman GS et al. Mitochondrial diseases. Nat Rev Dis Primers. 2016 Oct 20;2:16080. [PMID: 27775730]

Meyerson C et al. Leber hereditary optic neuropathy: current perspectives. Clin Ophthalmol. 2015 Jun 26;9:1165–76. [PMID: 26170609]

Parikh S et al. Diagnosis and management of mitochondrial disease: a consensus statement from the Mitochondrial Medicine Society. Genet Med. 2015 Sep;17(9):689–701. [PMID: 25503498]

Down Syndrome

Grieco J et al. Down syndrome: cognitive and behavioral functioning across the lifespan. Am J Med Genet C Semin Med Genet. 2015 Jun;169(2):135–49. [PMID: 25989505]

Taylor-Phillips S et al. Accuracy of non-invasive prenatal testing using cell-free DNA for detection of Down, Edwards and Patau syndromes: a systematic review and meta-analysis. BMJ Open. 2016 Jan 18;6(1):e010002. [PMID: 26781507]

Vermeesch JR et al. Prenatal and pre-implantation genetic diagnosis. Nat Rev Genet. 2016;17(10):643–56. [PMID: 27629932]

The Human Genome Project & Human Genetic Variation

Ashley EA. Towards precision medicine. Nat Rev Genet. 2016 Aug 16;17(9):507–22. [PMID: 27528417]

den Dunnen JT et al. HGVS recommendations for the description of sequence variants: 2016 update. Hum Mutat. 2016 Jun;37(6):564–9. [PMID: 26931183]

Goodwin S et al. Coming of age: ten years of next-generation sequencing technologies. Nat Rev Genet. 2016 May 17;17(6):333–51. [PMID: 27184599]

Richards S et al. Standards and guidelines for the interpretation of sequence variants: a joint consensus recommendation of the American College of Medical Genetics and Genomics and the Association for Molecular Pathology. Genet Med. 2015 May;17(5):405–24. [PMID: 25741868]

Vissers LE et al. Genetic studies in intellectual disability and related disorders. Nat Rev Genet. 2016 Jan;17(1):9–18. [PMID: 26503795]

Disorders of the Immune System

Jeffrey L. Kishiyama, MD, Jennifer J. Chang, MD, & Suzanne M. Donovan, MD, MPH

The function of the immune system is to protect the host from invasion of foreign organisms by distinguishing "self" from "non-self." A well-functioning immune system not only protects the host from external factors such as microorganisms or toxins but also prevents and repels attacks by endogenous factors such as tumors and participates in tissue repair. A normal immune response relies on the careful coordination of a complex network of biological factors, specialized cells, tissues, and organs necessary for the recognition of pathogens and subsequent elimination of foreign antigens. Dysfunction or deficiency of components of the immune system leads to a variety of clinical diseases of varying expression and severity, ranging from atopic disease to autoimmune disease, primary immunodeficiency, and cancer. This chapter introduces the intricate physiology of the immune system and abnormalities that lead to diseases of hypersensitivity and immunodeficiency.

The immune system consists of both antigen-specific and nonspecific components that have distinct yet overlapping functions. The antibody-mediated and cell-mediated immune systems are **adaptive**, providing **specificity** and memory of previously encountered antigens. The **nonspecific** or **innate** defenses include epithelial barriers, mucociliary clearance, phagocytes, dendritic cells, innate lymphoid cells, mast cells, and complement proteins. Despite being phylogenetically primitive and lacking specificity, these components are essential because they are largely responsible for natural immunity to a vast array of environmental threats and microorganisms. Knowledge of the components and physiology of normal immunity is essential for understanding the pathophysiology of diseases of the immune system.

NORMAL STRUCTURE & FUNCTION OF THE IMMUNE SYSTEM

ANATOMY

Cells of the Immune System

The major cellular components of the immune system consist of monocytes and macrophages, lymphocytes, and the family of granulocytic cells, including neutrophils, eosinophils, basophils, and mast cells. Derived from hematopoietic stem cells, these fully differentiated effector cells have membrane receptors for various chemoattractants, immunoglobulins, soluble mediators, and cell-surface proteins, which facilitate cellular homing, the activation or destruction of target cells. Furthermore, it is increasingly recognized that many immune cell-types have subsets, with distinct cytokine profiles and surface markers.

Mononuclear phagocytes play a central role in the immune response. **Tissue macrophages** are derived from blood monocytes and participate in antigen processing and secretion of mediators vital to initiating specific immune responses. Abundant near mucosal surfaces and recruited to sites of inflammation, these cells phagocytose and internalize microorganisms and debris, then travel to secondary lymphoid organs where they process and present that antigen in a form recognizable to T lymphocytes. In addition, macrophages function as effector cells for certain types of tumor immunity and participate in tissue repair through promotion of angiogenesis and fibrosis.

Macrophages are activated by binding of extracellular molecules to surface-bound receptors. Receptors for complement component C3b (bound fragments of complement, activated by microbes and antigen-bound immunoglobulins; ie,

ADA	Adenosine deaminase
ADCC	Antibody-dependent cell-mediated cytotoxicity
AIDS	Acquired immunodeficiency syndrome
APC	Antigen-presenting cell
ART	Antiretroviral therapy
BCR	B-cell receptor
BTK	Bruton tyrosine kinase
C1, C2, etc.	Complement factor 1, complement factor 2, etc.
cAMP	Cyclic adenosine monophosphate
CCR5	CC-subfamily chemokine receptor 5
CD	Clusters of differentiation
CD4	Helper T-cell subset
CD8	Cytotoxic T-cell subset
CGD	Chronic granulomatous disease
CMV	Cytomegalovirus
CNS	Central nervous system
CTLA-4	Cytotoxic lymphocyte antigen 4
CVID	Common variable immunodeficiency
CXCR5	CXC-subfamily chemoreceptor 5
EBV	Epstein–Barr virus
ECP	Eosinophil cationic protein
F(ab)	Antigen-binding fragment
Fc	Crystallizable fragment or C-terminal immunoglobulin domain
FcεRI	High-affinity IgE receptor
FcγR	Fc gamma receptor
FOXP3	Forkhead box P3
GALT	Gut-associated lymphoid tissue
GM-CSF	Granulocyte-macrophage colony-stimulating factor
H1, H2, H3	Histamine receptor type 1, 2, 3
HBV	Hepatitis B virus
HCV	Hepatitis C virus
HIES	Hyper-IgE syndrome
HIV	Human immunodeficiency virus
HPV	Human papillomavirus
HSV	Herpes simplex virus
HZV	Herpes zoster virus
ICAM-1	Intercellular adhesion molecule-1
IFN-γ	Interferon-γ
Ig	Immunoglobulin
IL-1, IL-2, etc.	Interleukin-1, interleukin-2, etc.
ILC	Innate lymphoid cell
IPEX	Immunodysregulation, polyendocrinopathy, enteropathy X-linked syndrome
IVIG	Intravenous immunoglobulin
JAK	Janus kinase
JC	Jakob-Creutzfeldt
LAK cell	Lymphokine-activated killer cell
LPS	Lipopolysaccharide
LT	Leukotriene
MAC	*Mycobacterium avium* complex
MBP	Major basic protein
MHC	Major histocompatibility complex
NADPH	Nicotinamide adenine dinucleotide phosphate
NHL	Non-Hodgkin lymphoma
NK	Natural killer cells
PAF	Platelet-activating factor
PCP	Pneumocystis pneumonia
PG	Prostaglandin
PNP	Purine nucleoside phosphorylase
PTK	Protein tyrosine kinase
RAG	Recombination-activating gene
RANTES	Chemokine regulated on activation, normal T expressed and secreted
RAST	Radioallergosorbent test
SCID	Severe combined immunodeficiency disease
STAT	Signal transducer and activator of transcription
TACI	Transmembrane activator and calcium-modulator and cyclophilin ligand interactor
TAME	N-α-p-tosyl-L-arginine methylester-esterase
TCR	T-cell receptor
T$_H$1	Helper T 1 subset
T$_H$2	Helper T 2 subset
T$_H$17	Helper T subset secreting IL-17
T$_{reg}$	Helper T subset with regulatory function
TGF-β	Transforming growth factor beta
TLR	Toll-like receptor
TNF	Tumor necrosis factor
TSH	Thyroid-stimulating hormone
TX	Thromboxane
VCAM-1	Vascular cell adhesion molecule-1
VDJ	Variable Diversity Joining gene recombination
VIP	Vasoactive intestinal peptide
XLA	X-linked agammaglobulinemia
XSCID	X-linked severe combined immunodeficiency disease
ZAP-70	Zeta-associated protein 70 tyrosine kinase

immune complexes) and the Fc portion of both immunoglobulins G and E (IgG and IgE) molecules facilitate activation and phagocytosis through both antigen-specific and nonspecific immune pathways. Constitutively expressing toll-like receptors (TLRs), macrophages also recognize pathogen-associated molecular patterns and bind associated pathogen components that augment macrophage activation against intracellular pathogens, enhancing microbial ingestion and killing through synthesis of proteolytic enzymes, arachidonic acid metabolites, and reactive oxygen metabolites. Activated macrophages can synthesize and release cytokines, such as tumor necrosis factor (TNF), IL-1, and IL-6, which shape immune responses but also trigger inflammation in both health and disease.

Dendritic cells share duties as sentinel and **antigen-presenting cells (APCs)** of the innate immune system. Many dendritic cells (eg, Langerhans cells, oligodendrocytes, Kupffer cells) encounter microbes at epithelial surfaces, share a common hematopoietic precursor, and function to process and transport antigen from skin, respiratory, and gastrointestinal (GI) surfaces to regional lymphoid tissues. Like macrophages, dendritic cells are highly efficient at presenting antigen to T lymphocytes, initiating adaptive immune responses and complementing their innate immune functions.

Lymphocytes express specialized receptors, responsible for the initial recognition and binding to specific antigens. They are functionally and phenotypically divided into B and T lymphocytes. Structurally, B and T lymphocytes cannot be distinguished visually from each other under the microscope. They can be enumerated by flow cytometric phenotyping or by immunohistochemical methods. Approximately 70–80% of circulating blood lymphocytes are T cells (CD3), and 10–15% are B cells (CD19); the remainder are referred to as **natural killer (NK) cells** (CD56, CD161; also known as NK cells or null cells). The thymus-derived cells (**T lymphocytes or T cells**) are involved in cellular immune responses. **B lymphocytes or B cells** are involved in humoral or antibody responses.

During embryonic development, T cell precursors migrate to the thymus, where they develop some of the functional and cell surface characteristics of mature T cells. Through positive and negative selection, clones of autoreactive T cells are eliminated, and mature T cells migrate to the peripheral lymphoid tissues. There, they enter the pool of long-lived lymphocytes that recirculate from the blood to the lymph. Immune tolerance may occur centrally in the thymus or peripherally through mechanisms of induced anergy (functional hyporesponsiveness), suppression by regulatory T cells (T_{reg}), or deletion through apoptosis (programmed cell death).

Numerous subpopulations of T cells are now appreciated, heterogeneous with respect to their cell surface markers and functional characteristics. The T-cell receptor (TCR) complex, expressed on **helper-inducer T cells (CD4$^+$)**, recognizes antigenic peptides, processed and presented on the surface of APCs. Modulated by a host of co-stimulatory factors, CD4$^+$ T cells enhance phagocytic cell function, amplify B-cell production of immunoglobulin, recruit leukocytes, regulate inflammation and promote **T cell (CD8$^+$)–mediated cytotoxicity**. Activated CD4$^+$ T cells regulate immune responses through cell-to-cell contact and by elaboration of soluble factors or cytokines.

Subsets of CD4$^+$ T cells are differentiated based on the cytokine milieu, antigen concentration, degree of TCR binding affinity, and nature of the APC and can be identified on the basis of their pattern of cytokine production. Often, CD4$^+$ T cell subsets display autocrine characteristics, promoting their own and reciprocally inhibiting other subset development. One subset, T_H1 cells, develop in the presence of IL-12, secreted from activated macrophages, especially in the presence of infection with intracellular organisms. T_H1 cells elaborate interferon-γ (IFN-γ) and TNF, stimulating macrophage ingestion and microbe killing. Pathogenetically, T_H1 cells contribute to type IV delayed hypersensitivity reactions, tuberculin granulomatous reactions, and autoimmune disorders such as rheumatoid arthritis and multiple sclerosis. T_H2 cell subsets develop in the presence of IL-4 and secrete IL-4, IL-5, and IL-13, which facilitate humoral responses and defense against helminths. T_H2 subsets also play a key role in atopic diseases. Because IL-4 and IL-13 promote IgE production, and IL-5 is a proliferation and differentiation factor for eosinophils, T_H2 cells have been implicated in eosinophil-mediated reactions and response to allergens. Via elaboration of IL-17, T_H17 cell subsets appear to boost early phagocytic cell responses by recruiting neutrophils to sites of infection and acute inflammation. In the primary immunodeficiency known as the **hyper-IgE syndrome**, defective development of T_H17 cells presents clinically with increased susceptibility to skin and pulmonary bacterial and fungal infections.

Cytotoxic or "**killer**" **T cells (CTLs)** are CD8$^+$ effector T cells, generated after interaction with certain foreign antigens, presented by dendritic cells, in the presence of CD4$^+$ T cell–derived cytokines. CTLs are responsible for defense against intracellular pathogens (eg, viruses), tumor immunity, and organ graft rejection. Most killer T cells exhibit the **CD8$^+$** phenotype, although in certain circumstances, CD4$^+$ T cells can also be cytotoxic. CTLs may kill their target through cell-to-cell adhesion, osmotic lysis, or by inducing apoptosis. CTLs participate in delayed hypersensitivity reactions and, in some cases, destroying infected cells. The resultant tissue damage may contribute to immunopathology.

A number of additional T-helper subsets have been discovered that contribute to immune regulation. **Regulatory T cells (T_{reg})** modulate and inhibit immune responses, thereby regulating homeostasis and tolerance versus inflammation, allergy, and autoimmunity. T_{reg} cells suppress activated T-effector cells by secreting transforming growth factor-β (TGF-β) and IL-10, both inhibitory cytokines. The best characterized T_{reg} cell expresses high-affinity receptors for IL-2 (CD25) and FOXP3, a transcription factor that may suppress autoimmune disease. On the surface of FOXP3$^+$ T_{reg} cells, CTLA-4 (cytotoxic T lymphocyte antigen 4) binds to B7, a co-receptor on APCs, leading to suppression of APC-mediated T cell responses. Mutations of FOXP3 have been associated with the unchecked inflammatory autoimmune disease, known as immunodysregulation, polyendocrinopathy, enteropathy X-linked syndrome (IPEX). Induction of antigen-specific T_{reg} may be a major mechanism of action of allergen immunotherapy for the treatment of allergic rhinitis, asthma, and food, and venom hypersensitivity. The major role of B cells is to differentiate into antibody-secreting plasma cells. **B-lymphocyte** maturation proceeds in antigen-independent and antigen-dependent stages. Antigen-independent development occurs in the marrow where pre-B cells mature into immunoglobulin-bearing naive B cells (cells that have not been exposed to antigen previously). Surface **immunoglobulin** functions as B cell antigen-binding receptors. During the maturation of lymphocyte-committed hematopoietic stem cells, the genes encoding the antigen-combining sites on immunoglobulin molecules are rearranged, generating the extreme immunologic diversity seen in pre-B cells. Immature B cells initially express IgM on their surface and later in development co-express IgD. While most naive B cells that do not encounter antigen survive only a matter of months, a portion of those activated through T cell–dependent processes become long-lived memory B cells.

Memory B cells and **plasma cells**, found predominantly in primary follicles and germinal centers of the lymph nodes and spleen, express other immunoglobulin isotypes, such as IgA and IgG, and possess the capacity for brisk **secondary immune responses** upon re-exposure to antigen. In addition to their role synthesizing both membrane-bound and soluble immunoglobulin, B cells may also release cytokines and function as antigen-presenting cells (APCs).

Null cells probably include a number of different cell types, including a group called **NK cells**. These cells appear distinct from other lymphocytes in that they are slightly larger, with a kidney-shaped nucleolus, have a granular appearance (large granular lymphocytes), and express distinct cell surface markers (CD56, CD161), but lack antigen-specific T-cell receptors (CD3, or TCRs). Recruited to sites of inflammation, NK cells possess membrane receptors for the IgG molecules (FcγR), facilitating antibody-dependent cell-mediated cytotoxicity (ADCC). Binding of an antibody-coated cell or foreign substance triggers release of perforin, a pore-forming protein that causes cytolysis. Other NK cell functions include antibody-independent cellular killing, inducing apoptosis in Fas-expressing cells, and immunomodulating responses to viruses, malignancy, and transplanted tissue through a potent release of IFN-γ, TNF, and other key cytokines. **Innate lymphoid cells (ILC)** morphologically and functionally resemble T cells but lack TCR and therefore also lack antigen-specificity. Producing cytokines, they contribute to innate immunity, with roles in defense against viruses and helminths, but may also be immunopathogenic in allergic inflammation and asthma.

Polymorphonuclear leukocytes (neutrophils) are granulocytes that phagocytose and destroy foreign antigens and microbial organisms. In acute inflammatory reactions, they are attracted to the site of antigen by **chemotactic** factors, including plasma-activated complement 5 (C5a), leukotriene B_4 (LTB_4), granulocyte colony-stimulating factor (G-CSF), granulocyte-macrophage colony-stimulating factor (GM-CSF), IL-8, and platelet-activating factor (PAF). The presence of receptors for complement C3b and invariant/constant regions of IgG molecules (Fcγ) on the surface of neutrophils also facilitates the clearance of opsonized microbes through the reticuloendothelial system. Smaller antigens are phagocytosed and destroyed by lysosomal enzymes. Locally released lysosomal enzymes destroy particles too large to be phagocytosed. Neutrophils contain or generate a number of **antimicrobial** factors, including oxidative metabolites, superoxide, and hydrogen peroxide, as well as myeloperoxidase, which catalyzes the production of hypochlorite, and proteolytic enzymes, including collagenase, elastase, and cathepsin B.

Eosinophils are often found in inflammatory sites or at sites of immune reactivity and play a crucial role in the host's defense against parasites. Despite many shared functional similarities to neutrophils, eosinophils are considerably less efficient than neutrophils at phagocytosis. Eosinophils play both a proactive and a modulatory role in inflammation. They are attracted to the site of the antigen–antibody reactions by PAF, C5a, chemokines, histamine, and LTB_4. When stimulated, they release numerous inflammatory factors, including major basic protein (MBP), eosinophil-derived neurotoxin, eosinophil cationic protein (ECP), eosinophil peroxidase, lysosomal hydrolases, and LTC_4. MBP destroys parasites, impairs ciliary beating, and causes exfoliation of respiratory epithelial cells; it may also trigger histamine release from mast cells and basophils. Eosinophil-derived products may play a role in the development of airway hyperreactivity. Interleukin-5 (IL-5) is a primary growth factor for eosinophils, and current pharmacologic IL-5 antagonists appear to be clinically useful in the treatment of eosinophil-derived asthma and airways diseases.

Mast cells, found chiefly in connective and subcutaneous tissue, are basophilic cells that interface with the environment (eg, skin, conjunctiva, respiratory and gastrointestinal tracts). They have prominent granules that are the source of many mediators of immediate hypersensitivity and have 30,000–200,000 cell surface membrane receptors for the Fc fragment of IgE. When an allergen molecule cross-links two adjacent mast cell surface–associated IgE antibodies, calcium-dependent cellular activation leads to the release of both preformed and newly generated mediators. Vasoactive mediators (eg, histamine), lipid mediators (eg, prostaglandins/leukotrienes), cytokines, and proteases contribute to the acute inflammation and tissue damage seen with mast cell activation. Beyond IgE, mast cells also have surface receptors for "anaphylatoxins" (activated complement fragments, C3a, C4a, and C5a), cytokines, and neuropeptides, such as substance P. Activation by these non–IgE-mediated mechanisms may contribute to host immunity and provide ties between the immune and neuroendocrine systems. Mast cell–deficient mice display a particular vulnerability to sepsis and rapid death after peritonitis, possibly owing to insufficient TNF production during bacterial infection. Mast cells also appear in areas of wound healing and in fibrotic lung disease. Experimentally, mast cell–derived mediators have been shown to promote angiogenesis and fibrogenesis, suggesting their presence in these sites is pathologically relevant.

Basophils are circulating granulocytes with properties similar to tissue mast cells. Possessing high-affinity receptors for IgE (FcεRI), they mediate both immediate- and late-phase allergic responses. These cells release many of the potent mediators of allergic inflammatory diseases, including histamine, leukotrienes (LTs), prostaglandins (PGs), and PAF, all of which have significant effects on the vasculature and on the inflammatory response.

Organs of the Immune System

Several tissues and organs play roles in host defenses and are functionally classified as the immune system. In mammals, the primary lymphoid organs are the thymus and the bone marrow. All cells of the immune system are originally derived from **bone marrow**. Pluripotent **stem cells** differentiate into lymphocyte, granulocyte, monocyte, erythrocyte, and megakaryocyte populations. Deficiency or dysfunction of the pluripotent stem cell or the various cell lines developing from it can result in immune deficiency disorders of varying expression and severity.

The **thymus**, derived from the third and fourth embryonic pharyngeal pouches, functions to produce T lymphocytes and is the site of initial T-lymphocyte differentiation. Its reticular structure allows a significant number of lymphocytes to migrate through it to become fully immunocompetent thymus-derived cells. Developing T cells in the thymic cortex are first **positively selected** for their ability to recognize self-peptides (ie, major histocompatibility complex, MHC). In subsequent **negative selection**, T cells that avidly recognize self-peptides are destroyed, thus removing deleterious self-reactive clones. In some murine models, autoimmune diseases such as systemic lupus erythematosus may develop in mice with defective apoptotic pathways in T cells recognizing self-antigen. The thymus also regulates immune function by secreting multiple bioactive substances that promote T-lymphocyte differentiation and are essential for T-lymphocyte–mediated immunity.

In mammals, the **lymph nodes**, **spleen**, and **gut-associated lymphoid tissue** are secondary lymphoid organs connected by blood and lymphatic vessels. Lymph nodes are strategically dispersed throughout the vasculature and are the principal organs of the immune system that deliver and localize antigen, promoting adaptive immunity through cell–cell interaction and lymphocyte activation. Lymph nodes have a framework of reticular cells and fibers that are arranged into a **cortex** and **medulla**. B lymphocytes, the precursors of antibody-producing cells, or **plasma cells**, are found in the cortex (the follicles and germinal centers), as well as in the medulla. T lymphocytes are found chiefly in the medullary and paracortical areas of the lymph node (Figure 3–1). The **spleen** filters and processes antigens from the blood and is functionally and structurally divided into B-lymphocyte and T-lymphocyte areas, similar to those of the lymph nodes. The spleen also removes damaged

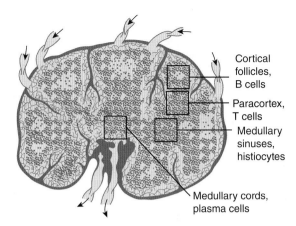

FIGURE 3–1 Anatomy of a normal lymph node. (Redrawn, with permission, from Chandrasoma P et al, eds. *Concise Pathology,* 3rd ed. Originally published by Appleton & Lange. Copyright © 1998 by The McGraw-Hill Companies, Inc.)

blood cells and immune complexes, including antibody-coated microbes. Loss of the spleen, through traumatic causes or therapeutic splenectomy, increases host susceptibility to encapsulated bacteria, which are normally cleared through opsonization and phagocytosis in splenic tissue.

Gut-associated lymphoid tissue, adjacent to the mucosal epithelium, includes the tonsils, the Peyer patches of the small intestine, and the appendix, all of which facilitate immune responses to the multitude of ingested antigens and commensal microbes. Like the lymph nodes and spleen, these tissues exhibit separation into B-lymphocyte–dependent and T-lymphocyte–dependent areas. Mucosal immune responses tend to generate antigen-specific IgA, and, with some orally administered antigens, T-cell anergy or tolerance may occur rather than immune stimulation. Increasingly, the commensal microbiome of the gastrointestinal tract has been recognized to shape both local and systemic innate and adaptive immune responses, influencing both health and disease (such as allergy or autoimmunity).

Inflammatory Mediators

Mediators are released or generated during immune responses to coordinate and regulate immune cell activities to generate physiological or cytotoxic responses. Targeting many diverse cell types, they can have antiviral, pro-inflammatory, or anti-inflammatory activities, can act locally or systemically, and can be redundant in their actions (Table 3–1). Mediators exist either in a preformed state in the granules of mast cells and basophils or are newly synthesized at the time of cellular activation. Increased awareness of the immunologic and physiologic effects of mediators has led to a better understanding of immunopathology and provides potential targets for future pharmacotherapies.

Preformed mediators include histamine, eosinophil and neutrophil chemoattractants, proteoglycans (heparin, chondroitin sulfate), and various proteolytic enzymes. **Histamine**

TABLE 3-1   Cytokines and their functions.

Cytokine	Major Cellular Source	Principal Effect
IFN-α	Macrophages, dendritic cells	Inhibit viral replication, activate NK cells
IFN-β	Virally infected cells	Inhibit viral replication, activate NK cells
IFN-γ	T cells, NK cells	Upregulate adhesion and MHC molecules, increase macrophage and antigen-presenting cell (APC) activity, promote T_H1 differentiation
IL-1	Macrophage, dendritic cells	Endogenous pyrogen, endothelial cell activation, induce acute-phase reactants
IL-2	T cells	T-cell growth factor *and* regulatory factor, B-cell and NK cell activation
IL-3	T cells	Hematopoietic growth factor
IL-4	T cells, mast cells	Induce IgE synthesis, T_H2 responses
IL-5	T_H2 cells, ILC	Eosinophil activation and growth factor, B-cell activation factor
IL-6	Macrophages, T cells, endothelial cells	Induce Ig synthesis and acute-phase reactants, T_H17 differentiation
IL-7	Bone marrow	B-cell and T-cell growth and differentiation factor
IL-8	Macrophages, neutrophils, endothelial and epithelial cells	Leukocyte chemotactic factor
IL-10	T cells, macrophages	Inhibit antigen presentation, cytokine responses
IL-12	Macrophages	Induce T_H1 responses
IL-13	T cells, mast cells	Induce immunoglobulin isotype switching to IgE
IL-17	T_H17	Activate CD4 T cells, stimulate neutrophilic inflammation
GM-CSF	Macrophages, T cells	Hematopoietic growth factor for neutrophils, eosinophils, and macrophages
TGF-β	Platelets	Immune modulator for leukocytes, tissue growth factor for wound healing
TNF	Macrophages, T cell	Endogenous pyrogen; activate neutrophils, endothelial cells, and acute-phase reactants; promote angiogenesis and coagulation

is a bioactive amine, packaged in dense intracellular granules, that when released binds to membrane-bound H_1, H_2, and H_3 receptors, resulting in significant physiologic effects. Binding to H_1 receptors causes smooth muscle contraction, vasodilatation, increased vascular permeability, and stimulation of nasal mucous glands. Stimulation of H_2 receptors causes enhanced gastric acid secretion, mucus secretion, and leukocyte chemotaxis. Histamine is important in the pathogenesis of allergic rhinitis, allergic asthma, and anaphylaxis.

Newly generated mediators include kinins, PAF, and arachidonic acid metabolites. In many immune cells, arachidonic acid, liberated from membrane phospholipid bilayers, is metabolized either by the lipoxygenase pathway to form **leukotrienes (LTs)** or by the cyclooxygenase pathway to form **prostaglandins (PGs)** and **thromboxanes** A_2 and B_2 (TXA_2 and TXB_2). LTB_4 is a potent chemoattractant for neutrophils. LTC_4, LTD_4, and LTE_4 constitute a slow-reacting substance of anaphylaxis, which has a bronchial smooth muscle spasmogenic potency 100–1000 times that of histamine, and which also causes vascular dilation and vascular permeability.

Almost all nucleated cells generate PGs. The most important are PGD_2, PGE_2, PGF_2, and PGI_2 (prostacyclin). Human mast cells produce large amounts of PGD_2, which causes vasodilatation, vascular permeability, and airway constriction. Activated polymorphonuclear neutrophils and macrophages generate $PGF_{2\alpha}$, a bronchoconstrictor, and PGE_2, a bronchodilator. PGI_2 causes platelet disaggregation. TXA_2 causes platelet aggregation, bronchial constriction, and vasoconstriction.

Macrophages, neutrophils, eosinophils, and mast cells generate **PAF**, which causes platelet aggregation, vasodilatation, increased vascular permeability, and bronchial smooth muscle contraction. PAF is the most potent eosinophil chemoattractant described and plays a role in anaphylaxis. The **kinins** are vasoactive peptides formed in plasma when kallikrein, released by basophils and mast cells, digests plasma kininogen. Kinins, including **bradykinin**, contribute to human angioedema and anaphylaxis by causing slow, sustained contraction of bronchial and vascular smooth muscle, vascular permeability, secretion of mucus, and stimulation of pain fibers. Bradykinin antagonists may be used therapeutically to treat life-threatening swelling in patients with hereditary angioedema.

Cytokines

Many immune functions are regulated or mediated by cytokines, which are soluble factors secreted by activated immune cells. Cytokines can be functionally organized into groups according to their major activities: (1) those that promote inflammation and mediate natural immunity, such as IL-1, IL-6, IL-8, TNF, and IFN-α; (2) those that support allergic inflammation, such as IL-4, IL-5, and IL-13; (3) those with immunoregulatory activity, such as IL-10, IL-12, TGF-β, and IFN-γ; and (4) those that act as hematopoietic growth factors, such as IL-3, IL-7, and GM-CSF (see Table 3–1). A group of chemotactic factors called **chemokines** regulate homing and migration of immune cells to sites of inflammation. Human immunodeficiency virus (HIV) may exploit certain chemokine receptors to infect host cells, and natural mutations in these same chemokine co-receptors may confer a susceptibility or resistance to infection. Targeting specific immune cells or pathogenetic mechanisms, therapeutic applications of cytokines are now available for a variety of autoimmune, inflammatory, atopic and hematologic disorders.

Complement Cascades

The complement system is a family of serum proteins, which, when activated through a series of proteolytic enzymes, enhances microbe opsonization, leukocyte recruitment, and target cell lysis. **Immune complex** formation (ie, the union of antigen with IgG or IgM antibody) initiates **classic complement pathway** activation. Complement-fixing sites on the Fc portion the immunoglobulin molecules are exposed, allowing binding of the first component of the complement sequence, C1q. Other components of the complement sequence are subsequently bound and activated, leading to significant amplification of the immune response. Important byproducts of the classic pathway include activated cleavage products, the anaphylatoxins C3a, C5a, and less-potent C4a. C5a is a potent leukocyte chemotactic factor that also causes mediator release from mast cells and basophils. C4b and C3b mediate immune complex binding to phagocytic cells, facilitating opsonization.

Activation of the complement sequence by the **alternative pathway** is initiated by a number of agents, including lipopolysaccharides (LPS; eg, bacterial endotoxin), trypsin-like molecules, aggregated IgA and IgG, and cobra venom. Activating the alternative pathway does not require the presence of antigen–antibody immune complexes or use the early components of the complement sequence, C1, C4, and C2. Ultimately, activating either the classic or alternative pathway leads to formation of the membrane attack complex, resulting in cell lysis, and/or tissue inflammation. Soluble inhibitors regulate the complement pathway to prevent unchecked activation and prolonged inflammation. Deficiency of one factor, C1-esterase inhibitor, leads to recurrent, potentially life-threatening attacks of facial, laryngeal, and gastrointestinal (GI) swelling in hereditary angioedema.

CHECKPOINT

1. What are the specific and nonspecific components of the cellular and noncellular limbs of the immune system?
2. What is the role of macrophages in the immune system, and what are some of the products they secrete?
3. What are the categories of lymphocytes, and how are they distinguished?
4. What is the role of lymphocytes in the immune system, and what are some of the products they secrete?
5. What is the role of eosinophils in the immune system, and what are some of the products they secrete?
6. What is the role of basophils in the immune system, and what are some of the products they secrete?
7. What is the role of epithelial cells in the immune system, and what are some of the products they secrete?
8. What are the primary and secondary lymphoid organs, and what roles do they play in the proper functioning of the immune system?

PHYSIOLOGY

1. Innate & Adaptive Immunity

Living organisms exhibit two levels of response against external invasion: an **innate system** of natural immunity and an **adaptive system** that is acquired. Innate immunity is present from birth, does not require previous antigenic exposure, and is nonspecific in its activity. The skin and epithelial surfaces serve as the first line of defense of the innate immune system, whereas enzymes, the alternative complement system pathway, acute-phase proteins, phagocytic, NK cells, and cytokines provide additional layers of protection.

Microbial cell walls or nucleic acids contain nonmammalian patterns or motifs that can bind to cell-associated pattern recognition receptors (ie, **Toll-like receptors [TLRs]**) on innate immune cells including macrophages and dendritic and epithelial cells. These structures are highly conserved, and different TLRs binds to specific pathogen-related products, such as LPS, viral RNA, microbial DNA, and fungal wall mannon proteins. Binding triggers transcription of proinflammatory factors and cytokine synthesis (TNF, IFNγ, IL-1, IL-6, and IL-12, among others) prior to adaptive responses. Some of these released cytokines are endogenous pyrogens, others antiviral, and still others shape adaptive immune responses by modulating the differentiation of naive T cells into specific T-helper subtypes or effector cells.

Through a series of proteolytic activations, the serum and membrane components of the **complement cascade** amplify and regulate microbial killing and inflammation. Despite the lack of specificity, innate immunity is largely responsible for protection against a vast array of environmental microorganisms and foreign substances.

Higher organisms have evolved an adaptive immune system, which is triggered by encounters with foreign agents that have evaded or penetrated the innate immune defenses. The adaptive immune system is characterized both by **specificity** for individual foreign agents and by **immunologic memory**, which makes possible an intensified response to subsequent encounters with the same or closely related agents. **Primary** adaptive immune responses require clonal expansion, leading to a delayed response to new exposures. **Secondary** immune responses are more rapid, larger, and more efficient. Stimulation of the adaptive immune system triggers a complex sequence of events that initiate the activation of lymphocytes, the production of antigen-specific antibodies (humoral immunity) and effector cells (cellular or cell-mediated immunity), and ultimately, the elimination of the inciting substance. Although adaptive immunity is antigen specific, the repertoire of responses is tremendously diverse, with an estimated 10^9 antigenic specificities.

2. Antigens (Immunogens)

Foreign substances that induce an immune response are called **antigens** or **immunogens**. Immunogenicity implies that the substance has the ability to react with antigen-binding sites on antibody molecules or TCRs. Complex foreign agents possess distinct and multiple antigenic determinants or "epitopes," dependent on the peptide sequence and conformational folding of immunogenic proteins. Most immunogens are proteins, although pure carbohydrates may be immunogenic as well. It is estimated that the human immune system can respond to 10^7–10^9 different antigens, an amazingly diverse repertoire.

3. Immune Response

The primary role of the immune system is to discriminate self from non-self and to eliminate foreign substances. The physiology of the normal immune response to antigen is summarized in Figure 3–2. A complex network of specialized cells, organs, and biologic factors is necessary for the recognition and subsequent elimination of foreign antigens. Both T and B cells need to migrate throughout the body to increase the likelihood that they will encounter an antigen to which they have specificity. Soluble antigens are transported to regional lymph tissues through afferent lymphatic vessels, while other antigens are carried by phagocytic dendritic cells. Regional, peripheral lymphoid organs and the spleen are sites for concentrated immune responses to antigen by recirculating lymphocytes and APCs. Antigens encountered via inhaled or ingested routes activate cells in the respiratory mucosa– or gut-associated lymphoid tissues. The major pathways of antigen elimination include the direct killing of target cells by cytotoxic T lymphocytes (CTLs; **cellular response**) and the elimination of antigen through antibody-mediated events arising from T- and B-lymphocyte interactions (**humoral response**). The series of events that initiate the immune response includes antigen processing and presentation, lymphocyte recognition and activation, cellular or humoral immune responses, and antigenic destruction or elimination.

Antigen Processing & Presentation

Most foreign immunogens are not recognized by the immune system in their native form and require capture and **processing** by professional **APCs**, which constitutively express class II MHC molecules and accessory **co-stimulatory molecules** on their surfaces. Such specialized cells include macrophages, dendritic cells in lymphoid tissue, Langerhans cells in the skin, Kupffer cells in the liver, microglial cells in the nervous system, and B lymphocytes.

Following an encounter with immunogens, the APCs internalize the foreign substance by phagocytosis or pinocytosis, modify the parent structure, and display antigenic fragments of the native protein on its surfaces in association with MHC class II molecules (see later discussion). T-cell–independent antigens such as polysaccharides can activate B cells without assistance from T cells by binding to B-cell receptors (BCRs, or surface-bound antibody), leading to rapid IgM responses, without generating memory cells or long-lived plasma cells. Most antigens, however, require internalization and processing by B cells or other APCs with subsequent recognition by CD4 T cells.

T-Lymphocyte Recognition & Activation

The recognition of processed antigen by specialized T lymphocytes known as **helper T (CD4) lymphocytes** and the subsequent activation of these cells constitute the critical events in the immune response. The helper T lymphocytes orchestrate the many cells and biologic signals (cytokines) necessary to carry out the immune response. Helper T lymphocytes recognize processed antigen displayed by APCs only in association with polymorphic cell surface proteins called the **major histocompatibility complex (MHC)**. With haplotypic mendelian inheritance, MHC genes are highly polymorphic. Known also as **human leukocyte antigens (HLAs)**, these proteins participate in the co-presentation of processed peptide antigens to T cells, thereby facilitating the essential distinction of "self" from "non-self." During cell-to-cell contact between T helper cells and APCs, the combined antigen–MHC complex functions as the binding epitope, interacting with the TCR and its associated accessory molecules, CD4 or CD8. Although HLA typing is used primarily for determining transplant compatibility, HLAs also determine immune responsiveness to foreign agents and confer susceptibility to certain autoimmune disorders. All somatic cells express MHC class I, whereas only the specialized APCs can express MHC class II. Exogenous foreign antigens are expressed in association with **MHC class II** structures, expressed only by specialized APCs.

Besides binding to modified antigen, T cell activation depends on the co-stimulation of **accessory molecules**. Accessory molecules on T cells bind to ligands found on APCs, epithelial cells, vascular endothelium, and extracellular

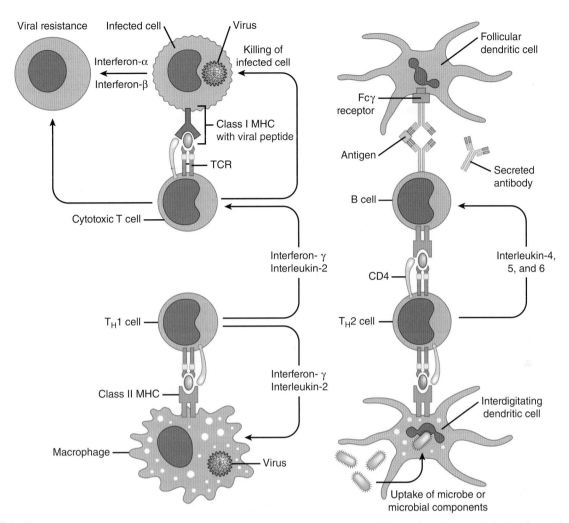

FIGURE 3-2 The normal immune response. Cytotoxic T-cell response is shown on the left side of the figure, and the helper T-cell response is shown on the right side. As depicted on the left, most CD8 T cells recognize processed antigen presented by MHC class I molecules and destroy infected cells, thereby preventing viral replication. Activated T cells secrete interferon-γ, which, along with interferon-α and interferon-β secreted by infected cells, produces cellular resistance to viral infection. On the right and at the bottom, CD4 helper (T$_H$1 and T$_H$2) cells recognize processed antigen presented by MHC class II molecules. T$_H$1 cells secrete interferon-γ and interleukin-2, which activate macrophages and cytotoxic T cells to kill intracellular organisms; T$_H$2 cells secrete interleukin-4, 5, and 6, which help B cells secrete protective antibodies. B cells recognize antigen directly or in the form of immune complexes on follicular dendritic cells in germinal centers.

matrix, controlling the subsequent T-cell function or homing (Table 3–2). In the absence of such signals, the T cell may be "tolerized" or may undergo apoptosis instead of being activated. Biologic products that block some of these co-stimulatory pathways are currently being investigated as potential therapeutic agents to prevent organ rejection in transplantation and in the management of some autoimmune diseases.

Before an activated T cell can differentiate, proliferate, produce cytokines, or participate in cell killing, the activation signal must be transduced into the cytoplasm or nucleus of the cell. The presence of **immunoreceptor tyrosine activation motifs** associated with each TCR complex facilitates and amplifies intracellular signaling. The binding of zeta-associated protein 70 (ZAP-70), a Syk-family protein tyrosine kinase (PTK), to CD3ε and ζ-subunits after they are phosphorylated is critical for downstream signaling. Another important

enzyme in the activation of T cells is CD45, a protein tyrosine phosphatase. The critical nature of these enzymes in lymphocyte development is underscored by the discovery of ZAP-70 and CD45 deficiency syndromes, disorders that result in various forms of severe combined immunodeficiency disease (SCID; see Primary Immunodeficiency Diseases).

T-cell activation does not occur in isolation but also depends on the cytokine milieu. In true autocrine fashion, the APCs involved in antigen presentation release **IL-1**, which induces the release of both **IL-2** and **IFN-γ** from CD4 cells. **IL-2** feeds back to stimulate the expression of additional **IL-2** receptors on the surface of the CD4 cells and stimulates the production of various cell growth and differentiation factors (**cytokines**) by the activated CD4 cells. Induction of IL-2 expression is particularly critical for T cells. Cyclosporine and tacrolimus, two immunosuppressive agents used to prevent organ transplant

TABLE 3–2   T-cell and APC surface molecules and their interactions.

T-Cell Surface Receptor	APC Counter-Receptor	Function and Effect
T-cell receptor (CD3)	Processed antigen + MHC complex	Antigen presentation
CD4	MHC class II	Presentation of antigen to helper T cell by APC
CD8	MHC class I	Presentation of antigen to cytotoxic T cell
CD40 ligand (CD154)	CD40	T-cell–induced B-cell activation
CD28	B7	T-cell proliferation and differentiation
CTLA-4	B7	T-cell anergy
LFA-1	ICAM-1	Adhesion

rejection, function by downregulating IL-2 production by T cells.

CD8 Effector Cells (Cellular Immune Response)

CTLs eliminate target cells (virally infected cells, tumor, or foreign tissues), thus constituting the cellular immune response. CTLs differ from helper T lymphocytes in their expression of the surface antigen CD8 and by the recognition of antigen complexed to cell surface proteins of **MHC class I**. All somatic cells can express MHC class I molecules. Pathogenic microorganisms, whose proteins gain access to the cell cytoplasm (eg, malarial parasites) or by de novo gene expression in the infected cell cytoplasm (eg, viruses) stimulate CD8 class I MHC-restricted T-cell responses. Killing of target cells by CTLs requires direct cell-to-cell contact. Two major mechanisms for killing target cells have been described: (1) CTL secretion of a pore-forming protein (perforin) that inserts in the plasma membrane of target cells along with serine proteases called granzymes, leading to osmotic lysis; and (2) expression of the Fas ligand on the surface of CTLs that bind to Fas on the target cell membrane inducing apoptosis. In addition to killing infected cells directly, CD8 T cells can elaborate a number of cytokines, including TNF and lymphotoxin. Memory CTLs may be long-lived to provide "recall" responses and immunity against latent or persistent viral infections.

Activation of B Lymphocytes (Humoral Immune Response)

The primary function of mature B lymphocytes is to synthesize antibodies. Like T-cell activation, B-lymphocyte activation is triggered after antigen binds to BCRs (ie, surface-bound immunoglobulin) and is regulated through concomitant co-receptor binding. In secondary lymphoid tissues, release of cytokines IL-2, IL-4, IL-5, and IL-6 by activated helper T lymphocytes promotes the proliferation and terminal differentiation of B cells into high-rate antibody-producing cells called plasma cells, which secrete antigen-specific **immunoglobulin**. If complement fragments bind B-cell surface complement receptors at the same time antigen engages BCRs, cellular responses are heightened. T cells also modulate humoral immunity through their activation-dependent membrane expression of **CD40 ligand** protein. During direct T- and B-cell contact, CD40 ligand binds to the **CD40 receptor** on the surface of B cells, inducing apoptosis or activation of immunoglobulin synthesis, depending on the situation. The importance of CD40 ligand–CD40 binding in normal humoral immunity is highlighted by the congenital immunodeficiency X-linked hyper-IgM syndrome. A defect in the synthesis of CD40 ligand on activated T cells results in impaired "isotype switching" and hyper-IgM, with subsequent deficient IgG and IgA production and impaired humoral immunity.

Although their primary function is immunoglobulin synthesis, B lymphocytes may also bind and internalize foreign antigen directly, process that antigen, and present it to CD4 T lymphocytes. A pool of activated B lymphocytes may differentiate into **memory cells**, which respond more rapidly and efficiently to subsequent encounters with identical or closely related antigenic structures.

Antibody Structure & Function

Antibodies (immunoglobulins) are proteins that possess "specificity," enabling them to combine with one particular antigenic structure. Antigen-binding sites for immunoglobulin will recognize three-dimensional structures, whereas TCRs bind short peptide segments without tertiary structure. Humoral (antibody-mediated) immune responses result in the production of a diverse repertoire (estimated 10^9–10^{11}) of antibody specificities, providing the ability to recognize and bind with a broad range of antigens. This diversity is a function of somatic recombination of gene segments within B lymphocytes early in ontogenetic development. Rearrangement occurs at the genetic loci for the immunoglobulin and TCR antigen binding sites through a process called **variable-diversity-joining (VDJ) gene recombination**. Somatic recombination, in both T cells and B cells, is dependent on **recombination-activating genes (RAG1 and RAG2)**, deficiency of which leads to a lack of T and B lymphocytes, an autosomal recessive form of SCID. Somatic mutations occurring after antigenic stimulation lead to a phenomenon called "affinity maturation," whereby the average affinity of antibody binding increases throughout the immune response.

All immunoglobulin molecules share a four-chain polypeptide structure consisting of two heavy and two light chains (Figure 3–3). Each chain includes an amino-terminal portion, containing the **variable (V) region**, and a carboxyl terminal portion, containing four or five **constant**

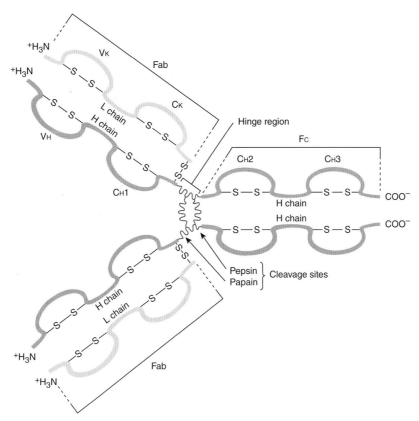

FIGURE 3-3 Structure of a human IgG antibody molecule. Depicted are the four-chain structure with two heavy chains (H) and two light chains (L). Each light chain consists of a variable and constant region. (V, variable region; C, constant region.) The sites of pepsin and papain cleavage are shown. (Reproduced, with permission, from Parslow TG, et al, eds. *Medical Immunology*, 10th ed. McGraw-Hill, 2001.)

(**C**) **regions**. V regions are highly variable structures that form the antigen-binding sites, whereas the C domains support effector functions of the molecules. The five classes (**isotypes**) of immunoglobulins are **IgG**, **IgA**, **IgM**, **IgD**, and **IgE** and are defined on the basis of differences in the C region of the heavy chains. The isotype expressed by a particular B lymphocyte depends on the state of cellular differentiation and "isotype switching," a process characterized by splicing of heavy chain mRNA prior to translation and leading to synthesis of different immunoglobulin classes. Different isotypes contribute to different effector functions on the basis of the ability of the molecule to bind to specific receptors and their efficiency in fixing serum complement. **IgG** is the predominant immunoglobulin in serum with the longest half-life. Four subclasses—IgG$_1$, IgG$_2$, IgG$_3$, and IgG$_4$—differ in their relative quantities and targets (protein vs. carbohydrate antigens). **IgA** is the predominant immunoglobulin on mucous membrane surfaces. It exists predominantly as a monomer in serum and as a dimer or trimer when secreted on mucous membrane surfaces. IgA antibodies protect the host from foreign antigens on mucous membrane surfaces, but they do not fix complement by the classic pathway. **IgM** is a pentamer found almost exclusively in the intravascular compartment. IgM is expressed early in immune responses, providing rapid adaptive immunity, and detection of antigen-specific IgM can be used diagnostically during certain infections. **IgD**

is a monomeric immunoglobulin. Its biological function is unknown. **IgE** is the heaviest immunoglobulin monomer, with a normal concentration in serum varying from 20 to 100 IU, but the concentration may be 5 times normal or even higher in an atopic individual. The Fc portion of IgE binds to receptors on the surfaces of mast cells and basophils. IgE antibodies play an important role in immediate hypersensitivity reactions.

Humoral Mechanisms of Antigen Elimination

Antibodies induce the elimination of foreign antigen through a number of different mechanisms. Binding of antibody to bacterial toxins or foreign venoms may cause neutralization or promote elimination of these antigen–antibody immune complexes through the reticuloendothelial system. Antibody-coated bacteria are more easily phagocytosed by macrophages in a process known as **opsonization**. Some classes of antibodies may complex with antigen and activate the complement cascade ("complement fixation"), culminating in lysis of the target cell. Finally, the major class of antibody, IgG, can bind to NK cells that subsequently complex with target cells and release cytotoxins (see prior discussion of antibody-dependent cellular cytotoxicity). IgG passes transplacentally, providing passive immunization of neonates.

After the successful elimination of antigen, the immune system uses several mechanisms to return to basal homeostasis. IgG can switch off its own response to antigen through the binding of immune complexes that transmit inhibitory signals into the nuclei of B cells.

Mechanisms of Inflammation

Elimination of foreign antigen by cellular or humoral processes is integrally linked to the inflammatory response, in which cytokines and antibodies trigger the recruitment of additional cells and the release of endogenous vasoactive and proinflammatory enzymatic substances (**inflammatory mediators**).

Inflammation may have both positive and deleterious effects. Tight control of inflammatory mechanisms promotes efficient elimination of foreign substances, killing microbes, infected cells, and tumors. Uncontrolled lymphocyte activation and unregulated antibody production, however, can lead to tissue damage and organ dysfunction. Pathogenic immune dysfunction is responsible for hypersensitivity reactions, immunodeficiency, and many of the clinical effects of autoimmunity. Imbalances in the inflammatory system may result from genetic defects, infection, neoplasms, and exposure to environmental triggers, although precise mechanisms that promote abnormal regulation and persistence of inflammatory processes are complex and poorly understood.

Hypersensitivity Immune Responses

Gell and Coombs classified the mechanisms of immune responses to antigen into four distinct types of reaction to allow for a clearer understanding of the immunopathogenesis of disease.

A. Type I

Clinical allergy represents an IgE-mediated hypersensitivity response arising from deleterious inflammation in response to the presence of normally harmless antigens, such as pollen, animal dander, or foods. Anaphylactic or immediate hypersensitivity reactions occur after binding of antigen to IgE antibodies attached to the surface of the mast cell or basophil and result in the release of preformed and newly generated inflammatory mediators that produce the clinical manifestations. Examples of type I–mediated reactions include anaphylactic shock, allergic rhinitis, allergic asthma, and allergic food and drug reactions.

B. Type II

Cytotoxic reactions involve the binding of either IgG or IgM antibody to antigens covalently bound to cell membrane structures. Antigen–antibody binding activates the complement cascade and results in destruction of the cell to which the antigen is bound. Examples of tissue injury by this mechanism include immune hemolytic anemia and Rh hemolytic disease in the newborn. An example of the type II–mediated disease

process without cell death is autoimmune hyperthyroidism, a disorder in which anti-thyroid antibodies bind to and stimulate thyroid tissue.

C. Type III

Antigen binding to antibodies with complement fixation forms immune complexes. Complement-bound immune complexes facilitate opsonization by phagocytes and ADCC. Complexes are usually cleared from the circulation in the reticuloendothelial system. However, deposition of these complexes in tissues or in vascular endothelium can produce immune complex–mediated tissue injury through complement activation, anaphylatoxin generation, polymorphonuclear leukocyte chemotaxis, mediator release, and tissue injury. Cutaneous Arthus reaction, systemic serum sickness, some aspects of clinical autoimmunity, and certain features of infective endocarditis are clinical examples of type III–mediated diseases. In the earliest reported cases of serum sickness, passive immunization with horse serum triggered the formation of human–anti-horse serum immune complexes, leading to fever, rash, renal dysfunction, and inflammatory arthritis.

D. Type IV

Cell-mediated immunity is responsible for host defenses against intracellular pathogenic organisms, although abnormal regulation of this system may result in delayed-type hypersensitivity. Type IV hypersensitivity reactions are mediated not by antibody but by antigen-specific T lymphocytes. Classic examples are tuberculin skin test reactions and contact dermatitis.

IgE Synthesis in Allergic Reactivity

Atopy or Ig-E–mediated immediate hypersensitivity results from the inappropriate and sustained production of IgE in response to allergen. T_H2 cytokines IL-4 and IL-13 are critical to isotype switching through induction of germline transcription of IgE heavy chain genes. IL-13 has about 30% structural homology with IL-4 and shares much of the activities of IL-4 on mononuclear cells and B lymphocytes. There is a strong genetic predisposition toward the development of atopic disease. Evidence has been found for the linkage of 5q31.1 and the IL-4, IL-5, IL-9, and IL-13 receptor genes, suggesting that a nearby gene in this chromosome locale regulates overall IgE production.

In contrast, T_H1-generated IFN-γ inhibits IL-4–dependent IgE synthesis in humans. Thus, an imbalance favoring IL-4 over IFN-γ may induce IgE formation. In one study, reduced cord blood IFN-γ at birth was found to be associated with clinical atopy at age 12 months.

In allergic inflammatory processes, T_H2 lymphocytes, innate lymphoid cells (ILCs), and follicular T cells represent a source of IL-4, as well as secondary signals necessary to drive the production of IgE by B lymphocytes. Another T_H2 cytokine, IL-5, promotes maturation, activation, chemotaxis, and prolongation of survival in eosinophils. In situ hybridization analyses of T-cell mRNA in airway mucosal biopsies from allergic rhinitis and asthma patients show a distinct T_H2 pattern. The demonstration of allergen-specific T-cell lines that proliferate and secrete large amounts of IL-4 on exposure to relevant antigen in vitro further supports the existence of specific T_H2-like clones. The original source of the IL-4 responsible for T_H2 differentiation is unclear, although some observations suggest that a T_H2 bias exists during fetal development in both atopic and nonatopic individuals. The "hygiene hypothesis" posits that environmental exposures, possibly to bacterial products, such as endotoxin, bacterial DNA, or the gut commensal microbiome, encourage a shift toward T_H1 and a subsequent reduced risk of clinical atopic disease. Mononuclear phagocytes are the major source of IL-12, suggesting a mechanism whereby antigens more likely to be processed by macrophages, including bacterial antigens and intracellular pathogens, produce T_H1 responses. Epidemiologic studies of children suggest those exposed to daycare at early ages and those with numerous siblings are at reduced risk for atopy and asthma.

Since the discovery of IgE more than 5 decades ago, scientists have considered various therapeutic strategies to selectively inhibit IgE antibody production and action. Recent data suggest that conventional and modified immunotherapy (allergy shots) eliminate ("anergize") rather than stimulate T_H2 responses to environmental allergen, potentially through generation of immunosuppressive T_{reg}. Current research has focused on understanding the mechanisms controlling IgE production, including the molecular events of B-cell switching to IgE synthesis, IL-4 and IL-13 signaling, T- and B-cell surface receptor interactions, and mechanisms driving T_H2

differentiation. Soluble cytokine receptors and genetically engineered monoclonal antibodies are currently under development for the purpose of cytokine neutralization in allergic diseases. The U.S. Food and Drug Administration (FDA) has approved several immunomodulatory agents, including omalizumab (anti-IgE), benralizumab, mepolizumab and reslizumab (all anti-IL-5 agents), and dupilumab (anti-IL-4 and anti-IL-13), for the treatment of severe refractory asthma and of atopic dermatitis.

CHECKPOINT

9. What are the components of and distinctions between the innate and adaptive forms of immunity?

10. Indicate the primary role of the immune system and the major classes of events by which this is accomplished.

11. What is the phenomenon of MHC restriction?

12. What signals are necessary to activate helper T lymphocytes?

13. What two signals are necessary to activate cytotoxic T lymphocytes?

14. What are the common structural features of antibodies?

15. Name four different mechanisms by which antibodies can induce the elimination of foreign antigens.

16. What are the four types of immune reactions in the Gell and Coombs classification scheme, and what are some examples of disorders in which each is involved?

17. What is the critical factor in switching Ig synthesis to the IgE isotype? What are some secondary factors that contribute to, or inhibit, IgE synthesis?

PATHOPHYSIOLOGY OF SELECTED IMMUNE DISORDERS

ALLERGIC RHINITIS

Clinical Presentation

Allergic airway diseases such as allergic rhinitis and asthma are characterized by local tissue damage and organ dysfunction in the upper and lower respiratory tract arising from an abnormal hypersensitivity immune response to normally harmless and ubiquitous environmental allergens. Allergens that cause airway disease are predominantly seasonal tree, grass, and weed pollens or perennial inhalants (eg, house dust mite or cockroach antigen, mold, animal dander, and some occupational protein antigens). Allergic disease is a common cause of pediatric and adult acute and chronic airway problems. Both allergic rhinitis and asthma account for significant morbidity, and atopic disorders have increased in prevalence over the past few decades. In a Danish survey, the prevalence

of skin test–positive allergic rhinitis in persons 15–41 years of age increased from 12.9% in 1990 to 22.5% in 1998. Allergic rhinitis is discussed here as a model for the pathophysiology of IgE-mediated allergic airway disease.

Etiology

Allergic rhinitis implies the existence of type I (IgE-mediated) immediate hypersensitivity to environmental allergens that impact the upper respiratory mucosa directly. Particles larger than 5 μm are filtered almost completely by the nasal mucosa. Because most pollen grains are at least this large, few intact particles would be expected to penetrate the lower airway when the nose is functioning normally. The allergic or atopic state is characterized by an inherited tendency to generate IgE antibodies to specific environmental allergens and the physiologic responses that ensue from inflammatory mediators released after the interaction of allergen with mast cell–bound IgE. The clinical presentation of allergic rhinitis includes nasal, ocular, and palatal pruritus, paroxysmal sneezing, rhinorrhea, and nasal congestion. A personal or family history of other allergic diseases such as asthma or atopic dermatitis supports a diagnosis of allergy. Confirmation of allergic rhinitis requires the demonstration of specific IgE antibodies to common allergens by in vitro immunoassay or in vivo (skin) testing in patients with a history of symptoms with relevant exposures.

Pathology & Pathogenesis

Inflammatory changes in the airways are recognized as critical features of both allergic rhinitis and chronic asthma. Cross-linking of surface-bound IgE by antigen activates tissue mast cells and basophils, inducing the immediate release of preformed mediators and the synthesis of newly generated mediators. Mast cells and basophils also have the ability to synthesize and release proinflammatory cytokines, growth and regulatory factors that interact in complex networks. The interaction of mediators with various target organs and cells of the airway can induce a **biphasic allergic response**: an early phase mediated chiefly by release of histamine and other stored mediators (tryptase, chymase, heparin, chondroitin sulfate, and TNF), whereas late-phase events are induced after generation of arachidonic acid metabolites (LTs and PGs) and PAF and de novo cytokine synthesis.

The **early-phase response** occurs within minutes after exposure to an antigen. After intranasal challenge or ambient exposure to a relevant allergen, the allergic patient begins sneezing and develops an increase in nasal secretions. After approximately 5 minutes, the patient develops mucosal swelling leading to reduced airflow. These changes are secondary to the effects of vasoactive and smooth muscle constrictive mediators, including histamine, N-α-p-tosyl-L-arginine methylesteresterase (TAME), LTs, PGD_2, and kinins and kininogens from mast cells and basophils. Histologically, the early response is characterized by vascular permeability, vasodilatation, tissue edema, and a mild cellular infiltrate of mostly granulocytes.

The **late-phase allergic response** may follow the early-phase response (dual response) or may occur as an isolated event. Late-phase reactions begin 2–4 hours after initial exposure to antigen, reach maximal activity at 6–12 hours, and usually resolve within 12–24 hours. If the exposure is frequent or ongoing, however, the inflammatory response becomes chronic. The late-phase response is characterized by erythema, induration, heat, burning, and itching and microscopically by a significant cellular influx of mainly eosinophils and mononuclear cells. Changes consistent with airway remodeling and tissue hyperreactivity may also occur.

Mediators of the early-phase response—except for PGD_2—reappear during the late-phase response in the absence of antigen re-exposure. Absence of PGD_2, an exclusive product of mast cell release, in the presence of continued histamine release suggests that basophils and not mast cells are an important source of mediators in the late-phase response.

There is an early accumulation of neutrophils and eosinophils, with later accumulation of activated T cells, synthesizing T_H2 cytokines. Inflammatory cells infiltrating tissues in the late-phase response may further elaborate cytokines and histamine-releasing factors that may perpetuate the response, leading to sustained hyperresponsiveness, mucus hypersecretion, IgE production, eosinophilia, and disruption of the target tissue (eg, bronchi, skin, or nasal mucosa).

There is strong circumstantial evidence that eosinophils are key proinflammatory cells in allergic airway disease. Eosinophils are frequently found in secretions from the nasal mucosa of patients with allergic rhinitis and in the sputum of asthmatics. Products of activated eosinophils such as MBP and eosinophilic cationic protein, which are destructive to airway epithelial tissue and predispose to persistent airway reactivity, have also been localized to the airways of patients with allergic disease.

The recruitment of eosinophils and other inflammatory cells to the airway is largely a product of activated **chemokines** and **adhesion molecules**. There are two subfamilies of chemokines, which differ in the cells they primarily attract and in the chromosome location of their genes. The C-C chemokines, including RANTES, MCP-1, MCP-3, and eotaxin, are located on chromosome segment 7q11-q21 and selectively recruit eosinophils. Leukocytes attach to vascular endothelial cells through receptor–ligand interaction of cell surface **adhesion molecules** of the integrin, selectin, and immunoglobulin supergene family. The interaction of these adhesion molecules and their counter-receptors mediates a sequence of events that includes margination of leukocytes along the walls of the microvasculature, adhesion of leukocytes to the epithelium, transmigration of leukocytes through vessel walls, and migration along a chemotactic gradient to reach tissue compartments. Both chemokine production and adhesion molecule expression are upregulated by soluble inflammatory mediators. For instance, endothelial cell adhesion molecule receptors, ICAM-1, VCAM-1, and E-selectin, are upregulated by IL-1, TNF, and LPS.

Clinical Manifestations

The clinical manifestations of allergic airway disease (Table 3–3) arise from the interaction of mast cell and basophil mediators with target organs of the upper and lower airway. The symptoms of allergic rhinitis appear immediately after exposure to a relevant allergen (early-phase response), although many patients experience chronic and recurrent symptoms on the basis of the late-phase inflammatory response. Complications of severe or untreated allergic rhinitis include sinusitis, auditory tube dysfunction, hyposmia, sleep disturbances, asthma exacerbations, and chronic mouth breathing.

A. Sneezing, Pruritus, and Mucus Hypersecretion

Patients with allergic rhinitis develop chronic or episodic paroxysmal sneezing; nasal, ocular, or palatal pruritus; and watery rhinorrhea triggered by exposure to a specific allergen. Patients may demonstrate signs of chronic pruritus of

TABLE 3–3 Clinical manifestations of allergic rhinitis.

Symptoms and Signs
Sneezing paroxysms
Nasal, ocular, palatal itching
Clear rhinorrhea
Nasal congestion
Pale, bluish nasal mucosa
Transverse nasal crease
Infraorbital cyanosis ("allergic shiners")
Serous otitis media
Laboratory Findings
Nasal eosinophilia
Evidence of allergen-specific IgE by skin or radioallergosorbent testing (RAST)

the upper airway, including a horizontal nasal crease from frequent nose rubbing ("allergic salute") and palatal "clicking" from rubbing the itching palate with the tongue. Many tissue mast cells are located near terminal sensory nerve endings. Pruritus and sneezing are caused by histamine-mediated stimulation of these c-fibers. Mucus hypersecretion results primarily from excitation of parasympathetic–cholinergic pathways. Early-phase symptoms are best treated with avoidance of relevant allergens and oral or topical antihistamines, which competitively antagonize H_1 receptor sites in target tissues. Anti-inflammatory treatment can reduce cellular inflammation during the late phase, providing more effective symptom relief than antihistamines alone. Allergen immunotherapy (hyposensitization) has shown effectiveness in reducing symptoms and airway inflammation by inhibiting both early- and late-phase allergic responses. Diverse mechanisms of immunotherapy have been observed, including reducing seasonal increases in IL-4 and allergen-specific IgE, inducing allergen-specific IgG_1 and IgG_4 (blocking antibodies), modulating T-cell cytokine synthesis by enhancing T_H1 and inhibiting T_H2 responses, and upregulating T_{reg} and downregulating eosinophilic and basophilic inflammatory responses to allergen. One trial found that immunotherapy administered to patients with grass-pollen allergy for 3–4 years induced prolonged clinical remission accompanied by a persistent alteration in immunologic reactivity that included sustained reductions in the late skin response and associated T-cell infiltration and IL-4 mRNA expression.

B. Nasal Stuffiness

Symptoms of nasal obstruction may become chronic as a result of persistent late-phase allergic mechanisms. Nasal mucous membranes may appear pale blue and boggy. Children frequently show signs of obligate mouth breathing, including long facies, narrow maxillae, flattened malar eminences, marked overbite, and high-arched palates (so-called adenoid facies). These symptoms are not mediated by histamine and are, therefore, poorly responsive to antihistamine therapy. Oral sympathomimetics that induce vasoconstriction by stimulating α-adrenergic receptors are often used in conjunction with antihistamines to treat nasal congestion. Topical decongestants may be used to relieve acute congestion but have limited value in patients with chronic allergic rhinitis because frequent use results in rebound vasodilation (rhinitis medicamentosa).

C. Airway Hyperresponsiveness

The phenomenon of heightened nasal sensitivity to reduced levels of allergen after initial exposures to the allergen is known as **priming**. Clinically, priming may be observed in patients who develop increased symptoms late in the pollen season compared with early in the season. Late-phase inflammation induces a state of nasal airway hyperresponsiveness to both irritants and allergens in patients with chronic allergic rhinitis and asthma. Airway hyperreactivity can cause heightened sensitivity to both environmental irritants such as tobacco smoke and noxious odors, as well as to allergens such as pollens. There are no standardized clinical tools to accurately assess late-phase hyperresponsiveness in allergic rhinitis as there are for asthma (methacholine or histamine bronchoprovocation challenge). Genetic markers for bronchial airway hyperresponsiveness, however, have been identified. It also appears that late-phase cellular infiltration and eosinophil byproducts may inflict airway epithelial damage, which in turn can predispose to upper and lower airways hyperreactivity.

Accumulating evidence supports a relationship between allergic rhinitis and asthma. Many patients with rhinitis alone demonstrate nonspecific bronchial hyperresponsiveness, and prospective studies suggest that nasal allergy may be a predisposing risk factor for developing asthma. Treatment of patients with allergic rhinitis may result in improvement of asthma symptoms, airway caliber, and bronchial hyperresponsiveness to methacholine and exercise. Finally, mechanistic studies of airway physiology have demonstrated that nasal disease may influence pulmonary function via both direct and indirect mechanisms. Such mechanisms may include the existence of a nasal–bronchial reflex (with nasal stimulation causing bronchial constriction), postnasal drip of inflammatory cells and mediators from the nose into the lower airways, absorption of inflammatory cells and mediators into the systemic circulation and ultimately to the lung, and nasal blockage and subsequent mouth breathing, which may facilitate the entry of asthmagenic triggers to the lower airway.

D. In Vivo or In Vitro Measurement of Allergen-Specific IgE

This is the primary tool for the confirmation of suspected allergic disease. In vivo **skin testing** with allergens suspected of causing hypersensitivity constitutes an indirect bioassay for the presence of allergen-specific IgE on tissue mast cells or basophils. Percutaneous or intradermal administration of dilute concentrations of specific antigens elicits an immediate wheal-and-flare response in a sensitized individual. This response marks a "local anaphylaxis" resulting from the controlled release of mediators from activated mast cells. Positive skin test results to airborne allergens, combined with a history and examination suggestive of allergy, strongly implicate the allergen as a cause of the patient's symptoms. Negative skin test results with an unconvincing allergy history argue strongly against an allergic origin. Major advantages to skin testing include simplicity, rapidity of performance, and low cost.

In vitro tests provide quantitative assays of allergen-specific IgE in the serum. In these assays, patient serum is reacted initially with antigen bound to a solid-phase material and then labeled with a radioactive or enzyme-linked anti-IgE antibody. These immunoallergosorbent tests show a 70–80% correlation with skin testing to pollens, dust mites, and danders and are useful in patients receiving chronic antihistamine therapy who are unable to undergo skin testing and in patients with extensive dermatitis.

E. Complications of Allergic Rhinitis

Serous otitis media and sinusitis are major comorbidities in patients with allergic rhinitis. Both conditions occur secondarily to the obstructed nasal passages and sinus ostia in patients with chronic allergic or nonallergic rhinitis. Complications of chronic rhinitis should be considered in patients with protracted rhinitis unresponsive to therapy, refractory asthma, or persistent cough. Serous otitis results from auditory tube obstruction by mucosal edema and hypersecretion. Children with serous otitis media can present with conductive hearing loss, delayed speech, and recurrent otitis media associated with chronic nasal obstruction.

Sinusitis may be acute, subacute, or chronic depending on the duration of symptoms. Obstruction of osteomeatal drainage in patients with chronic rhinitis predisposes to bacterial infection in the sinus cavities. Patients manifest symptoms of persistent nasal discharge, cough, sinus discomfort, and nasal obstruction. Examination may reveal chronic otitis media, infraorbital edema, inflamed nasal mucosa, and purulent nasal discharge. Radiographic diagnosis by x-ray film or computed tomographic (CT) scan reveals sinus opacification, membrane thickening, or the presence of an air-fluid level. Effective treatment of infectious complications of chronic rhinitis requires antibiotics, systemic antihistamine and decongestants, and perhaps intranasal or systemic corticosteroids.

CHECKPOINT

18. What are the major clinical manifestations of allergic rhinitis?
19. What are the major etiologic factors in allergic rhinitis?
20. What are the pathogenetic mechanisms in allergic rhinitis?

PRIMARY IMMUNODEFICIENCY DISEASES

There are many potential sites where developmental aberrations in the immune system can lead to abnormalities in immunocompetence manifesting as an increased susceptibility to infection (Figure 3–4; Tables 3–4 and 3–5). When these defects are genetic in origin, they are referred to as primary immunodeficiency disorders. This is in contrast to compromised immunity secondary to pharmacologic therapy, HIV, malnutrition, or systemic illnesses such as systemic lupus erythematosus or diabetes mellitus.

Clinical investigations of various congenital defects have helped characterize many aspects of normal immune physiology. Defects in host immunity place the susceptible individual at high risk for a variety of infectious, malignant, and autoimmune diseases and disorders. The nature of the specific functional defect will significantly influence the susceptibility to infections caused by specific pathogens and their associated clinical features. Table 3–5 lists some of the typical organisms causing infection in patients with various immunodeficiency disorders. Any immunopathogenic mechanism that impairs T-lymphocyte function, or **cell-mediated immunity**, predisposes the host to the development of serious chronic and potentially life-threatening opportunistic infections with viruses, mycobacteria, fungi, and protozoa involving any or all organ systems. Similarly, immunopathogenic dysfunction of B lymphocytes resulting in **antibody deficiency** will predispose the host to pyogenic sinopulmonary and mucosal infections. Defects in **innate immunity** adversely influence phagocytic function, leukocyte adhesion and migration, NK cell function, and/or TLR signaling, leading to ineffective microbial killing. As the molecular bases of many primary immunodeficiency disorders are being discovered, it has become apparent that different molecular defects can result in common clinical phenotypes.

As T lymphocytes play a central role in inducing and coordinating immune responses, dysfunction can be associated with an increased incidence of autoimmune phenomena. These include diseases clinically similar to rheumatoid arthritis, systemic lupus erythematosus, and immune hematologic cytopenias. Patients with impaired immune responses are also at greater risk for certain malignancies than the general

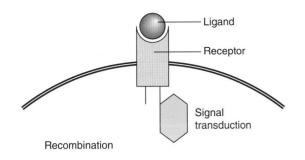

FIGURE 3–4 Simplified schema of defects in cell surface receptor–dependent activation leading to different primary immunodeficiency disorders. Table 3–4 lists the syndromes and immunologic deficits seen with a variety of these humoral, cellular, neutrophil, or combined immunodeficiency disorders.

population. The occurrence of cancer may be related to an underlying impairment of tumor surveillance, dysregulation of cellular proliferation and differentiation, chromosomal translocations during defective antigen receptor gene rearrangement, or the presence of infectious agents predisposing to or causing cellular transformation. Non-Hodgkin lymphoma or B-cell lymphoproliferative disease, skin carcinomas, and gastric carcinomas are the most frequently occurring tumors in patients with immunodeficiency.

Traditionally, the primary immunodeficiencies are classified according to which component of the immune response is principally compromised: the humoral response, cell-mediated immunity, innate immunity, complement, or phagocytic cell function (see Table 3–4). Distinct developmental stages characterize the maturation and differentiation of the cellular components of the immune system. The underlying

TABLE 3–4   Primary immunodeficiency disorders.

Combined Immunodeficiency		
XSCID	Deficiency of common γ chain of IL-2 receptor	Defective cytokine signaling
ZAP-70 deficiency	Defective TCR signaling	CD8 T-cell lymphopenia, CD4 T-cell dysfunction
SCID-ADA deficiency	Enzyme defect	T cell (–), B cell (–), NK cell (–)
P56^{lck} deficiency	Defective T-cell receptor–associated tyrosine kinase	T cell (+), B cell (+), NK cell (+)
JAK-3 deficiency	Defective cytokine signaling	T cell (–), B cell (+), NK cell (+)
RAG1 deficiency RAG2 deficiency	Recombination defect	T cell (–), B cell (–), NK cell (+)
PNP deficiency	Enzyme defect	T cell (–)
MHC class I deficiency	Defect in transporter associated with antigen presentation (TAP)	Bare lymphocyte syndrome, no MHC class I expression
MHC class II deficiency	Defective transcription of MHC class II genes	Bare lymphocyte syndrome, no MHC class II expression
Humoral Immunodeficiency		
X-linked agammaglobulinemia	Defect in BTK	Arrested maturation of B-cell lineage
Common variable immunodeficiency	Abnormal proliferation and differentiation of B cells or abnormal regulatory cell function[1]	Heterogeneous disorder with agammaglobulinemia
Hyper-IgM syndrome	Defective CD40-ligand binding	Abnormal immunoglobulin isotype switching
Cellular Immunodeficiency		
DiGeorge syndrome	Most have chromosome 22q11 deletion	Complete or partial T-cell deficiency
Phagocytic Cell Disorders		
Chronic granulomatous disease	Defective NADPH oxidase	Abnormal oxidative metabolism
Leukocyte adhesion deficiency	Defect in CD18 subunit of β$_2$-integrin molecule	
Disorders of Innate Immunity		
Hyper-IgE syndrome	Dysregulated cytokine response	Functional impairment in selected humoral, cellular, and neutrophilic responses
Toll-like receptor 3 deficiency	Impaired activation by pathogen-associated binding patterns	Impaired response to HSV

[1]Variable defects, although the most common is in terminal differentiation of B lymphocytes.

TABLE 3–5   Relationship of various pathogens to infection in primary immunodeficiency disorders.

	Pyogenic Bacteria	Mycobacteria	Fungi		Viruses	Parasites		
			Pneumocystis jiroveci	Other Fungi		*Giardia lamblia*	*Toxoplasma gondii*	*Cryptosporidium, Isospora*
SCID	+	+	+	+	+	–	–	–
Thymic hypoplasia	–	+	–	+	+	–	–	–
X-linked agammaglobulinemia	+	–	–	–	–	+	–	–
Common variable immunodeficiency	+	–	–	–	–	+	–	–
Complement deficiency	+	–	–	–	–	–	–	–
Phagocytic defects	+	–	–	–	–	–	–	–

Key: + = association; – = no association.

pathophysiologic abnormalities leading to primary immunodeficiency are diverse and include the following: (1) early developmental defects in cellular maturation; (2) specific enzyme defects; (3) abnormalities in cellular proliferation and functional differentiation; (4) abnormalities in cellular regulation; and (5) abnormal responses to cytokines.

COMBINED IMMUNODEFICIENCY

Severe Combined Immunodeficiency Disease

Clinical Presentation

Many primary immunodeficiency disorders present early in the neonatal period. In patients with severe combined immunodeficiency disease (SCID), there is an absence of normal thymic tissue, and the lymph nodes, spleen, and other peripheral lymphoid tissues are devoid of lymphocytes. In these patients, the complete or near-complete failure of development of both the cellular and the humoral component of the immune system results in severe infections. The spectrum of infections is broad because these patients may also suffer from overwhelming infection by opportunistic pathogens, disseminated viruses, and intracellular organisms. Failure to thrive may be the initial presenting symptom, but mucocutaneous candidiasis, chronic diarrhea, and pneumonitis are common. Vaccination with live viral vaccines or bacillus Calmette–Guérin (BCG) may lead to disseminated disease. Without immune reconstitution by bone marrow transplantation, SCID is inevitably fatal within 1–2 years.

Pathology and Pathogenesis

SCID is a heterogeneous group of disorders characterized by a failure in the cellular maturation of lymphoid stem cells,

resulting in reduced numbers and function of both B and T lymphocytes and hypogammaglobulinemia. The molecular basis for many types of SCID have been discovered (see Table 3–4). The genetic and cellular defects can occur at many different levels, starting with surface membrane receptors but also including deficiencies in signal transduction or metabolic biochemical pathways. Although the different molecular defects may cause clinically indistinguishable phenotypes, identification of specific mutations allows for improved genetic counseling, prenatal diagnosis, and carrier detection. Moreover, specific gene transfer offers hope as a future therapy.

1. Defective Cytokine Signaling—X-linked SCID (XSCID) is the most prevalent form of SCID, resulting from a genetic mutation in the common **γ chain** of the trimeric (αβγ) **IL-2 receptor**. This defective chain is shared by the receptors for IL-4, IL-7, IL-9, and IL-15, leading to dysfunction of all of these cytokine receptors. Defective signaling through the IL-7 receptor appears to block normal maturation of T lymphocytes. Circulating B-cell numbers may be preserved, but defective IL-2 responses inhibit proliferation of T, B, and NK cells, explaining the combined immune defects seen in XSCID patients. A defect in the α chain of the **IL-7 receptor** can also lead to an autosomal recessive form of SCID through mechanisms similar to XSCID but with intact NK cells.

2. Defective T-Cell Receptor and TCR signaling—The genetic defects for several other forms of autosomal recessive SCID have also been identified. A **deficiency of ZAP-70**, a protein tyrosine kinase important in signal transduction through the TCR, leads to a total absence of CD8 T lymphocytes. ZAP-70 plays an essential role in thymic selection during T-cell development. Consequently, these patients possess functionally defective CD4 T lymphocytes and no circulating CD8 T lymphocytes. B-lymphocyte and NK cell functions remain intact, but immunoglobulin production is impaired, in part owing to a lack of T-helper activity. **Mutations of CD3δ, CD3γ**, and **CD3ε** subunits may lead to partially arrested development of TCR expression and severe T-cell deficiency. **Deficiencies of both p56ˡᶜᵏ and Janus kinase 3 (Jak3)** can also lead to SCID through defective signal transduction. P56ˡᶜᵏ is a TCR-associated tyrosine kinase essential for T-cell differentiation, activation, and proliferation. Jak3 is a cytokine receptor–associated signaling molecule.

3. Defective Receptor Gene Recombination—Patients have been identified with defects in enzymes participating in VDJ recombination. **Recombination-activating genes (RAG1 and RAG2)** initiate recombination of antigen-binding receptor genes in both immunoglobulins and TCRs. Defects in RAG-1 and RAG-2 lead to a failure in VDJ receptor gene rearrangement and, subsequently, a severe quantitative and functional deficiency of T and B lymphocytes. NK cells are not antigen specific and for that reason are unaffected. **Artemis** and **DNA ligase-4** proteins are involved in double-stranded DNA breakage and repair during VDJ recombination of T-cell receptors and BCRs. Artemis mutations may also lead to increased sensitivity to ionizing radiation. Because NK cells are invariant, their numbers are typically preserved, even as T- and B-cell numbers are severely deficient.

4. Defective Nucleotide Salvage Pathway—Approximately 20% of SCID cases are caused by a **deficiency of adenosine deaminase (ADA)**, which is an enzyme in the purine salvage pathway, responsible for the metabolism of adenosine. Absence of the ADA enzyme results in an accumulation of toxic adenosine metabolites within the cells. These metabolites inhibit normal lymphocyte proliferation and lead to extreme cytopenia of both B and T lymphocytes. The combined immunologic deficiency and clinical presentation of this disorder, known as **SCID-ADA**, is identical to that of the other forms of SCID. Skeletal abnormalities and neurologic abnormalities may be associated with this disease. In similar fashion, **purine nucleoside phosphorylase deficiency** leads to an accumulation of toxic deoxyguanosine metabolites. T-cell development is impaired, possibly through induced apoptosis of double-positive thymocytes in the corticomedullary junction of the thymus. B-cell dysfunction is more variable.

CELL-MEDIATED IMMUNODEFICIENCY

DiGeorge Syndrome (22q11.2 Deletion Syndrome)

Clinical Presentation and Pathogenesis

The clinical manifestations of **DiGeorge syndrome** reflect the defective embryonic development of organs derived from the third and fourth pharyngeal arches, including the thymus, parathyroids, and cardiac outflow tract. Occasionally, the first and sixth pharyngeal pouches may also be involved. Cytogenetic abnormalities, most commonly chromosome 22q11

deletions, are associated with DiGeorge syndrome, especially in patients manifesting cardiac defects. DiGeorge syndrome is classified as complete or partial depending on the presence or absence of immunologic abnormalities. In this syndrome, the spectrum of immunologic deficiency is wide, ranging from immune competency to conditions in which there are life-threatening infections with organisms typically of low virulence. Patients affected by the complete syndrome have a profound T lymphocytopenia resulting from congenital **thymic aplasia** with impaired T-lymphocyte maturation, severely depressed cell-mediated immunity, and decreased suppressor T-lymphocyte activity. B lymphocytes and immunoglobulin production are unaffected in most patients, although in rare instances patients may present with mild hypogammaglobulinemia and absent or poor antibody responses to neoantigens. In this subset of patients, inadequate helper-T function as a result of dysfunctional T- and B-cell interaction and inadequate cytokine production leads to impaired humoral immunity.

DiGeorge syndrome is truly a developmental anomaly and can be associated with structural abnormalities in the cardiovascular system such as truncus arteriosus or right-sided aortic arch. Parathyroid abnormalities may lead to hypocalcemia, presenting with neonatal tetany or seizures. In addition, it is common for patients to exhibit facial abnormalities such as micrognathia, hypertelorism, low-set ears with notched pinnae, and a short philtrum.

HUMORAL IMMUNODEFICIENCY

X-Linked Agammaglobulinemia

Clinical Presentation

Formerly called Bruton agammaglobulinemia, **X-linked agammaglobulinemia (XLA)** is thought to be pathophysiologically and clinically more homogeneous than SCID. It is principally a disease of childhood, presenting clinically within the first year of life, after the disappearance of passively transferred maternal IgG, with multiple and recurrent sinopulmonary infections caused primarily by pyogenic bacteria and, to a much lesser extent, viruses. Because encapsulated bacteria require antibody binding for efficient opsonization, these humoral immune–deficient patients suffer from sinusitis, pneumonia, pharyngitis, bronchitis, and otitis media secondary to infection with *Streptococcus pneumoniae*, other streptococci, and *Haemophilus influenzae*. Although infections from fungal and opportunistic pathogens are rare, patients display a unique susceptibility to a rare but deadly enteroviral meningoencephalitis.

Pathology and Pathogenesis

Patients with XLA have pan-hypogammaglobulinemia, with decreased levels of IgG, IgM, and IgA. They exhibit poor to absent responses to antigen challenge, even though virtually all demonstrate normal functional T-lymphocyte responses to in vitro and in vivo tests (eg, delayed hypersensitivity skin reactions). The basic defect in this disorder appears to be arrested cellular maturation at the pre-B-lymphocyte stage. Indeed, normal numbers of pre-B lymphocytes can be found in the bone marrow, although in the circulation, B lymphocytes are virtually absent. Lymphoid tissues lack fully differentiated B lymphocytes (antibody-secreting plasma cells), and lymph nodes lack developed germinal centers. The gene defective in XLA has been isolated. The defective gene product, Bruton tyrosine kinase (BTK), is a B-cell–specific signaling protein belonging to the cytoplasmic tyrosine kinase family of intracellular proteins. Gene deletions and point mutations in the catalytic domain of the *BTK* gene block normal BTK function, necessary for B-cell maturation.

Common Variable Immunodeficiency Disease

Clinical Presentation

Common variable immunodeficiency disease is often referred to as acquired or adult-onset hypogammaglobulinemia. It is the most common serious primary immune deficiency disorder in adults. In North America, for example, it affects an estimated 1:100,000 to 1:10,000 individuals. The clinical spectrum is broad, and patients usually present within the first 2 decades of life. Affected individuals commonly develop recurrent sinopulmonary infections, including sinusitis, otitis, bronchitis, and pneumonia. Common pathogens are encapsulated bacteria such as *S pneumoniae*, *H influenzae*, and *Moraxella catarrhalis*. Bronchiectasis can be the result of recurrent serious respiratory infections, leading to infection with more virulent pathogens, including *Staphylococcus aureus* and *Pseudomonas aeruginosa*, which in turn can change the long-term prognosis. A number of important noninfectious disorders are commonly associated with common variable immunodeficiency, including GI malabsorption, autoimmune disorders, and neoplasms. The most frequently occurring malignancies are lymphoreticular, but gastric carcinoma and skin cancer also occur. Autoimmune disorders occur in 20–30% of patients and may precede the recurrent infections. Autoimmune cytopenias occur most frequently, but rheumatic diseases can also be seen. Serologic testing for infectious or autoimmune disease is unreliable in hypogammaglobulinemia. As in XLA, infusions of intravenous or subcutaneous immunoglobulin can reconstitute humoral immunity, decrease infections, and improve quality of life.

Pathology and Pathogenesis

Common variable immunodeficiency is heterogeneous disorder in which the primary immunologic abnormality is a marked reduction in antibody production. The vast majority of patients demonstrate an in vitro defect in terminal differentiation of B lymphocytes. Peripheral blood lymphocyte phenotyping demonstrates normal or reduced numbers of circulating B lymphocytes, but antibody-secreting plasma cells are conspicuously sparse in lymphoid tissues. In sharp contrast to XLA, no single gene defect can be held accountable for the multitude of defects known to cause common variable immunodeficiency. In many patients, the defect is intrinsic to the B-lymphocyte population. Approximately 15% of patients with common variable immunodeficiency disease demonstrate defective B-cell surface expression of transmembrane activator and calcium-modulator and cyclophilin ligand interactor (TACI), a member of the TNF receptor family. Lacking a functional TACI, the affected B cells will not respond to B-cell–activating factors, resulting in deficient immunoglobulin production. Another defect that may lead to common variable immunodeficiency disease involves deficient expression of B-cell surface marker CD19. When complexed with CD21 and CD81, CD19 facilitates cellular activation through BCRs. B-cell development is not affected, but humoral function is deficient. A variety of T-cell abnormalities may also lead to immune defects with subsequent impairment of B-cell differentiation. A mutation of inducible T-cell co-stimulator gene (ICOS), expressed by activated T cells and responsible for B-cell activation/antibody production, may be the molecular defect in some cases of common variable immunodeficiency disease. More than 50% of patients also have some degree of T-lymphocyte dysfunction as determined by absent or diminished cutaneous responses to recall antigens. Immune dysregulation may contribute to the morbidity and the myriad autoimmune manifestations associated with common variable immunodeficiency.

Hyper-IgM Immunodeficiency (CD40 and CD40 Ligand Deficiency)

Clinical Presentation

In patients with hyper-IgM immunodeficiency, serum levels of IgG and IgA are very low or absent, but serum IgM (and sometimes IgD) levels are normal or elevated. Inheritance of this disorder may be autosomal, although it is most often X-linked. Clinically, this syndrome is manifested by recurrent pyogenic respiratory infections, predisposition to *Pneumocystis jiroveci* pneumonia and an array of autoimmune phenomena such as Coombs-positive hemolytic anemia and immune thrombocytopenia.

Pathology and Pathogenesis

The principal abnormality is the defective expression of CD40-ligand (CD40L), a T-lymphocyte activation surface marker (also known as CD154 or gp39). In the course of normal immune responses, CD40L interacts with CD40 on B-cell surfaces during cellular activation, initiating proliferation and immunoglobulin isotype switching. In hyper-IgM syndrome, defective CD40 co-receptor stimulation during T- and B-cell interactions leads to impairment of B-cell isotype switching and subsequent production of IgM, but very low or no production of IgG, IgA, and IgE. CD40L–CD40 interaction also promotes dendritic cell maturation and IL-12 and IFN-γ secretion, so CD40L deficiency can be associated with impaired cell-mediated immunity and increased risk of opportunistic infection.

Selective IgA Deficiency

This is the most common primary immunodeficiency in adults, with a prevalence of 1:700 to 1:500 individuals. Most affected individuals have few or no clinical manifestations, but there is an increased incidence of upper respiratory tract infections, allergy, asthma, and autoimmune disorders. Whereas serum levels of the other immunoglobulin isotypes are typically normal, serum IgA levels in these individuals are markedly depressed, often less than 5 mg/dL.

As in common variable immunodeficiency, the primary functional defect is an inability of B cells to terminally differentiate to IgA-secreting plasma cells. An associated deficiency of IgG subclasses (mainly IgG_2 and IgG_4) and low-molecular-weight monomeric IgM is not uncommon and can be clinically significant. Because of the role of secretory IgA in mucosal immunity, patients with this immunodeficiency frequently develop significant infections involving the mucous membranes of the gut, conjunctiva, and respiratory tract. There is no specific therapy, but prompt antibiotic treatment is necessary in patients with recurrent infections. A subset of patients may recognize IgA as a foreign antigen. These patients are at risk for transfusion reactions to unwashed red blood cells or other blood products containing trace amounts of IgA.

DISORDERS OF PHAGOCYTIC CELLS & INNATE IMMUNITY

Defective phagocytic cell function presents with infections at sites of interface between the body and the outside world. Recurrent skin infections, abscesses, gingivitis, lymphadenitis, and poor wound healing are seen in patients with macrophage or neutrophil disorders. More difficult to assay, clinical immunodeficiency can occur through defects in phagocytic cell migration, adhesion, opsonization, or killing.

Chronic Granulomatous Disease

Clinical Presentation

Chronic granulomatous disease is typically X-linked and is characterized by impaired granulocyte function. This disorder of phagocytic cell function presents with recurrent skin infections, abscesses, and granulomas at sites of chronic inflammation. Abscesses can involve skin or viscera and may be accompanied by lymphadenitis. Catalase-positive organisms predominate; S aureus is thus the most common pathogen, although infections with Nocardia species, gram-negative Serratia marcescens, and Burkholderia cepacia can also occur. Aspergillus species and Candida represent common fungal pathogens in chronic granulomatous disease. Sterile

noncaseating granulomas resulting from chronic inflammatory stimuli can lead to GI or genitourinary tract obstruction. Chronic granulomatous disease typically presents in childhood, although cases presenting in adulthood are occasionally reported.

Pathology and Pathogenesis

Defects in the gene coding for nicotinamide adenine dinucleotide phosphate (NADPH) oxidase inhibit oxidative metabolism and severely compromise neutrophil-killing activity. NADPH oxidase is assembled from two membrane and two cytosolic components after phagocytic cell activation, leading to catalytic conversion of molecular oxygen into superoxide. Oxidative burst and intracellular killing rely on production of superoxide, which is later converted to hydrogen peroxide and sodium hypochlorite (bleach). In patients with chronic granulomatous disease, other neutrophil functions such as chemotaxis, phagocytosis, and degranulation remain intact, but microbial killing is deficient. Catalase-negative bacteria are effectively killed because microbes produce small amounts of peroxide, concentrated in phagosomes, leading to microbial death. Catalase-positive organisms scavenge these relatively small amounts of peroxide and are not killed without neutrophil oxidative metabolism. X-linked inheritance is most frequently seen, but autosomal recessive forms and spontaneous mutations can also lead to clinical disease.

Leukocyte Adhesion Deficiency, Type 1

Integrins and selectins are specialized molecules that play a role in leukocyte homing to sites of inflammation. These adhesion molecules facilitate cell–cell and cell–extracellular matrix interactions, allowing circulating leukocytes to stick and roll along endothelial cell surfaces prior to diapedesis into extravascular tissues. An autosomal recessive train, leukocyte adhesion deficiency type 1, and defective expression of β_2-integrin (CD11/CD18) adhesion molecules result in impaired leukocyte trafficking, leading to recurrent infections, lack of pus formation, and poor wound healing. Leukocytosis occurs because cells cannot exit the circulation, and recurrent infections of skin, airways, bowels, perirectal area, and gingival and periodontal areas are common.

Hyper-IgE Syndrome

Clinical Presentation

Hyper-IgE syndrome (HIES) is often referred to as "Job syndrome" because affected individuals suffer from recurrent boils as the tormented biblical figure did. The initial description of this immunodeficiency disorder was in two fair-skinned girls with recurrent staphylococcal "cold" skin abscesses associated with furunculosis, cellulitis, recurrent otitis, sinusitis, pneumatoceles, and a coarse facial appearance. The predominant organism isolated from sites of infection is

S aureus, although other organisms such as *H influenzae*, pneumococci, gram-negative organisms, *Aspergillus* sp., and *C albicans* are also often identified. Characteristically, patients have a chronic pruritic eczematoid dermatitis, defective shedding of primary teeth, growth retardation, coarse facies, scoliosis, osteopenia, vascular abnormalities, and hyperkeratotic fingernails. Extremely high IgE levels (>3000 IU/mL) have also been observed in patients' serum.

Pathology and Pathogenesis

The high IgE levels are thought to be a consequence of dysregulated immunologic responsiveness to cytokines, yet it is unclear whether the hyper-IgE contributes to the observed susceptibility to infection or is simply an immunologic epiphenomenon. Autosomal dominant forms have been associated with mutations in STAT3, a transcriptional factor involved in the activation of cytokine and growth factor receptors. Responses to numerous cytokines do appear impaired, along with decreased T_H17 function. Autosomal recessive forms have been associated with mutations in the dedicator of cytokinesis-8 (*DOCK8*) gene, which adds an increased susceptibility to cutaneous viruses and lymphopenia to the clinical presentation. A spectrum of immune abnormalities may be observed in HIES. Poor antibody responses to neoantigens, deficiency of IgA antibody against *S aureus*, and low levels of antibodies to carbohydrate antigens suggest humoral immunodeficiency. T-lymphocyte functional abnormalities are suggested by decreased absolute numbers of suppressor T lymphocytes, poor in vitro proliferative responses, and defects in cytokine production. Several reports have also documented highly variable abnormalities in neutrophil chemotaxis.

Toll-Like Receptor 3 Deficiency

Patients with toll-like receptor 3 (TLR3) deficiency have shown specific susceptibility to herpes simplex 1 (HSV1) encephalitis. Typically, binding of pathogen-associated molecular patterns to TLR will activate transcription factors, such as nuclear factor kappa beta (NF-κβ), IFN regulatory factors, and activator protein 1, leading to immune responsiveness. Defects in this pathway impair viral immunity. In TLR3 deficiency, defective IFN-α, IFN-β, and IFN-λ synthesis leads to uninhibited HSV1 replication in neurons and oligodendritic cells. A similar phenotype is seen in autosomal recessive UNC-93b deficiency. UNC-93b is required for TLR3 function, as it translocates TLR3 to its endosomal site of action.

CHECKPOINT

21. What are the major clinical manifestations of each of the five categories of primary immune deficiency?

22. What are the major pathogenetic mechanisms in each category of primary immune deficiency?

AIDS

Human immunodeficiency virus (HIV) infection is one of the greatest epidemics in human history. HIV is the agent responsible for acquired immunodeficiency syndrome (AIDS), the most common immunodeficiency disorder worldwide. AIDS, as the consequence of a chronic retroviral infection with HIV, produces severe, life-threatening CD4 helper T-lymphocyte dysfunction, opportunistic infections, and malignancies. AIDS is defined by serologic evidence of HIV infection in the presence of a variety of indicator diseases associated with clinical immunodeficiency. Tables 3–6 and 3–7 list criteria for defining and diagnosing AIDS. HIV is transmitted by exposure to infected body fluids or to sexual or even perinatal contact. Vertical transmission from mother to infant may occur in utero, during childbirth, and through breastfeeding. Transmissibility of the HIV virus is related to subtype virulence, viral load, and immunologic host factors.

Acute HIV infection may present as a self-limited, febrile viral syndrome characterized by fatigue, pharyngitis, myalgias,

TABLE 3–6 **Surveillance case definition for human immunodeficiency virus (HIV) infection among adults and adolescents (age ≥13 years), United States, 2008**

Stage	Laboratory Evidence[1]	Clinical Evidence
Stage 1	Laboratory confirmation of HIV infection and CD4+ T-lymphocyte count of ≥500 cells/μL or CD4+ T-lymphocyte percentage ≥29	None required (but no AIDS-defining condition)
Stage 2	Laboratory confirmation of HIV infection *and* CD4+ T-lymphocyte count of 200–499 cells/μL *or* CD4+ T-lymphocyte percentage of 14–28	None required (but no AIDS-defining condition)
Stage 3 (AIDS)	Laboratory confirmation of HIV infection *and* CD4+ T-lymphocyte count of <200 cells/μL *or* CD4+ T-lymphocyte percentage of <14[2]	Alternatively, documentation of an AIDS-defining condition (with laboratory confirmation of HIV infection)[1]
Stage unknown	Laboratory confirmation of HIV infection *and* no information on CD4+ T-lymphocyte count or percentage	Additionally, no information on presence of AIDS-defining conditions

[1]CD4+ T-lymphocyte percentage is the percentage of total lymphocytes. If the CD4+ T-lymphocyte count and percentage do not correspond to the same HIV infection stage, select the more severe stage.

[2]Documentation of an AIDS-defining condition supersedes a CD4+ T-lymphocyte count of ≥200 cells/μL and a CD4+ T-lymphocyte percentage of total lymphocytes of ≥14.

Centers for Disease Control and Prevention. Revised surveillance Case definitions for HIV infection among adults, adolescents, and children aged <18 months and for HIV infection and AIDS among children aged 18 months to <13 Years—United States, 2008. MMWR Recomm Rep. 2008 Dec 5;57(RR-10):1–14. [PMID: 19052530]

TABLE 3–7   AIDS-defining conditions.

Bacterial infections, multiple or recurrent[1]
Candidiasis of bronchi, trachea, or alveoli
Candidiasis of esophagus[2]
Cervical cancer, invasive[3]
Coccidioidomycosis, disseminated or extrapulmonary
Cryptococcosis, extrapulmonary
Cryptosporidiosis, chronic intestinal (>1 month's duration)
Cytomegalovirus disease (other than liver, spleen, or nodes), onset at age >1 month
Cytomegalovirus retinitis (with loss of vision)[1]
Encephalopathy, HIV-related
Herpes simplex: chronic ulcers (>1 month's duration) or bronchitis, pneumonitis, or esophagitis; onset at age >1 month
Histoplasmosis, disseminated or extrapulmonary
Isosporiasis, chronic intestinal (>1 month's duration)
Kaposi sarcoma[2]
Lymphoid interstitial pneumonia or pulmonary lymphoid hyperplasia complex[1,2]
Lymphoma, Burkitt (or equivalent term)
Lymphoma, immunoblastic (or equivalent term)
Lymphoma, primary, of brain
Mycobacterium avium complex or *Mycobacterium kansasii*, disseminated or extrapulmonary[2]
Mycobacterium tuberculosis at any site, pulmonary,[2,3] disseminated,[2] or extrapulmonary[2]
Mycobacterium, other species or unidentified species, disseminated[2] or extrapulmonary[2]
Pneumocystis jirovecii pneumonia[2]
Pneumonia, recurrent[2,3]
Progressive multifocal leukoencephalopathy
Salmonella septicemia, recurrent
Toxoplasmosis of brain, onset at age >1 month[2]
Wasting syndrome attributed to HIV

[1]Only among children aged <13 years.

[2]Condition that might be diagnosed presumptively.

[3]Only among adults and adolescents aged ≥13 years.

Centers for Disease Control and Prevention. Revised surveillance Case definitions for HIV infection among adults, adolescents, and children aged <18 months and for HIV infection and AIDS among children aged 18 months to <13 Years—United States, 2008. MMWR Recomm Rep. 2008 Dec 5;57(RR-10):1–18. [PMID: 19052530]

maculopapular rash, lymphadenopathy, and significant viremia, without detectable anti-HIV antibodies. Acute HIV infection may be detected with modern fourth- or fifth-generation immunoassays that utilize combination HIV p24 antigen and HIV antibody assays. These fourth- or fifth-generation immunoassays may detect acute HIV infection an average of 14 days following infection. Less commonly, primary HIV infection may also be associated with orogenital or esophageal ulcers, meningoencephalitis, or opportunistic infection. After an initial viremic phase, patients seroconvert and a period of clinical latency is usually seen. Lymph tissues become centers for massive viral replication during the latent, asymptomatic, stage of HIV infection. HIV viremia may be detectable by PCR assay; however, there may or may not be clinical symptoms of HIV infection until CD4 reserves become profoundly diminished. Over time, there is a progressive decline in CD4 T lymphocytes, a reversal of the normal CD4:CD8 T-lymphocyte ratio, and numerous other immunologic derangements. The clinical

manifestations are directly related to HIV tissue tropism and defective immune function. Marked immune deficiency is signaled by development of neurologic complications, opportunistic infections, or malignancies. The time course for progression is highly variable, but the median time before appearance of clinical disease is about 10 years in untreated individuals. Approximately 10% of those infected manifest rapid progression to AIDS (within 5 years after infection). A minority of individuals are termed "elite controllers" (HIV quantitative serum viral load <50/mL) or "viremic controllers" (detectable but low-level viral loads). In these individuals, genetic factors, host cytotoxic immune responses, viral load, and virulence appear to have an impact on susceptibility to infection and the rate of disease progression. Although not curative, modern antiretroviral therapies can suppress viral replication and restore immune function, leading to clinical recovery and markedly extended life expectancy.

Pathology and Pathogenesis

HIV is a single-stranded, positive-sense RNA lentivirus, whose RNA encodes for nine genes (Table 3–8). Chemokines (chemoattractant cytokines that regulate leukocyte trafficking to sites of inflammation) play a significant role in the pathogenesis of HIV disease. During the initial stages of infection and viral proliferation, virion entry and cellular infection require binding to two co-receptors on target T lymphocytes and monocyte/macrophages. All HIV strains express the envelope protein gp120, which binds to CD4 surface receptor molecules, but different viral strains display tissue "tropism" or specificity on the basis of the co-receptor they recognize. Changes in the viral phenotype during the course of an individual's HIV infection may lead to changes in tropism and cytopathology at different stages of their disease. Viral strains isolated in

TABLE 3–8   HIV genes and gene products.

Ltr	Long terminal repeat	Controls gene transcription
Gag	Polyprotein, processed into several gene products	Capsid, matrix, and nucleocapsid proteins
Pol	Polymerase	Encodes viral enzymes, including reverse transcriptase
Vif	Viral infectivity factor (p23)	Overcomes viral inhibitor
Vpr	Viral protein R	Participates in nuclear importation of viral prointegration complex
Rev	Regulator of viral gene expression	
Env	Envelope protein gp160	Cleaved into gp120, gp41, which mediate viral binding and fusion
Tat	Transcriptional activator	Increases viral gene expression
Nef	Negative effector (p24)	Regulates HIV replication

the early stages of infection and associated with mucosal and intravenous transmission (eg, R5-trophic viruses) bind macrophages expressing chemokine receptor CCR5. In the later stages of disease, CXCR-4-tropic strains of HIV are more commonly seen. X4-trophic viruses bind to chemokine receptor CXCR4, more broadly expressed on T cells, and are associated with syncytium formation. Since chemokine receptors play a role in viral cell entry, specific inherited polymorphisms of chemokine receptors influence susceptibility to infection and disease progression.

Following virion entry into the CD4 T lymphocyte, the reverse transcription step of HIV replication is error prone owing to a lack of proofreading mechanisms during and after viral reverse transcription. Mutations occur frequently, and even within an individual patient, HIV heterogeneity develops rapidly. Patients may be infected with more than one quasispecies, and through mechanisms of recombination, genes from separate strains may intermingle, contributing to genetic diversity. The development of antigenically and phenotypically distinct strains contributes to progression of disease, clinical drug resistance, and lack of efficacy of early vaccines.

Cellular activation is critical for viral infectivity and reactivation of integrated proviral DNA. After viral entry and capsid disassembly, HIV reverse transcriptase converts uncoated viral RNA into double-stranded viral DNA. Using several host proteins, including HIV integrase enzyme, the double-stranded viral DNA complex is transported into the host cell nucleus and integrates into the host chromosome. Integrated HIV DNA is referred to as "provirus" and may remain latent or become transcriptionally active, depending on the activation state of the host cell. Cellular activation triggers NF-κβ, a cytoplasmic transcription factor that migrates to the nucleus, initiating viral gene expression. HIV protein *Nef* enhances viral replication and reduces host antiviral immune responses. New infectious virions are assembled. Viral proteins and RNA are packaged at the infected cell's exterior membrane through a process called budding.

Although only 2% of mononuclear cells are found peripherally, lymph nodes from HIV-infected individuals can contain large amounts of virus sequestered among infected follicular dendritic cells in the germinal centers. For patients infected through vaginal or rectal mucosa, gut-associated lymphoid tissue is a major site of viral replication and persistence. Gut-associated lymphoid tissue harbors the majority of the host's T cells, and when HIV-infected epidermal Langerhans cells migrate to draining lymph nodes, large numbers of lymphocytes encounter surface-bound virus. The persistence of virus in these secondary lymphoid structures triggers cellular activation and massive, irrevocable depletion of CD4 T-lymphocyte reservoirs, as well as disease latency. The marked decline in CD4 T-lymphocyte counts is due to several mechanisms: (1) direct HIV-mediated infection and destruction of CD4 T lymphocytes during viral replication; (2) depletion by fusion and formation of multinucleated giant cells (syncytium formation); (3) toxicity of viral proteins to CD4 T lymphocytes and hematopoietic precursors; (4) loss of T-lymphocyte

co-stimulatory factors such as CD28; and (5) induction of apoptosis of uninfected T cells. CD8 CTL activity is initially brisk and effective at controlling viremia but later induces the generation of viral escape mutations. Ultimately, viral proliferation outstrips host responses, and HIV-induced immunosuppression leads to disease progression. Neutralizing antibodies are generated very late, but mutations in HIV-envelope proteins overcome protective humoral responses. Over time, the infection is characterized by systemic, generalized cytokine dysregulation and immune activation. Hyperactivity of the immune system increases naive T-cell infection. Ultimately, these events prove deleterious to maintenance of lymphatic organs, bone marrow integrity, and effective immune responses.

In addition to the cell-mediated immune defects, B lymphocyte function is altered such that many HIV-infected individuals have marked hypergammaglobulinemia but impaired specific antibody responses. Both anamnestic responses and those to neoantigens can be impaired.

The development of plasma HIV RNA quantification as an assay to measure viral burden has led to a better understanding of HIV dynamics and has provided a tool for assessing response to therapy. Despite viral suppression in peripheral blood, replication and activation of infected T-lymphocytes may continue within lymph nodes and the central nervous system (CNS), in a phenomenon referred to as "CNS escape." The risk of progression to AIDS appears correlated with an individual's viral load after seroconversion. Data from several large clinical cohorts have shown a direct correlation between the CD4 T-lymphocyte count and the risk of AIDS-defining opportunistic infections and malignancy. The viral load and the degree of CD4 T-lymphocyte depletion serve as important clinical indicators of immune status in HIV-infected individuals. The CD4 T-lymphocyte count is perhaps better for disease staging, and viral load better as a proxy measure for disease progression or monitoring response to therapy. Prophylaxis for opportunistic infections such as pneumocystis pneumonia (PCP) is recommended when the CD4 T-lymphocyte counts reach <200 cells/μL. Patients with HIV infection with a CD4 T lymphocyte count of <50 cells/μL are at significantly increased risk for cytomegalovirus (CMV) retinitis and *M avium* complex (MAC) infection. Unfortunately, some complications of HIV infection, including tuberculosis infection, non-Hodgkin lymphoma, and cardiovascular, hepatic, and neurocognitive diseases, may occur even with robust CD4 counts.

Monocytes, macrophages, and dendritic cells also express HIV receptors (CD4) and can be infected with HIV. This facilitates virus transfer to lymphoid tissues and immunoprivileged sites, such as the CNS. HIV-infected monocytes will also release large quantities of the acute-phase reactant cytokines, including IL-1, IL-6, and TNF, contributing to constitutional symptomatology. TNF, in particular, has been implicated in the severe wasting syndrome seen in patients with advanced disease. Concomitant infections may serve as cofactors for HIV infection, facilitate mucosal entry, and increase HIV expression through enhanced cytokine production, co-receptor surface expression, or increased cellular activation mechanisms. Epidemiologic studies of HSV-2–infected patients demonstrate a 2- to 7-fold increased risk of acquiring HIV compared with similar cohorts.

Clinical Manifestations

The clinical manifestations of AIDS are the direct consequence of the progressive and severe immunologic deficiency induced by HIV. Patients are susceptible to a wide range of atypical or opportunistic infections with bacterial, viral, protozoal, and fungal pathogens. Common nonspecific symptoms include fever, night sweats, and weight loss. Weight loss and cachexia can be due to nausea, vomiting, anorexia, or diarrhea. They often portend a poor prognosis.

The risk of opportunistic infections increases as the CD4 T-lymphocyte count declines. **Fungal pathogens** may affect immunocompetent hosts but frequently cause opportunistic infections in immunosuppressed HIV-infected patients. Infections with *Cryptococcus neoformans* meningoencephalitis, disseminated *Histoplasma capsulatum*, and disseminated *Coccidioides immitis* are typically seen in late stages of disease, when CD4 counts are below 200 cells/μL. Symptoms of *C. neoformans* meningoencephalitis include fever, malaise, headache, photophobia, and nausea. Presentation with altered mental status or elevated intracranial pressure is associated with a higher risk of death (or lifelong neurologic sequelae following survival). Occasionally, a cerebral cryptococcoma presents as a CNS mass lesion.

Found in regional soil contaminated with bird and bat droppings, *H capsulatum* infection is characterized by prominent constitutional symptoms, frequent pulmonary symptoms, and subacute meningoencephalitis symptoms. Disseminated disease may represent reactivation of latent disease when cellular immunity fails.

Previously thought to be a protozoan but now classified as a fungus, *Pneumocystis jirovecii* is one of the most common opportunistic infections in AIDS patients. Patients present clinically with fever, cough, shortness of breath, and hypoxemia, ranging in severity from mild to life-threatening. PCP may represent new acquisition of infection or reactivation of prior infection. A diagnosis of PCP can be made by substantiating the clinical and radiographic findings with direct fluorescent antibodies against PCP in expectorated sputum samples. Wright–Giemsa or silver methenamine staining of induced sputum samples may also be required for diagnosis. Further diagnostic testing such as bronchoalveolar lavage or fiberoptic transbronchial biopsy may be required to establish the diagnosis in the context of equivocal initial testing but strong suspicion of disease. Complications of PCP include pneumothoraces, progressive parenchymal disease with severe respiratory insufficiency, and, most commonly, adverse reactions to the medications used for treatment and prophylaxis.

As a consequence of chronic immune dysfunction, HIV-infected individuals are also at high risk for other pulmonary infections, including **bacterial pneumonias** with

S pneumoniae, H influenzae, and *P aeruginosa*; **mycobacterial infections** with *Mycobacterium tuberculosis* or *Mycobacterium avium-intracellulare* complex (MAC); and **fungal infections** with *C neoformans, H capsulatum, Aspergillus* sp., or *C immitis*. Clinical suspicion followed by early diagnosis of these infections should lead to aggressive treatment.

The risk of **M tuberculosis** reactivation is estimated to be 5–10% per year in HIV-infected patients compared with a lifetime risk of 10% in those without HIV. Furthermore, because of anergic skin responses, diagnosis of latent tuberculosis infection in the interest of prevention of active disease may be delayed. The development of active tuberculosis is significantly accelerated in HIV infection as a result of compromised cellular immunity. Respiratory symptoms of cough, dyspnea, or pleuritic chest pain may be associated with the insidious onset of fever, malaise, weight loss, and anorexia. Extrapulmonary manifestations occur in up to 70% of HIV-infected patients with tuberculosis, with miliary tuberculosis and tuberculous meningitis representing more serious complications. The emergence of multidrug resistance may compound the problem. **M avium-intracellulare** is a less virulent pathogen than *M tuberculosis*, and disseminated infections usually occur only with severe clinical immunodeficiency. *M avium-intracellulare* survives intracellularly within macrophages owing to defective cytokine (IFN-γ, IL-2, IL-12, TNF) synthesis, leading to impaired killing of phagocytosed organisms. Symptoms of MAC are nonspecific and typically consist of fever, weight loss, anemia, and GI distress with diarrhea.

The presence on physical examination of **oral candidiasis (thrush)** and **hairy leukoplakia** is highly correlated with HIV infection and portends rapid progression to AIDS. Oral candidiasis develops when reduced local and systemic immune function, sometimes combined with metabolic imbalances, contributes to opportunistic outgrowth of *Candida*, which is commonly a commensal organism. HIV-infected individuals with oral candidiasis are at much greater risk for **esophageal candidiasis**, which may present as substernal pain and dysphagia. This infection and its characteristic clinical presentation are so common that most practitioners treat these symptoms with empiric oral antifungal therapy. Should the patient not respond rapidly, other explanations for the esophageal symptoms should be explored, including **herpes simplex** and **CMV esophagitis**. Epstein–Barr virus (EBV) is the cause of hairy leukoplakia, another oral complication of HIV, manifested by white thickening of mucosal folds, most prominent on the buccal mucosa, the soft palate, and the floor of the mouth.

Diarrhea has been a hallmark feature of AIDS and leads to significant wasting, morbidity, and mortality. Persistent diarrhea, especially when accompanied by high fevers and abdominal pain, may signal **infectious enterocolitis**. The degree of CD4 lymphopenia is significantly correlated with the risk of opportunistic GI tract infections. The list of potential pathogens in such cases is long and includes bacteria, MAC, protozoans (*Cryptosporidium, Microsporidia, Isospora belli, Entamoeba histolytica, Giardia lamblia*), and even HIV itself. Because of their reduced gastric acid concentrations, patients also have an increased susceptibility to nonopportunistic infectious gastroenteritis with *Campylobacter*, *Salmonella*, and *Shigella*. Co-infection with viral hepatitis (HBV, HCV, CMV) can lead to accelerated cirrhosis and end-stage liver disease, but fortunately, instituting antiretroviral therapy can lead to a reduction in clinical disease.

Skin lesions commonly associated with HIV infection are typically classified as infectious (viral, bacterial, fungal), neoplastic, or nonspecific. **Herpes simplex virus (HSV)** and **herpes zoster virus (HZV)** may cause chronic persistent or progressive lesions in patients with compromised cellular immunity. HSV commonly causes oral and perianal lesions but can be an AIDS-defining illness when involving the lung or esophagus. The risk of disseminated HSV or HZV infection and the presence of **molluscum contagiosum** appear to be correlated with the extent of immunosuppression. **Seborrheic dermatitis** caused by *Pityrosporum ovale* and **fungal skin infections** (*C albicans*, dermatophyte species) are also common in HIV-infected patients. *Staphylococcus aureus* **infections**, including methicillin-resistant *S aureus*, can cause folliculitis, furunculosis, and bullous impetigo in HIV-infected patients and may require aggressive treatment to prevent dissemination and sepsis. **Bacillary angiomatosis** is a potentially fatal dermatologic disorder of tumor-like proliferating vascular endothelial cell lesions, the result of infection by *Bartonella quintana* or *Bartonella henselae*. The lesions may resemble those of **Kaposi sarcoma** but respond to treatment with tetracyclines.

CNS manifestations in HIV-infected patients include CNS infections and malignancies. **Toxoplasmosis** frequently presents with space-occupying lesions, causing headache, altered mental status, seizures, or focal neurologic deficits. **Cryptococcal meningitis** commonly manifests as headache and fever. Up to 90% of patients with cryptococcal meningitis exhibit a positive serum test for *C neoformans* antigen.

Patients with **HIV-associated neurocognitive disorder** typically have difficulty with cognitive tasks, poor short-term memory, slowed motor function, personality or affective changes, and waxing-and-waning dementia. In its severe form, **AIDS dementia** may be characterized by severe psychomotor retardation, akinesis, and language impairment, associated with widespread cortical atrophy and ventricular enlargement on imaging by CT or MRI. Up to 50% of patients with AIDS suffer from this disorder, perhaps caused by glial or macrophage infection by HIV resulting in destructive inflammatory changes within the CNS. R5 viruses are trophic for cells of monocytic lineage in the CNS. The differential diagnosis of CNS changes is broad and includes metabolic disturbances and toxic encephalopathy resulting from drugs. Other causes of altered mental status include neurosyphilis, CMV or herpes simplex encephalitis, mycobacterial or cryptococcal meningitis, lymphoma, and **progressive multifocal leukoencephalopathy**, a progressive demyelinating disease caused by a JC papovavirus.

Peripheral nervous system manifestations of HIV infection include **sensory, motor, and inflammatory polyneuropathies**. Almost 33% of patients with advanced HIV disease develop peripheral numbness, tingling, and pain in their extremities. These symptoms are likely a result of loss of nerve axons from direct neuronal infection by HIV. Alcoholism, thyroid disease, syphilis, vitamin B_{12} deficiency, drug toxicity (eg, stavudine or didanosine), **CMV-associated ascending polyradiculopathy**, and **transverse myelitis** also cause peripheral neuropathies. Less commonly, HIV-infected patients can develop an inflammatory demyelinating polyneuropathy similar to Guillain–Barré syndrome; however, unlike the sensory neuropathies, this inflammatory demyelinating polyneuropathy typically presents before the onset of clinically apparent immunodeficiency. The origin of this condition is not known, although an autoimmune reaction is suspected. **CMV retinitis** is the most common cause of rapidly progressive visual loss in HIV-infected patients. The diagnosis can be difficult to make because *Toxoplasma gondii* infection, microinfarction, and retinal necrosis can all cause visual loss.

HIV-related malignancies commonly seen in AIDS include Kaposi sarcoma, non-Hodgkin lymphoma, primary CNS lymphoma, invasive cervical carcinoma, and anal squamous cell carcinoma. Impairment of immune surveillance and defense and increased exposure to oncogenic viruses appear to contribute to the development of these neoplasms.

Kaposi sarcoma is the most common HIV-associated cancer. In San Francisco, 15–20% of HIV-infected men who have sex with men develop this tumor during the progression of their disease. For reasons that are unclear, Kaposi sarcoma is uncommon in women and children. Unlike classic Kaposi sarcoma, which affects elderly men in Africa and the Mediterranean region, the disease in HIV-infected patients may present with either localized cutaneous lesions or lymphatic or disseminated visceral involvement. It is often a progressive disease, and pulmonary involvement can be fatal. Histologically, the lesions of Kaposi sarcoma consist of a mixed cell population that includes vascular endothelial cells and spindle cells within a collagen network. Kaposi sarcoma is caused by human herpesvirus 8 (HHV-8), which in immunocompromised patients appears to promote angiogenesis through growth factor and proinflammatory gene product production. HIV itself appears to induce cytokines and growth factors that stimulate tumor cell proliferation rather than causing malignant cellular transformation. Clinically, cutaneous Kaposi sarcoma typically presents as a purplish nodular skin lesion or painless oral lesion. Sites of visceral involvement include the lung, lymph nodes, liver, and GI tract. In the GI tract, Kaposi sarcoma can result in either acute hemorrhage or chronic blood loss. In the lung, it often presents as bilateral coarse nodular infiltrates, frequently associated with pleural effusions.

Non-Hodgkin lymphoma is particularly aggressive in HIV-infected patients and is usually indicative of significant immune compromise. The majority of these tumors are high-grade B-cell lymphomas with a predilection for dissemination. Chronic B-cell stimulation, immune dysfunction, and loss of immunoregulation of EBV-infected cells are all risk factors for transformation of clonally selected cells and development of non-Hodgkin lymphoma. Large-cell and Burkitt-type lymphoma are often associated with EBV but only account for about half of cases. Many cases are diagnosed at advanced stages of disease, and the CNS is frequently involved either as a primary site or as an extranodal site of widespread disease.

Anal dysplasia and **anal squamous cell carcinoma** are more commonly found in HIV-infected men who have sex with men. These conditions are associated with concomitant anal or rectal infection with oncogenic types of human papillomavirus (HPV). In HIV-infected women, the incidence of HPV-related **cervical dysplasia** is as high as 40%, and dysplasia, and without proper screening for early detection and treatment, can progress to **invasive cervical carcinoma**.

In HIV-infected patients, adherence to multidrug treatment regimens remains a challenge, but clearly such antiretroviral therapy (ART) improves immune function. For reasons that are unclear, HIV-infected patients have an unusually high rate of adverse reactions to a wide variety of antibiotics and frequently develop severe, debilitating cutaneous reactions. Drug hypersensitivity and toxicity can be severe, potentially life-threatening, and life-limiting with certain agents.

Immune reconstitution syndrome is a reaction that occurs days to weeks after initiation of ART. Clinical relapse or worsening of mycobacterial, pneumocystis, hepatitis, or neurological infections occurs as a result of a resurgence of immune activity, causing paradoxical worsening of inflammation, possibly as residual antigens or subclinical pathogens are attacked.

Other complications of HIV infection include arthritides, myopathy, GI syndromes, dysfunction of the adrenal and thyroid glands, hematologic cytopenias, and nephropathy. As patients are living longer due to potent ART, cardiovascular complications have become more prominent. ART has been associated with dyslipidemia, insulin resistance, and other metabolic abnormalities. HIV infection itself may be atherogenic, both through effects on lipids and through proinflammatory mechanisms.

Since the disease was first described in 1981, medical knowledge of the underlying pathogenesis of HIV infection and AIDS has increased at a rate unprecedented in medical history. This knowledge has led to the rapid development of therapies directed at controlling HIV infection as well as the multitude of complicating opportunistic infections and cancers.

CHECKPOINT

23. What are the major clinical manifestations of AIDS?
24. What are the major steps in developing AIDS after infection with HIV?

CASE STUDIES

Yeong Kwok, MD

(See Chapter 25, p. 744–46 for Answers)

CASE 7

A 40-year-old woman comes to the clinic with a history of worsening nasal congestion and recurrent sinus infections. She had been healthy until about 1 year ago when she first noticed persistent rhinorrhea, sneezing, and stuffiness. She noted that when she went on a 2-week vacation to Mexico, her rhinorrhea disappeared, only to return when she came home again. She has lived in the same house for the past 5 years along with her husband and one child. They have had a dog for 4 years and a cat for 1 year. On physical examination, she has boggy, swollen nasal turbinates and a cobblestone appearance of her posterior pharynx.

Questions

A. What are the pathophysiologic mechanisms in allergic rhinitis?
B. What are the symptoms and signs of allergic rhinitis?
C. What are possible complications of allergic rhinitis?

CASE 8

A 2-month-old child is admitted to the ICU with fever, hypotension, tachycardia, and lethargy. The medical history is notable for a similar hospitalization at 2 weeks of age. Physical examination is notable for a temperature of 39°C, oral thrush, and rales in the right lung fields. Chest x-ray film reveals multilobar pneumonia. Given the history of recurrent severe infection, the pediatrician suspects an immunodeficiency disorder.

Questions

A. What is the most likely immunodeficiency in this child? Why?
B. What are the underlying genetic and cellular defects associated with this disease?
C. What is the overall prognosis for patients with this disorder?

CASE 9

An 18-month-old boy is brought to the emergency department by his parents with a high fever, shortness of breath, and cough. The boy was well until he was 6 months old. Since then, he has had four bouts of otitis media, and because of their severity and recurrence, he was placed on prophylactic antibiotics for several months. He was recently taken off the antibiotics to see how he would do. The day before presentation, he developed a cough that has quickly progressed into an illness with high fevers and lethargy. Both of his parents are healthy, and he has a healthy older sister. His father's family history is unremarkable, but his maternal uncle died of pneumonia in infancy. Examination is remarkable for a normally developed toddler who is lethargic and tachypneic. His temperature is 39°C, and he has decreased breath sounds at both lung bases. Chest x-ray film shows consolidation of the right and left lower lobes, as well as bilateral pleural effusions. He is admitted to the hospital, and the boy's blood cultures grow out *Streptococcus pneumoniae* the next day. Immunologic testing shows very low levels of IgG, IgM, and IgA antibodies in the serum, and flow cytometry shows the absence of circulating B lymphocytes.

Questions

A. What is the likely diagnosis in this patient? Why?
B. What is the primary pathophysiologic defect in the condition, and how does it lead to this clinical presentation?
C. Why are the affected children generally fine until they reach 4–6 months of age?

CASE 10

An 18-year-old man presents with complaints of fever, facial pain, and nasal congestion consistent with a diagnosis of acute sinusitis. His medical history is notable for multiple sinus infections, two episodes of pneumonia, and chronic diarrhea, all suggestive of a primary immunodeficiency syndrome. Workup establishes a diagnosis of common variable immunodeficiency syndrome.

Questions

A. What are the common infectious manifestations of common variable immunodeficiency syndrome?
B. What are the underlying immunologic abnormalities responsible for these infectious manifestations?
C. What other diseases is this patient at increased risk for?
D. What treatment is indicated?

CASE 11

A 2-year-old boy is hospitalized with recurrent *Staphylococcus aureus* abscesses. This is his fourth hospitalization; two previous hospitalizations were also with *S aureus* abscesses, and one was with *Serratia marcescens* pyelonephritis. His parents, sister, and brother have never been hospitalized for infections. The recurrent infections lead to a workup, and the boy is diagnosed with chronic granulomatous disease.

Questions

A. What is the likely mechanism of inheritance of chronic granulomatous disease?

B. What is the fundamental immune defect in chronic granulomatous disease?

C. Why are certain infections more common in individuals with this condition?

CASE 12

A 31-year-old male injection drug user presents to the emergency department with a chief complaint of shortness of breath. He describes a 1-month history of intermittent fevers and night sweats associated with a nonproductive cough. He has become progressively more short of breath, initially dyspneic only with exertion but now dyspneic at rest. He appears to be in moderate respiratory distress. His vital signs are abnormal, with a temperature of 39°C, heart rate of 112 bpm, respiratory rate of 20/min, and oxygen saturation of 88% on room air. Physical examination is otherwise unremarkable but notable for the absence of abnormal lung sounds. Chest x-ray film reveals a diffuse interstitial infiltrate characteristic of pneumocystis pneumonia, an opportunistic infection.

Questions

A. What is the underlying disease most likely responsible for this man's susceptibility to pneumocystis pneumonia?

B. What is the pathogenesis of the immunosuppression caused by this underlying disease?

C. What is the natural history of this disease? What are some of the common clinical manifestations seen during its progression?

REFERENCES

General

Abbas AK et al. *Basic Immunology: Functions and Disorders of the Immune System*, 5th ed. Elsevier, 2015.

Akdis M et al. Interleukins, from 1 to 38, interferons, transforming growth factor-β and TNF-α: receptors, functions, and roles in diseases. J Allergy Clin Immunol. 2016 138:984–1010.

DeFranco AL et al. *Immunity: The Immune Response in Infectious and Inflammatory Disease*. New Science Press Ltd, 2007.

Noval Rivas M et al. Regulatory T cells in allergic diseases. J Allergy Clin Immunol. 2016 Sep;138(3):639–52. [PMID: 27596705]

O'Shea JJ et al. JAKs and STATs in immunity, immunodeficiency, and cancer. N Engl J Med. 2013 Jan 10;368(2):161–70. [PMID: 23301733]

Schwartz RS. Shattuck lecture: diversity of the immune repertoire and immunoregulation. N Engl J Med. 2003 Mar 13;348(11):1017–26. [PMID: 12637612]

van de Veen W et al. Role of regulatory B cells in immune tolerance to allergens and beyond. J Allergy Clin Immunol. 2016 Sep;138(3):654–65. [PMID: 27596706]

Allergic Rhinitis

Adkinson FN et al, eds. *Middleton's Allergy Principles and Practice*, 8th ed. Mosby, 2013.

Akdis CA et al. Mechanisms and treatment of allergic disease in the big picture of regulatory T cells. J Allergy Clin Immunol. 2009 Apr;123(4):735–46. [PMID: 19348912]

Bernstein DI et al. Allergic rhinitis: mechanisms and treatment. Immunol Allergy Clin North Am. 2016 May;36(2):261–78. [PMID: 27083101]

Durham SR et al. Long-term clinical efficacy of grass-pollen immunotherapy. N Engl J Med. 1999 Aug 12;341(7):468–75. [PMID: 10441602]

Jutel M et al. International consensus on allergy immunotherapy. J Allergy Clin Immunol. 2015 Sep;136(3):556–68. [PMID: 26162571]

Kariyawasam HH et al. Allergic rhinitis, chronic rhinosinusitis and asthma: unravelling a complex relationship. Curr Opin Otolaryngol Head Neck Surg. 2013 Feb;21(1):79–86. [PMID: 23241653]

Wheatley LM et al. Clinical practice. Allergic rhinitis. N Engl J Med. 2015 Jan 29;372(5):456–63. [PMID: 25629743]

Primary Immunodeficiency Diseases

Bonilla FA et al. International Consensus Document (ICON): common variable immunodeficiency disorders. J Allergy Clin Immunol Pract. 2016 Jan-Feb;4(1):38–59. [PMID: 26563668]

Bousfiha A et al. The 2015 IUIS phenotypic classification for primary immunodeficiencies. J Clin Immunol. 2015 Nov;35(8): 727–38. [PMID: 26445875]

Notarangelo LD. Primary immunodeficiencies. J Allergy Clin Immunol. 2010 Feb;125(2 Suppl 2):S182–94. [PMID: 20042228]

Ochs HD et al, eds. *Primary Immunodeficiency Diseases: A Molecular and Genetic Approach*, 3rd ed. Oxford University Press, 2014.

Parvaneh N et al. Primary immunodeficiencies: a rapidly evolving story. J Allergy Clin Immunol. 2013 Feb;131(2):314–23. [PMID: 23374262]

Starr SP. Immunology update: primary immunodeficiency diseases. FP Essent. 2016 Nov;450:35–53. [PMID: 27869441]

Sullivan KE et al. *Stiehm's Immune Deficiencies*. Academic Press, 2014.

AIDS

Boassa A et al. Chronic innate immune activation as a cause of HIV-1 immunopathogenesis. Clin Immunol. 2008 Mar;126(3):235–42. [PMID: 17916442]

Cary DC et al. Molecular mechanisms of HIV latency. J Clin Invest. 2016 Feb;126(2):448–54. [PMID: 26731470]

Centers for Disease Control and Prevention. HIV/AIDS. https://www.cdc.gov/hiv/. Accessed April 2, 2018.

Centers for Disease Control and Prevention. Revised surveillance case definition for HIV infection—United States, 2014. MMWR Recomm Rep. 2014 Apr 11;63(RR-03):1–10. [PMID: 24717910]

Fauci AS. The acquired immune deficiency syndrome: the ever-broadening clinical spectrum. JAMA. 2016 Jul 12;316(2):230. [PMID: 27404204]

Jones RB et al. HIV-specific CD8+ T cells and HIV eradication. J Clin Invest. 2016 Feb;126(2):455–63. [PMID: 26731469]

Saag MS. *The Sanford Guide to HIV/AIDS Therapy 2017: Pocket Edition*, 25th ed. Antimicrobial Therapy, 2017.

Infectious Diseases

4

Christina T. Fiske, MD, MPH, & Karen C. Bloch, MD, MPH

Infectious diseases remain one of the leading causes of death in both developed and developing countries. Infections cause significant morbidity and mortality, especially in individuals who are most vulnerable to illness: the very young, the elderly, the immunocompromised, and the disenfranchised.

The pathogenesis of infectious diseases reflects the relationship among the human host, the infectious agent, and the external environment. Figure 4–1 portrays a host–agent–environment paradigm for the study of infectious diseases. The infectious agent can be either **exogenous** (ie, not normally found on or in the body) or **endogenous** (ie, one that may be routinely cultured from a specific anatomic site but that does not normally cause disease in the host). Infection results when an exogenous agent is introduced into a host from the environment or when an endogenous agent overcomes innate host immunity to cause disease. Host susceptibility plays an important role in both settings.

The environment includes **vectors** (insects and other carriers that transmit infectious agents) and **zoonotic hosts** or **reservoirs** (animals that harbor infectious agents and often act to amplify the infectious agent). For example, the white-footed mouse (*Peromyscus leucopus*) serves as an animal reservoir for *Borrelia burgdorferi*, the bacterium that causes Lyme disease. The *Ixodes* tick serves as an insect vector. Infection in the mouse is asymptomatic, and the bacteria can multiply to high levels in this animal. When the tick larva feeds on an infected mouse, it becomes secondarily infected with *B burgdorferi*, and this infection persists when the tick molts into a nymph. Subsequently, when an infected nymph feeds on a human, the bacterium is transmitted through infected saliva into the host bloodstream, causing disease.

The study of infectious diseases requires an understanding of pathogenesis at the level of the population, the individual, the cell, and the gene. For example, at the population level, the spread of tuberculosis in the community is related to the social interactions of an infectious human host. Outbreaks of tuberculosis have occurred in group settings such as homeless shelters, prisons, and nursing homes when an index case comes in close contact with susceptible persons. At the individual level, tuberculosis results from inhalation of respiratory droplets containing airborne tubercle bacilli. At the cellular level, these bacilli activate T cells, which play a critical role in containing the infection. Individuals with an impaired T-cell response (eg, those infected with human immunodeficiency virus [HIV]) are at particularly high risk for developing active tuberculosis at the time of the initial infection or for reactivation of latent tuberculosis as their immunity wanes. Finally, at the genetic level, individuals with specific polymorphisms in genes encoding inflammatory cytokines and macrophage proteins may be at significantly higher risk for tuberculosis.

Specific microorganisms have a tendency to cause certain types of infections: *Streptococcus pneumoniae* commonly causes pneumonia, meningitis, and bacteremia but rarely causes endocarditis (infection of the heart valves); *Escherichia coli* is a common cause of gastrointestinal (GI) and urinary tract infections; *Plasmodium* species infect red blood cells and liver cells to cause malaria; *Entamoeba histolytica* causes amebic dysentery, liver abscesses, and so on. Table 4–1 presents a clinical approach to taking a patient history that considers features of the host and the environment in identifying the most likely microorganisms associated with specific clinical syndromes.

HOST DEFENSES AGAINST INFECTION

Humans live in an environment brimming with microorganisms that have potential to cause disease. The human body has the ability to control infection through a number of

different mechanisms. Physical barriers impede the entry of bacteria from the external environment and from normally colonized sites in the body into sterile anatomic areas. When

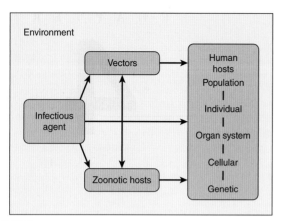

FIGURE 4–1 The fundamental relationships involved in the host–agent–environment interaction model. In the host, pathogenetic mechanisms extend from the level of populations (eg, person-to-person transmission) to the level of cellular and molecular processes (eg, genetic susceptibility).

these physical defenses are breached, the immune system is activated (Figure 4–2). **Innate immunity** (also called natural or native immunity), provided by preformed proteins (eg, complement) and immune cells (eg, phagocytes) that are activated by nonspecific foreign proteins, allows an immediate and rapid response to foreign material. **Adaptive immunity** (also called specific immunity) includes both early and late adaptive responses activated by specific antigenic proteins (eg, production of antibodies active against the specific strains of *S pneumoniae* contained in the pneumococcal vaccine in a previously vaccinated individual). Induction of these specific immune receptor cells may take several days in the immunologically naive host. **Protective immunity**, which occurs after initial exposure (via infection or vaccination) through generation of memory lymphocytes and pathogen-specific antibody, allows a much more rapid response to reinfection. These components of the immune response are discussed in detail later.

TABLE 4–1   Obtaining a history in the diagnosis of infectious diseases.

Component	Feature	Examples of Infection
History of present illness	Age	West Nile virus neuroinvasive disease much more common in the elderly
	Pregnancy	Pregnant women at increased risk for serious varicella pneumonia; risks to fetus with various infections or treatments
	Site of acquisition (eg, home, skilled nursing facility [SNF], hospital)	Multi-drug–resistant bacteria more commonly cultured from patient in an SNF or hospital
	Season	Influenza epidemics limited to fall through early spring
	Symptoms (duration, severity, pattern)	Bacterial meningitis excluded if symptoms last >1 week
Past medical history (including medications, allergies, and immunizations)	Immunocompromise (eg, HIV, organ transplant, corticosteroid use, chemotherapy, asplenia)	*Pneumocystis jirovecii* pneumonia in patients with AIDS
	Comorbid disease (eg, chronic obstructive pulmonary disease, diabetes mellitus, alcohol abuse)	Limb-threatening soft tissue infections in diabetic patients
	Transfusions	Blood-borne infections such as cytomegalovirus or hepatitis C virus
Habits and exposures	Substance use (eg, alcohol, cigarettes; type and route of illicit drug use)	Endocarditis associated with injection drug use due to seeding of bloodstream with skin bacteria
	Sexual contacts	Risk for sexually transmitted infections such as syphilis
	Outdoor activities	Arthropod-borne infections (eg, Rocky Mountain spotted fever)
	Pets	Zoonotic infections (eg, cat scratch disease)
Social history	Occupation	Q-fever in veterinarians
	Congregated living facility	Transmission of infection from an ill contact (eg, influenza, *Shigella*, norovirus)
	Homelessness	Tuberculosis, scabies
	Travel	Internationally acquired infections (eg, malaria)
Family history	Transmittable diseases	Tuberculosis
Review of systems	Symptoms by organ system	History of headache raises concern for central nervous system infection; diarrhea raises concern for gastroenteritis

FIGURE 4-2 Phases of the host response to infection. During the earliest stage of initial infection, nonspecific mediators (complement, phagocytes) predominate. Adaptive immunity (production of antibody, stimulation of lymphocytes) requires clonal expansion after recognition of specific antigens. Once immunity toward a specific agent is induced, the immune response remains primed so that the response to reinfection is much more rapid.

NORMAL MICROBIAL FLORA

Until recently, our view of human microbiology was shaped by what microorganisms were isolated from persons with acute infection. However, over time it has become apparent that the diversity of microorganisms observed from microscopy or genetic sequencing was far greater than the microorganisms that were isolated from traditional culture techniques. The human body harbors numerous species of bacteria, viruses, fungi, and protozoa, referred to as the human **microbiota** or **microbiome**. The great majority of these are **commensals**, defined as organisms that live symbiotically on or within the human host but rarely cause disease (Figure 4–3). Anatomic sites where bacteria are normally found include the skin (staphylococci and diphtheroids), oropharynx (streptococci, anaerobes), large intestine (enterococci, enteric bacilli), and vagina (lactobacilli).

Microbes do not exist in the human body in isolation but in complex communities and habitats. Imbalances in the composition of these habitats are associated with human infection

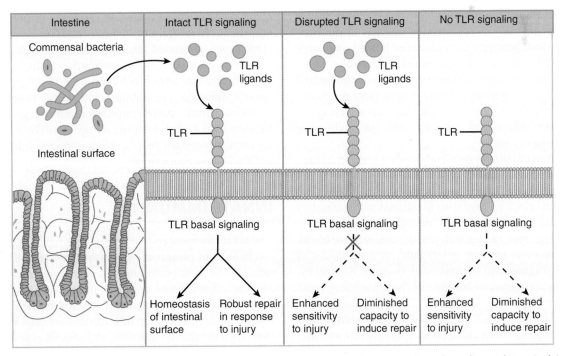

FIGURE 4-3 Commensal bacteria secrete toll-like receptor (TLR) ligands, which bind to TLR on the surface of normal intestinal tissue. This interaction stimulates basal signaling, which protects against cellular injury. Disruption of TLR signaling or antibiotic-associated eradication of commensal bacteria results in compromised ability of the intestinal epithelium to withstand injury and repair cell damage. (Redrawn, with permission, from Madara J. Building an intestine—architectural contributions of commensal bacteria. N Engl J Med. 2004;351:1686. Copyright © 2004 Massachusetts Medical Society. Reprinted with permission from Massachusetts Medical Society.)

and disease. One example of an infection that can result from a perturbed microbiota community is that caused by *Clostridium difficile*. *C difficile* is an anaerobic gram-negative rod that causes intestinal disease in the setting of antibiotic administration. Antibiotics alter the structure and function of an individual's gut microbiota, reducing the body's innate resistance to colonization with *C difficile* organisms (and other enteric pathogens) and providing them a niche to multiply and elaborate their enterotoxins. Similarly, broad-spectrum antibiotics will destroy normal vaginal flora, such as lactobacilli, and allow overgrowth of *Candida* (yeast) species, resulting in *Candida* vaginitis.

Determining when an isolate is a component of the normal flora rather than an invasive pathogen may be difficult. For example, culture of staphylococci from a blood sample may represent skin contamination at the time of phlebotomy or may indicate a potentially life-threatening bloodstream infection. Helpful clues include burden of organism (eg, number of positive blood cultures), symptoms and signs of infection (eg, cough, fever), and the presence of inflammatory cells (eg, polymorphonuclear cells in the sputum and an increased proportion of immature neutrophils in the blood). Isolation of an **obligate pathogen** such as *Mycobacterium tuberculosis* from any anatomic site is diagnostic of infection. Fortunately, few microorganisms are absolute pathogens. For example, *Neisseria meningitidis*, a major bacterial cause of meningitis, can be cultured from the oropharynx of as many as 10% of asymptomatic individuals, in which case it represents transient normal flora. Even if asymptomatic, the host can serve as a **carrier**, transferring bacteria to susceptible individuals. Infections resulting from commensals that rarely cause disease (eg, *Candida albicans*) or organisms ubiquitous in the environment that are generally not considered human pathogens (eg, *Aspergillus*) are termed **opportunistic infections**. These infections occur almost exclusively in **immunocompromised hosts**, such as HIV-infected patients or transplant recipients. The agents are opportunists in that they take advantage of impaired host immunity to cause infection but rarely cause disease in a healthy host.

The presence of bacteria on a body surface without causing disease is called **colonization**, whereas invasion of the tissues by a microorganism that causes disease is termed **infection**. The site from which an organism is cultured is important in differentiating colonization from infection. Growth of any microorganism from a normally sterile site such as blood, cerebrospinal fluid, synovial (joint) fluid, or deep tissues of the body is diagnostic of infection. For example, *Bacteroides*, the predominant genus of bacteria in the colon, may cause intra-abdominal abscesses and sepsis when the integrity of the colonic mucosa is breached. *Staphylococcus epidermidis*, a common skin commensal, can cause bacteremia after intravascular catheter placement. Knowledge of the common endogenous flora may be useful in determining the cause of an infection and may aid in the choice of empiric antibiotic therapy.

The normal flora prevent colonization through numerous mechanisms. Organisms comprising the normal flora often have a selective advantage over colonizers in that they are already established in an anatomic niche. Colonization of sites that are normally sterile or have very few microbes is generally easier because there is no competition for nutrients from endogenous flora. However, host defenses at these sites are often vigorous. For instance, the stomach is normally sterile because few microbes can survive at the normal gastric pH of 1.5 to 3.5. However, if antacids are used to decrease gastric acidity, colonization of the stomach and adjacent trachea with gram-negative bacteria occurs rapidly. Other host defense mechanisms that serve to inhibit colonization by pathogenic bacteria include (1) mechanical clearance; (2) phagocytic killing; and (3) deprivation of necessary nutrients. Successful colonizers have adapted the ability to evade or overcome these defenses. For example, gonococci, the bacteria that cause gonorrhea, avoid excretion in the urine by adhering to the mucosal epithelium of the urogenital tract with pili. Pneumococci resist phagocytosis by encapsulation within a slime layer that impairs uptake by neutrophils. Some staphylococci elaborate enzymes known as hemolysins, which destroy host red blood cells, thus giving them access to a needed source of iron.

When replacement of the normal flora occurs in the hospital environment, the organisms are said to be **nosocomially acquired**. The distinction between hospital-acquired and community-acquired infections has blurred in recent years, because of an increase in medical care in the home or skilled nursing facility among patients who previously would have required long-term hospitalization. For this reason, the broader term "health care–associated infections" is used to encompass both hospitalized patients and patients with frequent medical interactions (eg, residence in nursing home, outpatient hemodialysis, home intravenous antibiotics). Health care–associated infections are significant because the organisms involved are often resistant to multiple antibiotics. In the health care setting, colonization may progress to symptomatic infection. For example, individuals hospitalized for extended periods often become colonized with gram-negative bacteria such as *Pseudomonas aeruginosa*. These individuals are then at increased risk for life-threatening infections such as *Pseudomonas* pneumonia.

INNATE IMMUNITY

The innate immune system represents a rapid, multi-pronged mechanism to protect the host from infection. The components of the innate immune system are present at birth and not learned or adapted as a result of exposure to microorganisms. Innate immunity includes physical barriers to prevent microbial entry, activation of inflammatory cells and proteins that target the microorganisms, and activation of the adaptive immune system. The first line of defense are nonspecific barriers against infectious diseases that do not require prior contact with the microorganism. These defenses consist of simple physical (eg, skin) and chemical (eg, acidic gastric secretions) barriers that prevent easy entry of microorganisms into the body. Some infectious agents use a vector (such as an insect) to bypass structural barriers and gain direct access to the blood or subcutaneous tissues of the body. Once an agent has entered the body, the major innate defenses are the acute inflammatory response and the complement system. These defenses can neutralize the organism, recruit phagocytic cells, and induce a more specific response through humoral and cell-mediated immunity. The innate defenses of the body are important from an evolutionary perspective in enabling humans to encounter and adapt to a variety of new and changing environments.

Physical & Chemical Barriers to Infection

The squamous epithelium of the skin is the first line of defense against microorganisms encountered in the outside world. As keratinized epithelial surface cells desquamate, the skin maintains its protective barrier by generating new epithelial cells beneath the surface. The skin is also bathed with oils and moisture from the sebaceous and sweat glands. These secretions contain fatty acids that inhibit bacterial growth. Poor vascular supply to the skin may result in skin breakdown and increased susceptibility to infection. For example, chronically debilitated or bedridden patients may suffer from presacral pressure ulcers as a result of constant compression of this dependent body area; these ulcers allow direct entry of skin and enteric bacteria into previously sterile sites and predispose patients to severe infections.

The mucous membranes also provide a physical barrier to microbial invasion. The mucous membranes of the mouth, pharynx, esophagus, and lower urinary tract are composed of several layers of epithelial cells, whereas those of the lower respiratory tract, the GI tract, and the upper urinary tract are delicate single layers of epithelial cells. These membranes are covered by a protective layer of mucus, which traps foreign particles and prevents them from accessing the lining of epithelial cells. Because mucus is hydrophilic, many substances produced by the body easily diffuse to the surface, including enzymes with antimicrobial activity such as lysozyme and peroxidase.

Inflammatory Response

How host cells recognize invading organisms is an area of active research. Pattern recognition receptors (PRRs) in host cells include Toll-like receptors, nucleotide-binding oligomerization domain-like receptors, and other intracellular proteins. PRRs are activated when exogenous organisms interact with host cells through their sensing of pathogen-associated molecular patterns (PAMPs). Detection of PAMPs stimulates activation of a pro-inflammatory cascade that plays a key role in pathogen recognition and inactivation. Importantly, PRRs do not require prior contact with the organism to be activated. This response is usually tightly regulated through feedback mechanisms; however, when this goes awry, the immune cascade may lead to damage to host tissues, termed "autoimmune dysfunction."

Clinically, signs of inflammation (heat, erythema, pain, and swelling) are the characteristic features of localized infection, secondary tissue injury, and the body's response to this injury. Blood supply to the affected area increases in response to vasodilation, and the capillaries become more permeable, allowing antibodies, complement, and white blood cells to cross the endothelium and reach the site of injury. An important consequence of inflammation is that the pH of the inflamed tissues is lowered, creating an inhospitable environment for the microbe. The increased blood flow to the area allows continued recruitment of inflammatory cells as well as the necessary components for tissue repair and recovery.

When a microorganism enters host tissue, it activates circulating proteins including complement (see below) and induces the release of pro-inflammatory cytokines. These mediators result in the increased vascular permeability and vasodilation characteristic of inflammation. For example, the anaphylatoxins C3a, C4a, and C5a, produced by the activation of complement, stimulate the release of histamine from mast cells. Histamine dilates the blood vessels and further increases their permeability. Bradykinin is also released, increasing vascular permeability.

Pro-inflammatory cytokines include interleukin-1 (IL-1), IL-6, tumor necrosis factor, and interferon-γ. These factors, singly or in combination, promote fever, produce local inflammatory signs, and trigger catabolic responses. During severe infection, a change in hepatic synthesis of proteins occurs, resulting in an increase in some proteins and a decrease in others. Most notable is the increase in **acute-phase reactants**, which include rheumatoid factor, C-reactive protein (CRP), ferritin, and various proteinase inhibitors. The erythrocyte sedimentation rate (ESR), a nonspecific marker of inflammation, also increases, although in a slower fashion. A catabolic state is further augmented by simultaneous increases in levels of circulating cortisol, glucagon, catecholamines, and other hormones.

Mild to moderate inflammatory responses serve important host defense functions. For example, elevated body temperature may inhibit viral replication. Inflammatory hyperemia and systemic neutrophilia optimize phagocyte delivery to sites of infection. Decreased availability of iron inhibits the growth of microbes such as *Yersinia* that require this element as a nutrient. However, when the inflammatory responses become extreme, extensive tissue damage can result, as in the case of sepsis.

COMPLEMENT SYSTEM

The complement system is composed of a series of plasma protein and cell membrane receptors that are important mediators of host defenses and inflammation (Figure 4–4). Most of the biologically significant effects of the complement system are mediated by the third component (C3) and the terminal components (C5–9). These crucial proteins are activated through one of two mechanisms, termed the **classic** and **alternative**

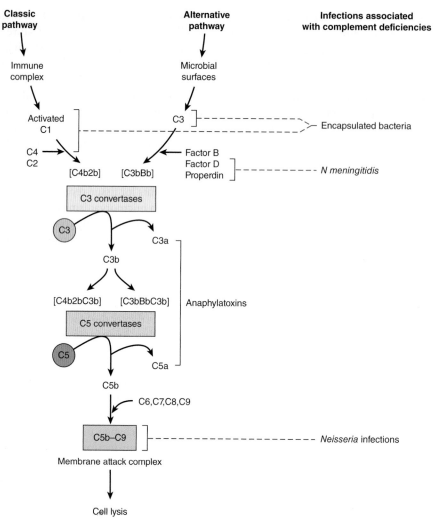

FIGURE 4–4 Complement reaction sequence and infections associated with deficiency states. (Redrawn, with permission, from Detrick B. Immunology. In: Carroll KC et al, eds. *Jawetz, Melnick, and Adelberg's Medical Microbiology*, 27th ed. McGraw-Hill, 2015.)

pathways. The classic pathway is activated by antigen–antibody complexes or antibody-coated particles, and the alternative pathway is activated by mechanisms independent of antibodies, usually by interaction with bacterial surface components. Both pathways form C3 convertase, which cleaves the C3 component of complement, a key protein common to both pathways. The two pathways then proceed in identical fashion to bind late-acting components to form a **membrane attack complex** (C5–9), which results in target cell lysis.

Once activated, complement functions to enhance the antimicrobial defenses in several ways. Complement facilitates phagocytosis by serving as an **opsonin**, binding to invading microorganisms and making them susceptible to engulfment and destruction by neutrophils and macrophages. The complement-derived membrane attack complex inserts itself into the membrane of a target organism, leading to increased permeability and subsequent lysis of the cell. Complement also acts indirectly by producing substances that are chemotactic for white blood cells.

Inherited disorders of complement are associated with an increased risk of bacterial infection. The specific infections seen in complement-deficient patients relate to the biologic functions of the missing component (see Figure 4–4). Patients with a deficiency of C3 or a component in either of the two pathways necessary for the activation of C3 typically have increased susceptibility to infections with encapsulated bacteria such as *S pneumoniae* and *Haemophilus influenzae*. In contrast, patients with deficiencies of C5–9 have normal resistance to encapsulated bacteria because C3b-mediated opsonization is intact. These patients, however, are unusually susceptible to infections with *N meningitidis* and *N gonorrhoeae* because they are unable to form a membrane attack complex and, therefore, cannot lyse the *Neisseria* cell membrane. Recurrent infection with encapsulated bacteria such as *Neisseria* is an indication for testing for complement deficiency, and if present, immunizations (with vaccines against *N meningitis*, *Haemophilus influenzae*, and *Streptococcus pneumoniae*) to protect against future infection with such encapsulated bacteria.

Phagocytosis

After the natural barriers of the skin or mucous membranes have been penetrated, the phagocytic cells—neutrophils, monocytes, and macrophages—constitute an important component of the innate immune system. The process of internalizing organisms by these cells (**phagocytosis**) involves attachment of the organism to the cell surface. This triggers extension of a pseudopod to enclose the bacterium in an endocytic vesicle, or **phagosome**.

The circulating polymorphonuclear neutrophil (PMN) is an important component of the host immune response that, in the absence of infection, circulates in a quiescent state. When chemotactic factors, arachidonic acid metabolites, or complement cleavage fragments interact with specific PMN membrane receptors, the neutrophil rapidly becomes activated and moves toward the chemoattractants. After phagocytosis, the mechanisms by which the phagolysosome destroys the microorganism can be divided into oxygen-independent and oxygen-dependent processes. Functional defects in circulating neutrophils or decreases in absolute number of neutrophils are important risk factors for infection.

Neutropenia, defined as an absolute neutrophil count of less than 1000 cells/μL, is a predisposing factor for life-threatening bacterial and fungal infections. The risk of infection is inversely proportionate to the number of neutrophils, rising significantly with neutrophil counts less than 500 cells/μL, termed "severe neutropenia." The longer the duration of profound neutropenia, the greater is the risk of infection. At the first sign of infection (eg, fever), these patients should be given broad-spectrum antibacterial agents to cover gram-negative bacterial pathogens. In addition to impaired immunity, neutropenic hosts often have additional risk factors for infection, such as the need for long-term indwelling central venous catheters (predisposing to infection with skin bacteria) and the frequent use of parenteral nutrition (predisposing to fungal infection).

Several inherited disorders of neutrophil function have been described. **Chédiak–Higashi syndrome** is a rare autosomal recessive hereditary disorder in which the neutrophils have a profound defect in the formation of intracellular granules. Opsonized bacteria such as *Staphylococcus aureus* are ingested normally, but viable bacteria persist intracellularly, presumably because of the inability of the neutrophil's intracellular granules to fuse with phagosomes to form phagolysosomes. Patients with Chédiak–Higashi syndrome typically present in childhood with recurrent bacterial infections involving the skin and soft tissues and the upper and lower respiratory tracts.

Myeloperoxidase deficiency is the most common neutrophil disorder, with a prevalence of one case per 2000 individuals. In this autosomal recessive disorder, phagocytosis, chemotaxis, and degranulation are normal, but metabolic pathways are impaired, leading to delayed microbicidal activity. Most patients with this defect are asymptomatic. In contrast, **chronic granulomatous disease** is a genetically heterogeneous group of inherited disorders characterized by the failure of phagocytic cells to produce superoxides. The defect involves neutrophils, monocytes, eosinophils, and some macrophages. Oxygen-dependent intracellular killing is impaired, and these patients are susceptible to recurrent, often life-threatening infections. Patients with chronic granulomatous disease also tend to form granulomas in tissues, particularly in the lungs, liver, and spleen. Chronic granulomatous disease is usually diagnosed in childhood after recurrent severe infections with *S aureus* and *Aspergillus* species, and affected patients benefit from prophylactic antimicrobials.

INDUCED DEFENSES OF THE BODY

Although innate host defenses against infectious agents are generally nonspecific and do not require prior exposure to the invading agent, induced defenses are highly specific and are qualitatively and quantitatively altered by prior antigenic exposure. Details of the pathophysiology of the host immune system are covered in Chapter 3. Recurrent infections or infections with unusual organisms may be clues to an underlying defect in the induced immune response (Table 4–2).

TABLE 4–2 **Infections associated with common defects in humoral and cellular immune response.**

Host Defect	Examples of Related Immunodeficiency States	Commonly Associated Infections
T-lymphocyte deficiency or dysfunction	AIDS Solid organ transplant Corticosteroid use Idiopathic CD4$^+$ leukopenia	Viral: reactivation of herpes group viruses (HSV, VZV, CMV) Bacterial: *Listeria monocytogenes*, *Mycobacterium tuberculosis* Fungal: Candida esophagitis, *Aspergillus*, cryptococcal meningitis Parasitic: *Toxoplasma gondii*
B-cell deficiency or dysfunction	Common variable immunodeficiency Agammaglobulinemia Chronic lymphocytic leukemia (secondary hypogammaglobulinemia)	Viral: enteroviruses Bacteria: *Streptococcus pneumoniae*, *Haemophilus influenzae*, *Neisseria meningitidis*, *Mycoplasma pneumonia* Parasites: *Giardia lamblia*
Mixed T- and B-cell deficiency or dysfunction	Ataxia-telangiectasia Severe combined immunodeficiency	Recurrent sinopulmonary infections Chronic diarrhea Mucocutaneous candidiasis Viral: respiratory viruses, herpes group viruses

ESTABLISHMENT OF INFECTION

An infectious disease occurs when a pathogenic organism causes inflammation or organ dysfunction. This may be caused directly by the infection itself, as when the etiologic agent replicates in the host, or indirectly as a result of the host's inflammatory response. Many infections are subclinical, not producing any obvious manifestations of disease. To cause overt infection, all microorganisms must go through the following stages: The microorganism must (1) encounter the host; (2) gain entry into the host; (3) multiply and spread from the site of entry; and (4) cause host tissue injury, either directly (eg, cytotoxins) or indirectly (host inflammatory response). The severity of infection ranges from asymptomatic to life-threatening, and the course may be characterized as acute, subacute, or chronic. Whether infection is subclinical or overt, the outcome is either (1) resolution (eg, eradication of the infecting pathogen); (2) chronic active infection (eg, HIV, hepatitis); (3) prolonged asymptomatic excretion of the agent (eg, carrier state with *Salmonella typhi*); (4) latency of the agent within host tissues (eg, latent tuberculosis or varicella zoster virus); or (5) host death from infection.

Except for **congenital infections** (acquired in utero), humans first encounter microorganisms at birth. During parturition, the newborn comes into contact with microorganisms present in the mother's vaginal canal and on her skin. Most of the bacteria the newborn encounters do not cause harm, and for those that might cause infection, the newborn usually has **passive immunity** through maternal antibodies. For example, neonates are protected against infection with *H influenzae* by maternal antibodies for the first 6 months of life until passive immunity wanes and the risk of infection with this bacterium increases. On the other hand, newborns whose mothers are vaginally colonized with group B streptococci are at increased risk in the perinatal period for serious infections such as sepsis or meningitis with this organism. For this reason, it is recommended that (1) vaginal cultures be done to screen for group B streptococci for all pregnant women; and (2) intrapartum antibiotic prophylaxis be administered to those with positive detection of group B streptococci.

Direct entry of microorganisms into the host (ie, bypassing the usual chemical and physical barriers) may occur when (1) an insect vector directly inoculates the infectious agent into the host (eg, a mosquito transmitting malaria); (2) bacteria gain direct access to host tissues through loss of integrity of the skin or mucous membranes (eg, trauma, surgical wounds); or (3) microbes gain access via instruments or catheters that allow communication between usually sterile sites and the outside world (eg, indwelling venous catheters).

Ingression occurs when an infectious agent enters the host via an orifice contiguous with the external environment. This primarily involves inhalation of infectious aerosolized droplets (eg, *M tuberculosis*) or ingestion of contaminated foods (eg, *Salmonella*, hepatitis A virus). Other infectious agents directly infect mucous membranes or cross the epithelial surface to cause infection. This commonly occurs in sexually transmitted diseases. For example, HIV can cross vaginal mucous membranes via penetration of virus-laden macrophages from semen. After the initial encounter with the host, the infectious agent must successfully multiply at the site of entry. The process whereby the newly introduced microorganism successfully competes with normal flora and is able to multiply is termed **colonization** (eg, pneumococci colonizing the upper respiratory tract). When the microorganism multiplies at a normally sterile site, it is termed **infection** (eg, pneumococci multiplying in the alveoli, causing pneumonia). Factors that facilitate the multiplication and spread of infection include inoculum size (the quantity of infectious organisms introduced), host anatomic factors (eg, impaired ciliary function in children with cystic fibrosis), availability of nutrients for the microbe, physicochemical factors (eg, gastric pH), microbial virulence factors, and anatomic sanctuaries (eg, abscesses). An abscess is a special case in which the host has contained the infection but is unable to eradicate it, and these localized infections generally require surgical drainage. Once introduced, infections can spread along the epidermis (eg, impetigo), along the dermis (eg, erysipelas), along subcutaneous tissues (eg, cellulitis), along fascial planes (eg, necrotizing fasciitis), into muscle tissue (eg, myositis), along veins (eg, suppurative thrombophlebitis), into the blood (eg, bacteremia, fungemia, viremia), along lymphatics (eg, lymphangitis), and into organs (eg, pneumonia, brain abscesses, hepatitis).

Infections cause direct injury to the host through a variety of mechanisms. If organisms are present in sufficient numbers and are of sufficient size, **mechanical obstruction** can occur (eg, children with roundworm gastrointestinal infections may present with bowel obstruction). More commonly, pathogens cause an intense secondary **inflammatory response**, which may result in life-threatening complications (eg, children with *H influenzae* epiglottitis may present with mechanical airway obstruction secondary to intense soft tissue swelling of the epiglottis). Some bacteria produce **neurotoxins** that affect host cell metabolism rather than directly causing cell damage (eg, tetanus toxin antagonizes inhibitory neurons, causing unopposed motor neuron stimulation, manifested clinically as sustained muscle rigidity). Host cell death can occur by a variety of mechanisms. *Shigella* produces a **cytotoxin** that causes death of large intestine enterocytes, resulting in the clinical syndrome of dysentery. Poliovirus-induced cell lysis of the anterior horn cells of the spinal cord causes flaccid paralysis. Gram-negative bacterial **endotoxin** can initiate a cascade of cytokine release, resulting in sepsis syndrome and septic shock.

Many infections that begin as mild and easily treatable conditions readily progress without prompt treatment. Small, seemingly insignificant skin abrasions superinfected with toxic shock syndrome toxin (TSST-1)–producing *S aureus* can result in fulminant infection and death. Even indolent infections, such as infective endocarditis caused by viridans group streptococci can be fatal unless recognized and appropriately treated.

There are three potential outcomes of infection: recovery, chronic infection, and death. Most infections resolve, either spontaneously (eg, rhinovirus, the leading cause of the common cold) or with medical therapy (eg, streptococcal pharyngitis after treatment with penicillin). Chronic infections may be either **saprophytic**, in which case the organism does not adversely affect the health of the host, or **parasitic**, causing tissue damage to the host. An example of a saprophytic infection is *Salmonella typhi*, which may be harbored asymptomatically in the gallbladder of about 2% of individuals after acute infection. Chronic infection with the hepatitis B virus may be either saprophytic, in which case the human host is infectious for the virus but has no clinical evidence of liver damage, or parasitic, with progressive liver damage and cirrhosis. A final form of chronic infection is tissue **latency**. Varicella-zoster virus, the agent causing chicken pox, survives in the dorsal root ganglia, with reactivation causing a dermatomal eruption with vesicles or shallow ulcerations, commonly known as shingles or zoster. When the ability of the immune system to control either the acute or chronic infection is exceeded, the infection may result in **host death**.

All infectious agents, regardless of specific mechanisms, must successfully reproduce and evade host defense mechanisms. This knowledge helps the physician to prevent infections (eg, vaccinate against influenza virus); to treat and cure infection (eg, administer antibiotic for *E coli* urinary tract infection); and to prevent further transmission, recurrence, or reactivation (eg, advise use of barrier protection to reduce the sexual spread of genital herpes simplex infection).

CHECKPOINT

1. By what three general mechanisms do hosts resist colonization by pathogenic bacteria?
2. What are three ways in which the normal flora contributes to the balance between health and disease?
3. Which specific host defenses against infection do not require prior contact with the infecting organism?
4. What are the categories of outcomes from an infection?

PATHOPHYSIOLOGY OF SELECTED INFECTIOUS DISEASE SYNDROMES

INFECTIVE ENDOCARDITIS

Clinical Presentation

Infective endocarditis refers to a bacterial or, rarely, a fungal infection of the cardiac valves. Infection of extracardiac endothelium is termed "endarteritis" and can cause disease that is clinically similar to endocarditis. The most common predisposing factor for infective endocarditis is the presence of structurally abnormal cardiac valves. Consequently, patients with a history of rheumatic or congenital heart disease, a prosthetic heart valve, or a history of prior endocarditis are at increased risk for infective endocarditis. Infection involves the left side of the heart (mitral and aortic valves) almost exclusively, except in patients who are injection drug users or, less commonly, in patients with valve injury from a pulmonary artery (Swan–Ganz) catheter, in whom infection of the right side of the heart (tricuspid or pulmonary valve) may occur.

Etiology

The most common infectious agents causing native valve infective endocarditis are gram-positive bacteria, including viridans group streptococci, *S aureus*, and enterococci. The specific bacterial species causing endocarditis can often be anticipated on the basis of epidemiologic factors. Injection drug users commonly introduce skin bacteria such as *S aureus* into the blood when nonsterile needles are used or the skin is not adequately cleaned before needle insertion. Patients with recent dental work are at risk for transient bacteremia with normal oral flora, particularly viridians group streptococci, with secondary seeding of endovascular tissue. Genitourinary tract infections with enterococci may lead to bacteremia and subsequent seeding of heart valves. Patients with prosthetic heart valves are also at increased risk for infective endocarditis resulting from skin flora such as *S epidermidis* or *S aureus*. Before the availability of antibiotics, infective endocarditis was a uniformly fatal disease. Even with antibiotics, the case fatality rate for left-sided *S aureus* endocarditis exceeds 25%, and definitive cure often requires both prolonged intravenous antibiotic administration and urgent surgery to replace infected cardiac valves.

Pathogenesis

Endothelial damage is a common predisposing factor for the development of endocarditis. This may result from turbulent blood flow, as occurs with valvular regurgitation, or from micro-abrasion, common with injection drug use. In this latter setting, it is thought that impurities present in the injected material cause repeated injury to the tricuspid valve endothelium, or less frequently, pulmonary valve endothelium, before being cleared from the bloodstream by the pulmonary circulation. Denuded endothelium results in exposure of extracellular matrix proteins expressing fibronectin, leading to a sticky matrix composed of fibrin, platelets, and adhesion proteins. Infective endocarditis occurs when microorganisms are deposited onto these sterile thrombi during the course of bacteremia (Figure 4–5). Not all bacteria adhere equally well

FIGURE 4–5 Pathogenesis of bacterial valve colonization. Viridans group streptococci adhere to fibrin-platelet clots that form at the site of damaged cardiac endothelium (**A**). The fibrin-adherent streptococci activate monocytes to produce tissue factor activity (TFA) and cytokines (**B**). These mediators activate the coagulation pathway, resulting in further recruitment of platelets and growth of the vegetation (**C**). (Redrawn, with permission, from Moreillon P et al. Pathogenesis of streptococcal and staphylococcal endocarditis. Infect Dis Clin North Am. 2002;16:297. Copyright © Elsevier.)

to these sites. For example, *E coli*, a frequent cause of urosepsis, is rarely implicated as a cause of endocarditis. Conversely, virulent organisms such as *S aureus* can invade intact endothelium, causing endocarditis in the absence of preexisting valvular abnormalities

Once infected, these vegetations enlarge through further deposition of platelets and fibrin, providing the bacteria a sanctuary from host defense mechanisms such as polymorphonuclear leukocytes and complement. Consequently, once infection takes hold, the infected vegetation continues to grow in a largely unimpeded fashion. Infected vegetations also act as mechanical barriers to antibiotic penetration, necessitating the prolonged administration of intravenous (rather than oral) antibiotics that kill (**bacteriocidal agents**) rather than inhibit (**bacteriostatic agents**) the responsible organism. Surgical removal of the infected valve is sometimes required for cure, particularly if there is mechanical valve dysfunction with resultant decompensated heart failure, abscess formation around the valve ring, or prosthetic valve infection.

A hallmark of infective endocarditis is sustained high-grade bacteremia, which stimulates both the humoral and cellular immune systems. A variety of immunoglobulins are expressed, resulting in immune complex formation, increased serum levels of rheumatoid factor, and nonspecific hypergammaglobulinemia. Immune complex deposition along the renal glomerular basement membrane may result in the development of acute glomerulonephritis and renal failure.

Clinical Manifestations

Infective endocarditis is a multisystem disease with protean manifestations. Table 4–3 summarizes the important features of the history, physical examination, laboratory results, and complications of infective endocarditis. Cutaneous findings suggestive of endocarditis include Osler nodes, painful papules on the pads of the fingers and toes thought to be secondary to deposition of immune complexes; and Janeway lesions, painless hemorrhagic lesions on the palms and soles caused by septic microemboli (Figure 4–6). Symptoms and signs of endocarditis may be acute, subacute, or chronic. The clinical manifestations reflect primarily (1) hemodynamic changes from valvular damage; (2) end-organ symptoms and signs from septic emboli (right-sided emboli to the lungs, left-sided emboli to the brain, spleen, kidney, and extremities); (3) end-organ symptoms and signs from immune complex deposition; and (4) persistent bacteremia with metastatic seeding of infection (abscesses or septic joints). Death is usually caused by hemodynamic collapse or by septic emboli to the central nervous system, resulting in brain abscesses or mycotic aneurysms and intracerebral hemorrhage. Adverse outcomes are more common among older patients, those with *S aureus* infections, and those with prosthetic valve infections. Outcomes are also worse in patients with complications from endocarditis (heart failure, valve ring abscess, or emboli) and in patients who have experienced a delay in receiving valvular surgery (those with large vegetations and significant valvular destruction).

CHECKPOINT

5. Which patients are at highest risk for infective endocarditis?

6. What are the leading bacterial agents of infective endocarditis?

7. What features characterize infective endocarditis in intravenous drug users? In patients with prosthetic heart valves?

8. What hemodynamic features predispose to infective endocarditis?

9. What is the outcome of untreated bacterial endocarditis?

10. What are the risk factors for a fatal outcome? What are the most common causes of death in untreated infective endocarditis?

TABLE 4-3   Features of infective endocarditis.

Organ System	History	Physical Examination	Laboratory or Radiographic Data
General	Fever Chills Fatigue Malaise	Fever Tachycardia Diaphoresis Rigors	Positive blood cultures ↑ White blood cell count ↑ Rheumatoid factor
Head, eyes, ears, nose, and throat (HEENT)	Blurred vision	Subconjunctival hemorrhage Roth spots (funduscopic examination) Endophthalmitis	
Respiratory	Shortness of breath Pleuritic chest pain	Diminished breath sounds Crackles	Pleural-based cavitary lesions (septic pulmonary emboli) Pulmonary edema (heart failure)
Cardiac	Shortness of breath	Murmur (systolic or diastolic) ↑ Jugular venous pressure Lower extremity edema	Vegetation on echocardiogram Prolonged PR interval on electrocardiogram (heart block with myocardial ring abscess)
Gastrointestinal	Abdominal pain	Splenomegaly	Splenic infarct or abscess on CT scan
Genitourinary	Flank pain Blood in urine	Costovertebral angle tenderness	↑ Blood urea nitrogen ↑ Serum creatinine Hematuria ↓ Serum complement levels (C3, C4, CH50) due to immune-complex glomerulonephritis
Musculoskeletal	Joint pain Back pain	Joint effusion, erythema, warmth Spinal tenderness to palpation	Arthrocentesis (↑ white blood cell count; bacteria on Gram stain; positive cultures) MRI of spine (discitis, osteomyelitis, epidural abscess)
Cutaneous	Rash	Splinter hemorrhages (nail beds) Janeway lesions (painless hemorrhagic macules on palms and soles) Petechiae Osler nodes (painful nodules on fingers and toes)	
Neurologic	Headache Confusion Seizure	Altered consciousness Focal weakness	MRI of brain (septic emboli, mycotic aneurysm)

MENINGITIS

Clinical Presentation

Symptoms commonly associated with both bacterial and viral meningitis include acute onset of fever, headache, neck stiffness (**meningismus**), photophobia, and confusion. Bacterial meningitis causes significant morbidity (neurologic sequelae, particularly sensorineural hearing loss) and mortality and thus requires immediate antibiotic therapy. With rare exceptions, only supportive care with analgesics is necessary for viral meningitis.

Because the clinical presentations of bacterial and viral meningitis may be indistinguishable, laboratory studies of the cerebrospinal fluid are critical in differentiating these entities. Cerebrospinal fluid leukocyte **pleocytosis** (white blood cells in the cerebrospinal fluid) is the hallmark of meningitis. Bacterial meningitis is generally characterized by neutrophilic pleocytosis (predominance of polymorphonuclear neutrophils in the cerebrospinal fluid). Common causes of lymphocytic pleocytosis include viral infections (eg, enterovirus, West Nile virus), fungal infections (eg, cryptococcus in HIV-infected persons), and spirochetal infections (eg, neurosyphilis or Lyme neuroborreliosis). Noninfectious causes such as cancer, connective

FIGURE 4–6 Osler node causing pain within pulp of the big toe in a woman hospitalized with acute bacterial endocarditis. (Osler nodes are painful: remember "O" for "ouch" and "Osler.") Note the multiple painless flat Janeway lesions over the sole of the foot. (Used, with permission, from David A. Kasper, DO, MBA. Originally published in: Chumley H. Bacterial endocarditis. In: Usatine RP et al, eds. *The Color Atlas of Family Medicine*, 2nd ed. McGraw-Hill, 2013.)

tissue diseases, and hypersensitivity reactions to drugs can also cause lymphocytic pleocytosis. The cerebrospinal fluid in bacterial meningitis is generally characterized by marked elevations in protein concentration, an extremely low glucose level, and, in the absence of previous antibiotic treatment, a positive Gram stain for bacteria. However, there is often significant overlap between the cerebrospinal fluid findings in bacterial and nonbacterial meningitis, and differentiating these entities at presentation is a significant clinical challenge.

Etiology

Bacterial agents causing meningitis vary according to host age (Table 4–4). Infections in neonates are typically caused by translocation of vaginal flora during birth. Post-neonatal meningitis is most frequently caused by encapsulated bacteria, specifically *S pneumoniae* and *N meningitidis*, although the introduction of a conjugate vaccine against the former has led to a decline in the incidence of *S pneumoniae* meningitis (in both pediatric and adult populations). *Listeria monocytogenes* is a food-borne pathogen that has a particular predilection for causing meningitis in elderly, immunocompromised, or pregnant patients. The microbiology of bacterial meningitis varies for postneurosurgery patients (*S aureus*, gram-negative bacilli, *P aeruginosa*), patients with ventricular shunts (*S epidermidis*, *S aureus*, gram-negative bacilli), and neutropenic patients (gram-negative bacilli, including *P aeruginosa*), with important implications for empiric therapy. Subacute or chronic meningitis may be caused by *M tuberculosis*, fungi (eg, *Coccidioides immitis*, *Cryptococcus neoformans*), and spirochetes such as *Treponema pallidum* (the bacterium causing syphilis) or *Borrelia burgdorferi* (the bacterium causing Lyme disease). The diagnosis of meningitis caused by these organisms may be delayed because many of these pathogens are difficult to culture and require special serologic or molecular diagnostic techniques.

Pathogenesis

The pathogenesis of bacterial meningitis involves a sequence of events in which virulent microorganisms overcome the host defense mechanisms (Table 4–5).

Most cases of bacterial meningitis begin with bacterial colonization of the nasopharynx (Figure 4–7, panel A). An exception is *Listeria*, which enters the bloodstream through ingestion of contaminated food. Pathogenic bacteria such as *S pneumoniae* and *N meningitidis* secrete an IgA protease that inactivates host antibody and facilitates mucosal attachment. Many of the causal pathogens also possess surface characteristics that enhance mucosal colonization. *N meningitidis* binds to nonciliated epithelial cells by finger-like projections known as **pili**.

TABLE 4–4 Proportion of cases of bacterial meningitis in the United States by host age, 2003–2007.

Pathogen	Age			
	<2 Months	**2 Months–17 Years**	**18–50 Years**	**>50 Years**
Group B streptococci	>85%	~5%	<5%	<5%
H influenzae	<5%		<5%	<5%
Listeria monocytogenes	<5%	<5%	<5%	~10%
N meningitidis		~40%	~20%	~5%
S pneumoniae	<5%	~50%	~65%	~75%

TABLE 4–5   Pathogenetic sequence of bacterial neurotropism.

Neurotropic Stage	Host Defense	Strategy of Pathogen
1. Colonization or mucosal invasion	Respiratory mucus	Enzymatic degradation
	Secretory IgA	IgA protease secretion
	Ciliary activity	Ciliostatic enzymes
	Mucosal epithelium	Binding molecules and adhesive pili
2. Intravascular survival	Complement	Production of polysaccharide capsule and enzymatic degradation
3. Crossing of blood–brain barrier	Cerebral endothelium	Binding to endothelial receptors and adhesive pili
4. Survival within cerebrospinal fluid	Complement and antibodies (low levels in uninfected patients)	Rapid bacterial replication prior to complement production and recruitment of neutrophils

Once the mucosal barrier is breached, bacteria gain access to the bloodstream, where they must overcome host defense mechanisms to survive and invade the central nervous system (CNS) (Figure 4–7, panel B). The bacterial capsule, a feature common to *N meningitidis*, *H influenzae*, and *S pneumoniae*, is the most important virulence factor in this regard. Host defenses counteract the protective effects of the pneumococcal polysaccharide capsule by activating the alternative complement pathway, resulting in C3b activation, opsonization, phagocytosis, and intravascular clearance of the organism.

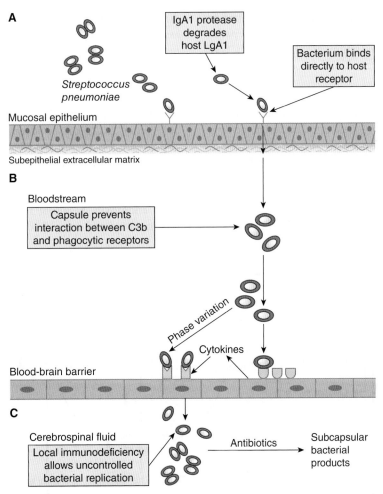

FIGURE 4–7 Pathogenic steps leading to pneumococcal meningitis. The pneumococcus adheres to and colonizes the nasopharynx. IgA1 protease protects the pneumococcus from host antibody (**A**). Once in the bloodstream, the bacterial capsule helps the pneumococcus to evade opsonization (**B**). The pneumococcus accesses the cerebrospinal fluid through receptors on the endothelial surface of the blood–brain barrier (**C**). (Redrawn, with permission, from Koedel U et al. Pathogenesis and pathophysiology of pneumococcal meningitis. Lancet Infect Dis. 2002;2:731.)

This defense mechanism is impaired in patients who have undergone splenectomy, and such patients are predisposed to the development of overwhelming bacteremia and meningitis with encapsulated bacteria. Activation of the complement system membrane attack complex is an essential host defense mechanism against invasive disease by *N meningitidis*, and patients with deficiencies of the late complement components (C5–9) are at increased risk for meningococcal meningitis.

The blood–brain barrier consists of endothelial cells joined by intercellular tight junctions that prevent access of intravascular organisms into the CNS. The exact mechanism of how pathogens transverse the blood–brain barrier is incompletely understood (Figure 4–7, panel C). Possible routes include (1) transport by infected leukocytes (the "Trojan Horse" hypothesis); and (2) opening of the intercellular junctions following cytokine release. Invasion of the spinal fluid by a meningeal pathogen results in increased permeability of the blood–brain barrier, where local host defense mechanisms are inadequate to control the infection. Normally, complement components are minimal or absent in the cerebrospinal fluid. Meningeal inflammation leads to increased, but still low, concentrations of complement, inadequate for opsonization, phagocytosis, and removal of encapsulated meningeal pathogens. Immunoglobulin concentrations are also low in the cerebrospinal fluid, with an average blood-to-cerebrospinal-fluid IgG ratio of 800:1.

The ability of meningeal pathogens to induce a marked subarachnoid space inflammatory response contributes to many of the pathophysiologic consequences of bacterial meningitis. Although the bacterial capsule is largely responsible for intravascular and cerebrospinal fluid survival, the subcapsular surface components (ie, the cell wall and lipopolysaccharide) of bacteria are more important determinants of meningeal inflammation. The major mediators of the inflammatory process are thought to be IL-1, IL-6, matrix metalloproteinases,

and tumor necrosis factor (TNF). Within 1–3 hours after intracisternal inoculation of purified lipopolysaccharide in an animal model, there is a brisk release of TNF and IL-1 into the cerebrospinal fluid, preceding the development of inflammation. Indeed, direct inoculation of TNF and IL-1 into the cerebrospinal fluid produces an inflammatory cascade identical to that seen with experimental bacterial infection. In contrast, experimental injection of purified pneumococcal capsular polysaccharide proteins directly into the cerebrospinal fluid does not result in significant inflammation in animals.

Cytokine and proteolytic enzyme release leads to loss of membrane integrity, with resultant cellular swelling. The development of cerebral edema contributes to an increase in intracranial pressure, resulting in potentially life-threatening cerebral herniation (Figure 4–8). **Vasogenic cerebral edema** is principally caused by the increase in blood–brain barrier permeability. **Cytotoxic cerebral edema** results from swelling of the cellular elements of the brain because of toxic factors released by bacteria or neutrophils. **Interstitial cerebral edema** reflects obstruction in the flow of cerebrospinal fluid, as in hydrocephalus. Neuronal cell death, or **apoptosis**, is caused both by the immune inflammatory response and by direct toxicity of bacterial components, and clinically may be associated with cognitive impairment as a long-term sequela of meningitis. Cerebrovascular complications including infarction or hemorrhage are common and may be due to localized intravascular coagulation.

Understanding the pathophysiology of bacterial meningitis has therapeutic implications. Although bactericidal antibiotic therapy is critical for adequate treatment, rapid bacterial killing releases inflammatory bacterial fragments, potentially exacerbating inflammation and abnormalities of the cerebral microvasculature. In animal models, antibiotic therapy has been shown to cause rapid bacteriolysis and release of bacterial endotoxin, resulting in increased cerebrospinal fluid inflammation and cerebral edema.

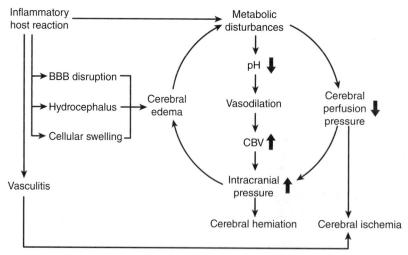

FIGURE 4–8 Pathophysiological alterations leading to neuronal injury during bacterial meningitis. (BBB, blood–brain barrier; CBV, cerebral blood volume.) (Redrawn, with permission, from Koedel U et al. Pathogenesis and pathophysiology of pneumococcal meningitis. Lancet Infect Dis. 2002;2:731.)

The importance of the immune response in triggering cerebral edema has led researchers to study the role of adjuvant anti-inflammatory medications for bacterial meningitis. Studies evaluating the role of corticosteroids have shown variable results. A meta-analysis has shown a slight decrease in the risk of sensorineural hearing loss and in mortality among adults with pneumococcal meningitis when glucocorticoids are given contemporaneously with the first dose of antibiotics. Most authorities recommend the use of adjuvant corticosteroids for patients in high-income settings with suspected bacterial meningitis. (The benefits of corticosteroids for patients from low-income areas is less clear.)

Clinical Manifestations

Among patients who develop community-acquired bacterial meningitis, an antecedent upper respiratory tract infection is common. Patients with a history of head injury or neurosurgery, especially those with a persistent cerebrospinal fluid leak, are at particularly high risk for meningitis. Manifestations of meningitis in infants may be difficult to recognize and interpret; therefore, the physician must be alert to the possibility of meningitis in the evaluation of any febrile neonate.

Most patients with meningitis have a rapid onset of fever, headache, and neck stiffness or pain (meningismus). Nuchal rigidity is frequently noted on physical examination. Other clues seen in a variable proportion of cases include nausea or vomiting, photophobia, **Kernig sign** (resistance to passive extension of the flexed leg with the patient lying supine), and **Brudzinski sign** (involuntary flexion of the hip and knee when the examiner passively flexes the patient's neck). More than half of patients with meningococcemia develop a characteristic petechial or purpuric rash, predominantly on the extremities, although onset of skin lesions may lag behind other symptoms.

Although a change in mental status (lethargy, confusion) is common in bacterial meningitis, up to one-third of patients present with normal mentation. Between 10% to 30% of patients have cranial nerve dysfunction, focal neurologic signs, or seizures. Coma, papilledema, and the Cushing triad (bradycardia, respiratory depression, and hypertension) are ominous signs of impending **herniation** (brain displacement through the foramen magnum with brainstem compression), heralding imminent death.

Despite advances in treatment, the case fatality rate of meningitis remains high, and neurologic impairment is common among survivors. Morbidity and mortality may be decreased by rapid initiation of appropriate antibiotics. Any patient suspected of having meningitis requires prompt medical assessment and emergent lumbar puncture for Gram stain and culture of the cerebrospinal fluid, followed immediately by the administration of antibiotics (and consideration of corticosteroids if the cerebrospinal fluid results support bacterial meningitis).

CHECKPOINT

11. What is the typical presentation of bacterial meningitis?
12. What are the major etiologic agents of meningitis, and how do they vary with age or other host characteristics?
13. What is the sequence of events in development of meningitis, and what features of particular organisms predispose to meningitis?
14. What are the diverse causes of cerebral edema in patients with meningitis?
15. Why is rapid bacteriolysis theoretically dangerous in meningitis?
16. What are the associated clinical manifestations of untreated bacterial meningitis?

PNEUMONIA

Clinical Presentation

The respiratory tract is the most common site of infection by pathogenic microorganisms. Pneumonia accounts for >1 million hospitalizations each year in the United States, and >50,000 deaths. Pneumonia, together with influenza, is the leading cause of death from an infectious disease in the United States.

Diagnosis and management of pneumonia require knowledge of host risk factors, potential infectious agents, and environmental exposures. Pneumonia is an infection of the lung tissue caused by a number of different bacteria, viruses, and fungi, resulting in inflammation of the lung parenchyma and accumulation of an inflammatory exudate in the airways. Infection typically begins in the alveoli, with secondary spread to the interstitium, resulting in consolidation and impaired gas exchange. Infection can also extend to the pleural space, causing **pleuritis** (inflammation of the pleura, characterized by pain on inspiration). The exudative inflammatory response of the pleura to pneumonia is termed a **parapneumonic effusion**; when bacterial infection is present in the pleura, this is termed **empyema**.

Etiology

Despite technologic advances in diagnosis, no causative agent is identified in more than 50% of cases of community-acquired pneumonia. Even in cases in which a microbiologic diagnosis is made, there is usually a delay of several days before the pathogen can be identified and antibiotic susceptibility determined. Symptoms are nonspecific and do not reliably differentiate the various causes of pneumonia. Therefore, knowledge of the most common etiologic organisms is crucial in determining rational empiric antibiotic regimens. Bacterial causes of community-acquired pneumonia vary by comorbid disease and severity of pulmonary infection (Table 4–6).

TABLE 4–6 Common etiologic agents of community-acquired pneumonia as determined by severity of illness.

Etiologic Agent	Outpatient	Hospitalized	
		Mild to Moderate Infection (Not in ICU)	Severe Infection (Requiring ICU)
S pneumoniae	X	X	X
M pneumoniae	X	X	
C pneumoniae	X	X	
H influenzae	X	X	X
Respiratory viruses[1]	X	X	
Legionella species		X	X
Gram-negative bacilli			X
Anaerobes (aspiration)		X	
S aureus			X

[1]Influenza A and B, adenovirus, respiratory syncytial virus, and parainfluenza.

Data from Mandell LA et al. Infectious Diseases Society of America/American Thoracic Society consensus guidelines on the management of community-acquired pneumonia in adults. Clin Infect Dis. 2007;44:227–72.

Pneumonia can be divided into two categories depending on where the infection was acquired: community-acquired or hospital-acquired (nosocomial). Nosocomial pneumonia is defined as pneumonia that occurs 48 hours or more after admission to the hospital and that did not appear to be incubating at the time of admission. The distinction of where the infection was acquired is important because nosocomial pneumonia is more likely to be caused by multidrug-resistant bacteria such as methicillin-resistant *S aureus* (MRSA) or *Pseudomonas*. Knowledge of where and when the patient became ill with pneumonia can be a clue as to which microorganisms should be empirically treated while awaiting definitive culture results.

Traditionally, *S pneumoniae* has been the most common organism isolated in community-acquired pneumonia in both immunocompetent and immunocompromised individuals. However, viral pathogens such as influenza and respiratory syncytial virus (RSV) have increasingly been recognized as significant pathogens contributing to community-acquired pneumonia. Several additional organisms require special consideration in specific hosts or because of public health importance (Table 4–7). Understanding and identifying patient risk factors (eg, smoking, HIV infection) and host defense mechanisms (cough reflex, cell-mediated immunity) focus attention on the most likely etiologic agents, guide empiric therapy, and suggest possible interventions to decrease further risk. For example, patients who have suffered strokes and have impaired ability to protect their airways are at risk for aspirating oropharyngeal secretions. Precautions such as avoiding thin liquids in these patients may decrease the risk of future lung infections. Likewise, an HIV-infected patient with a low CD4 lymphocyte count is at risk for pneumocystis pneumonia and should be given prophylactic antibiotics.

Pathogenesis

Pneumonia is disproportionally a disease of the elderly and impaired host; it occurs infrequently in immunocompetent individuals. This can be attributed to the effectiveness of host defenses, including anatomic barriers and cleansing mechanisms in the nasopharynx and upper airways and local humoral and cellular factors in the alveoli.

The lung is constantly exposed to a mixture of particulate matter and microbes that are present in inspired air. Pulmonary pathogens reach the lungs by one of three routes: (1) direct inhalation of infectious respiratory droplets into the lower airways; (2) aspiration of oropharyngeal contents; or (3) hematogenous spread. Acute pneumonia occurs when there is a defect in the host defenses, infection with a particularly virulent microorganism, or exposure to a large inoculum. The pulmonary antimicrobial defense mechanisms consist of innate and adaptive immunity (Figure 4–9). Incoming air with suspended particulate matter is subjected to turbulence in the nasal passages and then to abrupt changes in direction as the airstream is diverted through the pharynx and along the branches of the tracheobronchial tree. Particles larger than 10 mm are trapped in the nose or pharynx; those with diameters of 2–9 mm are deposited on the mucociliary blanket; only smaller particles reach the alveoli. *M tuberculosis* and *Legionella pneumophila* are examples of bacteria that are deposited directly in the lower airways through inhalation of small airborne particles.

The respiratory epithelium that lines the airways and alveoli is an important component of the host defense against respiratory pathogens. Epithelial cells are covered with beating cilia blanketed by a layer of mucus. Each cell has about 200 cilia that beat up to 500 times/min, moving the mucus

TABLE 4-7 Common risk factors and causes of pneumonia in specific adult hosts.

Risk Factor	Etiologic Agents		Pathogenetic Mechanism
	Acute Symptoms	**Subacute or Chronic Symptoms**	
HIV infection	S pneumoniae	Fungi (eg, Aspergillus, Histoplasma, Cryptococcus)	Cell-mediated immune dysfunction
	H influenzae	M tuberculosis, atypical mycobacteria	Impaired humoral response
	P jirovecii		
Solid organ or bone marrow transplantation	Cytomegalovirus	Nocardia	Cell-mediated immune dysfunction
		Fungi	Neutropenia (bone marrow transplant)
	Legionella species	M tuberculosis	
	P jirovecii		
	P aeruginosa		
Chronic obstructive pulmonary disease or smoking	S pneumoniae		Decreased mucociliary clearance
	H influenzae		
	Moraxella catarrhalis		
	P aeruginosa		
Structural lung disease (bronchiectasis)	P aeruginosa		
	Burkholderia cepacia		
	S aureus		
Alcoholism	K pneumoniae	Mixed anaerobic infection (lung abscess)	Aspiration of oropharyngeal contents
	Oral anaerobes		
Injection drug abuse	S aureus		Hematogenous spread
Environmental or animal exposure	Legionella species (infected water)	C immitis (Southwest United States)	Inhalation
	C psittaci (birds)	H capsulatum (east of Mississippi)	
	C burnetii (animals)	C neoformans (birds)	
	Hanta virus (rodents)		
Institutional exposure (eg, hospital, nursing home)	Gram-negative bacilli		Microaspirations
	P aeruginosa		Bypass of upper respiratory tract defense mechanisms (eg, intubation)
	S aureus		
	Acinetobacter species		Hematogenous spread (eg, intravenous catheters)
Post-influenza	S aureus		Disruption of respiratory epithelium
	S pyogenes		Ciliary dysfunction
			Inhibition of polymorphonuclear neutrophils

layer upward toward the larynx. The mucus itself contains antimicrobial compounds such as lysozyme and lactoferrin.

Most bacteria are 0.5–2 μm in size and can reach the terminal bronchioles, alveolar ducts, and alveoli. Upon their arrival, they are opsonized by surfactant, complement, and antibodies. Macrophages recognize the pathogen via pattern recognition receptors such as Toll-like receptors, which leads to generation of inflammatory cytokines such as TNF-α and IL-1. This signaling cascade recruits neutrophils and, ultimately, antigen-specific T and B lymphocytes into the area. Lymphocytes produce antibody and have cytotoxic ability (eg, ability to kill virally infected cells) to further defend

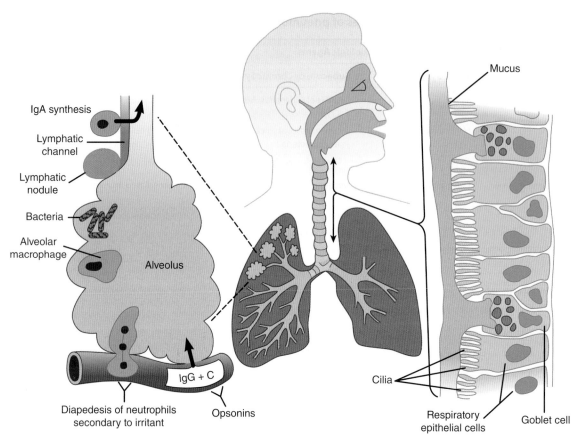

FIGURE 4–9 Pulmonary defense mechanisms. Abrupt changes in direction of airflow in the nasal passages can trap potential pathogens. The epiglottis and cough reflex prevent introduction of particulate matter in the lower airway. The ciliated respiratory epithelium propels the overlying mucous layer (right) upward toward the mouth. In the alveoli, cell-mediated immunity, humoral factors, and the inflammatory response defend against lower respiratory tract infections. (C, complement.) (Redrawn, with permission, from Storch GA. Respiratory system. In: Schaechter M et al, eds. *Mechanisms of Microbial Disease*, 4th ed. Lippincott Williams & Wilkins, 2007.)

against ongoing infection. Another important role of the immune response is the activation of anti-inflammatory mediators, which ensures that the inflammatory response is held in check and that noninvolved areas of the lung are not injured. Impairment at any level of host defenses increases the risk of developing pneumonia. Alteration in the level of consciousness (eg, stroke, alcohol abuse) can compromise epiglottic closure leading to aspiration of bacteria that have colonized the oropharynx. Chronic cigarette smokers have decreased mucociliary clearance secondary to cilia damage and therefore compensate using the cough reflex to clear aspirated material, excess secretions, and foreign bodies. Children with cystic fibrosis have defective ciliary activity and are prone to develop recurrent sinopulmonary infections, particularly with *S aureus* and *P aeruginosa*. Patients with neutropenia, whether acquired or congenital, are also susceptible to lung infections with gram-negative bacteria and fungi. HIV-infected patients have depleted CD4 T lymphocyte counts and are predisposed to a variety of bacterial (including mycobacterial) and fungal infections. Respiratory viruses may destroy epithelium, disrupt normal ciliary activity, and cause abnormal neutrophil and macrophage function.

Clinical Manifestations

Most patients with pneumonia have fever, cough (usually productive), tachypnea, tachycardia, and an infiltrate on chest x-ray. Extrapulmonary manifestations that may provide clues to the etiologic agents include pharyngitis (*Chlamydia pneumoniae*), erythema nodosum rash (fungal and mycobacterial infections), and diarrhea (*Legionella*).

The following considerations aid in guiding empiric therapy for a patient who presents with symptoms consistent with pneumonia: (1) Is this pneumonia community acquired or hospital acquired? (2) Is this patient immunocompromised (eg, HIV infected, a transplant recipient)? (3) Is this patient an injection drug user? (4) Has this patient had a recent alteration in consciousness (suggestive of aspiration)? (5) Are the symptoms acute (days) or chronic (weeks to months)? (6) Has this patient lived in or traveled through geographic areas associated with specific endemic infections (eg, histoplasmosis, coccidioidomycosis)? (7) Has this patient had recent zoonotic exposures associated with pulmonary infections (eg, psittacosis, Q fever)? (8) Could this patient have a contagious infection of public health importance (eg, tuberculosis)? (9) Could this patient's pulmonary infection be associated with a common source exposure (eg, *Legionella* or influenza outbreak)? (10) Does the illness necessitate hospitalization or intensive care admission (eg, pneumonia due to *Legionella*, *S pneumonia*, or *S aureus*)?

CHECKPOINT

17. What are the important pathogens for patients with community-acquired pneumonia based on severity of illness and site of care?
18. What host features influence the likelihood of particular causes of pneumonia?
19. What are the four mechanisms by which pathogens reach the lungs?
20. What are the defenses of the respiratory epithelium against infection?

INFECTIOUS DIARRHEA

Clinical Presentation

Each year throughout the world, more than 5 million people—most of them children younger than 1 year—die of acute infectious diarrhea (see also Chapter 13). Although death is a rare outcome of infectious diarrhea in the United States, morbidity is substantial. It is estimated that there are more than 200 million episodes each year, resulting in 1.8 million hospitalizations at a cost of $6 billion per year. The morbidity and mortality attributable to diarrhea are largely due to loss of intravascular volume and electrolytes, with resultant cardiovascular failure. For example, adults with cholera can excrete more than 1 L of fluid per hour. Contrast this with the normal volume of fluid lost daily in the stools (150 mL), and it is clear why massive fluid losses associated with infectious diarrhea can lead to dehydration, cardiovascular collapse, and death.

GI tract infections can present with primarily upper tract symptoms (nausea, vomiting, crampy epigastric pain), small intestine symptoms (profuse watery diarrhea), or large intestine symptoms (tenesmus, fecal urgency, bloody diarrhea). Diarrhea with visible blood or mucus is termed invasive diarrhea (or dysentery). Sources of infection include person-to-person transmission (fecal–oral spread of *Shigella*), water-borne transmission (*Cryptosporidium*), food-borne transmission (*Salmonella* or *S aureus* food poisoning), and overgrowth after antibiotic administration (*C difficile* infection). Diarrhea can also be defined in terms of duration: acute (14 days or fewer), persistent diarrhea (14–30 days), or chronic (more than 30 days).

Etiology

A wide range of viruses, bacteria, fungi, and protozoa can infect the GI tract. Most cases of acute infectious gastroenteritis are due to viral pathogens. However, the majority of cases of diarrhea are self-limited, and diagnostic evaluation is not performed. Patients presenting to medical attention are biased toward the subset with more severe symptoms (eg, high fevers, hypotension, bloody diarrhea), immunocompromise (eg, HIV, neutropenia), or prolonged duration. An exception is large outbreaks of food-borne illness, in which epidemiologic investigations may detect patients with milder variants of disease.

Pathogenesis

A comprehensive approach to GI tract infections starts with the classic host–agent–environment interaction model. A number of host factors influence GI tract infections. Patients at extremes of age and with comorbid conditions (eg, HIV infection) are at higher risk for symptomatic infection. Medications that alter the GI microenvironment or destroy normal bacterial flora (eg, antacids, antibiotics) also predispose patients to infection. Microbial agents responsible for GI illness can be categorized according to type of organism (bacterial, viral, protozoal), propensity to attach to different anatomic sites (stomach, small bowel, colon), and pathogenesis (enterotoxigenic, cytotoxigenic, enteroinvasive). Environmental factors can be divided into three broad categories based on mode of transmission: (1) water borne; (2) food borne; and (3) person to person. Table 4–8 summarizes these relationships and provides a framework for assessing the pathogenesis of GI tract infections.

The spectrum of diarrheal infections is typified by the diverse clinical manifestations and mechanisms through which *E coli* can cause diarrhea. Colonization of the human GI tract by *E coli* is universal, typically occurring within hours after birth. However, when the host organism is exposed to pathogenic strains of *E coli* not normally present in the bowel flora, localized GI disease or even systemic illness may occur. There are five major classes of diarrheogenic *E coli* (and several newer proposed subgroups): enterotoxigenic (ETEC), enteropathogenic (EPEC), enterohemorrhagic (EHEC), enteroaggregative (EAEC), and enteroinvasive (EIEC) (Table 4–9). Features common to all pathogenic *E coli* are evasion of host defenses, colonization of intestinal mucosa, and multiplication with host cell injury. This organism, like all GI pathogens, must survive transit through the acidic gastric environment and be able to persist in the GI tract despite the mechanical force of peristalsis and competition for scarce nutrients from existing bacterial flora. Adherence can be nonspecific (at any part of the intestinal tract) or, more commonly, specific, with attachment occurring at well-defined anatomic areas.

The term "gastroenteritis" classically denotes infection of the stomach and proximal small bowel. Symptoms and signs include a combination of diarrhea, vomiting, and abdominal pain. The most common cause is viruses, such as rotavirus and norovirus. Decreasing rates of rotavirus-associated gastroenteritis have been observed among adults due to the rotavirus vaccine being used in children. Other causative organisms include *Bacillus cereus*, *S aureus*, and *Campylobacter*. These

TABLE 4–8   Approach to gastrointestinal tract infections.

Paradigm	Category	Epidemiology	Example
Environment	Water borne	Fecal contamination of water supply	*Vibrio cholerae*
	Food borne	Contaminated food (bacteria or toxin)	*S aureus*
			Salmonella
	Person to person (eg, fecal–oral spread)	Child care centers	*Shigella*
			Rotavirus
Agent	Bacterial		*Campylobacter*
	Viral		*Norovirus*
	Parasitic		*Entamoeba histolytica*
Host	Age	Infants, elderly	Enterohemorrhagic *E coli*
	Comorbidity	HIV	*Cryptosporidium*
	Gastric acidity	Antacid use	*Salmonella*
	GI flora	Antibiotic use	*Clostridium difficile*
Site	Stomach	Gastroenteritis	*B cereus*
	Small intestine	Secretory diarrhea	*V cholerae*
	Large intestine	Inflammatory diarrhea	*Shigella*

bacterial organisms, as well as norovirus, are major causes of food-borne-related gastroenteritis. *B cereus* and *S aureus* both produce preformed toxins that, even in the absence of viable bacteria, are capable of causing food-borne disease, often within a few hours of the offending meal. Food poisoning by *B cereus* causes vomiting and diarrhea, whereas that caused by *S aureus* is usually associated with vomiting and abdominal cramps. With both, symptoms typically resolve within about 24 hours.

Infectious diarrhea involving the small and large bowel is clinically differentiated into secretory, inflammatory, and hemorrhagic types, with different pathophysiologic mechanisms accounting for these diverse presentations. **Secretory** (watery) diarrhea is caused by a number of bacteria (eg, *Vibrio cholerae*, ETEC, EAEC), viruses (eg, rotavirus, norovirus), and protozoa (eg, *Giardia*, *Cryptosporidium*). These organisms attach superficially to enterocytes in the lumen of the small bowel. Stool examination is notable for the absence of fecal leukocytes, although in rare cases there is occult blood in the stools. Some of these pathogens elaborate **enterotoxins**, proteins that increase intestinal cyclic adenosine monophosphate (cAMP) production, leading to net fluid secretion. The classic example is cholera. The bacterium *V cholerae* attaches to the epithelium of the small intestine and produces cholera toxin, which causes prolonged activation of epithelial adenylyl cyclase and increased intracellular cyclic AMP. The high cAMP levels cause a dramatic efflux of water and secretion of sodium, chloride, and potassium and bicarbonate ions by intestinal villi, leading to profuse watery diarrhea (Figure 4–10). Clinically, the patient presents with copious diarrhea ("rice-water stools"), progressing to dehydration and vascular collapse, sometimes within 12 hours, unless given vigorous

TABLE 4–9   *Escherichia coli* in diarrheal disease.

	Susceptible Populations				
Class	Developed Countries	Developing Countries	Clinical Syndrome	Site	Toxins
ETEC	Returning travelers	Age <5 years	Watery diarrhea	Small intestine	Heat-labile and heat-stable toxin
EIEC	Rare	All ages	Dysentery (bloody diarrhea, mucus, fever)	Large intestine > small intestine	*Shigella*-like enterotoxin
EHEC	Children, elderly	Rare	Hemorrhagic colitis; hemolytic uremic syndrome	Large intestine	Shiga toxins (Stx1 and Stx2)
EPEC	Rare	Age <2 years	Watery diarrhea	Small intestine	Unknown
EAEC	Rare	Children	Persistent watery diarrhea	Small intestine	Enteroaggregative heat-stable enterotoxin

FIGURE 4-10 Pathogenesis of *Vibrio cholerae* and enterotoxigenic *E coli* (ETEC) in diarrheal disease. *V cholerae* and ETEC share similar pathogenetic mechanisms in causing diarrheal illness. The bacteria gain entry to the small intestinal lumen through ingestion of contaminated food (**left**). They elaborate an enterotoxin that is composed of one A subunit and five B subunits. The B subunits bind to the intestinal cell membrane and facilitate entry of part of the A subunit (**right**). Subsequently, this results in a prolonged activation of adenylyl cyclase and the formation of cyclic adenosine monophosphate (cAMP), which stimulates water and electrolyte secretion by intestinal endothelial cells. (Redrawn, with permission, from Vaughan M. Cholera and cell regulation. Hosp Pract. 1982;17(6):145–52.)

volume resuscitation. ETEC, a common cause of acute diarrheal illness in young children and the most common cause of diarrhea in travelers returning to the United States from developing countries, produces two enterotoxins. The heat-labile toxin (LT) activates adenylyl cyclase, whereas the heat-stable toxin (ST) activates guanylyl cyclase activity. Activation of both enzymes leads to secretion of massive amounts of fluid and electrolytes into the intestinal lumen, similar to the action of the cholera toxin.

Inflammatory diarrhea is a result of bacterial invasion of the mucosal lumen, with resultant cell death. Patients with this syndrome are usually febrile, with complaints of crampy lower abdominal pain as well as diarrhea, which may contain visible mucus. The term **dysentery** is used when significant numbers of fecal leukocytes and gross blood are present. Pathogens associated with inflammatory diarrhea include EIEC, *Shigella*, *Salmonella*, *Campylobacter*, and *Entamoeba histolytica*. *Shigella*, the prototypical cause of bacillary dysentery, is transmitted via direct person–person contact or from contaminated food or water. *Shigella* invades the colonic enterocyte through formation of an endoplasmic vacuole, which is lysed intracellularly. Bacteria then proliferate in the cytoplasm and invade adjacent epithelial cells causing cell death. Production of a **cytotoxin**, the Shiga toxin, leads to local cell destruction and death. EIEC resembles *Shigella* both clinically and with respect to the mechanism of invasion of the enterocyte wall through a similar toxin, termed Shigella-like enterotoxin.

Hemorrhagic diarrhea, a variant of inflammatory diarrhea, is primarily caused by EHEC. Infection with *E coli* O157:H7 has been associated with a number of deaths from the hemolytic-uremic syndrome, with several well-publicized outbreaks related to contaminated foods. EHEC causes a broad spectrum of clinical disease, with manifestations including (1) asymptomatic infection; (2) watery (nonbloody) diarrhea; (3) hemorrhagic colitis (bloody, inflammatory diarrhea); and (4) hemolytic-uremic syndrome (an acute illness, primarily of children, characterized by anemia and renal failure). EHEC does not invade enterocytes; however, it does produce two Shiga-like toxins (Stx1 and Stx2) that closely resemble the Shiga toxin in structure and function. After binding of EHEC to the cell surface receptor, the A subunit of the Shiga toxin catalyzes the destructive cleavage of ribosomal RNA and halts protein synthesis, leading to cell death. Shiga toxin can enter the systemic circulation and is phagocytosed by neutrophils, which are in turn endocytosed by target endothelial cells. This leads to vascular damage and in some patients, a prothrombotic state that precedes the hemolytic-uremic syndrome.

Clinical Manifestations

Clinical manifestations of GI tract infections vary depending on the site of involvement (see Table 4–9). For instance, in staphylococcal food poisoning, symptoms develop several hours after ingesting food contaminated with toxin-producing *S aureus*. The symptoms of staphylococcal food poisoning are profuse vomiting, nausea, and abdominal cramps. Diarrhea is variably present with agents causing gastroenteritis. Profuse watery (noninflammatory, nonbloody) diarrhea is associated with bacteria that have infected the small intestine and elaborated an enterotoxin (eg, *Clostridium perfringens, V cholerae*). In contrast, colitis-like symptoms (lower abdominal pain, tenesmus, fecal urgency) and inflammatory or bloody diarrhea occur with bacteria that more commonly infect the large intestine. The incubation period is generally longer (>3 days) for bacteria that localize to the large intestine, and colonic mucosal invasion can occur, causing fever, bacteremia, and systemic symptoms.

CHECKPOINT

21. How many individuals in the world die yearly of infectious diarrhea?

22. What are different modes of spread of infectious diarrhea? Give an example of each.

23. What are the different mechanisms by which infectious organisms cause diarrhea?

SEPSIS & SEPTIC SHOCK

Clinical Presentation

Sepsis is a clinical syndrome characterized by a dysregulated inflammatory response to infection. It is a leading cause of morbidity and mortality in the United States, with an estimated incidence rate of 300 cases per 100,000 population and a case fatality rate of 20–50%. The medical costs of sepsis in the United States exceed $17 billion annually. Rates of sepsis continue to rise secondary to medical advances such as the widespread use of indwelling intravascular catheters, increased implantation of prosthetic material (eg, cardiac valves and artificial joints), and administration of immunosuppressive drugs and chemotherapeutic agents. These interventions serve to increase the risk of infection and subsequent sepsis.

Sepsis is a continuum of conditions, from infection and bacteremia to sepsis and septic shock. The study of sepsis has been facilitated by the establishment of a standardized case definition. Patients with **early sepsis** have infection and bacteremia and are at risk for progressing to sepsis and septic shock. **Sepsis** is defined as life-threatening organ dysfunction caused by a dysregulated immune response to infection. Critical care experts have developed a severity score, called the Sequential (Sepsis-related) Organ Failure Assessment (SOFA) score, to predict which patients are at highest risk of dying of sepsis. The score is calculated 24 hours after admission to the ICU and every 48 hours thereafter. **Septic shock** includes patients who, despite fluid resuscitation, require vasopressor support and exhibit signs of organ dysfunction (SOFA score ≥2). Patients with septic shock have a predicted mortality of 40%. Another commonly used term is **systemic inflammatory response syndrome (SIRS)**. SIRS is a clinical syndrome that is a form of dysregulated inflammation and may be seen with infection as well as with noninfectious states such as

pancreatitis, pulmonary embolism, and myocardial infarction. Leukopenia and hypothermia, included in the SIRS case definition, are predictors of a poor prognosis when associated with sepsis.

Etiology

Although evidence of infection is a diagnostic criterion for sepsis, only 28% of patients with sepsis have bacteremia, and slightly more than 10% will have **primary bacteremia**, defined as positive blood cultures without an obvious source of bacterial seeding. Common sites of infection among patients with sepsis syndrome (in decreasing order of frequency) include the respiratory tract, the genitourinary tract, abdominal sources (eg, gall bladder, colon), device-related infections, and wound or soft tissue infections.

The bacteriology of sepsis has evolved in the last decade. Gram-negative bacteria (*Enterobacteriaceae* and *Pseudomonas*), previously the most common cause of sepsis, have been supplanted by gram-positive organisms, which now cause more than 50% of cases. Staphylococci are the most common bacteria cultured from the bloodstream, presumably because of an increase in the prevalence of chronic indwelling venous access devices and implanted prosthetic material. The incidence of fungal sepsis has risen dramatically owing to an increase in immunosuppressed and neutropenic patients. Sepsis associated with *P aeruginosa*, *Candida*, or mixed (polymicrobial) organisms is an independent predictor of mortality.

Pathogenesis

The normal host response to infection is recognition via pathogen recognition receptors (eg, Toll-like receptors) and immune cell migration, primarily by neutrophils, to the site of infection, where they release inflammatory mediators. The process is highly regulated, with anti-inflammatory cytokines such as IL-10 suppressing release of inflammatory cytokines (eg, TNF-α). Sepsis occurs when the inflammatory response overwhelms the local environment and becomes systemic. The cause of the systemic reaction is likely multifactorial and may include the effect of the microorganism, the release of large quantities of pro-inflammatory mediators, and even the genetic susceptibility of the individual. The different stages of sepsis (early sepsis to septic shock) represent a continuum, with patients often progressing from one stage to the next within days or even hours after admission.

Sepsis generally starts with a localized infection. Bacteria may then invade the bloodstream directly (leading to bacteremia and positive blood cultures) or may proliferate locally and release toxins into the bloodstream. These toxins can arise from a structural component of the bacteria (eg, endotoxin) or may be exotoxins, which are proteins synthesized and released by the bacteria. **Endotoxin** is defined as the **lipopolysaccharide (LPS)** moiety contained in the outer membrane of gram-negative bacteria. Endotoxin is composed of an outer polysaccharide chain (the **O side chain**), which varies between species and is not toxic, and a highly conserved lipid portion (**lipid A**), which is embedded in the outer bacterial membrane. Injection of either purified endotoxin or lipid A is highly toxic in animal models, causing a syndrome analogous to septic shock in the absence of viable bacteria.

Sepsis was initially considered largely to be a result of overstimulation of the host inflammatory response and uncontrolled release of inflammatory mediators. The failure of a number of pharmacologic interventions aimed at blocking endotoxin or the resultant inflammatory cascade suggests that other factors, such as host immunosuppression, play a critical role. Specific stimuli such as organism, inoculum, and site of infection stimulate **CD4 T cells** to secrete cytokines with either inflammatory (type 1 helper T-cell) or antiinflammatory (type 2 helper T-cell) properties (Figure 4–11). Among patients who die of sepsis, there is significant loss of cells essential for the adaptive immune response (B lymphocytes, CD4 T cells, dendritic cells). Genetically programmed cell death, termed **apoptosis**, is thought to play a key role in

the decrease in these cell lines and downregulates the surviving immune cells. The clinical consequences of sepsis include hemodynamic changes (tachycardia, tachypnea), inappropriate vasodilation, and poor tissue perfusion, with resultant organ dysfunction (see Figure 4–11).

A. Hemodynamic Alterations

All forms of shock result in inadequate tissue perfusion and subsequent cell dysfunction and death (see Chapter 11). In noninfectious forms (such as cardiogenic shock and hypovolemic shock), **systemic vascular resistance** is elevated as a compensatory mechanism to maintain blood pressure. In the hypoperfused tissues, there is enhanced extraction of oxygen from circulating red blood cells, leading to decreased pulmonary artery oxygenation. In contrast, vasodilation leads to hypotension and hypoperfusion in septic shock. This is an unintended consequence of vasoactive mediators such as nitric oxide, which is released from endothelial cells in

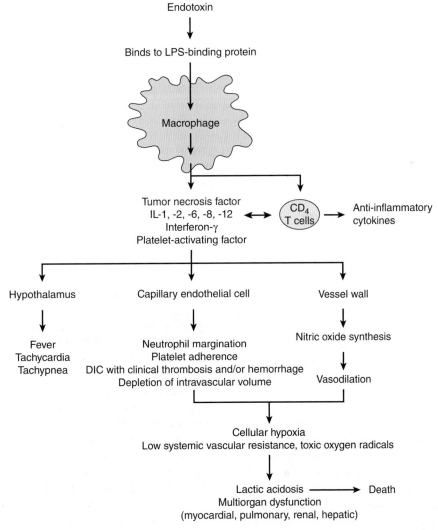

FIGURE 4–11 Pathogenic sequence of the events in septic shock. Activation of macrophages by endotoxin and other proteins leads to release of inflammatory mediators and immune modulation resulting in host tissue damage and, in some cases, death. (Redrawn and modified, with permission, from Horn DL et al. What are the microbial components implicated in the pathogenesis of sepsis? Clin Infect Dis. 2000;31:852.)

response to bacterial endotoxin. Hypovolemia results from inappropriate arterial and venous dilation and leakage of plasma into the extravascular space as a result of increased endothelial permeability. Even with fluid resuscitation, systemic vascular resistance remains low despite a compensatory increase in **cardiac output**. Inefficient oxygen extraction and tissue hypoperfusion result in an increased pulmonary artery oxygen content.

A hyperdynamic circulatory state, described as **distributive shock** to emphasize the maldistribution of blood flow to various tissues, is the common hemodynamic finding in sepsis. Distributive shock is characterized by a loss of normal mechanisms of vascular autoregulation, producing imbalances in blood flow with regional shunting and relative hypoperfusion of some organs. Animal studies have documented predictable changes in organ blood flow, with a marked reduction in blood flow to the stomach, duodenum, small bowel, and pancreas; a moderate reduction in blood flow to the myocardium and the skeletal muscles; and relative preservation of perfusion to the kidneys and CNS.

Myocardial depression is a common finding in early septic shock. Initially, patients have low cardiac filling pressures and low cardiac output secondary to volume depletion resulting from vasodilation. After fluid replacement, cardiac output is normal or increased, but ventricular function is abnormal. From 24 to 48 hours after the onset of sepsis, left and right ventricular ejection fractions are reduced, and end-diastolic and end-systolic volumes are increased. This myocardial depression has been attributed to direct toxic effects of nitric oxide, TNF-α, and IL-1. Reduced ejection fraction and consequent myocardial depression are reversible in patients who survive the initial period of septic shock.

B. Vascular and Multiorgan Dysfunction

Most patients who die of septic shock have either refractory hypotension or multiple-organ failure. Refractory hypotension can occur from two mechanisms. First, some patients cannot sustain high cardiac output in response to the septic state and develop progressive high-output cardiac failure. Second, circulatory failure may be associated with severe vasodilation and hypotension refractory to intravenous fluid resuscitation and vasopressor therapy.

The development of multiple-organ failure represents the terminal phase of a hypermetabolic process that begins during the initial stages of shock. Organ failure results from microvascular injury induced by local and systemic inflammatory responses to infection. Maldistribution of blood flow is accentuated by impaired erythrocyte deformability, with microvascular obstruction. Sepsis is associated with a decrease in the number of functional capillaries, which causes an inability to extract oxygen maximally. Aggregation of neutrophils and platelets may also reduce blood flow. Demargination of neutrophils from vascular endothelium results in a further release of inflammatory mediators and subsequent migration of neutrophils into tissues. Components of the complement system are activated, attracting more neutrophils and releasing locally active substances such as prostaglandins and leukotrienes. The net result of all of these changes is microvascular collapse and, ultimately, organ failure.

The outcome of sepsis depends on the number of organs that fail: Mortality among patients with multiorgan failure (three or more organ systems) averages 70%. Respiratory failure develops in 18% of patients with sepsis. At the most severe end of the spectrum is **acute respiratory distress syndrome** (**ARDS**), characterized by endothelial injury in the pulmonary microvasculature. The injury disturbs capillary blood flow and increases endothelial permeability leading to noncardiogenic pulmonary edema, decreased lung compliance, and refractory hypoxia. Renal failure, seen in 15% of cases, is usually a multifactorial process, with additive injury from intra-renal shunting, renal hypoperfusion, and administration of nephrotoxic agents (antibiotics and radiologic imaging dye). Other organs affected by sepsis include the CNS (altered mentation, coma) and the blood (disseminated intravascular coagulation).

Clinical Manifestations

The clinical manifestations of sepsis include those related to the systemic response to infections (tachycardia, tachypnea, alterations in temperature and leukocyte count) and those related to specific organ system dysfunction (cardiovascular, respiratory, renal, hepatic, and hematologic abnormalities). Sepsis sometimes begins with very subtle clues that can be easily confused with more common and less serious illnesses. Awareness of these early signs of sepsis can lead to early recognition and intervention. Clinical guidelines emphasize the use of a systematic approach to the recognition and early treatment of sepsis. Initial responses should include obtaining cultures of blood and other body fluids, empiric administration of broad-spectrum antibiotics, determination of serum lactate as a marker of hypoperfusion, and use of intravenous fluid and vasopressor therapy for patients with sustained hypotension.

CHECKPOINT

24. What is the mortality rate of sepsis and septic shock in the United States?
25. What factors contribute to hospital-related sepsis?
26. Which organisms are most commonly associated with sepsis?
27. What is the role of the host immune system in the pathogenesis of sepsis?
28. What activates the immune response?
29. What are some distinctive hemodynamic features of septic shock versus noninfectious shock syndromes?

CASE STUDIES

Yeong Kwok, MD

(See Chapter 25, p. 746–49 for Answers)

CASE 13

A 55-year-old man who recently emigrated from China presents to the emergency department with fever. He states that he has had recurring fevers over the past 3 weeks, associated with chills, night sweats, and malaise. Today he developed new painful lesions on the pads of his fingers, prompting him to come to the emergency department. His medical history is remarkable for "being very sick as a child after a sore throat." He has recently had several teeth extracted for severe dental caries. He is taking no medications. On physical examination, he has a fever of 38.5°C, blood pressure of 120/80 mm Hg, heart rate of 108 bpm, and respiratory rate of 16/min, with an oxygen saturation of 97% on room air. Skin examination is remarkable for painful nodules on the pads of several fingers and toes. He has multiple splinter hemorrhages in the nail beds and painless hemorrhagic macules on the palms of the hands. Ophthalmoscopic examination is remarkable for retinal hemorrhages. Chest examination is clear to auscultation and percussion. Cardiac examination is notable for a grade 3/6 holosystolic murmur heard loudest at the left lower sternal border, with radiation to the axilla. Abdominal and back examinations are unremarkable.

Questions

A. What is the likely diagnosis? What are some common predisposing factors to this disease? Which is most likely in this patient?

B. Which infectious agents are most likely to be involved?

C. What is the name given to the various lesions found on this man's hands and feet? What is the pathogenetic mechanism responsible for their formation?

D. What are some other common clinical manifestations of this disease? What are the most common causes of death in this disease? What factors are predictive of a fatal outcome?

E. Why does treatment of endocarditis require prolonged courses of antibiotics to succeed?

CASE 14

A 25-year-old man presents to the emergency department with fever and in a confused, irrational state. He is accompanied by his wife, who provides the history. She states that he had been well until approximately 1 week ago, when he developed symptoms of upper respiratory tract infection that were slow to improve. On the morning of admission, he complained of progressive severe headache and nausea. He vomited once. He became progressively lethargic as the day progressed, and she brought him to the hospital. He has no other medical problems and takes no medications.

On examination, he is febrile to 39°C, with a blood pressure of 95/60 mm Hg, heart rate of 100 bpm, and respiratory rate of 18/min. He is lethargic and confused, lying with his hand over his eyes. Funduscopic examination shows no papilledema. The neck is stiff, with a positive Brudzinski sign. Heart, lung, and abdominal examinations are unremarkable. Neurologic examination is limited by the patient's inability to cooperate but appears to be nonfocal. The Kernig sign (resistance to passive extension of the flexed leg with the patient lying supine) is negative.

Questions

A. What infectious diagnosis is suggested? What are the most likely etiologic agents in this patient? What would they be if he were a newborn? If he were a child?

B. What is the pathophysiologic sequence of events in the development of this disease? What features of the pathogens involved facilitate their ability to produce this disease?

C. What are the possible causes of cerebral edema in this patient?

D. What tests should be performed to confirm the diagnosis? What kinds of treatments should be started or considered? Why?

CASE 15

A 68-year-old man presents to the hospital emergency department with acute fever and persistent cough. He has had cough productive of green sputum for 3 days, associated with shortness of breath, left-sided pleuritic chest pain, fever, chills, and night sweats. His medical history is notable for chronic obstructive pulmonary disease (COPD), requiring intermittent oral glucocorticoid use. His medications include albuterol, ipratropium bromide, and corticosteroid inhalers. The patient lives at home and is active. On examination, he is febrile to 38°C, with a blood pressure of 110/50 mm Hg, heart rate of 98 bpm, and respiratory rate of 20/min. Oxygen saturation is 92% on room air. He is a thin man in moderate respiratory distress, speaking in sentences of three or four words. Lung examination is notable for rales in the left lung base and left axilla and diffuse expiratory wheezes. The remainder of the examination is unremarkable. Chest x-ray film reveals left lower lobe and lingular infiltrates. A diagnosis of pneumonia is made, and the patient is admitted to the hospital for administration of intravenous antibiotics.

Questions

A. On the basis of this patient's underlying condition and severity of illness, what are the likely pathogens involved in this case? How would your differential change if he required ICU admission?

B. What are the mechanisms by which pathogens reach the lungs?

C. What are the normal host defenses against pneumonia?

D. What are some common host risk factors for pneumonia? What are the pathogenetic mechanisms by which they increase the risk of pneumonia? Which of these risk factors are present in this patient?

CASE 16

A 21-year-old woman presents with a complaint of diarrhea. She returned from Mexico the day before her visit. The day before that, she had an acute onset of profuse watery diarrhea. She denies blood or mucus in the stools. She has had no associated fever, chills, nausea, or vomiting. She has no other medical problems and is taking no medications. Examination is remarkable for diffuse, mild abdominal tenderness to palpation without guarding or rebound tenderness. Stool is guaiac negative. Infectious diarrhea is suspected.

Questions

A. What are the different modes of spread of infectious diarrhea? Give an example of each.

B. What is the likely anatomic site of infection in this case? Why?

C. What is the most likely pathogen in this case? What is the pathogenetic mechanism by which it causes diarrhea?

CASE 17

A 65-year-old woman is admitted to the hospital with community-acquired pneumonia. She is treated with intravenous antibiotics and is given oxygen by nasal cannula. A Foley catheter is placed in her bladder. On the third hospital day she is switched to oral antibiotics in anticipation of discharge. On the evening of hospital day 3, she develops fever and tachycardia. Blood and urine cultures are ordered. The following morning, she is lethargic and difficult to arouse. Her temperature is 35°C, blood pressure is 85/40 mm Hg, heart rate is 110 bpm, and respiratory rate is 20/min. Oxygen saturation is 94% on room air. Head and neck examinations are unremarkable. Lung examination is unchanged from admission, with rales in the left base. Cardiac examination is notable for a rapid but regular rhythm, without murmurs, gallops, or rubs. Abdominal examination is normal. Extremities are warm. Neurologic examination is nonfocal. The patient is transferred to the ICU for management of presumed sepsis and given intravenous fluids and antibiotics. Blood and urine cultures are positive for gram-negative rods.

Questions

A. What factors contribute to hospital-related sepsis?
B. By what mechanism do gram-negative rods result in sepsis? What role does the immune response play in the pathogenesis of sepsis?
C. Describe the hemodynamic changes that result in septic shock.
D. By what mechanisms does sepsis result in multiorgan failure?
E. What factors predict a poor outcome in patients with sepsis?

REFERENCES

General

Ahlers LR et al. Nucleic acid sensing and innate immunity: signaling pathways controlling viral pathogenesis and autoimmunity. Curr Clin Microbiol Rep. 2016 Sep;3(3):132–41. [PMID: 27857881]

Kumar S et al. Recognition of bacterial infection by innate immune sensors. Crit Rev Microbiol. 2013 Aug;39(3):229–46. [PMID: 22866947]

Lewis LA et al. Meningococcal disease and the complement system. Virulence. 2014 Jan 1;5(1):98–126. [PMID: 24104403]

Lynch SV et al. The human intestinal microbiome in health and disease. N Engl J Med. 2016 Dec 15;375(24):2369–79. [PMID: 27974040]

Theriot CM et al. Interactions between the gastrointestinal microbiome and *Clostridium difficile*. Ann Rev Microbiol. 2015;69:445–61. [PMID: 26488281]

Yim JJ et al. Genetic susceptibility in tuberculosis. Respirology. 2010 Feb;15(2):241–56. [PMID: 20199642]

Infective Endocarditis

Ambrosioni J et al; Hospital Clinic Infective Endocarditis Investigators. The changing epidemiology of infective endocarditis in the twenty-first century. Curr Infect Dis Rep. 2017 May;19(5):21. [PMID: 28401448]

Baddour LM et al; American Heart Association Committee on Rheumatic Fever, Endocarditis, and Kawasaki Disease of the Council on Cardiovascular Disease in the Young, Council on Clinical Cardiology, Council on Cardiovascular Surgery and Anesthesia, and Stroke Council. Infective endocarditis in adults: diagnosis, antimicrobial therapy, and management of complications: a scientific statement for healthcare professionals from the American Heart Association. Circulation. 2015 Oct 13;132(15):1435–86. [PMID: 26373316]

Cahill TJ et al. Infective endocarditis. Lancet. 2016 Feb 27;387(10021):882–93. [PMID: 26341945]

Cresti A et al. Epidemiological and mortality trends in infective endocarditis, a 17-year population-based prospective study. Cardiovasc Diagn Ther. 2017 Feb 7;7(1):27–35. [PMID: 28164010]

Meningitis

Castelblanco RL et al. Epidemiology of bacterial meningitis in the USA from 1997 to 2010: a population-based observational study. Lancet Infect Dis. 2014 Sep;14(9):813–9. [PMID: 25104307]

Klein RS et al. Protective and pathological immunity during central nervous system infections. Immunity. 2017 Jun 20;46(6):891–909. [PMID: 28636958]

McGill F et al. Acute bacterial meningitis in adults. Lancet. 2016 Dec 17;388(10063):3036–47. [PMID: 27265346]

van Ettekoven CN et al. Update on community-acquired bacterial meningitis: guidance and challenges. Clin Microbiol Infect. 2017 Sep;23(9):601–6. [PMID: 28478238]

Pneumonia

Jain S et al; CDC EPIC Study Team. Community-acquired pneumonia requiring hospitalization. N Engl J Med. 2015 Jul 30;373(5):415–27. [PMID: 26172429]

Mandell LA et al. Infectious Diseases Society of America/American Thoracic Society consensus guidelines on the management of community-acquired pneumonia in adults. Clin Infect Dis. 2007 Mar 1;44(Suppl 2):S27–72. [PMID: 17278083]

National Center for Health Statistics. Health, United States, 2014: with special feature on adults aged 55–64. 2015 May. Hyattsville, MD. Report No. 2015-1232. https://www.ncbi.nlm.nih.gov/pubmed/26086064.

Prina E et al. Community-acquired pneumonia. Lancet. 2015 Sep 12;386(9998):1097–108. [PMID: 26277247]

Quinton LJ et al. Dynamics of lung defense in pneumonia: resistance, resilience, and remodeling. Annu Rev Physiol. 2015;77:407–30. [PMID: 25148693]

Infectious Diarrhea

Bresee JS et al. The etiology of severe acute gastroenteritis among adults visiting emergency departments in the United States. J Infect Dis. 2012 May 1:205(9):1374–81. [PMID: 22454468]

Clements A et al. Infection strategies of enteric pathogenic *Escherichia coli*. Gut Microbes. 2012 Mar–Apr;3(2):71–87. [PMID: 22555463]

Dupont HL. Acute infectious diarrhea in immunocompetent adults. N Engl J Med. 2014 Apr 17;370(16):1532–40. [PMID: 24738670]

Giddings SL et al. Traveler's diarrhea. Med Clin North Am. 2016 Mar;100(2):317–30. [PMID: 26900116]

Sepsis, Sepsis Syndrome, and Septic Shock

Angus DC et al. Epidemiology of severe sepsis in the United States: analysis of incidence, outcome, and associated costs of care. Crit Care Med. 2001 Jul:29(7):1303–10. [PMID: 11445675]

Hotchkiss RS et al. Immunosuppression in sepsis: a novel understanding of the disorder and a new therapeutic approach. Lancet Infect Dis. 2013 Mar;13(3):260–8. [PMID: 23427891]

Rhodes A et al. Surviving sepsis campaign: international guidelines for management of sepsis and septic shock: 2016. Intensive Care Med. 2017 Mar:43(3):304–77. [PMID: 28101605]

Singer M et al. The third international consensus definitions for sepsis and septic shock (Sepsis-3). JAMA. 2016 Feb 23;315(8):801–10. [PMID: 26903338]

Neoplasia

Mark M. Moasser, MD, & Weiyun Z. Ai, PhD, MD

Cell growth and maturation are normal events in organ development during embryogenesis, growth, and tissue repair, and in remodeling after injury. Disordered regulation of these processes can result in loss of control over cell growth, differentiation, and spatial confinement. Human neoplasia collectively represents a spectrum of diseases characterized by abnormal cell growth, loss of tissue homeostasis, and distorted architecture. Such new growth is called a **neoplasm** or **tumor** and can sometimes be a proliferative process confined to one specific tissue site with little systemic manifestations and no threat to the overall state of health. The term "**benign**" is often used to describe such low-impact tumors, which include many common growths such as dermal nevi, warts, and uterine fibroids. The term "**cancer**" or "**malignant** tumor" is used to describe a more advanced form of neoplasia that involves tissue invasion and destruction and defines an inherently progressive biologic process that can culminate in systemic disease and host death. The process of tumorigenesis involves a series of stochastic events in a proliferative context that can generate unlimited diversity in the molecular and phenotypic attributes of tumor cells, both among affected individuals and within a single affected individual. Classification schemes have been devised to provide a framework to reduce this complexity and capture many of the shared attributes of cancers, which are largely based on tissue type and organ of origin. Each type of cancer can exhibit a diversity of biologic behaviors among different patients, and molecular or histologic attributes are used to further sub-classify cancers and identify patterns of behavior.

The recognition of overt malignancy by symptoms or physical examination findings defines the clinical phase of disease. The clinical phase is preceded by a **preclinical phase**, which is usually unknown to the patient but may sometimes be identified by screening interventions. Preclinical signs and potential precursors of colon cancer and breast cancer may consist of polyps in the colon and proliferative abnormalities of the breast, respectively. Such precursor lesions usually harbor molecular genetic abnormalities and exhibit features of abnormal cell proliferation without demonstrating invasiveness and may precede the development of an invasive cancer by months to years; or they may not progress to an invasive cancer within the individual's lifetime. More commonly, the preclinical phase goes undetected until an invasive cancer is present, occasionally with regional or distant metastases. Our understanding of the pathophysiology of various neoplasma is based on clinical and pathologic observations of large series of patients, along with a more recently gained understanding of the cellular and molecular underpinnings of these disorders.

THE CELLULAR & MOLECULAR BASIS OF NEOPLASIA

Neoplasia is a result of stepwise alterations in cellular function. These phenotypic alterations produce morphologic changes that are readily evident by microscopy and may predate tumor development by many years. Morphologic abnormalities may include enlargement of the cell, called cell **hypertrophy**, reflecting too much protein and membrane synthesis. It may include crowding owing to too much cell division, called cell **hyperplasia**. It may include cell **dysplasia**, which reflects a reversion to a more immature cell without a committed identity. It may include **metaplasia**, which reflects abnormal cell reprogramming to appear and function like a cell of a different type. Such changes in cell behavior and function are a result of molecular abnormalities involving cell signaling that can arise owing to defects in the execution of instructions encoded in the cellular genome. Of these various types of abnormalities, the proliferative abnormalities are the primary forces underlying the progressive nature of many forms of neoplasia that may ultimately lead to uncontrolled growth, invasion, and metastasis, which are the hallmarks of cancer.

Underlying the pathophysiology of neoplasia are changes in the cellular genome that underlie all cellular and biochemical aberrations responsible for the malignant phenotype. While the process of DNA replication is designed to ensure that all cells of the human body maintain an exact copy of the human genome, this process is ultimately imperfect. With the passing of time, and with stochastic occurrence of errors in DNA replication, accelerated by exposure to environmental carcinogens, cells in various tissues of the body acquire mutations in their genomes. The number of such mutations in various tissues increases with age. Some mutations have no phenotypic consequences for the cells, others may induce changes that lead to cell death, others may induce cellular dysplasia or metaplasia, and yet others may induce changes that lead to increased proliferation. The proliferative phenotype passes the mutated genome to more cells, beginning a self-perpetuating process. Cells that have acquired a growth advantage owing to DNA mutation may repopulate the tissue over time, and additional DNA mutations may select for yet another cell population within this population with even higher growth rates. Repeated cycles of clonal and subclonal selection, called **clonal evolution**, may eventually lead to a cellular clone with a growth pattern that defies the normal tissue architecture and appears as an outgrowth or new growth in microscopic sections, typically called a **neoplasm** or **tumor** (Figure 5–1). Therefore, this process of new growth, called **neoplasia**, is actually preceded by a years-long process of molecular evolution at the cellular DNA level, which is not apparent by microscopy. A microscopically normal-appearing tissue that bears a high proportion of cells with genetic mutations is sometimes referred to as having a **genetic field defect** and is considered to have a high risk for

the future development of cancer. With increasing age, biopsies of many normal tissues in healthy humans confirm the presence of increasing mutations in cellular DNA. Because of this, it is generally accurate to consider adult cancer as a disease of aging. The pathophysiology of childhood cancer is not as well understood and may be different from that of adult cancer. Childhood cancer may be the endpoint of a series of molecular genetic changes that began very early with errors during the highly proliferative process of development that begins in utero.

In addition to genetic changes involving the nucleic acid sequence of the cellular genome, epigenetic changes are also commonly seen in neoplasia and contribute to the malignant phenotype. Epigenetic phenomena involve chemical modifications of the DNA/protein complex without changes in the genetic sequence. An increasing number of genetic, epigenetic, and proteomic changes are being cataloged from the study of cancer cells, both in vivo, from primary tumors of patients, and in vitro, from established cancer cell lines grown in tissue culture. Some of these changes are specific to a certain tumor type, whereas others are seen more generally across different tumor types. In certain types of cancer, a particular genetic alteration is etiologically linked with, and is pathognomonic of, that cancer type. It may play a significant role as a molecular marker of that disease and as a target for drug development. However, most types of cancers do not have unifying molecular characteristics. Although many of the most common types of cancer are categorized by their primary organ site, such as breast or prostate, an organ-based classification system belies the heterogeneous nature of cancers; thus, in actuality, what is currently called "breast cancer" is in fact a constellation of many diseases with diverse molecular and phenotypic characteristics. Technological advances in high-throughput analysis of the entire cellular genome and of the total cellular

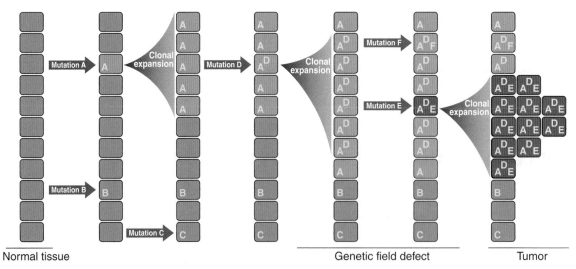

FIGURE 5–1 Schematic depiction of the clonal evolution of cancer. Mutations occur stochastically in the tissue. While many are inconsequential, some can contribute to a proliferative phenotype that can expand to form a subclone. Additional mutations within this subclone can confer higher proliferative potential, and sequential cycles of such growth-promoting mutations can eventually repopulate the tissue, creating a genetic field defect in a normal-appearing tissue. Ultimately, mutations that promote continued growth beyond tissue boundaries can lead to the formation of a tumor with morphological and clinical consequences.

TABLE 5–1 Examples of repositories of mass cancer mutation data

Database	Sponsor	Website
Public Databases		
Catalogue of Somatic Mutations in Cancer (COSMIC)	Wellcome Sanger Institute, Hinxton, Cambridgeshire, UK	https://cancer.sanger.ac.uk/cosmic
The Cancer Genome Atlas	National Cancer Institute, Bethesda, MD	https://cancergenome.nih.gov/
ClinVar	National Institutes of Health, Bethesda, MD	https://www.ncbi.nlm.nih.gov/clinvar/
cBioPortal for Cancer Genomics	Multi-institutional consortium led by Memorial Sloan Kettering Cancer Center, NY	http://www.cbioportal.org/
International Cancer Genome Consortium	Worldwide consortium	http://icgc.org/
Commercial Databases		
Oncomine	Thermo Fisher Scientific, Waltham, MA	https://www.oncomine.org/
BioExpress Suite	Ocimum Biosolutions, Hyderabad, India	https://ocimumbio.com/
OncoLand	OmicSoft Corporation, Cary, NC	http://www.omicsoft.com/

gene transcription profiles have allowed the characterization of tumors by in-depth analyses of their genetic (DNA) and transcriptomic (RNA) features (the **transcriptome** being the sum of all of the RNA transcripts in the cancer). Such molecular signatures provide important predictive and prognostic clinical information, superior to that provided by simple histologic characterization. The technologies underlying the molecular analysis of tumors are rapidly evolving, both in the depth and scale of the analysis and in their cost and speed. Tens of thousands of different types of cancer have undergone in-depth genomic and transcriptomic analyses, and the data output is expanding exponentially, creating considerable challenges in mass data deposition, organization, sharing, and mining. Reconciling the mass data emerging from the analyses of human cancers is one of the principal challenges in what is being called the **Era of Big Data**. Numerous repositories have been developed with portals constructed to enable academic and commercial entities to mine these massive data sets. Some of the common databases are listed in Table 5–1. Although molecular profiling of cancers has already led to new classification systems for several types of cancer, these may soon become redundant in favor of a complete individualized molecular tumor characterization for every single patient's tumor in real time. Many academic institutions and commercial entities are beginning to develop the capabilities to offer such individualized tumor characterization in real time.

Although the progressive phenotypic characteristics of neoplasia result predominantly through sequential molecular alterations and abnormal function of the proliferating tumor cells, it is now clear that at some level abnormal function of the host stromal cells is fundamentally involved in continued tumor progression. These cells include connective tissue cells, hematopoietic and bone marrow compartment cells, immune system cells, and adipose tissue cells. Also involved are various secreted juxtacrine and paracrine growth factors, matrix proteins, and other soluble factors in the tumor microenvironment. Stromal cell abnormalities can be nonproliferative, such as secretion of requisite growth factors, or proliferative, such as expansion of the blood vessel network to support the growth of enlarging tumors or expansion of the extracellular matrix compartment.

CHECKPOINT

1. What is the preclinical phase of cancer?
2. What causes mutations in the genome?
3. What is a genetic field defect?
4. What is the source of the mass data from human cancers?

GENETIC AND EPIGENETIC CHANGES IN NEOPLASIA

Maintaining genomic integrity is a fundamental cellular task. A complex cellular apparatus serves to recognize DNA damage or errors in DNA replication and to correct them, to activate checkpoints to halt further cell replication while corrective measures take place, or to signal suicidal cell death (apoptosis) if repairs cannot be made. These mechanisms, while extremely competent, are ultimately imperfect, and uncorrected errors lead to the acquisition and accumulation of mutations in the genomic DNA in many cells throughout the human body. The accumulation of such mutations is subject to many influences, including inheritable genetic factors, environmental factors, and stochastic factors. Inherited defects in the very genes involved in the machinery that guards the genome can greatly increase the spontaneous rate at which genomic mutations or structural alterations occur, accelerating the accumulation of mutations. Exposure to the environmental factors of ionizing radiation and chemical carcinogens may initiate or accelerate the accumulation of genomic mutations. Gene mutations inherited from parents that are present in all the cells in the body are called **germline** mutations; gene mutations acquired during life in specific cells are called **somatic** mutations. The frequency of somatic mutations in tumor cells, referred to as the mutational burden, varies greatly among different types of cancer. The relative mutational burden of many cancer types is shown in Figure 5–2.

Melanomas, lung and oropharyngeal cancers, and cancers of the gastrointestinal (GI) tract have the highest mutational burden of all cancers. This is due to the direct exposure of these tissues to the outside environment and exposure to mutagenic insults such as ultraviolet (UV) light (skin), inhaled carcinogens (lung and oropharynx), and ingested carcinogens and products of endogenous bacterial flora (GI tract). Cancers of mesenchymal tissues and organs without direct environmental exposure have lower mutational burdens. Specific types of DNA mutation (specific nucleotide changes) are linked with specific environmental insults, and such environmental footprints are evident in the altered tumor genome. For example, melanomas of the skin have a high number of specific types of mutation typically induced by UV light. Cancers of the oropharynx and lung have a high number of mutations typically induced by tobacco carcinogens. Some types of mutation are due to overactivity of the APOBEC family of enzymes (ABOBEC being an acronym for "apolipoprotein B mRNA editing enzyme catalytic polypeptide-like") and likely represent collateral damage from these enzymes of the innate immune system, whose mutagenic functions are intended to infect viruses. Other types of mutation are a result of spontaneous errors that occur in all normal cells and that accumulate with advancing age. Mutation in DNA can occur in various ways. It can be a change in a single base or in two bases, it can be a deletion of one or a few bases, or it can be insertion of extra bases. Alterations of the genome can also occur in larger ways, with DNA segments as large as kilobases or megabases entirely deleted from the genome, or alternatively, recopied many times (so-called amplification).

Defects in DNA Sequence

DNA can incur many types of damage, including chemical modifications or breakages, either to a single strand or to both strands. Cells are endowed with a repertoire of DNA repair mechanisms, each designed for a specific type of damage, to repair and restore the DNA's nucleotide sequence. Malfunction in one or more of these DNA repair mechanisms is one of the fundamental hallmarks of cancer and is often an early event in tumorigenesis. Faulty DNA repair leads to much more rapid accumulation of genetic defects, providing a genetic diversity that propels a selection process leading to a proliferation of tumor cells with better survival, higher proliferative rates, and

more invasive and metastatic phenotypes. The major DNA repair mechanisms implicated in tumorigenesis are summarized in Table 5–2 and discussed below.

The nucleotides in genome DNA can be chemically altered by exogenous or endogenous carcinogens, radiation, UV light, and other mutagens. Single-strand defects are typically repaired by the nucleotide-excision repair (NER) and base-excision repair (BER) mechanisms. BER typically repairs bulky DNA lesions caused by oxidation, alkylation, or deamination, whereas NER typically repairs non-bulky lesions such as thymidine dimers caused by UV light. Loss of genes involved in these pathways increases the mutation rate of the genome and, if defective in the germline, may increase the risk of cancers. In particular, germline defects in many of the genes involved in NER lead to the clinical syndrome of xeroderma pigmentosum. Affected individuals are intolerant to sunlight and have a 1000-fold-higher risk of developing UV-induced skin cancers.

Homologous recombination is the preferred and most accurate mode of repairing double-strand breaks in DNA because it uses the identical second copy of the DNA template (available in the G2 phase) to repair the DNA break with complete fidelity. Malfunction in this important DNA repair mechanism (called homologous recombination deficiency [HRD]) can develop as a result of the loss of one of its critical genes (see Table 5–2). Such malfunction forces cells to use more error-prone mechanisms to repair double-strand DNA breaks. Tumors with HRD, such as *BRCA1*- and *BRCA2*-deficient tumors, typically have large numbers of structural abnormalities in the tumor genome with many copy number variations. Identifying tumors with HRD has become clinically important because there are specific therapies that are effective in treating HRD tumors. Many commercial assays of HRD have been developed for clinical use in patient samples. The genes involved in homologous recombination repair are sometimes defective in the germline, accounting for familial cancer susceptibility syndromes; others can be somatically inactivated in developing tumors.

Non-homologous end-joining (NHEJ) mechanisms are important in repairing double-strand breaks when an identical chromosome copy is unavailable, such as in the G1 phase of the cell cycle. In addition to its role in correcting insult-induced DNA breaks, NHEJ plays a normal physiologic role in mediating V(D)J recombination, which promotes massive diversity in T-cells and B-cells through genomic rearrangements at the T-cell and B-cell receptor genes. As such, patients with germline defects in genes critical for NHEJ have dysfunctional T cells and B cells, leading to the clinical syndrome of severe combined immunodeficiency (SCID). Since NHEJ joins ends without a template for the correct DNA sequence, it is prone to error and can sometimes join DNA ends that do not belong to each other. This can result in chromosomal rearrangements including chromosomal translocations, in which a segment of one chromosome is fused to a segment of another chromosome. This imperfect function of NHEJ likely accounts for a large proportion of the chromosomal translocations found in cancer cells. Other mechanisms for repairing

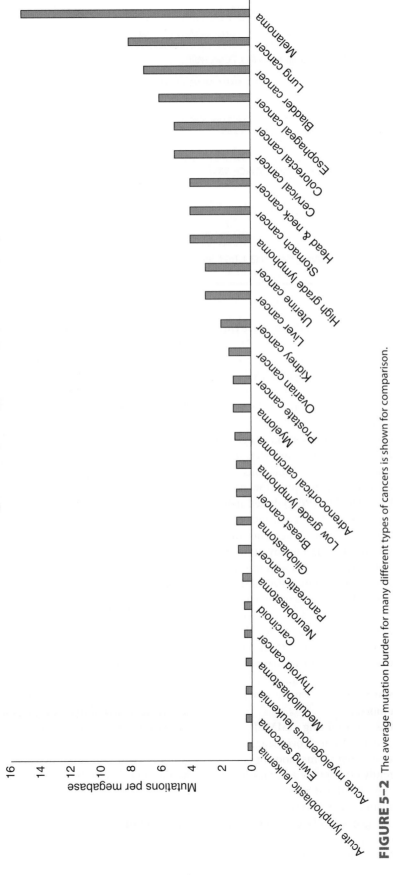

FIGURE 5–2 The average mutation burden for many different types of cancers is shown for comparison.

TABLE 5–2 DNA repair mechanisms and cancer pathogenesis.

Cellular DNA Repair Mechanism	Genes Required or Involved	Examples of Defects in Various Cancers
Base excision repair	OGG1, NEIL1, MBD4, MUTYH, UNG, SMUG1, MPG, TDG, APE1, XRCC1, PNKP, TDP1, APTX, DNA polymerases beta, delta, epsilon, FEN1, PCNA, PARP	Germline MUTYH mutation associated with colon cancer risk. Somatic mutations in different cancers, including colon and gastric cancers.
Mismatch repair	MLH1, MLH3, MSH2, MSH3, MSH4, MSH5, MSH6, PMS1, PMS2, PMS2L3	Germline mutation in Lynch syndrome. Somatic mutations in gastrointestinal, uterine, and other cancers.
Nucleotide excision repair	RAD23B, XPC, CEN2, CSA, CSB, TFIIH, XBP, XPD, XPA, RPA, XPG, ERCC1, ERCC4, XAB2	Germline mutations in xeroderma pigmentosum.
Homologous recombination repair	MRE11, RAD50, RAD51, RAD52, RAD54, BRCA1, BRCA2, ATM, XRCC2, XRCC3, FANCF, NBS1	Germline mutations in several cancer-risk syndromes, including breast/ovarian cancer syndrome. Somatic mutations in many types of cancer.
Non-homologous end-joining	KU70, KU80, DNA-PKcs, Artemis, XRCC4, LIG4, XLF	Germline mutations in severe combined immunodeficiency disease (SCID). Somatic mutations in different cancers.
Microhomology-mediated end-joining	MRE11, PARP1, FEN1, XRCC1, LIG3, NBS1	Increased expression in cancers.

double-strand breaks are also error prone and may cause chromosomal translocations.

The process of DNA replication commonly incurs errors in incorporating nucleotides into the newly synthesized DNA strand, leading to mismatches in the double-strand DNA. A family of proteins constitutes the mechanism of DNA mismatch repair that routinely repairs these errors (see Table 5–2). Defects in mismatch repair genes lead to insertion or deletion errors during correction, and tumors with mismatch repair deficiency have tens of thousands of such mutations. This hypermutable phenotype has a genomic footprint that can be detected by **polymerase chain reaction (PCR)**–based methods, called microsatellite instability (MSI) assays, which detect and measure variations in small genome fragments called microsatellites. These are of uniform length in any individual patient, but they are highly variable in tumors with mismatch repair deficiency, and such tumors are thus called MSI high (whereas most other tumors are MSI low). Commercial assays have been developed to detect MSI in clinical tumor samples because the MSI status of a tumor has prognostic significance and also predicts response or resistance to certain types of therapy. Once again, the genes involved in mismatch repair are sometimes defective in the germline, accounting for familial cancer susceptibility syndromes, or genes can be somatically inactivated in developing tumors.

Microhomology-mediated end-joining (MMEJ) is a mechanism that relies on homology to small overhangs in broken DNA ends to mediate end-joining. This mode of double-strand break repair is inherently error prone and may lead to deletion mutations and chromosomal rearrangements. MMEJ is mostly a back-up mechanism for DNA repair. But in many cancers, overexpression of the genes involved in MMEJ leads to its inappropriate function as a primary mechanism, overriding high-fidelity repair mechanisms and ultimately leading to

more mutations. Thus, in contrast to high-fidelity DNA repair mechanisms that are typically dysfunctional in cancers, the error-prone MMEJ mechanism is often overactive in cancers.

CHECKPOINT

5. What is the source of a germline mutation in a patient?
6. What type of cancer has the highest mutation rate?
7. Name several DNA repair mechanisms that can be dysfunctional in cancers.
8. What is the preferred and most accurate mode of repairing double-strand breaks in DNA, and what is the name given to its malfunction?
9. What is microsatellite instability?

Defects in Chromatin Structure and Dynamics

In addition to the repertoire of DNA repair mechanisms available to correct errors, the integrity of the genome is also preserved and protected by a mega-structural framework consisting of a densely packaged complex of the genome DNA and histone proteins referred to as **chromatin**. Chromatin is highly structured into repeating units called nucleosomes, and the packing of these units provides protection to the DNA and a mode of regulation that determines access to it. This process is under tight regulation by epigenetic mechanisms that can modify and alter the biochemical properties of the histone proteins. Such epigenetic mechanisms determine whether certain regions of the genome are loosened to provide access for gene transcription or for DNA replication or repair, or tightened for transcriptional silencing, genome protection, or chromosome condensation during mitotic separation (Figure 5–3).

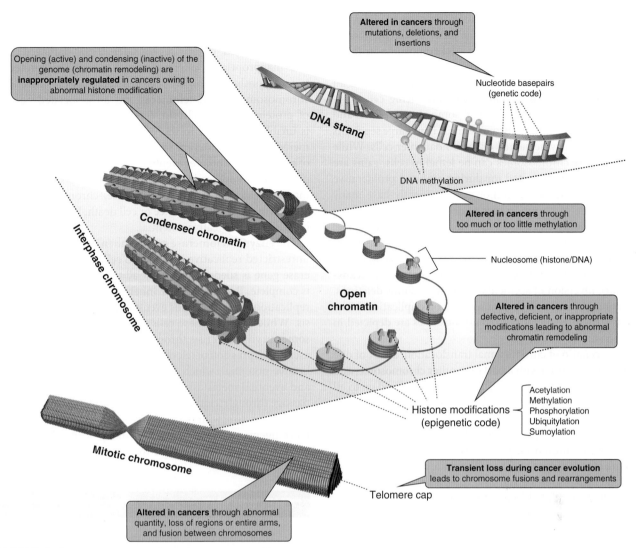

FIGURE 5–3 There are multiple dimensions in the structure and regulation of the genome: the specific nucleotide sequence code; the condensing of genomic regions to keep genes silent and protected; the opening of genomic regions to enable transcriptional activity, replication, or repair; and the complete condensation of the chromosome to prepare for mitosis. The structure and regulation of each dimension of genome integrity and control are frequently altered in cancers. The various types of alteration are reported in the callouts.

Loss of the epigenetic control of chromatin is commonly seen in cancer cells, leading to abnormal expression of many genes, increased susceptibility to DNA damage, and errors in mitotic separation. Alterations in chromatin structure are often visible under light microscopy, and the degree of observed abnormalities in chromatin allows pathologists to assign a nuclear grade when performing a histologic characterization of cancer cells. Underlying the epigenetic deregulation of the genome are defects in the molecular mechanisms that function to regulate chromatin structure. Epigenetic mechanisms involved in chromatin remodeling include the so-called **BAF complexes** (SWI/SNF proteins) and the **polycomb repressive complexes**; many of these are known to be mutated, abnormally expressed, or otherwise dysfunctional in cancer cells, underlying the observed epigenetic abnormalities. Another epigenetic mechanism that functions to regulate the expression of genes is the direct methylation of DNA, frequently at promoter regions. DNA methylation suppresses gene transcription and functions to silence certain areas of the genome, while other areas remain transcriptionally active. Abnormal methylation or demethylation of the genome is commonly found in cancer cells. This abnormality constitutes yet another epigenetic mechanism by which some genes are silenced and other genes are activated to promote the tumorigenic phenotype.

Defects in Genome Content

Maintaining the integrity of the genome also requires preserving its entire content, despite the fact that the human genome is split into 46 fragments (46 chromosomes). As such, a complex cellular machinery is in place to preserve the integrity of each chromosome, to orchestrate the proper duplication of each of the chromosomes in every S phase, and the proper allocation and distribution of a full set of chromosomes to each daughter cell during every mitosis. In neoplasia, these mechanisms can fail, leading to abnormalities in the structure or number of chromosomes, which is referred to as **chromosome instability**. Errors in orchestrating replication or in properly separating and allocating chromosomes during mitosis results in an uneven distribution to daughter cells, producing cell progeny that have increased numbers of some chromosomes and reduced numbers of other chromosomes. Thus, large segments of the genome may be gained or lost in daughter cells. While losses of entire chromosomes can be lethal to cells, gains are often tolerated and selected for during repeated proliferative cycles. As a consequence, tumor cells frequently have many more than the 46 chromosomes of normal cells, an attribute called **aneuploidy**. In addition to abnormal numbers of whole, intact chromosomes, errors in repairing DNA breaks often lead to chromosome rearrangements, including fusion events between different chromosomes (called **chromosomal translocation**), inversion of segments of a chromosome, deletions, truncations (shortened chromosomes), or duplications. The various structural alterations of chromosomes are depicted in Figure 5–4.

In the scenario of chromosomal translocation, a part of one chromosome is fused with a part of another chromosome, and the resulting abnormal hybrid chromosome is passed on to all tumor cell progeny thereafter. A chromosomal translocation can be a random event seen in one cancer only, or it can be a specific and recurring event seen in multiple cancers. In fact, a very specific chromosomal translocation can be the defining attribute of some types of cancer. For example, a translocation between chromosomes 9 and 22 creates a shortened chromosome called the Philadelphia chromosome, a defining attribute of chronic myelogenous leukemia.

Defects in Protecting Chromosome Ends

The fact that the diploid human genome is fragmented into 46 chromosomes means that there are 92 ends in the human genomic DNA. There are cellular mechanisms in place to hide and protect these loose ends from the DNA repair machinery that would otherwise consider them damaged DNA and inappropriately attempt to fuse them. This protection is accomplished by highly repeated sequences at the ends of chromosomes called **telomeres** and an associated complex of proteins called **shelterin**. Since normal DNA replication is unable to proceed to the very end of the telomeres, telomeres shorten with every replication. With continuous cycles of replication, telomeres eventually shorten to nothing; a loss of protective telomeres leads to a **telomere crisis** consisting of inappropriate DNA damage response, chromosome fusion, and ultimately cell senescence or cell death. Indeed, most cells have limited replicative potential.

The enzyme **telomerase** can lengthen telomeres and confer unrestricted replicative potential to cells; however, the telomerase gene is silenced in almost all tissues after development is complete. Because of their inherent property of continuous replication, neoplastic cells eventually encounter telomere crisis. While many of these cells may become senescent or die, some survive the crisis through the re-expression of telomerase. The expression of telomerase then allows unrestricted replicative potential, which accounts for the continuous growth and eventual metastasis of malignant tumors. However, with passage through telomere crisis, significant damage to genome integrity occurs, with many chromosome fusions, breaks, and rearrangements; this accounts for many of the chromosomal rearrangements and much of the aneuploidy seen in cancer cells.

CHECKPOINT

10. What regulates chromatin structure?
11. What are some of the chromosomal abnormalities that occur in cancers?
12. What is telomere crisis?

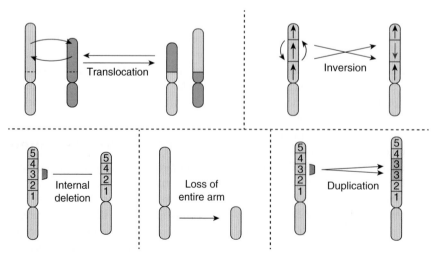

FIGURE 5–4 Various types of structural chromosomal rearrangements that occur in tumors.

SPECIFIC GENE MUTATIONS IN NEOPLASIA

A principal deleterious effect of DNA mutations is their effects on the functions of the genes encoded by the genome. The cataloging of mutated genes has been a fundamental task of molecular oncology because it identifies genes whose functions are relevant to tumor cells. Genes that confer an advantage to tumor cells through a loss-of-function alteration are named **tumor suppressor genes**. Genes that confer an advantage through a gain-of-function alteration are named **proto-oncogenes**, and their altered counterparts are named **oncogenes**. Tumor suppressor genes are much more common because many types of gene mutation can cause loss of function or loss of expression of the protein product, whereas an increase in the activity of a proto-oncogene protein product requires very specific changes in the amino acid sequence. Mutations that can disrupt tumor suppressor genes include mutations that create a premature stop codon (**nonsense mutation**), mutations that change the open reading frame of the transcript (**frame-shift mutations**), and mutations that delete critical parts of the gene (**deletion mutations**). Alternatively, the gene can be silenced by promoter methylation or can be entirely or partially lost by **deletion**. Proto-oncogenes can be activated through **mutation**, gene **amplification** and **overexpression**, **chromosomal translocation**, and possibly other mechanisms. Tables 5–3 and 5–4 provide examples of oncogenes and tumor suppressor genes, respectively. In general, during the gain-of-function alteration of a proto-oncogene, mutation of only one allele is sufficient to produce the gain of function. In contrast, during the loss-of-function alteration of a tumor suppressor gene, both alleles must be inactivated. In certain cases, loss of one allele can result in a reduction of gene expression. For some genes, this gene-dosage reduction is sufficient to promote tumorigenic growth. In addition to being generated through the mutation of cellular proto-oncogenes, oncogenes can also be acquired through the introduction of foreign genomic material, typically transmitted by viruses. The topic of oncogenic viruses is discussed in more detail later in this chapter.

The diploid human genome naturally contains defective alleles of many genes, and although defective alleles are for the most part biologically silent, in the case of tumor suppressor genes, a defective allele can confer significant cancer risk to an individual and all family members harboring such an allele. The loss of function of a gene in adult tissues is statistically much more probable when only one functional allele exists in all cells from the beginning of life, and inherited susceptibility to cancer is almost always a result of germline passage of a defective tumor suppressor gene allele. Many of the identified tumor suppressor genes that are frequently inactivated in sporadic human tumors have also been linked to specific hereditary cancer syndromes. In families with these syndromes, a defective allele of the responsible tumor suppressor gene is passed in the germline, and members who harbor this heterozygous genotype inherit a high risk for tumors in which the second allele has also been lost. An inherited mutation in one allele of the *TP53* gene can cause the rare Li–Fraumeni syndrome, characterized by the early development of bone, breast, brain, and soft tissue tumors (sarcomas), along with other organ-specific tumors (such as adrenal cancer). Inherited mutations

TABLE 5–3 **Representative oncogenes activated in human cancers.**

Oncogene	Cellular Function	Tumor Types Activated	Mechanism of Activation
EGFR (HER1)	Growth factor receptor	Glioblastoma, breast and lung cancer	Mutation, amplification
ERBB2 (HER2)	Growth factor receptor	Breast, gastric, bladder, and colon cancer	Amplification
ALK	Growth factor receptor	Lung cancer, lymphoma	Gene fusion
KRAS, NRAS, HRAS	G protein, signal transduction	Multiple tumor types	Mutation
BRAF	Signal transduction	Melanomas; thyroid, colon, and lung cancer	Mutation, gene fusion
ABL1	Signal transduction	Leukemia	Gene fusion
MYC	Transcription factor	Multiple tumor types	Amplification, mutation
MYB	Transcription factor	Leukemia	Amplification, overexpression
FOS	Transcription factor	Multiple tumor types	Overexpression
PIK3CA	Signal transduction	Breast, endometrial, and colon cancer	Mutation
FGFR1	Growth factor receptor	Breast and lung cancer, leukemia	Amplification, gene fusion
FL1	Transcription factor	Ewing sarcoma	Gene fusion
RET	Growth factor receptor	Parathyroid and medullary thyroid carcinoma, pheochromocytoma	Mutation

TABLE 5–4   Representative tumor suppressor genes inactivated in human tumors or the human germline.

Tumor Suppressor Gene	Cellular Function	Tumor Types with Inactivated Alleles	Mechanism of Inactivation	Hereditary Syndromes with a Germline-Inactivated Allele
TP53	DNA protection, cell cycle regulator	Multiple tumor types	Mutation	Li–Fraumeni
RB1	Cell cycle regulator	Retinoblastoma, small-cell lung cancer, sarcoma	Deletion, mutation	Familial retinoblastoma
APC	Cell adhesion, signal transduction	Colon cancer	Deletion, mutation	Familial adenomatous polyposis
PTEN	Signal transduction	Glioblastomas, prostate and breast cancers	Deletion, mutation	Cowden
MSH2	DNA mismatch repair	Endometrial, colon, and other GI cancers	Mutation	Hereditary nonpolyposis colon cancer (Lynch syndrome)
MLH1	DNA mismatch repair	Endometrial, colon, and other GI cancers	Mutation	Hereditary nonpolyposis colon cancer (Lynch syndrome)
BRCA1	DNA ds-break repair	Breast and ovarian cancers	Mutation	Familial breast/ovarian cancer
BRCA2	DNA ds-break repair	Breast and ovarian cancers	Mutation	Familial breast/ovarian cancer
WT1	Transcription factor	Wilms tumor	Deletion, mutation	Childhood Wilms tumor
NF1	GTPase activator	Sarcoma, glioma	Deletion, mutation	Neurofibromatosis
NF2	Cytoskeletal protein	Schwannoma	Mutation	Neurofibromatosis
VHL	Ubiquitin ligase	Kidney cancer, multiple tumor types	Mutation	Von Hippel–Lindau disease
CDKN2A(p16)	Cell cycle regulator	Melanoma, pancreatic and esophageal cancers	Deletion, mutation, methylation	Familial melanoma

in single alleles of the *BRCA1* or *BRCA2* gene confer a high risk for breast or ovarian cancers. Table 5–4 lists some hereditary cancer syndromes linked with tumor suppressor genes. The list includes predominantly **high-penetrance** genes, which confer a very high risk of disease when inherited. Families carrying these alleles are noticeable for their high incidences of cancers associated with these genes. However, many human cancers, possibly a majority, are etiologically linked with germline alleles of moderate- or low-penetrance genes, or possibly a combination of two or more low-penetrance genes. Cancers arising from such genes do not cluster as tightly within families and therefore are not as frequently noted to be clinical familial syndromes. Rather, they are being increasingly recognized by modern-day large-scale germline sequencing efforts.

In contrast to single alleles of defective tumor suppressor genes, single alleles of mutationally activated oncogenes are not biologically silent and, if present in the germline, can have profound clinical manifestations, including even embryonic demise. Because of this fact, inherited syndromes involving the germline transmission of activated oncogenes are rare. One example, however, is the familial syndrome of **multiple endocrine neoplasia type II**, in which heterozygotes carrying an activated *RET* oncogene on chromosome 10 are at increased risk of developing pheochromocytoma, medullary carcinoma of the thyroid, and parathyroid tumors (see Table 5–3).

CHECKPOINT

13. What is the difference between an oncogene and a tumor suppressor gene?
14. What are the genetic mechanisms by which oncogenes are activated and tumor suppressor genes are inactivated?
15. What is the molecular basis for most inherited susceptibilities to certain cancers?

PROTO-ONCOGENES & TUMOR SUPPRESSOR GENES IN NORMAL PHYSIOLOGY & IN NEOPLASIA

Proteins encoded by proto-oncogenes and tumor suppressor genes perform diverse cellular functions. Not surprisingly, they include proteins that recognize and repair DNA damage, proteins that regulate the cell cycle, proteins that mediate growth factor signal transduction pathways and regulate programmed cell death, proteins involved in cell adhesion to matrix or in cell-to-cell communication, and proteins that regulate the metabolic needs and biomass production of cells.

The deregulation of these pathways through mutational events results in increased genomic instability, overactive growth factor signaling, unrestricted proliferation, inactivation of programmed cell death (apoptosis), decreased dependency on cell adhesion, increased energy supplies and protein synthesis, and extracellular proteolysis. Many of these functions may be altered simultaneously through deregulation of transcription factors that regulate many genes.

Examples of tumor suppressor proteins include both the **retinoblastoma protein** and the **p16 cell cycle inhibitor**, which function in restricting proliferation at the G1 checkpoint of the cell cycle. Loss of the genes encoding these proteins can result in unchecked progression through the G1/S checkpoint. The *TP53* tumor suppressor gene encodes the **p53 protein**, which is a critical guardian of genomic integrity and serves to recognize DNA damage and consequently to inhibit cell cycle progression and to induce apoptosis. Loss of the p53 protein can result in continued cell replication despite DNA damage and failure to activate apoptosis. The fundamental importance of p53 function and of genomic stability in the oncogenic process is underscored by the fact that *TP53* mutations are the most common mutations in human cancers, being found in more than half of all human tumors. The *PTEN* tumor suppressor gene encodes the **PTEN phosphatase protein**, which is involved in the regulation of the Akt and mTor signaling

pathway. This protein underlies many cellular functions and reconciles the proliferative, metabolic, and synthetic activities of the cell with inputs including nutrient and energy supply and growth factor signals; thus, it can enable cells to survive periods of stress or starvation. Loss of PTEN can enable sustained proliferative and synthetic activities despite shortages in nutrients and energy supply. **Cadherins** are proteins involved in cell–cell adhesion. Loss of cadherins can result in reduced cell adhesion, cell detachment, and metastasis. Table 5–4 presents a partial list of examples of tumor suppressor genes. When all human tumor suppressor genes have been fully identified, the list will be much larger.

Proto-oncogenes include proteins involved in various steps of the extracellular growth factor signaling pathway from the membrane receptors to the membrane intermediates to the proteins mediating the cytoplasmic signaling cascades. The **receptor tyrosine kinases** (RTKs) are some of the most important signaling proteins in cells because they regulate cell behavior in response to extracellular ligands. The RTKs exert their effects through two important downstream signaling pathways: the Ras–Raf–MAPK pathway and the PI3K–Akt pathway. Many, if not most, cancers activate this pathway by one mechanism or another, and indeed many of the genes encoding these signaling proteins are oncogenes or tumor suppressor genes (Figure 5–5).

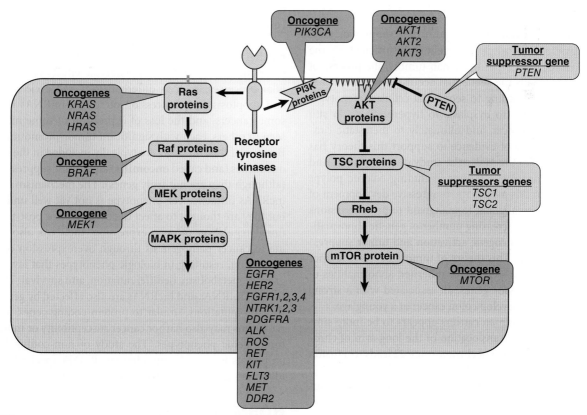

FIGURE 5–5 Membrane-bound receptor tyrosine kinases (RTKs) activate two important cytoplasmic signaling cascades to affect numerous biological phenotypes, including proliferation, differentiation, survival, protein synthesis, metabolism, and others. Many of the genes involved in this pathway are oncogenes. These are highlighted in the red callouts; when mutationally activated in cancers, they promote excessive signaling. Some of the genes that negatively regulate the pathway are tumor suppressor genes. These are highlighted in the blue callouts; when they are lost in cancers, they allow for unrestricted pathway signaling.

The epidermal growth factor receptor (**EGFR**) is an RTK that binds a number of extracellular ligands and, in cooperation with its homolog, **HER2**, signals proliferative and apoptotic pathways. Overactivity of EGFR or HER2 can lead to unregulated growth. The *EGFR* gene is mutated or amplified in many cancers, including nearly half of all glioblastomas, as well as subsets of lung, breast, oropharyngeal, and other epithelial cancers. The *HER2* gene is amplified in 20% of breast cancers and subsets of gastric, esophageal, bladder, and colon cancers; its amplification confers an aggressive phenotype. **Ras** proteins are a family of membrane-bound signaling switches that function immediately downstream of membrane receptors at a key branch point of cytoplasmic signaling. Mutational activation of Ras proteins causes overactive cytoplasmic signaling and deregulation of proliferative and apoptotic pathways. Ras appears to be critically important in tumorigenesis because nearly one-third of all human tumors harbor mutationally activated forms of the *KRAS*, *NRAS*, or *HRAS* genes. **Raf** proteins are a family of serine-threonine kinases that function downstream of Ras proteins. Mutational activation of the *BRAF* gene can lead to overactive signaling and deregulation of proliferative and apoptotic pathways; its activation is commonly found in many tumors. Table 5–3 presents a partial list of oncogenes identified in human malignancies, along with the tumor types in which they are commonly observed and the cellular function encoded by their proto-oncogene counterparts.

Since the inactivation of a single tumor suppressor gene or the activation of a single oncogene is insufficient for the development of most types of human tumors, the process of tumorigenesis entails the sequential acquisition of a number of "hits" over time leading to sequential cellular phenotypic changes—from atypia to dysplasia to hyperplasia to in situ cancer to invasive cancer, and ultimately to metastatic cancer. The largest body of evidence to support this theory has been generated from the molecular study of colon cancer and identifiable pre-neoplastic lesions, including colonic polyps and adenomas. In this model, the progressive development of neoplasia from premalignant to malignant to invasive lesions is associated with an increasing number of genetic abnormalities, including both oncogene activation and tumor suppressor gene inactivation. This theory of tumorigenesis is further supported by the identification of inherited abnormalities of several tumor suppressor genes, all associated with a strong familial tendency to develop colon cancer at a young age.

A small subset of human cancers appears to be more simplistic in evolution. A translocation of the long arm of chromosome 9 to the long arm of chromosome 22 leads to a fusion of the *BCR* gene with the *c-Abl* gene and results in expression of the **BCR-Abl** oncoprotein seen in chronic myelogenous leukemia (CML). The expression of this oncogene in hematopoietic cells of animal models reproduces the disease. This oncogenic event is seen in virtually 100% of cases of this disease, and a treatment that inhibits the kinase activity of this oncoprotein produces remissions in nearly 100% of affected patients. Thus, in contrast to the multistep process involved in most types of carcinogenesis, the steps necessary for the development of CML may be much simpler.

The identification of tumor suppressor genes and oncogenes as the fundamental enablers of tumorigenesis has led to the hypothesis that cancer can be successfully treated by treatments that counteract the biochemical sequelae of these molecular abnormalities. This hypothesis has fueled attempts to develop therapeutic agents that can inhibit the function of activated oncoproteins or restore the function of inactivated tumor suppressor proteins. Current pharmaceutical technologies have enabled the development of drugs targeting gain-of-function mutations, and many oncogenes can now be inhibited by such drugs. However, it is not yet possible to restore the function of a lost tumor suppressor gene. But since normal cells may use alternative pathways to compensate for the loss of a tumor suppressor gene, activating the functions of such alternative pathways is a roundabout way to kill cancer cells. Such collateral target genes utilized for therapeutic purposes are called **synthetic lethal genes**.

NON-CODING RNAs IN NEOPLASIA

In addition to transcribing mRNAs encoding protein products, the genome also transcribes many forms of RNA that do not encode protein products, but rather function to regulate the expression of many other genes. These include **microRNAs (miRNAs)** and **long non-coding RNAs (lncRNAs)**, both of which are implicated in the pathogenesis of cancer. A single miRNA can target and destabilize many protein-coding genes and can have broad phenotypic effects on diverse cellular processes, such as differentiation, cell cycle regulation, and apoptosis. Overexpression of certain miRNAs is seen in some cancers, and the loss of expression of some miRNAs is seen in others, each with significant tumor-promoting effects. Because of this, miRNAs are typically included in the family of oncogenes (and called **oncomiRs**) and tumor suppressor genes (although they are not truly genes). The mechanism by which lncRNAs influence cell phenotype is not yet well understood, but they are thought to affect the epigenetic or post-transcriptional regulation of gene expression. lncRNAs also contribute to cancer pathogenesis through overexpression or loss of expression, resulting in biologic phenotypes that favor tumor growth, metabolism, dedifferentiation, and survival. The functions of miRNAs and lncRNAs are also affected by germline or somatic mutations, similar to protein-coding genes, and such mutations may also harbor cancer susceptibility or more direct tumorigenic phenotypes. The study of non-coding RNAs is only in its infancy. Many other small RNA species have been identified and may be important in cancer pathogenesis.

HORMONES AND GROWTH FACTORS IN NEOPLASIA

Although structurally altered genes, classified as oncogenes or tumor suppressor genes, are key mediators of neoplasia, the role of unaltered genes is not to be dismissed, as such genes are likely equally important in carcinogenesis. The oncogenic process may be driven through abnormalities in signaling of all kinds: abnormal time, duration, or intensity; abnormal tissue expression; or abnormal subcellular compartment localization. The regulation of growth in complex organisms requires specialized proteins for the normal growth, maturation, development, and function of cells and specialized tissues. The complexity of the human organism requires that these proteins be expressed at precisely coordinated points in space and time. An essential component of this regulation is the system of hormones, growth factors, and growth inhibitors. On binding to specific receptor proteins on the cell surface or in the cytoplasm, these factors lead to a complex set of signals that can result in a variety of cellular effects, including mitogenesis, growth inhibition, changes in cell cycle regulation, apoptosis, differentiation, and induction of a secondary set of genes. The actual end effects depend not only on the particular type of interacting factor and receptor, but also on the cell type and milieu in which factor–receptor coupling occurs. This system allows for cell-to-cell interactions, whereby a factor secreted by one cell or tissue can enter the bloodstream and influence another set of distant cells (endocrine action) or act on adjacent cells (paracrine action). An autocrine action is also possible when a cell produces a factor that binds to a receptor on or in the same cell. An altered concentration of these growth factors or receptor overexpression or mutation can change the signaling behavior, contributing to a malignant phenotype. Only a subset of growth factor receptors are proto-oncogenes. However, many additional **growth factors** and **growth factor receptors** appear to be important in tumor growth and progression, although they are not classified as proto-oncogenes because they serve tumorigenic causes without incurring mutations or without overexpression.

An important class of growth factor signaling molecules are the RTKs. A number of RTK families exist, and in experimental models, most are capable of transforming cells if activated or overexpressed. Although all of these abnormalities are not necessarily seen in naturally occurring human tumors, the experimental data highlight the potential inherent in these proteins and the important role they may be playing in tumor cells despite lacking the "oncogene" label. Members of the HER family of RTKs are commonly mutated or amplified in human tumors and exemplify the important role of RTKs in human neoplasia. And despite having a normal sequence and expression level, they likely play an important role in other tumors. For example, HER1 (also called EGFR) is not mutated or overexpressed in colon cancers but is sometimes activated by autocrine signaling in the cancer cells, and EGFR-targeted therapies are used to treat this type of cancer. Other families of RTKs, such as the platelet-derived growth factor (PDGF) receptors, fibroblast growth factor (FGF) receptors, vascular endothelial growth factor (VEGF) receptors, and insulin-like growth factor (IGF) receptors, function similarly to the HER family of RTKs. In general, these receptors are not reported to

be mutated or amplified in human tumors. However, there is increased expression in many tumors or aberrant expression in tumors from tissue types that ordinarily do not to express that receptor. Alternatively, there may be excessive production of receptor ligands owing to a variety of mechanisms (eg, loss of epigenetic silencing of the gene coding for the ligand or excessive gene transcription of the same gene). In experimental systems, each of these RTK systems has oncogenic potential, building a circumstantial case that they may be important players in human tumors.

Some growth factor signaling pathways function to inhibit cell growth and provide negative regulation in response to extracellular stimuli. Desensitization of cells to such growth inhibitors is common in tumors. An example of this is the **transforming growth factor-β (TGF-β)**. TGF-β has diverse biological effects. It potently inhibits cell proliferation but also stimulates the production and deposition of extracellular matrix (ECM) and adhesion factors. These functions are important in tissue remodeling during embryogenesis and wound repair. In some tumor types, the anti-proliferative response to TGF-β is lost early on because of mutations in its downstream signaling components. However, continued secretion, and often over-secretion, of TGF-β by the tumor and stromal tissues leads to an increase in the production of ECM and adhesion factors and promotes the invasive and metastatic property of tumors.

Another important class of receptors is the large superfamily of **nuclear hormone receptors**. These include the cellular receptors for a variety of hormones, among them estrogen and progesterone, androgens, glucocorticoids, thyroid hormone, and retinoids. The actions of estrogen are fundamentally important in the development of breast cancer. In women, oophorectomy early in life offers substantial protection against its development. (In animal models, too, mammary carcinogenesis is significantly retarded in the absence of estrogen.) More than half of all breast cancers are dependent on estrogen for proliferation. Although these data clearly implicate the estrogen signaling pathway in breast carcinogenesis, specific abnormalities of the **estrogen receptor (ER)** are not seen in breast cancers; therefore, the ER does not qualify as a tumor suppressor protein or oncoprotein. Although the loss of certain tumor suppressor genes or the activation of certain oncogenes leads to the development of breast cancer, it is possible that continued ER function is essential throughout this process and that, without ER function, it cannot proceed. Alternatively, it is possible that abnormal ER signaling, perhaps as a result of altered cofactors, cross-talk, or phosphorylation status, drives breast carcinogenesis. Although the mechanism by which estrogen and its receptor drive breast cancers has not yet been determined, the fundamental role of estrogen in this disease is well established. Furthermore, treatments that work through inhibiting the production of the active ligand or that inhibit the function of the ER are the most effective therapies for breast cancer yet developed and are highly active in the prevention and treatment of breast cancer. The **androgen receptor (AR)**, similarly, plays a critical role in the development of prostate cancer, although only occasional activating mutations and amplification of the AR have been reported in this cancer.

On the other hand, retinoids (ligands for retinoic acid receptors) are well known to participate in the differentiation of a variety of tissues during development and to cause the differentiation of certain tumors in tissue culture models. These observations have been exploited as a treatment approach for acute promyelocytic leukemia (APL). APL is characterized by a t(15;17) chromosomal translocation resulting in the fusion of the *PML* gene with the **retinoic acid receptor-α** (*RAR-α*) gene. The resulting fusion protein blocks the differentiation of hematopoietic progenitor cells and eventually leads to the development of APL. While this fusion protein is not by itself transforming in experimental models and cannot be categorized as a classic oncogene or tumor suppressor gene, it is etiologically involved in the pathogenesis of APL. Because the fusion protein contains the ligand-binding domain of RAR-α, it remains sensitive to ligand, and treatment with the ligand all-*trans* retinoic acid results in differentiation of tumor cells and complete remission in most patients with this form of leukemia.

CONTROL OF THE CELL CYCLE IN NEOPLASIA

A hallmark of neoplasia is excessive proliferation inappropriate for the tissue context, which thus leads to architectural distortion and tissue destruction. Several molecular mechanisms contribute to the unrestricted proliferative capacity of tumor cells. First, excessive growth factor or hormonal signaling stimulates proliferation. Second, telomerase gene activation lifts the natural replicative ceiling pre-existing in most cells. Third, the orderly progression of the phases of the cell cycle is strictly regulated by a large family of cell cycle machinery proteins that can halt cell replication if precise conditions are not met. At the heart of cell cycle regulation are complexes of cyclins and cyclin-dependent kinases (CDKs) that drive the forward direction of cell cycle progression. These are under both positive and negative regulation by a plethora of other proteins and a highly complex, intertwined signaling network that functions to ensure that cell cycle progression proceeds in a desired and healthy manner (Figure 5–6). At each phase of the cell cycle, certain checkpoints are in place to ensure that the tasks of that phase have been properly met. Typically, most

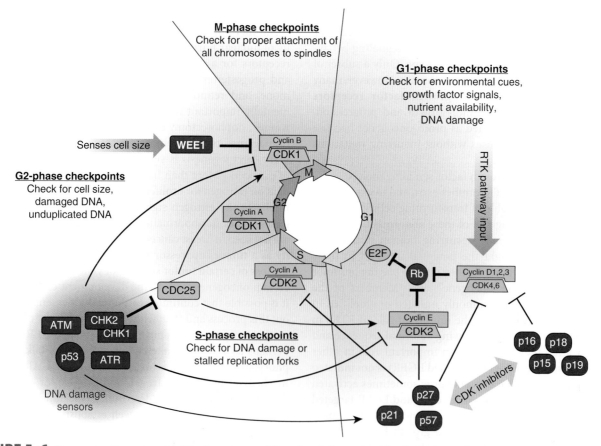

FIGURE 5–6 Progression through each of the four phases of the cell cycle is regulated by distinct sets of cyclin–CDK complexes. These are in turn negatively and positively regulated by a number of cell cycle inhibitors and activators, as shown in the figure. The proteins whose functions promote cell cycle progression, many of which are oncogenes, are shown in green. The proteins whose functions inhibit cell cycle progression, many of which are tumor suppressor genes, are shown in red.

non-neoplastic cells proliferate only when instructed to do so by growth factor signals in G1 phase, and only when nutrients and environmental conditions are appropriate. In S-phase, the cell must ensure that DNA replication is completed without damage or errors. In G2 phase, the cell must double its mass by protein and lipid synthesis in preparation for division. In M-phase, the cell must orchestrate the proper spindle attachment and alignment of all the chromosomes in preparation for mitotic separation. This cell cycle machinery is under tight regulation by proteins that function to sense DNA damage, and that can exert a hold on cell cycle progression while DNA is being repaired. In cancers, deregulation of the cell cycle machinery is almost universal, and many cell cycle regulators are oncogenes or tumor suppressor genes that exhibit a gain-of-function or loss-of-function, respectively. Indeed, cell cycle regulators are some of the most frequently mutated, amplified, or otherwise altered genes in tumors of all kinds. In fact, the *p53* gene is the single most common tumor suppressor gene; it is mutated in approximately half of all human tumors. The consequences of dysfunctional cell cycle regulation are many. Cells will proliferate with damaged DNA, leading to the accumulation of more and more errors in their genome. They will proliferate despite lack of sufficient nutrients or physical space. They will divide without proper duplication and separation of all chromosomes, such that daughter cells will have abnormal genome content. The RTK signaling pathway, apoptotic pathway, metabolic pathways, and other efferent and afferent biologic signaling pathways that communicate with the cell cycle machinery are also each deregulated in human cancers.

CONTROL OF THE APOPTOTIC PROGRAM IN NEOPLASIA

Despite the extensive mechanisms that exist to protect and repair genomic DNA, and to regulate cell proliferation and maintain metabolic homeostasis, cells invariably experience scenarios in which these imperfect mechanisms fail, leaving no path forward for the proper execution of replicative or metabolic programs. When such scenarios develop, a cell death program is triggered, called **apoptosis**. The regulation and execution of apoptosis involves a large number of proteins and mitochondria. These are in communication with many input signals that function to report DNA damage, metabolic stress, or other malfunctioning programs, or with extracellular ligands that instruct a cell to undergo apoptosis. Some integral proteins of the apoptotic machinery are the protease family of **caspases** and the **Bcl-2 family of BH domain proteins**. The signaling network that regulates the execution of apoptosis is complex and only partially understood at this time. A number of proteins function to promote apoptosis, and a number of proteins function to inhibit it (Figure 5–7). Whether apoptosis occurs depends greatly on the balance of these stimulatory and inhibitory proteins.

Cancer cells are frequently faced with unrepaired DNA, metabolic stress, hypoxia, and other scenarios that would ordinarily trigger apoptosis. The apoptotic program is in fact a tumor-suppressing mechanism. However, one of the hallmarks of cancer cells is their acquisition of methods to disrupt the apoptotic mechanism so as to escape the lethal fate it bestows; thus, cancer cells survive through repeated cycles of DNA damage, metabolic stress, and other stressors. These methods include the upregulation of the inhibitors of apoptotic proteins and the downregulation of their promoters (see Figure 5–7). In particular, upregulation of Bcl-2 is frequently seen in many cancers, and it accounts for the survival potential of these cancers, including their resistance to chemotherapeutic drugs. Many lymphomas have excessive levels of Bcl-2. In follicular lymphomas, for example, a chromosomal translocation places the Bcl-2 gene next to the immunoglobulin gene, leading to excessively high transcriptional levels of Bcl-2. Another common abnormality in cancer (seen in approximately 50% of all cancers) is loss of the tumor suppressor gene *p53* and thus loss of the p53 protein. Since the p53 protein functions to sense DNA damage and trigger activation of the apoptotic cascade, its loss is a key step in allowing cancer cells to survive despite the presence of unrepaired DNA damage.

CHECKPOINT

16. What are some of the oncogenes in the RTK pathway?
17. Is the estrogen receptor an oncogene?
18. Can miRNA be oncogenes?
19. How is cell cycle regulation altered in cancers?
20. How is the apoptotic program affected in cancers?
21. How is apoptosis deregulated in follicular lymphomas?

STROMAL INTERACTIONS & INFLUENCES IN NEOPLASIA

Normal tissues exhibit an orderly architectural structure that supports proper organ function. The establishment and maintenance of this high-level order is governed by two-way communication between the principal cellular components of the specific tissue and numerous stromal elements in their surrounding microenvironment. These stromal interactions ensure the proper initial construction of the tissue architecture during embryogenesis and thus enable tissue remodeling and repair after any damage or wounding. Stromal elements include mesenchymal cells and extracellular matrix proteins and fibrils that provide structural tissue support, stiffness or elasticity, and a skeletal framework for anchorage and adhesion; proteinaceous membrane barriers that separate tissue compartments; and cells of the hematopoietic system that are "on call" to recognize tissue injury or infection and respond by secreting growth factors to initiate necessary immunologic and inflammatory responses. In normal tissues, these stromal interactions function to establish or restore tissue homeostasis and to reach a resting state of equilibrium, but in neoplasms, these two-way interactions continue and proceed in a way that never reaches homeostasis or equilibrium. Thus, tumors are in

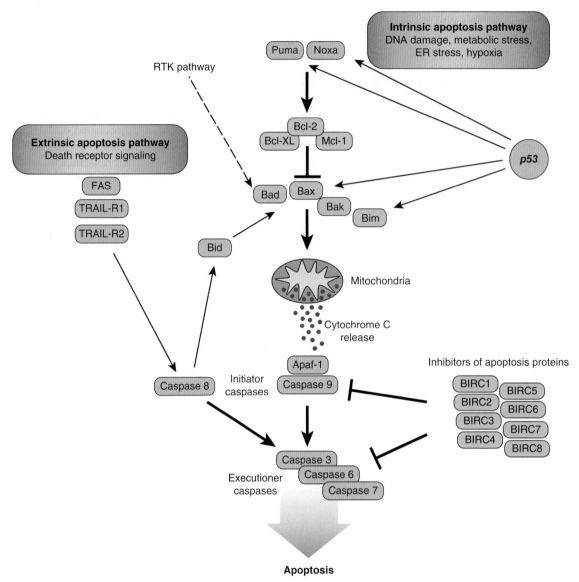

FIGURE 5-7 The decision to execute apoptosis (programmed cell death) is governed by a complex signaling network of proteins. Those that function to promote apoptosis are shown in red, and those that function to oppose apoptosis are shown in green. Apoptosis can be activated by the intrinsic pathway in response to stressful or catastrophic cellular events or by the extrinsic pathway in response to a signaling instruction from cell death receptors. Cancer cells frequently suppress the apoptotic response by upregulating the anti-apoptotic proteins or downregulating the pro-apoptotic proteins.

effect "wounds that do not heal." Tumor–stromal relationships involve a complex series of molecular and cellular interactions that are not entirely understood, but which involve tumor cell mechanisms to (1) capitalize on stromal influences beneficial to tumor growth and (2) evade stromal influences detrimental to tumor growth.

The **extracellular matrix (ECM)** is composed of physically robust fibrillary proteins that provide a skeletal framework for cell anchorage. A number of protein families serve to constitute the ECM, to attach cells to the ECM, to attach cells to each other, and to dissolve and re-establish the ECM when necessary. Abnormalities of these proteins frequently occur in later stages of tumorigenesis, accounting for the loss of architecture,

and can mediate the invasive and metastatic phenotype of tumor cells. **Integrins** are a large family of membrane proteins that anchor cells to the ECM and activate intracellular signaling pathways in response to ECM attachment. Cells have the ability to express any of a large repertoire of integrin combinations, but the specificity of integrin expression is not well understood. However, tumor cells can reshuffle their integrin expression profiles in favor of an invasive or metastatic phenotype. **Cadherins** are a family of membrane proteins that function in epithelial cell-to-cell adhesion. Loss of E-cadherin expression is seen in some human epithelial tumors, leading to a more invasive phenotype. The expression and activity of many secreted and membrane-anchored proteases are increased in tumor cells. These proteases include the **matrix metalloprotease** family and the **serine protease** family of proteins. Increased protease activity leads to ECM degradation, triggering of the plasminogen activation cascade, and activation of transmembrane receptors through cleavage and shedding of their extracellular domains. Through abnormalities in ECM deposition, cell adhesion protein expression, and membrane and secreted protease activity, cancer cells develop an invasive and ultimately a metastatic phenotype.

CANCER AND THE IMMUNE SYSTEM

The process of tumorigenesis is inherently and intricately intertwined with many facets of the immune system. The interactions and relationships are complex and only partially understood at this time. The complexity begins with the causality relationship and extends to the minutiae of cellular and molecular components involved in the interface between a tumor and the host immune system. The complexity in the causal relationship is that the immune system can play a role in causing or preventing cancer, and it can promote the progression or suppress the growth of an existing cancer. The cancer itself can also stimulate or suppress elements of the immune system. As such, the relationship between cancer and the immune system is impossible to define in simple or causal terms; this relationship is best considered a delicate balance of dynamic tumor-promoting and tumor-suppressing forces governed by an amalgam of variables that can change over time.

Tissue injury stimulates the recruitment and activity of numerous elements of the immune system's process of inflammation (Figure 5–8). The inflammatory response includes innate immune system cells such as resident macrophages, which function to engulf debris or microbes, secrete cytokines to attract other cells of the innate and adaptive immune system, and generate signals to begin the tissue repair process, including both proliferative and angiogenic growth factors. Neutrophils are recruited to secrete a variety of products to kill bacteria and remodel the matrix. This constitutes the normal process of inflammation, which typically reaches its endpoint with the repair and return of the injured tissue to homeostasis. However, homeostasis is not always achieved, and inflammation can sometimes continue for prolonged periods. It is well recognized that chronic inflammation can promote the development of cancer. Examples include inflammatory bowel diseases such as ulcerative colitis and Crohn's disease, which can lead to the development of colon cancer. The mechanism by which chronic inflammation promotes tumorigenesis is not entirely understood. The inflammatory

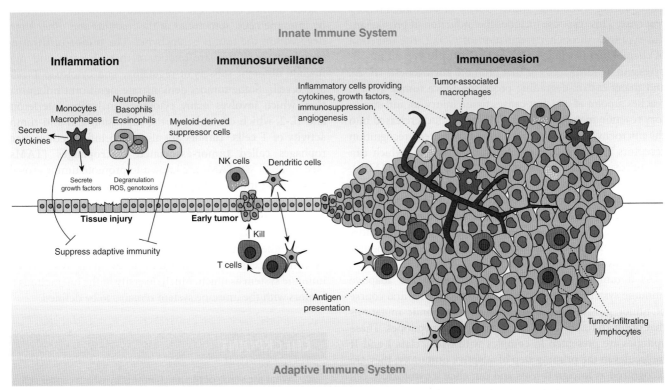

FIGURE 5–8 The engagement of immune cells with injured epithelium or tumor cells is shown here, summarized and simplified according to a hypothetical timeline. Inflammation of normal tissues, if prolonged, can promote tumorigenesis. Tumors are frequently engaged with elements of the innate and adaptive immune system throughout their existence. But through the balancing of many factors, some tumors escape from the eradicative effects of immunosurveillance and develop into clinical disease states, albeit in continuous confrontation with many elements of the immune system that exert both anti-tumor and pro-tumor effects. The inflammatory response can also contribute to tumorigenic growth once a tumor has developed.

microenvironment contains many growth factors that induce proliferative and migratory activities in the wounded epithelium, as well as cytokines such as IL-6, which can induce proliferative and migratory responses. Neutrophils secrete many factors that generate reactive oxygen and nitrogen species, which can not only activate tumorigenic signaling pathways in epithelial cells, but can also induce DNA damage and promote mutagenesis. Neutrophils also secrete products that can affect the epigenetic regulation of epithelial cells, inducing abnormalities in gene expression and genome protection. **Myeloid-derived suppressor cells** are recruited to sites of inflammation and function to suppress the activation of an adaptive immune response, which can enable the tumorigenic process to evade detection. These inflammatory conditions, by promoting proliferative and genotoxic and immuno-evasive events, can lead to cancer development. But not all inflammatory conditions are cancer promoting; therefore, there is some level of specificity, not yet understood, in chronic inflammation that is associated with tumorigenesis.

Inflammation can precede and promote tumorigenesis, but the reverse also holds: tumors can induce the inflammatory response. Many tumors arise in tissues without a preceding period of inflammation, and in these tissues, the early events in tumor cells can initiate an inflammatory response. The activation of many oncogenes in epithelial cells leads to the activation of signaling pathways that would normally be activated during wounding, which results in an inflammatory response. This response includes the induction of prostaglandin synthesis through upregulation of COX2, the secretion of chemokines (such as CCL2 or CCL20) that recruit monocytes and dendritic cells or that promote angiogenesis (IL-8), and many matrix-degrading proteases. Once tumor growth reaches a point at which it causes tissue injury, an inflammatory reaction may be initiated. Cellular products released into the microenvironment are recognized by pattern recognition receptors (PRRs) of the innate immune system, which can recognize damage-associated molecular patterns (DAMPs). DAMPs, which are stress signals, include ATP and purine metabolites, DNA or RNA, certain chromatin-associated proteins, and certain heat shock proteins, released into the extracellular microenvironment. PRRs include Toll-like receptors (on macrophages and dendritic cells), which can recognize these stress signals and activate adaptive immune responses.

As a tumor develops, the engagement of the adaptive immune system becomes more relevant to the natural course of tumor growth and progression. The genomic mutations that occur in tumor cells lead to new protein epitopes. These epitopes are presented in complex with MHC class I and II molecules in the priming step of adaptive immunity; they are recognized as foreign threats and can elicit a cytotoxic T-cell response. However, not all mutations are equally immunogenic; the degree of immunogenicity likely depends on the extent of sequence divergence of the mutated region, as well as the affinity of the mutated region to bind MHC molecules for presentation. The mutational burden of the cancer cell also determines the potency of the adaptive response, and

cancers with many mutated genes are typically more immunogenic. However, the adaptive immune system is regulated by a number of checkpoints designed to avert over-aggressive or autoimmune responses. Among these are the expression of the PD-L1 receptor, which can suppress the actions of cytotoxic T cells (Figure 5–9). Tumor cells commonly demonstrate increased expression of PD-L1, which enables them to evade being targeted by T cells. Tumor cells also downregulate their expression of MHC class I molecules, which also averts recognition and targeting by cytotoxic T cells. Downregulation of MHC molecules can enable tumor cells to evade the adaptive immune system, but the absence of these "self" identifiers comes at the cost of increased susceptibility to natural killer cells of the innate immune system; tumor cells thus walk a fine line in the regulation of their MHC proteins. It is believed that many tumor cells are cleared by these components of the innate and adaptive immune system early in their evolution through a process called **immunosurveillance**. However, some tumors eventually develop mechanisms to survive and are able to balance the pro-tumorigenic and anti-tumorigenic elements of the immune system in their favor, enabling them to escape this policing step. This process of immuno-evasion eventually leads to the development of clinical cancers (see Figure 5–8). Reverting the balance between pro-tumorigenic and anti-tumorigenic factors has become the mainstay of modern immunotherapy approaches.

Well-formed tumors are sometimes significantly infiltrated by immune cells, sometimes at the margins and other times deep within the tumor parenchyma. The **tumor-infiltrating lymphocytes** (TILs) are important in such cases and may include different subsets of regulatory and cytotoxic T cells and B cells. Some tumors demonstrate significant inflammation, which involves many cytokines, including interferons and IL-2, which can enhance the expansion and anti-tumor activity of T cells. Tumors are also often infiltrated by macrophages called **tumor-associated macrophages** (TAMs) (see Figure 5–8). TAMs are known to promote tumor growth by secreting immunosuppressive factors that inhibit effector T cells, by secreting growth factors that promote tumor growth or stimulate angiogenesis, and by secreting factors and proteases that facilitate matrix remodeling (see Figure 5–9). On the other hand, some tumors experience less infiltration by immune cells and appear not to engage the activities of the immune system as much. Much diversity in the interactions of tumors with the immune system remains to be defined.

CHECKPOINT

22. What are some of the mechanisms by which cancer cell adhesion is altered?

23. What role do tumor-associated macrophages play in tumor biology?

24. How can tumor cells evade being killed by primed cytotoxic T cells?

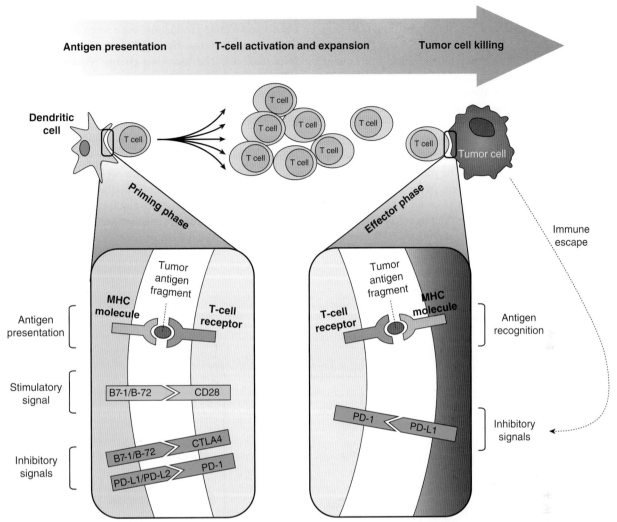

FIGURE 5–9 The immune system can recognize foreign peptides such as mutated residues from cancer cells. Presentation of the peptide results in priming of T cells, as shown on the left. Activated cytotoxic T cells can then identify tumor cells expressing the mutated residue and kill them. This system has checkpoints built in to restrain the immune system from over-aggressive targeting. Both stimulatory and inhibitory interactions are involved in this regulation. Upregulation of PD-L1 by many tumor cells is a mechanism that enables them to suppress the cytotoxic actions of activated T cells and escape the immune system.

ALTERATIONS IN METABOLISM & OXYGENATION IN NEOPLASIA

In addition to abnormalities in cell proliferation and survival, signal transduction, adhesion, and migration, tumor cells exhibit changes in metabolic pathways to meet their increased metabolic requirements. Oxygen pressure is reduced in tumor tissues, and tumor hypoxia signals change in gene expression, mediated through the **hypoxia-inducible factor-1 alpha (HIF1α)** transcription factor for adaptation to the hypoxic environment. Tumor cells secrete **angiogenic growth factors**, which signal the proliferation of vascular structures into tumor tissue for nutrition and oxygenation. The identification of tumor factors that signal pathologic neovascularization has been of particular interest because such factors could be targets for therapeutic drug development for treatments that inhibit tumor angiogenesis. The best-studied pro-angiogenic factor is the **vascular endothelial growth factor (VEGF)**, a mitogen to endothelial cells often secreted by tumor cells that activates the VEGF receptors in endothelial cells, leading to de novo vascularization. Although most cells do not ordinarily express VEGF, malignant transformation often results in the induction of VEGF expression by tumor cells, either directly through the effects of oncogenes or the loss of tumor suppressor genes or indirectly as a result of hypoxia and the induction of hypoxia-induced gene transcription. Other growth factors also have pro-angiogenic effects, including epidermal growth factor, fibroblast growth factor, PDGF, transforming growth factor-α, and others.

Tumor cells needs to generate energy and synthesize biomass at rates much higher than normal cells to sustain their high proliferation rates. As a result, tumor cells frequently have high rates of protein synthesis to supply all the structural and signaling proteins, high rates of fatty acid synthesis to supply structural membrane lipids and signaling lipids, and high rates of nucleotide synthesis to supply enough DNA and RNA. And they need to do this despite reduced nutrient availability owing to lessened and disrupted vascular supplies. In particular, glucose metabolism is uniquely altered in tumor cells. In normal cells, glucose generates some ATP in the initial metabolic steps of glycolysis to generate pyruvate. The resulting pyruvate is then transported to mitochondria, where it undergoes oxidative phosphorylation along the electron transport chain to generate many more ATP molecules. The metabolism of glucose by oxidative phosphorylation requires oxygen but is a highly efficient mode of generating energy from glucose. When oxygen availability is low, cells increase the rate of glycolysis, with ultimate conversion to lactate, to generate ATP. Tumor cells

preferentially metabolize glucose through high rates of glycolysis and lactate production, even when oxygen is abundant. This counterintuitive finding is named the **Warburg effect** (Figure 5–10). The increased energy requirements of tumor cells and their less efficient means of glucose metabolism account for the substantially increased uptake of glucose by tumor cells compared with normal cells. This wide differential in glucose uptake forms the basis for radiologic imaging modalities that can detect tumors by imaging the accumulation of injected radiolabeled glucose analogs at tumor sites throughout the body. One example of this is positron emission tomography (PET) scanning using [^{18}F]-fluorodeoxyglucose as the radiotracer. This imaging technique is widely used in clinical oncology to locate tumors much more specifically than is possible with conventional computed tomography (CT) scanning.

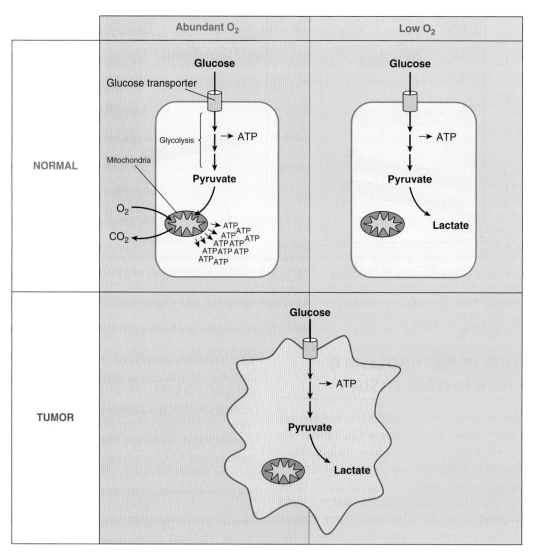

FIGURE 5–10 Normal cells metabolize glucose using glycolysis followed by oxidative phosphorylation in the mitochondria when oxygen is abundant. This highly efficient mode of metabolism generates plenty of ATP molecules from glucose. If the oxygen supply is limited, cells instead convert the pyruvate to lactate and increase the rate of glycolysis to generate ATP, although this is a far less efficient mode of generating energy. Tumor cells are observed to use this same, less efficient pathway of glycolysis converting pyruvate to lactate even when oxygen is abundant and thus have high glycolytic rates to meet their energy demands. This observation is called the Warburg effect.

The amino acid serine is uniquely important for tumor cells. In addition to its role in protein synthesis, serine is metabolized by cells to provide one-carbon units that can support the synthesis of nucleotides required for DNA and RNA. The amino acid glutamine is also uniquely important for tumor cells. In addition to its role in protein synthesis, glutamine plays an important role in energy generation, since it is abundant in serum and tissues, it can be readily transported into cells, and its metabolites can generate energy for tumor cells via the Krebs cycle. Although serine and glutamine are not essential amino acids, tumor cells rely heavily on their uptake to meet their enormous needs for synthesis and energy. In addition to avid uptake of these amino acids from serum, another way tumor cells deal with threatened nutrient deprivation is through **autophagy**, which involves the breakdown of cellular organelles in autophagosomes to generate amino acids and other metabolites.

Tumor cells reprogram their metabolic circuitry primarily to meet their synthesis and energy needs. However, this reprogramming has widespread secondary effects far beyond the production of biomass and energy. Many of the metabolites used to generate biomass or energy are also substrates for the post-translational modification of proteins, including acetylations, methylations, and glycosylations. Such post-translational modifications are the backbone of chromatin modification and form the basis for the epigenetic regulation of the genome. As such, altered tumor metabolism is invariably linked with the epigenetic deregulation of the tumor genome, with widespread consequences for gene expression and genome integrity. Some of the metabolites that are substantially increased in tumor cells and promote tumorigenic properties have been termed **oncometabolites** (Table 5–5). Pharmacologic approaches to reduce oncometabolite levels are providing a new direction for cancer therapeutics.

Another consequence of altered metabolic programming in cancer cells is a deregulation of reactive oxygen species (ROS) homeostasis. Normal cells use protective mechanisms to minimize ROS levels produced by the electron transport chain, since excessive ROS levels can damage proteins, DNA, and lipids. Increased ROS levels, which create a situation referred to as **oxidative stress**, are commonly found in tumor cells and appear to play a pro-tumorigenic role. Oxidative stress can function to promote tumorigenesis by increasing DNA damage and genomic instability and by inhibiting protein phosphatases, thus promoting tumorigenic signaling. However, high enough ROS levels can damage proteins and lead to apoptosis. As such, tumor cells also have increased levels of antioxidant proteins to protect against lethal levels of oxidative stress. Neoplastic cells must walk a fine line in the regulation of oxidative stress.

CHECKPOINT

25. What makes tumor cells react to hypoxia?
26. How do tumor cells stimulate the growth of blood vessels?
27. What is the Warburg effect?
28. What is autophagy?
29. What do oncometabolites do that is detrimental?

THE ROLE OF THE MICROBIOME IN NEOPLASIA

The human body encompasses both sterile tissue compartments and a number of nonsterile anatomic compartments. The latter harbor gigantic numbers of bacterial organisms.

TABLE 5–5 Oncometabolites commonly found at high levels in cancers.

Oncometabolite	Role in Normal Physiology	Mechanism of Increase in Tumors	Role in Tumor Cells
Glucose	Source of energy and carbon	Increased glucose uptake	Feeds aerobic glycolysis, is an essential carbon source
Fumarate	Krebs cycle intermediate	Inactivating mutation in fumarate hydratase gene	Inhibits many metabolic enzymes, interferes with epigenetic modifications
Succinate	Krebs cycle intermediate	Inactivating mutation in succinate dehydrogenase gene	Inhibits many metabolic enzymes, interferes with epigenetic modifications
(D)-2-hydroxy-glutarate	Unknown, very low levels	Gain-of-function mutation in isocitrate dehydrogenase genes	Inhibits α-KG-dependent enzymes, interferes with epigenetic modifications
Lactate	Product of glycolysis	Increased aerobic glycolysis	Lowers extracellular pH, causes immunosuppression
Glutamine	Protein synthesis, source of nitrogen and energy	Increased glutamine uptake	Supports anabolic and energy needs
Serine	Protein synthesis, source of carbon and energy	Increased serine uptake	Supports anabolic and energy needs
Choline	Synthesis of membrane and signaling lipids, methyl donor for DNA methylation	Increased choline uptake, increased lipid catabolism	Supports lipid anabolic needs, alters DNA methylation

Indeed, their number vastly exceeds the number of human cells in the body. These nonsterile sites include the skin, oral cavity and nostrils, GI tract, lung, vagina, uterus, and urogenital tract, with the largest population of bacteria residing in the GI tract. The so-called **microbiome** often engages in a symbiotic relationship with the human host; for example, in facilitating digestion by detoxifying dietary components or by breaking down otherwise indigestible carbohydrates. However, it is now evident that the microbiome also engages in activities relevant to the development of human diseases, including cancer. These activities increase the incidence of certain cancers and reduce the incidence of others.

The microbiome is highly diverse in its content but is also incredibly diverse among individuals. This diversity is associated with dietary, hygienic, behavioral, and environmental factors. This diversity may also account for the large differences observed in cancer incidences among populations from different nations, cultures, continents, and time periods. In addition, the frequent use of antibiotics may alter the composition of the microbiome, which may affect the incidence of various cancers.

The precise mechanisms by which resident bacteria may promote tumorigenesis are not completely understood, but several mechanisms have been proposed. Bacteria can secrete a number of genotoxic products, inducing DNA damage in adjacent epithelial cells. Bacteria can generate metabolites that affect epigenetic programming in nearby epithelial cells. They can secrete factors that directly interact with proteins on the surface of or inside epithelial cells. They can influence cell signaling in ways that promote the development of neoplastic change. And they can secrete factors that interfere with immune system surveillance in an unfavorable manner, perhaps inhibiting immune effector cells that function to detect and eliminate tumor cells.

The most definitive example linking the microbiome to cancer has been the bacterial species *Helicobacter pylori*. *H pylori* colonizes the gastric mucosa of a large subset of the human population, and its presence is associated with the development of gastritis and an increased risk of developing gastric epithelial cancer and one type of gastric lymphoma. This is largely attributed to a number of virulence factors secreted by *H pylori* that can damage the gastric epithelium as well as to an increased production of free radicals that can damage cell DNA. The microbiome can contribute to cancer development not only by containing a specific cancer-promoting species such as *H pylori*, but also by altering the relative abundance of various species. For example, an increase in abundance of *Fusobacterium* species has been linked to the development of colorectal cancers, although the mechanisms are not yet well understood.

VIRAL CAUSES OF NEOPLASIA

Viruses carry genetic material and express their genes when they infect host cells. The expression of these genes in infected cells can lead to proliferative phenotypes that span the

TABLE 5–6   Oncogenic human viruses.

Virus Type	Virus Family	Associated Cancer Type
HTLV-I	Retrovirus (RNA virus)	T-cell leukemia/lymphoma
HBV (hepatitis B virus)	Hepadnavirus (hepatotropic DNA virus)	Hepatocellular carcinoma
HCV (hepatitis C virus)	Hepacivirus (RNA virus)	Hepatocellular carcinoma
EBV (Epstein–Barr virus)	Herpesvirus (DNA virus)	Nasopharyngeal carcinoma Burkitt lymphoma Immunoblastic lymphoma Hodgkin disease
HHV-8 (KSHV)	Herpesvirus (DNA virus)	Kaposi sarcoma Body cavity lymphoma
HPV (specific high-risk serotypes)	Papillomavirus (DNA virus)	Cervical carcinoma Anal carcinoma Oropharyngeal carcinoma
Merkel cell polyomavirus	Polyomavirus	Skin cancer

HHV-8, human herpesvirus-8; HPV, human papillomavirus; HTLV, human T-cell leukemia/lymphoma virus; KSHV, Kaposi sarcoma herpesvirus.

spectrum from benign growths to malignant cancers. Different classes of viruses have been associated with human tumorigenesis, including viruses carrying DNA or RNA (Table 5–6). Some of these viruses are highly prevalent and even endemic in certain areas of the world. For example, the hepatitis B and C viruses and the human papillomavirus (HPV) are among the most prevalent; together, they account for a significant burden of global cancer mortality. It is hoped that viral causes of cancer mortality can be reduced by effective vaccination strategies.

Viruses can promote tumorigenesis through different mechanisms. Some viruses carry genes encoding proteins that target and inactivate human tumor suppressor genes. The best studied example is HPV, which is transmitted by sexual contact. HPV accounts for many cancers of the oropharynx and genital regions, particularly cancers of the uterine cervix and anus. Although the HPV genome encodes many genes, among them are two genes, E6 and E7, which are oncoproteins. These oncoproteins interfere with many cellular pathways. For example, the E6 protein can bind and inactivate the *p53* tumor suppressor gene in human cells, and the E7 protein can bind and inactivate the *Rb* tumor suppressor gene. This oncoprotein interference represents a mechanism other than genomic mutation for the inactivation of tumor suppressors in human cells. The E6 and E7 proteins likely interfere with other cellular pathways as well. There are more than 100 strains of HPV, and only a few are considered "high risk" in terms of promoting cancer. The differences between the "low-risk" and "high-risk" types of HPV appear to be related to differences in the E6 and E7 genes carried by the different types of HPV and perhaps also in their level of expression. Many low-risk types of HPV cause neoplastic growths such as benign warts in the skin, feet, or genital areas but do not cause malignancy. The high-risk types of HPV cause pre-cancerous changes in the cervical epithelium and invasive cancers of the cervix, anus, and oropharynx.

Although some viruses, such as HPV, can promote tumorigenesis directly through oncogenes encoded in their genome, other viruses can promote tumorigenesis indirectly. The hepatitis C virus (HCV) does not encode a protein that inactivates host tumor suppressors. However, its cytotoxicity to hepatocytes leads to chronic inflammation, oxidative stress, and eventual fibrosis and cirrhosis; in this case, it is thought that tumorigenesis is promoted indirectly through persistent chronic inflammation.

CANCER METASTASIS

The growth of a malignant tumor at its primary site can induce local tissue destruction, obstruction, and various other associated symptoms. But, since the primary tumor can often be surgically removed, these problems usually do not account for the cancer's lethality. Instead, the most lethal attribute of cancer is its propensity for **metastasis**; that is, the spread of the cancer to other areas of the body where it can generate new tumors. Metastasis does not follow a random distribution pattern; rather, each type of cancer favors metastasis to specific organs. Prostate cancers almost always metastasize to bone. Melanomas have a predilection for the liver and brain. Even for a given cancer, different subtypes typically metastasize to different organs. For example, luminal-type breast cancers (those with cells resembling the inner [luminal] epithelial cells lining the mammary ducts) typically metastasize to bone, whereas basal-like breast cancers (those with cells resembling the basal cells that line the ducts) metastasize to the liver and lung.

The mechanisms that underlie the metastasis of tumor cells to distant organs are not entirely clear. Tumor cells can acquire increased motility, which enables them to separate from the primary tumor mass. Such rogue cells can then travel through lymphatic channels, through the bloodstream, or directly through connective tissues. Some epithelial tumor cells may undergo a process that fundamentally changes their cytoskeletal and signaling protein expression patterns to temporarily resemble more flexible mesenchymal cells. This reversible process, called **epithelial-to-mesenchymal transition**, may enable them to traverse the extracellular matrix better by squeezing through tight openings such as in between endothelial cells, effectively enabling them to enter the vasculature and to exit at distant sites, and subsequently to return to their original epithelial state. The reason some tumors appear to prefer certain distant sites of metastasis is not well understood.

But it is thought that certain factors at specific sites of metastasis provide a fruitful microenvironment for certain tumor cells. This has been called the "**seed-and-soil hypothesis**" for the pathogenesis of tumor metastasis. However, the specific elements that constitute the "seed" and the "soil" are not yet well defined. Tumor cells may express certain chemokine receptors, driving them to sites where their chemokine ligands are abundant. Some tumor cells may home into certain distant sites seeking specific growth factors for support. The expression of specific integrin receptors may favor their binding to matrix proteins at specific organ sites. The bone marrow is a common site for the metastasis of many tumors, possibly because of the rich growth factor milieu and easy access from the bloodstream.

While the mechanisms that enable the traveling and homing of tumor cells to specific distant sites are fundamentally important in mediating metastasis, these mechanisms make up only half the metastatic process. Once a tumor cell has arrived at a distant site, its proliferative capacity alone is insufficient to generate a new tumor at the site of metastasis. In fact, most tumor cells are incapable of generating a new tumor at a distant site. The ability to do so is found in only a very small subset of tumor cells, typically called **cancer stem cells** or **tumor-initiating cells**. Defining and identifying tumor-initiating cells and determining the mechanisms that enable them to generate an entirely new tumor is a matter of ongoing study.

The process of metastasis follows a continuous pattern of branching and cross-seeding (Figure 5–11). Multiple metastases may originate from a single ancestral clone of cells within a primary tumor or from different ancestral clones within the primary tumor. An established metastasis may then seed many new metastases, essentially serving as a branch point in metastatic dissemination. This process may then proceed with multiple metastases seeding additional generations of metastases. In addition, cells from one metastasis may travel and land at a site of another pre-existing metastasis, which is referred to as a cross-seeding of metastases. These patterns of tumor dissemination, suspected for decades, have only recently been confirmed by phylogenetic analysis of tumor genomic samples obtained from many different anatomic sites in autopsy studies of deceased patients.

CELLULAR HETEROGENEITY IN NEOPLASIA

The molecular changes of neoplastic cells and their phenotypic behavior is a constantly evolving process. Every cell division can result in additional genomic abnormalities with a variety of phenotypic consequences. Certain genotypes result in proliferative, survival, or other biological attributes that favor clonal expansion. Such neoplastic clones can eventually overtake the tumor cell population and change its clinical behavior. This remodeling process occurs repetitively with recurrent cell divisions, recreating a process akin to evolution, albeit in a much shorter time frame. Attributes acquired early

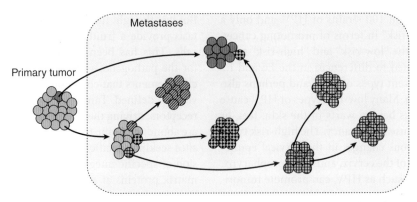

FIGURE 5−11 Selected tumor cell clones from a primary tumor can seed new sites of metastasis. Selected tumor cell clones from these metastases can, in turn, seed additional sites of metastasis, and the formation of new metastases can proceed in a branched fashion, with independent lineages harboring different mutational ancestries. In addition to seeding new metastases, tumor cells disseminating from one metastatic site can cross-seed another already established metastatic site.

in the evolution of a cancer include enhanced proliferation and survival. Changes acquired at the midpoint of evolution include the ability to overcome spatial limitations by invading surrounding tissues, the ability to survive under conditions of low oxygen and few nutrients, and the ability to evade host immune defenses. Changes acquired later in the progression of neoplasia are the ability to travel to distant organs and the ability to resist anti-cancer treatments.

The evolving nature of a cancer with repeated cell proliferation cycles along constantly expanding cell lineages creates heterogeneity in the whole tumor cell population. Tumor cell heterogeneity is a common characteristic of many types of cancer and introduces significant complexity in the molecular or histologic characterization of cancers. Tumors may have some areas with poor differentiation and other areas that are more differentiated. Certain regions may harbor mutational activation of one oncogene, whereas other regions may demonstrate activation of a different oncogene. Some areas of the tumor may be hypermetabolic or hyperproliferative, whereas other areas may have reduced metabolic or proliferative activities. The inherent heterogeneity of a cancer is a considerable barrier to its effective treatment since each type of treatment may affect only one subpopulation of tumor cells. At one extreme end of tumor heterogeneity is the existence of tumor cells with such low metabolic and proliferative activity that they are considered to be in a state of **dormancy**. Such tumor

cell dormancy can last for a period of many years, after which the cells may recover, leading to late relapses of tumors previously thought to have been eradicated.

Although many (or most) of the cells that arise from cancer cell division themselves proceed to multiply, the changes with repeated cycles of cell division often lead to the loss of some of the more fundamental properties of the ancestral cancer cells. For example, many tumor cells are unable to give rise to a new tumor if isolated and re-implanted. In fact, only a small proportion of cancer cells appear to be capable of starting new colonies of cancer cells if isolated and implanted in, or metastasized to, a new site in the body. Such cells, named **cancer stem cells**, typically do not proliferate as quickly as most other tumor cells but are capable of self-renewal and of generating daughter cells that can proliferate more quickly and produce new tumors.

CHECKPOINT

30. What are cancer stem cells?
31. What is an example of a bacterial cause of human cancer?
32. How do viruses cause tumors?
33. Can metastases metastasize?

NEOPLASIA CLASSIFICATION

The terms "neoplasia" and "neoplasm" describe a large number of human diseases with extremely diverse characteristics. At the first level of classification, neoplasms can be benign or malignant. Benign neoplasms are relatively straightforward to name and classify, since they are easily identified as an overgrowth of the readily identifiable normal tissue within which they arise. The suffix "-oma" is typically applied to the primary

tissue name to describe the benign overgrowth of the tissue. Examples include "lipoma" to describe a benign neoplasm of adipose tissue, "osteoma" to describe a benign neoplasm of bone, and "adenoma" to describe a benign neoplasm of a wide variety of glandular epithelial tissues such as colon, breast, and lung. The classification of malignant neoplasms is much more complex, since their morphology often does not resemble their tissue of origin, and they may also appear at anatomic sites of metastasis not reflecting their organ of origin. Therefore, the classification of malignant neoplasms (cancers) into categories and subcategories is of great value in diagnosing, studying, understanding, and developing treatments for them. Malignant transformation involves the development of abnormal cellular behavior. In some cancers, the abnormalities are subtler and the cancer cells retain many of their specialized tissue functions. These cancers are referred to as "well differentiated." In other cancers, the abnormalities are extreme, such that the cancer cells bear little resemblance to the normal cells in their primary tissue. Such cancers referred to as "poorly differentiated" if it is difficult to identify their tissue of origin by microscopic examination. In such cases, molecular markers may be required to identify a cancer's origin.

The broadest classification of tumors relies on the most fundamental characterization of cell types based on their primitive embryologic origins. During early embryonic development, three cell lineages are established: ectoderm, endoderm, and mesoderm. All subsequent cells, including those of adult tumors, can be traced to one of these three cellular origins. As such, tumors are broadly classified into the categories of **carcinoma** if they originate from **ectodermal** or **endodermal** tissues, or **sarcomas** if they originate from **mesodermal** tissues. Even if completely unrecognizable by morphologic analysis, fundamental differences in the expression of certain proteins, especially intermediate filaments such as keratins and vimentin, will identify the lineage of origin. Fundamental differences in the biology of endodermal or ectodermal tissues from that of mesenchymal tissues underlie the vast differences in the cancers that arise from these different cell types. Endodermal and ectodermal origin tissues form much of the "front-line" tissues of the body (eg, skin, GI tract, respiratory tract) that are exposed to the outside environment; are in contact with the microbiome; and have cell structures, polarity, and adhesive functions critical for their "border control" functions. (A notable exception is the nervous system, which also arises early from the ectoderm). On the other hand, mesenchymal origin tissues are sterile tissues, are generally not exposed to the environment, and are more focused toward bodily functions not directly related to the environment.

Carcinomas are the most common type of cancer and include all the common epithelial tissue cancers such as lung, colon, breast, and prostate cancers. **Sarcomas** arise from mesenchymal cell types, predominantly in the connective tissues. Further classification of carcinomas and sarcomas is based on the organ of origin. In the growing infant and child, mesenchymal tissues are very active in growth and remodeling, and mesenchymal tumors are common (eg, in the muscle, cartilage, bone, and blood). In adults, the mesenchymal tissues are not very active, and epithelial tumors are by far the most common (eg, in the lung, breast, prostate, and colon). Malignancies of blood cells, including leukemias and lymphomas, are technically a subtype of sarcomas because they are of mesenchymal origin. However, because of the highly specialized nature of hematologic cell types, they are generally grouped together under the entity of "hematologic neoplasms." Developments in the gene expression profiling of tumors have enabled tumor classification based on characteristic molecular portraits, and further work in this area may result in an entirely new classification of human tumors based on their gene expression profiles.

EPITHELIAL NEOPLASIA

Epithelial cells are in constant turnover, arising from a basal layer that continually generates new cells. The mature and functional layer of cells performs specialized tissue or organ functions and, with senescence, is eventually sloughed off. Proliferating epithelial cells normally observe anatomic boundaries such as the basement membrane that underlies the basal layer of cells in the epithelium. The potential to divide, migrate, and differentiate is tightly controlled. The stimulus to divide may be autonomous or exogenous as a response to factors from adjacent or distant cells. Inhibitory signals and factors may also be present and serve to function as negative regulators to check uncontrolled growth. The neoplastic phenotype of epithelial cells can be seen as a spectrum from **hyperplastic** to **pre-invasive** to frankly **invasive** and **metastatic** neoplasia, as illustrated in Figure 5–12. Because of their embryonic origins, malignancies of epithelial origin are termed carcinomas. Hyperplasia can be a normal physiologic response in some situations, such as that which occurs in the lining of the uterus in response to estrogens before the ovulatory phase of the menstrual cycle. It can also be a pathologic finding associated with a predisposition to progress to invasive carcinoma. In such instances of hyperplasia, there are usually accompanying disorders of maturation that may be recognizable by microscopic examination. These changes are termed **dysplasia**, **atypical hyperplasia**, or **metaplasia**, depending on the type of epithelium in which they are observed. More aggressive proliferation without the ability to invade through the basement membrane is termed **pre-invasive carcinoma** or **carcinoma in situ**. Technically, these cells do not have the capacity to invade the basement membrane and metastasize, although they may over time progress to **invasive carcinoma**. The term "invasive carcinoma" implies that tissue boundaries, especially the basement membrane, have been breached. **Metastatic carcinoma** occurs via the lymphatic system to regional lymph nodes and via the bloodstream to distant organs and other tissues. This pattern of metastasis, however, is not unique to epithelial malignancies. In general, epithelial neoplasms have a (variable) propensity to spread to regional nodes as well as to distant sites.

From a pathophysiologic standpoint, certain structural and functional characteristics are acquired by malignant cells in the course of their evolution, as outlined in Table 5–7. What follows in the next section is a more in-depth discussion of three epithelial cancers to illustrate some of the pathophysiological principles underlying their development. Colon cancer is an example of an epithelial neoplasm for which stepwise

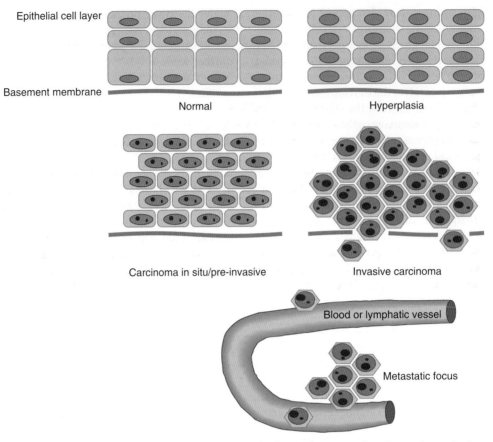

FIGURE 5–12 The phenotypic transition of epithelial cells from normal to hyperplasia to pre-invasive carcinoma in situ to invasive carcinoma to metastatic carcinoma.

molecular evolution has been well documented, as colonoscopy has enabled precursor lesions to be readily identified, biopsied, and studied. Breast cancer is a type of neoplasm with distinct subtypes driven by distinct biologic drivers. And lung cancer is an epithelial neoplasm directly associated with environmental mutagens and driven by mutationally activated oncogenes.

CHECKPOINT

34. What is the difference between carcinoma and sarcoma?
35. What is carcinoma in situ?

1. Colon Carcinoma

The model of stepwise genetic alterations in cancer is best illustrated by observation of colonic lesions at different stages of progression to malignancy. Certain genetic alterations are found commonly in early-stage adenomas, whereas others tend to occur more frequently at later stages of tumorigenesis or after the development of invasive carcinoma. The timeline of genotypic and phenotypic changes during the development of colon cancer are shown in Figure 5–13. These changes are in keeping with the concept that serial phenotypic changes, driven by serial genetic alterations, must occur in a cell for it to exhibit full malignant (invasive and metastatic) properties.

The earliest molecular defect in the pathogenesis of colon cancer is activation of the Wnt signaling pathway, which occurs through the development of somatic mutations in the **APC tumor suppressor gene** in the normal colonic mucosa. This leads to abnormal cell proliferation and the initial steps in neoplasia that lead to formation of polyps in the colon. At an early point in polyp formation, growth factor receptor signaling pathways are activated. This occurs through mutational activation of the **KRAS**, **NRAS**, or **BRAF signal transduction oncogenes**, which further remove restraints on cell proliferation and enable polyps to grow bigger. The next step in tumorigenesis are mutations in genes involved in the TGF-β signaling pathway. This further deregulates growth patterns and properties of enlarging polyps. Deletion or loss of expression of the **DCC** gene is common in the progression to invasive colon cancers. The DCC protein is a transmembrane protein of the immunoglobulin superfamily and may be a receptor for certain extracellular molecules that guide cell growth and/or apoptosis. Mutational inactivation of **TP53** disrupts cell cycle checkpoints, staves off apoptosis, and occurs at a late stage in the progression to an invasive cancer phenotype. The genes specifically responsible for subsequent progression to a metastatic phenotype are not yet well understood.

TABLE 5–7   Phenotypic changes in the progression of neoplasia.

1. Genomic instability
   Impaired DNA repair
   Aberrant cell cycle checkpoint control

2. Enhanced proliferation
   Autonomous growth
   Abnormalities of cell cycle control
   Exaggerated response to hormonal or growth factor stimuli
   Lack of response to growth inhibitors or cell contact inhibition

3. Evasion of immune system
   Antigen modulation and masking
   Elaboration of immune response antagonistic molecules

4. Invasion of tissue and stroma
   Attachment to extracellular matrix
   Secretion of proteolytic enzymes
   Recruitment of stromal cells to produce proteolytic enzymes
   Loss of cell cohesion

5. Ability to gain access to and egress from lymphatics and blood vessels
   Enhanced cell motility
   Recognition of endothelial protein sequences
   Cytoskeletal modifications

6. Establishment of metastatic foci
   Cell adhesion and attachment
   Tissue-specific tropism

7. Ability to recruit vascularization to support growth of primary or metastatic tumor

8. Drug resistance
   Altered drug metabolism and drug inactivation
   Increased synthesis of targeted enzymes
   Enhanced drug efflux
   Enhanced DNA damage repair

In parallel to these sequential abnormalities in the regulation of cell proliferation, colon cancers also acquire defects in mechanisms that protect genomic stability. These generally occur along one of two mechanisms. In some colon cancers, the abnormalities are a result of mutations in mismatch repair genes. **Mismatch repair genes** are a family of genes involved in "proofreading" DNA and correcting incorporation errors during replication; they include *MSH2, MLH1, PMS1,* and *PMS2*. Tumors with mutations in mismatch repair genes perform DNA replication with many errors, and thus these tumors develop thousands of mutations, resulting in what is referred to as a hypermutator phenotype. This phenotype can be detected by a PCR-based **microsatellite instability (MSI)** assay in which the hypermutator tumor phenotype will test **MSI high**. In colon cancers that are not MSI high, genomic instability occurs as a result of mutations in **chromosomal instability (CIN) genes**. Because of their impaired ability to preserve chromosome structure and content, these tumors have losses or gains of large segments of chromosomes or entire chromosomes and are highly aneuploid.

The stepwise acquisition of genetic abnormalities described above is associated with alterations in the phenotypic behavior of the colonic mucosa. The earliest change in the progression to colon cancer is an increase in cell number (hyperplasia) on the epithelial (luminal) surface. This produces an adenoma, which is characterized by gland-forming cells exhibiting increases in size and cell number but no invasion of surrounding structures (Figure 5–14). Presumably, these changes are a result of enhanced proliferation and loss of cell cycle control but occur before acquisition of the capacity to invade the ECM. Additional dysplastic changes, such as loss of mucin production and altered cell polarity, may be present to a variable degree. Some adenomas may continue to enlarge and ultimately progress to invasive carcinoma. An early feature associated with disrupted architecture even before invasion occurs is the development of fragile new vessels or the destruction of existing vessels, which can cause microscopic bleeding. This can be screened for clinically with the fecal occult blood tests used for early diagnosis of pre-invasive and invasive colon cancer. All phenotypic changes cannot be explained by a known genetic abnormality, nor do all identified genetic alterations have a known phenotypic result. However, the stepwise nature of genotypic and phenotypic abnormalities is well established and strongly supports the mechanistic link between these parallel processes.

Further functional changes in the cell and surrounding tissue are also manifested in the pre-invasive and invasive stages. Once the basement membrane is penetrated by invasive malignant cells, access can be gained to the regional lymphatics and spread to regional pericolic lymph nodes can occur. Entry of cells into the bloodstream can lead to distant spread in a pattern that reflects venous drainage. Therefore, hematogenous spread from primary colon tumors to the liver is common, whereas rectal tumors usually disseminate to the liver, lung, and bone. In addition to anatomic considerations, there may exist specific tropism of malignant cells mediated by surface proteins that cause the cells to preferentially home in on certain organs or sites.

Colonic epithelium is specialized to secrete mucus proteins and to absorb water and electrolytes (Chapter 13). The maintenance of a tight luminal barrier, intracellular charge differences, and the ability to exclude toxins are additional specialized functions. Some of these functions are maintained in the progression to neoplasia and may contribute to a specific phenotype of the malignant cell. One example is the expression of a **transporter membrane protein, MDR-1**, present on several types of epithelium, including the colon. MDR-1 is known to cause efflux of several compounds out of the cells, presumably as a protective mechanism to exclude toxins. In advanced colon cancer, this protein may contribute to the relative resistance of this and other tumor types to a variety of chemotherapeutic agents transported by MDR-1. In some cases, the activation of a latent gene-encoding **carcinoembryonic antigen (CEA)** can result in measurable levels of the CEA

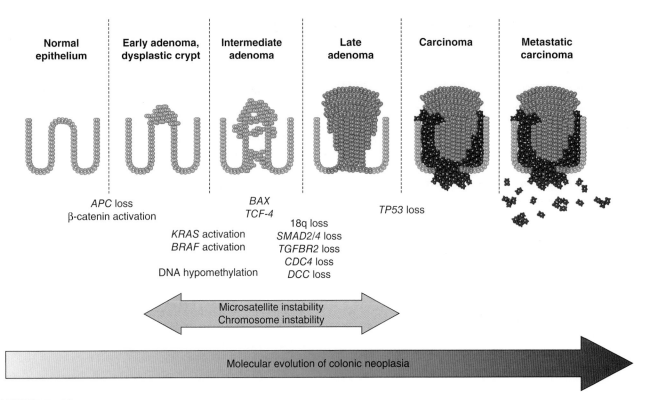

FIGURE 5–13 The sequential phases of cellular abnormalities and polyp formation in the colon are shown on a timeline that also depicts the corresponding genetic events associated with each cellular landmark.

protein in the serum of patients with localized or metastatic colon cancer (as well as other adenocarcinomas).

The timeline and frequency for the transformation of normal colon epithelial cells to colon cancer is determined by the stochastic nature of genetic mutations and the multitude

FIGURE 5–14 Edge of an adenomatous polyp, showing adenomatous change (left), compared with normal mucosal glands (right). Adenomatous change is characterized by increased size and stratification of nuclei and loss of cytoplasmic mucin. Note the arrangement of nuclei of the adenoma perpendicular to the basement membrane (polarity). (Reproduced, with permission, from Chandrasoma P et al. *Concise Pathology*, 3rd ed. Originally published by Appleton & Lange. Copyright © 1998 by The McGraw-Hill Companies, Inc.)

of such mutations required for the full malignant phenotype to become manifest. This process can be accelerated by both endogenous and exogenous events. Endogenous events account for the inherited susceptibility to colon cancer, whereas exogenous events account for the dietary and environmental contributors to colon cancer.

Endogenously, if one of the required mutations is preexisting in the germline DNA acquired at conception, then that individual begins life with colon epithelial cells already well along the pathway of tumorigenesis. As an example, the *APC* gene, which is one of the earliest genes mutated during colon tumorigenesis, is genetically mutated in the germline of some families. Family members who inherit this mutated *APC* gene develop the clinical syndrome of **familial adenomatous polyposis (FAP)**, characterized by the development of extremely numerous colon polyps and eventual development of colon cancer at a very young age. Mutations in other genes, such as **MSH2** or **MLH1**, which are involved in DNA mismatch repair, are also seen in the germline of some families. Family members who inherit these mutated genes develop the clinical syndrome of **hereditary non-polyposis colorectal cancer (HNPCC)**. This syndrome is also characterized by a high frequency of developing colon cancer, although with fewer polyps and an older age at onset than seen in FAP.

Exogenously, the development of mutations in the colon epithelial cells can also be accelerated by chemical compounds within the lumen of the gut or within the bloodstream. These include chemical substances derived from bacterial colonic flora, from ingested foods, or from endogenous metabolites such as fecapentaenes, 3-ketosteroids, and benzo[α]pyrenes, which are mutagenic. Levels of these substances can be reduced by low-fat, high-fiber diets; several epidemiologic studies confirm that such diets reduce the risk of colon cancer.

Dietary and environmental factors may also interact with inherited genetic changes to promote the development of colon cancers. In particular, there may be inherited genes, which, by themselves, cause only a slight increase in colon cancer incidence and thus do not create familial clusters of colon cancer cases. But these genes may promote the development of colon cancer in specific individuals exposed to certain dietary or environmental risk factors.

CHECKPOINT

36. What are some of the genes mutated in the evolution of colon cancers?

37. How does mismatch repair deficiency occur in colon cancers?

38. What causes familial adenomatous polyposis?

2. Breast Carcinoma

The female breast is a specialized gland that undergoes repeated cycles of growth factor– and hormone-induced changes that define the different stages of breast development (ie, fetal, pubertal, menstrual, pregnancy-associated, lactational growth, and postlactational involution). Deregulation of this complex biology leads to a diverse group of neoplastic breast diseases inherently connected with growth factor or hormonal signaling. These range from benign fibrocystic changes of the breast to malignant tumors of the breast. Three broadly defined molecular pathways appear to be relevant to the pathophysiology of breast cancers: hormone signaling, growth factor signaling, and DNA repair pathways.

Hormone Signaling

The prolonged use of exogenous estrogen and progesterone therapies, typically used to postpone menopause, is a breast cancer risk factor that clearly implicates the hormonal signaling pathway. In contrast, reduced exposure to estrogen and progesterone protects against the development of breast cancer. This has been demonstrated in ovariectomized animal models of breast carcinogenesis and confirmed by clinical studies demonstrating that women who have undergone oophorectomy at a young age have a significant reduction in their lifetime risk of developing breast cancer. The clinical success of anti-estrogen therapies provides proof of principle of the essential role of estrogen signaling in the pathogenesis of breast cancer. Agents that inhibit the production of estrogen or the ability of estrogen to activate the nuclear estrogen receptor (ER) are highly effective in reducing the development of breast cancer, or in stopping the progression of pre-invasive, invasive, or metastatic breast cancers. However, although the central roles of estrogen

and the ER in the pathogenesis of breast cancer are now well established, the evidence to date does not etiologically implicate genetic abnormalities of estrogen, the ER, or downstream ER target genes in the development of breast cancer, and thus neither estrogen nor the ER is considered an oncogene. It appears that ER signaling is a physiological pathway existing in breast epithelial cells whose continued signaling activity is favorable to, or perhaps even necessary for, the transformational steps triggered by as yet unknown drivers of the neoplastic process. However, unlike oncogenes, estrogen signaling is clearly insufficient to initiate tumorigenesis, as the breasts of all healthy women are constantly under active estrogenic signaling without the development of tumors.

The importance of the estrogen signaling pathway does not extend to all breast cancers, however, since half of all breast cancers seem to demonstrate loss of activity of this signaling pathway or no expression of the ER. Some investigators believe that ER-negative breast cancer is a different disease with an alternative pathophysiology. Most likely, there are common early molecular steps in the development of ER-positive and ER-negative breast cancers; however, at an early or intermediate step, these pathways diverge, leading to the development of breast cancers with distinctly different phenotypes.

Growth Factor Signaling

A number of growth factor signaling pathways are implicated in the pathophysiology of breast cancers. The growth factor IGF-1 is an important regulator of mammary gland biology, and elevated serum IGF-1 levels are associated with an increased risk of breast cancers. However, abnormalities of the IGF1 receptor are not seen in breast cancers. Much more directly implicated are the growth factor receptors of the human epidermal growth factor receptor (HER) family. Amplification of the ERBB2 (aka HER2) gene and overexpression of the HER2 protein are common in pre-invasive and invasive breast cancers. Overexpression of the EGFR (aka HER1) gene is also seen with less frequency. The HER family receptors activate a number of downstream signaling pathways, including proliferative, apoptotic, and metabolic pathways. An important downstream pathway is the PI3K/Akt signaling pathway. Components of this pathway are also mutationally activated in breast cancers. In fact, the proto-oncogene PIK3CA, encoding the catalytic subunit of PI3K, is the most commonly mutated gene in breast cancers. The proto-oncogene AKT1 and the tumor suppressor gene PTEN are also mutationally or epigenetically altered in breast cancers, activating this important signaling pathway. The growth factor receptor signaling pathway intermediates are mostly oncogenes and, because of their abnormal activities, are not typically seen in their mutated form in the germline of individuals. However, mutated alleles of the tumor suppressor gene PTEN can be seen in the germline of some familial lineages, causing Cowden syndrome, with its high risk of breast cancer and other tumors.

DNA Repair Pathways

The loss of genomic stability is also a common event in the pathogenesis of many breast cancers. Many of the genes involved in maintaining DNA integrity are tumor suppressor genes and thus are involved both in the pathogenesis of breast cancers at the familial level through germline transmission of mutated alleles, and also in the pathogenesis of sporadic breast cancers through the somatic mutation at the tissue level. The *BRCA1* and *BRCA2* genes account for a majority of familial breast cancers. Mutated alleles of these genes are seen in 0.2–2% of various ethnic populations and confer a lifetime risk of developing breast cancer of up to 70%. Mutations in these genes are also associated with a high incidence of ovarian cancer in women and increased incidences of prostate cancer, melanomas, and breast cancer in men. Both of these genes function as tumor suppressor genes such that breast tumors contain both the inherited abnormality in one allele and a somatic loss of the remaining allele. Sporadic (nonfamilial) cases of breast cancer may also contain *BRCA1* mutations or may have abnormalities in other proteins that interact with BRCA1 to perform DNA repair functions involving double-strand breaks in DNA. The *TP53* gene, also involved in the detection and response to DNA damage, is also frequently mutated in *BRCA1*- or *BRCA2*-defective cancers. The existence of a mutated *TP53* gene in the germline also carries with it a very high risk and early onset of breast cancer, defining a familial clustering of cancers known as Li–Fraumeni syndrome. Other tumor suppressor genes involved in the detection of or response to DNA damage are also involved in the pathogenesis of breast cancers. The *PALB2* gene, which works in partnership with *BRCA2* in the repair of DNA, is also mutated in the germline of other familial lineages, conferring a high risk of cancers of the breast and pancreas. The *ATM* gene, also involved in the response to DNA damage, is mutated in some other breast cancers, and when inactivated in the germline, leads to the clinical syndrome of ataxia-telangiectasia, characterized by extreme sensitivity to radiation and predisposition to cancer. There are many other genes involved in DNA repair, which, when mutated, can contribute to the pathogenesis of breast cancers. However, many of these have only modest or low **penetrance** (ie, confer only a modest or slight increase in breast cancer risk), and thus their identification and association with cancer risk is more difficult to establish, and it will take many years to identify all such genes. Some that have been identified thus far include *RAD51C*, *CHEK2*, and *BRIP1*.

The Cellular Evolution of Breast Cancer

Cancer of the breast is almost always a result of the malignant transformation of secretory epithelial cells. The normal secretory breast epithelium consists of two layers: the basal myoepithelial layer and the luminal epithelial layer. These layers can be identified by their characteristic patterns of expression of keratin filaments. The identity of the cell of origin of breast cancers has been debated for decades and has not yet been completely defined. Our current understanding suggests that all breast cancers arise from a cell subset within the luminal epithelial layer. However, in the course of tumorigenesis, some breast cancers can de-differentiate and ultimately develop characteristic features of the basal layer cells.

Abnormalities in the ductal epithelium are evident even before the onset of hyperproliferative states that exhibit excessive numbers and layers of luminal cells. Genetic abnormalities likely underlie the earliest form of ductal pathology, called flat atypia, wherein the normal single-layered epithelium architecture is preserved, although the cell population is replaced by atypical cells. Further molecular evolution leads to hyperplasia, carcinoma in situ, and invasive cancer (Figure 5–15).

Breast Cancer Subtyping by Morphology or Receptor Expression

Breast cancers are extremely heterogeneous in their morphology and biology. Such a diverse disease requires classification systems to better understand and manage it. Indeed, many classification systems have been proposed. Figure 5–16 depicts the three most common: the histologic subtypes classification, the clinical subtypes classification, and based on gene expression profiles, the biological ("intrinsic subtypes") characterization. These different classifications reflect different biologies, prognoses, and responses to specific therapies.

Normal ductal epithelium   Flat epithelial atypia   Atypical ductal hyperplasia   Ductal carcinoma in situ   Invasive ductal carcinoma

FIGURE 5–15 Early genetic events lead to proliferative ductal epithelial replacement, but not overgrowth. Additional genetic events lead to progressively increased and abnormal overgrowth (hyperplasia, then carcinoma in situ) and eventually to invasive ductal carcinoma. Changes in chromatin are evident in the nuclei early on and are one of the features of atypia.

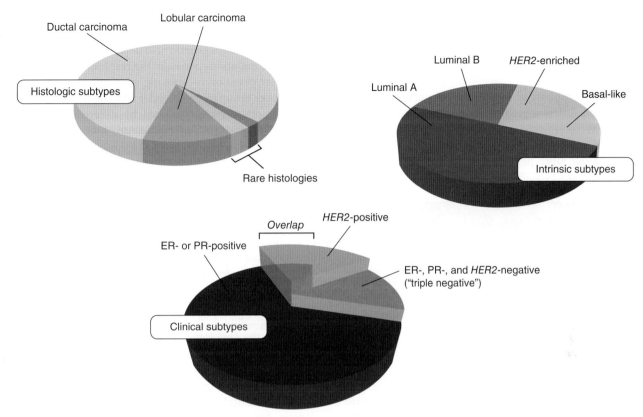

FIGURE 5–16 Breast cancers are frequently classified using different classification systems. Three are shown here—histologic subtypes (top left), intrinsic subtypes (top right), and clinical subtypes (bottom)—with their proportional incidences shown via pie chart. The clinical subtypes, widely used in clinical management, do not divide breast cancers into exclusive categories, such that a cancer can be both ER/PR positive and HER2 positive (ie, HER2 amplified), as shown by the overlapping area in the bottom pie chart.

The oldest system is the **histologic subtypes** classification of breast cancer. By their distinct morphologies, the majority of breast cancers can be classified as ductal carcinomas, a minority as lobular carcinomas, and a few percent as other rare subtypes. Both in situ and invasive cancers fall into these two subtypes. Ductal carcinomas exhibit varying degrees of tubule formation, but lobular carcinomas have lost the ability to form tubules. This is due to a failure in cell–cell attachment as a consequence of the mutational loss of the cell adhesion protein E-cadherin. While ductal carcinomas make dense solid tumors, lobular carcinomas often do not. Instead, lobular carcinomas grow as disconnected and diffuse infiltrates of cells; consequently, they are typically much harder to detect manually and radiographically.

Another system to classify breast cancers is according to their expression of ER or PR and amplification of HER2. This **clinical subtypes** system is favored by clinicians because it is directly linked with treatment options. ER- or PR-positive breast cancers are amenable to treatment with anti-estrogen therapies. HER2-amplified breast cancers are clinically labelled HER2 positive and are amenable to treatment with therapies targeting HER2. Breast cancers that lack all three features are called "triple-negative" breast cancers; they are important to identify because there are as yet no targeted therapy options for them. The clinical subtyping by receptor expression does not define exclusive subtypes, since hormone receptor expression and HER2 amplification can be present in the same cancer; thus, the ER-positive, PR-positive, and HER2-amplified subtypes overlap.

Breast Cancer Subtyping by Transcriptomic Analysis

The development of techniques to simultaneously determine the expression of 10,000 or more genes has revolutionized the way cancers can be classified. This kind of genome-wide transcriptome analysis reveals that breast cancers can be classified by molecular signatures into at least four **intrinsic subtypes:** basal-like, luminal A, luminal B, and HER2-enriched. These molecular subtypes have strong prognostic significance, with the luminal A subtype having the best prognosis and the basal-like subtype the worst prognosis. The subtypes are also linked with specific mechanistic characteristics. The basal-like subtype lacks a unifying molecular attribute, but its hallmark is a significant amount of genomic instability. The HER2-enriched subtype is linked with the amplification and overexpression of the *ERBB2* (*HER2*) oncogene and the consequent downstream signaling events related to it. The two luminal subtypes are characterized by the expression of ER-linked genes, and ER function plays an important role in these cancers.

The four intrinsic subtypes loosely simulate the clinical subtypes of breast cancer since the gene expression profiles are largely driven by ER or HER2.

In addition to its prognostic significance, this analysis of breast cancers by molecular signatures has predictive value regarding the sensitivity of each to various anti-cancer treatments. Indeed, different predictive gene signatures have been developed as commercial assays for clinical breast cancer samples and can provide validated prognostic and predictive scores, enabling more personalized treatment planning for individual patients.

CHECKPOINT

39. What are some of the molecular pathways involved in breast cancer pathogenesis?
40. What are some of the germline genes that cause familial breast cancers?
41. How many types of breast cancer are there?
42. What is the role of HER2 in breast cancer?

3. Lung Carcinoma

Lung cancer is the greatest cause of cancer mortality worldwide. This is because the lung epithelium is highly exposed to environmental carcinogens, in particular those in tobacco smoke. Exposure to these carcinogens induces gene mutations in the epithelium along the entire respiratory tract. In fact, in smokers, even normal-appearing respiratory epithelium harbors gene mutations long before the onset of lung cancer. As such, lung cancer is an example of a cancer that is preceded by and arises from a genetic field defect (see Figure 5–1). And since gene mutations persist in the respiratory epithelium for years after cessation of smoking, smokers remain at risk for lung cancer for up to two decades after smoking cessation.

The respiratory tract is lined by different epithelial cell types, with bronchiolar epithelium lining the conducting and protective passages of the upper airways and lower bronchioles, and alveolar epithelium lining the distal alveoli (Figure 5–17). At least four distinct types of cancer develop in the lung, arising from distinct cells of origin in the bronchiolar and alveolar respiratory epithelium. Squamous-cell lung cancers are thought to arise from basal progenitor cells lining the bronchiolar epithelium. These undergo metaplastic change to develop squamous differentiation. Small-cell lung cancers are thought to arise from pulmonary neuroendocrine cells found scattered in the bronchioles. Adenocarcinomas are thought to arise from alveolar type 2 cells, which are thought to have progenitor capability. Large-cell lung cancer is a collective term applied to the remaining rarer subtypes of lung cancer. Consistent with the location of their cells of origin, squamous-cell and small-cell lung cancers are frequently found in more central areas of the lungs, whereas adenocarcinomas frequently arise in the distal regions of the lungs. Since small-cell lung cancers arise from a distinctly different (neuroendocrine) cell of origin and their biologic behavior is also very different, the other three types are usually collectively referred to as non-small-cell lung cancers to clearly differentiate them from small-cell lung cancer.

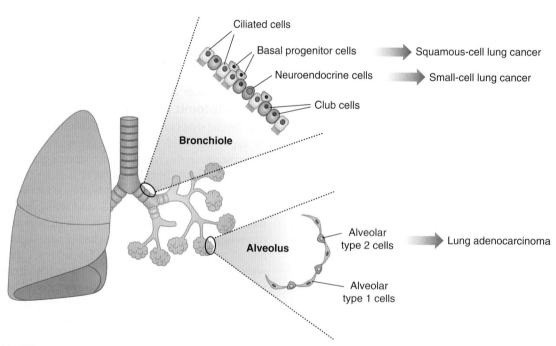

FIGURE 5–17   The repertoire of cells lining the respiratory system changes from the proximal airways to the distal alveoli. The proximal airways are involved in the passage of air, protection, and drainage of secretions, whereas the distal alveoli are involved in gas exchange. According to our current understanding, the different types of lung cancer arise from different types of cells within the respiratory system.

In contrast to colon cancer, in which gene mutations occur in a specific temporal sequence and govern the development of progressive stages of cellular pathology, the mutations incurred in the process of lung tumorigenesis do not follow a sequential order; instead, the pre-neoplastic respiratory epithelium is perhaps best described as experiencing an accumulation of mutations. For example, lung adenocarcinomas are frequently preceded by pre-neoplastic lesions called atypical adenomatous hyperplasia; their cells frequently harbor the same oncogene mutations found in the later adenocarcinomas.

Numerous oncogenes that are disease drivers for subsets of adenocarcinomas and squamous-cell lung cancers have been identified. These subsets are exclusive of one another, each defining a true molecular subtype of lung cancer (Figure 5–18). Each of these oncogenes is activated by different genomic events, such as gene fusions occurring as a result of chromosome translocation, internal deletions, point mutations, or gene amplifications. The development of the KRAS-mutated molecular subtype is strongly associated with smoking, whereas the development of EGFR- and other kinase-mutated molecular subtypes is more commonly seen in nonsmokers. Tobacco carcinogens induce point mutations in DNA, and the activation of KRAS occurs through such point mutation. Other oncogenes typically require deletions or fusion events in the DNA to become activated, but these are not typical of tobacco-induced damage. The tumor-driving nature of many of these oncogenes has now been confirmed by the dramatic response to therapy with selective inhibitors of them. Work is ongoing to discover yet other molecular subtypes of lung cancers. Many of these oncogene-defined subtypes of lung cancer are quite rare in incidence, but their identification is critical, since it can lead to rational therapies with substantial therapeutic benefits. Thus, the current diagnostic and therapeutic management of lung cancer is a prime example of personalized medicine.

CHECKPOINT

43. What is the principal cause of lung cancer?
44. What are some of the oncogenes that drive the biology of lung cancer?

MESENCHYMAL, NEUROENDOCRINE & GERM CELL NEOPLASIA

Mesenchymal, neuroendocrine, and germ cell neoplasms account for a large proportion of the tumors of childhood and young adulthood, ostensibly because these cells are actively dividing and more subject to mutational events. Table 5–8 provides a representative list of mesenchymal, neuroendocrine, and germ cell tumors, as well as the embryologic cell groups from which they arise. Owing to the extensive migration and convolution of embryonic cell layers during early development, these tumor types may not evolve in specific anatomic sites. Neuroendocrine tumors (NETs) are derived from cells that migrate throughout the body and have developed specific enzymatic capabilities and accumulated cytoplasmic proteins that serve a secretory function. As such, they are frequently identified by certain enzymatic markers, in particular nonspecific esterase. Although they were all originally thought to arise from the neural crest, not all NETs

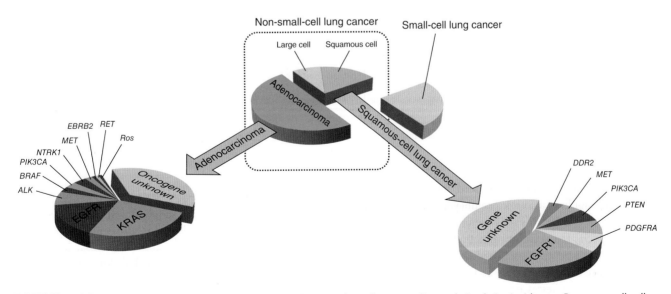

FIGURE 5–18 The four types of lung cancer are shown in the central pie chart according to their relative incidences. Because small-cell lung cancers derive from a distinctly different cellular origin than the other three types, the other three are collectively called non-small-cell lung cancer. Of these types, adenocarcinomas and squamous-cell lung cancers are driven by any of a number of different oncogenes, as depicted in their respective pie charts. The proportion of these cancers with unknown oncogenes may diminish as more discoveries are made. The relative incidences shown are generalizations, since the actual proportional incidences vary substantially depending on demographics.

TABLE 5–8   Mesenchymal, neuroendocrine, and germ cell neoplasia.

Neoplasia Type	Embryonic Derivation	Neoplasia Type	Embryonic Derivation
Wilms tumor	Metanephric blastemal	Germ cell tumors	
Neuroblastoma	Neuroblasts	Teratoma (benign)	Germ cell
Retinoblastoma		Germinoma, dysgerminoma	
Ganglioneuroma		Testicular, extragonadal germ cell tumors	
Neural crest–derived tumors	Neural crest	Seminoma	
Small-cell carcinoma		Choriocarcinoma	
Ewing sarcoma		Embryonal carcinoma	
Primitive neuroectodermal tumor		Endodermal sinus, yolk sac tumors	
Malignant melanoma		Ovarian germ cell tumors	
Pheochromocytoma		Sarcomas	Mesenchymal cell
Neuroendocrine tumors		Rhabdomyosarcoma	Striated muscle
GI endocrine tumors		Leiomyosarcoma	Smooth muscle
Insulinoma		Liposarcoma	Adipocyte
Glucagonoma		Osteosarcoma	Osteoblast
Somatostatinoma		Chondrosarcoma	Chondrocyte
Gastrinoma		Malignant fibrous histiocytoma	Fibroblast
GRFoma		Synovial sarcoma	Synovial cell
VIPoma		Lymphangiosarcoma	Lymphatic endothelium
Pituitary tumors		Hemangiosarcoma	Blood vessel endothelium
Intracranial brain tumors		Kaposi sarcoma	Endothelial cell + fibroblasts?
Glioblastoma/astrocytoma	Glial precursors	Hepatoblastoma	Mesenchymal cell + hepatocytes
Ependymoma, oligodendroglioma, medulloblastoma		Mesothelioma	Mesothelial cell
Adrenocortical carcinoma	Mesonephric mesenchyme	Schwannoma	Peripheral nerve sheath
Somatic (non–germ cell) testicular and ovarian cancers	Mesonephric mesenchyme	Meningioma	Arachnoidal fibroblast

GRF, growth hormone–releasing factor; VIP, vasoactive intestinal peptide.

can be traced to the neural crest. Indeed, tumors of this classification may not have a common embryonic ancestry. However, this tumor classification has been maintained because of its unique specialized secretory functions. NETs can secrete biologically active peptides and produce specific clinical syndromes because of their secretory activities. Germ cell tumors can arise within the testes or in extragonadal sites through which germ cells migrate during development. Mesenchymal cells, by virtue of their function, are distributed throughout the body, and mesenchymal tumors can thus arise at any anatomic site.

1. Neuroendocrine Tumors

NETs arise from neural crest tissue and, more specifically, from enterochromaffin cells, whose final resting place after embryonic migration is along the submucosal layer of the intestines and pulmonary bronchi. Reflecting this embryonic origin, neuroendocrine cells can at times express the necessary enzymes to produce bioactive amines, as well as a variety of small peptide hormones. A low-grade NET is classified as a **carcinoid tumor** (regardless of any hormonal secretion). Cytoplasmic granules typical of neuroendocrine cells are also commonly seen. These features may also be shared by other

TABLE 5–9 Neuroendocrine tumor location by site of embryonic origin.

Foregut	Midgut	Hindgut
Esophagus	Jejunum	Rectum
Stomach	Ileum	
Duodenum	Appendix	
Pancreas	Colon	
Gallbladder and bile duct	Liver	
Ampulla of Vater	Ovary	
Larynx	Testes	
Bronchus	Cervix	
Thymus		

TABLE 5–10 Peptides and amines secreted by neuroendocrine tumor cells.

Adrenocorticotropic hormone (ACTH)
Calcitonin
Gastrin
Glicentin
Glucagon
Growth hormone
Insulin
Melanocyte-stimulating hormone (β-MSH)
Motilin
Neuropeptide K
Neurotensin
Serotonin
Somatostatin
Pancreatic polypeptide
Substance K
Substance P
Vasoactive intestinal peptide

tumors of neural crest origin. In contrast to epithelial neoplasms, morphologic changes observed with the light microscope do not distinguish between malignant and benign cells. The anatomic distribution of primary NETs is consistent with embryonic development patterns, as shown in Table 5–9. NETs and other mesenchymal neoplasms demonstrate similar patterns of tissue invasion followed by local and distant spread to regional lymph nodes and distant organs. The characteristics of increased mitotic count (an indicator of rapid proliferation), nuclear pleomorphism, lymphatic and vascular invasion, and an undifferentiated growth pattern are associated with a higher rate of metastases and a less favorable clinical prognosis.

A frequent site of NET metastasis is the liver. In this setting, especially with midgut NETs, there can be a constellation of symptoms as a consequence of the secretion of vasoactive substances (including **serotonin**) into the bloodstream, producing the **carcinoid syndrome** (Table 5–10). These vasoactive substances reflect the neuroendocrine origin of NETs and the latent machinery that can be activated inappropriately in the malignant state. The serotonin and other peptides secreted can cause intermittent flushing from vasodilation, secretory diarrhea, wheezing, and excessive salivation or lacrimation. Long-term tissue damage can occur by exposure to these substances and their metabolites. Fibrosis of the pulmonary and tricuspid heart valves, mesenteric fibrosis, and hyperkeratosis of the skin have all been reported in patients with carcinoid syndrome. A urinary marker commonly used to aid in the diagnosis or to monitor patients being treated is a metabolite of serotonin: **5-hydroxyindoleacetic acid (5-HIAA)**.

2. Testicular Cancer and Other Germ Cell Neoplasms

Testicular cancer arises chiefly from germ cells within the testes. Germ cells are the population of cells that give rise to spermatozoa through meiotic division and can, therefore,

theoretically retain the ability to differentiate into any cell type. Some testicular neoplasms arise from remnant tissue outside the testes owing to the midline migration of germ cells that occurs during early embryogenesis. This is followed by the formation of the urogenital ridge and eventually by the aggregation of germ cells in the ovary or testis. As predicted by this pattern of migration, **extragonadal germ cell neoplasms** are found in the midline axis of the lower cranium, mediastinum, or retroperitoneum. The pluripotent ability of the germ cell (ie, the ability of one cell to give rise to an entire organism) is most evident in benign germ cell tumors such as **mature teratomas**. These tumors often contain differentiated elements from all three germ cell layers, including teeth and hair in lesions termed **dermoid cysts**. Malignant teratomas can also exist as a spectrum bridging other germ cell layer–derived neoplasms such as sarcomas and epithelium-derived carcinomas. Malignant testicular cancers may coexist with benign mature teratomas, and the benign component sometimes becomes apparent only after the malignancy has been eradicated with chemotherapy.

Proteins expressed during embryonic or trophoblastic development, such as alpha-fetoprotein and human chorionic gonadotropin, can be secreted and measured in the serum. Testicular carcinoma follows a lymphatic and hematogenous pattern of spread to regional retroperitoneal nodes and distant organs such as the lung, liver, bone, and brain. The exquisite sensitivity of even advanced testicular cancers to radiation and chemotherapy may be a result of the foreign nature of malignant germ cells when present in a mature organism. This foreign nature may create more specific activity of cytotoxic insults and stimulate a more vigorous immune rejection of the tumor.

CHECKPOINT

45. What products of neuroendocrine tumors reflect their embryonic origin?

46. From what cellular elements of the testes does testicular cancer generally arise?

47. What are some characteristic markers that may be monitored in testicular tumor progression?

3. Sarcomas

The sarcomas consist of a family of neoplasms arising from tissues of mesenchymal origin. They can arise within structures of mesenchymal tissue, such as bone, muscle, cartilage, and connective tissues, or they can arise in areas without a defined tissue from cells that came to rest at such spots during embryonic migration. Compared with epithelial cancers, sarcomas are quite rare, accounting for less than 1% of adult cancers. The reasons for this are not entirely clear, but it may be because tissues of mesenchymal origin have far less proliferative activity than epithelial tissues in adults, have less need to replenish their tissues with new cells, and are thus less prone to DNA replication errors that can introduce mutations or structural alterations in genes. Sarcomas are much more common during childhood, when these tissues do experience proliferative activity to support the growing body.

Although sarcomas are rare in incidence, they are extremely heterogeneous in histologic appearance and biologic behavior and thus represent a challenging case for accurate classification with more than 50 subtypes recognized. Most tumors arising in tissues of mesenchymal origin are benign. Examples of these are lipomas, tumors of adipose tissue very common in adults; hemangiomas, abnormal growths of blood vessels in the skin or various organs; schwannomas, benign growths of schwann cells of peripheral nerves; and myxomas, benign growths within muscle. The distinction of benign versus malignant is more challenging in tumors deriving from mesenchymal tissues than it is for those deriving from epithelial tissues. This is because epithelial tissues have distinct cellular architecture, including ducts, tubules, and alveoli lined by single or double layers of cells exhibiting polarity, adhesion, and enclosure. Such highly ordered architecture is perceptibly disrupted in neoplasia, and malignancy is readily evident at the microscopic level in the form of architectural distortion and invasion of the surrounding connective tissues. Mesenchymal tissues have less complex micro-architecture and no polarity, and the concept of invasion and destructiveness by a tumor is more difficult to assess from examination of microscopic

sections. The microscopic characteristic most often used to distinguish benign from malignant tumors of mesenchymal tissue is proliferative activity. This characteristic correlates with the propensity for metastasis and helps guide the management of these tumors. While epithelial tumors can often be seen to metastasize via lymphatic channels to local lymph nodes, sarcomas do not generally migrate via lymphatics. Instead, they metastasize via the systemic blood vessels, most often to the lung.

Sarcomas have a wide range of biologic behavior. Some, such as desmoid tumors, can grow to a large size and cause local problems owing to their size and pressure but have little capacity for distant metastasis; thus, they are generally considered to be benign. Others, such as Ewing sarcoma, are highly aggressive and metastasize early. The subtyping of sarcomas involves identifying the type of mesenchymal tissue it would most resemble if it were differentiated (see Table 5–8). Sarcoma of bone (osteosarcoma) is generally considered a separate category from all other sarcomas. The remainder, arising in non-bone sites, are collectively called **soft-tissue sarcomas**. Whereas some sarcomas readily show differentiation toward a particular tissue such as skeletal muscle (rhabdomyosarcoma), smooth muscle (leiomyosarcoma), or fat cells (liposarcoma), other sarcomas show no resemblance to normal tissues and are difficult to classify.

Genomic alterations are common in sarcomas and appear to follow several patterns. Some sarcomas have complex karyotypes with no recurring patterns, implicating genomic instability in their underlying pathophysiology. Other sarcomas have defined and recurrent genomic alterations that implicate specific genes in their pathophysiology. Some of these sarcomas have characteristic chromosomal translocations, whereas others have characteristic activating mutations within specific oncogenes. Chromosomal translocations create gene fusions and consequent novel fusion oncoproteins or increased expression of specific genes. Many of the gene fusion events seen in sarcomas involve a member of the TET family of genes (eg, *EWSR1*, *FUS*, *TAFII68*) fused to a transcription factor. A prototype is Ewing sarcoma in which a chromosomal translocation fuses the *EWSR1* gene with a gene from the ETS family of transcription factors. Most of these fusions occur with the *FL1* gene and the remainder with other members of the ETS family. Fusion of the *EWSR1* gene with non-ETS family genes also occurs and causes other types of sarcoma. Specific gene fusion events have been documented for specific types of sarcomas; occasionally, when subtyping of the sarcoma is difficult by histologic analysis, molecular genomic analysis can identify characteristic gene fusion events that specify the sarcoma subtype. Other sarcomas have characteristic gene mutation events. The best-known examples are the **gastrointestinal stromal tumors (GISTs)**. These sarcomas of the GI tract have characteristic mutations in one of three oncogenes—*KIT*, *PDGFRA*, or *BRAF*—and are typically treated by inhibitors of these oncogenes. Desmoid fibromatosis is often associated with activation of the Wnt signaling pathway, with mutations in the *APC* or *β-catenin* genes. Mutational inactivation of the

TP53 tumor suppressor gene also occurs in sarcomas, causing increased genomic instability but is so widespread that it does not define a specific subtype of sarcoma. The *NF1* tumor suppressor gene is sometimes mutated in sarcomas, causing excessive G-protein signaling. Mutations of either of these tumor suppressor genes, when present in the germline, cause inheritable syndromes of cancer risk that include sarcomas.

As with carcinomas, sarcomas can be induced by tumor viruses. The best documented example of this is Kaposi sarcoma, a malignant tumor arising in connective tissues of the skin or internal organs, caused by the human herpesvirus type 8 (HHV-8). Kaposi sarcoma predominantly occurs in immunosuppressed patients with HIV infection.

CHECKPOINT

48. Are sarcomas more common in children or adults?
49. Are sarcomas more or less likely to directly invade tissues compared with epithelial malignancies?
50. To what sites do sarcomas commonly metastasize?
51. What is the genetic lesion found in Ewing sarcoma?
52. What are the oncogenes that have characteristic mutations in gastrointestinal stromal tumors?

CANCER STAGING AND GRADING

Once cancer is diagnosed, a myriad of decision algorithms come into consideration, including decisions regarding surgical resection, chemotherapy, radiation therapy, molecular targeted therapy, immunotherapy, and other forms of therapy. The presentation of cancer is highly variable, potentially different in every patient, and the success and outcomes of therapy can vary significantly among patients with the same type of cancer. Furthermore, since treatments for cancer are currently imperfect and many patients ultimately die from it, the treatment of cancer is in continuous evolution, with many improved therapies replacing existing treatments. The enormous diversity of patients and of treatment options has over time made for very complex decision making regarding the optimal treatment of an individual patient. To reduce this complexity, most cancers are generally categorized according to stage (and sometimes according to grade). Most clinical research trials are conducted in patients with particular stages of specific cancers so that clinicians can readily extrapolate the resulting data, conclusions, and recommendations to their own patients with similar stages of those cancers. Other cancers are now also categorized according to specific molecular and/or genetic markers. This additional categorization will undoubtedly increase in the future.

Cancer Staging

For solid tumors, the stage of a cancer describes the anatomic extent of the cancer at and beyond its site of origin. This information has significant prognostic value for most types of solid-tumor cancers. To provide a uniform method of describing the extent of a cancer, a well-defined staging system, referred to as tumor–node–metastasis (TNM) staging, is used. The disease in any given patient is assigned three numbers: T (for tumor stage), N (for node stage), and M (for metastasis stage). The T number describes the size and extent of the tumor. The N number describes the extent of lymph node metastases. The M stage is usually simply 0, if there are no distant metastases, or 1, if distant metastases are present. The numbering system for TNM staging is different for each type of cancer and is defined, revised, and published every few years by the American Joint Committee on Cancer (AJCC). Cancer presentation varies widely among patients and may involve up to 30 different combinations of T, N, and M numbers. Thus, for each cancer type, the various TNM staging numbers are grouped together into four prognostic staging groups denoted by Roman numerals I–IV and alphabetical substages. Categorization into stages is done to reflect the expected prognosis for that stage of disease. Stage I cancers typically have an excellent prognosis, often requiring no treatment other than surgical excision, whereas stage IV cancers have a dismal prognosis with very few long-term survivors despite the use of all available therapies. The staging system can be applied at the time of presentation based on physical examination and radiographic findings; this is called **clinical staging**. A more accurate staging can be applied after surgical resection of the primary tumor and sampling of the regional lymph nodes. This involves a much more reliable examination of the tissues by pathologists and is called **pathologic staging**. The N stage is sometimes different for clinical staging and pathologic staging to allow clinicians to stage the disease based on their lymph node palpation findings and pathologists to stage the disease based on their microscopic examination of them. As an example, Figure 5–19 illustrates the system used for breast cancer staging. The current eighth edition of the TNM staging system is being released by the AJCC in 2018.

Cancers of the blood and bone marrow cannot be staged by the TNM system given their tissue of origin. Consequently, each type of hematologic malignancy has its own staging system.

Cancer Grading

Cancer grading describes the appearance and behavior of the tumor cells. This information has significant prognostic value of its own, independent of the cancer's stage. To minimize variability among different pathologists, well-defined criteria have been developed for the tissue analysis of each type of cancer. Unlike the TNM staging of cancers, there is no national or global authority governing all grading systems. Rather, the grading system for each type of cancer has been proposed by specific pathologists and by general consensus has been adopted over time by others in the field. Often the grade assessment is broken down into different categories and independently scored. The degree of differentiation or

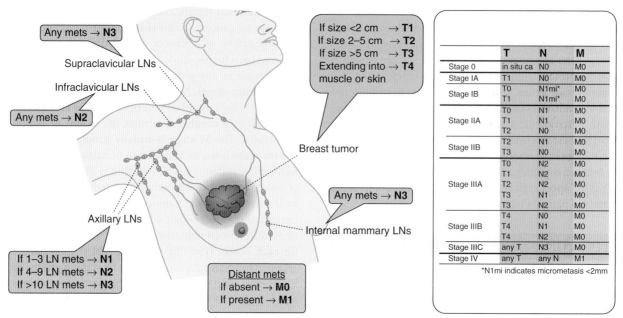

FIGURE 5–19 The pathologic tumor–node–metastasis (TNM) staging system for breast cancer is shown here in its simplest form, according to the AJCC seventh edition from 2010. (A new 2018 edition is pending.) The detailed staging manual defines many more subdivisions of the T and N stages (eg, T1a, T1b), as well as a clinical staging system. Similar staging systems are defined for all types of solid-tumor cancer.

de-differentiation is the most common category and reflects how much the biologic behavior of the cancer cell has departed from its normal cellular ancestor. Poorly differentiated cancers may have no resemblance to their tissue of origin at all. Another category is the quality of nuclear chromatin, which, if significantly altered, can reflect highly aggressive biologic behavior. Another category is a quantitative assessment of the proliferative rate, typically in the form of number of observed mitoses within a predefined area. For the management of some cancers, the assessment of grade has only modest value, whereas for other cancers, the assessment of grade is critical for management decisions. For example, in the management of early-stage prostate cancer, the grading system used, the Gleason grading system, is absolutely critical (Figure 5–20). This system is named after the pathologist who developed it in the 1960s, and it is now universally used by pathologists and clinicians today to estimate mortality risk in early-stage prostate cancer and to assist in making treatment decisions.

Personalized Definitions of Cancer

While describing the cancer affecting a patient by its type, stage, and grade establishes a context that provides considerable prognostic information, there remains considerable heterogeneity in disease biology. There can be vast differences in the behavior and treatment responsiveness of the disease among different patients. Additional information in the form of receptor markers (for breast cancers), MSI status (for colon cancers), karyotypes (for many blood cancers), and other biomarkers is used in various diseases to predict disease behavior with even more precision. However, it is understood that disease heterogeneity is potentially infinite in scope; in fact, every

single patient with cancer has a different, unique disease. An ideal of clinical oncology is to characterize the attributes of each patient's tumor to such a degree that it defines the unique identity of that individual's disease. This has become the principal goal of the current era, often labelled "personalized medicine," "precision medicine," or "genomic medicine." A number of technologies are available and many others are in development to characterize a tumor in more depth, including full genomic sequencing, full RNA transcriptomic analysis, and multiplex proteomic analysis. While such technologies to deeply annotate a single tumor are currently available, the predictive and prognostic information they provide to enable the physician to make reliable treatment decisions is still very primitive. Currently, however, a number of commercial tumor genomic and tumor transcriptomic assays are in use, and they are becoming increasingly adopted by clinical oncologists. It is distinctly possible that the molecular definition of a cancer will eventually replace both stage and grade as the principal basis for planning its treatment.

CHECKPOINT

53. What are the three categories involved in staging solid-tumor cancers?
54. What is the system used for grading prostate cancer?

HEMATOLOGIC NEOPLASMS

Hematologic neoplasms are malignancies of cells derived from hematopoietic precursors. The true hematopoietic stem cell

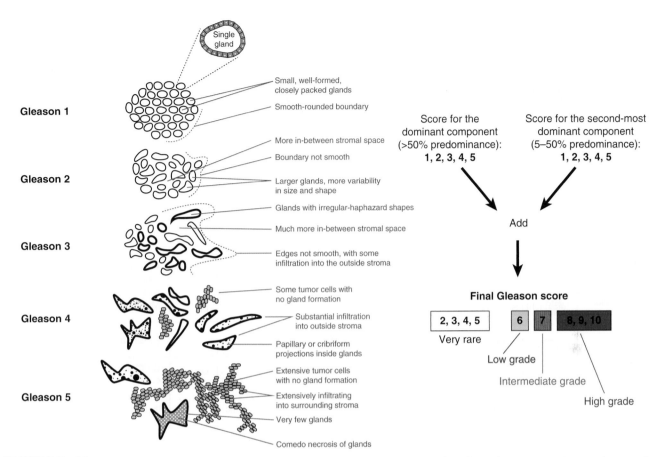

FIGURE 5-20 The Gleason grading system for prostate cancers. The system is largely based on the uniformity, compactness, shape, and infiltrating features of the malignant glandular structures. Specific morphologic features are used to define scores from 1 to 5. Tumors are often heterogeneous in appearance; in such cases, the two most predominant patterns are scored and combined into a single final score from 2 to 10.

has the capacity for self-renewal and the ability to give rise to precursors (**colony-forming units**) that proliferate and terminally differentiate toward one of any lineage (Figure 5–21). Distinct hematologic neoplasms can arise from each of the cell types along the differentiation process. Many of these arise in the bone marrow, circulate in the bloodstream, and can infiltrate certain organs and tissues. Others may form tumors in lymphoid tissue, particularly lymphomas, which arise from lymphoblasts. The lineage of a hematopoietic cell and the degree of differentiation along that lineage are associated with the cell surface expression of characteristic proteins, many of which are receptors, others adhesion molecules and proteases, and still others of unknown function. These clusters of differentiation (CD) antigens have become essential diagnostic tools in the management of hematologic neoplasms, and some types of malignancy are defined by characteristic CD expression patterns.

The cellular ultrastructure and machinery of the malignant cell can somewhat resemble those of its cell of origin. A markedly enhanced proliferative rate and arrest of differentiation are the hallmarks of these neoplasms. Examination of the interphase nucleus of cells, an analysis called cytogenetics, can sometimes reveal chromosomal abnormalities such as

deletions (monosomy), duplications (trisomy), or balanced translocations. Certain types of hematologic neoplasms tend to have stereotypic chromosomal abnormalities. Given their clonal nature, these abnormalities will be evident on all malignant cells. In some cases of chromosomal translocation, a new fusion gene is formed and can result in the production of a fusion protein possessing abnormal function compared with the original gene products (Table 5–11). This function usually involves loss of cell cycle control, abnormal signal transduction, or reprogrammed gene expression as a result of an aberrant transcription factor. In contrast to solid tumors, many hematologic malignancies are specifically linked to certain chromosomal translocations; therefore, karyotype studies are essential in the diagnosis of hematologic malignancies. Other genetic changes described in hematologic malignancies include mutations or deletions of the *p53*, retinoblastoma (*Rb*), and Wilms tumor (*WT1*) suppressor genes and the activation of mutations in the *N-ras* oncogene. Additional genetic changes can be detected in the clonal evolution of leukemias as disease progresses to a more aggressive form in the patient's course. This finding lends further support to the theory that neoplasia is the result of stepwise genetic alterations that correspond to the sequential acquisition of additional phenotypic

FIGURE 5–21 Classification of leukemias according to cell type and lineage. (Redrawn, with permission, from Chandrasoma P et al. *Concise Pathology*, 3rd ed. Originally published by Appleton & Lange. Copyright © 1998 by The McGraw-Hill Companies, Inc.)

TABLE 5–11   Chromosomal translocations of hematologic neoplasms.

Neoplasm	Chromosomal Translocation	Fusion Gene Resulting from Translocation	Fusion Protein Function
Follicular lymphoma	t(14;18)	IgH-*bcl*-2	Inhibitor of apoptosis
Mantle cell lymphoma	t(11;14)	IgH-*bcl*-1	Cyclin
Follicular lymphoma	t(14;19)	IgH-*bcl*-3	Transcription repressor
Diffuse large-cell lymphoma	t(3;14)	IgH/K/L-*bcl*-6	Transcription repressor
Burkitt lymphoma	t(8;14)	IgH-*myc*	Transcription factor
Anaplastic large T-/null-cell lymphoma	t(2;5)	*NPM-ALK*	Tyrosine kinase
CML	t(9;22)	*bcr-abl*	Tyrosine kinase
AML M3	t(15;17)	*PML-RAR*	Transcription factor
AML	t(8;21)	*AML1*	Transcription factor
T-cell ALL	t(1;14)	*tal*-1-TCR	Transcription factor

ALL, acute lymphocytic leukemia; AML, acute myelogenous leukemia; CML, chronic myelogenous leukemia; IgH, immunoglobulin heavy chain enhancer; RAR, retinoic acid receptor; TCR, T-cell receptor.

changes that favor abnormal growth, invasion, and resistance to normal host defenses.

1. Lymphoid Neoplasms

Lymphoid neoplasms consist of B-cell, T-cell, or natural killer (NK) cell types. The malignant cells arise from mature and immature B or T cells at different stages of normal maturation. In general, leukemias are derived from immature lymphocytes, lymphomas from mature lymphocytes, and plasma cell (formerly "multiple") myeloma and related neoplasms from plasma cells (terminally differentiated B lymphocytes).

Acute lymphocytic leukemia (ALL) is a rapidly progressive neoplasm derived from immature lymphocytes named lymphoblasts, which overtake the bone marrow and sometimes infiltrate other organs. Genetic events are common in ALL, and these are linked with biological outcome and used for prognostication. The previous morphologic classification of ALL, used for many years, is now being revised in favor of classification according to B-cell or T-cell lineage and encompassing the spectrum of cytogenetic abnormalities. A distinct genetic alteration, the Philadelphia chromosome [t(9;22)], which is almost universal in CML, can also be seen in some cases of ALL, but its biological role may be different from that in CML because the targeted therapies that block it in ALL are not as effective as they are in CML.

Malignant lymphomas are a diverse group of cancers that result from neoplastic proliferation of mature B or T lymphocytes. These tumors may arise anywhere in the body, most commonly within lymph nodes and occasionally in bone marrow and other organs in which lymphoid elements reside. One subtype of lymphoma composed of malignant cells in a mixture of benign inflammatory cell types with a unique biology is called Hodgkin lymphoma. Hodgkin lymphoma is distinguished by the presence of giant Reed–Sternberg cells of B-cell lineage, which are considered the malignant cells in this neoplasm. The Reed–Sternberg cell constitutes only 1–10% of the total number of cells in pathologic specimens from patients with this disease. It is associated with the infiltration of nonneoplastic inflammatory cells.

All other types of lymphoma are referred to as non-Hodgkin lymphomas. Several factors are associated with their development. These include congenital or acquired immunodeficiency states such as AIDS or iatrogenic immunosuppression (eg, in organ transplantation). Virus infections are associated with some types. For example, most cases of Burkitt lymphoma that occur in Africa (endemic form) are associated with Epstein–Barr virus (EBV) infection (although Burkitt lymphomas that occur in temperate zones are associated with EBV in only 30% of cases). Human T-cell leukemia/lymphoma virus I (HTLV-I) plays a causative role in the genesis of adult T-cell leukemia/lymphoma, and the malignant cells contain the integrated virus. Human herpesvirus-8 (HHV-8) is associated with body cavity–based lymphoma, a rare B-cell lymphoma that occurs predominantly in patients with HIV infection. Chronic immune stimulation may be a causal mechanism in the development of lymphomas as well. For example, chronic gastritis secondary to *Helicobacter pylori* infection may give rise to gastric mucosa–associated lymphoid tissue (MALT) lymphomas. Indeed, resolution of gastric MALT lymphoma may occur in the majority of patients with localized disease who are treated with antibiotics effective against *H pylori*.

The classification of lymphomas has evolved over several decades, as their distinguishing molecular characteristics have been better characterized. The latest classification was devised in 2016 by an international group of lymphoma specialists for the World Health Organization. This scheme characterizes non-Hodgkin lymphomas according to their B-cell or T-cell origin using a combination of criteria: clinical and morphologic features, immunoreactivity with monoclonal antibodies that recognize surface antigens, and specific molecular characteristics including expression of certain genes and characteristic genetic alterations including gene rearrangements and gene mutations. Additionally, precursor-undifferentiated B-cell and T-cell lymphoblastic lymphomas are in a separate class from the more mature B-cell and T-cell lymphomas. Most non-Hodgkin lymphomas originate in B cells and express a B-cell marker, CD20, on their surface. Their monoclonal origin can be inferred by characterization of the specific class of light chain they express. Kappa and lambda B-cell lymphomas are further classified as malignant expansions of cells from the germinal center, mantle zone, or marginal zone of normal lymph nodes. The mature B-cell non-Hodgkin lymphoma classification encompasses more than 20 classes (and smaller subtypes within some of these classes).

Somatic gene rearrangements occur normally during B-cell and T-cell differentiation to form a B-cell or T-cell receptor that serves as a unique identifier for each tumor cell. The B-cell receptor is composed of the immunoglobulin heavy and light chains, both of which are composed of constant and variable regions. The genes for the variable and constant regions of the B-cell receptor are discontinuous in the B-cell germline DNA but are combined by somatic rearrangement to produce a functional antibody molecule. The T-cell receptor gene is analogous to the immunoglobulin molecule in that discontinuous segments of this gene also undergo somatic rearrangement early in T-cell development. Polymerase chain reaction (PCR) and flow cytometry are two common techniques to recognize B-cell or T-cell receptors on each lymphocyte. These techniques allow separation of monoclonal malignant lymphocytes from normal (polyclonal) lymphocytes. DNA hybridization by Southern blot analysis is another technique that permits recognition of a band of electrophoretic mobility that serves as a "fingerprint" for a monoclonal population of lymphoma cells.

Many non-Hodgkin lymphomas exhibit karyotypic abnormalities. The most prevalent translocations include t(8;14), t(14;18), and t(11;14) (see Table 5–11). Each translocation involves an oncogene with the immunoglobulin heavy-chain gene locus at chromosome 14q32. Identification and cloning of the breakpoints have identified 8q24 as *c-myc*, 18q21 as *bcl-2*, and 11q13 as *bcl-1*. The proximity of these oncogenes to the immunoglobulin gene results in deregulation and increased expression of the oncogene product.

Representative subtypes of non-Hodgkin lymphoma include the indolent lymphomas, such as follicular and marginal zone lymphomas, and the aggressive lymphomas, such as mantle cell, diffuse large-cell, and Burkitt lymphomas.

Follicular lymphomas are low-grade tumors that may be insidious in their presentation and clinical course. The translocation t(14;18)(q32;q21) is found in more than 90% of follicular lymphomas. Mutation of the *bcl-2* oncogene that codes for the bcl-2 protein, which blocks apoptosis when overexpressed, results in its overexpression by these cells. In patients whose lymphomas harbor this translocation, the absence of bcl-2 translocation as assessed by the highly sensitive polymerase chain reaction test may be a marker for complete remission status. Spontaneous regression of lymph node size is common in patients with follicular lymphomas. However, follicular lymphomas are not curable with standard chemotherapy, and although patients with it tend to have an indolent clinical course, transformation to a more aggressive grade of lymphoma occurs in 40–50% of them by 10 years.

An important subtype of marginal zone lymphomas are the MALT lymphomas, which may originate in the stomach, lungs, skin, parotid gland, thyroid, breasts, or other extranodal sites, where they characteristically align themselves with epithelial cells. As noted, there is a close association between gastric MALT lymphomas and *H pylori* infection.

Another indolent B-cell neoplasm is chronic lymphocytic leukemia (CLL) (and its lymphoma equivalent, small lymphocyte lymphoma [SLL]). These are neoplasms of mature B cells. CLL is the most common leukemia in adults. Because CLL results in increased numbers of lymphocytes in the peripheral blood that may not exhibit morphologic abnormalities, assays of clonality are essential in its diagnosis. The disease involves expansion of a neoplastic clone, and clonality can be easily assayed by the exclusively expressed antibody light chains normally present in B cells. CLL and SLL are actually the same disease; they differ only in where the neoplastic cells accumulate—predominantly in the blood and bone marrow in CLL, and in the lymph nodes and bone marrow in SLL.

In contrast to indolent lymphomas, diffuse large B-cell lymphoma, mantle-cell lymphoma, and Burkitt lymphoma have aggressive clinical courses but are curable diseases. Mantle-cell lymphoma presents histologically as a monotonous population of small- to medium-sized atypical lymphoid cells with irregular nuclear outlines and arrayed in a nodular or diffuse pattern. The diagnosis of mantle-cell lymphoma is based on morphologic criteria with confirmation by monoclonal antibody staining against cyclin D1 (bcl-1) and SOX11. The t(11;14) translocation found in 90% of cases of mantle-cell lymphoma results in juxtaposition of the *PRAD1* gene on chromosome 11 with the immunoglobulin heavy chain gene on chromosome 14. This results in overexpression of the *PRAD1* gene product, cyclin D1. Cyclin D1 binds to and activates cyclin-dependent kinases, which are thought to facilitate cell cycle progression through the G1 phase. This disease occurs more commonly

among older males and presents with adenopathy and hepatosplenomegaly. Mantle-cell lymphomas are significantly more resistant to treatment with combination chemotherapy than follicular lymphomas. They also are incurable.

Diffuse large-cell lymphoma is the most prevalent subtype of non-Hodgkin lymphoma in adults. One-third of patients present with lymphoma involvement of extranodal sites, particularly the head and neck, stomach, skin, bone, testis, and nervous system. Diffuse large B-cell lymphomas commonly harbor mutations or rearrangements of the *BCL6* gene.

Virtually all cases of Burkitt lymphoma are associated with alterations of chromosome 8q24, resulting in overexpression of *c-myc*, an oncogene that encodes a transcriptional regulator of cell proliferation, differentiation, and apoptosis. Adults with Burkitt lymphoma who present with high tumor burdens and elevated serum lactate dehydrogenase levels have a poor prognosis. The high tumor burden may be associated with a hypermetabolic state that can be triggered by treatment as the tumor undergoes sudden lysis. This tumor lysis syndrome can cause life-threatening hyperkalemia, hyperphosphatemia, hyperuricemia, and hypocalcemia.

Like mature B-cell lymphomas, T-cell lymphomas are a group of heterogeneous diseases with many subtypes. Anaplastic large-cell lymphoma is characterized by the proliferation of highly atypical cells that express the CD30 antigen. These tumors have a T-cell phenotype, and more than 50% of cases are associated with the chromosomal translocation t(2;5)(p23;q35), resulting in the nucleophosmin-anaplastic lymphoma kinase (NPM-ALK) fusion protein. Activation of the ALK receptor tyrosine kinase results in an unregulated mitogenic signal.

Another type of T-cell lymphoma is the adult T-cell leukemia/lymphoma, an aggressive disease associated with HTLV-I infection characterized by generalized adenopathy, polyclonal hypergammaglobulinemia, hypercalcemia, and lytic bone lesions.

Plasma Cell ("Multiple") Myeloma

Plasma cell myeloma (formerly "multiple myeloma") is a special type of lymphoid neoplasm that results from malignant proliferation of terminally differentiated B cells (plasma cells) that secrete a monoclonal immunoglobulin called the M protein. Almost all cases of myelomas are preceded by a pre-malignant condition called monoclonal gammopathy of undetermined significance (MGUS). MGUS is, by definition, an asymptomatic, benign condition. But some patients with MGUS do produce a small amount of the monoclonal immunoglobulin M protein. MGUS is quite prevalent, found in 3% of the general population older than 50 years of age. MGUS and myeloma also share certain genetic abnormalities, supporting the notion that myeloma evolves from MGUS. It appears that MGUS progresses to myeloma at a constant rate of about 1% per year. Thus, the pathogenesis of plasma cell myeloma appears to be a two-step process: establishment of the premalignant condition, MGUS, followed by progression to the malignant disease, myeloma.

MGUS appears to result from a variety of cytogenetic abnormalities. For example, approximately half of MGUS cases are found to have chromosome translocation involving the immunoglobulin heavy chain IgH on chromosome 14. In the other half of cases, an increased number of chromosomes (hyperdiploidy) is found. In 40% of myeloma cases, translocation of chromosome 14 brings IgH into juxtaposition with one or more of five oncogenes, leading to overexpression of these oncogenes. Hyperdiploidy is another mechanism to overexpress certain genes important in generating clonal plasma cells in MGUS. Only a small percentage of MGUS will ever progress to myeloma. The constant annual rate of progression from MGUS to myeloma seems to suggest that this progression is instigated by a "random second hit" rather than an accumulation of "hits." The events that can serve as the "second hit" include additional genetic changes, dysregulation of proliferation, and/or apoptosis and alteration of tumor microenvironment, among others.

Myeloma cells present a unique challenge among cancers. Since they are neoplasms of immunoglobulin-secreting plasma cells, they place a heavy burden on cell homeostatic mechanisms. The secretion of immunoglobulins proceeds along the secretory pathway and requires their synthesis at the ribosomes, proper folding and maturation by molecular chaperones within the endoplasmic reticulum, and ultimate transport to the membrane for export. When the volume of protein secretion exceeds the capacity of the endoplasmic reticulum to properly fold and maintain them, unfolded or misfolded proteins accumulate. Such dysfunctional proteins are sticky; when they aggregate, they disrupt endoplasmic reticulum function, a condition referred to as **endoplasmic reticulum stress** (Figure 5–22). Endoplasmic reticulum stress is detected by specific receptors in the endoplasmic reticulum membrane that function to activate a response mechanism called the **unfolded protein response**. The unfolded protein response exerts many effects to reduce ER stress, including slowing protein translation, slowing cell proliferation, increasing the expression of chaperone proteins and improving protein quality control, inducing the degradation of unfolded proteins, and inducing autophagy, the process by which cellular debris and organelles are digested within lysosomes. If these adaptational responses are unable to sufficiently relieve endoplasmic reticulum stress, the unfolded protein response can alternatively activate apoptosis. The pathogenesis of myeloma frequently involves the activation of the unfolded protein response to enable the neoplastic plasma cells to cope with the high secretory demand in addition to the many metabolic and energetic challenges associated with neoplastic growth. Although some of the effects of the unfolded protein response are beneficial to them, other physiologic effects, including anti-proliferative, anti-synthetic, and pro-apoptotic effects, are detrimental to them. As such, myeloma cells "walk a fine line" in activating the unfolded protein response. We are only now beginning to understand how the unfolded protein response is altered in myeloma cells to enable them to procure its benefits but escape its detriments. To accomplish this, a number of the genes involved in the unfolded protein response are mutated in myeloma plasma cells. Manipulating the unfolded protein response has been one of the most effective strategies in the pharmacologic treatment of myeloma. For example, inhibiting the proteasome in myeloma cells eliminates one of their adaptational mechanisms, increasing endoplasmic reticulum stress beyond their capacity for adaptation and leading to apoptosis.

2. Myeloid Neoplasms

Myeloid neoplasms are derived from hematopoietic precursors. Depending on the precise step in hematopoiesis that is disrupted by the molecular genetic abnormalities, the cellular expansion can involve cells with features resembling any phase of myelocytic maturation. These cells can be cytologically normal or dysplastic. Myeloid neoplasms are broadly divided into three groups: myeloproliferative neoplasms, myelodysplastic syndromes, and acute myelogenous leukemia (AML). Myeloproliferative neoplasms are marked by proliferation of one or more of the myeloid lineages, such as granulocytes, erythroid cells, and megakaryocytes. Myelodysplastic syndromes are characterized by both the proliferation and apoptosis of hematopoietic cells; affected patients usually present with a hypercellular bone marrow but cytopenias in the peripheral bloodstream. AML is a rapidly progressive neoplasm derived from hematopoietic precursors, or myeloid stem cells, that give rise to granulocytes, monocytes, erythrocytes, and platelets. There are several lines of evidence that genetic events occurring early in stem cell maturation can lead to leukemia. First, there is a lag time of 5–10 years in the development of leukemia after exposure to known causative agents such as chemotherapy, radiation, and certain solvents. Second, many cases of secondary leukemia evolve out of a prolonged "preleukemic phase," manifested as a **myelodysplastic syndrome** of hypoproduction with abnormal maturation without actual malignant behavior. Finally, examination of precursor cells at a stage earlier than the malignant expanded clone in any given type of leukemia can reveal genetic abnormalities such as monosomy or trisomy of different chromosomes. Additional genetic changes can be found in the malignant clone compared with the morphologically normal stem cell that developmentally precedes it.

Acute myelogenous leukemias have been traditionally classified by morphology and cytochemical staining, as shown in Table 5–12. **Auer rods** are crystalline cytoplasmic inclusion bodies characteristic of, though not uniformly seen in, all myeloid (but not lymphoid) leukemias. In contrast to mature myeloid cells, leukemic cells have large immature nuclei with open chromatin and prominent nucleoli. The appearance of the individual cell types of AML mirrors the cell type from which they derive. M1 leukemias originate from early myeloid precursors with no apparent maturation toward any terminal myeloid cell type. This is apparent in the lack of granules or other features that mark more mature myeloid cells. M3 leukemias are a neoplasm of promyelocytes, precursors

FIGURE 5-22 The secretory pathway ensures proper translation, folding, and protein secretion through the endoplasmic reticulum (ER) and Golgi apparatus. When protein secretion is taking place at a high output, such as in myeloma cells, the secretory machinery may not be able to keep up with the volume. This can result in unfolded or misfolded proteins accumulating in the ER, which can aggregate and disrupt ER function. This is called ER stress and is sensed by the three receptors, IRE1, PERK, and ATF6, which proceed to activate the unfolded protein response. The unfolded protein response can promote many adaptive responses (shown with pink labels) to enable cells to adapt to the high secretory demand. Alternatively, if the ER stress is beyond the capacity for adaptation, the unfolded protein response can trigger apoptosis. The unfolded protein response is very active in myeloma plasma cells, which are constantly making and secreting immunoglobulins. (ERAD, endoplasmic reticulum–associated degradation.)

of granulocytes, and M3 cells exhibit abundant azurophilic granules typical of normal promyelocytes. M4 leukemias arise from myeloid precursors that can differentiate into granulocytes or monocytes, whereas M5 leukemias derive from precursors already committed to the monocyte lineage. Therefore, M4 and M5 cells both contain the characteristic folded nucleus and gray cytoplasm of monocytes, whereas M4 cells also contain granules of a granulocytic cytochemical staining pattern. M6 and M7 leukemias cannot be readily identified on morphologic grounds, but immunostaining for erythrocytic

proteins is positive in M6 cells, and staining for platelet glycoproteins is apparent in M7 cells.

Before the introduction of molecular genetic techniques, chromosomal deletions, duplications, and balanced translocations had been noted in the leukemic cells of some patients. Cloning of the regions where balanced translocations occur has, in some cases, revealed a preserved translocation site that reproducibly fuses one gene with another, resulting in the production of a new fusion protein. Acute promyelocytes leukemia is marked by the t(15;17) translocation that juxtaposes

TABLE 5–12 Morphologic classification of acute myelogenous leukemias.

M1	Myeloblasts without differentiation
M2	Myeloblasts with some degree of differentiation
M3	Acute promyelocytic leukemia
M4	Acute myelomonocytic leukemia
M5	Acute monocytic leukemia
M6	Erythroleukemia
M7	Megakaryoblastic leukemia

TABLE 5–13 Molecular classification of acute myelogenous leukemias.

Acute myeloid leukemia with recurrent genetic abnormalities
AML with t(8;22); RUNX1-RUNX1T1
AML with inv(16) or t(16;16); CBFB-MYH11
APL with t(15;17); PML-RARA
AML with t(9;11); MLLT3-MLL
AML with t(6;9); DEK-NUP214
AML with inv(3) or t(3;3); RPN1-EVI1
AML (megakaryoblastic) with t(1;22); RBM15-MKL1
Provisional entity; AML with mutated NPM1
Provisional entity; AML with mutated CEBPA
Acute myeloid leukemia with myelodysplastic-related changes
Therapy-related myeloid neoplasms
Acute myeloid leukemia, not otherwise specified
Myeloid sarcoma
Myeloid proliferation related to Down syndrome
Blastic plasmacytoid dendritic cell neoplasms

the *PML* gene with the *RAR-α* gene. *RAR-α* encodes a retinoic acid steroid hormone receptor, and *PML* encodes a transcription factor. The fusion protein possesses novel biologic activity that results in enhanced proliferation and a block of differentiation. Interestingly, administration of all-trans retinoic acid (ATRA) can restore differentiation of leukemic cells and induce a temporary remission of acute promeylocytic leukemia L, supporting the importance of the *RAR-α–PML* fusion protein. Monosomy of chromosome 7 can be seen in leukemias arising out of the myelodysplasia syndrome or in de novo leukemias, and in both cases, this finding is associated with a worse clinical prognosis. Monosomy of chromosome 7 and other serial cytogenetic changes can also be seen with relapse of treated leukemia, a situation characterized by a more aggressive course and resistance to therapy. With increasing knowledge of the various genetic alterations that dominate the behavior, prognosis, and treatment responses of different forms of AML, the classification of this disease is gradually shifting towards a genetic classification scheme (Table 5–13). This reclassification will continue to evolve as new genetic–clinical links are recognized and established.

As hematopoietic neoplasms, acute leukemias involve both abnormal bone marrow and (frequently) abnormal circulating leukemic (blast) cells. Occasionally, extramedullary leukemic infiltrates known as **chloromas** can be seen in other organs and on mucosal surfaces. A marked increase in the number of circulating blasts can sometimes cause vascular obstruction accompanied by hemorrhage and infarction in the cerebral and pulmonary vascular beds. This **leukostasis** results in complications such as stroke, retinal vein occlusion, and pulmonary infarction. In most cases of AML and other leukemias, peripheral blood counts of mature granulocytes, erythrocytes, and platelets are decreased. This is probably due to crowding of the bone marrow by blast cells and the elaboration of inhibitory substances by leukemic cells, or due to alteration of the bone marrow stromal microenvironment and cytokine milieu necessary for normal hematopoiesis. Susceptibility to infections as a result of depressed granulocyte number and function and abnormal bleeding as a result of low platelet counts are common presentations in patients with leukemia.

Chronic myelogenous leukemia (CML) is the most well-known myeloproliferative neoplasm. It is an indolent leukemia manifested by an increased number of immature granulocytes in the marrow and peripheral circulation. One of the hallmarks of CML is the **Philadelphia chromosome**, a cytogenetic feature that is a result of the balanced translocation of chromosomes 9 and 22, resulting in a fusion gene, *bcr-abl*, that encodes a kinase that phosphorylates several key proteins involved in cell growth and apoptosis. CML eventually transforms into acute leukemia (blast crisis), accompanied by further cytogenetic changes. Targeted therapies that inhibit the enzymatic function of the bcr-abl kinase by competing with the ATP-binding site induce remissions in most patients in the chronic phase of CML. Furthermore, resistance to these *bcr-abl* inhibitors can involve amplification of the bcr-abl breakpoint, as well as development (or clonal expansion) of mutations in the ATP-binding pocket of bcr-abl, which prohibit the binding of inhibitors.

THE SYSTEMIC EFFECTS OF NEOPLASIA

Many effects of malignancies are mediated not by the tumor cells themselves but by direct and indirect effects, as outlined in Tables 5–14 and 5–15, respectively. Direct effects (see Table 5–14) include compression or invasion of vital

TABLE 5–14   Direct systemic effects of neoplasms.

Effect	Clinical Syndrome(s)
Vessel compression	Edema, superior vena cava syndrome
Vessel invasion and erosion	Bleeding
Lymphatic invasion	Lymphedema
Nerve invasion	Neuropathic pain, numbness, dysesthesia
Brain metastases	Weakness, numbness, headache, coordination and gait abnormalities, visual changes
Spinal cord compression	Back pain, paralysis, incontinence
Bone invasion and destruction	Pain, fracture
Bowel obstruction and perforation	Nausea, vomiting, pain, ileus
Airway obstruction	Dyspnea, pneumonia, lung volume loss
Ureteral obstruction	Renal failure, urinary infection
Liver invasion and metastases	Hepatic insufficiency
Lung and pleural metastases	Dyspnea, chest pain
Bone marrow infiltration	Pancytopenia, infection, bleeding

structures, such as blood and lymphatic vessels, nerves, spinal cord or brain, bone, airways, GI tract, and urinary tract. These may cause a typical pain pattern, as well as dysfunction of the involved organ and obstruction of a conduit. On occasion, an inflammatory or desmoplastic host response rather than the tumor itself can result in the same effect.

Indirect effects (see Table 5–15) are heterogeneous and poorly understood. Likewise, the onset and clinical course of these effects are unpredictable. When affecting distant targets uninvolved by tumor, they are collectively termed **paraneoplastic syndromes**. Some of these effects are stereotypic syndromes resulting from the elaboration of peptide hormones or cytokines with specific biologic activity, as shown in Table 5–15.

The peptides secreted by a given neoplasm may reflect the tissue of origin or may be the result of activation of latent genes not normally expressed. Common examples of paraneoplastic phenomena include the syndrome of inappropriate antidiuretic hormone (SIADH), occurring most often in small-cell lung cancer. The result of ectopic ADH production is retention of free water and hyponatremia, which can result in altered sensorium, coma, and death. Another peptide secreted in small-cell lung cancer is ACTH, which can cause Cushing syndrome from adrenocorticosteroid excess, with skin fragility, central redistribution of body fat, proximal myopathy, and other features. Hypercalcemia can occur in many types of malignancies. It has several causes, including secretion of a parathyroid hormone–like peptide as a result of activation of the parathyroid hormone–related protein gene (*PTHrP*), as well as elaboration of locally acting cytokines that increase bone uptake in areas of tumor infiltration of bone. Some paraneoplastic syndromes, particularly those involving the nervous system, are related to antibodies generated in response to cancer cells that cross-react with normal cells in the nervous system.

In some malignancies, such as NETs, several active peptides may act in concert to produce a constellation of symptoms and tissue effects. Cytokines, such as the interleukins and tumor necrosis factor, may be responsible for tumor-related fevers and weight loss. Some paraneoplastic syndromes are associated with the development of autoantibodies. These can derive from an immune response to tumor-associated antigens or from an inappropriate production of antibody, as can occur in lymphoid neoplasms. Finally, the nucleic acid, cytoplasmic, and membrane products of cell breakdown can result in electrolyte and other metabolic abnormalities, as well as coagulopathic disorders, resulting in clotting or bleeding.

CHECKPOINT

55. What are the hallmarks of hematologic malignancies?
56. What are some characteristics of low-grade lymphomas?
57. What are some characteristics of high-grade lymphomas?

TABLE 5–15   Paraneoplastic syndromes (indirect systemic effects of neoplasms).

Tumor Type	Cause of Indirect Effect	Clinical Syndrome(s)
Effects of Hormone or Peptide Secretion		
Lung	ACTH	Cushing syndrome
Lung, breast, kidney, others	PTH or PTH-related protein	Hypercalcemia
Lung	ADH, ANP	SIADH, hyponatremia
Germ cell, trophoblastic, hepatoblastoma	Gonadotropins (FSH, LH, β-hCG)	Gynecomastia, precocious puberty
Lung, gastric	Growth hormone	Acromegaly
Neuroendocrine (eg, carcinoid)	Various vasoactive peptides	Flushing, wheezing, diarrhea
Sarcoma, mesothelioma, insulinoma	Insulin, insulin-like growth factor	Hypoglycemia
Cutaneous Effects		
GI	Unknown	Acanthosis nigricans (hyperkeratosis and hyperpigmentation in skin folds)
GI, lymphoma	Unknown	Leser–Trélat (large seborrheic) keratoses
Lymphoma, hepatoma, melanoma	Melanin deposits	Melanosis (skin darkening)
Lymphoma	Autoantibodies to subepidermal proteins	Skin bullae (blisters)
Myeloid leukemia	Neutrophilic skin infiltrates	Sweet syndrome
Neurologic Effects		
Lung, prostate, colorectal, ovarian, cervical, others	Unknown	Subacute cerebellar degeneration
Lung, testicular, Hodgkin lymphoma	Unknown	Limbic encephalitis
Lung	Unknown	Dementia
Lung, others	Unknown	Amyotrophic lateral sclerosis
Lung, others	Unknown	Peripheral sensory or sensorimotor neuropathy
Lymphoma	Unknown, possible autoantibodies	Ascending radiculopathy (Guillain–Barré syndrome)
Lung, GI	Autoantibodies to voltage-gated Ca^{2+} channels	Eaton–Lambert (myasthenia-like) syndrome
Hematologic and Coagulopathic Effects		
Several	Unknown	Anemia
Adenocarcinomas (especially gastric)	Unknown	Microangiopathic hemolytic anemia
Several	Interleukin-1, -3, and hematopoietic growth factors	Granulocytosis
Hodgkin lymphoma, others	Eosinophilic hematopoietic growth factors	Eosinophilia
Several	Unknown	Thrombocytosis
Adenocarcinomas (especially pancreatic), others	Unknown, possible exposed phospholipids from cell membranes	Thrombosis
Adenocarcinoma (especially prostate)	Urokinase, other mediators of fibrinolysis	Disseminated intravascular coagulation
Metabolic Effects		
Various	Interleukin-1, tumor necrosis factor	Cachexia, anorexia
Lymphoma, others	Interleukins-1, -6	Fever
Hematologic neoplasms	Hypermetabolism/cell breakdown products	Tumor lysis syndrome: hyperuricemia, hyperkalemia, hyperphosphatemia, hypocalcemia
Lymphoma, others	Tumor hypoxia	Lactic acidosis

ACTH, adrenocorticotropic hormone; ADH, antidiuretic hormone (arginine vasopressin); ANP, atrial natriuretic protein; FSH, follicle-stimulating hormone; GI, gastrointestinal; β-hCG, human chorionic gonadotropin; LH, luteinizing hormone; PTH, parathyroid hormone; SIADH, syndrome of inappropriate secretion of antidiuretic hormone.

CASE STUDIES

Yeong Kwok, MD

(See Chapter 25, p. 749–51 for Answers)

CASE 18

A 54-year-old man presents with several weeks of facial flushing and diarrhea. His symptoms began intermittently but are becoming more constant. A 24-hour urine collection reveals an elevated level of 5-hydroxyindoleacetic acid (5-HIAA), a metabolite of serotonin. An abdominal CT scan shows a 2 cm mesenteric mass in the ileum and likely metastatic tumors in the liver.

Questions

A. This patient has the malignant carcinoid syndrome. From what type of tissue do carcinoid tumors arise, and how does this account for the body site where they first appear?

B. What accounts for the frequent association of systemic symptoms, the so-called carcinoid syndrome, with carcinoid tumors?

C. Why is the 24-hour urine collection for 5-HIAA useful in the diagnosis of carcinoid syndrome?

CASE 19

A 54-year-old man presents to the clinic for a routine check-up. He is well, with no physical complaints. The history is remarkable only for a father with colon cancer at age 55 years. Physical examination is normal. Cancer screening is discussed, and the patient is sent home with fecal occult blood testing supplies and scheduled for a colonoscopy. The fecal occult blood test results are positive. The colonoscopy reveals a villous adenoma and a 2 cm carcinoma.

Questions

A. How are the two lesions—adenoma and carcinoma—thought to be related?

B. What are the two principal lines of evidence in favor of such a model?

C. Describe the genetic alterations in the stepwise progression of colon cancer and the phenotypic changes associated with these alterations.

D. What is the explanation for the presence of occult blood in stools of patients with early colorectal cancer?

CASE 20

A 40-year-old woman presents for the evaluation of a left-sided breast lump. She does have a strongly positive family history, with her mother and one older sister both having had breast cancer. Physical examination is notable for a 2 cm lump in the left breast. A biopsy shows invasive ductal carcinoma. The tumor is positive for estrogen receptor expression and *HER2* gene amplification.

Questions

A. What genetic factors may have been involved in this patient's risk for developing breast cancer?

B. What are the two major subtypes of breast cancer?

C. Describe the distinction between invasive breast cancer and carcinoma in situ.

D. How is our knowledge of the tumor receptors used in the treatment of breast cancer?

CASE 21

A 25-year-old man presents with a complaint of testicular enlargement. Examination reveals a hard nodule on the left testicle, 2 cm in diameter. Orchiectomy is diagnostic of testicular cancer.

Questions

A. From what cellular elements of the testes does testicular cancer generally arise? What is the normal development of these cells?
B. In addition to the testes, where else might testicular cancer arise? What is the explanation for this distribution?
C. What serum markers might be monitored to evaluate disease progression and response to therapy?

CASE 22

A 16-year-old previously healthy teenager presents with a 2-month history of pain and swelling of his knee. He thought it began after a soccer game, but it has not gotten better. Physical examination shows marked swelling of the knee and the distal thigh. Radiographs show a 3 cm partially calcified mass in the distal femur, just above the knee joint. A biopsy reveals an osteosarcoma.

Questions

A. From which tissues do sarcomas arise?
B. Why are many sarcomas more common in children, adolescents, and young adults than in older adults?
C. What accounts for the calcifications that can be seen in osteosarcomas?

CASE 23

A 28-year-old woman presents to her primary care physician with complaints of fatigue, intermittent fevers, and 5 pounds of weight loss over a 6-week period. Her medical history is remarkable for a renal transplantation at age 15 years performed for end-stage renal disease as a result of post-streptococcal glomerulonephritis. Physical examination reveals two enlarged, matted, nontender lymph nodes in the left anterior cervical chain; a firm, nontender 1.5 cm lymph node in the right groin; and an enlarged liver. Biopsy of the lymph nodes in the cervical region reveals follicular, cleaved-cell lymphoma.

Questions

A. One theory states that chronic immune stimulation or modulation may be an early step in lymphomagenesis. What observations support this view?
B. How would one classify this patient's lymphoma? What are some characteristics of this grade of lymphoma?
C. From which cell line do follicular lymphomas originate? What are some of the common genetic mutations seen with this type of lymphoma? How might one of these mutations contribute to the formation of lymphoma?
D. What is the pathophysiologic mechanism causing this patient's fever and weight loss?

CASE 24

A 22-year-old woman presents with a 2-week history of fatigue, bleeding from her gums, and very heavy menstrual bleeding. Physical examination reveals a pale woman with an enlarged spleen and petechiae on her legs. A complete blood cell count shows a markedly elevated white cell count (WBC 178,000) with severe anemia (hemoglobin 7.8) and thrombocytopenia (platelet count 25,000). Blast cells (abnormally immature leukemic cells) comprise 30% of the total white cell count. A bone marrow biopsy is positive for AML of the M1 type.

Questions

A. How are leukemias classified in general? More specifically, how are AMLs classified?
B. What accounts for the patient's symptoms and physical findings? What other major symptoms or signs may be present?
C. What types of genetic abnormalities are responsible for the development of leukemias? How can this knowledge be used to treat some leukemias?

CASE 25

A 64-year-old man is brought to the emergency room by his family for evaluation of mental status changes. They noticed that he was becoming somewhat confused the day before presentation, describing him as "just not acting like his usual self." That morning, he was barely arousable and even more confused. He had previously been feeling a bit tired but was otherwise without complaint except for a nagging cough. He had had no falls or head trauma. He had a greater than 50-pack-year smoking history and currently smokes one pack per day. A chest x-ray shows a 3 cm mass in his right upper lung field. Blood chemistries show a serum calcium level of 14 mg/dL. A computed tomography scan of the head is normal.

Questions

A. What is the likely cause of the patient's mental status changes?
B. What can explain the high serum calcium level?
C. What is another possible electrolyte abnormality found in individuals with malignancy that can also lead to a decreased level of consciousness?

REFERENCES

General

DeVita VT et al. *Cancer: Principles and Practice of Oncology*, 10th ed. Lippincott Williams & Wilkins, 2014.
Hanahan D et al. Hallmarks of cancer: the next generation. Cell. 2011 Mar 4;144(5):646–74. [PMID: 21376230]
Mendelsohn J et al. *The Molecular Basis of Cancer*, 4th ed. WB Saunders, 2014.

Cancer Genetics and Epigenetics

Corces MR et al. The three-dimensional cancer genome. Curr Opin Genet Dev. 2016 Feb;36:1–7. [PMID: 26855137]
Dawson MA. The cancer epigenome: concepts, challenges, and therapeutic opportunities. Science. 2017 Mar 17;355(6330):1147–52. [PMID: 28302822]
Jeggo PA et al. DNA repair, genome stability and cancer: a historical perspective. Nat Rev Cancer. 2016;16:35–42. [PMID: 26667849]
Kinnaird A et al. Metabolic control of epigenetics in cancer. Nat Rev Cancer. 2016 Nov;16(11):694–707. [PMID: 27634449]

Koschmann C et al. Mutated chromatin regulatory factors as tumor drivers in cancer. Cancer Res. 2017 Jan 15;77(2):227–33. [PMID: 28062403]
Martincorena I et al. Somatic mutation in cancer and normal cells. Science. 2015 Sep 25;349(6255):1483–9. [PMID: 26404825]
Torgovnick A et al. DNA repair mechanisms in cancer development and therapy. Front Genet. 2015 Apr 23;6:157. [PMID: 25954303]

Cancer Metabolism

DeBerardinis RJ et al. Fundamentals of cancer metabolism. Sci Adv. 2016 May 27;2(5):e1600200. [PMID: 27386546]
Pavlova NN et al. The emerging hallmarks of cancer metabolism. Cell Metab. 2016 Jan 12;23(1):27–47. [PMID: 26771115]

Tumor Stroma and Host Factors

Bhome R et al. A top-down view of the tumor microenvironment: structure, cells and signaling. Front Cell Dev Biol. 2015 May 29;3:33. [PMID: 26075202]
Rajaqapala SV et al. The human microbiome and cancer. Cancer Prev Res (Phila). 2017 Apr;10(4):226–34. [PMID: 28096237]

Turley SJ et al. Immunological hallmarks of stromal cells in the tumour microenvironment. Nat Rev Immunol. 2015 Nov;15(11):669–82. [PMID: 26471778]

Weis SM et al. Tumor angiogenesis: molecular pathways and therapeutic targets. Nat Med. 2011 Nov 7;17(11):1359–70. [PMID: 22064426]

Tumor Heterogeneity and Stem Cells

Brown DV et al. Insights into the next generation of cancer stem cell research. Front Biosci. 2014 Jun 1;19:1015–27. [PMID: 24896333]

Kreso A et al. Evolution of the cancer stem cell model. Cell Stem Cell. 2014 Mar 6;14(3):275–91. [PMID: 24607403]

McGranahan N et al. Clonal heterogeneity and tumor evolution: past, present, and the future. Cell. 2017 Feb 9;168(4):613–28. [PMID: 28187284]

Tumor Immunology

Chen DS et al. Elements of cancer immunity and the cancer-immune set point. Nature. 2017 Jan 18;541(7637):321–30. [PMID: 28102259]

Munn LL. Cancer and inflammation. Wiley Interdiscip Rev Syst Biol Med. 2017 Mar;9(2). [Epub ahead of print] [PMID: 27943646]

Colon Cancer

Gelsomino F et al. The evolving role of microsatellite instability in colorectal cancer: a review. Cancer Treat Rev. 2016 Dec;51:19–26. [PMID: 27838401]

Grady WM et al. The molecular pathogenesis of colorectal cancer and its potential application to colorectal cancer screening. Dig Dis Sci. 2015 Mar;60(3):762–72. [PMID: 25492499]

Mahasneh A et al. Molecular biomarkers for an early diagnosis, effective treatment and prognosis of colorectal cancer: current updates. Exp Mol Pathol. 2017 Jun;102(3):475–83. [PMID: 28506769]

Okugawa Y et al. Epigenetic alterations in colorectal cancer: emerging biomarkers. Gastroenterology. 2015 Oct;149(5):1204–25. [PMID: 26216839]

Sepulveda AR et al. Molecular biomarkers for the evaluation of colorectal cancer: guideline from the American Society for Clinical Pathology, College of American Pathologists, Association for Molecular Pathology, and American Society of Clinical Oncology. J Mol Diagn. 2017 Mar;19(2):187–225. [PMID: 28185757]

Breast Cancer

Afghahi A et al. The changing landscape of genetic testing for inherited breast cancer predisposition. Curr Treat Options Oncol. 2017 May;18(5):27. [PMID: 28439798]

Kleibl Z et al. Women at high risk of breast cancer: molecular characteristics, clinical presentation and management. Breast. 2016 Aug;28:136–44. [PMID: 27318168]

Roulot A et al. Tumoral heterogeneity of breast cancer. Ann Biol Clin (Paris). 2016 Dec 1;74(6):653–60. [PMID: 27848916]

Skol AD et al. The genetics of breast cancer risk in the post-genome era: thoughts on study design to move past BRCA and towards clinical relevance. Breast Cancer Res. 2016 Oct 3;18(1):99. [PMID: 27716388]

Lung Cancer

Chen Z et al. Non-small-cell lung cancers: a heterogeneous set of diseases. Nat Rev Cancer. 2014 Aug;14(8):535–46. [PMID: 25056707]

Kadara H et al. Early events in the molecular pathogenesis of lung cancer. Cancer Prev Res (Phila). 2016 Jul;9(7):518–27. [PMID: 27006378]

Wood SL et al. Molecular histology of lung cancer: from targets to treatments. Cancer Treat Rev. 2015 Apr;41(4):361–75. [PMID: 25825324]

Neuroendocrine Tumors

Kunz PL. Carcinoid and neuroendocrine tumors: building on success. J Clin Oncol. 2015 Jun 1;33(16):1855–63. [PMID: 25918282]

Testicular Cancer and Other Germ Cell Tumors

Gonzalez-Exposito R et al. Molecular biology of testicular germ cell tumors. Clin Transl Oncol. 2016 Jun;18(6):550–6. [PMID 26482724]

Hematologic Neoplasms

Bianchi G et al. Pathogenesis beyond the cancer clone(s) in multiple myeloma. Blood. 2015 May 14;125(20):3049–58. [PMID: 25838343]

De Kouchkovsky J et al. Acute myeloid leukemia: a comprehensive review and 2016 update. Blood Cancer J. 2016 Jul 1;6(7):e441. [PMID: 27367478]

Fabbri G et al. The molecular pathogenesis of chronic lymphocytic leukaemia. Nat Rev Cancer. 2016 Mar;16(3):145–62. [PMID: 26911189]

Hunger SP et al. Redefining ALL classification: toward detecting high-risk ALL and implementing precision medicine. Blood. 2015 Jun 25;125(26):3977–87. [PMID: 25999453]

Nogal H et al. Pathogenesis of non-Hodgkin's lymphoma. J Clin Oncol. 2011 May 10;29(14):1803–11. [PMID: 21483013]

Spivak JL. Myeloproliferative neoplasms. N Engl J Med. 2017 Jun 1;376(22):2168–81. [PMID: 28564565]

Blood Disorders

6

J. Ben Davoren, MD, PhD, & Gerald Hsu, MD, PhD

NORMAL STRUCTURE & FUNCTION

Blood is an extremely complex fluid, composed of both formed elements (red cells, white cells, platelets) and plasma. Red blood cells (**erythrocytes**) are the most common formed elements, carrying oxygen to the cells of the body via their main component, **hemoglobin**. White blood cells are generally present at about 1/700th the number of erythrocytes and function as mediators of immune responses to infection or other stimuli of inflammation. Platelets are the formed elements that participate in coagulation. Plasma is largely water, electrolytes, and plasma proteins. The plasma proteins most important in blood clotting are the coagulation factors. Because blood circulates throughout the body, alterations in normal blood physiology—either formed elements or plasma proteins—may have widespread adverse consequences.

FORMED ELEMENTS OF BLOOD

Anatomy

A. Bone Marrow and Hematopoiesis

Although the mature formed elements of blood are quite different from each other in both structure and function, all of these cells develop from a common hematopoietic **stem cell** population, which resides in the bone marrow. The developmental process is called **hematopoiesis** and represents an enormous metabolic task for the body. More than 100 billion cells are produced every day. This makes the bone marrow one of the most active organs in the body. In adults, most of the active marrow resides in the vertebrae, sternum, and ribs. In children, the marrow is more active in the long bones.

The process of differentiation from stem cell to mature erythrocyte, granulocyte, lymphocyte, monocyte, or platelet is shown in Figure 6–1. It is not clear exactly what early events

lead dividing stem cells down a particular path of development, but many different peptides, called **cytokines**, are clearly involved (Table 6–1; see also Chapter 3). Perhaps because mature white blood cells have a much shorter half-life in the circulation, white blood cell precursors usually outnumber red blood cell precursors by a ratio of 3:1 in the bone marrow.

The major hormone that stimulates the production of **erythrocytes** (**erythropoiesis**) is **erythropoietin**. This peptide is produced by the kidneys and regulates red blood cell production by a feedback system: When blood hemoglobin levels fall (**anemia**), oxygen delivery to the kidneys falls, and the kidneys produce more erythropoietin, causing the marrow to produce more red cells. When hemoglobin levels rise, the kidneys produce less erythropoietin and the marrow fewer red cells.

For white blood cells, the situation is more complex. The most common cells are the **granulocytes**, so named because their cytoplasms are filled with granules. Of these, the neutrophils are the most prevalent and the most important cells in producing inflammation. Granulocyte production (**myelopoiesis**) can be affected by many cytokines at different stages of development. Figure 6–1 shows that interleukin-3 (IL-3), granulocyte colony-stimulating factor (G-CSF), and granulocyte–macrophage colony-stimulating factor (GM-CSF) are the most important. All three proteins have been purified, sequenced, and cloned. The latter two proteins are used therapeutically. Unlike G-CSF, GM-CSF also stimulates the maturation of a different white blood cell line, the **monocyte-macrophage line**. These cells are part of the immune system as well (ie, they ingest foreign bacteria) and can reside in skin and other tissues, not just blood. Their function, along with that of the B- and T-lymphocyte populations, is discussed more fully in Chapter 3.

Platelets are not cells but fragments of larger multinucleated cells in the marrow called **megakaryocytes**. Platelets are

FIGURE 6–1 Hematopoiesis: development of the formed elements of blood from bone marrow stem cells. Cells below the horizontal line are found in normal peripheral blood. The principal cytokines that stimulate each cell lineage to differentiate are shown. (CSF, colony-stimulating factor; EPO, erythropoietin; G, granulocyte; IL, interleukin; M, macrophage; SCF, stem cell factor; TPO, thrombopoietin) See Table 6–1 for details. (Redrawn, with permission, from Ganong WF. *Review of Medical Physiology*, 22nd ed. McGraw-Hill, 2005.)

crucial to normal blood clotting. Platelet production is also stimulated by multiple cytokines but depends mainly on the action of IL-3, IL-6, IL-11, and **thrombopoietin (TPO)**. This peptide is produced by the liver, kidney, skeletal muscle, and marrow stroma. One model of **thrombopoiesis** proposes that the production of TPO occurs at a constant rate. However, the amount of this hormone free to interact with platelet precursors rises and falls, probably as a result of uptake by TPO

receptors (c-Mpl) on existing platelets in the blood. Therefore, a low platelet count (with a lower mass of c-Mpl) stimulates thrombopoiesis as a result of increased circulating levels of TPO. A second model proposes that low platelet levels can induce increased production of TPO in marrow stromal cells via various cytokines, including platelet-derived growth factor (PDGF) and fibroblast growth factor (FGF). These two models are not necessarily mutually exclusive. Inflammation

TABLE 6–1 **Cytokines that regulate hematopoiesis.**

Cytokine	Cell Lines Stimulated	Cytokine Source
IL-1	Erythrocyte Granulocyte Megakaryocyte Monocyte	Multiple cell types
IL-3	Erythrocyte Granulocyte Megakaryocyte Monocyte	T lymphocytes
IL-4	Basophil	T lymphocytes
IL-5	Eosinophil	T lymphocytes
IL-6	Erythrocyte Granulocyte Megakaryocyte Monocyte	Endothelial cells Fibroblasts Macrophages
IL-11	Erythrocyte Granulocyte Megakaryocyte	Fibroblasts Osteoblasts
Erythropoietin	Erythrocyte	Kidney Kupffer cells of liver
SCF	Erythrocyte Granulocyte Megakaryocyte Monocyte	Multiple cell types
G-CSF	Granulocyte	Endothelial cells Fibroblasts Monocytes
GM-CSF	Erythrocyte Granulocyte Megakaryocyte	Endothelial cells Fibroblasts Monocytes T lymphocytes
M-CSF	Monocyte	Endothelial cells Fibroblasts Monocytes
Thrombopoietin	Megakaryocyte	Liver, kidney

CSF, colony-stimulating factor; G, granulocyte; IL, interleukin; M, macrophage; SCF, stem cell factor.

FIGURE 6–2 Normal thin blood smear, seen at low power (40×) with Wright stain. Erythrocytes predominate and can be seen to be thin disks with central pallor (see text). Platelets are the numerous small, dark bodies. Larger cells with lobulated nuclei are mature neutrophils. Lymphocytes and monocytes are not present on this smear.

Examination of the appropriateness of blood cell development is best undertaken with the microscope, using the **thin blood smear** (Figure 6–2). Modern technical equipment, which can optically sort cells by size and various optical reflective parameters, gives important information, especially about whether cell numbers are out of the normal ranges (Table 6–2). However, microscopic examination of the blood smear, usually using Wright stain, gives additional information once an abnormality is detected and should always be done when a blood disorder is suspected on clinical grounds.

Physiology

A. Erythrocytes

Mature red blood cells are biconcave, disk-shaped cells filled with hemoglobin, which function as the oxygen-carrying component of the blood. In contrast to most other cells, they do not have nuclei at maturity; their nuclei are extruded during the final phase of erythrocyte development. The presence of erythrocytes with nuclei in the peripheral blood smear suggests an underlying disease state. Normal red cells are about 8 µm in diameter, a size that is larger than the smallest capillaries. However, their biconcave shape gives them enough

can also lead to thrombocytosis via IL-6-mediated increases in TPO production by the liver.

For all the marrow's complexity and metabolic activity, there is tremendous regulation of the marrow through the interaction of various cytokines. Normally, only the most mature elements in each cell lineage are released into the general circulation, demonstrating this exquisite control over development. Complex negative-feedback mechanisms must be at work to maintain circulating quantities of each formed element at the consistent levels at which they are found.

TABLE 6–2   Normal values obtained on automated blood count—formed elements of blood.

Element	Male Adult	Female Adult
Hemoglobin	14–18 g/dL	12–16 g/dL
Hematocrit (percentage of blood that is erythrocytes)	42–50%	37–47%
Red cell count	$4.6–6 \times 10^6/\mu L$	$4.2–5.4 \times 10^6/\mu L$
Mean corpuscular volume (MCV)	80–100 fL	80–100 fL
White blood cell (total) count	4000–11,000/μL	4000–11,000/μL
Neutrophils	2500–7500/μL	2500–7500/μL
Lymphocytes	1500–3500/μL	1500–3500/μL
Monocytes	200–800/μL	200–800/μL
Eosinophils	60–600/μL	60–600/μL
Basophils	<100/μL	<100/μL
Platelets	150,000– 400,000/μL	150,000– 400,000/μL

flexibility to slip through small capillaries and deliver oxygen to the tissues. Once extruded from the bone marrow, individual erythrocytes function for about 120 days before they are removed from the circulation by the spleen.

In a typical blood smear (stained with Wright stain), erythrocytes dominate the microscopic field, and their biconcave disk shape resembles that of a doughnut. There is a thicker outer rim that appears red owing to the hemoglobin present and an area of central pallor where the disk is thinnest. Young erythrocytes (reticulocytes) appear bluer (basophilic) because they still contain some ribosomes and mitochondria for a few days after the nuclei are extruded.

Hemoglobin is the most important substance in the erythrocyte. This protein is actually a tetramer, made of two α-protein subunits and two β-protein subunits (in normal adult hemoglobin, called hemoglobin A). Each α- or β-subunit contains the actual oxygen-binding portion of the complex, **heme**. Heme is a compound whose centrally important atom is iron; it is this atom that binds oxygen in the lungs and subsequently releases it in the tissues of the body. A low level of hemoglobin in the blood, from a variety of causes (see later discussion), is **anemia**, the most common general blood disorder.

B. Granulocytes: Neutrophils, Eosinophils, and Basophils

The granulocytes are the most common white blood cells; of these, neutrophils are most abundant, followed by eosinophils and basophils (see Table 6–2). Developmentally, all three types are similar: As they mature, their nuclei become more convoluted and multilobed, and each develops a cytoplasm filled with granules. These granules contain a variety of enzymes, prostaglandins, and mediators of inflammation, with specific factors dependent on the cell type. Early progenitor cells for each type of granulocyte ("blasts") are indistinguishable on microscopic examination of the bone marrow, but under the influence of different cytokines, they become morphologically distinct cell types.

Basophils contain very dark blue or purple granules when stained with either Giemsa or Wright stain. Basophil granules are large and usually obscure the nucleus because of their density. Normally, basophils function in hypersensitivity reactions (as described in Chapter 3). However, their numbers can be increased in diseases not associated with hypersensitivity, such as chronic myelogenous leukemia.

Eosinophils contain large, strikingly "eosinophilic" granules (staining red with Wright or Giemsa stain). Eosinophil nuclei are usually bilobed. Normally, eosinophils function as part of the inflammatory response to parasites too large to be engulfed by individual immune cells. They are also involved in some allergic reactions.

Neutrophils contain granules that are "neutrophilic" (ie, neither eosinophilic nor basophilic). Although they predominate in the blood, their major function is actually in the tissues; they must leave the blood by inserting themselves between the endothelial cells of the vasculature to reach sites of injury or infection. Their granules contain highly active enzymes such as **myeloperoxidase**, which, along with the free radical oxygen ions produced by membrane enzymes such as **nicotinamide adenine dinucleotide phosphate (NADPH) oxidase**, kill bacteria that neutrophils ingest via endocytosis or phagocytosis. They are the "first line of defense" against bacterial pathogens, and low numbers of them (leukopenia) lead directly to a high incidence of significant bacterial infections (see later discussion). Of all the cells produced by the bone marrow, the neutrophils comprise the greatest fraction. Their life span in blood, only 8 hours, is much shorter than that of any other cell type. Evidence of their importance and their short survival is commonly manifested, because microscopic examination of a blood smear from a patient with an active infection may show not only increased numbers of mature, multilobed neutrophils (neutrophilia), but also increased numbers of less mature cells. These less mature cells, released from a large storage pool in the bone marrow, are called **bands** and have a characteristic horseshoe-shaped nucleus that is not yet fully lobulated. The phenomenon of finding these cells in the peripheral blood is called a **left shift** of the granulocyte lineage.

C. Other White Blood Cells: Monocytes and Lymphocytes

Both monocytes and lymphocytes arise from the common stem cell. It is the widespread **pluripotential** ability of stem cells to differentiate into these cells, in addition to the granulocytes, erythrocytes, and platelets, that makes bone marrow transplantation a therapeutic option for immune system disorders

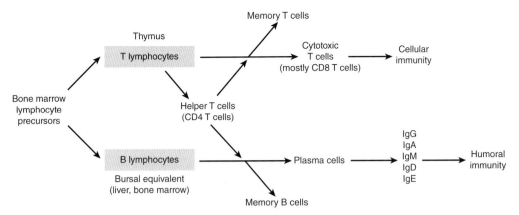

FIGURE 6–3 Development of the immune system from the common bone marrow stem cell. (Redrawn, with permission, from Ganong WF. *Review of Medical Physiology*, 22nd ed. McGraw-Hill, 2005.)

and malignancies. Monocytes have a very long life span, probably several months, but spend only about 3 days in the circulation. They mostly reside in tissues and act there as immune cells that engulf (**phagocytose**) bacteria and subsequently can "present" components of these bacteria to lymphocytes in a way that further amplifies and refines the immune response (see Chapter 3). On blood smear evaluation, monocytes are the largest cells seen, with irregular but not multilobed nuclei and pale blue cytoplasm, often with prominent vacuoles.

Lymphocyte precursors leave the marrow early and require extramedullary (outside of the marrow) maturation to become normally functioning immune cells in either the blood or the lymphatic system (Figure 6–3). Their crucial roles in recognizing "self" versus "nonself" and in modulating virtually all aspects of the immune response are described in Chapter 3. On microscopic examination of the blood smear, lymphocytes are small cells, slightly larger than an erythrocyte, with dark nuclei essentially filling the entire cell; only a thin rim of light blue cytoplasm is normally seen. Granules are sparse or absent.

D. Platelets

Platelets are the smallest formed elements in the blood. They are fragments of larger, multinucleated cells, which are the largest discrete constituents of the bone marrow (**megakaryocytes**), but platelets have no nuclei of their own. Most platelets remain in the circulation, but a substantial minority is trapped in the spleen; this phenomenon becomes important in a variety of immune-mediated decreases in platelet count (**thrombocytopenia**; see later discussion). In the setting of a normal platelet count, they have a circulatory half-life of about 10 days. In cases of thrombocytopenia, their half-life decreases, as they are consumed in the routine maintenance of vascular integrity.

Platelets are integral components of the coagulation system. Their membranes provide an important source of phospholipids (PLs), which are required for the function of the coagulation system proteins (Figure 6–4), and contain important receptors that allow attachment to endothelial cells (**platelet adhesion**) so that a **platelet plug** can be formed in response to blood vessel injury. This prevents further blood loss after

trauma and limits the coagulation response to the site of injury rather than letting coagulation proceed inappropriately.

The cytoplasm is also important for platelet function, particularly the intracellular **dense granules** and **alpha granules**. The phenomenon of platelet activation is also called "degranulation" and can be initiated by exposure of platelets to the activated blood coagulation factor **thrombin**, adenosine 5′-diphosphate (ADP), or collagen. This last reaction is probably the most important, occurring when collagen, normally in the basement membrane below the endothelial cells, is exposed to the blood after injury. Platelet activation can also be induced by exposure to **platelet-activating factor** (**PAF**) (a neutrophil-derived phospholipid cytokine), thromboxane A2, serotonin, and epinephrine.

During platelet activation, the dense and alpha granules release further activators of platelet activity, such as ADP, and platelet factor 4, which can also bind to endothelial cells. Platelet factor 4 is clinically relevant because it binds to the most commonly used therapeutic anticoagulant, heparin (see later discussion). After activation, platelets change shape from discoid to spherical with filopodial extensions and finally to a flat shape that allows for adequate coverage of the site of vessel injury. The last step in platelet activity is platelet aggregation, in which platelets stick to each other, firming up the platelet plug. On examination of the blood smear, platelets are small, irregularly shaped blue or purple granular bodies. In conditions in which platelet numbers are rising as a result of increased marrow activity, the more immature platelets can be identified by their larger size.

CHECKPOINT

1. What is the ratio of red blood cells to white blood cells in the bloodstream?
2. What is the number of cells produced daily by the bone marrow?
3. What are the different formed elements of blood, and how can they and their subtypes be distinguished?

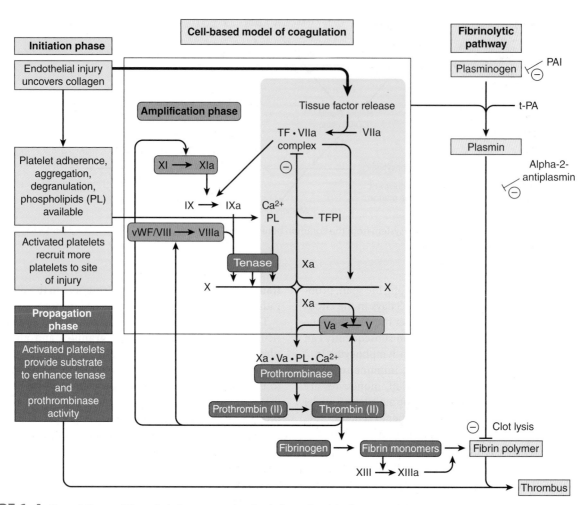

FIGURE 6–4 Coagulation and thrombolytic systems, showing balanced activity between them. (Ca^{2+}, calcium; PAI, plasminogen activator inhibitor; PL, phospholipids; TF, tissue factor [thromboplastin]; TFPI, tissue factor pathway inhibitor; t-PA, tissue plasminogen activator; vWf, von Willebrand factor. All clotting factors are shown as Roman numerals and the addition of an "a" indicates "activated.")

COAGULATION FACTORS & THE COAGULATION SYSTEM

Anatomy

The **coagulation system**, diagrammed in Figure 6–4, is a highly complex, regulated interaction of cells and plasma proteins. The coagulation system provides for immediate activation when control of bleeding (**hemostasis**) is required and confines its activity to the site of blood loss. Otherwise, coagulation might occur throughout the entire circulatory system, which would be incompatible with life.

The major components of hemostasis are platelets (discussed previously), endothelial cells (lining the blood vessels), other tissue factor (TF)–bearing cells, and the coagulation factors, which are plasma proteins. The end result of the activated coagulation system is the formation of a complex of cross-linked **fibrin** molecules and platelets that terminate hemorrhage after injury. To maintain a well-regulated balance between prothrombotic and antithrombotic factors, the sophisticated coagulation system provides several points of control (see Figure 6–4).

The coagulation factors do not generally circulate in active forms. Most of them are enzymes (serine proteases) and remain dormant until needed. This is accomplished by having other enzymes (the other proteases in the coagulation system) available that can cleave the inactive factors into active ones. All factors have roman numerals, and the inactive forms are written without annotation (eg, factor II, also known as prothrombin). The activated forms of the factors are signified by the letter "a" (eg, factor IIa, also known as thrombin).

Most of the coagulation factors are made by the liver, but factor XIII derives from platelets, and factor VIII is made by endothelial cells. Factors II, VII, IX, and X are particularly important factors (Table 6–3) because they are all dependent on the liver enzyme γ-carboxylase. Gammacarboxylase is dependent on vitamin K, and the oral anticoagulant **warfarin** acts by interfering with vitamin K activity. Two of the anticoagulant proteins, protein S and protein C (see later discussion), are also vitamin K dependent.

Physiology

Hemostasis is divided into three major processes: primary hemostasis, secondary hemostasis, and fibrinolysis.

TABLE 6–3   Coagulation factors of plasma.

Name	Production Source
Procoagulant Factors	
Factor I (fibrinogen)	Liver
Factor II (prothrombin)	Liver
Factor III (tissue thromboplastin)	Tissue
Factor IV (calcium)	...
Factor V (proaccelerin)	Liver
Factor VI (obsolete = factor Va)	...
Factor VII (proconvertin)	Liver
Factor VIII (antihemophilic factor)	Endothelial cells
Factor IX (Christmas factor)	Liver
Factor X (Stuart–Prower factor)	Liver
Factor XI (plasma thromboplastin antecedent)	Liver
Factor XII (Hageman factor)	Liver
Factor XIII (fibrin-stabilizing factor)	Platelets
Anticoagulant Factors	
Antithrombin	Liver
Protein C	Liver
Protein S	Liver
Plasminogen	Liver
Tissue factor pathway inhibitor	Endothelial cells

Primary hemostasis involves vasoconstriction and platelet adhesion and activation at sites of endothelial injury. Collagen and thrombin activate platelets, leading to an increase in intracellular calcium, secretion of platelet granules, and activation of various signaling pathways.

Secondary hemostasis is the process whereby fibrin is formed. The classical coagulation cascade, involving the intrinsic, extrinsic, and common pathways, better describes coagulation in vitro, as tested by the coagulation assays: activated partial thromboplastin time (aPTT) and prothrombin time (PT). The cell-based model of coagulation has replaced the coagulation cascade as a more accurate depiction of the in vivo coagulation process (see Figure 6–4). Secondary hemostasis is further divided into three overlapping phases: initiation, amplification, and propagation.

Initiation occurs at the surface of injured cells. It starts with the release of TF by the injured cells. TF, also called **thromboplastin**, is a lipid-rich protein material exposed to plasma upon injury to the vascular wall. It directly activates factor VII, forming the complex TF-VIIa, which activates both factor IX

and factor X. Together on the surface of the injured cell, factors Xa (an enzyme) and Va (a cofactor, activated from factor V by factor Xa) catalyze the conversion of prothrombin (II) to thrombin (IIa). Thrombin, a serine protease, cleaves the ubiquitous plasma protein fibrinogen into fibrin monomers, small insoluble proteins that can polymerize with each other to form the complex fibrin; however, the amount of thrombin formed at the site of the injured cell is insufficient by itself to produce enough fibrin to stabilize the platelet plug.

Amplification, unlike the initiation phase, occurs at the surface of platelets. During this phase, thrombin produced in the initiation phase activates platelets and coagulation factors V, VIII, and XI found on the platelet surface. Factor VIII is normally complexed to **von Willebrand factor (vWF)**, the protein that allows platelets to adhere to endothelial cells. Thrombin activates factor VIII by releasing it from vWF. It also activates both V and XI, which allows them to bind to the platelet surface. Factor XIa then catalyzes the activation of IX to IXa, providing supplemental factor IXa at the platelet surface.

Propagation involves activated platelets recruiting other circulating platelets to the site of vessel injury and the formation of two major complexes: tenase and prothrombinase, which are crucial to fibrin production. Factors VIIIa and IXa form the tenase complex on the surface of platelets in the presence of PLs and calcium (VIIIa-IXa-Ca^{2+}-PL). Together, they activate factor X on the platelet surface. Factor Xa then forms the prothrombinase complex with factor Va on the platelet surface, again in the presence of PLs and calcium (Xa-Va-Ca^{2+}-PL). This complex catalyzes the cleavage of prothrombin (II) to thrombin (IIa) and can convert multiple molecules per complex. As the activated platelets recruit more circulating platelets to the site of injury, a critical mass of platelets leads to a surge of thrombin generation. This, in turn, leads to enough fibrin formation to stabilize the platelet plug. This fibrin polymer is further solidified by chemical cross-links catalyzed by factor XIIIa, which itself is activated by thrombin. Factor XIIIa also incorporates α_2-antiplasmin into the clot to protect it from fibrinolytic proteases.

Fibrinolysis involves the process of breaking down fibrin into its degradation products. **Plasmin** is the main catalytic enzyme in this process. It is a serum protease that cleaves fibrin, resulting in breakup of the clot and creating fibrin degradation products that inhibit thrombin. Thrombin, working in a negative feedback fashion, actually helps catalyze the formation of plasmin from the inactive precursor protein, **plasminogen**. Plasminogen can also be cleaved by **tissue plasminogen activator (t-PA)** to form plasmin; t-PA and related proteins are used clinically to break up clots that form in coronary arteries in patients with a new myocardial infarction, as well as in the cerebral arteries of patients with a new stroke. Inhibitors of fibrinolysis include plasminogen activator inhibitor and α_2-antiplasmin.

In addition to the fibrinolytic pathway, checks on the coagulation system (ie, the anticoagulant system) also involve various feedback loops and inhibitors. Factor Xa binds to another plasma (and lipid-bound) protein called **tissue factor pathway**

inhibitor (**TFPI**). TFPI not only inhibits further activity of factor Xa itself but also prevents Xa from binding to the platelet surface, and the combination of factor Xa and TFPI greatly inhibits the TF-VIIa complex. Furthermore, downstream prothrombinase activity can be sustained only if the initial injury continues to generate enough factor IXa and VIIIa (in the form of the tenase complex) to activate more factor X on platelet surfaces.

Other anticoagulants include a group of inhibitors of the coagulation factors. They are composed of antithrombin (AT), protein S, and protein C (see later discussion). AT is a protease inhibitor and physically blocks the action of the serine proteases in the coagulation system. Its activity is enhanced up to 2000-fold by heparin. Protein C, activated by thrombin, cleaves factor Va into an inactive form so that the prothrombinase complex cannot cleave prothrombin (II) into thrombin. Protein C requires protein S as a cofactor. This complex also inactivates factor VIIIa.

LABORATORY TESTING OF THE COAGULATION PROCESS

Assays are available to determine both the absolute level and the activity of each of the coagulation factors, but in practice there are two common in vitro tests of coagulation function, both reported in terms of "seconds required to form a clot": the PT and the aPTT. The tests are designed in such a way that the results will be prolonged out of the normal range in different pathologic states, but significant alterations in the coagulation pathway inevitably lead to changes in both tests because of the multiple interactions of the involved factors.

PT assesses the "extrinsic" TF-dependent and common pathways of the classical coagulation cascade and is used clinically to monitor the effects of warfarin. Because all vitamin K–dependent factor levels are lowered by warfarin, eventually the aPTT will also become abnormal with high enough doses; but factor VII has the shortest half-life of those factors, so its levels fall first. Because of its critical role in clotting, thrombin is the principal factor whose activity must be reduced to achieve and maintain therapeutic anticoagulation. PT is reported clinically with its companion test, the **international normalized ratio** (**INR**), which removes the impact of different prothrombin batch purity on the PT result.

The aPTT assesses the "intrinsic" non-TF-dependent and common pathways and is prolonged most easily when there are reduced levels of factor VIII or factor IX activity, regardless of whether these factors are present at low concentrations or are present at normal concentrations but are being actively inhibited by other molecules. The aPTT is also very sensitive to the presence of heparin bound to AT and is used to monitor the anticoagulant effects of unfractionated heparin. Low-molecular-weight heparins (a specific purified subset of unfractionated heparin) in combination with AT preferentially inhibit factor Xa. In the doses of low-molecular-weight heparins usually given for prevention or treatment of thrombosis, the aPTT will not be prolonged (at least not into the usual "therapeutic range" for unfractionated heparin) despite good evidence of anticoagulation efficacy if factor Xa activity is measured directly. Newer **direct oral anticoagulants** (thrombin or factor Xa inhibitors) affect aPTT or PT/INR less reproducibly, and drug-specific anti-Xa assays or the **thrombin time** may be needed in cases in which there are concerns about under- or over-anticoagulation with these agents.

CHECKPOINT

4. Name the vitamin K–dependent clotting factors and the organ in which they are synthesized.
5. What are the two major complexes found on the surface of activated platelets that are important to the surge in thrombin production? Describe the coagulation factors that form these complexes and what the complexes specifically activate.
6. What is the main catalytic enzyme in fibrinolysis? Name two inhibitors of fibrinolysis.

OVERVIEW OF BLOOD DISORDERS

FORMED ELEMENT DISORDERS

Disorders of red cells, white cells, and platelets are separated for discussion because one or the other is found to be the most abnormal during laboratory testing. However, because of the clonal nature of hematopoiesis, many disorders affect all the formed elements of the blood. This is perhaps best demonstrated in the "blast crisis" phase of chronic myelogenous leukemia, in which the majority of both myeloid and lymphoid cells in the blood may be shown to express an identical gene rearrangement, called *bcr-abl* or the Philadelphia chromosome, that has arisen in a single abnormal progenitor cell.

1. Red Cell Disorders

There are many red cell abnormalities, but the principal ones are a variety of anemias. **Anemia** is defined as an abnormally low hemoglobin concentration in the blood. There are several methods of classification, but the prevailing systems are based on red cell size and shape.

In normal persons, erythrocytes are of uniform size and shape, and the automated blood count shows a mean corpuscular volume (MCV) near 90 fL, which is the estimated volume of a single cell. Automated systems usually report abnormalities of red cells as changes in hemoglobin concentration, red cell number, and MCV. Small cells (with low MCVs) are termed **microcytic**, and cells larger than normal are termed **macrocytic**. The relative nonuniformity of cell shapes (**poikilocytosis**) or sizes (**anisocytosis**) can further aid in subclassifying erythrocyte disorders.

The morphologic classification of anemias is set forth in Table 6–4 and Figure 6–5. In general, the microcytic anemias are a result of abnormalities in hemoglobin production, either in number of hemoglobin molecules per cell or in type of hemoglobin molecules (**hemoglobinopathies**). **Iron deficiency anemia** resulting from chronic blood loss and the **thalassemias** are examples of microcytic anemia.

The macrocytic anemias reflect either abnormal nuclear maturation or a higher fraction of young, large red cells (reticulocytes). When the nuclei of maturing red cells appear too young and large for the amount of hemoglobin in the cytoplasm, the macrocytic anemia is termed **megaloblastic**. These anemias are most often a result of either vitamin deficiencies (vitamin B_{12} or folic acid) or drugs that interfere with DNA synthesis. Abnormal nuclear maturation can also be a result of clonal proliferation in the bone marrow, producing preleukemic states termed the **myelodysplastic syndromes**.

The normocytic anemias can result from multiple causes: decreased numbers of red cell precursors in the marrow (primary failure called aplastic anemia, replacement of marrow elements with cancer, certain viral infections, or autoimmune inhibition called **pure red cell aplasia**), low levels

TABLE 6–4   Morphologic classification and common causes of anemia.

Type	MCV	Common Causes
Macrocytic	Increased	Folic acid deficiency
		Vitamin B_{12} deficiency
		Liver disease
		Alcohol
		Hypothyroidism
		Drugs (sulfonamides, zidovudine, antineoplastic agents)
		Myelodysplastic syndromes
Microcytic	Decreased	Iron deficiency
		Thalassemias
Normocytic	Normal	Aplastic anemia
		Anemia of chronic disease
		Chronic kidney disease
		Hemolytic anemia
		Spherocytosis

MCV, mean corpuscular volume.

of erythropoietin (resulting from chronic kidney disease), or chronic inflammatory diseases that affect the availability of iron in the marrow. Other normocytic anemias can be

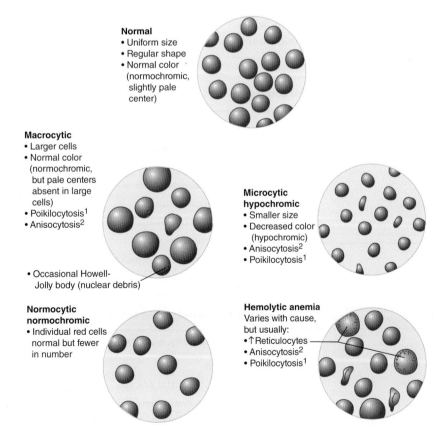

Normal
- Uniform size
- Regular shape
- Normal color (normochromic, slightly pale center)

Macrocytic
- Larger cells
- Normal color (normochromic, but pale centers absent in large cells)
- Poikilocytosis[1]
- Anisocytosis[2]

- Occasional Howell-Jolly body (nuclear debris)

Microcytic hypochromic
- Smaller size
- Decreased color (hypochromic)
- Anisocytosis[2]
- Poikilocytosis[1]

Normocytic normochromic
- Individual red cells normal but fewer in number

Hemolytic anemia
Varies with cause, but usually:
- ↑Reticulocytes
- Anisocytosis[2]
- Poikilocytosis[1]

FIGURE 6–5 Thin blood smear appearance of erythrocytes in the different morphologic types of anemias. (1, poikilocytosis [variation in shape]; 2, anisocytosis [variation in size].) (Redrawn, with permission, from Chandrasoma P et al. *Concise Pathology*, 3rd ed. Originally published by Appleton & Lange. Copyright © 1998 by The McGraw-Hill Companies, Inc.)

secondary to decreased life span of the cells that are produced. Examples of this phenomenon are acute blood loss; **autoimmune hemolytic anemias**, in which antibodies or complement bind to red cells and cause their destruction; **sickle cell anemia**, in which the abnormal hemoglobin polymerizes and obliterates the usual resilience of the red cell; and **hereditary spherocytosis** or **hereditary elliptocytosis**, in which defects in the erythrocyte membrane affect their ability to squeeze through the capillary microcirculation.

Anemias are very common. In contrast, an elevated hemoglobin concentration, termed **erythrocytosis**, is uncommon. Elevations in hemoglobin concentration can occur as a secondary phenomenon because of increased erythropoietin levels, such as that found in smokers or people who live at high altitudes (whose low blood oxygen levels stimulate erythropoietin production). Some tumors, especially renal tumors, can also make erythropoietin. Primary **polycythemia** is an abnormality of the bone marrow itself. This myeloproliferative syndrome leads to an increased red cell mass and consequent low erythropoietin levels by the negative-feedback mechanism discussed previously.

2. White Blood Cell Disorders

Abnormalities in white cell numbers occur commonly (Table 6–5), whereas abnormalities of function are rare. Neoplastic transformation in the form of leukemia (granulocytes and monocytes) or lymphoma (lymphocytes) is fairly common. The leukemias are discussed in Chapter 5.

Changes in neutrophil count are the most common white cell abnormality detected on the automated blood count. Increased numbers of neutrophils (**leukocytosis**) suggest acute or chronic infection or inflammation but can be a sign of many conditions. These include stress, because adrenal corticosteroids cause **demargination** of neutrophils from blood vessel walls.

Decreased numbers of neutrophils (**neutropenia**) can be seen in overwhelming infection and benign diseases such as **cyclic neutropenia** (see later discussion) but can also be seen when the bone marrow is infiltrated with tumor or involved by the myelodysplastic syndromes. Many drugs can also directly suppress marrow production, and because neutrophils have the shortest half-life in the blood of any cell produced by the marrow, their numbers may fall quickly.

Lymphocyte numbers can vary substantially (Table 6–6). Lymphocyte counts are classically elevated in viral infections, such as infectious mononucleosis. However, persistent elevations suggest malignancies, particularly **chronic lymphocytic leukemia**, which may not cause any symptoms and be incidentally discovered on a routine blood count.

Decreased lymphocyte counts (**lymphopenia**) are a common complication of corticosteroid therapy but are most worrisome for immunodeficiency states; HIV directly infects lymphocytes, and the likelihood of opportunistic infections increases as lymphocyte counts fall, resulting in progression from HIV infection to full-blown AIDS.

3. Platelet Disorders

Abnormalities in platelet number are fairly common, particularly low counts (**thrombocytopenia**). Causes are listed

TABLE 6–5   Causes of abnormal neutrophil counts.

Neutrophilia	Neutropenia
Increased Marrow Activity	*Decreased Marrow Activity*
Bacterial infections	Drugs (antineoplastic agents, antibiotics, gold, certain diuretics, antithyroid agents, antihistamines, antipsychotics)
Acute inflammation	Radiation exposure
Leukemia and myeloproliferative disorders	Megaloblastic anemia
Release from Marrow Pool	Cyclic neutropenia
	Kostmann (infantile) neutropenia
Stress (catecholamines)	Aplastic anemias
Corticosteroids	Myelodysplastic syndromes
Endotoxin exposure	Marrow replacement by tumor
Demargination into Blood	*Decreased Neutrophil Survival*
Bacterial infections	Sepsis
Hypoxemia	Viral or rickettsial infection
Stress (catecholamines)	Immune destruction associated with drugs
Corticosteroids	Immune destruction associated with autoantibodies (systemic lupus erythematosus, Felty syndrome)
Exercise	Hypersplenism

TABLE 6–6 Causes of abnormal lymphocyte counts.

Lymphocytosis
Medium to large, atypical lymphocytes predominant
Viral infections (mononucleosis, mumps, measles, hepatitis, rubella)
Active immune responses, particularly in children
Toxoplasmosis
Lymphoma with circulating cells
Chronic lymphocytic leukemia
Small, mature lymphocytes predominant
Chronic infections (tuberculosis)
Autoimmune diseases (myasthenia gravis)
Metabolic diseases (Addison disease)
Lymphoma with circulating cells
Chronic lymphocytic leukemia
Immature cells predominant
Acute lymphocytic leukemia
Lymphoblastic lymphoma
Lymphopenia
Immunodeficiency states (AIDS)
Corticosteroid therapy
Toxic drugs
Cushing syndrome

TABLE 6–7 Causes of platelet abnormalities.

Thrombocytosis
Myeloproliferative disorders, especially essential thrombocythemia
Postsplenectomy
Reactive (postsurgical, posthemorrhage, anemias)
Inflammatory disorders
Malignancies
Thrombocytopenia
Decreased Production
Aplastic anemia
Marrow infiltration
Vitamin B_{12} and folate deficiencies
Radiation or chemotherapy
Hereditary
Infection (HIV, parvovirus, CMV)
Cirrhosis (low thrombopoietin levels)
Decreased Survival
Immune mediated (idiopathic, systemic lupus erythematosus, drug induced, neonatal from maternal IgG)
Hypersplenism
Disseminated intravascular coagulation
Thrombotic thrombocytopenic purpura, hemolytic uremic syndrome
Prosthetic valves
Qualitative Platelet Disorders
Inherited
Bernard–Soulier syndrome (adhesion defect)
Glanzmann thrombasthenia (aggregation defect)
Storage pool disease (granule defect)
Von Willebrand disease
Wiskott–Aldrich syndrome
Acquired
Uremia
Dysproteinemias
Chronic liver disease
Drug induced (especially aspirin)

in Table 6–7. Decreased production of platelets occurs when the marrow is affected by a variety of diseases or when TPO production by the liver is impaired, as in cirrhosis. Increased destruction of platelets is much more prevalent. There are three general mechanisms. Because a significant number of platelets normally reside in the spleen, any increase in spleen size or activity (**hypersplenism**) leads to lower platelet counts. Platelet consumption as a result of ongoing clotting will also lower counts. Most common, however, is immune-mediated consumption caused either by drugs or autoantibodies. The latter are usually directed against the platelet membrane antigen gpIIb/IIIa.

Functional platelet disorders are common, especially the acquired disorders resulting from uremia (renal failure) or aspirin, which inhibits the platelet enzyme cyclooxygenase and decreases platelet aggregability. Inherited abnormalities are unusual with the exception of **von Willebrand disease**, which results from either quantitative or qualitative defect of vWF, the carrier protein for factor VIII. vWF also acts as a bridge between platelets and the endothelium and thus is crucial for the formation of the platelet plug in the coagulation cascade.

Elevations in the platelet count above normal (**thrombocytosis**) are relatively common and are especially apt to occur in recovery from iron deficiency anemia upon iron repletion. In the myeloproliferative disorders, such as polycythemia, platelet counts are often high. In **essential thrombocythemia**, platelet counts may be higher than 1,000,000/μL.

COAGULATION FACTOR DISORDERS

The most important coagulation factor disorders are quantitative rather than qualitative and usually hereditary rather than acquired (Table 6–8). Exceptions to this rule are **acquired factor inhibitors**, which are antibodies that bind to one of

TABLE 6–8   Coagulation factor deficiencies.

Factor	Disease	Inheritance Pattern	Frequency	Disease Severity
Fibrinogen	Afibrinogenemia	Autosomal recessive	Rare	Variable
	Dysfibrinogenemia	Autosomal dominant	Rare	Variable
Factor V	Parahemophilia	Autosomal recessive	Very rare	Moderate to severe
Factor VII		Autosomal recessive	Very rare	Moderate to severe
Factor VIII	Hemophilia A	X-linked recessive	Common	Mild to severe
vWF	von Willebrand disease	Autosomal dominant	Common	Mild to moderate
Factor IX	Hemophilia B	X-linked recessive	Uncommon	Mild to severe
Factor X		Autosomal recessive	Rare	Variable
Factor XI	Rosenthal syndrome	Autosomal recessive	Uncommon	Mild
Factor XII	Hageman trait	Autosomal recessive or dominant	Rare	Asymptomatic
Factor XIII		Autosomal recessive	Rare	Severe

the coagulation factors, most often factor VIII. These may or may not cause clinical bleeding problems, but they can be extremely difficult to treat. The quantitative disorders that most commonly cause bleeding are **hemophilia A** (deficiency of factor VIII) and **hemophilia B** (deficiency of factor IX). Both are X chromosome–linked recessive traits, and affected males have very low levels of factor VIII or IX. It is not clear why all affected males do not have a complete absence of factor VIII or IX activity. Hemophilia A is more common, with a prevalence of 1:10,000 males worldwide. Both disorders lead to spontaneous and excessive post-traumatic bleeding, particularly into joints and muscles. Females with the trait have 50% of the normal amount of either factor and tend not to have any bleeding problems; in general, one needs only half of the normal quantities of most coagulation factors to clot normally. The aPTT test is usually designed to become abnormal when factor VIII or IX activities fall below 50% of normal.

Vitamin K deficiency also leads to quantitative declines in the levels of factors II, VII, IX, and X and proteins C and S; prolongation of the prothrombin time may result.

Quantitative inherited abnormalities of the anticoagulation systems also occur. Protein S deficiency, protein C deficiency,

and AT deficiency all occur and lead to abnormal clotting problems, as discussed in the next section.

Finally, the condition of **consumptive coagulopathy** or **disseminated intravascular coagulation** (**DIC**) needs to be included. This condition is generally a result of overwhelming infection, specific leukemias or lymphomas, or massive hemorrhage. In DIC, the coagulation factors become depleted. Often the fibrinolytic system is simultaneously activated, and uncontrolled bleeding may occur throughout the entire circulatory system. PT and aPTT are usually both abnormal.

CHECKPOINT

7. Define anemia, and suggest three causes each for macrocytic and microcytic anemia.
8. What are some categories of explanations for a white blood cell count that is substantially increased or decreased compared with the normal range?
9. What are the three general mechanisms of thrombocytopenia?
10. What is the nature of the defects in hemophilia A and B?

PATHOPHYSIOLOGY OF SELECTED BLOOD DISORDERS

RED CELL DISORDERS

1. Iron Deficiency Anemia

Etiology

Iron deficiency anemia is the most common form of anemia. Although in many developing countries dietary deficiency of

iron can occur, in developed nations the main cause is loss of iron, almost always through blood loss from the GI or genitourinary tracts.

Because of recurrent menstrual blood loss, premenopausal women represent the population with the highest incidence of iron deficiency. The incidence in this group is even higher because of iron losses during pregnancy, because the developing fetus efficiently extracts maternal iron for use in its own hematopoiesis. In men or in postmenopausal women with iron deficiency, GI bleeding is usually the cause. Blood loss in this case may result from relatively benign disorders, such as peptic ulcer, arteriovenous malformations, or angiodysplasia (small vascular abnormalities along the intestinal walls). More serious causes are inflammatory bowel disease and malignancy. Endoscopic investigation to exclude malignancy is mandatory in patients without a known cause of iron deficiency.

There are other less common causes of iron deficiency, but most are related to blood loss: Bleeding disorders and hemoptysis are the chief possibilities. When no source of bleeding is uncovered, insufficient dietary intake (eg, vegetarian diets) and GI malabsorption should be considered as a possible cause of iron deficiency anemia. Such malabsorption occurs in patients with celiac disease, *Helicobacter pylori* infection, partial gastrectomy, or gastric bypass surgery. Other mechanisms of iron deficiency anemia include intravascular hemolysis (paroxysmal nocturnal hemoglobinuria or cardiac valvular disease) and iron depletion in response to erythropoietin treatment.

Pathogenesis

Body iron stores are generally sufficient to last several years, but there is a constant loss of iron in completely healthy persons, such that iron balance depends on adequate intake and absorption. Dietary iron is primarily absorbed in the duodenum (Figure 6–6). Absorption is increased in the setting of anemia, hypoxia, and systemic iron deficiency. Iron is also recycled from senescent erythrocytes via macrophage

phagocytosis and lysis. The export of iron to plasma from these cellular sites is regulated by **hepcidin**, a 25–amino acid peptide produced by the liver. Hepcidin binds to ferroportin, a transmembrane protein, inducing its internalization and lysosomal degradation. When iron stores are low, hepcidin production is reduced and ferroportin molecules are expressed on the basolateral membrane of enterocytes, where they transfer iron from the cytoplasm of enterocytes to plasma **transferrin**. Conversely, when iron stores are adequate or elevated, hepcidin production is increased, resulting in the internalization of ferroportin and reduced export of iron into plasma. In inflammatory states, hepcidin production is increased, leading to the internalization of **ferroportin** on macrophages and the trapping of recycled iron within macrophage stores.

Iron is stored in most body cells as **ferritin**, a combination of iron and the protein apoferritin. It is also stored as **hemosiderin**, which is ferritin partly stripped of the apoferritin protein shell. Iron is transported in blood bound to its carrier protein, transferrin. Because of the complex interactions between these molecules, a simple measurement of serum iron rarely reflects body iron stores (see later discussion).

Iron is found predominantly in hemoglobin and is also present in **myoglobin**, the oxygen-storing protein of skeletal muscle. The main role for iron is as the ion in the center of the body's oxygen-carrying molecule, **heme**. Held stably in the ferrous form by the other atoms in heme, iron reversibly binds oxygen. Each protein subunit of hemoglobin contains one heme molecule; because hemoglobin exists as a tetramer, four iron molecules are needed in each hemoglobin unit. In iron deficiency, the final step in heme synthesis is interrupted

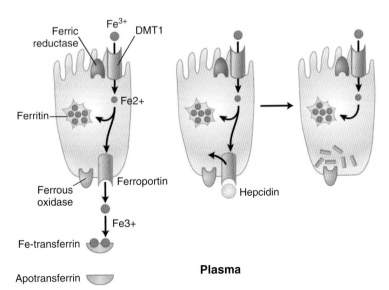

FIGURE 6-6 Iron transport and regulation in the duodenal enterocyte. Under normal conditions (left), iron (Fe) transits from the intestinal lumen into the enterocyte through divalent metal transporter 1 (DMT1) and is either stored intracellularly bound to ferritin or exported through ferroportin where it is bound to plasma transferrin. Hepcidin (middle and right) binds to ferroportin resulting in its internalization and degradation, thereby decreasing iron export from intracellular stores. (Reproduced, with permission, from Aster JC et al. *Pathophysiology of Blood Disorders*, 2nd ed. McGraw-Hill, 2017, Figure 5–2.)

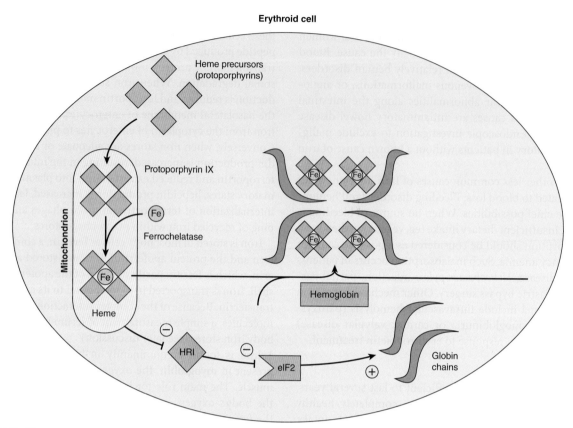

FIGURE 6–7 Heme synthesis, emphasizing the role of iron and the insertion of heme into individual globin chains to make hemoglobin, and the role of the heme-regulated translational inhibitor (HRI) of globin synthesis. Normal concentrations of heme keep the activity of HRI low, preserving normal globin synthesis.

(Figure 6–7). In this step, ferrous iron is inserted into protoporphyrin IX by the enzyme ferrochelatase; when heme synthesis is interrupted, there is inadequate heme production. Globin biosynthesis is inhibited by heme deficiency through a **heme-regulated translational inhibitor (HRI)**. Elevated HRI activity (a result of heme deficiency) inhibits a key transcription initiation factor for heme synthesis, eIF2. Thus, less heme and fewer globin chains are available in each red cell precursor. This directly causes anemia, a decrease in the hemoglobin concentration of the blood.

As noted, heme is also the oxygen acceptor in myoglobin; therefore, iron deficiency will also lead to decreased myoglobin production. Other proteins also depend on iron; most of these are enzymes. Many use iron in the heme molecule, but some use elemental iron. Although the exact implications of iron deficiency on their activity is not known, these enzymes are crucial to metabolism, energy production, DNA synthesis, and even brain function.

Pathology

As iron stores are depleted, the peripheral blood smear pattern evolves. In early iron deficiency, the hemoglobin level of the blood falls, but individual erythrocytes appear normal. In response to a falling oxygen level, erythropoietin levels rise and

stimulate the marrow, but the hemoglobin level cannot rise in response because of the iron deficiency. Other hormones are presumably also stimulated, however, and the resulting "revved-up" marrow usually causes an elevated blood platelet count. An elevated white cell count is less common. Reticulocytes are notably absent.

Eventually, the hemoglobin concentration of individual cells falls, leading to the classic picture of microcytic, hypochromic erythrocytes (see Figure 6–5). This is most commonly found as an abnormally low MCV of red cells on the automated hemogram. There is also substantial anisocytosis and poikilocytosis, seen on the peripheral smear, and **target cells** may be seen. The target shape occurs because there is a relative excess of red cell membrane compared with the amount of hemoglobin within the cell, so that the membrane bunches up in the center.

Laboratory results are often confusing. A low serum ferritin level is diagnostic of iron deficiency, but even in obvious cases, levels can be normal; ferritin levels rise in acute or chronic inflammation or significant illnesses, which can themselves be the cause of iron (blood) loss. Serum iron levels fall in many illnesses, and levels of its serum carrier, transferrin, fluctuate as well, so neither is a consistent indicator of iron deficiency, nor is their ratio, the transferrin saturation. Nevertheless, serum ferritin is the most sensitive and specific test for iron deficiency. If ferritin levels are not diagnostic, measuring serum-soluble transferrin receptor (sTfR) can help. TfRs are membrane glycoproteins that facilitate iron transport from plasma transferrin into body cells. Erythroid precursors increase their expression of membrane TfR in the setting of iron deficiency but not anemia of chronic disease. Some membrane TfR is released into the serum as sTfR. The amount of sTfR in the serum reflects the amount of membrane TfR. A high ratio of sTfR to ferritin predicts iron deficiency when ferritin is not diagnostically low. Though helpful, this test has had limited adoption in clinical practice.

Other than observing a hematologic response to empiric iron supplementation, bone marrow biopsy can confirm a diagnosis of iron deficiency. Iron is normally found in the macrophages of the marrow, where it supplies erythrocyte precursors; intracellular hemosiderin is easily visualized with Prussian blue stain. These macrophages do not stain at all if there is iron deficiency.

Clinical Manifestations

All anemias lead to classic symptoms of decreased oxygen-carrying capacity (ie, fatigue, weakness, and shortness of breath, particularly dyspnea on exertion), and iron deficiency is no exception. Decreased oxygen-carrying capacity leads to decreased oxygen delivery to metabolically active tissues, which nonetheless must have oxygen; this leads directly to fatigue. The compensatory mechanisms of the body lead to additional symptoms and signs of anemia. Some patients appear pale not only because there is less hemoglobin per unit of blood (oxygenated hemoglobin is red and gives color to the skin), but also because superficial skin blood vessels constrict, diverting blood to more vital structures. Patients may also respond to the anemia with tachycardia. This increased cardiac output is appropriate because one way to increase oxygen delivery to the tissues is to increase the number of times each hemoglobin molecule is oxygenated in the lungs every hour. This tachycardia may cause benign cardiac murmurs due to the increased blood flow.

Abnormalities of the GI tract occur because iron is also needed for proliferating cells. **Glossitis**, in which the normal tongue papillae are absent, can occur, as can gastric atrophy with **achlorhydria** (absence of stomach acid). The achlorhydria may compound the iron deficiency because iron is best absorbed in an acidic environment, but this complication is quite unusual.

In children, there may be significant developmental problems, both physical and mental. Iron-deficient children, mostly in developing regions, perform poorly on tests of cognition compared with iron-replete children. Iron therapy can reverse these findings if started early enough in childhood. The exact mechanism of cognitive loss in iron deficiency is not known. Another unexplained but often observed phenomenon in severe iron deficiency is **pica**, a craving for non-nutritive substances such as clay or dirt.

Many patients have no specific symptoms or findings at all, and their iron deficiency is discovered because of anemia noted on a blood count obtained for another purpose. It is of interest that mild anemias (hemoglobins of 11–12 g/dL) may be tolerated very well because they develop slowly. In addition to the physiologic compensatory mechanisms discussed previously (increased cardiac output, diversion of blood flow from less metabolically active areas), there is a biochemical adaptation as well. The ability to transfer oxygen from hemoglobin to cells depends partly on a small molecule in erythrocytes called **2,3-biphosphoglycerate (2,3-BPG)**. In high concentrations, the ability to unload oxygen in the tissues is increased. Chronic anemia leads to elevated 2,3-BPG concentrations in erythrocytes.

Other patients who do not present with symptoms directly related to the anemia present instead with symptoms or signs related directly to blood loss. Because the most common site of unexpected (nonmenstrual) blood loss is the GI tract, patients often have visible changes in the stool. There may be gross blood (**hematochezia**), which is more common with bleeding sites near the rectum, or black, tarry, metabolized blood (**melena**) from more proximal sites. Significant blood loss from the urinary tract is very uncommon.

CHECKPOINT

11. What is the most common form of anemia and its most likely cause in a premenopausal woman? In a man?
12. In what situations might the serum ferritin level be normal or elevated in a patient with iron deficiency?
13. What are some disorders associated with iron deficiency anemia?
14. What are the physiologic adaptations to slowly developing iron deficiency anemia?

2. Pernicious Anemia

Etiology

Pernicious anemia is a megaloblastic anemia in which there is abnormal erythrocyte nuclear maturation. Unlike in many other types of anemia, such as that resulting from iron deficiency, hemoglobin synthesis is normal. Pernicious anemia is the end result of a cascade of events that are autoimmune in origin. The ultimate effect is a loss of adequate stores of vitamin B_{12} (cobalamin), which is a cofactor involved in DNA synthesis. Rapidly proliferating cells are those most often affected, predominantly bone marrow cells and those of the GI epithelium. The nervous system is also affected, demonstrating that this is a systemic disease. Anemia is merely the most common manifestation.

Besides pernicious anemia, cobalamin deficiency can also be a result of bacterial overgrowth in the intestine (because bacteria compete with the host for cobalamin), intestinal malabsorption of vitamin B_{12} involving the terminal ileum (such as in Crohn's disease), surgical removal of the antrum of the stomach (gastrectomy), and, rarely, dietary deficiency, which occurs only in strict vegetarians (vegans). In the diet, cobalamin is found mostly in animal products.

Pernicious anemia is most common in older patients of Scandinavian descent and is more commonly found in those of European and African than Asian descent. In the United States, black females are one of the most common groups. Pernicious anemia accounts for only a small percentage of patients with anemia, however.

Pathogenesis

The initial events in the pathogenetic cascade begin in the stomach (Figure 6–8). The gastric parietal cells are initially affected by an autoimmune phenomenon that leads to two discrete effects: loss of gastric acid (**achlorhydria**) and loss of **intrinsic factor**. Pernicious anemia interferes with both the initial availability and the absorption of vitamin B_{12}: Stomach acid is required for the release of cobalamin from foodstuffs, and intrinsic factor is a glycoprotein that binds cobalamin and is required for the effective absorption of cobalamin in the terminal ileum. Both stomach acid and intrinsic factor are made exclusively by parietal cells.

Evidence for the autoimmune destruction of parietal cells is strong: Patients with pernicious anemia have atrophy of the gastric mucosa, and pathologic specimens show infiltrating lymphocytes, which are predominantly antibody-producing B cells. In addition, 90% or more of patients have antibodies in their serum directed against parietal cell membrane proteins. The major protein antigen appears to be H^+-K^+ ATPase, the **proton pump**, which is responsible for the production of stomach acid. Cytotoxic T cells whose receptors recognize H^+-K^+ ATPase may also contribute to the gastric atrophy. More than half of patients also have antibodies to intrinsic factor itself or the intrinsic factor–cobalamin complex. Furthermore, patients with pernicious anemia have a higher incidence of other autoimmune diseases, such as Graves disease. Lastly, corticosteroid therapy, used as first-line therapy for many autoimmune disorders, may reverse the pathologic findings in pernicious anemia. Despite this evidence, the exact mechanism of the inciting event remains unknown.

Complete vitamin B_{12} deficiency develops slowly, even after total achlorhydria and loss of intrinsic factor occur. Liver stores of vitamin B_{12} are adequate for several years. However, the lack of this vitamin eventually leads to alterations in DNA synthesis and, in the nervous system, altered myelin synthesis.

FIGURE 6–8 Pathogenesis and effects of pernicious anemia (autoimmune atrophic gastritis). (Redrawn, with permission, from Chandrasoma P et al. *Concise Pathology*, 3rd ed. Originally published by Appleton & Lange. Copyright © 1998 by The McGraw-Hill Companies, Inc.)

FIGURE 6-9 Role of cobalamin (vitamin B_{12}) and folic acid in nucleic acid and myelin metabolism. Lack of either cobalamin or folic acid retards DNA synthesis (**A**), and lack of cobalamin leads to loss of folic acid, which cannot be held intracellularly unless polyglutamated. Lack of cobalamin also leads to abnormal myelin synthesis, probably via a deficiency in methionine production (**B**). (Redrawn, with permission, from Chandrasoma P et al. *Concise Pathology*, 3rd ed. Originally published by Appleton & Lange. Copyright © 1998 by The McGraw-Hill Companies, Inc.)

In DNA synthesis, cobalamin, along with folic acid, is crucial as a cofactor in the synthesis of deoxythymidine from deoxyuridine (Figure 6-9). Cobalamin accepts a methyl group from methyltetrahydrofolate, which leads to the formation of two important intracellular compounds. The first is methylcobalamin, which is required for the production of the amino acid methionine from homocysteine. The second is reduced tetrahydrofolate, which is required as the single-carbon donor in purine synthesis. Thus, cobalamin deficiency depletes stores of reduced tetrahydrofolate and impairs DNA synthesis because of lowered purine production. In cobalamin deficiency, other reduced folates may substitute for tetrahydrofolate (and may explain why pharmacologic doses of folic acid can partially reverse the megaloblastic blood cell changes, but not the neurologic changes, seen in pernicious anemia). However, methyltetrahydrofolate, normally the methyl donor to cobalamin, accumulates. This folate cannot be retained intracellularly because it cannot be **polyglutamated**; the addition of multiple glutamate residues leads to a charged compound that does not freely diffuse out of the cell. Therefore, there is relative folate deficiency in pernicious anemia as well. In addition, methionine may serve as a principal donor of methyl groups to these other "substituting" reduced folates; because methionine cannot be produced in cobalamin deficiency, this compounds the problems in purine synthesis.

The exact mechanism of the neurologic consequences of pernicious anemia, with **demyelination** (loss of the myelin sheaths around nerves), is unknown. Defects in the methionine synthase pathway have been suggested but not proven experimentally. Instead, observations in cobalamin-deficient gastrectomized rats implicate an imbalance of cytokines and growth factors as a potential mediator of nerve damage. The synthesis of the cytokine **tumor necrosis factor** (**TNF**) is regulated by S-adenosyl-methionine, a product of methionine. Deficiency of methionine may indirectly lead to neuropathy via unregulated production of TNF, a myelinolytic cytokine, among other mechanisms.

The production of succinyl-coenzyme A (CoA) also depends on the presence of cobalamin. It is unclear whether a decrease in the production of succinyl-CoA, which may affect fatty acid synthesis, is also involved in the demyelinating disease.

Pathology

The gastric disorders associated with pernicious anemia are dominated by the picture of **chronic atrophic gastritis** (see Figure 6-8). The normally tall columnar epithelium is replaced by a very thin mucosa, and there is obvious infiltration of plasma cells and lymphocytes. Pernicious anemia also increases the risk for gastric adenocarcinoma. Thus, pathologic examination may also reveal cancer.

The peripheral blood smear picture (see Figure 6-5) varies, depending on the length of time the patient has been cobalamin deficient. In early stages, the patient may have mild macrocytic anemia, and large ovoid erythrocytes (**macro-ovalocytes**) are commonly seen. In full-blown megaloblastic anemia, however, there are abnormalities in all cell lines. The classic picture reveals significant anisocytosis and poikilocytosis of the red cell line, and there are hypersegmented neutrophils, revealing the nuclear dysgenesis from abnormal DNA synthesis (Figure 6-10). In severe cases of pernicious anemia, the red and white cell series are easily mistaken for acute leukemia because the cells look so atypical.

Bone marrow aspiration and biopsy are not necessary in the diagnosis and results from them may be misleading because the marrow pathology can be confused with acute leukemia, hypercellularity, increased erythroblasts, and even cytogenetic changes. Typical findings in B_{12} deficiency include

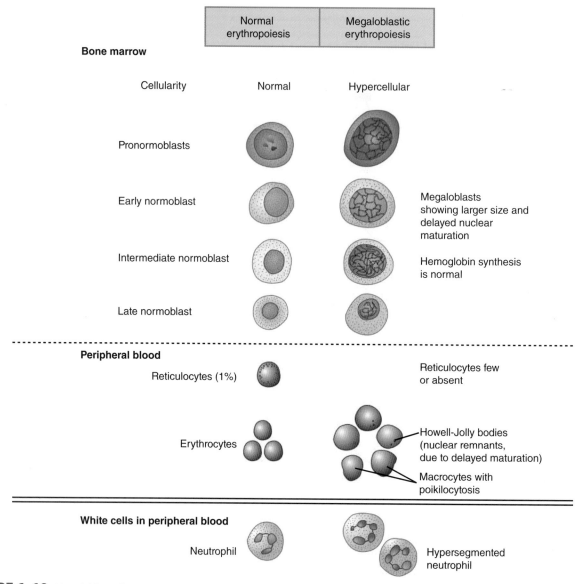

	Normal erythropoiesis	Megaloblastic erythropoiesis

Bone marrow

Cellularity	Normal	Hypercellular

Pronormoblasts

Early normoblast — Megaloblasts showing larger size and delayed nuclear maturation

Intermediate normoblast — Hemoglobin synthesis is normal

Late normoblast

Peripheral blood

Reticulocytes (1%) — Reticulocytes few or absent

Erythrocytes — Howell-Jolly bodies (nuclear remnants, due to delayed maturation)

— Macrocytes with poikilocytosis

White cells in peripheral blood

Neutrophil — Hypersegmented neutrophil

FIGURE 6–10 Megaloblastic hematopoiesis: morphologic changes visible on microscopic examination of bone marrow or peripheral blood. (Redrawn, with permission, from Chandrasoma P et al. *Concise Pathology*, 3rd ed. Originally published by Appleton & Lange. Copyright © 1998 by The McGraw-Hill Companies, Inc.)

megaloblastic changes—nuclei that are too large and immature in cells with mature, hemoglobin-filled cytoplasm—that are seen at each stage of erythrocyte development. These cells are not seen in the peripheral blood because the abnormal erythrocytes generally are destroyed in the marrow (**intramedullary hemolysis**) by unexplained processes. This compounds the anemia. Megaloblastic changes can be seen in the marrow even in the absence of obvious changes on the peripheral blood smear.

Spinal cord abnormalities consist of demyelination of the posterolateral spinal columns, called **subacute combined degeneration**. Peripheral nerves may also show demyelination. Demyelination eventually results in neuronal cell death, which is also obvious on pathologic examination. Because neurons do not divide, new neurons cannot replace the dead ones.

Laboratory findings include elevated lactate dehydrogenase (LDH) and, sometimes, indirect bilirubin consistent with the hemolysis occurring in the bone marrow. LDH is directly released from lysed red cells, and free hemoglobin is metabolized to bilirubin. Serum vitamin B_{12} levels are usually low, revealing the deficient state. Yet there remain high rates of both false positive and false negative test results because only 20% of total measured serum B_{12} is bound to the cellular delivery protein, transcobalamin; the rest is bound to haptocorrin, which is not available for cells to use. Antibodies to intrinsic factor are usually detectable. Serum elevations of methylmalonic acid (MMA) and/or homocysteine (see Figure 6–9) are highly predictive of B_{12} deficiency. The Schilling test, which assesses the oral absorption of vitamin B_{12} with and without added intrinsic factor, is no longer used, because of lack of availability of radioactively labeled vitamin B_{12}. Typically, the approach is to first measure serum B_{12} and, if results are equivocal, to obtain serum levels of MMA and/or homocysteine.

Clinical Manifestations

The clinical presentation consists of one or more symptoms related to the underlying deficiency. Anemia is the most commonly encountered abnormality and is often very severe; hemoglobin levels of 4 g/dL (less than a third of normal) can be seen. This degree of anemia is rare with other causes, such as iron deficiency. Typical symptoms are fatigue, dyspnea, or dizziness because a decreased red cell mass equals a decreased oxygen-carrying capacity of the blood. High-output heart failure is relatively common, with tachycardia and signs of left ventricular failure (see Chapter 10). Because oxygen demands are constant (or rise with exercise) and oxygen-carrying capacity is falling, the only way to maintain tissue oxygenation in anemia is to increase cardiac output (ie, the number of times per minute each red cell is fully oxygenated by the lungs). Eventually, however, the left ventricle fails.

However, symptoms may be mild because the anemia develops slowly as a result of the extensive liver storage of vitamin B_{12}. Patients with anemia usually adapt over time to slow changes in oxygen-carrying capacity. The same changes in 2,3-BPG that encourage oxygen delivery to the tissues from the hemoglobin in red cells in other anemias occur in vitamin B_{12} deficiency.

GI symptoms are less prevalent and include malabsorption, muscle wasting (unusual), diarrhea (more common), and **glossitis** (most common). In glossitis, the normal tongue papillae are absent regardless of whether the tongue is painful, red, and "beefy" or pale and smooth.

Neurologic symptoms are least likely to improve with cobalamin replacement therapy. As with other neuropathies involving loss of myelin from large peripheral sensory nerves, numbness and tingling (**paresthesias**) occur frequently and are the most common symptoms. Demyelination and neuronal cell death in the posterolateral "long tracts" of the spinal cord interfere with delivery of positional information to the brainstem, cerebellum, and sensory cortex. Patients, therefore, complain of loss of balance and coordination. Examination reveals impaired **proprioception** (position sense) and vibration sense. True dementia may also occur when demyelination involves the brain. Importantly, but somewhat unexpectedly, neurologic symptoms may occur in the absence of any changes in the peripheral blood smear suggestive of pernicious anemia.

Less commonly, vitamin B_{12} deficiency can manifest with thrombosis and possibly at unusual sites such as cerebral venous sinuses. The prothrombotic state may be secondary to hyperhomocysteinemia seen in severe vitamin B_{12} deficiency.

CHECKPOINT

15. Name two crucial cofactors in DNA synthesis whose deficiency results in pernicious anemia. In what specific biochemical pathways do they participate?

16. What neurologic defects are observed in prolonged pernicious anemia?

17. What symptoms of pernicious anemia are usually relatively mild?

18. Are changes in the peripheral blood smear necessary for neurologic effects of vitamin B_{12} deficiency?

WHITE CELL DISORDERS

1. Malignant Disorders

The most important leukocyte abnormalities are the malignant disorders leukemia and lymphoma. They are discussed in Chapter 5.

2. Cyclic Neutropenia

Absolute neutropenia, characterized by neutrophil counts less than 1500–2000/μL (>2 SD below the mean in normals), is a commonly encountered problem in medicine and can result from a large number of disease entities (see Table 6–5). Cyclic neutropenia, however, is rare. It is of interest because it provides insight into normal neutrophil production and function. It is characterized by a lifetime history of neutrophil counts that decrease to zero or near zero for 3–5 days at a time every 3 weeks and then rebound. Interestingly, the peripheral blood neutrophil counts and monocyte counts oscillate in opposite phases on this 3-week cycle.

Etiology

Classic, childhood-onset cyclic neutropenia results from heterozygous germline mutations in the gene *ELANE* (*ELAstase, neutrophil expressed*), formerly known as *ELA2*, which encodes for a single enzyme, neutrophil elastase (NE). NE is found in the primary azurophilic granules of neutrophils and monocytes. There are approximately 100 cases of childhood cyclic neutropenia in the literature, most of which are consistent with an autosomal dominant inheritance. However, sporadic adult cases also occur, and these are associated with neutrophil elastase mutations. There does not seem to be a racial predilection or gender bias in incidence.

Pathogenesis

The neutrophil count in blood is stable in normal individuals, reflecting the fact that there is a large storage pool of granulocytes in the marrow. The marrow reserve exceeds the circulating pool of neutrophils by 5- to 10-fold. This large pool is necessary because it takes nearly 2 weeks for the full development of a neutrophil from an early stem cell within the bone

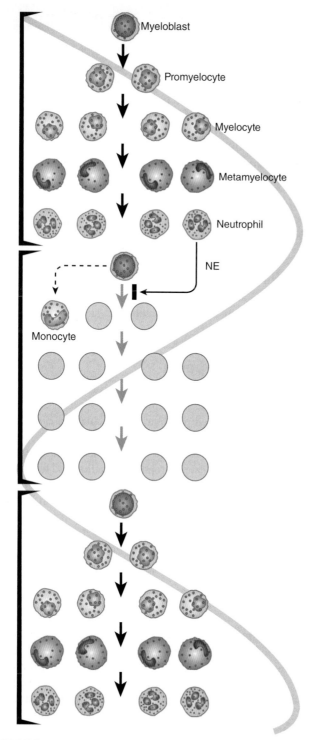

FIGURE 6–11 Feedback loop hypothesis to explain hematopoietic cycling. Neutrophil elastase (NE) is postulated to inhibit further differentiation by a myeloblast. Gray sine wave denotes neutrophil count oscillations. In this model, NE is produced by the terminally differentiating cohort of neutrophils and ultimately feeds back to inhibit further production of neutrophils, which results in loss of the inhibitory cycle—at least for a while, until production of the neutrophils resumes, followed again by the inhibitory action of NE in a cyclic manner. (Redrawn from Horwitz MS et al. Neutrophil elastase in cyclic and severe congenital neutropenia. Blood. 2007 Mar 1;109(5):1817–24. Copyright American Society of Hematology.)

marrow, yet the average life span of a mature neutrophil in blood is less than 12 hours.

In cyclic neutropenia, the storage pool is not adequate. Daily measurements of neutrophil counts in the blood reveal striking variations in their number. Studies of neutrophil kinetics in affected patients reveal that the defect is in abnormal production, rather than abnormal disposition, of neutrophils. Neutrophil production occurs in discrete waves even in normal individuals. As neutrophils differentiate from an early progenitor cell, they produce neutrophil elastase, which is thought to inhibit the differentiation of myeloblasts in a negative feedback loop. This results in an oscillatory wave with peaks and troughs of neutrophil production. As neutrophil numbers increase in the marrow, a peak is obtained in which enough neutrophil elastase causes a drop in neutrophil differentiation. Then, as the number of neutrophils drops again to a nadir, the production of neutrophil elastase also declines, allowing the number of neutrophils to climb once again. In cyclic neutropenia, it is hypothesized that the mutant neutrophil elastase may have an excessive inhibitory effect, causing prolonged trough periods and inadequate storage pools to maintain a normal peripheral neutrophil count. However, once they are extruded from the marrow, the neutrophils appear to have a normal life span (Figure 6–11).

The myeloid progenitor for neutrophils can also produce monocytes. Therefore, during neutrophil nadirs, the myeloid progenitor cell can preferentially differentiate to the monocyte lineage, giving rise to the opposing oscillatory waves of neutrophils and monocytes seen in these patients (Figure 6–12).

The waves are remarkably constant in their periodicity. Almost every patient has a cycle between 19 and 22 days, and each patient's cycle length is constant during his or her lifetime. Neutrophils and monocytes are not the only marrow elements that cycle. Platelet and reticulocyte counts also cycle with the same cycle length, but in contrast to the blood neutrophil count, clinically significant decreases are not observed.

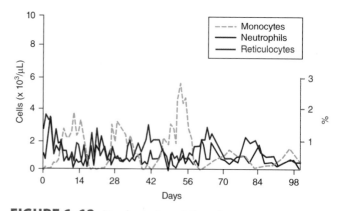

FIGURE 6–12 Regular cyclic variation of monocytes, reticulocytes, and neutrophils in a patient with cyclic neutropenia. Note that monocytes and reticulocytes tend to rise when neutrophils fall. (Redrawn, with permission, from Dale D et al. Cyclic neutropenia: a clinical review. Blood Rev. 1988;2:178. Copyright © Elsevier.)

This is presumably because the blood life spans of these elements are so much longer than the life span of neutrophils. Because multiple cell lines are seen to cycle, it is believed that neutrophil elastase mutations accelerate the process of **apoptosis** (programmed cell death) in early progenitor cells, as well, unless they are "rescued" by G-CSF.

Clinically, administration of pharmacologic doses of G-CSF (filgrastim) to affected individuals has three interesting effects that partially overcome the condition. First, although cycling continues, mean neutrophil counts increase at each point in the cycle, such that patients are rarely neutropenic. Second, cycling periodicity decreases immediately from 21 days to 14 days. Third, other cell line fluctuations change in parallel; their cycle periodicity also decreases to 14 days, suggesting that an early progenitor cell is indeed at the center of this illness. However, the fact that cycling does not disappear demonstrates that there are other abnormalities yet to be discovered. It also suggests that there may be an inherent cycling of all stem cells in normal individuals that is modulated by multiple cytokines in the marrow.

Pathology

The pathologic features of cyclic neutropenia are seen mostly in the laboratory. The peripheral blood smear appears normal except for the paucity of neutrophils—mature or immature—during the nadirs of each cycle. Individual neutrophils appear normal. The bone marrow, however, shows striking differences depending on the day of the cycle on which it is examined. During the nadir of each cycle, there are increased numbers of early myeloid precursors such as promyelocytes and myelocytes, and mature neutrophils are rare. This picture is similar to that seen in acute leukemia, but 10 days later, as circulating neutrophil counts are rising, an entirely normal-appearing marrow is typical.

Clinical Manifestations

In general, neutropenia from any cause places patients at risk for severe bacterial infections, generally from enteric organisms, because of the alteration in host defenses in the GI tract. This is especially true when the neutropenia results from administration of chemotherapeutic agents, because chemotherapy also affects the lining of the GI tract. Neutrophils, with their ability to engulf bacteria and deliver toxic enzymes and oxidizing free radicals to sites of infection, normally serve as the first line of host defense against the bacteria that inhabit the gut. Such patients are also at risk for fungal infections if the neutropenia lasts more than several days; this is because it takes longer for fungi to reproduce and invade the bloodstream. Untreated infections of either type can be rapidly fatal, particularly if the neutrophil count is less than about 250/μL.

In cyclic neutropenia, then, recurrent infections are to be expected, and deaths from infections with intestinal organisms have been reported. Each cycle is characterized by malaise and fever coincident with the time neutrophil counts are falling. Cervical lymphadenopathy is almost always present, as are oral ulcers. These symptoms usually last for about 5 days and then subside until the next cycle.

When infections occur, the site is usually predictable. Skin infections, specifically small, superficial pyogenic abscesses (**furunculosis**) or bacterial invasion of the dermis or epidermis (**cellulitis**), are the most common and respond to antibiotic therapy with few sequelae. The next most common infection site is usually the gums, and chronic gingivitis is evident in about half of patients. It is also the most noticeably improved problem when patients receive therapy with filgrastim. Other infections are unusual, but any neutropenic patient is at risk for infection from organisms that reside in the GI system. In the few patients who have required abdominal surgery during their neutropenia, ulcers similar to those seen in the mouth have been noted; this destruction of the normal mucosal barrier presumably eases entry of intestinal bacteria into the bloodstream. Because the period of greatest susceptibility to infection is only a few days in each cycle, most patients grow and develop normally.

CHECKPOINT

19. How long does it take for a neutrophil to develop from a stem cell in the bone marrow? Once fully mature, what is its life span?

20. At what level of neutropenia does the incidence of infection dramatically increase?

21. What are the most common sites and types of infections observed in neutropenic patients?

22. What is the probable underlying abnormality in cyclic neutropenia?

PLATELET DISORDERS

1. Drug-Associated Immune Thrombocytopenia

Etiology

Thrombocytopenia, defined as the occurrence of platelet levels below the normal laboratory range, is a commonly encountered abnormality. Although there are many causes (see Table 6–7), the possibility of a drug-induced immune thrombocytopenia should always be considered.

Many drugs have been associated with this phenomenon, and the most common ones are listed in Table 6–9. In practice, the association between a given drug and thrombocytopenia is usually made clinically rather than with specific tests. Thrombocytopenia usually occurs at least 5–7 days after exposure to the drug, if given for the first time. The suspect drug is stopped, and platelet counts rebound within a few days. Rechallenge with the drug, which is rarely done, almost always reproduces the thrombocytopenia.

Heparin is the most important cause of thrombocytopenia because of its frequent use in hospitalized patients; its use also

TABLE 6–9   Common drugs that may cause thrombocytopenia.

Abciximab	Heparin
Acetaminophen	Hydrochlorothiazide
Acetazolamide	Indinavir
Allopurinol	Interferon alfa
Amiodarone	Iodinated contrast agents
Amphotericin B	Linezolid
Aspirin	Methyldopa
Atorvastatin	Nonsteroidal anti-inflammatory drugs (NSAIDs)
Captopril	Ondansetron
Carbamazepine	Penicillins
Cephalosporins	Pentoxifylline
Chlorothiazide	Phenothiazines
Chlorthalidone	Phenytoin
Cimetidine	Prednisone
Clopidrogel	Procainamide
Cocaine	Quinidine
Danazol	Quinine
Digoxin	Ranitidine
Eptifibatide	Rifampin
Ethanol	Sulfonamides (antibiotics and hypoglycemics)
Famotidine	Ticlopidine
Fluconazole	Tirofiban
Furosemide	Valproic acid
Gold salts	Vancomycin

carries the potential to cause a life-threatening thrombotic syndrome. The pathophysiology of the thrombocytopenia caused by heparin is also the most completely described.

Pathogenesis

Although the phenomenon of drug-induced thrombocytopenia has been known for decades to be immune in nature, the specific mechanisms have long been controversial. The association of antibodies with platelets leads to their destruction via the spleen. The spleen acts as the major "blood filter" and recognizes platelets bound to antibodies as abnormal and thus removes them. Spleen removal also occurs in autoimmune (idiopathic) thrombocytopenia, which is relatively common and difficult to distinguish clinically from drug-induced thrombocytopenia.

There are various mechanisms underlying drug-induced immune thrombocytopenia. Quinine- or NSAID-induced thrombocytopenia involves the tight binding of antibody to normal platelets only in the presence of the sensitizing drug. The antibody usually targets epitopes on the glycoprotein IIb/IIIa or Ib/IX complexes, the major platelet receptors for fibrinogen and vWF, respectively. Penicillin and cephalosporin antibiotics are believed to lead to platelet destruction via hapten-dependent antibodies. The drug acts as a hapten, a small molecule that elicits an immunologic response only when bound to a large carrier molecule or protein. Some drugs (gold salts, procainamide, and possibly sulfonamides) can induce autoantibodies capable of binding to and destroying platelets even in the absence of the sensitizing drug. Finally, antithrombotic agents that block the binding of fibrinogen to gpIIb/IIIa receptors (abciximab, tirofiban, or eptifibatide) can cause an acute immune-mediated thrombocytopenia, in which patients develop severe thrombocytopenia within hours of exposure. The mechanism involves either naturally occurring antibodies that recognize the murine component of abciximab or structural changes to the gpIIb/IIIa receptor caused by the binding of tirofiban or eptifibatide.

For heparin, there is clear evidence of binding to a platelet protein, platelet factor 4 (PF4). PF4 resides in the alpha granules of platelets and is released when they are activated. It binds back onto the platelet surface through a specific PF4 receptor molecule, further increasing platelet activation. It also binds with high affinity to heparin and to heparin-like glycosaminoglycan molecules present on the vascular endothelium. This non-immune-based adhesion to PF4 can lead to mild thrombocytopenia via promotion of platelet binding to fibrinogen and subsequent aggregation, known as **heparin-induced thrombocytopenia (HIT) type I**. This can happen in 30% of patients exposed to heparins without clinical sequelae. However, the combination of heparin with PF4 can also act as an antigenic stimulus that provokes the production of immunoglobulin G (IgG) directed against the combination. This immunologic response is known as **heparin-induced thrombocytopenia (HIT) type II**. About 10–20% of these patients with heparin-PF4 antibodies will develop the serious clinical syndrome of heparin-induced thrombocytopenia (and thrombosis) (HIT[T]), which paradoxically involves both thrombocytopenia 5–10 days after drug exposure and a prothrombotic state via increased platelet activation. There is a 10-fold increased risk for HIT in patients receiving unfractionated heparin (UFH) compared with those receiving low-molecular-weight heparins. Cardiac or orthopedic surgery patients are at higher risk for clinical HIT (1–5%) than medical or obstetric patients (0.1–1%) when receiving UFH. Women are at twice the risk for HIT as men.

Thrombocytopenia occurs in HIT type II after a series of steps. First, PF4 is released from platelets either by heparin itself or by other stimuli. Heparin then binds to PF4, forming an antigenic complex that results in the production of IgG antibodies that can bind directly to this compound. The new complex of IgG–heparin–PF4 binds to platelets through the platelet Fc receptor, via its IgG end. Platelets bound with this antibody complex are then destroyed by the spleen.

Despite the resulting thrombocytopenia, HIT type II leads to a prothrombotic state via the additional binding of the heparin–PF4 portion to the PF4 receptor on platelets, promoting platelet cross-linking, activation, and aggregation (Figure 6–13).

Because each end of this IgG–heparin–PF4 molecule can bind to a platelet, it is possible that platelets can become cross-linked by a single molecule. Many platelets could actually interact in this fashion, leading to further platelet aggregation and activation. Clinically, this decreases the numbers of circulating platelets, but it may also lead to the creation of a thrombus at the site of activation. Thus, despite the fact that heparin is the most commonly used anticoagulant, in this case it may actually provoke coagulation. Furthermore, the activation of platelets via this mechanism leads to increased amounts of circulating PF4, which can bind to more heparin and thus continue the cycle. The excess PF4 can also bind to the endothelial surface via the heparin-like glycosaminoglycans described earlier. It is thus possible that the antibodies to the heparin–PF4 construct could bind to the endothelial

cells as well, which may lead to endothelial cell injury, further increasing the risk of local thrombosis by releasing TF and ultimately thrombin. Lastly, there is some evidence that macrophages may release TF in response to these antibodies, further stimulating coagulation.

Pathology

The peripheral blood smear is not strikingly abnormal unless platelet counts are less than about 75,000/μL, and then it is usually abnormal only because relatively few platelets are seen. Platelet morphology is usually normal, although large platelets can be seen. These large platelets are less mature and are a bone marrow compensation for a low peripheral platelet count, with platelet production from megakaryocytes being increased. Although drugs—heparin in particular—may cause platelet aggregation in vivo and in vitro, this is usually not apparent on review of the blood smear.

The bone marrow usually appears normal, although the megakaryocyte number may be relatively increased, presumably reflecting an attempt to increase the number of platelets (megakaryocyte fragments) in the circulation. In a few cases

FIGURE 6–13 Pathogenesis of heparin-induced thrombocytopenia (HIT). IgG is the autoantibody against the heparin–PF4 complex. Platelets can bind to each other and become activated via the IgG–Fc receptor interaction, the PF4–PF4 receptor interaction, or both. Aggregation and thrombus formation may thus occur. Furthermore, IgG may bind to the endothelial cell–bound heparin–PF4 construct and cause vascular damage, which may also provoke thrombus formation.

of immune-mediated thrombocytopenia, however, there may be decreased numbers of megakaryocytes. There are many hypotheses as to why this may occur, but it most likely means that the antigenic combination of drug–platelet protein is also occurring on megakaryocytes, so that they and the platelets in the peripheral circulation are being immunologically destroyed. This destruction would not involve the spleen, of course, but would require antibody-dependent cell killing.

In patients who develop heparin-induced thrombocytopenia and thrombosis, thrombi are seen that are relatively rich in platelets when compared with "typical" thrombi seen in other situations. They are described as "white clots." The thrombi may be either arterial or venous.

Clinical Manifestations

Despite the fact that the platelet count in immune-mediated thrombocytopenia can be extremely low (<10,000/μL, compared with a normal value of over 150,000/μL), severe bleeding is unusual. More often, there is easy bruising with minimal trauma. With platelet counts of less than about 5000/μL, pinpoint hemorrhages (**petechiae**) may spontaneously occur in the skin or mucous membranes. These are self-limited because the plasma coagulation factors are still intact, and only a small number of aggregated platelets are needed to provide adequate phospholipids for clotting.

The relationship between the likelihood of bleeding and the platelet count is not linear. The **bleeding time**, a test used clinically to evaluate platelet function, does not even begin to be abnormally prolonged until the platelet count is less than 90,000/μL. Spontaneous bleeding is unlikely until platelet counts are less than 20,000/μL but is still uncommon until counts are less than about 5000/μL, assuming that patients do not have other abnormalities of hemostasis. For example, aspirin inhibits platelet aggregation and increases the likelihood of bleeding. When bleeding from thrombocytopenia does occur, it is most often mucosal or superficial in the skin. This is most commonly seen as a nose bleed (epistaxis), but bleeding of the gums, GI tract, or bladder mucosa may also be seen.

As mentioned, however, when immune thrombocytopenia occurs as a result of heparin, paradoxical clotting may occur instead of bleeding. This may create a very confusing picture, because the heparin may have been given therapeutically for another thrombosis; it may be difficult to determine whether the new thrombosis is an extension of the initial clot or a new one resulting from the heparin exposure. However, the occurrence of the simultaneous thrombocytopenia provides a clue.

When heparin-induced thrombocytopenia and thrombosis do occur, the clinical manifestation of the new thrombosis will depend on the site of the thrombus. Most studies of this disorder suggest that when thrombosis occurs, it is at the site of previous vascular injury or abnormality. Thus, in patients with atherosclerotic vascular disease, arterial thromboses are much more common than venous clots. Patients experience a rapid onset of severe pain, usually in an extremity, with a cool, pale limb. Pulses are absent. This can be life-threatening

(5–10% mortality rate) or at least extremity threatening because oxygen flow to the affected area is cut off, and emergency clot removal or vascular bypass surgery may be necessary. Venous clots also occur in a manner similar to typical venous clots (see later discussion). In addition to stopping heparin, patients with type II HIT need anticoagulation to prevent and treat thrombosis formation. Direct thrombin inhibitors (argatroban, lepirudin, or bivalirudin) provide a direct means of blocking the effects of thrombin, a primary mediator of the coagulation system.

CHECKPOINT

23. What is the most common category of cause of thrombocytopenia?
24. Name the platelet protein antibodies implicated in the pathogenesis of heparin-induced thrombocytopenia.
25. By what mechanism can heparin-induced thrombocytopenia actually increase clot formation?
26. Why is major bleeding unusual in drug-induced thrombocytopenia?

COAGULATION DISORDERS

1. Inherited Hypercoagulable States
Etiology

The formation of blood clots in otherwise normal vessels is distinctly abnormal because the coagulation system in mammalian species is both positively and negatively balanced by so many factors. Nonetheless, there are a number of diseases that result in abnormal clotting (**thrombosis**). Abnormal clotting states may be either primary, in that the abnormalities result from genetic predispositions involving the coagulation factors themselves, or secondary (ie, acquired) because of changes in coagulation factors, blood vessels, or blood flow.

As first noted by the pathologist Virchow more than 150 years ago, there are three possible contributors to the formation of an abnormal clot (thrombus): decreased blood flow, vessel injury or inflammation, and changes in the intrinsic properties of the blood. Persistent physiologic changes in any of these three factors (the Virchow triad) are referred to as the "hypercoagulable states."

The primary, or inherited, hypercoagulable states are all autosomal dominant genetic defects. This means that carriers (heterozygotes) are affected. Except for hyperprothrombinemia, all lead only to moderate (50%) decreases in the levels of the relevant factors. Despite the relatively modest fall, affected individuals are predisposed to abnormal thrombosis. These disorders are relatively rare in the general population, but they do account for a significant percentage of young patients who come to medical attention with thromboses. The specific states to be discussed are activated protein C (APC) resistance (the most commonly encountered abnormality), protein C deficiency, protein S deficiency, AT deficiency, and the pro-thrombin 20210 AG abnormality. Hyperhomocystinemia, an inborn error of metabolism, is also an inherited hypercoagulable state, but because it does not involve the coagulation cascade, it is not further discussed here.

Pathogenesis

In the coagulation cascade, activated factor V (Va) plays a pivotal role (Figure 6–14). It is required for the formation of the prothrombinase complex with factor Xa, which leads to the thrombin burst and fibrin generation during hemostasis. Factor Va thus makes an excellent negative control point, so that once clot formation has begun, it does not go on unchecked.

Protein C is the major inhibitor of factor Va. Although it is an anticoagulation factor, its production is contingent on vitamin K–dependent γ-carboxylation, just like the coagulation factors II, VII, IX, and X. Protein C, when activated by the presence of clotting that generates thrombin, cleaves factor Va into an inactive form, and activation of factor X is thus slowed. By itself, however, protein C only weakly influences factor Va; its negative effect on factor Va is enhanced by a protein cofactor, protein S.

Factor V does not provide the only negative control point, however. Protein C also inhibits activated factor VIIIa, which is critical to forming the tenase–factor IXa complex, which is needed to activate factor X on activated platelets leading to prothrombinase generation (see Figure 6–4). Factors II, IX, X, and XI (the serine proteases) are inhibited by a different molecule, AT. The action of AT itself is also regulated and highly dependent on the binding of an accelerator, heparin, or similar molecules present in abundance along the endothelial cells that line the vasculature. Evidence suggests that AT may also inhibit the TF–VIIa complex.

The fact that deficiencies of protein S, protein C, and AT activity cause clinically significant thrombosis demonstrates an important concept: It is the lack of adequate anticoagulant activity, rather than the overproduction of procoagulant activity, that characterizes most of the hypercoagulable states.

A. Activated Protein C Resistance—APC resistance is the most common inherited hypercoagulable state, with as many as 3–7% of the general population heterozygous for the abnormality. Up to 25% of patients who have venous thrombosis without an inciting event are found to have APC resistance in a large patient series. Most cases result from a single DNA base-pair mutation in the factor V gene, where guanine (G) is replaced by adenine (A). This single base change leads to substitution of the amino acid glutamine for arginine at position 506, and the altered factor V is referred to as "factor V Leiden," named for the town in the Netherlands where it was discovered. This amino acid change alters the three-dimensional conformation of the cleavage site within factor Va, where APC normally binds to inactivate it. Thus, factor Va molecules can continue to enhance factor Xa's conversion of prothrombin to thrombin (factor IIa), via the prothrombinase complex, and coagulation is not inhibited. This mutation also leads to loss of a cleavage product normally formed when factor V is inactivated by APC, a cofactor important in APC's inactivation of factor VIIIa. Therefore, loss of this cofactor leads to decreased anticoagulant activity and contributes to the hypercoagulable state.

B. Protein C Deficiency—Protein C deficiency is common; up to 1 of every 200 individuals in the population is a heterozygote. Yet, thrombosis is uncommon among these individuals. The families that are thrombosis prone are thought to carry additional genetic factors, in addition to protein C deficiency, that increase their risk for thrombosis.

As noted earlier, protein C inactivates factors Va and VIIIa but requires protein S for its own action. Protein C also depends on the presence of platelet PL and calcium. In protein C deficiency, there is less inhibition of the prothrombinase complex, leading to relatively unrestricted clot formation. Normally, some of the thrombin generated binds to an endothelial cell protein, thrombomodulin, and this complex activates protein C in the first place. This "negative feedback loop" is thus lost in protein C deficiency.

Protein C deficiency is not all one disease, however, unlike the factor V Leiden abnormality. Type I deficiency refers to individuals with decreased levels of protein C. Type II deficiency denotes cases with normal protein C levels but low protein C activity.

C. Protein S Deficiency—Protein S deficiency is also an uncommon heterogeneous disorder. Type I protein S deficiency refers to cases with low free and total protein S levels. Type II deficiency, which is the least encountered, refers to an abnormally functioning protein S. Type III deficiency refers only to low levels of free protein S. In the coagulation cascade, when factors Va and Xa are complexed together, the inactivation site on factor Va is "hidden" from protein C. Protein S, not a protease itself, exposes this site so that protein C can cleave

FIGURE 6–14 The central role of factor V in the control of the coagulation cascade. The action of each of the negative control factors—protein S, protein C, and antithrombin—is shown in color.

Va. Because protein S is so crucial, deficiency of protein S also leads to the unregulated procoagulant action of factor Xa.

D. Antithrombin Deficiency

—AT deficiency is less common than any of the previously discussed disorders, with approximately 1 in 2000 cases in the general population. AT binds to and inhibits not just thrombin (thus its name), but also the activated forms of factors IX, X, XI, and XII, and perhaps the factor VII–TF complex as well. Unlike protein C's proteolytic cleavage of factor Va, AT binds to each factor, directly blocking their activity; it is not an enzyme. This action is accelerated—up to 2000 times—in a reversible manner by the anticoagulant molecule heparin, which binds to AT via its pentasaccharide sequence. The anticoagulant fondaparinux is a synthetic version of this five-saccharide sequence, and thus it can also bind to AT. In AT deficiency, then, multiple coagulation steps are unbalanced, and the coagulation cascade may proceed unrestrained. More than 100 different AT mutations have been reported. Type I molecular defects involve a parallel decrease in antigen and activity, whereas type II defects involve a dysfunctional molecule with decreased activity but normal or near-normal antigen levels.

E. Hyperprothrombinemia

—A mutation in the untranslated region of the prothrombin gene (a single base-pair mutation, called 20210 AG) is associated with elevated plasma prothrombin (II) levels and an increased risk of thrombosis. Presumably, this leads to excess thrombin generation when the prothrombinase complex is activated. This is probably the second most common hereditary hypercoagulable state after factor V Leiden. It is the first hereditary thrombophilia associated with overproduction of procoagulant factors.

Pathology

The pathologic features of thrombi in hypercoagulable states are indistinguishable from those of genetically normal individuals on a gross anatomic or microscopic basis, except that there is a greater likelihood in hypercoagulable states of having a clot in unusual sites (see Clinical Manifestations section).

Most of the pathologic features of the hereditary hypercoagulable states consist of laboratory abnormalities. In the evaluation of patients suspected of having a hereditary hypercoagulable state, there are two basic types of laboratory abnormalities. The first type is quantitative: Specific immunologic assays can define the relative amount of protein C, protein S, AT, or fibrinogen present in a given patient's serum, but they do not evaluate the function of any of these molecules. The second type is qualitative: The assays for protein C or protein S activity (rather than amount) measure the ability (or inability) of the patient's protein C or S to prolong a clotting time in vitro. APC resistance can be evaluated with a different clotting assay, but generally the presence of the specific mutation in factor V Leiden is assessed by the polymerase chain reaction because the full sequence of the molecule is known. The polymerase chain reaction is also used for detecting the 20210 AG prothrombin abnormality. Prothrombin levels can also be measured and are consistently in the highest quartile of prothrombin levels found.

Clinical Manifestations

Most thromboembolic events encountered in clinical practice are secondary, not primary. Patients have blood clots usually in the deep veins of the legs for two reasons: (1) because of sluggish blood flow (in high-capacity, low-flow veins) compared with other sites, particularly when inactive (eg, bedridden after surgery or as a result of illness); and (2) because the extremities are more likely to sustain injury than the trunk. Trauma causes blood vessel compression or injury; thus, two elements of the Virchow triad are more readily observed in the legs than elsewhere.

These venous clots in the legs (commonly referred to as deep venous thromboses [DVTs]) usually present with pain, swelling, and redness below the level of the thrombus, with normal arterial pulses and distal extremity perfusion. Because blood return to the central circulation is blocked in these high-capacity vessels, superficial collateral veins just under the skin may be prominent and engorged. The swelling is mechanical, because normal arterial blood flow continues to the extremity while venous return is compromised, leading to engorgement. Pain occurs primarily as a result of the swelling alone but can also occur from lactic acid buildup in the muscles of the legs. This happens when the pressure in the legs increases to the point that it compromises arterial blood flow and adequate oxygen delivery to those muscles.

Pulmonary emboli, the major source of morbidity and mortality after DVT of the lower extremity, typically present with acute-onset shortness of breath, hypoxemia, and a history suggesting an initial DVT that has now broken off and migrated through the right side of the heart to the pulmonary arterial system. The clot blocks blood flow from the heart to a portion of lung, leading to hypoxemia, which can be exacerbated by underlying lung disease.

The clinical presentations of all hypercoagulable states are similar, but there are some interesting differences. DVTs tend to occur (whether there is a hypercoagulable state or not) in patients with a history of trauma, pregnancy, oral contraceptive use, or immobility, but rarely in adolescents or young adults. Inherited hypercoagulable states are suspected in patients who present with a thromboembolic event, usually because they are young or experience recurrent clots. Events that occur without any specific risks are particularly suspect. Because of the dominant pattern of inheritance, suspicion is aroused when other family members have had clotting problems, underscoring the importance of taking a family history.

Despite the distinct coagulation abnormalities, most thromboses still occur in usual sites (ie, the deep veins of the legs with or without pulmonary embolism). Other unusual sites (eg, the sagittal sinus of the skull or the mesenteric veins in the abdomen) are more likely to be found in patients with underlying coagulation disorders than in those without. Arterial thromboses, however, are extremely rare.

Interestingly, only a minority of patients with an inherited hypercoagulable state develop symptomatic thromboses; this is particularly true for heterozygotes. Each disorder is slightly different, presumably because of the redundancy of the factors in the coagulation cascade. And undoubtedly the penetrance of each state varies in individual patients because of factors we do not yet understand. Heterozygotes who develop thrombosis usually present in the setting of a "typical" risk factor: sustaining an injury, having an extremity immobilized, having surgery, or being pregnant.

Homozygous protein C or protein S deficiencies present the highest likelihood of causing illness. Both conditions usually result in thrombosis, which is fatal in early life (neonatal purpura fulminans), although some patients may not present until their teens. Heterozygotes for protein C deficiency are unlikely to develop a thrombosis over their lifetimes, although they are about 4–6 times more likely to do so than members of the general population. Heterozygotes for protein S deficiency have a 1- to 10-fold increased relative risk of thrombosis.

AT deficiency is another significant defect in terms of the likelihood of developing thrombosis. These patients have a lifetime 5- to 10-fold increased relative risk for thrombosis.

The situation is complex in the case of APC resistance. Heterozygotes for APC resistance probably represent more than one-third of all patients with familial thromboses. Although there is a 3- to 5-fold increased relative risk of thrombosis for heterozygotes of this mutation, heterozygosity rarely leads to thrombosis unless there is an additional risk factor for hypercoagulability. In heterozygotes, proteins C and S can still cleave factor VIIIa, and the factor V abnormality is a relative rather than absolute insensitivity to APC. There is still negative control of the clotting cascade at the factor X step by TFPI as well.

Even homozygous factor V Leiden does not inevitably cause thrombosis. Families in which homozygous females have had repeated pregnancies without difficulty have been carefully described. This is somewhat surprising because pregnancy, a hypercoagulable state itself, leads to decreases in protein S concentration, which would be expected to amplify the resistance to protein C. Nevertheless, there is at least a 20- to 50-fold increased risk of thrombosis versus the general population for homozygotes for factor V Leiden.

Persons with the prothrombin 20210 AG mutation are nearly all heterozygotes, with about a 2- to 3-fold higher risk of thrombosis than the general population.

CHECKPOINT

27. What constitutes the Virchow triad of factors predisposing to the formation of intravascular clots?
28. Deficiencies in which proteins can result in clinically significant thromboses?
29. What is the basis for activated protein C resistance?

CASE STUDIES

Yeong Kwok, MD

(See Chapter 25, p. 751–55 for Answers)

CASE 26

A 65-year-old previously well man presents to the clinic with complaints of fatigue of 3 months' duration. Questioning reveals diffuse weakness and feeling winded when walking uphill or climbing more than one flight of stairs. All symptoms have slowly worsened over time. There are no other complaints, and the review of systems is otherwise negative. The patient has no significant medical history, social history, or family history. On physical examination, he appears somewhat pale, with normal vital signs. The physical examination is unremarkable except for his rectal examination, which reveals brown, guaiac-positive stool (suggesting the presence of blood in the stool). A blood test reveals anemia.

Questions

A. What is the most likely form of anemia in this man? What is the probable underlying cause?
B. What is the mechanism by which this disorder results in anemia?
C. What might one expect to see in the peripheral blood smear?
D. What other tests might be ordered to confirm the diagnosis?
E. What is the pathophysiologic mechanism of this patient's fatigue, weakness, and shortness of breath? Why is he pale?

CASE 27

A 58-year-old black woman presents to the emergency department with complaints of progressive fatigue and weakness for the past 6 months. She is short of breath after walking several blocks. On review of systems, she mentions mild diarrhea. She has noted intermittent numbness and tingling of her lower extremities and a loss of balance while walking. She denies other neurologic or cardiac symptoms and has no history of black or bloody stools or other blood loss. On physical examination, she is tachycardic to 110 bpm; other vital signs are within normal limits. The head-and-neck examination is notable for pale conjunctivas and a beefy red tongue with loss of papillae. Cardiac examination shows a rapid, regular rhythm with a grade 2/6 systolic murmur at the left sternal border. Lung, abdominal, and rectal examination findings are normal. Neurologic examination reveals decreased sensation to light touch and vibration in the lower extremities. The hematology consultant on call is asked to see this patient because of a low hematocrit level.

Questions

A. What vitamin deficiency is the probable cause of this woman's anemia? How does this result in anemia?
B. What might one expect the peripheral blood smear to look like? What other blood tests may be ordered, and what results would be anticipated? What test might differentiate the various causes of this vitamin deficiency?
C. The workup reveals pernicious anemia. What is the pathogenesis of this disease? What is the evidence to support an autoimmune origin?
D. What is the pathophysiologic mechanism of this woman's symptoms of tachycardia, paresthesias, and impaired proprioception?

CASE 28

A 6-year-old boy presents to the pediatric emergency department. His mother states that he has had 3 days of general malaise and fevers to 38.5°C. He has no other localizing symptoms. The medical history is remarkable for multiple febrile illnesses. His mother says, "It seems like he gets sick every month." The physical examination is notable for cervical lymphadenopathy and oral ulcers. Blood tests reveal a neutrophil count of 200/μL. The patient is admitted to the hospital. Blood, urine, and cerebrospinal fluid cultures are negative, and over 48 hours, the patient's neutrophil counts return to normal. He is then discharged.

Questions

A. What is the likely pathogenesis of cyclic neutropenia? What evidence supports this theory?
B. What aspects of this case presentation support the diagnosis of cyclic neutropenia? What is the expected clinical course?
C. Assuming that the diagnosis of cyclic neutropenia is correct, what would one expect the peripheral blood smear to look like? What would you expect the bone marrow examination results to show at admission? What would you expect them to be in 2 weeks?

CASE 29

A 36-year-old man was admitted to hospital after sustaining multiple fractures to the lower extremities after jumping from a three-story building in a suicide attempt. His fractures required surgical repair. He has no significant medical history. Current medications include morphine for pain and subcutaneous heparin for prophylaxis against deep venous thrombosis. Consultation with a hematologist is requested because of a dropping platelet count. On physical examination, the patient has multiple bruises, and his lower extremities are casted bilaterally. Examination is otherwise normal. Laboratory tests from the last several days reveal a platelet count that has dropped from 170,000/μL on admission to 30,000/μL 5 days later.

Questions

A. What is the most likely cause of this man's thrombocytopenia?
B. By what mechanisms does heparin sometimes cause thrombocytopenia?
C. What are the possible clinical consequences of this patient's thrombocytopenia?

CASE 30

A 23-year-old woman presents to the emergency department with a chief complaint of acute onset of shortness of breath. It is associated with right-sided chest pain, which increases with inspiration. The patient denies fever, chills, cough, and other respiratory symptoms. She has had no lower extremity swelling. She has not been ill, bedridden, or immobile for prolonged periods. Her medical history is notable for an episode about 2 years ago of deep venous thrombosis in the right lower extremity while taking oral contraceptives. She has been otherwise healthy and is currently taking no medications. The family history is notable for a father who died of a pulmonary embolism. On physical examination, she appears anxious and in mild respiratory distress. She is tachycardic to 110 bpm, with a respiratory rate of 20/min. She has no fever, and blood pressure is stable. The remainder of the physical examination is normal. Chest x-ray film is normal. Ventilation-perfusion scan reveals a high probability of pulmonary embolus. Given her history of deep vein thrombosis, a hypercoagulable state is suspected.

Questions

A. What constitutes the Virchow triad of predisposing factors for venous thrombosis? Which components of the triad may be present in this patient?

B. What are some causes of inherited hypercoagulable states specifically associated with the coagulation cascade? How do they result in hypercoagulability?

C. How might this woman be evaluated for the presence of an inherited hypercoagulable state?

REFERENCES

General

Hoffman R et al. *Hematology: Basic Principles and Practice*, 7th ed. Elsevier, 2017.

Kaushansky K et al. *Williams Hematology*, 9th ed. McGraw-Hill, 2015.

Marder VK et al. *Hemostasis ad Thrombosis: Basic Principles and Clinical Practice*, 6th ed. Lippincott Williams & Wilkins, 2012.

Iron-Deficiency Anemia

Camaschella C. Iron-deficiency anemia. N Engl J Med. 2015 May 7;372(19):1832–43. [PMID: 25946282]

Camaschella C. New insights into iron deficiency and iron deficiency anemia. Blood Rev. 2017 Jul;31(4):225–33. [PMID: 28216263]

DeLoughery TG. Iron deficiency anemia. Med Clin North Am. 2017 Mar;101(2):319–32. [PMID: 28189173]

Dev S et al. Overview of iron metabolism in health and disease. Hemodial Int. 2017 Jun;21(Suppl 1):S6–S20. [PMID: 28296010]

Gozzelino R et al. Iron homeostasis in health and disease. Int J Mol Sci. 2016 Jan 20;17(1).pii: E130. [PMID: 26805813]

Kim A et al. New insights into iron regulation and erythropoiesis. Curr Opin Hematol. 2015 May;22(3):199–205. [PMID: 25710710]

Liu J et al. Hepcidin: a promising therapeutic target for iron disorders: a systematic review. Medicine (Baltimore). 2016 Apr;95(14):e3150. [PMID: 27057839]

Peng YY et al. Ferritin and iron studies in anaemia and chronic disease. Ann Clin Biochem. 2017 Jan;54(1):43–8. [PMID: 27701066]

Sangkhae V et al. Regulation of the iron homeostatic hormone hepcidin. Adv Nutr. 2017 Jan 17;8(1):126–36. [PMID: 28096133]

Silva B et al. An overview of molecular basis of iron metabolism regulation and the associated pathologies. Biochim Biophys Acta. 2015 Jul;1852(7):1347–59. [PMID: 25843914]

Pernicious Anemia

Green R. Vitamin B_{12} deficiency from the perspective of a practicing hematologist. Blood. 2017 May 11;129(19):2603–11. [PMID: 28360040]

Green R et al. Megaloblastic anemias: nutritional and other causes. Med Clin North Am. 2017 Mar;101(2):297–317. [PMID: 28189172]

Minalyan A et al. Autoimmune atrophic gastritis: current perspectives. Clin Exp Gastroenterol. 2017 Feb 7;10:19–27. [PMID: 28223833]

Osborne D et al. Autoimmune mechanisms in pernicious anaemia & thyroid disease. Autoimmun Rev. 2015 Sep;14(9):763–8. [PMID: 25936607].

Shipton MJ et al. Vitamin B_{12} deficiency—a 21st century perspective Clin Med (Lond). 2015 Apr;15(2):145–50. [PMID: 25824066]

Stabler SP. Clinical Practice. Vitamin B_{12} deficiency. N Engl J Med. 2013 Jan 10;368(2):149–60. [PMID: 23301732]

Wong CW. Vitamin B_{12} deficiency in the elderly: is it worth screening? Hong Kong Med J. 2015 Apr;21(2):155–64. [PMID: 25756278]

Cyclic Neutropenia

Makaryan V et al. The diversity of mutations and clinical outcomes for ELANE-associated neutropenia. Curr Opin Hematol. 2015 Jan;22(1):3–11. [PMID: 25427142]

Drug-Induced Thrombocytopenia

Al-Nouri ZL et al. Drug-induced thrombotic microangiopathy: a systematic review of published reports. Blood. 2015 Jan 22;125(4):616–8. [PMID: 25414441]

Arman M et al. Human platelet IgG Fc receptor FcγRIIA in immunity and thrombosis. J Thromb Haemost. 2015 Jun;13(6):893–908. [PMID: 25900780]

Greinacher A. Clinical Practice. Heparin-induced thrombocytopenia. N Engl J Med. 2015 Jul 16;373(3):252–61. [PMID: 26176382]

Junqueira DR et al. Unfractionated heparin versus low molecular weight heparins for avoiding heparin-induced thrombocytopenia in postoperative patients. Cochrane Database Syst Rev. 2017 Apr 21;4:CD007557. [PMID: 28431186]

Krzych ŁJ et al. Heparin-induced thrombocytopenia. Anaesthesiol Intensive Ther. 2015;47(1):63–76. [PMID: 25751293]

Nagler M et al. Diagnostic value of immunoassays for heparin-induced thrombocytopenia: a systematic review and meta-analysis. Blood. 2016 Feb 4;127(5):546–57. [PMID: 26518436]

Qiao J et al. The platelet Fc receptor, FcγRIIa. Immunol Rev. 2015 Nov;268(1):241–52. [PMID: 26497525]

Staibano P et al. The unique immunological features of heparin-induced thrombocytopenia. Br J Haematol. 2017 Apr;177(2):198–207. [PMID: 28369702]

Warkentin TE. Heparin-induced thrombocytopenia. Curr Opin Crit Care. 2015 Dec;21(6):576–85. [PMID: 26539932]

Warkentin TE. Heparin-induced thrombocytopenia in critically ill patients. Semin Thromb Hemost. 2015 Feb;41(1):49–60. [PMID: 25590528]

Hypercoagulable States

Bauer KA et al. Issues in the diagnosis and management of hereditary antithrombin deficiency. Ann Pharmacother. 2016 Sep;50(9):758–67. [PMID: 27281301]

MacCallum P et al. Diagnosis and management of heritable thrombophilias. BMJ 2014;349:g4387. [PMID: 25035247]

Middeldorp S. Inherited thrombophilia: a double-edged sword. Hematology Am Soc Hematol Educ Program. 2016 Dec 2;2016(1):1–9. [PMID: 27913455]

Pazzola G et al. The challenge of bleeding in antiphospholipid antibody-positive patients. Curr Rheumatol Rep. 2015 Feb;17(2):7. [PMID: 25618573]

Rhéaume M et al. Pregnancy-related venous thromboembolism risk in asymptomatic women with antithrombin deficiency: a systematic review. Obstet Gynecol. 2016 Apr;127(4):649–56. [PMID: 26959206]

Spychalska-Zwolińska M et al. Thrombophilia diagnosis: a retrospective analysis of a single-center experience. Blood Coagul Fibrinolysis. 2015 Sep;26(6):649–54. [PMID: 26083989]

Van Cott EM et al. Factor V Leiden. Am J Hematol. 2016 Jan;91(1):46–9. [PMID: 26492443]

Nervous System Disorders

Vikram G. Shakkottai, MD, PhD, &
Catherine Lomen-Hoerth MD, PhD

The major functions of the nervous system are to detect, analyze, and transmit information. Information is gathered by sensory systems, integrated by the brain, and used to generate signals to motor and autonomic pathways for control of movement and of visceral and endocrine functions. These actions are controlled by neurons, which are interconnected to form signaling networks that compose motor and sensory systems. In addition to neurons, the nervous system contains neuroglial cells that serve a variety of immunologic and support functions and modulate the activity of neurons. Understanding the pathophysiology of nervous system disease requires knowledge of neural and glial cell biology and the anatomy of neural networks. The first part of this chapter reviews several basic aspects of histology, cellular physiology, and anatomy of the nervous system.

Understanding the causes of neurologic diseases requires knowledge of molecular and biochemical mechanisms. Discoveries in the fields of molecular biology and genetics have made available important information about the mechanisms of several disease states. Several neurologic disorders for which some of the molecular mechanisms of pathogenesis are known are discussed later in this chapter, including cerebellar ataxia, motor neuron disease, Parkinson disease, myasthenia gravis, epilepsy, Alzheimer disease, and stroke. Exciting advances in our understanding of these diseases, including how they overlap, are leading to new therapeutic targets and the hope of better treating these devastating diseases.

NORMAL STRUCTURE & FUNCTION OF THE NERVOUS SYSTEM

HISTOLOGY & CELL BIOLOGY

Neurons

The major function of neurons is to receive, integrate, and transmit information to other cells. Neurons consist of three parts: **dendrites**, which are elongated processes that receive information from the environment or from other neurons; the **cell body**, which contains the nucleus; and the **axon**, which may be up to 1 m long and conducts impulses to muscles, glands, or other neurons (Figure 7–1). Most neurons are multipolar, containing one axon and several dendrites. Bipolar neurons have one dendrite and one axon and are found in the cochlear and vestibular ganglia, retina, and olfactory mucosa. Spinal sensory ganglia contain pseudounipolar neurons that have a single process that emanates from the cell body and divides into two branches, one extending to the spinal cord and the other extending to the periphery. Axons and dendrites usually branch extensively at their ends. Dendritic branching can be very complex, with the result that a single neuron may receive thousands of inputs. Axon branching allows several target cells to simultaneously receive a message from one neuron. Each branch of the axon terminates on the next cell at a **synapse**, which is a structure specialized for information transfer from the axon to muscle, glands, or another neuron. Synapses between neurons most often occur between axons and dendrites but may occur between an axon and a cell body, between two axons, or between two dendrites.

Signals are propagated electrically along axons. Like other cells, neurons maintain cell size and osmolarity primarily through the action of Na^+-K^+ ATPase, which actively pumps Na^+ out of cells in exchange for K^+. This results in the formation of concentration gradients for Na^+ and K^+ across the cell membrane. The membrane is practically impermeable to Na^+, but the presence of K^+ leak channels permits the flow of K^+ out of cells. This produces a difference in electrical charge across the membrane that counters transport of K^+ from the cell. The flow of ions continues until the opposing electrical

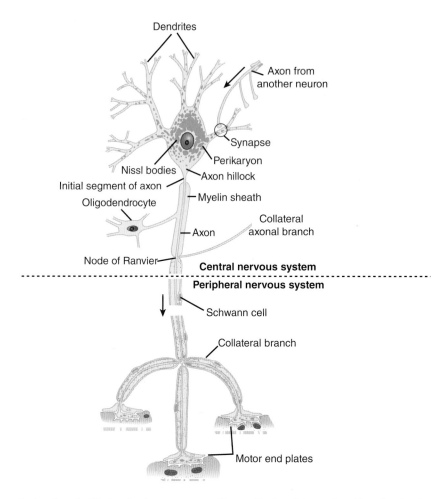

FIGURE 7-1 Schematic drawing of a Nissl-stained motor neuron. The myelin sheath is produced by oligodendrocytes in the central nervous system and by Schwann cells in the peripheral nervous system. Note the three motor end plates, which transmit the nerve impulse to striated skeletal muscle fibers. (Redrawn, with permission, from Junqueira LC et al, eds. *Basic Histology*, 11th ed. McGraw-Hill, 2005.)

force reaches a value that balances the diffusional force and the membrane reaches the **equilibrium potential** for K⁺ (E_K). E_K is calculated by the Nernst equation:

$$E_K = 2.3 \frac{RT}{F} \log \frac{[K^+]_o}{[K^+]_i}$$

where

R = gas constant (2 kcal mol⁻¹°K⁻¹)

T = absolute temperature (°K)

F = Faraday constant (2.3×10^4 kcal V⁻¹ mol⁻¹)

$[K^+]_o$ = concentration of K^+ outside the cell

$[K^+]_i$ = concentration of K^+ inside the cell

In most neurons, the resting membrane potential (E_m) is –50 to –100 mV and lies close to E_K since the leak of K⁺ is the major determinant of the charge difference across the membrane.

The membrane potential may be altered by increasing the permeability of the membrane to another ion, which drives the resting membrane potential toward the equilibrium potential

for that ion. Neurons are highly specialized to use rapid changes in membrane potential to generate electrical signals. This is accomplished by **ligand-gated** and **voltage-gated ion channels** that allow the passage of Na⁺, K⁺, Ca²⁺, or Cl⁻ ions in response to electrical or chemical stimuli. These channels are composed of protein complexes embedded in the lipid membrane to form aqueous pores to the inside of the cell. In general, channels are selective for a particular species of ion. An array of charged amino acids within voltage-dependent channels detects changes in voltage and induces a conformational change in the channel to alter ion permeability. Binding sites for **neurotransmitters**, such as glutamate, γ-aminobutyric acid (GABA), glycine, and acetylcholine, exist on ligand-gated channels and, when occupied, induce a conformational change to open the channel.

Electrical signals are propagated in neurons because a voltage change across the membrane in one part of a neuron is propagated to other parts. Passive spread of a voltage disturbance weakens with increasing distance from the source unless energy-dependent processes amplify the signal. Passive spread of electrical signals works well over short distances and is a major mechanism of signal propagation in dendrites. However, long-distance communication down axons to nerve terminals requires amplification. This is accomplished through the generation of self-propagating waves of excitation known as **action potentials**.

An action potential arises primarily from voltage-dependent changes in membrane permeability to Na$^+$ and K$^+$ (Figure 7–2). If a depolarizing stimulus raises the membrane potential to about –45 mV, voltage-gated Na$^+$ channels open, allowing an influx of Na$^+$ and further depolarization toward E$_{Na}$ (±50 mV). Nearby areas of membrane are depolarized to the threshold for Na$^+$ channel activation, propagating a wave of depolarization from the initial site. The resting potential is restored quickly by a combination of events. First, Na$^+$ channels close rapidly and remain in an inactive state until the membrane potential returns to negative levels for several milliseconds. Voltage-dependent K$^+$ channels open as the membrane potential becomes more depolarized, speeding the efflux of K$^+$ from cells and driving the membrane potential back to E$_K$. K$^+$ channels that participate in the action potential also inactivate, but more slowly than Na$^+$ channels, thereby allowing cell repolarization. Plasma membrane ion exchangers and ion pumps ensure that ionic gradients across the membrane continue to be maintained, by counteracting the ion fluxes that occur in the course of the generation of action potentials.

Neurons transmit signals chemically to other cells at synapses (Figure 7–3). Presynaptic and postsynaptic cells are electrically isolated from each other and separated by a narrow synaptic cleft. Signaling across the cleft occurs through the release of neurotransmitters from the terminal of the presynaptic neuron. Most neurotransmitters are stored in membrane-bound synaptic vesicles and are released into the synaptic cleft by Ca^{2+}-dependent exocytosis. Depolarization of the nerve terminal opens voltage-gated Ca^{2+} channels, stimulating Ca^{2+} influx and neurotransmitter release. Neurotransmitters diffuse across the cleft and bind to receptors on ligand-gated ion channels concentrated at the postsynaptic membrane. This produces local permeability changes, altering the membrane potential of the postsynaptic cell. If the response is depolarizing, an action potential may be generated if there are enough voltage-gated Na$^+$ channels nearby and the membrane potential has been raised to the threshold for their activation. Receptor-gated ion channels are highly selective for a particular neurotransmitter and for the type of ions they pass, which determines whether they generate excitatory or inhibitory responses. In general, **excitatory neurotransmitters**, such as glutamate, open cation channels that allow influx of Na$^+$ or Ca^{2+} and generate a depolarizing **excitatory**

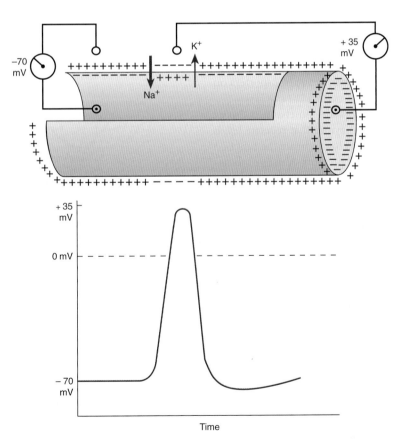

FIGURE 7–2 Conduction of the nerve impulse through an unmyelinated nerve fiber. In the resting axon, there is a difference of 70 mV between the interior of the axon and the outer surface of its membrane (resting potential). During the impulse passage, more Na$^+$ (thick arrow) passes into the axon interior than the amount of K$^+$ (thin arrow) that migrates in the opposite direction. In consequence, the membrane polarity changes (the membrane becomes relatively positive on its inner surface), and the resting potential is replaced by an action potential (+35 mV here). (Redrawn, with permission, from Junqueira LC et al, eds. *Basic Histology*, 10th ed. McGraw-Hill, 2003.)

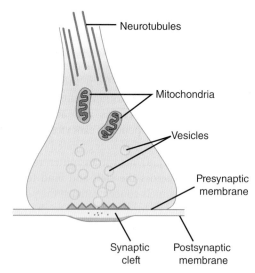

FIGURE 7–3 Schematic drawing of a synaptic terminal. Vesicles pass through the presynaptic membrane and release a transmitter substance into the synaptic cleft. (Redrawn, with permission, from Waxman SG. *Clinical Neuroanatomy*, 28th ed. McGraw-Hill, 2017.)

postsynaptic potential. **Inhibitory neurotransmitters**, such as GABA and glycine, open Cl⁻ channels and generate an **inhibitory postsynaptic potential**, keeping the postsynaptic membrane near E_{Cl} (= –70 mV). Termination of the signal is achieved by removal of the neurotransmitter from the synaptic cleft. Acetylcholine is hydrolyzed by acetylcholinesterase at the postsynaptic membrane. Other neurotransmitters such as glutamate are removed by specific membrane transporters on nerve terminals or glial cells.

Not all neurotransmitter receptors are ion channels. Many receptors are coupled to cellular enzymes that regulate levels of **intracellular second messengers** to modulate the function of ion channels and many other cell proteins. A major mechanism by which messengers regulate ion channels is promoting **phosphorylation** of channel subunits. For example, binding of the neurotransmitter norepinephrine to β-adrenergic receptors activates the enzyme **adenylyl cyclase** and stimulates the production of cyclic adenosine monophosphate (**cAMP**). The cAMP, in turn, activates a cAMP-dependent protein kinase that can phosphorylate voltage-gated calcium channels. In many cases, this increases the duration of time the channel remains open once it is activated, resulting in increased Ca²⁺ influx through the channel. Other neurotransmitter receptors, such as α₁-adrenergic, muscarinic cholinergic, or metabotropic glutamate receptors, are coupled to the enzyme **phospholipase C**, which catalyzes the hydrolysis of the membrane lipid phosphatidylinositol-4,5-bisphosphate. Binding of neurotransmitter to the receptor activates phospholipase C to produce two second messengers: **1,2-diacylglycerol** and **inositol-1,4,5-trisphosphate**. Diacylglycerol activates several enzymes of the protein kinase C family, some of which phosphorylate ion channels and either enhance or suppress their function. Inositol-1,4,5-trisphosphate binds an intracellular receptor that is itself a calcium ionophore, allowing release of calcium from intracellular stores into the cytosol. This calcium signal activates several calcium-dependent enzymes, including phosphatases and kinases that can alter the phosphorylation state and function of several ion channels and other cell proteins.

Astrocytes

Astrocytes serve a variety of metabolic, immunologic, structural, and nutritional support functions required for the normal function of neurons. They possess numerous processes that radiate from the cell body, surrounding blood vessels and synapses, and fill the space between neurons in the brain and spinal cord (Figure 7–4). Astrocytes express voltage- and ligand-gated ion channels and regulate K⁺ and Ca²⁺ concentrations within the interstitial space. Many synapses are invested with astrocytic processes, and this allows astrocytes to modulate neurotransmission by regulating extracellular concentrations of these cations. Astrocytes provide structural and trophic support for neurons through the production of extracellular matrix molecules such as laminin and through

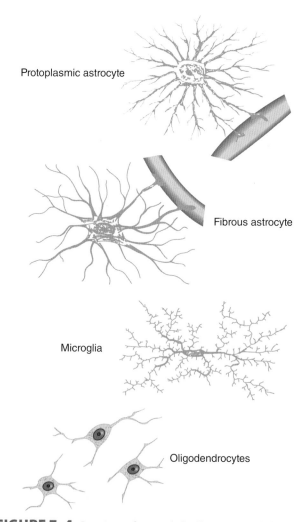

FIGURE 7–4 Drawings of neuroglial cells as seen in slides stained by metallic impregnation. Observe that only astrocytes exhibit vascular end-feet, which cover the walls of blood capillaries. (Redrawn, with permission, from Mescher AL. *Junqueira's Basic Histology*, 14th ed. McGraw-Hill, 2016.)

the release of growth factors such as nerve growth factor, fibroblast growth factors, and brain-derived neurotrophic factor. End-feet of astrocytic processes at blood vessels provide sites for the release of cytokines and chemoattractants during central nervous system (CNS) injury. Astrocytes respond to brain injury by increasing in size—and in some cases in number—through a process called **reactive astrocytosis**. This phenotypic change is characterized by an increase in cells expressing glial-fibrillary acidic protein and by synthesis and release of cytokines that regulate inflammatory responses and entry of hematogenous cells into the CNS. Astrocytes also play an important role in terminating neuronal responses to glutamate, the most abundant excitatory neurotransmitter in the brain. In cell cultures, neurons die in the presence of high levels of glutamate unless astrocytes are present. Glutamate transporters present on astrocyte cell membranes remove glutamate from the synapse. Astrocytes also contain glutamine synthase, which converts glutamate to glutamine, detoxifying the CNS of both glutamate and ammonia.

Oligodendrocytes & Schwann Cells

Plasma membranes of oligodendrocytes in the CNS and Schwann cells in the peripheral nervous system envelop axons. For many axons, the membranes of these glial cells are wrapped layer on layer around the axon, forming a myelin sheath (Figure 7–5). Gaps form between myelin sheaths from neighboring glia and produce **nodes of Ranvier** where a small portion of the axon is exposed to the interstitial space and where voltage-dependent Na⁺ channels are clustered in the axonal membrane. Between the nodes, myelin insulates the axon from the extracellular space, allowing efficient spread of depolarization from one node to another. This allows action potentials to propagate rapidly by jumping from node to node in a process called **saltatory conduction**.

Microglia

Although peripheral blood lymphocytes and monocytes enter from the circulation and patrol the CNS, microglia, which reside in the CNS, function as the main immune effector cells. They appear to be derived from bone marrow precursors of macrophage-monocyte lineage and invade the CNS during the perinatal period. Microglia cells are activated by brain injury,

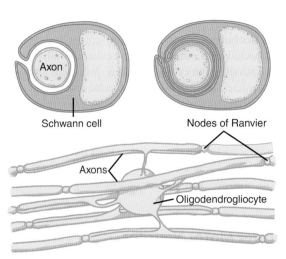

FIGURE 7–5 Myelination of axons. **Top left:** Unmyelinated axon. **Top right:** Myelinated axon. Note that the cell membrane of the Schwann cell has wrapped itself around the axon. **Bottom:** Myelination of several axons in the CNS by an oligodendrogliocyte. (Redrawn, with permission, from Ganong WF. *Review of Medical Physiology*, 22nd ed. McGraw-Hill, 2005.)

infection, or neuronal degeneration. Activation is characterized by proliferation; migration into damaged tissue; increased or de novo expression of surface receptors, including CD45 (leukocyte common antigen), MHC class I and class II, and immunoglobulin Fc receptors; and secretion of several cytokines, reactive oxygen intermediates, and proteinases. This response functions to remove dead tissue and destroy invading organisms but may contribute to CNS damage, particularly in certain inflammatory and degenerative CNS diseases.

CHECKPOINT

1. What are the primary functions of neurons, astrocytes, and microglia?
2. What role does myelin play in axonal conduction?
3. What is responsible for the resting membrane potential and for the generation of action potentials?
4. What are some of the major neurotransmitters in the nervous system, and what effects do they produce when they bind to their receptors?

FUNCTIONAL NEUROANATOMY

To understand neuroanatomy, it is useful to study structures as parts of functional systems.

MOTOR SYSTEM

Large **alpha motor neurons** of the spinal cord ventral horns and brainstem motor nuclei (facial nucleus, trigeminal motor nucleus, nucleus ambiguus, hypoglossal nucleus) extend axons into spinal and cranial nerves to innervate skeletal muscles. Damage to these **lower motor neurons** results in loss of all voluntary and reflex movement because they compose the output of the motor system. Neurons in the precentral gyrus and neighboring cortical regions (**upper motor neurons**) send axons to synapse with lower motor neurons. Axons from these upper motor neurons compose the **corticospinal** and **corticobulbar tracts**. The motor cortex and spinal cord are connected with other deep cerebral and brainstem motor nuclei, including the caudate nucleus, putamen, globus pallidus, red nuclei, subthalamic nuclei, substantia nigra, reticular nuclei, and neurons of the cerebellum. Neurons in these structures are distinct from cortical motor (**pyramidal**) neurons and are referred to as **extrapyramidal** neurons. Many parts of the cerebral cortex are connected by fiber tracts to the primary motor cortex. These connections are important for complex patterns of movement and for coordinating motor responses to sensory stimuli.

1. Lower Motor Neurons & Skeletal Muscles

Anatomy

Each alpha motor neuron axon contacts up to about 200 muscle fibers, and together they constitute the **motor unit** (Figure 7–6). Axons of the motor neurons intermingle to form spinal ventral roots, plexuses, and peripheral nerves. Muscles are innervated from specific segments of the spinal cord, and each muscle is supplied by at least two roots. Motor fibers are rearranged in the plexuses so that most muscles are supplied by one peripheral nerve. Thus, the distribution of muscle weakness differs in spinal root and peripheral nerve lesions.

Physiology

The lower motor neurons are the final common pathway for all voluntary movement. Therefore, damage to lower motor neurons or their axons causes flaccid weakness of innervated muscles. In addition, muscle tone or resistance to passive movement is reduced, and deep tendon reflexes are impaired or lost. Tendon reflexes and muscle tone depend on the activity of alpha motor neurons (Figure 7–7), specialized sensory

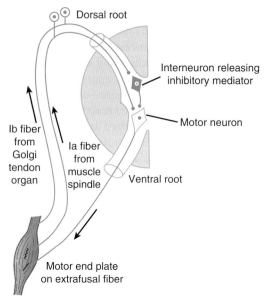

FIGURE 7–7 Diagram illustrating the pathways responsible for the stretch reflex and the inverse stretch reflex. Stretch stimulates the muscle spindle, and impulses pass up the Ia fiber to excite the motor neuron. It also stimulates the Golgi tendon organ, and impulses passing up the Ib fiber activate the interneuron to release the inhibitory mediator glycine. With strong stretch, the resulting hyperpolarization of the motor neuron is so great that it stops discharging. (Redrawn, with permission, from Barrett KE et al, eds. *Ganong's Review of Medical Physiology*, 25th ed. McGraw-Hill, 2016.)

receptors known as muscle spindles, and smaller **gamma motor neurons** whose axons innervate the spindles. Some gamma motor neurons are active at rest, making the spindle fibers taut and sensitive to stretch. Tapping on the tendon stretches the spindles, which causes them to send impulses that activate alpha motor neurons. These in turn fire, producing the brief muscle contraction observed during the **myotactic stretch reflex**. Alpha motor neurons of antagonist muscles are simultaneously inhibited through the phenomenon of reciprocal inhibition. Both alpha and gamma motor neurons are influenced by descending fiber systems, and their state of activity determines the level of tone and activity of the stretch reflex.

Each point of contact between nerve terminal and skeletal muscle forms a specialized synapse known as a **neuromuscular junction** composed of the presynaptic motor nerve terminal and a postsynaptic motor end plate (Figure 7–8). Presynaptic terminals store synaptic vesicles that contain the neurotransmitter acetylcholine. The amount of neurotransmitter within a vesicle constitutes a quantum of neurotransmitter. Action potentials depolarize the motor nerve terminal, opening voltage-gated calcium channels and stimulating calcium-dependent release of neurotransmitter from the terminal. Released acetylcholine traverses the synaptic cleft to the postsynaptic membrane (end plate), where it binds to nicotinic cholinergic receptors. These receptors are ligand-gated cation channels, and, on binding to acetylcholine, they allow

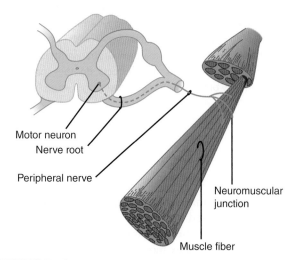

FIGURE 7–6 Anatomic components of the motor unit. (Redrawn, with permission, from Aminoff MJ et al, eds. *Clinical Neurology*, 9th ed. McGraw-Hill, 2015.)

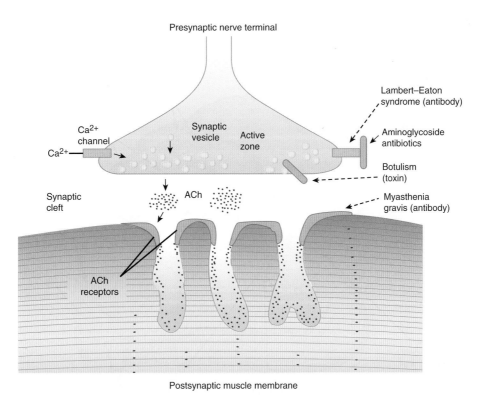

Presynaptic nerve terminal

Lambert–Eaton syndrome (antibody)

Aminoglycoside antibiotics

Botulism (toxin)

Myasthenia gravis (antibody)

Ca²⁺ channel

Ca²⁺

Synaptic vesicle

Active zone

Synaptic cleft

ACh

ACh receptors

Postsynaptic muscle membrane

FIGURE 7–8 Sites of involvement in disorders of neuromuscular transmission. **Left:** Normal transmission involves depolarization-induced influx of calcium (Ca²⁺) through voltage-gated channels. This stimulates release of acetylcholine (ACh) from synaptic vesicles at the active zone and into the synaptic cleft. ACh binds to ACh receptors and depolarizes the postsynaptic muscle membrane. **Right:** Disorders of neuromuscular transmission result from blockage of Ca²⁺ channels (Lambert–Eaton syndrome or aminoglycoside antibiotics), impairment of Ca²⁺-mediated ACh release (botulinum toxin), or antibody-induced internalization and degradation of ACh receptors (myasthenia gravis). (Redrawn, with permission, from Aminoff MJ et al, eds. *Clinical Neurology*, 9th ed. McGraw-Hill, 2015.)

entry of extracellular sodium into the motor end plate. This depolarizes the motor end plate, which in turn depolarizes the muscle fiber through activation of voltage-gated sodium channels. After activation, cholinergic receptors are rapidly inactivated, reducing sodium entry. They remain inactive until acetylcholine dissociates from the receptor. This is facilitated by the enzyme acetylcholinesterase, which hydrolyzes acetylcholine and is present in the postsynaptic zone.

Neuromuscular transmission may be disturbed in several ways (see Figure 7–8). In **Lambert–Eaton myasthenic syndrome**, antibodies to calcium channels inhibit calcium entry into the nerve terminal and reduce neurotransmitter release. In these cases, repetitive nerve stimulation facilitates calcium accumulation in the nerve terminal and increases acetylcholine release. Clinically, limb muscles are weak, but if contraction is maintained, power increases. Electrophysiologically, the amplitude of the muscle response increases to repetitive nerve stimulation. **Aminoglycoside antibiotics** also impair calcium channel function and cause a similar syndrome. Proteolytic toxins produced by *Clostridium botulinum* cleave specific presynaptic proteins, preventing neurotransmitter release at both neuromuscular and parasympathetic cholinergic synapses. As a result, patients with **botulism** develop weakness, blurred vision, diplopia, ptosis, and large unreactive pupils. In **myasthenia gravis**, autoantibodies to the nicotinic acetylcholine receptor (AChR) block neurotransmission by inhibiting receptor function and activating complement-mediated lysis of the postsynaptic membrane. Myasthenia gravis is discussed in greater detail later in this chapter.

Motor nerves exert trophic influences on the muscles they innervate. Denervated muscles undergo marked atrophy, losing more than half of their original bulk in 2–3 months. Nerve fibers are also required to organize the muscle end plate and to cluster cholinergic receptors to that region. Receptors in denervated fibers fail to cluster and become spread across the muscle membrane. Muscle fibers within a denervated motor unit may then discharge spontaneously, giving rise to a visible twitch (**fasciculation**) within a portion of a muscle. Individual fibers may also contract spontaneously, giving rise to **fibrillations**, which are not visible to the examiner but can be detected by electromyography. Fibrillations usually appear 7–21 days after damage to lower motor neurons or their axons.

CHECKPOINT

5. From where do lower motor neurons emanate, and to where do they send axons?
6. Describe four mechanisms that can disturb the function of the neuromuscular junction.

FIGURE 7–9 Lateral aspect of the cerebrum. The cortical areas are shown according to Brodmann, with functional localizations. (Redrawn, with permission, from Waxman SG. *Clinical Neuroanatomy*, 28th ed. McGraw-Hill, 2017.)

2. Upper Motor Neurons

Anatomy

The motor cortex is the region from which movements can be elicited by electrical stimuli (Figure 7–9). This includes the primary motor area (Brodmann area 4), premotor cortex (area 6), supplementary motor cortex (medial portions of 6), and primary sensory cortex (areas 3, 1, and 2). In the motor cortex, groups of neurons are organized in vertical columns, and discrete groups control contraction of individual muscles. Planned movements and those guided by sensory, visual, or auditory stimuli are preceded by discharges from prefrontal, somatosensory, visual, or auditory cortices, which are then followed by motor cortex pyramidal cell discharges that occur several milliseconds before the onset of movement.

Cortical motor neurons contribute axons that converge in the corona radiata and descend in the posterior limb of the internal capsule, cerebral peduncles, ventral pons, and medulla. These fibers constitute the **corticospinal** and **corticobulbar tracts** and together are known as upper motor neuron fibers (Figure 7–10). As they descend through the diencephalon and brainstem, fibers separate to innervate extrapyramidal and cranial nerve motor nuclei. The lower brainstem motor neurons receive input from crossed and uncrossed corticobulbar fibers, although neurons that innervate lower facial muscles receive primarily crossed fibers.

In the ventral medulla, the remaining corticospinal fibers course in a tract that is pyramidal in shape in cross-section—thus, the name **pyramidal tract**. At the lower end of the medulla, most fibers decussate, although the proportion of crossed and uncrossed fibers varies somewhat among individuals. The bulk of these fibers descend as crossed fibers in the lateral corticospinal tract of the spinal cord.

Different groups of neurons in the cortex control muscle groups of the contralateral face, arm, and leg. Neurons near the ventral end of the central sulcus control facial muscles, whereas neurons on the medial surface of the hemisphere control leg muscles (see Figure 7–10). Because the movements of the face, tongue, and hand are complex in humans, a large share of the motor cortex is devoted to their control. A somatotopic organization is also apparent in the lateral corticospinal tract of the cervical cord, where fibers to motor neurons that control leg muscles lie laterally and fibers to cervical motor neurons lie medially.

Physiology

Upper motor neurons are the final common pathway between cortical and subcortical structures, such as the basal ganglia, in the planning, initiation, sequencing, and modulation of all voluntary movement. Much has been learned about the normal function of upper motor neurons through the study of animals and humans with focal brain lesions. Upper motor

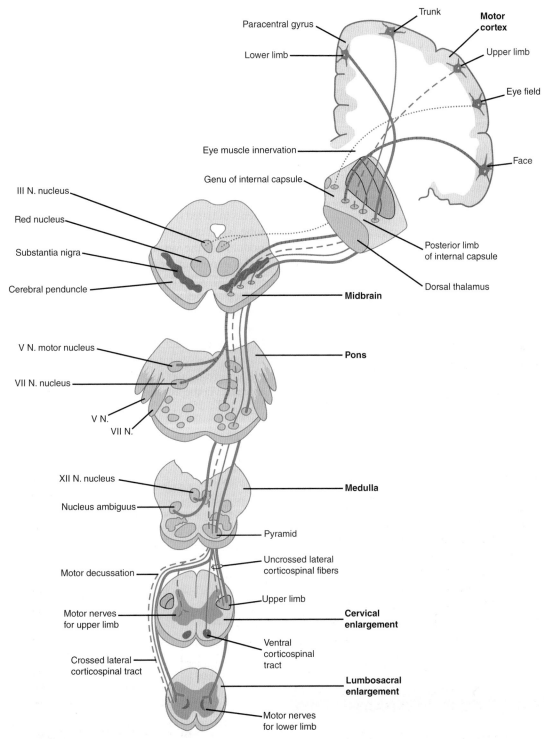

FIGURE 7–10 Schematic illustration of upper motor neuron pathways. (Redrawn, with permission, from Ropper AH et al, eds. *Adams and Victor's Principles of Neurology*, 10th ed. McGraw-Hill, 2014.)

neuron pathways can be interrupted in the cortex, subcortical white matter, internal capsule, brainstem, or spinal cord. Unilateral upper motor neuron lesions spare muscles innervated by lower motor neurons that receive bilateral cortical input, such as muscles of the eyes, jaw, upper face, pharynx, larynx, neck, thorax, and abdomen. Unlike paralysis resulting from lower motor neuron lesions, paralysis from upper motor neuron lesions is rarely complete for a prolonged period of time. Acute lesions, particularly of the spinal cord, often cause flaccid paralysis and absence of spinal reflexes at all segments below the lesion. With spinal cord lesions, this state is known as **spinal shock**. After a few days to weeks, a state known as **spasticity** appears, which is characterized by increased tone and hyperactive stretch reflexes. A similar but less striking sequence of events can occur with acute cerebral lesions.

Upper motor neuron lesions cause a characteristic pattern of limb weakness and change in tone. Antigravity muscles of the limbs become more active relative to other muscles. The arms tend to assume a flexed, pronated posture, and the legs become extended. In contrast, muscles that move the limbs out of this posture (extensors of the arms and flexors of the legs) are preferentially weakened. Tone is increased in antigravity muscles (flexors of the arms and extensors of the legs), and if these muscles are stretched rapidly, they respond with an abrupt catch, followed by a rapid increase and then decline in resistance as passive movement continues. This sequence constitutes the **"clasp knife" phenomenon**. **Clonus**—a series of involuntary muscle contractions in response to passive stretch—may be present, especially with spinal cord lesions.

Pure pyramidal tract lesions in animals cause temporary weakness without spasticity. In humans, lesions of the cerebral peduncles also cause mild paralysis without spasticity. It appears that control of tone is mediated by other tracts, particularly corticorubrospinal and corticoreticulospinal pathways. This may explain why the degrees of weakness and spasticity often do not correspond in patients with upper motor neuron lesions.

The distribution of paralysis resulting from upper motor neuron lesions varies with the location of the lesion. Lesions above the pons impair movements of the contralateral lower face, arm, and leg. Lesions below the pons spare the face. Lesions of the internal capsule often impair movements of the contralateral face, arm, and leg equally, because motor fibers are packed closely together in this region. In contrast, lesions of the cortex or subcortical white matter tend to differentially affect the limbs and face because the motor fibers are spread over a larger area of brain. Bilateral cerebral lesions cause weakness and spasticity of cranial, trunk, and limb muscles, which leads to dysarthria, dysphonia, dysphagia, bifacial paresis, and sometimes reflexive crying and laughing (**pseudobulbar palsy**).

CHECKPOINT

7. Define the motor cortex, and describe its organization.
8. Fibers from which nuclei and in which tracts constitute upper motor neurons? What is their path?
9. Describe the somatotopic organization of motor neurons in the cortex.
10. What are the characteristics of weakness and tone in upper motor neuron lesions?
11. How is the distribution of paralysis and spasticity affected by the location of an upper motor neuron lesion?

3. Cerebellum

Anatomy

The cerebellar cortex can be divided into three anatomic regions (Figures 7–11A and 7–11B). The **anterior lobe** lies rostral to the primary fissure and includes the remainder of the vermis. It receives proprioceptive input from muscles and tendons via the dorsal and ventral spinocerebellar tracts and influences posture, muscle tone, and gait. The **posterior lobe**, which composes the remainder of the cerebellar hemispheres, receives major input from the cerebral cortex via the pontine nuclei and middle cerebellar peduncles and is important for the coordination and planning of voluntary skilled movements initiated from the cerebral cortex. The **flocculonodular lobe** (see Figure 7–11B), composed of the flocculus and the nodulus of the vermis, has connections to vestibular nuclei and is important for the control of posture and eye movement.

The majority of efferents from the cerebellar cortex project to deep cerebellar nuclei, which in turn project to the cerebrum and brainstem through two main pathways (Figure 7–12). Direct projections from the flocculus and nodule to the vestibular nuclei calibrate vestibulocular responses. The fastigial nucleus receives input from the vermis and sends fibers to bilateral vestibular nuclei and reticular nuclei of the pons and medulla via the inferior cerebellar peduncles. Other regions of

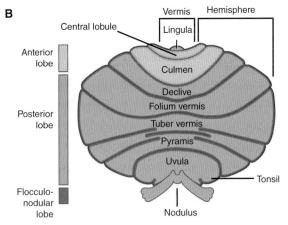

FIGURE 7–11 Anatomic divisions of the cerebellum in midsagittal view: (**A**) unfolded (arrows) and (**B**) viewed from behind. (Redrawn, with permission, from Aminoff MJ et al, eds. *Clinical Neurology*, 9th ed. McGraw-Hill, 2015.)

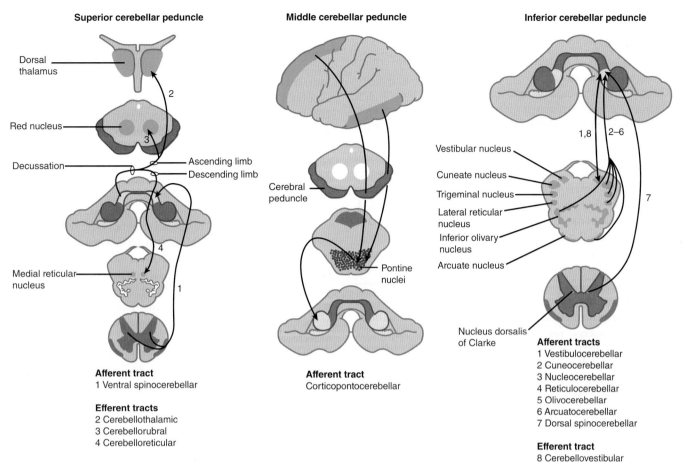

Superior cerebellar peduncle

- Dorsal thalamus
- Red nucleus
- Decussation
  - Ascending limb
  - Descending limb
- Medial reticular nucleus

Afferent tract
1 Ventral spinocerebellar

Efferent tracts
2 Cerebellothalamic
3 Cerebellorubral
4 Cerebelloreticular

Middle cerebellar peduncle

- Cerebral peduncle
- Pontine nuclei

Afferent tract
Corticopontocerebellar

Inferior cerebellar peduncle

- Vestibular nucleus
- Cuneate nucleus
- Trigeminal nucleus
- Lateral reticular nucleus
- Inferior olivary nucleus
- Arcuate nucleus
- Nucleus dorsalis of Clarke

1,8   2–6   7

Afferent tracts
1 Vestibulocerebellar
2 Cuneocerebellar
3 Nucleocerebellar
4 Reticulocerebellar
5 Olivocerebellar
6 Arcuatocerebellar
7 Dorsal spinocerebellar

Efferent tract
8 Cerebellovestibular

FIGURE 7–12 Cerebellar connections in the superior, middle, and inferior cerebellar peduncles. The peduncles are indicated by dark brown shading, and the areas to and from which they project by blue shading. (Redrawn, with permission, from Aminoff MJ et al, eds. *Clinical Neurology*, 9th ed. McGraw-Hill, 2015.)

the cerebellar cortex send fibers to the **dentate, emboliform**, and **globose nuclei**, whose efferents form the superior cerebellar peduncles, enter the upper pons, decussate completely in the lower midbrain, and travel to the contralateral red nucleus. At the red nucleus, some fibers terminate, whereas others ascend to the ventrolateral nucleus of the thalamus, where thalamic neurons send ascending efferent fibers to the motor cortex of the same side. A smaller group of fibers descend after decussation in the midbrain and terminate in reticular nuclei of the lower brainstem. Thus, the cerebellum controls movement through connections with cerebral motor cortex and brainstem nuclei.

Physiology

The cerebellum is responsible for the coordination of muscle groups, control of stance and gait, and regulation of muscle tone. Rather than causing paralysis, damage to the cerebellum interferes with the performance of motor tasks. The major manifestation of cerebellar disease is **ataxia**, in which simple movements are delayed in onset and their rates of acceleration and deceleration are decreased, resulting in **intention tremor** and **dysmetria** ("overshooting"). Lesions of the cerebellar

hemispheres affect the limbs, producing limb ataxia, whereas midline lesions affect axial muscles, causing truncal and gait ataxia and disorders of eye movement. Cerebellar lesions are often associated with **hypotonia** as a result of decreased activity of alpha and gamma motor neurons. If a lesion of the cerebellum or cerebellar peduncles is unilateral, the signs of limb ataxia appear on the same side as the lesion. However, if the lesion lies beyond the decussation of efferent cerebellar fibers in the midbrain, the clinical signs are on the side opposite the lesion.

CHECKPOINT

12. What is the overall role of the cerebellum?
13. What are the anatomic regions of the cerebellum, what do they control, and through which other regions of the brain do they make connections?
14. What are the consequences of damage to the cerebellum, and what symptoms and signs are seen in patients with cerebellar lesions?
15. Below which point do unilateral cerebellar lesions manifest on the opposite side?

4. Basal Ganglia

Anatomy

Several subcortical, thalamic, and brainstem nuclei are critical for regulating voluntary movement and maintaining posture. These include the basal ganglia (ie, the caudate nucleus and putamen [corpus striatum]) (Figure 7–13), globus pallidus, substantia nigra, and subthalamic nuclei. They also include the red nuclei and the mesencephalic reticular nuclei. The major pathways that involve the basal ganglia form three neuronal circuits. The first is the cortical–basal–ganglionic–thalamic–cortical loop. Inputs mainly from premotor, primary motor, and primary sensory cortices (see Figure 7–9, areas 1, 2, 3, 4, and 6) project to the corpus striatum, which sends fibers to the medial and lateral portions of the globus pallidus. Fibers from the globus pallidus form the ansa and fasciculus lenticularis, which sweep through the internal capsule and project onto ventral and intralaminar thalamic nuclei. Axons from these nuclei project to the premotor and primary motor cortices (areas 4 and 6), completing the loop. In the second loop, the substantia nigra sends dopaminergic fibers to the corpus striatum, which has reciprocal connections with the substantia nigra. The substantia nigra also projects to the ventromedial thalamus. The third loop is composed of reciprocal connections between the globus pallidus and the subthalamic nucleus. The subthalamic nucleus also sends efferents to the substantia nigra and corpus striatum.

Physiology

Basal ganglia circuits regulate the initiation, amplitude, and speed of movements. Diseases of the basal ganglia cause abnormalities of movement and are collectively known as **movement disorders**. They are characterized by motor deficits (bradykinesia, akinesia, loss of postural reflexes) or abnormal activation of the motor system, resulting in rigidity, tremor, and involuntary movements (chorea, athetosis, ballismus, and dystonia).

Several neurotransmitters are found within the basal ganglia, but their role in disease states is only partly understood. **Acetylcholine** is present in high concentrations within the corpus striatum, where it is synthesized and released by large Golgi type 2 neurons (Figure 7–14). Acetylcholine acts as an excitatory transmitter at medium-sized spiny striatal neurons that synthesize and release the inhibitory neurotransmitter **GABA** and project to the globus pallidus. **Dopamine** is synthesized by neurons of the substantia nigra, whose axons form the nigrostriatal pathway that terminates in the corpus striatum. Dopamine released by these fibers inhibits striatal GABAergic neurons. In Parkinson disease, degeneration of nigral neurons leads to loss of dopaminergic inhibition and a relative excess of cholinergic activity. This increases GABAergic output from the striatum and contributes to the paucity of movement that is a cardinal manifestation of the disease. Anticholinergics and dopamine agonists tend to restore the normal balance of striatal cholinergic and dopaminergic inputs and are effective in treatment. The pathogenesis of Parkinson disease is discussed later in this chapter.

Huntington disease is inherited as an autosomal dominant disorder. When disease onset occurs later in life, patients develop involuntary, rapid, jerky movements (**chorea**) and slow writhing movements of the proximal limbs and trunk (**athetosis**). When disease onset occurs earlier in life, patients develop signs of parkinsonism with tremor (cogwheeling) and stiffness. The spiny GABAergic neurons of the striatum preferentially degenerate, resulting in a net decrease in GABAergic

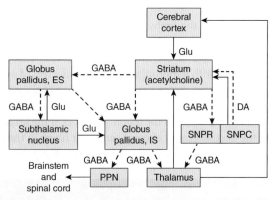

FIGURE 7–13 Diagrammatic representation of the principal connections of the basal ganglia. Solid lines indicate excitatory pathways; dashed lines indicate inhibitory pathways. The transmitters are indicated in the pathways, where they are known. (DA, dopamine; Glu, glutamate.) Acetylcholine is the transmitter produced by interneurons in the striatum (ie, the putamen and the caudate nucleus, which have similar connections). (ES, external segment; IS, internal segment; SNPC, substantia nigra, pars compacta; SNPR, substantia nigra, pars reticulate.) The subthalamic nucleus also projects to the pars compacta of the substantia nigra; this pathway has been omitted for clarity. (Redrawn, with permission, from Barrett KE et al, eds. *Ganong's Review of Medical Physiology*, 25th ed. McGraw-Hill, 2016.)

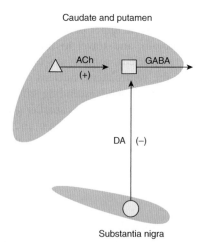

FIGURE 7–14 Simplified neurochemical anatomy of the basal ganglia. Dopamine (DA) neurons exert a net inhibitory effect, and acetylcholine (ACh) neurons exert a net excitatory effect on the GABAergic output from the striatum. In Parkinson disease, DA neurons degenerate. The net effect is an increase in GABAergic output from the striatum. (Redrawn, with permission, from Greenberg DA et al, eds. *Clinical Neurology*, 5th ed. McGraw-Hill, 2002.)

output from the striatum. This contributes to the development of chorea and athetosis. Dopamine antagonists, which block inhibition of remaining striatal neurons by dopaminergic striatal fibers, reduce the involuntary movements. Neurons in deep layers of the cerebral cortex also degenerate early in the disease, and later this extends to other brain regions, including the hippocampus and hypothalamus. Thus, the disease is characterized by cognitive deficits and psychiatric disturbances in addition to the movement disorder.

The gene for Huntington disease is located on chromosome 4p and encodes for a 3144-amino acid protein, **huntingtin**, which is widely expressed and interacts with several proteins involved in intracellular trafficking and endocytosis, gene transcription, and intracellular signaling. The protein contains a trinucleotide (CAG) repeat of 11–34 copies that encodes a polyglutamine domain and is expanded in patients with the disease. Deletion of the gene in mice causes embryonic death, whereas heterozygous animals are healthy. Transgenic mice with an expanded repeat develop a neurodegenerative disorder, suggesting that the disease results from the toxic effect of a gain-of-function mutation.

The mechanisms by which mutant huntingtin causes disease are not certain. The mutant protein is degraded, and the resulting fragments that contain the glutamine repeats form aggregates, which are deposited in nuclear and cytoplasmic inclusions. These fragments may bind abnormally to other proteins and interfere with normal protein processing or disrupt mitochondrial function. Nuclear fragments may interfere with nuclear functions such as gene expression. For example, in the cerebral cortex, mutant huntingtin reduces the production of brain-derived neurotrophic factor by suppressing its transcription. In addition, normal huntingtin is protective for cortical and striatal neurons and blocks the processing of procaspase 9, thereby reducing **apoptosis** (programmed cell death). Therefore, both loss of neurotrophic support and enhanced caspase activity could promote striatal cell loss in Huntington disease.

CHECKPOINT

16. Which are the component nuclei of the basal ganglia, and what is their functional role?
17. What are the clinical consequences of lesions in the basal ganglia?
18. What are some of the neurotransmitters within the basal ganglia, and what is their role in disorders of basal ganglia function?

SOMATOSENSORY SYSTEM

Somatosensory pathways confer information about touch, pressure, temperature, pain, vibration, and the position and movement of body parts. This information is relayed to thalamic nuclei and integrated in the sensory cortex of the parietal lobes to provide conscious awareness of sensation. Information is also relayed to cortical motor neurons to adjust fine movements and maintain posture. Some ascending sensory fibers, particularly pain fibers, enter the midbrain and project to the amygdala and limbic cortex, where they contribute to emotional responses to pain. In the spinal cord, painful stimuli activate local pathways that induce the firing of lower motor neurons and cause a reflex withdrawal. Thus, somatosensory pathways provide tactile information, guide movement, and serve protective functions.

Anatomy

A variety of specialized end organs and free nerve endings transduce sensory stimuli into neural signals and initiate the firing of sensory nerve fibers. Fibers that mediate cutaneous sensation from the trunk and limbs travel in sensory or mixed sensorimotor nerves to the spinal cord (Figure 7–15). Cutaneous sensory nerves contain small myelinated Aδ fibers that transmit information about pain and temperature, larger myelinated fibers that mediate touch and pressure sensation, and more numerous unmyelinated pain and autonomic C fibers. Myelinated proprioceptive fibers and afferent and efferent muscle spindle fibers are carried in the larger sensorimotor nerves. The cell bodies of the sensory neurons are in the dorsal root ganglia, and their central projections enter the spinal cord via the dorsal spinal roots. Innervation of the skin, muscles, and surrounding connective tissue is segmental, and each root innervates a region of skin known as a **dermatome** (Figure 7–16). Cell bodies of the sensory neurons that innervate the face reside in the trigeminal ganglion and send their central projections in the trigeminal nerve to the brainstem. The trigeminal innervation of the face is subdivided into three regions, each innervated by one of the three divisions of the trigeminal nerve.

The dorsal roots enter the dorsal horn of the spinal cord (see Figure 7–15). Large myelinated fibers divide into ascending and descending branches and either synapse with dorsal gray neurons within a few cord segments or travel in the **dorsal columns**, terminating in the gracile or cuneate nuclei of the lower medulla on the same side. Secondary neurons of the dorsal horn also send axons up the dorsal columns. Fibers in the dorsal columns are displaced medially as new fibers are added, so that in the cervical cord, leg fibers are located medially and arm fibers laterally (see Figure 7–15). The gracile and cuneate nuclei send fibers that cross the midline in the medulla and ascend to the thalamus as the **medial lemniscus** (Figure 7–17). The dorsal column–lemniscal system carries information about pressure, limb position, vibration, direction of movement, recognition of texture and shape, and two-point discrimination.

Thinly myelinated and unmyelinated fibers enter the lateral portion of the dorsal horn and synapse with dorsal spinal neurons within one or two segments. The majority of secondary fibers from these cells cross in the anterior spinal commissure and ascend in the anterolateral spinal cord as the **lateral**

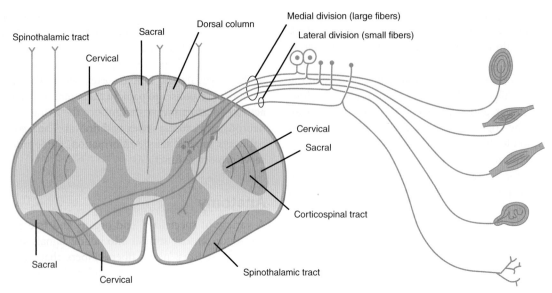

FIGURE 7–15 Schematic illustration of a spinal cord segment with its dorsal root, ganglion cells, and sensory organs. Sensory organs shown (from top to bottom) are the pacinian corpuscle, muscle spindle, tendon organ, encapsulated ending, and free nerve endings. The somatotopic arrangement of fibers in the dorsal columns, spinothalamic tract, and corticospinal tract is also shown. (Redrawn, with permission, from Waxman SG. *Clinical Neuroanatomy*, 28th ed. McGraw-Hill, 2017.)

spinothalamic tracts. Crossing fibers are added to the inner side of the tract, so that in the cervical cord, the leg fibers are located superficially and the arm fibers deeper. These fibers carry information about pain, temperature, and touch sensation.

Sensation from the face is carried by trigeminal sensory fibers that enter the pons and descend to the medulla and upper

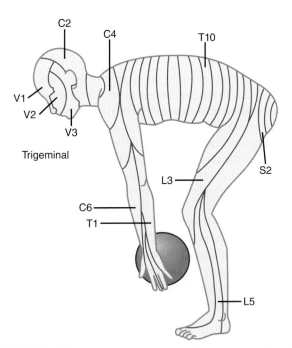

FIGURE 7–16 Segmental distribution of the body viewed in the approximate quadruped position, including sensory distribution of the trigeminal (V) cranial nerve. (Redrawn, with permission, from Waxman SG. *Clinical Neuroanatomy*, 28th ed. McGraw-Hill, 2017.)

FIGURE 7–17 Sensory pathways conveying touch, pressure, vibration, joint position, pain, and temperature sensation. (Redrawn, with permission, from Aminoff MJ et al, eds. *Clinical Neurology*, 9th ed. McGraw-Hill, 2015.)

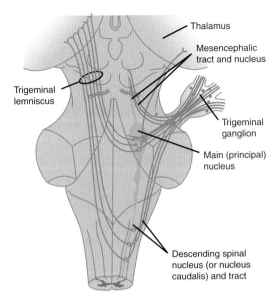

FIGURE 7–18 Schematic drawing of the trigeminal system. (Redrawn, with permission, from Waxman SG. *Clinical Neuroanatomy*, 28th ed. McGraw-Hill, 2017.)

cervical cord (Figure 7–18). Fibers carrying information about pain and temperature sensation terminate in the **nucleus of the spinal tract of cranial nerve V**, which is continuous with the dorsal horn of the cervical cord. Touch, pressure, and postural information is conveyed by fibers that terminate in the **main sensory** and **mesencephalic nuclei of the trigeminal nerve**. Axons arising from trigeminal nuclei cross the midline and ascend as the **trigeminal lemniscus** just medial to the spinothalamic tract. Fibers from the spinothalamic tract, medial lemniscus, and trigeminal lemniscus merge in the midbrain and terminate, along with sensory fibers ascending from the spinal cord, in the posterior thalamic nuclei, mainly in the nucleus ventralis posterolateralis. These thalamic nuclei project to the primary somatosensory cortex (see Figure 7–9, areas 3, 1, and 2) and to a second somatosensory area on the upper bank of the Sylvian fissure (lateral cerebral sulcus). The primary somatosensory region is organized somatotopically like the primary motor cortex.

Physiology

A. Pain

Free nerve endings of unmyelinated C fibers and small-diameter myelinated Aδ fibers in the skin convey sensory information in response to chemical, thermal, and mechanical stimuli. Intense stimulation of these nerve endings evokes the sensation of pain. In contrast to skin, most deep tissues are relatively insensitive to chemical or noxious stimuli. However, inflammatory conditions can sensitize sensory afferents from deep tissues to evoke pain on mechanical stimulation. This sensitization appears to be mediated by bradykinin, prostaglandins, and leukotrienes released during the inflammatory response. Information from primary afferent fibers is relayed via sensory ganglia to the dorsal horn of the spinal cord and

then to the contralateral spinothalamic tract, which connects to thalamic neurons that project to the somatosensory cortex.

Damage to these pathways produces a deficit in pain and temperature discrimination and may also produce abnormal painful sensations (**dysesthesias**), usually in the area of sensory loss. Such pain is termed **neuropathic pain** and often has a strange burning, tingling, or electric shock–like quality. It may arise from several mechanisms. Damaged peripheral nerve fibers become highly mechanosensitive and may fire spontaneously without known stimulation. They also develop sensitivity to norepinephrine released from sympathetic postganglionic neurons. Electrical impulses may spread abnormally from one fiber to another (**ephaptic conduction**), enhancing the spontaneous firing of multiple fibers. Neuropeptides released by injured nerves may recruit an inflammatory reaction that stimulates pain. In the dorsal horn, denervated spinal neurons may become spontaneously active. In the brain and spinal cord, synaptic reorganization occurs in response to injury and may lower the threshold for pain. In addition, inhibition of pathways that modulate transmission of sensory information in the spinal cord and brainstem may promote neuropathic pain.

Pain-modulating circuits exert a major influence on the perceived intensity of pain. One such pathway (Figure 7–19) is composed of cells in the periaqueductal gray matter of the midbrain that receive afferents from the frontal cortex and hypothalamus and project to rostroventral medullary neurons. These in turn

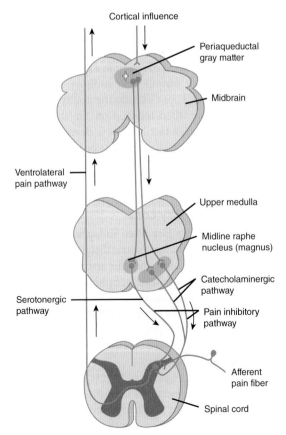

FIGURE 7–19 Schematic illustration of the pathways involved in pain control. (Used with permission of A. Basbaum.)

project in the dorsolateral white matter of the spinal cord and terminate on dorsal horn neurons. Additional descending pathways arise from other brainstem nuclei (locus ceruleus, dorsal raphe nucleus, and nucleus reticularis gigantocellularis). Major neurotransmitters used by these systems include endorphins, serotonin, and norepinephrine, providing the rationale for the use of opioids, serotonin agonists, and serotonin and norepinephrine reuptake inhibitors in the treatment of pain.

B. Proprioception and Vibratory Sense

Receptors in the muscles, tendons, and joints provide information about deep pressure and the position and movement of body parts. This allows one to determine an object's size, weight, shape, and texture. Information is relayed to the spinal cord via large Aα and Aβ myelinated fibers and to the thalamus by the dorsal column–lemniscal system. Detecting vibration requires sensing touch and rapid changes in deep pressure. This depends on multiple cutaneous and deep sensory fibers and is impaired by lesions of multiple peripheral nerves, the dorsal columns, medial lemniscus, or thalamus, but rarely by lesions of single nerves. Vibratory sense is often impaired together with proprioception.

C. Discriminative Sensation

The primary sensory cortex provides awareness of somatosensory information and the ability to make sensory discriminations. Touch, pain, temperature, and vibration sense are considered the primary modalities of sensation and are relatively preserved in patients with damage to the sensory cortex or its projections from the thalamus. In contrast, complex tasks that require the integration of multiple somatosensory stimuli and of somatosensory stimuli with auditory or visual information are impaired. These include the ability to distinguish two points from one when touched on the skin (**two-point discrimination**), localize tactile stimuli, perceive the position of body parts in space, recognize letters or numbers drawn on the skin (**graphesthesia**), and identify objects by their shape, size, and texture (**stereognosis**).

D. Anatomy of Sensory Loss

The patterns of sensory loss often indicate the level of nervous system involvement. Symmetric distal sensory loss in the limbs, affecting the legs more than the arms, usually signifies a generalized disorder of multiple peripheral nerves (**polyneuropathy**). Sensory symptoms and deficits may be restricted to the distribution of a single peripheral nerve (**mononeuropathy**) or two or more peripheral nerves (**mononeuropathy multiplex**). Symptoms limited to a dermatome indicate a spinal root lesion (**radiculopathy**).

In the spinal cord, segregation of fiber tracts and the somatotopic arrangement of fibers give rise to distinct patterns of sensory loss. Loss of pain and temperature sensation on one side of the body and of proprioception on the opposite side occurs with lesions that involve one half of the cord on the side of the proprioceptive deficit (**Brown–Séquard syndrome;**

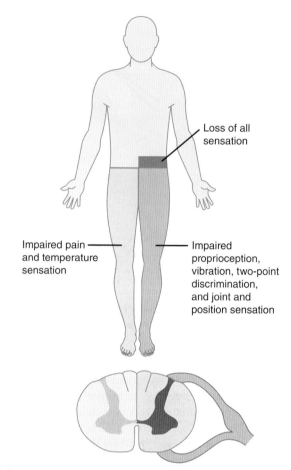

FIGURE 7–20 Brown–Séquard syndrome with lesion at the left tenth thoracic level (motor deficits not shown). (Redrawn, with permission, from Waxman SG. *Clinical Neuroanatomy*, 28th ed. McGraw-Hill, 2017.)

Figure 7–20). Compression of the upper spinal cord causes loss of pain, temperature, and touch sensation first in the legs, because the leg spinothalamic fibers are most superficial. More severe cord compression compromises fibers from the trunk. In patients with spinal cord compression, the lesion is often above the highest dermatome involved in the deficit. Thus, radiographic studies should be tailored to visualize the cord at and above the level of the sensory deficit detected on examination. Intrinsic cord lesions that involve the central portions of the cord often impair pain and temperature sensation at the level of the lesion because the fibers crossing the anterior commissure and entering the spinothalamic tracts are most centrally situated. Thus, enlargement of the central cervical canal in **syringomyelia** typically causes loss of pain and temperature sensation across the shoulders and upper arms (Figure 7–21).

Brainstem lesions involving the spinothalamic tract cause loss of pain and temperature sensation on the opposite side of the body. In the medulla, such lesions can involve the neighboring spinal trigeminal nucleus, resulting in a "crossed" sensory deficit involving the ipsilateral face and contralateral limbs. Above the medulla, the spinothalamic and trigeminothalamic tracts lie close together, and lesions there cause contralateral sensory loss of the face and limbs. In the midbrain and thalamus, medial

FIGURE 7–21 Syringomyelia (the presence of a cavity in the spinal cord resulting from the breakdown of gliomatous new formations, presenting clinically with pain and paresthesias followed by muscular atrophy of the hands) involving the cervicothoracic portion of the cord. (Redrawn, with permission, from Waxman SG. *Clinical Neuroanatomy*, 28th ed. McGraw-Hill, 2017.)

lemniscal fibers run together with pain and temperature fibers, and lesions are more likely to impair all primary sensation contralateral to the lesion. Because sensory fibers converge at the thalamus, lesions there tend to cause fairly equal loss of pain, temperature, and proprioceptive sensation on the contralateral half of the face and body. Lesions of the sensory cortex in the parietal lobe impair discriminative sensation on the opposite side of the body, whereas detection of the primary modalities of sensation may remain relatively intact.

CHECKPOINT

19. Which fibers carry pain, and how are they segregated from fibers that carry proprioception information in the spinal cord?

20. What are the differences in characteristics of sensory loss at different levels of the nervous system?

21. What is the function of the sensory cortex in the parietal lobe, and what are the clinical features of damage to this region?

VISION & EYE MOVEMENT CONTROL

The visual system provides our most important source of sensory information about the environment. The visual system and pathways for the control of eye movements are among the best characterized pathways in the nervous system. Familiarity with these neuroanatomic features is often extremely valuable in localization of neurologic disease.

Anatomy

The cornea and lens of the eye refract and focus images on the photosensitive posterior portion of the retina. The posterior retina contains two classes of specialized photoreceptor cells, **rods** and **cones**, which transduce photons into electrical signals. At the retina, the image is reversed in the horizontal and vertical planes so that the inferior visual field falls on the superior portions of the retina and the lateral field is detected by the nasal half of the retina.

Fibers from the nasal half of the retina traverse the medial portion of the optic nerve and cross to the other side at the **optic chiasm** (Figure 7–22). Each **optic tract** contains fibers from the same half of the visual field of both eyes. The optic tracts terminate in the **lateral geniculate nuclei** of the thalamus. Lateral geniculate neurons send fibers to the primary visual cortex in the occipital lobe (**calcarine cortex**, area 17 of Figure 7–9). These fibers form the **optic radiations**, which extend through the white matter of the temporal lobes and the inferior portion of the parietal lobes.

Eye movements are produced by the extraocular muscles, which function in pairs to move the eyes along three axes (Figure 7–23). These muscles are innervated by the **oculomotor** (III), **trochlear** (IV), and **abducens** (VI) nerves. The oculomotor nerve innervates the ipsilateral **medial**, **superior**, and **inferior rectus muscles** and the **inferior oblique muscles**. It also supplies the ipsilateral levator palpebrae, which elevates the eyelid. The oculomotor nerve also carries parasympathetic fibers that mediate pupillary constriction (see later discussion). Trochlear nerve fibers decussate before leaving the brainstem, and each trochlear nerve supplies the contralateral **superior oblique muscle**. The abducens nerve innervates the **lateral rectus muscle** of the same side.

Cortical and brainstem gaze centers innervate the extraocular motor nuclei and provide for supranuclear control of gaze. A **vertical gaze center** is located in the midbrain tegmentum, and **lateral gaze centers** are present in the pontine paramedian reticular formation. Each lateral gaze center sends fibers to the neighboring ipsilateral abducens nucleus and, via the **medial longitudinal fasciculus**, to the contralateral oculomotor nucleus. Therefore, activation of the right lateral gaze center stimulates conjugate deviation of the eyes to the right. Rapid **saccadic eye movements** are initiated by the **frontal eye fields** in the premotor cortex, which stimulate conjugate movement of the eyes to the opposite side. Slower eye movements involved in pursuit of moving objects are controlled by parieto-occipital gaze centers, which stimulate conjugate gaze

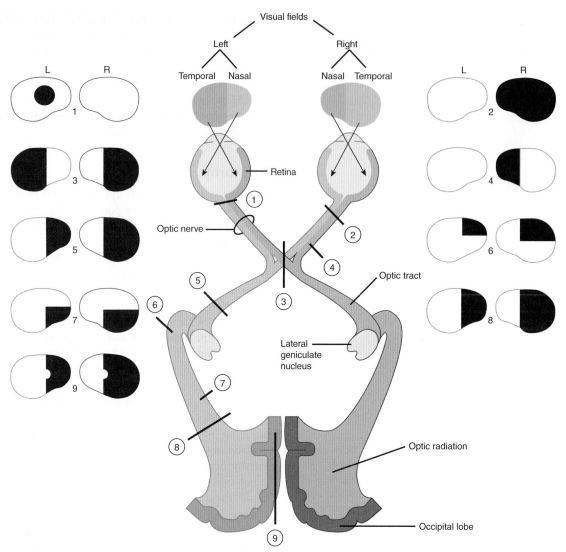

FIGURE 7–22 Common visual field defects and their anatomic bases. (1) Central scotoma caused by inflammation of the left optic disk (optic neuritis) or optic nerve (retrobulbar neuritis). (2) Total blindness of the right eye from a complete lesion of the right optic nerve. (3) Bitemporal hemianopia caused by pressure exerted on the optic chiasm by a pituitary tumor. (4) Right nasal hemianopia caused by a perichiasmal lesion (eg, calcified internal carotid artery). (5) Right homonymous hemianopia from a lesion of the left optic tract. (6) Right homonymous superior quadrantanopia caused by partial involvement of the optic radiation by a lesion in the left temporal lobe (Meyer loop). (7) Right homonymous inferior quadrantanopia caused by partial involvement of the optic radiation by a lesion in the left parietal lobe. (8) Right homonymous hemianopia from a complete lesion of the left optic radiation. (A similar defect may also result from lesion 9.) (9) Right homonymous hemianopia (with macular sparing) resulting from posterior cerebral artery occlusion. (Redrawn, with permission, from Simon RP et al, eds. *Clinical Neurology*, 10th ed. McGraw-Hill, 2018.)

to the side of the gaze center. These cortical areas control eye movements through their connections with the brainstem gaze centers.

The size of the pupils is determined by the balance between parasympathetic and sympathetic discharge to the pupillary muscles. The parasympathetic oculomotor **nuclei of Edinger–Westphal** send fibers in the oculomotor nerves that synapse in the ciliary ganglia within the orbits and innervate the pupillary constrictor muscles.

The motor portion of pupillary dilation is controlled by a three-neuron system (Figure 7–24). It is composed of axons from neurons in the posterolateral hypothalamus that descend

through the lateral brainstem tegmentum and the intermediolateral column of the cervical spinal cord to the level of T1. There they terminate on preganglionic sympathetic neurons within the lateral gray matter of the thoracic cord. These neurons send axons that synapse with postganglionic neurons in the superior cervical ganglion. Postganglionic neurons send fibers that travel with the internal carotid artery and the first division of the trigeminal nerve to innervate the iris. The fibers also innervate the tarsal muscles of the eyelids. Damage to these pathways causes **Horner syndrome**, which consists of miosis, ptosis, and sometimes impaired sweating ipsilateral to the lesion.

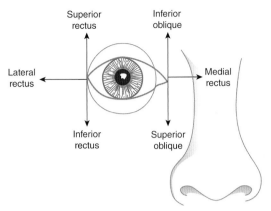

FIGURE 7-23 Extraocular muscles subserving the six cardinal positions of gaze. The eye is adducted by the medial rectus and abducted by the lateral rectus. The adducted eye is elevated by the inferior oblique and depressed by the superior oblique; the abducted eye is elevated by the superior rectus and depressed by the inferior rectus. (Redrawn, with permission, from Simon RP et al, eds. *Clinical Neurology*, 10th ed. McGraw-Hill, 2018.)

Physiology

A. Vision

The rods are sensitive to low levels of light and are most numerous in the peripheral regions of the retina. In retinitis

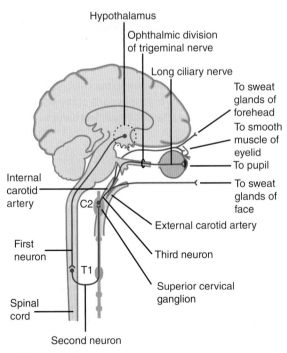

FIGURE 7-24 Oculosympathetic pathways. This three-neuron pathway projects from the hypothalamus to the intermediolateral column of the spinal cord, then to the superior cervical (sympathetic) ganglion, and finally to the pupil, the smooth muscle of the eyelids, and the sweat glands of the forehead and face. Interruption of these pathways results in Horner syndrome. (Redrawn, with permission, from Simon RP et al, eds. *Clinical Neurology*, 10th ed. McGraw-Hill, 2018.)

pigmentosa, there is degeneration of the retina that begins in the periphery. Poor twilight vision is thus an early symptom of this disorder. Cones are responsible for perception of stimuli in bright light and for discrimination of color. They are concentrated in the macular region, which is crucial for visual acuity. In disorders of the retina or optic nerve that impair acuity, diminished color discrimination is often an early sign.

Visual processing begins in the retina, where information gathered from rods and cones is modified by interactions among bipolar, amacrine, and horizontal cells. Amacrine and bipolar cells send their output to ganglion cells, whose axons compose the optic nerve. Photoreceptors convey information about the absolute level of illumination. Retinal processing renders ganglion cells sensitive to simultaneous differences in contrast for detection of edges of objects.

Ganglion cell axons terminate in a highly ordered fashion in well-defined layers of the lateral geniculate nuclei. Because of the separation of fibers in the optic chiasm, the receptive fields of cells in the lateral geniculate lie in the contralateral visual field. Geniculate neurons are arranged in six layers, and ganglion cell axons from each eye terminate in separate layers. Cells in different layers are in register, so that the receptive fields of cells in the same part of each layer are in corresponding regions of the two retinas. A greater proportion of cells are devoted to the macular region of both retinas. This reflects use of the central retina for high acuity and color vision. Some visual processing occurs in the geniculate, particularly for contrast and edge perception and movement detection.

In the primary visual cortex, visual fields from the eyes are also represented in a topographic projection. Cortical neurons are functionally organized in columns perpendicular to the cortical surface. Geniculate fibers terminate within layer IV of the visual cortex, and cells within a column above and below layer IV show the same eye preference and similar receptive fields. Narrow alternating columns of cells supplied by one eye or the other lie next to each other (**ocular dominance columns**). A tremendous amount of visual processing occurs in the primary visual cortex, including the synthesis of complex receptive fields and the determination of axis orientation, position, and color. The retina is not simply represented as a map on the cortex; rather, each area of the retina is represented in multiple columns and analyzed with respect to the position, color, and orientation of objects. As in the geniculate, a major portion of the primary visual cortex is devoted to analyzing information derived from the macular regions of both retinas. Cortical areas 18 and 19 (and many other areas) provide higher levels of visual processing.

The anatomic organization of the visual system is useful for localizing neurologic disease (see Figure 7-22). Lesions of the retina or optic nerves (**prechiasmal lesions**) impair vision from the ipsilateral eye. Lesions that compress the central portion of the chiasm, such as pituitary tumors, disrupt crossing fibers from the nasal halves of both retinas, causing **bitemporal hemianopia**. Lesions involving structures behind the chiasm (**retrochiasmal lesions**) cause visual loss in the contralateral field of both eyes. Lesions that completely destroy the optic tract, lateral geniculate nucleus, or optic radiations on one side produce a contralateral **homonymous hemianopia**. Selective destruction of temporal lobe optic radiations causes **superior quadrantanopia**, and lesions of the parietal optic radiations cause **inferior quadrantanopia**. The posterior portions of the optic radiations and the calcarine cortex are supplied mainly by the posterior cerebral artery, although the macular region of the visual cortex receives some collateral supply from the middle cerebral artery. Therefore, a lesion of the primary visual cortex generally causes contralateral homonymous hemianopia, but if it is due to posterior cerebral artery occlusion, it may spare macular vision. In rare cases of bilateral cortical blindness, patients may be unaware of their lack of vision.

B. Eye Movement

Conjugate eye movements are regulated by proprioceptive information from neck structures and information about head movement and position from the vestibular system. This information is used to maintain fixation on a stationary point when moving the head. In a comatose patient, the integrity of these oculovestibular and oculocephalic pathways can be assessed by the "doll's eye" or vestibulo-ocular reflex maneuver. This is elicited by briskly turning the head, which normally results in conjugate movement of the eyes in the opposite direction in a comatose patient. Irrigation of the ear with 10–20 mL of cold water reduces the activity of the labyrinth on that side and elicits jerk nystagmus, with the fast component away from the irrigated ear in a conscious individual. In coma, the fast saccadic component is lost, and the vestibular influence on eye movements dominates. Cold-water irrigation then results in deviation of the eyes toward the irrigated ear. These caloric responses are lost with midbrain or pontine lesions, with damage to the labyrinths, or with drugs that inhibit vestibular function.

C. Pupillary Function

The size of the pupils is controlled by the amount of ambient light sensed by the retina (Figure 7–25). Fibers from each retina terminate within midbrain pretectal nuclei that send fibers to both Edinger–Westphal nuclei. The fibers mediate pupillary constriction in bright light. In dim light, this reflex is inhibited and the influence of sympathetic fibers predominates, causing pupillary dilatation. The pupillary constrictor fibers release acetylcholine, which activates muscarinic AChRs and thus stimulates contraction of the pupillary sphincter muscle of the iris. Sympathetic pupillary fibers release norepinephrine, which activates α_1-adrenergic receptors, causing contraction of the radial muscle of the iris. Drugs that inhibit muscarinic receptors, such as atropine, or that stimulate α_1-adrenergic receptors, such as epinephrine, dilate the pupils, whereas drugs that stimulate muscarinic receptors or block α_1-adrenergic receptors cause pupillary constriction.

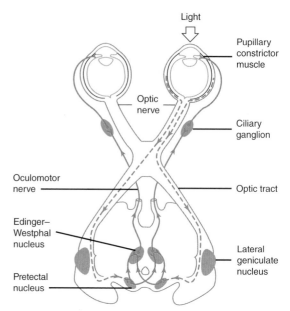

FIGURE 7–25 Anatomic basis of the pupillary light reflex. The afferent visual pathways from the retina to the pretectal nuclei of the midbrain are represented by dashed lines, the efferent pupilloconstrictor pathways from the midbrain to the retinas by solid lines. Note that illumination of one eye results in bilateral pupillary constriction. (Redrawn, with permission, from Simon RP et al, eds. *Clinical Neurology*, 10th ed. McGraw-Hill, 2018.)

CHECKPOINT

22. What is the pathway of fibers from the retina to the visual cortex?
23. What is the innervation of the extraocular muscles?
24. Describe how lesions in various parts of the visual pathways produce characteristic visual field defects.

HEARING & BALANCE

Anatomy

Structures of the middle ear serve to amplify and transmit sounds to the cochlea, where specialized sensory cells (hair cells) are organized to detect ranges in amplitude and frequency of sound. The semicircular canals contain specialized hair cells that detect movement of endolymphatic fluid contained within the canals. Similar hair cells in the saccule and utricle detect movement of the otolithic membrane, which is composed of calcium carbonate crystals embedded in a matrix. The semicircular canal hair cells detect angular acceleration, whereas the hair cells of the utricle and saccule detect linear acceleration. Axons from auditory and vestibular neurons compose the eighth cranial nerve, which traverses the petrous bone, is joined by the facial nerve, and enters the posterior fossa through the auditory canal. Auditory fibers terminate in the cochlear nuclei of the pons, and vestibular fibers terminate in the vestibular nuclear complex.

Cochlear neurons send fibers bilaterally to a network of auditory nuclei in the midbrain, and impulses are finally relayed through the medial geniculate thalamic nuclei to the auditory cortex in the superior temporal gyri. Vestibular nuclei have connections with the cerebellum, red nuclei, brainstem gaze centers, and brainstem reticular formation. The vestibular nuclei exert considerable control over posture through descending vestibulospinal, rubrospinal, and reticulospinal pathways.

Physiology

A. Hearing

There are three types of hearing loss: (1) **conductive deafness**, resulting from diseases of the external or middle ear that impair conduction and amplification of sound from the air to the cochlea; (2) **sensorineural deafness**, resulting from diseases of the cochlea or eighth cranial nerve; and (3) **central deafness**, resulting from diseases affecting the cochlear nuclei or auditory pathways in the CNS. Because of the redundancy of central pathways, almost all cases of hearing loss are due to conductive or sensorineural deafness. Besides hearing loss, auditory diseases may cause **tinnitus**, the subjective sensation of noise in the ear. Tinnitus resulting from disorders of the cochlea or eighth cranial nerve sounds like a constant nonmusical tone and may be described as ringing, whistling, hissing, humming, or roaring. Transient episodes of tinnitus occur in most individuals and are not associated with disease. When persistent, tinnitus is often associated with hearing loss.

Conductive and sensorineural deafness may be distinguished by examining hearing with a vibrating 512 Hz tuning fork. In the **Rinne test**, the tuning fork is held on the mastoid process behind the ear and then placed at the auditory meatus. If the sound is louder at the meatus, the test is positive. Normally the test is positive because sound transmitted through air is amplified by middle-ear structures. In sensorineural deafness, although sound perception is reduced, the Rinne test is still positive because middle-ear structures are intact. In conductive deafness, sounds are heard less well through air, and the test is negative. In the **Weber test**, the tuning fork is applied to the forehead at the midline. In conductive deafness, the sound is heard best in the abnormal ear, whereas with sensorineural deafness, the sound is heard best in the normal ear. **Audiometry** can distinguish types of hearing loss. In general, sensorineural deafness causes greater loss of high-pitched sounds, whereas conductive deafness causes more loss of low-pitched sounds.

B. Vestibular Function

In contrast to hearing, vestibular function is commonly disturbed by small brainstem lesions. The vestibular nuclei occupy a large portion of the lateral brainstem, extending from the medulla to the midbrain. Although there are extensive bilateral connections between vestibular nuclei and other motor pathways, these connections are not redundant but highly lateralized and act in concert to control posture, balance, and conjugate eye movement.

Patients with diseases of the vestibular system complain of disequilibrium and dizziness. Cerebellar disease also causes disequilibrium, but this is often described as a problem with coordination rather than a feeling of dizziness in the head. Interpretation of the complaint of dizziness can often be difficult. Many patients use the term loosely to describe sensations of light-headedness, weakness, or malaise. Directed questioning is often required to establish whether there is truly an abnormal sensation of movement (**vertigo**).

Vertigo may be due to disease of the labyrinth or vestibular nerve (peripheral vertigo) or to dysfunction of brainstem and CNS pathways (central vertigo). In general, peripheral vertigo is more severe and associated with nausea and vomiting, especially if the onset is acute. Diseases of the semicircular canal neurons or their fibers frequently cause rotational vertigo, whereas diseases involving the utricle or saccule cause sensations of tilting or listing, as on a boat. Traumatic and ischemic lesions may cause associated hearing loss. Dysfunction of one labyrinth often causes horizontal and rotatory **jerk nystagmus**. The slow phase of the nystagmus is caused by the unopposed action of the normal labyrinth, which drives the eyes to the side of the lesion. The fast-jerk phase is due to a rapid saccade, which maintains fixation.

Vertigo resulting from lesions of the CNS is usually less severe than peripheral vertigo and is often associated with other findings of brainstem dysfunction. In addition, nystagmus associated with central lesions may be present in vertical or multiple directions of gaze. Common causes of central vertigo include brainstem ischemia, brainstem tumors, and multiple sclerosis.

CONSCIOUSNESS, AROUSAL & COGNITION

Anatomy

Consciousness is awareness of self and the environment. It has two aspects: **arousal**, which is the state of wakefulness, and **cognition**, which is the sum of mental activities. This distinction is useful because neurologic disorders can affect arousal and cognition differently. Arousal is generated by activity of the ascending reticular activating system (Figure 7–26), which is composed of neurons within the central mesencephalic brainstem, the lateral hypothalamus, and the medial, intralaminar, and reticular nuclei of the thalamus. Widespread projections from these nuclei synapse on distal dendritic fields of large pyramidal neurons in the cerebral cortex and generate an arousal response. Cognition is the chief function of the cerebral cortex, particularly of the prefrontal cortex and cortical association areas of the occipital, temporal, and parietal lobes. Some specialized mental functions are localized to specific cortical regions. Several subcortical nuclei in the basal ganglia

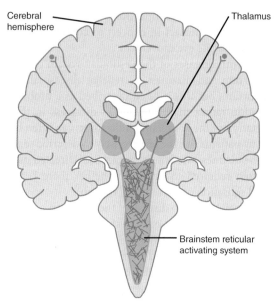

FIGURE 7–26 Brainstem reticular activating system and its ascending projections to the thalamus and cerebral hemispheres. (Redrawn, with permission, from Aminoff MJ et al, eds. *Clinical Neurology*, 9th ed. McGraw-Hill, 2015.)

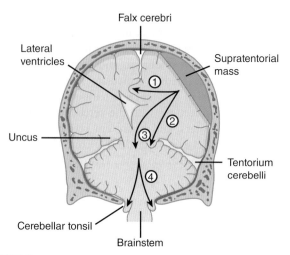

FIGURE 7–27 Anatomic basis of herniation syndromes. An expanding supratentorial mass lesion may cause brain tissue to be displaced into an adjacent intracranial compartment, resulting in (1) cingulate herniation under the falx cerebri; (2) downward transtentorial (central) herniation; (3) uncal herniation over the edge of the tentorium; or (4) cerebellar tonsillar herniation into the foramen magnum. Coma and ultimately death result when (2), (3), or (4) produces brainstem compression. (Redrawn, with permission, from Greenberg DA et al, eds. *Clinical Neurology*, 5th ed. McGraw-Hill, 2002.)

and thalamus are intimately linked with cortical association areas, and damage to these nuclei or their interconnections with the cortex may give rise to cognitive deficits similar to those observed with cortical lesions.

Physiology

A. Arousal

The reticular activating system is excited by a wide variety of stimuli, especially somatosensory stimuli. It is most compact in the midbrain and can be damaged by central midbrain lesions, resulting in failure of arousal, or **coma**. Higher nuclei and projections are less localized, and lesions rostrad to the midbrain, therefore, must be bilateral to cause coma.

Less severe dysfunction causes **confusional states** in which consciousness is clouded and the patient is sleepy, inattentive, and disoriented. Alertness is reduced, and the patient appears drowsy or falls asleep easily without frequent stimulation. More awake patients perceive stimuli slowly but are distractible, assigning important and irrelevant stimuli equal value. Perceptions may be distorted, leading to **hallucinations**, and the patient may be unable to organize and interpret a complex set of stimuli. The inability to perceive properly interferes with learning, memory, and problem solving. Thoughts become disorganized and tangential, and the confused patient may maintain false beliefs even in the face of evidence of their falsity (**delusions**). In some cases, the confusional state presents as **delirium**, which is characterized by heightened alertness, disordered perception, agitation, delusions, hallucinations, convulsions, and autonomic hyperactivity (sweating, tachycardia, hypertension).

Coma may result from structural or metabolic causes. Some structural lesions of the cerebral hemispheres, such as

hemorrhages, large areas of ischemic infarction, abscesses, or tumors, can expand over minutes or a few hours and cause brain tissue to herniate into the posterior fossa (Figure 7–27). If lateral within the temporal lobe, the expanding mass may drive the uncus of the temporal lobe into the ambient cistern surrounding the midbrain, compressing the ipsilateral third cranial nerve (**uncal herniation**). This causes pupillary dilation and impaired function of eye muscles innervated by that nerve. Continued pressure distorts the midbrain, and the patient lapses into coma with posturing of the limbs. With continued herniation, pontine function is impaired, causing loss of oculovestibular responses. Eventually, medullary function is lost and breathing ceases. Hemispheric lesions closer to the midline compress the thalamic reticular formation structures and can cause coma before eye findings develop (**central herniation**). With continued pressure, midbrain function is affected, causing the pupils to dilate and the limbs to posture. With progressive herniation, pontine vestibular and then medullary respiratory functions are lost.

Several nonstructural disorders that diffusely disturb brain function can produce a confusional state or, if severe, coma (Table 7–1). Most of these disorders are acute, and many, particularly those caused by drugs and metabolic toxins, are reversible. Clues to the cause of these "metabolic" encephalopathies are provided by general physical examination, drug screens, and certain blood studies. When these disorders cause coma, pupillary light responses are usually preserved despite impaired oculovestibular or respiratory function. This finding is of great help in distinguishing metabolic from structural causes of coma.

TABLE 7–1 Nonstructural causes of confusional states and coma.

Drugs (sedative-hypnotics, ethanol, opioids)
Global cerebral ischemia
Hepatic encephalopathy
Hypercalcemia
Hyperosmolar states
Hyperthermia
Hypoglycemia
Hyponatremia
Hypoxia
Hypothyroidism
Meningitis and encephalitis
Seizure or prolonged postictal state
Subarachnoid hemorrhage
Thyrotoxicosis
Uremia
Wernicke encephalopathy

Neurons in the dorsal midbrain and especially nuclei within the pontine reticular formation are important for **sleep**. Thus, lesions involving the pons may preserve consciousness but disturb sleep. In contrast, diffuse lesions of the neocortex, such as those resulting from global cerebral ischemia, may preserve the reticular activating system and brainstem sleep centers, resulting in a patient with preserved sleep–wake cycles who cannot interact in any meaningful way with the environment (coma vigil or apallic state).

B. Cognition

Several disorders disturb cognition rather than level of consciousness. Specific cortical regions generally mediate different cognitive functions, although there is considerable overlap and interconnection between cortical and subcortical structures in all mental tasks. When several of these abilities are impaired, the patient is said to suffer from **dementia**. Dementia is discussed in more detail later in this chapter.

The prefrontal cortex (see Figure 7–9) generally refers to areas 9, 10, 11, 12, 45, 46, and 47 of Brodmann on the superior and lateral surfaces of the frontal lobes and the anterior cingulate, parolfactory, and orbitofrontal cortex inferiorly and mesially. These regions are essential for orderly planning and sequencing of complex behaviors, attending to several stimuli or ideas simultaneously, concentrating and flexibly altering the focus of concentration, grasping the context and meaning of information, and controlling impulses, emotions, and

thought sequences. Damage to the frontal lobes or connections to the caudate and dorsal medial nuclei of the thalamus causes **frontal lobe syndrome**. Patients may suffer dramatic alterations in personality and behavior, whereas most sensorimotor functions remain intact. Some patients become vulgar in speech, slovenly, grandiose, and irascible, whereas others lose interest, spontaneity, curiosity, and initiative. The affect may become apathetic and blunted (**abulia**). Some patients lose the capacity for creativity and abstract reasoning and the ability to solve problems while becoming excessively concrete in their thinking. Often, they are distractible and unable to focus attention when presented with multiple stimuli. The most dramatic manifestations are seen after bilateral frontal lobe damage; unilateral damage can lead to subtle alterations in behavior that may be difficult to detect. Involvement of premotor areas may lead to incontinence, the inability to perform learned motor tasks (**apraxia**), variable increases in muscle tone (**paratonia**), and the appearance of primitive grasp and oral reflexes (sucking, snouting, and rooting).

In about 90% of people, **language** is a function of the left hemisphere. Whereas 99% of right-handed people are left hemisphere dominant, about 40% of left-handed people are right hemisphere dominant for language. In most left-handed people, hemispheric dominance for language is incomplete, and damage to the dominant hemisphere tends to disturb language less severely than in right-handed individuals. The cortical regions most critical for language include Broca area (area 44), Wernicke area (area 22), the primary auditory cortex (areas 41 and 42), and neighboring frontal and temporoparietal association areas (see Figure 7–9). Injury to these areas or their connections to other cortical regions results in **aphasia**. Lesions in the frontal speech areas cause nonfluent, dysarthric, halting speech, whereas lesions of the temporal speech area cause fluent speech that contains many errors or may be totally devoid of understandable words. Patients with damage to temporal speech areas also lack comprehension of spoken words. Isolation of the temporal speech area from the occipital lobes causes an inability to read (**alexia**). Portions of the parietal lobe adjacent to the temporal lobe are important for retrieval of previously learned words, and damage here may result in **anomia**. The inferior parietal region is important for the translation of linguistic messages generated in the temporal language areas into visual symbols. Damage to this region may result in an inability to write (**agraphia**).

Memory requires that information be registered by the primary somatosensory, auditory, or visual cortex. Posterior cortical areas involved in language comprehension are needed for the immediate processing and recall of spoken or written events. The hippocampi and their connections to the dorsal medial nuclei of the thalamus and the mammillary nuclei of the hypothalamus constitute a limbic system network crucial for learning and processing events for long-term storage. When these areas are damaged, the patient is unable to learn new material or retrieve memories from the recent past. The most severe symptoms occur with bilateral lesions; unilateral disease causes subtler learning deficits. Memories that remain with a person for years are considered remote memories and are stored in corresponding association cortex areas (eg, visual cortex for scenes). Remote memories remain intact in patients with damage to limbic structures required for learning. However, they may be lost by damage to cortical association areas. Understanding the mechanisms by which recent memories are transferred from the limbic memory network to the association cortex for long-term storage is a major goal of current research.

The parietal association cortex is the region principally involved in the visuomotor integration of constructional tasks. The visual cortex is required for observation, whereas the auditory cortex and the temporal language cortex are necessary for drawing objects on command. The inferior parietal cortex (areas 39 and 40) integrates visual and auditory information, and the output from this region is translated into motor patterns by the motor cortex. Thus, lesions to the parietal lobes commonly cause constructional impairment. Damage to either hemisphere may result in constructional errors. Drawings may show rotation of objects, disorientation of objects on the background, fragmentation of design, inability to draw angles properly, or omission of parts of a figure presented for copying. It is often difficult to determine which side is damaged, although if language is preserved, a nondominant parietal deficit is more likely.

Calculation ability, abstract reasoning, problem solving, and several other aspects of intelligence are difficult to localize because they require the integration of several cortical regions. They are frequently disturbed by diseases that cause widespread cortical dysfunction, such as those that cause dementia.

CHECKPOINT

25. What is the network of neurons that maintains normal arousal and consciousness?
26. What are the symptoms and signs of cerebral herniation caused by focal brain lesions?
27. Which cognitive functions are controlled by the frontal lobes and by the parietal association cortex?
28. Which regions of the cortex are important for language and memory?

PATHOPHYSIOLOGY OF SELECTED NEUROLOGIC DISORDERS

Nervous system disease may be caused by a wide variety of degenerative, metabolic, structural, neoplastic, or inflammatory conditions that affect neurons, glia, or both. The resultant dysfunction is expressed by either neuronal hyperactivity, as seen during seizures, or decreased neuronal activity, as observed after a stroke. The specific functional abnormalities observed depend on the network of neurons affected. For example, because amyotrophic lateral sclerosis is a disorder of upper and lower motor neurons, neurologic deficits are limited to the motor system. In Parkinson disease, dopaminergic neurons of the substantia nigra degenerate, causing symptoms of extrapyramidal motor system dysfunction. In patients with ischemic stroke, the particular constellation of deficits is determined by the vascular territory affected. Therefore, an understanding of the pathophysiology of neurologic disease requires an analysis of events occurring at both the cellular level and the level of neural networks.

CEREBELLAR ATAXIA

Clinical Presentation

Cerebellar ataxia is a heterogenous group of disorders that affect the cerebellum and its connections. It is estimated that cerebellar ataxias affect up to 150,000 people in the United States. Clinical features of cerebellar ataxia include the following: (1) **ataxic gait**, which results in a widened base, staggering, falls, and, if severe, wheelchair confinement; (2) **truncal ataxia**, which can result in the inability to sit unsupported by the arms; (3) **dysmetria**, an impaired ability to perform accurate movements during ballistic movements owing to a faulty estimation of distance; (4) **limb ataxia**, which results in difficulty with coordinated tasks; (5) **vertigo** with nausea and vomiting, resulting from damage to the vestibulocerebellum; (6) **static and kinetic tremor**, also called intention tremor; (7) **cerebellar dysarthria**, also termed scanning speech, which results in slurred speech and, in severe cases, rendering speech unintelligible; and (8) **nystagmus and ocular dysmetria**, abnormalities in eye movements.

The causes of ataxia are varied. Ataxia may result from **vascular insults** to the cerebellum, **toxic insults** (including alcohol), **infections**, **autoimmune disorders**, **vitamin deficiency** (eg, thiamine, vitamin E), and **degenerative disorders** (inherited or sporadic). The prevalence of inherited ataxias, as a group, may be as high as 25–30 per 100,000 persons. The most common sporadic form of degenerative cerebellar ataxia is **multiple system atrophy of the cerebellar type (MSA-C)**. The heritable ataxias may be inherited in a dominant fashion (the so-called **spinocerebellar ataxias [SCAs]**) or in a recessive manner. Although mutations in more than 450 genes are associated with cerebellar ataxia, the role of most of these genetic variants in ataxia is unknown. Moreover, although individual genetic causes of ataxia are rare, understanding the basis for cerebellar dysfunction and degeneration in ataxia can give us insight into the disease pathogenesis of other neurodegenerative diseases.

Polyglutamine Ataxia

The largest group of dominantly inherited ataxias result from glutamine-encoding CAG repeats in various disease genes. These include SCA types 1, 2, 3, 6, 7, and 17. The pathogenesis of the dominant polyglutamine ataxias is thought to be a gain-of-function mutation causing an expanded number of glutamine repeats in the respective disease proteins. Although the putative roles of these different proteins are diverse, the clinical features of the polyglutamine SCAs are remarkably similar, and it is thus difficult to clinically distinguish one type of SCA from another. The mechanism by which polyglutamine expansion leads to ataxia remains unknown. Several mechanisms have been proposed, including the following:

- Altered protein function owing to polyglutamine expansion
- Formation of toxic oligomeric complexes
- Transcriptional dysregulation
- Aberrant neuronal signaling, including excitotoxicity
- Mitochondrial dysfunction
- Impaired axonal transport
- Impairment in cellular protein homeostasis
- RNA toxicity

Recent work in mouse models of SCA1 and SCA2 has suggested that similar transcriptional modules are altered in both disorders, which may account for the similarity in neuronal vulnerability and, hence, phenotypes. It remains to seen whether the convergence of pathological and clinical phenotypes in other cerebellar ataxias is accounted for by a similar downstream effect on transcripts that are particularly important for cerebellar function.

Autoimmune and Paraneoplastic Ataxia

Autoimmune cerebellar syndromes represent a small subset of ataxias. However, they are important to recognize for two reasons. First, some of the autoimmune ataxias can help us to understand disease pathogenesis; second, these disorders are treatable, particularly when recognized early. A subset of autoimmune ataxias is associated with an underlying, often occult, malignancy. The ataxia in these cases is thought to be a result of immune cross-reactivity between tumor and cerebellar antigens. The new onset of the neurological symptoms may suggest the presence of a previously unidentified tumor. As a remote effect of an underlying malignancy, the ataxia can thus be considered a paraneoplastic syndrome.

Other immune ataxias that have a parallel genetic etiology are outlined below.

Gluten Ataxia

Cerebellar ataxia is a neurological manifestation of celiac disease, a disorder associated with gluten sensitivity. Clinically, gastrointestinal symptoms of diarrhea, bloating, and malabsorption occur following gluten ingestion, along with characteristic pathologic changes in villus and crypt morphology and inflammation in the epithelium on duodenal biopsies. Antibodies directed against tissue transglutaminase 6 is a serologic marker of the disease. Interestingly, a rare genetic form of cerebellar ataxia results from mutations in the gene encoding transglutaminase 6 (TGM6). Importantly, a gluten-free diet reduces antibody levels over time, causing resolution of gastrointestinal symptoms and improvement of neurological symptoms.

Cerebellar Ataxias Resulting from Ion-Channel Antibodies

Patients with elevated levels of antibodies directed against calcium channels (P/Q- and N-type) and voltage-gated potassium channels may present with cerebellar ataxia. P/Q-type calcium channels are highly expressed in cerebellar Purkinje neurons, and, in mouse models, reduced channel activity is associated with ataxia. In humans, mutations in CACNA1A, the gene encoding the P/Q calcium channel, results in episodic spinocerebellar ataxia type 2 (SCA2) and spinocerebellar ataxia type 6 (SCA6).

CHECKPOINT

29. What are the clinical features of cerebellar ataxia?
30. Which class of disease genes or proteins is responsible for the most common dominantly inherited ataxias?
31. What mechanisms may play a role in degeneration in the polyglutamine spinocerebellar ataxias (SCAs)?

MOTOR NEURON DISEASE

Clinical Presentation

Motor neuron diseases predominantly affect the anterior horn cells of the spinal cord and are characterized by wasting and skeletal muscle weakness. Spontaneous discharges of degenerating motor nerve fibers occur, giving rise to muscle twitches known as **fasciculations** (see prior discussion). Electromyography characteristically shows features of denervation, including increased numbers of spontaneous discharges (**fibrillations**) in resting muscle and a reduction in the number of motor units detected during voluntary contraction. Sprouting of remaining healthy motor fibers may occur, leading to the appearance of large, polyphasic motor unit potentials (reinnervation).

The **spinal muscular atrophies** (**SMAs**) are a heterogeneous group of genetic diseases characterized by the selective degeneration of lower motor neurons. The most common form is autosomal recessive with childhood onset and has a frequency of between 1:6000 and 1:10,000. Childhood SMA has been divided into three types depending on age of onset and clinical progression. SMA I is infantile spinal muscular atrophy (**Werdnig–Hoffmann disease**), a disorder that usually manifests within the first 3 months of life. Infants with this condition have difficulty sucking, swallowing, and breathing. Atrophy and fasciculations are found in the tongue and limb muscles. SMA I is rapidly progressive, leading to death from respiratory complications usually by the age of 3 years. SMA II begins in the latter half of the first year of life. It progresses more slowly than the infantile form, and patients may survive into adulthood. SMA III (**Kugelberg–Welander disease**) is a juvenile form that develops after age 2. Patients develop weakness of the proximal limb muscles with relative sparing of bulbar muscles. The pattern of weakness can falsely suggest a myopathy such as limb-girdle dystrophy rather than a motor neuron disease. The course is gradually progressive, leading to disability in adulthood. All three forms of SMA result from deletions or mutations in the survival motor neuron 1 (*SMN1*) gene on chromosome 5q13. The SMN gene product is expressed in all tissues and appears to be involved in RNA metabolism. Loss of SMN function promotes apoptosis of lower motor neurons. It is not yet known why motor neurons are selectively affected. Some clinical trials have looked at adjusting the levels of the SMN protein in an attempt to modulate disease progression using drugs such as hydroxyurea and valproic acid, but unfortunately these studies failed to show any improvement in the disease. Recent focus has turned to antisense oligonucleotides and stem cell therapies to attempt to slow disease progression.

In adults, motor neuron disease usually begins between the ages of 20 and 80 years, with an average age at onset of 56 years. It is commonly sporadic but is familial in up to 10% of cases. Several varieties have been described, depending on the relative involvement of upper or lower motor neurons and bulbar or spinal anterior horn cells. For example, X-linked spinobulbar atrophy is an X-linked recessive disorder that typically manifests clinically in the fourth or fifth decade and is associated with an expanded CAG repeat in the androgen receptor gene. As with other genetic disorders associated with triplet repeat expansions, the neurodegeneration is associated with neuronal inclusions. Testosterone promotes the development of inclusions, and women homozygous for the mutation develop only mild symptoms. Moreover, female mice carrying the mutation show motor impairment after testosterone administration, whereas castration reduces impairment in male mice. These findings led to testing the use of gonadotropin-releasing hormone antagonists, which reduce testosterone release from the testes, as treatments for the disease. Unfortunately, the treatments did not improve function and resulted in significantly reduced quality of life secondary to the low testosterone. Current work is focusing on RNAi targeting of the polyQ-AR transcript to reduce the expression and toxicity of the expanded repeat.

The most common form of motor neuron disease in adults is **amyotrophic lateral sclerosis** (**ALS**), in which mixed upper and lower motor neuron deficits are found in limb and bulbar muscles. In 80% of patients, the initial symptoms result from weakness of limb muscles. Complaints are often bilateral but asymmetric. Involvement of bulbar muscles causes difficulty with swallowing, chewing, speaking, breathing, and coughing. Neurologic examination reveals a mixture of upper and lower motor neuron signs. There is usually no involvement of extraocular muscles or sphincters. The disease is progressive and generally fatal within 3–5 years, with death usually resulting from pulmonary infection and respiratory failure.

Pathology & Pathogenesis

In ALS, there is selective degeneration of motor neurons in the primary motor cortex and the anterolateral horns of the spinal cord. Many affected neurons show cytoskeletal disease with accumulations of intermediate filaments in the cell body and axons. There is only a subtle glial cell response and little evidence of inflammation. The cause is unknown, but biochemical and genetic studies have provided several clues.

A. Glutamate Signaling and RNA Processing

Glutamate (Figure 7–28) is the most abundant excitatory neurotransmitter in the CNS. Glutamate activates a large family of receptors that either open cation channels (ionotropic receptors) or activate phospholipase C (metabotropic receptors), which catalyzes the formation of the second messenger inositol-1,4,5-trisphosphate (IP_3). Influx of Na^+ and Ca^{2+} through glutamate-gated cation channels depolarizes cells, whereas IP_3 stimulates the release of Ca^{2+} from intracellular storage sites. The net effect of these events is to generate an excitatory postsynaptic potential and raise the concentration of free intracellular Ca^{2+} in the cytosol of the postsynaptic neuron. This Ca^{2+} signal activates calcium-sensitive enzymes and is quickly terminated by the removal of glutamate from the synapse and by mechanisms for calcium sequestration and extrusion in the postsynaptic cell. A breakdown of normal mechanisms for terminating the excitatory signal leads to sustained elevations of intracellular Ca^{2+}, which cause cell death.

Glutamate is removed from synapses by transport proteins on surrounding astrocytes and nerve terminals. In astrocytes, it is metabolized to glutamine and can be shuttled back to neurons for reconversion into glutamate. In 60% of patients with sporadic ALS, there is a large decrease in glutamate transport activity in the motor cortex and spinal cord but not in other regions of the CNS. This has been associated with a loss of the astrocytic glutamate transporter protein excitatory amino acid transporter 2 (EAAT2), perhaps resulting from a defect in splicing of its messenger RNA. In cultured spinal cord slices, the pharmacologic inhibition of glutamate transport induces motor neuron degeneration. Thus, selective loss of a glutamate transporter may cause excitotoxicity in ALS by increasing extracellular levels of glutamate.

A second alteration in glutamate signaling has been found recently in spinal motor neurons from five patients with ALS. RNA editing is a process whereby gene-specified codons are altered by RNA-dependent deaminases. In GluR2 receptor subunits, this process is virtually 100% efficient, resulting in conversion of glutamine to arginine in the second transmembrane domain of this subunit, which markedly reduces the calcium permeability of a major subclass of glutamate receptors. Editing efficiency was reduced in more than 50% of neurons from the patients with ALS. Because transgenic mice that

FIGURE 7-28 Glutamatergic neurotransmission. Depolarization stimulates release of glutamate from presynaptic terminals into the synaptic cleft, where it binds to ionotropic or metabotropic glutamate receptors, stimulating Ca^{2+} influx and activation of phospholipase C (PLC). PLC catalyzes hydrolysis of phosphatidylinositol-4,5-bisphosphate (PIP_2) to produce inositol-1,4,5-trisphosphate (IP_3), which causes release of Ca^{2+} from storage sites in smooth endoplasmic reticulum (SER). Synaptic actions of glutamate are terminated mainly by uptake through Na^+-dependent glutamate transporters (GT) on glia. In astrocytes, glutamate is converted into glutamine by glutamine synthetase.

express GluR2 made artificially more permeable to calcium develop a motor neuron disease late in life, it is possible that defective editing of GluR2 contributes to ALS pathogenesis. These findings suggest that sporadic ALS may be caused by a defect in RNA metabolism.

B. Free Radicals

About 10% of ALS cases are familial, and 20% of these familial cases result from missense mutations in the **cytosolic copper-zinc superoxide dismutase (SOD1)** gene on the long arm of chromosome 21. SOD1 catalyzes the formation of hydrogen peroxide from superoxide anions. Hydrogen peroxide is then detoxified by catalase or glutathione peroxidase to form water. Not all mutations reduce *SOD1* activity, and the disorder is typically inherited as an autosomal dominant trait, suggesting that familial ALS results from a gain, rather than loss, of function. This is supported by the finding that transgenic mice expressing mutant *SOD1* develop motor neuron disease analogous to human familial ALS, whereas mice lacking SOD1 do not develop motor neuron disease. One hypothesis suggests that the mutant enzyme has an altered substrate specificity catalyzing the reduction of hydrogen peroxide to yield hydroxyl radicals and using peroxynitrite to produce nitration of tyrosine residues in proteins. This is consistent with the findings of elevated levels of carbonyl proteins in the brain and elevated levels of free nitrotyrosine in the spinal cord of ALS patients. EAAT2 may also be inactivated by mutant SOD1, thereby promoting excitotoxicity. Some mutations also promote the formation of SOD aggregates, which may be neurotoxic.

C. Cytoskeletal Proteins

Motor neurons tend to be very large, with extremely long axons, and cytoskeletal proteins that maintain axonal structure may be critical targets for motor neuron injury. A role for neurofilament dysfunction in ALS is supported by the finding that neurofilamentous inclusions in cell bodies and proximal axons are an early feature of ALS pathology. In addition, mutations in the heavy chain neurofilament subunit (NF-H) have been detected in some patients with sporadic ALS, suggesting that NF-H variants may be a risk factor for ALS. Peripherin is another intermediate filament protein found with neurofilaments in neuronal inclusions in ALS and in mice with *SOD1* mutations. Peripherin expression is increased in response to cell injury, and overexpression of peripherin causes a late-onset motor neuron disease in mice. Inclusions containing peripherin and neurofilaments may interfere with axonal transport, resulting in failure to maintain axonal structure and transport of macromolecules such as neurotrophic factors required for motor neuron survival.

D. TDP-43

An exciting discovery of the protein transactive response DNA-binding protein 43 (TDP-43) may offer new clues to the etiology of this disorder. This newly discovered protein is the major component of the ubiquitinated, tau-negative inclusions that are the pathological hallmark of sporadic and familial ALS and frontotemporal dementia (FTD). It is also found in some cases of Alzheimer disease and Parkinson disease. Mutations in this gene, located on chromosome 1, co-segregate with disease in familial forms of ALS and FTD and are not found in *SOD1* familial ALS. FTD and ALS overlap in approximately 15–25% of cases, and these disorders are starting to be referred to as "TDP-43 proteinopathies." Several other genes and gene regions have been identified to cause both FTD and ALS, including *TARDBP* on chromosome 1p36.2, *MAPT* on chromosome *7q21*, and *DCTN1* on chromosome 2p13.

E. C9ORF72

The major genetic cause of ALS and/or FTD was recently discovered. Two independent research teams have identified hexanucleotide repeats in an intron of C9ORF72 on chromosome 9 in 34% of familial ALS cases, 6% of sporadic ALS cases, 26% of familial FTD cases, and 5% of sporadic FTD cases. The protein is of unknown function. These mutations likely induce a gain-of-function mutation similar to other noncoding repeat expansion disorders. This discovery of another disorder caused by nucleotide repeats may provide an additional rationale for a new drug development paradigm focused on decreasing expression of these toxic repeats.

CHECKPOINT

32. What are the clinical features of motor neuron disease?
33. Which gene is responsible for some cases of familial ALS, and what is a postulated molecular mechanism by which the mutation causes disease?
34. What two other mechanisms may play a role in motor neuron degeneration?

PARKINSON DISEASE

Clinical Presentation

Parkinsonism is a clinical syndrome of rigidity, bradykinesia, tremor, and postural instability. Most cases are due to Parkinson disease, an idiopathic disorder with a prevalence of about 1–2 per 1000. In the first half of the last century, parkinsonism was a common sequela of von Economo encephalitis. Parkinsonism can also result from exposure to certain toxins such as manganese, carbon disulfide, 1-methyl-4-phenyl-1,2,3,6-tetrahydropyridine (MPTP), and carbon monoxide. Several drugs, particularly butyrophenones, phenothiazines, metoclopramide, reserpine, and tetrabenazine, can cause reversible parkinsonism. Parkinsonism may also result from repeated head trauma or may be a feature of several basal ganglia diseases, including Wilson disease, some cases of early-onset Huntington disease, multiple system atrophy (MSA), and progressive supranuclear palsy. In these disorders, other symptoms and signs are present along with parkinsonism.

Pathology & Pathogenesis

In Parkinson disease, there is selective degeneration of monoamine-containing cell populations in the brainstem and basal ganglia, particularly of pigmented dopaminergic neurons of the substantia nigra. In addition, scattered neurons in the basal ganglia, brainstem, spinal cord, and sympathetic ganglia contain eosinophilic, cytoplasmic inclusion bodies (**Lewy bodies**). These contain filamentous aggregates of α-synuclein, along with parkin, synphilin, neurofilaments, and synaptic vesicle proteins.

Important clues about the pathogenesis of Parkinson disease have been discovered through study of the potent neurotoxin MPTP. MPTP is a byproduct of synthesis of a synthetic opioid derivative of meperidine. Illicit use of opioid preparations heavily contaminated with MPTP led to several cases of parkinsonism in the early 1980s. MPTP selectively injures dopaminergic neurons in the brain and produces a clinical syndrome very similar to Parkinson disease.

MPTP enters the brain (Figure 7–29) and is converted by monoamine oxidase B present in glia and serotonergic nerve terminals to *N*-methyl-4-phenyldihydropyridine (MPDP$^+$), which diffuses across glial membranes and then undergoes nonenzymatic oxidation and reduction to the active metabolite *N*-methyl-4-phenylpyridinium (MPP$^+$). Plasma membrane transporters that normally act to terminate the action of monoamines by removing them from synapses take up MPP$^+$. Internalized MPP$^+$ inhibits oxidative phosphorylation by interacting with complex I of the mitochondrial electron transport chain. This inhibits ATP production and reduces metabolism of molecular oxygen, allowing for increased formation of peroxide, hydroxyl radicals, and superoxide radicals that react with lipids, proteins, and nucleic acids that cause cell injury. In support of a role for mitochondrial dysfunction and oxidative damage in the pathogenesis of Parkinson disease is evidence that the insecticide rotenone, which inhibits mitochondrial complex I, produces parkinsonism in animals with degeneration of nigrostriatal dopaminergic neurons and cytoplasmic inclusions that resemble Lewy bodies. Exposure to paraquat, a common herbicide structurally similar to MPP$^+$ that also inhibits complex I, can lead to selective degeneration of dopaminergic neurons and aggregation of α-synuclein.

FIGURE 7–29 Proposed mechanism of MPTP-induced parkinsonism. MPTP enters brain astrocytes and is converted to MPDP$^+$ through the action of monoamine oxidase type B (MAO-B). MPDP$^+$ is then metabolized extracellularly to MPP$^+$, which is taken up through dopamine uptake sites on dopamine nerve terminals and concentrated in mitochondria. The resulting disturbance of mitochondrial function can lead to neuronal death. (Redrawn, with permission, from Greenberg DA et al, eds. *Clinical Neurology*, 5th ed. McGraw-Hill, 2002.)

Furthermore, impaired complex I activity has been observed in cell lines derived from Parkinson disease patients, and one genetic variant of NADH dehydrogenase 3 in complex I is associated with a reduced risk of the disease among Caucasians. Thus, alterations in mitochondrial complex I activity appear to play an important role in the pathogenesis of Parkinson disease.

The reasons dopaminergic neurons appear selectively vulnerable to complex I inhibition are unclear. Although controversial, some evidence suggests that dopamine can promote neurotoxicity. Addition of exogenous dopamine is toxic to neurons in culture. Dopamine undergoes auto-oxidation to generate superoxide radicals or is metabolized by monoamine oxidase to generate hydrogen peroxide. Superoxide dismutase catalyzes the conversion of superoxide to H_2O_2, which is converted by glutathione peroxidase and catalase to water. However, H_2O_2 can also react with ferrous iron to form highly reactive hydroxyl radicals. Thus, dopamine within dopaminergic neurons may provide a source of reactive oxygen species, which, when coupled with reduced complex I function, may promote cell death.

Approximately 5% of Parkinson disease cases are familial. Genetic studies that have identified causative mutations in five genes provide important information about molecular pathways involved in the disease. These genes include the genes for α-synuclein (*PARK1*), parkin (*PARK2*), DJ-1 (*PARK7*), ubiquitin-C-hydrolase-L1 (*PARK5*), PTEN (phosphatase and tensin homolog deleted on chromosome 10)–induced kinase 1 (*PINK1*), and leucine-rich repeat kinase 2 (*LRRK2*).

Mutations in the gene for α-synuclein on chromosome 4q21-23 cause autosomal dominant Parkinson disease. Alpha-synuclein is found in nerve terminals in close proximity to synaptic vesicles. Its normal function is not known. Overexpression of nonmutant human α-synuclein in transgenic mice results in the formation of Lewy bodies, reduced dopaminergic terminals in the striatum, and impaired motor performance resulting from the formation of abnormal complexes at the synapse with SNARE proteins. Genomic triplication of α-synuclein leading to overexpression has been documented in a human family with autosomal dominant Parkinson disease. This suggests that it is the production of neuronal inclusions containing α-synuclein, rather than a change in α-synuclein function, that contributes to the degeneration of dopaminergic neurons. Interestingly, mice lacking α-synuclein are resistant to the toxic effects of the complex I inhibitor MPTP, suggesting that mitochondrial dysfunction generates an environment that favors α-synuclein aggregation and neurodegeneration.

Misfolded, damaged, or unassembled proteins are generally degraded by a process involving covalent attachment of ubiquitin. Ubiquitin is a 76-residue protein that marks proteins for processing by a proteolytic complex (**proteasome**). A missense mutation in one component of the ubiquitin–proteasome system, ubiquitin carboxyl terminal hydrolase L1, has been found in one family with autosomal dominant Parkinson disease. Mutations in *parkin* on chromosome 6q25 have been identified in cases of autosomal recessive juvenile parkinsonism. Parkin is an E3 ubiquitin ligase that catalyzes the addition of ubiquitin to specific proteins to target them for degradation. Known *parkin* mutations cause loss of function, which presumably leads to a disturbance in protein degradation. However, most patients with *parkin* mutations lack Lewy bodies, suggesting that other mechanisms, such as increased oxidative stress, cause neurodegeneration in these patients. In support of this mechanism is the finding that *Drosophila* mutants that lack parkin show mitochondrial pathology.

The most common known genetic form of Parkinson disease was recently discovered. Mutations in the glucocerebrosidase (GCase) enzyme account for 3% of sporadic Parkinson disease cases and 25% of juvenile-onset Parkinson disease cases. This enzyme is involved in lysosomal processing. Enzyme activity is reduced by 58% in the substantia nigra of heterozygous patients and by 33% in patients with sporadic Parkinson disease. Inhibiting this enzyme leads to the accumulation of α-synuclein, which leads to further inhibition of this enzyme.

CHECKPOINT

35. What are the clinical features of parkinsonism?
36. What are some of the causes of this syndrome?
37. What are two major mechanisms proposed to explain the pathophysiology of Parkinson disease?

MYASTHENIA GRAVIS

Clinical Presentation

Myasthenia gravis is an autoimmune disorder of neuromuscular transmission. The major clinical features are fluctuating fatigue and weakness that improve after a period of rest and after administration of acetylcholinesterase inhibitors. Muscles with small motor units, such as ocular muscles, are most often affected. Oropharyngeal muscles, flexors and extensors of the neck, proximal limb muscles, and the erector spinae muscles are involved less often. In severe cases, all muscles are weak, including the diaphragm and intercostal muscles, and death may result from respiratory failure.

About 5% of patients have coexistent hyperthyroidism. Rheumatoid arthritis, systemic lupus erythematosus, and polymyositis are also more common in patients with myasthenia gravis than in the general population, and up to 30% of patients have a maternal relative with an autoimmune disorder. These associations suggest that patients with myasthenia gravis share a genetic predisposition to autoimmune disease.

Pathology & Pathogenesis

The major structural abnormality in myasthenia gravis is a simplification of the postsynaptic region of the neuromuscular synapse. The muscle end plate shows sparse, shallow, and abnormally wide or absent synaptic clefts. In contrast, the number and size of the presynaptic vesicles are normal. Scattered collections of lymphocytes, some within the vicinity of motor end plates, may be present. IgG and the C3 component of complement are present at the postsynaptic membrane.

Electrophysiologic studies indicate that the postsynaptic membrane has a decreased response to applied acetylcholine. Studies with iodine-125–labeled α-bungarotoxin, which binds with high affinity to muscle nicotinic AChRs, show a 70–90% decrease in the number of receptors per end plate in affected muscles. Circulating antibodies to the receptor are present in 90% of patients, and the disorder may be passively transferred to animals by administering IgG from affected patients. Moreover, immunization with AChR protein from muscle can produce myasthenia in experimental animals. The antibodies block acetylcholine binding and receptor activation (Figure 7–30). In addition, the antibodies cross-link receptor molecules, increasing receptor internalization and degradation. Bound antibody also activates complement-mediated destruction of the postsynaptic region, resulting in simplification of the end plate. Many patients who lack antibodies to AChR have autoantibodies instead against the muscle-specific receptor tyrosine kinase (MuSK), which is an important mediator of AChR clustering at the end plate. These antibodies inhibit clustering of receptors in muscle cell culture.

During repetitive stimulation of a motor nerve, the number of quanta released from the nerve terminal declines with successive stimuli. Normally, this causes no clinical impairment because a sufficient number of AChR channels are opened by the reduced level of neurotransmitter. However, in myasthenia gravis, in which there is a deficiency in the number of functional receptors, neuromuscular transmission fails at lower levels of quantal release. Electrophysiologically, this is measured as a decremental decline in the compound muscle action potential during repetitive stimulation of a motor nerve. Clinically, this is manifested by muscle fatigue with sustained or repeated activity.

Treatment has reduced the mortality rate from approximately 30% to 5% in generalized myasthenia gravis. The two basic strategies for treatment that stem from knowledge of the pathogenesis are to increase the amount of acetylcholine at the neuromuscular junction and to inhibit immune-mediated destruction of AChRs.

By preventing acetylcholine metabolism, cholinesterase inhibitors can compensate for the normal decline in released neurotransmitter during repeated stimulation. Therapy with cholinesterase inhibitors can also cause a paradoxical increase in weakness known as a **cholinergic crisis**, which results from an excess of acetylcholine. At the molecular level, acetylcholine binding first opens nicotinic cation channels, but with continued exposure to the agonist, the channels desensitize and shut down again. The desensitized channels recover their sensitivity to acetylcholine only after the neurotransmitter is removed. Removal of acetylcholine is impaired when cholinesterase activity is inhibited. This can result in a depolarization block of neurotransmission similar to the effect of the depolarizing paralytic agent succinylcholine or organophosphate insecticides and nerve gases that markedly inhibit acetylcholinesterase. Therefore, the dose of cholinesterase inhibitors must be carefully regulated to reduce myasthenia but avoid a cholinergic crisis.

Plasmapheresis, corticosteroids, and immunosuppressant drugs are effective in reducing levels of autoantibody to AChRs and suppressing disease. The thymus is thought to play an important role in the pathogenesis of the disease by supplying helper T cells sensitized against thymic proteins that cross-react with AChRs. In most patients with myasthenia gravis, the thymus is hyperplastic, and 10–15% have thymomas. Thymectomy is indicated if a thymoma is suspected. In patients with generalized myasthenia without thymoma, thymectomy induces remission in 35% and improves symptoms in another 45% of patients.

For patients with AChR antibody–negative myasthenia gravis who test positive for the MuSK antibody, the clinical features and treatment are different. Patients tend to be younger women with bulbar weakness, and muscle atrophy is often seen, particularly in the tongue, making it difficult to distinguish from motor neuron disease. Results of repetitive stimulation studies and single-fiber electromyography (EMG) studies in the limbs are often normal, necessitating facial studies to make a diagnosis. Cholinesterase inhibitors often make these patients worse, but plasma exchange is very effective, as is less conventional immunosuppressive therapy. Thymectomy is not clearly beneficial in this population.

Lastly, there are myasthenia gravis patients with no antibodies for either AChR antibodies or MuSK, referred to as double sero-negative patients. Recently, a new antibody has been found in 50% of these patients. Antibodies to lipoprotein-related

- Y Antiacetylcholine-receptor antibody
- ◇ Acetylcholine
- ⌄ Acetylcholine receptors

FIGURE 7–30 Pathogenesis of myasthenia gravis. Acetylcholine released at the nerve ending by the nerve impulse normally binds with acetylcholine receptors. This evokes the action potential in the muscle. In myasthenia gravis, antiacetylcholine receptor antibody binds to the acetylcholine receptor and inhibits the action of acetylcholine. Bound antibody evokes immune-mediated destruction of the end plate. (Redrawn, with permission, from Chandrasoma P et al, eds. *Concise Pathology*, 3rd ed. Originally published by Appleton & Lange. Copyright © 1998 by The McGraw-Hill Companies, Inc.)

protein 4 (LRP4), which is the agrin-binding receptor of the MuSK complex, disrupt agrin-induced AChR clustering, causing the disease symptoms. The clinical presentation of these patients is similar to that of those with AChR–myasthenia gravis without thymoma.

CHECKPOINT

38. What is the clinical presentation of myasthenia gravis?
39. What causes this disorder?
40. What is the pathophysiology of symptoms in myasthenia gravis?

EPILEPSY

Clinical Presentation

Seizures are paroxysmal disturbances in cerebral function caused by an abnormal synchronous discharge of cortical neurons. The epilepsies are a group of disorders characterized by recurrent seizures. Approximately 0.6% of people in the United States suffer from recurrent seizures, and idiopathic epilepsy accounts for more than 75% of all seizure disorders. In some forms of idiopathic epilepsy, a genetic basis is apparent. Other forms are secondary to brain injury from stroke, trauma, a mass lesion, or infection. About two-thirds of new cases arise in children, and most of these cases are idiopathic or caused by trauma. In contrast, seizures or epilepsy with onset in adult life is more often due to underlying brain lesions or metabolic causes.

Seizures are classified by behavioral and electrophysiologic data (Table 7–2). **Generalized tonic-clonic seizures** are attacks characterized by a sudden loss of consciousness followed rapidly by tonic muscle contraction, causing limb extension and arching of the back. The tonic phase lasts 10–30 seconds and is followed by a clonic phase of limb jerking. The

TABLE 7–2   Simplified classification of seizures.

I. Partial (focal seizures)
A. Simple partial seizures with motor, sensory, psychic, or autonomic symptoms
B. Complex partial seizures
C. Partial seizures with secondary generalization
II. Generalized seizures
A. Absence seizures
B. Tonic-clonic seizures
C. Other (myoclonic, tonic, clonic, atonic)

jerking builds in frequency to a peak after 15–30 seconds and then slows gradually over another 15–30 seconds. Thereafter, the patient remains unconscious for several minutes. As consciousness is regained, there is a period of postictal confusion lasting several minutes. In patients with recurrent seizures or an underlying structural or metabolic abnormality, confusion may persist for a few hours. Focal abnormalities may be present on neurologic examination during the postictal period. Such findings suggest a focal brain lesion requiring further laboratory and radiologic study.

Typical **absence seizures** begin in childhood and usually remit by adulthood. Seizures are characterized by brief lapses in consciousness lasting several seconds without loss of posture. These spells may be associated with eyelid blinking, slight head movement, or brief jerks of limb muscles. Immediately after the seizure, the patient is fully alert. The spells may occur several times throughout the day and impair school performance. The electroencephalogram (EEG) shows characteristic runs of spikes and waves at a rate of three per second, particularly after hyperventilation (Figure 7–31). The disorder is transmitted as an autosomal dominant trait with incomplete penetrance.

FIGURE 7–31 EEG of a patient with typical absence (petit mal) seizures, showing a burst of generalized 3 Hz spike-and-wave activity (center of record) that is bilaterally symmetric and bisynchronous. Odd-numbered leads indicate electrode placements over the left side of the head; even numbers, those over the right side. (Redrawn, with permission, from Aminoff MJ et al, eds. *Clinical Neurology*, 9th ed. McGraw-Hill, 2015.)

Some forms of epilepsy cause seizures with only a tonic or clonic phase. In others, the seizure is manifested by sudden loss of muscle tone (atonic seizures). In myoclonic epilepsy, sudden, brief contractions of muscles occur. Myoclonic seizures are found in certain neurodegenerative diseases or after diffuse brain injury, as occurs during global cerebral ischemia.

Focal seizures are caused by focal brain disease. Therefore, in general, patients with simple or focal dyscognitive seizures should be investigated for underlying brain lesions. **Simple focal seizures** begin with motor, sensory, visual, psychic, or autonomic phenomena depending on the location of the seizure focus. Consciousness is preserved unless the seizure discharge spreads to other areas, producing a tonic-clonic seizure (**secondary generalization**). **Focal dyscognitive seizures** are characterized by the sudden onset of impaired consciousness with stereotyped, coordinated, involuntary movements (**automatisms**). Immediately before impairment of consciousness, there may be an aura consisting of unusual abdominal sensations, olfactory or sensory hallucinations, unexplained fear, or illusions of familiarity (déjà vu). Seizures usually last for 2–5 minutes and are followed by postictal confusion. Secondary generalization may occur. The seizure focus usually lies in the temporal or frontal lobe.

Pathogenesis

Normal neuronal activity occurs in a nonsynchronized manner, with groups of neurons inhibited and excited sequentially during the transfer of information between different brain areas. Seizures occur when neurons are activated synchronously. The kind of seizure depends on the location of the abnormal activity and the pattern of spread to different parts of the brain.

Interictal spike discharges are often observed on EEG recordings from patients with epilepsy. These are due to the synchronous depolarization of a group of neurons in an abnormally excitable area of brain. Experimentally, this is known as the **paroxysmal depolarizing shift** and is followed by a hyperpolarizing afterpotential that is the cellular correlate of the slow wave that follows spike discharges on the EEG. The shift is produced by depolarizing currents generated at excitatory synapses and by the subsequent influx of sodium or calcium through voltage-gated channels.

Normally, discharging excitatory neurons activate nearby inhibitory interneurons that suppress the activity of the discharging cell and its neighbors. Most inhibitory synapses use the neurotransmitter GABA. Voltage-gated and calcium-dependent potassium currents are also activated in the discharging neuron to suppress excitability. In addition, adenosine generated from adenosine triphosphate (ATP) released during excitation further suppresses neuronal excitation by binding to adenosine receptors present on nearby neurons. Disruption of these inhibitory mechanisms by alterations in ion channels, or by injury to inhibitory neurons and synapses, may allow for the development of a seizure focus. In addition, groups of neurons may become synchronized if local excitatory circuits

are enhanced by the reorganization of neural networks after brain injury.

Spread of a local discharge occurs by a combination of mechanisms. During the paroxysmal depolarizing shift, extracellular potassium accumulates, depolarizing nearby neurons. Increased frequency of discharges enhances calcium influx into nerve terminals, increasing neurotransmitter release at excitatory synapses by a process known as **post-tetanic potentiation**. This involves increased calcium influx through voltage-gated channels and through the N-methyl-D-aspartate (NMDA) subtype of glutamate receptor–gated ion channels. NMDA receptor–gated channels preferentially pass calcium ions but are relatively quiescent during normal synaptic transmission because they are blocked by magnesium ions. Magnesium block is relieved by depolarization. In contrast, the effect of inhibitory synaptic neurotransmission appears to decrease with high-frequency stimulation. This may be partly due to rapid desensitization of GABA receptors at high concentrations of released GABA. The net effect of these changes is to recruit neighboring neurons into a synchronous discharge and cause a seizure.

In secondary epilepsy, loss of inhibitory circuits and sprouting of fibers from excitatory neurons appear to be important for the generation of a seizure focus. In several of the idiopathic epilepsies, genetic studies have identified mutations in ion channels. In severe myoclonic epilepsy of infancy, an early-onset form of epilepsy, mutations are most commonly found in *SCN1A*, an Na+ channel subunit. Benign familial neonatal convulsions have been linked to mutations in two homologous voltage-gated K+ channels: KCNQ2 encoded by a gene on chromosome 20q13.3 and KCNQ3 encoded by a gene on chromosome 8q24. Generalized epilepsy associated with febrile seizures has been linked to mutations in *SCN1A* and *SCN1B*, both of which are voltage-gated Na+ channel subunits, and *GABRG2*, a GABA$_A$ receptor subunit gene. Another rare condition, autosomal dominant nocturnal frontal lobe epilepsy, is associated with mutations on chromosome 20q13.2 in the gene for the α4 subunit of neuronal nicotinic cholinergic receptors. Lastly, a genome-wide association study in idiopathic generalized epilepsy revealed the first common genetic risk variants. These variants were found in genes with both known and largely unknown pathways, such as *CHRM3*, *VRK2*, *ZEB2*. Mutations of *PNPO* result in pyridoxamine 5'-phosphate oxidase (PNPO) deficiency, causing a form of neonatal epileptic encephalopathy. And, as noted above, mutations of *SCN1A* are present in severe myoclonic epilepsy of infancy.

Animal models have provided clues to the pathogenesis of absence seizures. Absence seizures arise from synchronous thalamic discharges mediated by activation of low-threshold calcium currents (T or "transient" currents) in thalamic neurons. The anticonvulsant ethosuximide blocks T channels and suppresses absence seizures in humans. T channels are more likely to be activated after hyperpolarization of the cell membrane. Activation of GABA$_B$ receptors hyperpolarizes thalamic neurons and facilitates T-channel activation. Lethargic (lh/lh)

TABLE 7-3 Known mechanisms of action of some anticonvulsant drugs.

Drug	Main Indications	Mechanisms of Action
Phenytoin	Generalized tonic-clonic and partial seizures	Inhibits voltage-gated sodium and calcium channels
Carbamazepine	Generalized tonic-clonic and partial seizures	Inhibits voltage-gated sodium and calcium channels
Phenobarbital	Generalized tonic-clonic and partial seizures	Enhances $GABA_A$ receptor function
Valproate	Generalized tonic-clonic, absence, myoclonic, and partial seizures	Increases levels of GABA by inhibiting succinic semialdehyde dehydrogenase
Ethosuximide	Absence seizures	Inhibits low-threshold (T-type) voltage-gated calcium channels
Felbamate	Generalized tonic-clonic and partial seizures	Antagonist of NMDA subtype of glutamate receptors; enhances action of GABA at $GABA_A$ receptors
Lamotrigine	Generalized tonic-clonic and partial seizures	Inhibits voltage-gated sodium channels
Vigabatrin	Partial and secondarily generalized seizures	Increases GABA levels by inhibiting GABA transaminase
Tiagabine	Partial seizures	Increases GABA levels by inhibiting GABA reuptake

mice demonstrate frequent absence spells accompanied by 5 to 6 Hz spike-wave discharges on the EEG and respond to drugs used in human absence epilepsy. A single mutation in a gene on chromosome 2 results in this autosomal recessive disorder. There is an increase in the number of $GABA_B$ receptors in the cerebral cortex in mice with this disorder, and the $GABA_B$ agonist baclofen worsens the seizures, whereas antagonists alleviate them. This suggests that abnormal regulation of $GABA_B$ receptor function or expression may be important in the pathogenesis of absence seizures. This is supported by the finding that γ-hydroxybutyrate, which causes behavioral and electroencephalographic alterations similar to those seen during absence attacks, activates $GABA_B$ receptors and that $GABA_B$ agonists increase and $GABA_B$ antagonists reduce spike-wave discharges in rats genetically susceptible to absence seizures (GAERS rats).

The main targets for currently available anticonvulsants are (1) voltage-gated sodium and calcium channels that are involved in the generation of action potentials and neurotransmitter release; and (2) ligand-gated channels that modulate synaptic excitation and inhibition. Many agents act by more than one mechanism. Several anticonvulsants and some of their presumed mechanisms of action are listed in Table 7-3.

CHECKPOINT

41. What is the clinical presentation of the major types of seizures?

42. What are some disorders that lead to secondary epilepsy, and what changes in brain structure lead to secondary epilepsy?

43. What kinds of mutations have been associated with idiopathic epilepsies?

DEMENTIA & ALZHEIMER DISEASE

1. Clinical Features of Dementia

Dementia is an acquired decline in intellectual function resulting in loss of social independence. Patients experience impairment of memory and at least one other area of cortical function, such as language, calculation, spatial orientation, decision making, judgment, or abstract reasoning. In contrast to patients with confusional states, symptoms progress over months to years, and alertness is preserved until the very late stages of disease. Dementia affects 5–20% of persons over age 65, and, although not part of normal aging, its incidence increases with age. The most common causes, listed in Table 7-4, account for almost 90% of cases. Treatable causes are important to recognize and include hypothyroidism, vitamin B_{12} deficiency, neurosyphilis, brain tumor, normal pressure (communicating) hydrocephalus, and chronic subdural hematoma. In addition, although not curable, dementia associated with HIV infection may be slowed by antiretroviral treatment. About 10–15% of patients referred for evaluation of dementia suffer from depression ("**pseudodementia**"), which may also respond to treatment.

Cerebrovascular disease is the second most common cause of dementia (after Alzheimer disease). In such cases, dementia results from either multiple infarctions in the territory of major cerebral vessels (**multi-infarct dementia**) or from subcortical infarctions in the distributions of deep penetrating arterioles (**lacunar state**, **Binswanger disease**, **subcortical arteriosclerotic encephalopathy**). There is usually a history of stepwise progression of neurologic deficits, focal signs on neurologic examination, and multiple infarctions on brain imaging studies. Patients generally have a history of hypertension or other risk factors for atherosclerosis.

Chronic drug intoxication is often listed as a cause of dementia but actually produces a confusional state. The existence of

TABLE 7–4   Major causes of dementia.

Alzheimer disease (>50% of cases)
Multiple cerebral infarcts
Dementia with Lewy bodies
Alcoholism
Normal pressure hydrocephalus
Primary or metastatic CNS neoplasms
Frontotemporal dementia
Parkinson disease
Huntington disease
Pick disease
Prion diseases (eg, Creutzfeldt–Jakob disease)
Neurosyphilis
HIV infection
Hypothyroidism
Deficiency of vitamins B_{12}, B_6, B_1, or niacin
Chronic meningitis
Subdural hematoma

alcohol-induced dementia is controversial. Although animal and cell culture studies provide evidence for a direct neurotoxic effect of alcohol, dementia in patients with alcoholism also results from associated nutritional deficiency, recurrent head trauma, and (rarely) acquired hepatocerebral degeneration, a complication of chronic hepatic insufficiency caused by alcoholic cirrhosis.

2. Alzheimer Disease

Clinical Features

Alzheimer disease is the most common cause of dementia and accounts for more than 50% of cases. It is a slowly progressive disorder that runs a course of 5–10 years, typically beginning with impairment of learning and recent memory. Anomia, aphasia, and acalculia eventually develop, causing loss of employability and inability to manage finances. Spatial disorientation causes patients to become lost easily, and apraxias lead to difficulty with cooking, cleaning, and self-care. A frontal lobe gait disorder may appear, with short, shuffling steps, flexed posture, difficulty turning, and a tendency to fall backward (**retropulsion**) similar to that seen in Parkinson disease. In later stages, social graces are lost, and psychiatric symptoms such as paranoia, hallucinations, and delusions may appear. Cholinesterase treatments such as donepezil, rivastigmine, and galantamine may help for a couple of years to improve

Amyloid plaques

FIGURE 7–32 Amyloid plaques in the cerebral cortex in Alzheimer disease.

memory, but eventually the neuronal degeneration progresses and these medications are no longer effective. Terminally ill patients are bedridden, mute, and incontinent.

Pathology

The pathology of Alzheimer disease is characterized by extracellular neuritic plaques in the cerebral cortex and in the walls of meningeal and cerebral blood vessels (Figure 7–32). These plaques contain a dense core of amyloid material surrounded by dystrophic neurites (axons and dendrites), reactive astrocytes, and microglia. Other structural changes include the formation of intraneuronal neurofibrillary tangles, neuronal and synaptic loss, reactive astrocytosis, and microglial proliferation. Controversy exists as to which features are most related to the pathogenesis of the disease. The formation of neuritic plaques is particularly characteristic of Alzheimer disease, but there is little evidence that the course or onset of disease correlates with plaque number. Neurofibrillary tangles are paired helical filaments composed of a hyperphosphorylated form of the microtubule protein tau. They are not specific for Alzheimer disease and occur in several other neurodegenerative disorders. In general, all pathologic changes are most prominent in the hippocampus, entorhinal cortex, association cortex, and basal forebrain. This accounts for the early symptoms of memory loss and disturbance of higher cortical functions, with preservation of primary sensory and motor function until later in the course of the disease.

Pathophysiology

A. Amyloid β-Peptide—The major protein in neuritic plaques is **amyloid β-peptide (Aβ)**, which is proteolytically derived from a membrane protein, the **β-amyloid precursor protein (APP)** encoded by a gene on chromosome 21q21.3-22.05. APP interacts with extracellular matrix and supports the growth of neurites in neuronal cultures. Genetic evidence implicates Aβ in the pathogenesis of Alzheimer disease. Almost all patients with trisomy 21 (Down syndrome) develop pathologic changes indistinguishable from those seen in Alzheimer disease, suggesting that having an increased copy of the *APP* gene increases the metabolism of APP to Aβ. About 10% of cases of Alzheimer disease are familial, with early onset (before age 65 years) and autosomal dominant inheritance. In approximately 5% of these families, Alzheimer disease is strongly linked to missense mutations immediately flanking the Aβ sequence in the *APP* gene. Transgenic mice expressing human APP with these mutations show elevated levels of Aβ, behavioral abnormalities, and neuritic plaques. The APP mutations result in either increased production of all forms of Aβ or mainly in the long 42-amino-acid form, $A\beta_{42}$, which self-aggregates and promotes plaque formation. Aβ is toxic to cultured neurons and stimulates production of cytokines from microglial cells. Aβ also triggers the release of glutamate from glial cells and may injure neurons through excitotoxicity. This evidence links an increased production of Aβ, particularly $A\beta_{42}$, to Alzheimer disease and suggests that Aβ causes the neurodegeneration. Transgenic mice that express mutant forms of familial human APP develop synaptic dysfunction before plaque deposition, indicating that diffusible forms of Aβ are neurotoxic. This may explain why plaque number and disease severity correlate poorly.

B. Presenilins—The enzymatic pathways that regulate Aβ formation are critical areas of current research that may lead to new treatments. Some clues have come from analysis of additional families with Alzheimer disease. APP is cleaved at the amino terminal of the Aβ sequence by the membrane-anchored protease beta-amyloid precursor protein cleaving enzyme (BACE), also known as beta-secretase. This cleavage generates a 99–amino acid carboxyl terminal fragment. A second enzymatic activity termed γ-secretase cleaves this fragment to yield Aβ. Almost 70% of familial cases of Alzheimer disease have been linked to missense mutations in the gene **PS-1/S182**, on chromosome 14q24.3, which encodes a seven-trans-membrane protein (**presenilin 1**). Another 20% of cases have been linked to mutations in another gene, **STM2** (**presenilin 2**), on chromosome 1q31-42. The proteins encoded by these genes are 67% identical in amino acid sequence and presumably have similar functions. Current evidence indicates that the presenilins are subunits of γ-secretase, because mutant mice lacking either presenilin show reduced γ-secretase function, and mutations designed to inhibit the predicted aspartyl protease function of presenilins eliminate γ-secretase activity. Mutant variants of presenilins associated with familial Alzheimer disease increase the production of $A\beta_{42}$. This suggests that these mutations produce Alzheimer disease by selectively altering γ-secretase activity to favor production of the longer, amyloid-producing form of Aβ. In addition, γ-secretase is important for processing Notch proteins and other substrates critical for neuronal function, and mice deficient in presenilins show deficiencies in spatial memory and synaptic plasticity. Thus, γ-secretase deficiency may contribute to neurodegeneration in patients with presenilin mutations.

C. Apolipoprotein E—The majority of patients with Alzheimer disease are older than 60 years, and in about 50% of these patients, the e4 isoform of **apolipoprotein E (apoE4)** has been identified as a risk factor. ApoE is a 34-kDa protein that mediates the binding of lipoproteins to the low-density lipoprotein (LDL) receptor and the LDL receptor-related protein (LRP). It is synthesized and secreted by astrocytes and macrophages and is thought to be important for mobilizing lipids during normal development of the nervous system and during regeneration of peripheral nerves after injury. There are three major isoforms (apoE2, apoE3, and apoE4), which arise from different alleles (e2, e3, and e4) of a single gene on chromosome 19q13.2. The e3 allele is the most common, accounting for about 75% of all alleles, whereas e2 and e4 account for roughly 10% and 15%, respectively. The e4 allele is associated with increased risk and earlier onset of both familial and sporadic late-onset Alzheimer disease. In contrast, inheritance of e2 is associated with decreased risk and later onset. It is important to note that Alzheimer disease develops in the absence of e4 and also that many persons with e4 escape disease. Therefore, genotyping is not currently recommended as a useful genetic test.

The mechanism by which apoE alleles alter disease risk is uncertain. In cultured neurons, apoE3 increases neurite outgrowth in the presence of very low-density lipoproteins, whereas apoE4 inhibits outgrowth. Alzheimer patients homozygous for the e4 allele have larger and denser senile plaques than patients homozygous for the e3 allele. ApoE is found in neuritic plaques, and apoE4 binds Aβ more readily than does apoE3. Therefore, apoE4 may facilitate plaque formation or reduce the clearance of Aβ from brain tissue. In addition, apoE enters neurons and binds the microtubule-associated protein tau, which is the major constituent of neurofibrillary tangles. ApoE3 binds tau much more avidly than apoE4. Binding of apoE3 to tau may prevent the formation of neurofibrillary tangles and support the normal microtubule assembly required for neurite outgrowth.

CHECKPOINT

44. What are the treatable causes of dementia?
45. What are the clinical features of Alzheimer disease?
46. In which proteins are there mutations associated with familial forms of Alzheimer disease?
47. What is the association between apolipoprotein E and Alzheimer disease?

STROKE

Clinical Presentation

Stroke is a clinical syndrome characterized by the sudden onset of a focal neurologic deficit that persists for at least 24 hours and results from an abnormality of the cerebral circulation.

It is the third leading cause of death in the United States. The incidence of stroke increases with age and is higher in men than in women. Significant risk factors include hypertension, hypercholesterolemia, diabetes, smoking, heavy alcohol consumption, and oral contraceptive use. Advances in neuroimaging have had a great impact on treatment and outcomes.

Pathophysiology

A. Vascular Supply

The focal symptoms and signs that result from stroke correlate with the brain area supplied by the affected blood vessel. There are two major categories of stroke, based on pathogenesis: ischemic and hemorrhagic (Table 7–5). In ischemic stroke, vascular occlusion interrupts blood flow to a specific brain region, producing a fairly characteristic pattern of neurologic deficits resulting from loss of functions controlled by that region. The pattern of deficits resulting from hemorrhage is less predictable because it depends on the location of the bleed and also on factors that affect the function of brain regions distant from the hemorrhage (eg, increased intracranial pressure, brain edema, compression of neighboring brain tissue, rupture of blood into ventricles or subarachnoid space).

B. Ischemic Stroke

Ischemic strokes result from thrombotic or embolic occlusion of cerebral vessels. Neurologic deficits caused by the occlusion of large arteries (Figure 7–33) result from focal ischemia to the area of brain supplied by the affected vessel (Figure 7–34) and produce recognizable clinical syndromes (Table 7–6). Not all signs are present in every patient because the extent of the

TABLE 7–5   Classification of stroke.

Ischemic Stroke
Thrombotic Occlusion
Large vessels (major cerebral arteries)
Small vessels (lacunar stroke)
Venous occlusion
Embolic Occlusion
Artery to artery
Cardioembolic
Hemorrhage Stroke
Intraparenchymal hemorrhage
Subarachnoid hemorrhage
Subdural hemorrhage
Epidural hemorrhage
Hemorrhagic ischemic infarction

deficit depends on the presence of collateral blood flow, individual variations in vascular anatomy, blood pressure, and the exact location of the occlusion. Thrombosis usually involves the internal carotid, middle cerebral, or basilar arteries. Symptoms typically evolve over several minutes and may be preceded by brief episodes of reversible focal deficits known as **transient ischemic attacks**. Emboli from the heart, aortic arch, or carotid arteries usually occlude the middle cerebral artery because it carries more than 80% of blood flow to the cerebral hemisphere. Emboli that travel in the vertebral and basilar arteries commonly lodge at the apex of the basilar artery or in one or both posterior cerebral arteries.

Ischemic strokes involving occlusion of small arteries occur at select locations, where perfusion depends on small vessels that are end arteries. Most result from a degenerative change in the vessel, described pathologically as **lipohyalinosis**, which is caused by chronic hypertension and predisposes to occlusion. The most common vessels involved are the lenticulostriate arteries, which arise from the proximal middle cerebral artery and perfuse the basal ganglia and internal capsule. Also commonly affected are small branches of the basilar and posterior cerebral arteries that penetrate the brainstem and thalamus. Occlusion of these vessels causes small areas of tissue damage known as **lacunar infarctions**. These typically occur in the putamen, caudate, thalamus, pons, and internal capsule and less commonly in subcortical white matter and the cerebellum. Lacunar infarctions produce several fairly stereotyped clinical syndromes. The two most common are pure motor stroke and pure sensory stroke. In pure motor stroke, the infarction is usually within the internal capsule or pons contralateral to the weak side. In pure sensory stroke, the infarction is usually in the contralateral thalamus.

Several vascular, cardiac, and hematologic disorders can cause focal cerebral ischemia (Table 7–7). The most common is **atherosclerosis** of the large arteries of the neck and base of the brain (Figure 7–35). Atherosclerosis is thought to arise from injury to vascular endothelial cells by mechanical, biochemical, or inflammatory insults (see Chapter 11). Endothelial injury stimulates the attachment of circulating monocytes and lymphocytes, which migrate into the vessel wall and stimulate proliferation of smooth muscle cells and fibroblasts. This leads to the formation of a fibrous plaque. Damaged endothelial cells also provide a nidus for platelet aggregation and activation. Activated platelets secrete growth factors that encourage further proliferation of smooth muscle and fibroblasts. The plaque may eventually enlarge to occlude the vessel or may rupture, releasing emboli.

C. Hemorrhage Stroke

Epidural and **subdural hematomas** typically occur as sequelae of head injury. Epidural hematomas arise from damage to an artery, typically the middle meningeal artery, which can be ruptured by a blow to the temporal bone. Blood dissects the dura from the skull and compresses the hemisphere lying below. Initial loss of consciousness from the injury results from concussion and may be transient. Neurologic symptoms

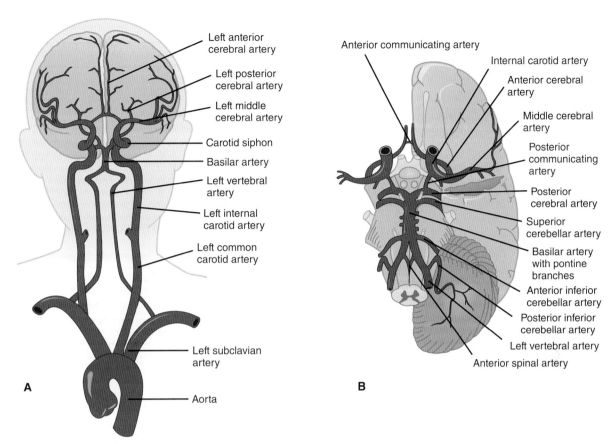

FIGURE 7-33 Major cerebral arteries. **A:** Anterior view. **B:** Inferior view showing the circle of Willis and principal arteries of the brainstem. (Redrawn, with permission, from Waxman SG. *Clinical Neuroanatomy*, 28th ed. McGraw-Hill, 2017.)

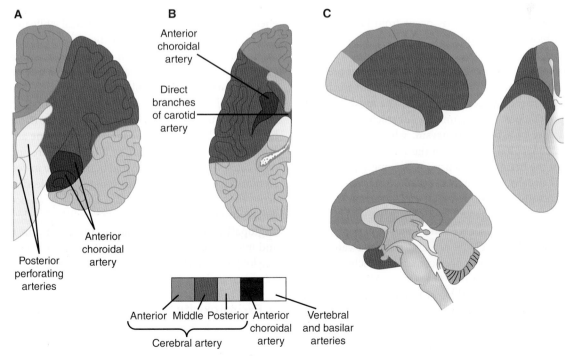

FIGURE 7-34 Vascular territories of the major cerebral arteries. **A:** Coronal section through the cerebrum. **B:** Horizontal section through the cerebrum. **C:** Vascular supply to the cerebral cortex. (Redrawn, with permission, from Chusid JG. *Correlative Neuroanatomy and Functional Neurology*, 19th ed. Originally published by Appleton & Lange. Copyright © 1985 by The McGraw-Hill Companies, Inc.)

TABLE 7–6   **Vascular territories and clinical features in ischemic stroke.**

Artery	Territory	Symptoms and Signs
Anterior cerebral	Medial frontal and parietal cortex, anterior corpus callosum	Paresis and sensory loss of contralateral leg and foot
Middle cerebral	Lateral frontal, parietal, occipital, and temporal cortex and adjacent white matter, caudate, putamen, internal capsule	Aphasia (dominant hemisphere), neglect (nondominant hemisphere), contralateral hemisensory loss, homonymous hemianopia, hemiparesis
Vertebral (posterior inferior cerebellar)	Medulla, lower cerebellum	Ipsilateral cerebellar ataxia, Horner syndrome, crossed sensory loss, nystagmus, vertigo, hiccup, dysarthria, dysphagia
Basilar (including anterior inferior cerebellar, and superior cerebellar)	Lower midbrain, pons, upper and mid cerebellum	Nystagmus, vertigo, diplopia, skew deviation, gaze palsies, hemi- or crossed sensory loss, dysarthria, hemi- or quadriparesis, ipsilateral cerebellar ataxia, Horner syndrome, coma
Posterior cerebral	Distal territory: medial occipital and temporal cortex and underlying white matter, posterior corpus callosum	Contralateral homonymous hemianopia, dyslexia without agraphia, visual hallucinations and distortions, memory defect, cortical blindness (bilateral occlusion)
	Proximal territory: upper midbrain, thalamus	Sensory loss, ataxia, third nerve palsy, contralateral hemiparesis, vertical gaze palsy, skew deviation, hemiballismus, choreoathetosis, impaired consciousness

return a few hours later as the hematoma exerts a mass effect that may be severe enough to cause brain herniation (see Figure 7–27). Subdural hematomas usually arise from venous blood that leaks from torn cortical veins bridging the subdural space. These may be ruptured by relatively minor trauma, particularly in the elderly. The blood is under low pressure, and symptoms resulting from mass effect may not appear for several days.

Subarachnoid hemorrhage may occur from head trauma, extension of blood from another compartment into the subarachnoid space, or rupture of an arterial aneurysm. Cerebral dysfunction occurs because of increased intracranial pressure and from poorly understood toxic effects of subarachnoid blood on brain tissue and cerebral vessels. The most common cause of spontaneous (nontraumatic) subarachnoid hemorrhage is rupture of a **berry aneurysm**, which is thought to arise from a congenital weakness in the walls of large vessels at the base of the brain. The aneurysms become symptomatic in adulthood, usually after the third decade. Rupture suddenly elevates intracranial pressure, which can interrupt cerebral blood flow and cause a generalized concussive injury. This results in loss of consciousness in about half of patients. With very large hemorrhages, global cerebral ischemia can cause severe brain damage and prolonged coma. Focal ischemia may later result from vasospasm of arteries at or near the site of rupture. Recurrence of hemorrhage within the first few days is a common and often fatal complication.

Intraparenchymal hemorrhage may result from acute elevations in blood pressure or from a variety of disorders that weaken vessels. The resultant hematoma causes a focal neurologic deficit by compressing adjacent structures. In addition, metabolic effects of extravasated blood disturb the function of surrounding brain tissue, and nearby vessels are compressed, causing local ischemia. Chronic hypertension is the most common predisposing factor. In hypertensive patients, small **Charcot–Bouchard aneurysms** appear in the walls of small penetrating arteries and are thought to be the major sites of rupture. Most vulnerable are the small vessels also involved in lacunar infarction. Hypertensive hemorrhages occur mainly in the basal ganglia, thalamus (Figure 7–36), pons, and cerebellum and less commonly in subcortical white matter. Other causes of intraparenchymal hemorrhage include **vascular malformations**, which contain abnormally fragile vessels susceptible to rupture at normal arterial pressures, and certain **brain tumors**, such as glioblastoma multiforme, which induce proliferation of fragile vessels within the tumor. Certain **platelet** and **coagulation disorders** may predispose to intracerebral hemorrhage by inhibiting coagulation. **Cocaine** and **amphetamines** cause rapid elevation of blood pressure and are common causes of intraparenchymal hemorrhage in young adults. Hemorrhage may be related to spontaneous bleeding from the acute elevation in blood pressure, rupture of an occult vascular abnormality, or drug-induced vasculitis. **Cerebral amyloid angiopathy** is a disorder that occurs mainly in the elderly and may be associated with Alzheimer disease. Deposition of amyloid weakens the walls of small cortical vessels and causes lobar hemorrhage, often at several sites.

D. Excitotoxicity

Most efforts to intervene in stroke have focused on the vasculature. In ischemic stroke, these efforts include restoring circulation through surgical endarterectomy and reducing thrombosis with anticoagulant, antiplatelet, and thrombolytic drugs. A complementary approach is to attempt to reduce the

TABLE 7–7 Conditions associated with focal cerebral ischemia.

Vascular Disorders
Atherosclerosis
Fibromuscular dysplasia
Vasculitis
Systemic (polyarteritis nodosa, lupus, giant cell arteritis, granulomatosis with polyangiitis [formerly Wegner granulomatosis], Takayasu arteritis)
Primary CNS
Meningitis (syphilis, tuberculosis, fungal, bacterial, herpes zoster)
Drug induced (cocaine, amphetamines)
Carotid or vertebral artery dissection
Lacunar infarction
Migraine
Multiple progressive intracranial occlusions (moyamoya syndrome)
Venous or sinus thrombosis
Cardiac Disorders
Mural thrombus
Rheumatic heart disease
Arrhythmias
Endocarditis
Mitral valve prolapse
Paradoxical embolus
Atrial myxoma
Prosthetic heart valves
Hematologic Disorders
Thrombocytosis
Polycythemia
Sickle cell disease
Leukocytosis
Hypercoagulable states (homocysteinemia, protein S deficiency, antiphospholipid syndrome, sickle cell disease)

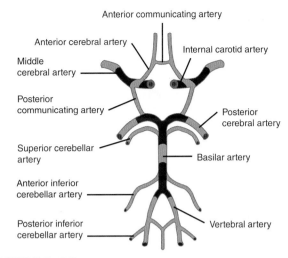

FIGURE 7–35 Sites of predilection (dark red areas) for atherosclerosis in the intracranial arterial circulation. (Redrawn, with permission, from Aminoff MJ et al, eds. *Clinical Neurology*, 9th ed. McGraw-Hill, 2015.)

receptors (Figure 7–37). As noted, glutamate is released at excitatory synapses, and glutamate levels in the extracellular space are normally tightly regulated by sodium-dependent reuptake systems in neurons and glia. In glia, glutamate is further detoxified by conversion to glutamine via the ATP-dependent enzyme glutamine synthetase. Glutamine is then released by glia and taken up by neurons, where it is repackaged into synaptic vesicles for subsequent release. Ischemia

FIGURE 7–36 CT scan in hypertensive intracerebral hemorrhage. Blood is seen as a high-density signal at the site of hemorrhage in the thalamus (left arrow) and in its extension into the third ventricle (top arrow) and the occipital horns of the ipsilateral (bottom arrow) and contralateral (right arrow) lateral ventricles. (Reproduced, with permission, from Greenberg DA et al, eds. *Clinical Neurology*, 8th ed. McGraw-Hill, 2012.)

vulnerability of brain tissue to ischemic damage. This is based on observations that CNS glutamate homeostasis is markedly altered during ischemia, leading to increased and toxic levels of extracellular glutamate.

Neurons deep within an ischemic focus die from energy deprivation. However, at the edge of the ischemic region, neurons appear to die because of excessive stimulation of glutamate

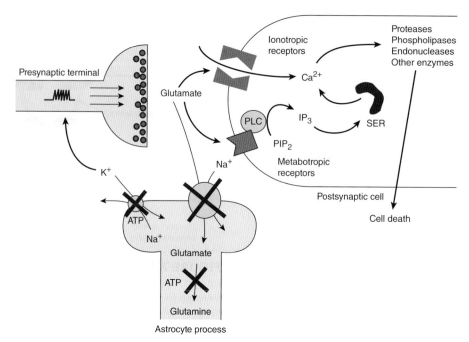

FIGURE 7–37 Excitotoxicity in neuronal ischemia. Depletion of energy supplies inhibits Na+-K+ ATPase, leading to accumulation of extracellular K+ and a decline in extracellular Na+. The increase in extracellular K+ depolarizes nerve terminals, causing release of glutamate. The reduction in extracellular Na+ reduces Na+-dependent glutamate uptake, potentiating synaptic effects of released glutamate. This generates a sustained increase in intracellular Ca2+ in the postsynaptic cell, leading to cell death. The bold, red "X" denotes inhibition of Na+-K+ ATPase (**left**), glutamate transporters (**right**), and glutamine synthetase (**bottom**). Other abbreviations are defined in the legend to Figure 7–28.

deprives the brain of oxygen and glucose, and the resultant disruption in cellular metabolism depletes neurons and glia of energy reserves required to maintain normal transmembrane ion gradients. This leads to the accumulation of intracellular Na+ and the collapse of the transmembrane Na+ gradient, which in turn inhibits glutamate uptake. Declining energy reserves also reduce conversion of glutamate to glutamine in glia. Both events promote accumulation of extracellular glutamate, which stimulates glutamate receptors on surrounding neurons, causing entry of Ca2+ and Na+. The influx of cations depolarizes these neurons, stimulating additional Ca2+ influx through voltage-gated channels.

Ischemia also disrupts K+ homeostasis, leading to an increase in the concentration of extracellular K+ ($[K^+]_o$). Neuronal activity can rapidly increase $[K^+]_o$, and one major function of glial cells is to keep $[K^+]_o$ at about 3 mmol/L to help neurons maintain their resting membrane potential. Two energy-dependent transporters are particularly important for removal of extracellular K+ by glia: an Na+-K+ ATPase and an anion transporter that cotransports K+ and Na+ with Cl-. In ischemia, these energy-dependent mechanisms fail, and K+ released into the extracellular space can no longer be taken up by glia. This depolarizes neurons because the gradient of K+ across neuronal membranes determines the level of the resting

membrane potential. Depolarization activates the release of neurotransmitters, increasing the accumulation of glutamate at excitatory synapses and in the extracellular space.

The net effect of these events is a tremendous influx of Na+ and Ca2+ into neurons through glutamate- and voltage-gated ion channels. The resultant overload in intracellular Ca2+ appears to be especially toxic and may exceed the ability of the neuron to extrude or sequester the cation. This results in sustained activation of a variety of calcium-sensitive enzymes, including proteases, phospholipases, and endonucleases, leading to cell death. In support of an excitotoxic mechanism of cell death in stroke are animal studies that demonstrate a reduction in the size of ischemic lesions after treatment with glutamate receptor antagonists.

CHECKPOINT

48. What are the differences between the clinical presentation of stroke resulting from ischemia and stroke caused by spontaneous hemorrhage?

49. What are the most common causes of stroke?

50. What role does glutamate play in neuronal injury during ischemia?

CASE STUDIES

Yeong Kwok, MD

(See Chapter 25, p. 755–58 for Answers)

CASE 31

A 70-year-old woman is brought to the emergency department after a fall. She lives alone and was found by a neighbor who overheard her screams. Her neighbor helped her get up, but she found that she could not walk and had trouble maintaining her balance. Her neighbor also noted that there were many empty bottles of vodka in her apartment. On examination, the patient is alert and cooperative. She has an unsteady, wide-based gait and a positive Romberg test. She has obvious dysmetria on finger-to-nose and heel-to-shin testing. Her x-rays show osteopenia, and her head magnetic resonance imaging shows mild cerebral and cerebellar atrophy. Her blood alcohol level is 0.08%; other laboratory test results are normal.

Questions

A. What is the likely cause of the patient's fall and neurologic findings?
B. What are the common clinical features of this condition?
C. If many members of her family, including individuals who never used alcohol, had similar symptoms, what neurologic disorder might you suspect?

CASE 32

A 43-year-old right-handed man presents to the clinic with gradual onset of right hand and arm weakness. He had been in good health and an avid golfer until a few weeks ago when he noted that he was having trouble keeping his club steady during his swing. His driving distance had markedly decreased, and he had begun to drop things that he was holding with his right hand. He had no numbness or other sensory symptoms. On physical examination, he appears well and has normal vital signs. He has mild wasting and fasciculations along his right brachioradialis muscle. His grip strength is 4 out of 5 on the right and 5 out of 5 on the left. He has absent reflexes in his right arm and 1+ reflexes on the left. An electromyelogram shows features of denervation, including increased numbers of spontaneous discharges in resting muscle, and a reduction in the number of motor units detected during voluntary contraction. A diagnosis of amyotrophic lateral sclerosis (ALS) is entertained.

Questions

A. What are the presenting clinical symptoms and progression of the clinical course in ALS?
B. Which cells are affected in ALS?
C. What are some possible molecular mechanisms responsible for the pathologic changes?

CASE 33

A 63-year-old man comes to the clinic with a several-month history of difficulty with his gait and coordination. He finds walking difficult and has almost fallen on a number of occasions, especially when trying to change directions. He has also found that using his hands is difficult, and other people have noticed that his hands shake. Physical examination is notable for a resting tremor in the hands that disappears with intentional movement. He has a shuffling gait with difficulty turning. There is so-called cogwheeling rigidity in his arms, a jerky sensation with passive flexion and extension of the arms.

Questions

A. What is the likely diagnosis? What clinical features make this diagnosis likely?
B. What are the underlying pathologic changes responsible for the clinical presentation?
C. What are some possible molecular mechanisms responsible for the pathologic changes?

CASE 34

A 35-year-old woman presents to the clinic with a chief complaint of double vision. She reports intermittent and progressively worsening double vision for approximately 2 months, rarely at first but now every day. She works as a computer programmer, and the symptoms increase the longer she stares at the computer screen. She has also noted a drooping of her eyelids, which seems to worsen with prolonged working at the screen. Both symptoms subside with rest. She is generally fatigued but has noted no other weakness or neurologic symptoms. Her medical history is unremarkable. Physical examination is notable only for the neurologic findings. Cranial nerve examination discloses impaired lateral movement of the right eye and bilateral ptosis, which worsen with repetitive eye movements. Motor, sensory, and reflex examinations are otherwise unremarkable.

Questions

A. What is the likely diagnosis? What is the pathogenesis of this disease?
B. What other neurologic manifestations might you expect to see?
C. What is the mechanism by which this patient's ocular muscle weakness increases with prolonged activity?
D. What associated conditions should be investigated in this patient?
E. What treatments should be considered?

CASE 35

A 73-year-old man is brought in by his wife with concerns about his worsening memory. He is a retired engineer who has recently been getting lost in the neighborhood where he has lived for 30 years. He has been found wandering and has often been brought home by neighbors. When asked about this, he becomes upset and defensive and states that he was just trying to get some exercise. He has also had trouble dressing himself and balancing his checkbook. A physical examination is unremarkable, except that he scores 12 points out of 30 on the Mini-Mental State Examination, a test of cognitive function. A metabolic workup is normal. A computed tomography scan of the head shows generalized brain atrophy, though perhaps only what would be expected for his age. He is diagnosed with dementia, likely from Alzheimer disease.

Questions

A. If a brain biopsy is done, what is likely to be found?
B. Where in the brain are the changes characteristic of Alzheimer disease most prominent, and how does that explain the progression of symptoms?
C. What is the role of the amyloid peptide in Alzheimer disease?
D. Is there a role for genetic testing to determine risk for developing Alzheimer disease at this time?

CASE 36

A middle-aged man is transported to the emergency department unconscious and accompanied by a nurse from the medical floor. The nurse states that the patient was in line in front of her in the hospital cafeteria when he suddenly fell to the floor. He then had a "generalized tonic-clonic seizure." She called for assistance and accompanied him to the emergency department. No other historical information is available. On physical examination, the patient is confused and unresponsive to commands. He is breathing adequately and has oxygen in place via nasal prongs. His vital signs are as follows: temperature, 38°C; blood pressure, 170/90 mm Hg; heart rate, 105 bpm; respiratory rate, 18/min. Oxygen saturation is 99% on 2 L of oxygen. Neurologic examination is notable for reactive pupils of 3 mm, intact gag reflex, decreased movement of the left side of the body, and Babinski reflexes bilaterally. Examination is otherwise unremarkable.

Questions

A. Describe what is meant by a generalized tonic-clonic seizure.

B. What are some of the underlying causes of seizure disorders? Which cause might you be most concerned about in this patient?

C. What is the likely pathophysiology of the seizure in this patient?

CASE 37

A 72-year-old man presents to the emergency department with acute onset of right-sided weakness. The patient was eating breakfast when he suddenly lost strength on the right side of his body such that he was unable to move his right arm or leg. He also noted a loss of sensation in the right arm and leg and difficulty speaking. His wife called 911, and he was brought to the emergency department. His medical history is remarkable for long-standing hypertension, hypercholesterolemia, and recently diagnosed coronary artery disease. On physical examination, his blood pressure is 190/100 mm Hg. Neurologic examination is notable for right facial droop and a dense right hemiparesis. A Babinski reflex is present on the right. CT scan of the brain shows no evidence of hemorrhage. The patient is admitted to the neurologic ICU.

Questions

A. What is the diagnosis? Which artery or vascular territory is apt to be involved?

B. What are some risk factors for this condition?

C. What are the possible mechanisms by which this man developed these focal neurologic deficits? Which are most likely in this patient? Why?

D. What underlying disorder may be responsible? How does it result in stroke?

REFERENCES

General

Kandel ER et al. *Principles of Neural Science*, 5th ed. McGraw-Hill, 2012.

Ropper A et al. *Adams and Victor's Principles of Neurology*, 10th ed. McGraw-Hill, 2014.

Functional Neuroanatomy

Aminoff M et al. *Clinical Neurology*, 9th ed. McGraw-Hill, 2015.

Campbell WW. *DeJong's The Neurologic Examination*, 7th ed. Lippincott Williams and Wilkins, 2012.

Cerebellar Ataxia

Maas RP et al. The preclinical stage of spinocerebellar ataxias. Neurology. 2015 Jul 7;85(1):96–103. [PMID: 26062625]

Paulson et al. Polyglutamine spinocerebellar ataxias—from genes to potential treatments. Nat Rev Neurosci. 2017 Oct;18(10):613–26. [PMID: 28855740]

Perucca G et al. Role of neuroimaging in the diagnosis of hereditary cerebellar ataxias in childhood. J Neuroradiol. 2016 Jun;43(3):176–85. [PMID: 27126632]

Ramirez-Zamora A et al. Treatable causes of cerebellar ataxia. Mov Disord. 2015 Apr 15;30(5):614–23. [PMID: 25757427]

Rossi M et al. Autosomal dominant cerebellar ataxias: a systematic review of clinical features. Eur J Neurol. 2014 Apr;21(4):607–15. [PMID: 24765663]

Shakkottai VG et al. Clinical neurogenetics: autosomal dominant spinocerebellar ataxia. Neurol Clin. 2013 Nov;31(4):987–1007. [PMID: 24176420]

Storey E. Genetic cerebellar ataxias. Semin Neurol. 2014 Jul;34(3):280–92. [PMID: 25192506]

Todd P et al. Overview of cerebellar ataxia in adults. Up to Date. 2017 Jan 20. https://www.uptodate.com/contents/overview-of-cerebellar-ataxia-in-adults.

Motor Neuron Disease

Kaur SJ et al. Mutant *SOD1* mediated pathogenesis of amyotrophic lateral sclerosis. Gene. 2016 Feb 15;577(2):109–18. [PMID: 26657039]

Laferriere F et al. Advances and challenges in understanding the multifaceted pathogenesis of amyotrophic lateral sclerosis. Swiss Med Wkly. 2015 Jan 30;145:w14054. [PMID: 25635517]

Mavlyutov TA et al. Role of the sigma-1 receptor in amyotrophic lateral sclerosis (ALS). J Pharmacol Sci. 2015 Jan;127(1):10–6. [PMID: 25704013]

Peters OM et al. Emerging mechanisms of molecular pathology in ALS. J Clin Invest. 2015 May;125(5):1767–79. Erratum in: J Clin Invest. 2015 Jun;125(6):2548. [PMID: 25932674]

Saberi S et al. Neuropathology of amyotrophic lateral sclerosis and its variants. Neurol Clin. 2015 Nov;33(4):855–76. [PMID: 26515626]

Taylor JP et al. Decoding ALS: from genes to mechanism. Nature. 2016 Nov 9;539(7628):197–206. [PMID: 27830784]

Therrien M, Dion PA, Rouleau GA. ALS: Recent developments from genetics studies. Curr Neurol Neurosci Rep. 2016 Jun;16(6):59. [PMID: 27113253]

Trias E et al. Significance of aberrant glial cell phenotypes in pathophysiology of amyotrophic lateral sclerosis. Neurosci Lett. 2017 Jan 1;636:27–31. [PMID: 27473942]

Parkinson Disease

Amalric M. Targeting metabotropic glutamate receptors (mGluRs) in Parkinson's disease. Curr Opin Pharmacol. 2015 Feb;20:29–34. [PMID: 25462289]

Ambrosi G et al. A further update on the role of excitotoxicity in the pathogenesis of Parkinson's disease. J Neural Transm (Vienna). 2014 Aug;121(8):849–59. [PMID: 24380931]

Fernandez HH. 2015 Update on Parkinson disease. Cleve Clin J Med. 2015 Sep;82(9):563–8. [PMID: 26366951]

Ferreira M et al. An updated review of Parkinson's disease genetics and clinicopathological correlations. Acta Neurol Scand. 2017 Mar;135(3):273–84. [PMID: 27273099]

Gardoni F et al. Targeting glutamatergic synapses in Parkinson's disease. Curr Opin Pharmacol. 2015 Feb;20:24–8. [PMID: 25462288]

Reichmann H et al. The nonmotor features of Parkinson's disease: pathophysiology and management advances. Curr Opin Neurol. 2016 Aug;29(4):467–73. [PMID: 27262147]

Schneider SA et al. Clinical and pathological features of Parkinson's disease. Curr Top Behav Neurosci. 2015;22:205–20. [PMID: 24850081]

Zhu M et al. Sensory symptoms in Parkinson's disease: clinical features, pathophysiology, and treatment. J Neurosci Res. 2016 Aug;94(8):685–92. [PMID: 26948282]

Myasthenia Gravis

Avidan N et al. Genetic basis of myasthenia gravis - a comprehensive review. J Autoimmun. 2014 Aug;52:146–53. [PMID: 24361103]

Aydin Y et al. Thymectomy in myasthenia gravis. Eurasian J Med. 2017 Feb;49(1):48–52. [PMID: 28416933]

Berrih-Aknin S et al. Myasthenia gravis: a comprehensive review of immune dysregulation and etiological mechanisms. J Autoimmun. 2014 Aug;52:90–100. [PMID: 24389034]

Gilhus NE et al. Myasthenia gravis - autoantibody characteristics and their implications for therapy. Nat Rev Neurol. 2016 May;12(5):259–68. [PMID: 27103470]

Gilhus NE et al. Myasthenia gravis: subgroup classification and therapeutic strategies. Lancet Neurol. 2015 Oct;14(10):1023–36. [PMID: 26376969]

Ha JC et al. Myasthenia gravis and related disorders: pathology and molecular pathogenesis. Biochim Biophys Acta. 2015 Apr;1852(4):651–7. [PMID: 25486268]

Hurst RL et al. Muscle-specific receptor tyrosine kinase (MuSK) myasthenia gravis. Curr Neurol Neurosci Rep. 2016 Jul;16(7):61. [PMID: 27170368]

Keijzers M et al. Clinical and scientific aspects of acetylcholine receptor myasthenia gravis. Curr Opin Neurol. 2014 Oct;27(5):552–7. [PMID: 25105461]

Phillips WD et al. Pathogenesis of myasthenia gravis: update on disease types, models, and mechanisms. F1000Res. 2016 Jun 27;5. [PMID: 27408701]

Reddel SW et al. Clinical and scientific aspects of muscle-specific tyrosine kinase-related myasthenia gravis. Curr Opin Neurol. 2014 Oct;27(5):558–65. [PMID: 25159928]

Taioli E et al. Comparison of conservative treatment and thymectomy on myasthenia gravis outcome. Ann Thorac Surg. 2016 Dec;102(6):1805–13. [PMID: 28148454]

Epilepsy

Gavvala JR et al. New-onset seizure in adults and adolescents: a review. JAMA. 2016 Dec 27;316(24):2657–68. [PMID: 28027373]

Orsini A et al. Recent advances in epilepsy genetics. Neurosci Lett. 2018 Feb 22;667:4–9. [PMID: 28499889]

Sands TT. Genetic testing in pediatric epilepsy. Curr Neurol Neurosci Rep. 2017 May;17(5):45. [PMID: 28405954]

Walker MC. Pathophysiology of status epilepticus. Neurosci Lett. 2018 Feb 22;667:84–91. [PMID: 28011391]

Wang J et al. Epilepsy-associated genes. Seizure. 2017 Jan;44:11–20. [PMID: 28007376]

Dementia and Alzheimer Disease

Birch AM. The contribution of astrocytes to Alzheimer's disease. Biochem Soc Trans. 2014 Oct;42(5):1316–20. [PMID: 25233409]

Bozzali M et al. Quantitative MRI to understand Alzheimer's disease pathophysiology. Curr Opin Neurol. 2016 Aug;29(4):437–44. [PMID: 27228309]

Chouraki V et al. Genetics of Alzheimer's disease. Adv Genet. 2014;87:245–94. [PMID: 25311924]

Dzamba D et al. Glial cells - the key elements of Alzheimer's disease. Curr Alzheimer Res. 2016;13(8):894–911. [PMID: 26825092]

Hernández-Zimbrón LF et al. Deciphering an interplay of proteins associated with amyloid β 1-42 peptide and molecular mechanisms of Alzheimer's disease. Rev Neurosci. 2014;25(6):773–83. [PMID: 25010778]

Iqbal K et al. Tau and neurodegenerative disease: the story so far. Nat Rev Neurol. 2016 Jan;12(1):15–27. [PMID: 26635213]

Kumar A et al. A review on Alzheimer's disease pathophysiology and its management: an update. Pharmacol Rep. 2015 Apr;67(2):195–203. [PMID: 25712639]

Mendez MF. Early-onset Alzheimer disease. Neurol Clin. 2017 May;35(2):263–81. [PMID: 28410659]

Pierce AL et al. Late-onset Alzheimer disease. Neurol Clin. 2017 May;35(2):283–93. [PMID: 28410660]

Raman MR et al. Imaging markers of cerebrovascular pathologies: pathophysiology, clinical presentation, and risk factors. Alzheimers Dement (Amst). 2016 Dec 18;5:5–14. [PMID: 28054023]

Stroke

Caplan LR et al. Basic pathology, anatomy, and pathophysiology of stroke. In: *Caplan's Stroke: A Clinical Approach*, 4th ed. Cambridge University Press, 2016.

Chen R et al. Diabetes and stroke: epidemiology, pathophysiology, pharmaceuticals and outcomes. Am J Med Sci. 2016 Apr;351(4):380–6. [PMID: 27079344]

Chen Y et al. Stroke event rates and the optimal antithrombotic choice of patients with paroxysmal atrial fibrillation: a systematic review and meta-analysis of randomized controlled trials. Medicine (Baltimore). 2015 Dec;94(52):e2364. [PMID: 26717376]

Dalen JE et al. Silent atrial fibrillation and cryptogenic strokes. Am J Med. 2017 Mar;130(3):264–67. [PMID: 27756556]

Ettehad D et al. Blood pressure lowering for prevention of cardiovascular disease and death: a systematic review and meta-analysis. Lancet. 2016 Mar 5;387(10022):957–67. [PMID: 26724178]

Lip GY et al. Stroke prevention in atrial fibrillation: a systematic review. JAMA. 2015 May 19;313(19):1950–62. Erratum in: JAMA. 2015 Aug 25;314(8):837. [PMID: 25988464]

Xie X et al. Effects of intensive blood pressure lowering on cardiovascular and renal outcomes: updated systematic review and meta-analysis. Lancet. 2016 Jan 30;387(10017):435–43. [PMID: 26559744]

Yew KS et al. Diagnosis of acute stroke. Am Fam Physician. 2015 Apr 15;91(8):528–36. [PMID: 25884860]

Diseases of the Skin

Laura B. Pincus, MD, & Timothy H. McCalmont, MD

NORMAL SKIN

The skin is the most accessible organ of the human body. Its most basic function is simply a protective one. As a barrier, the skin holds off desiccation and disease by keeping moisture in and pathogens out. Nevertheless, characterization of the skin as mere "plastic wrap" is a gross underestimation of the anatomic and physiologic complexity of this vital structure.

Unlike parenchymal organs, end-organ dysfunction or failure is not a prerequisite for the diagnosis of a skin disease, because all skin diseases can be observed clinically irrespective of their functional effects. Among the spectacular array of neoplastic, inflammatory, infectious, and genetic cutaneous disorders, some elicit only trivial aberrations in skin structure or function, whereas others lead to profound and morbid consequences.

ANATOMY

The integumentary system consists of a layer of tissue, 1–4 mm thick, that covers all exposed surfaces of the body. The skin merges uninterruptedly with the structurally similar envelope of the mucous membranes, but skin is distinct from mucosa in that it contains adnexal structures such as the eccrine units that exude sweat and the folliculosebaceous apocrine units that produce hairs and oils. There is considerable variation in skin thickness and composition, depending on the requirements of a particular body site. For example, the thinnest skin overlies the eyelids, where delicacy and mobility are essential. The thickest skin is present on the upper trunk, where sturdiness exceeds mobility in importance. The surfaces of the palms and soles are characterized by a high density of eccrine sweat units, reflecting the importance of this region in temperature regulation; an absence of hairs, which would interfere with sensation; and an accentuation of the cornified layer (see later discussion), contributing to the tackiness needed to

handle objects deftly. The size of the structures between sites can also vary greatly, best illustrated by the contrast between the large terminal hair follicles found on the scalp, bearded areas, and genital skin and the small vellus hair follicles found at most other sites.

HISTOLOGY

Using a light microscope, two important skin layers are easily identifiable: a stratified squamous epithelium, the **epidermis**; and a layer of connective tissue, the **dermis**. The subjacent adipose tissue is considered a third layer by some and is referred to as the **subcutis**.

The epidermis consists of keratinocytes arrayed in four distinct substrata: the basal, spinous, granular, and cornified layers (Figure 8–1). Basal keratinocytes include the proliferative pool of keratinocytes. These cells divide, giving rise to progeny that are displaced toward the skin surface. As the keratinocytes move outwardly, they progressively flatten and accumulate keratin filaments within their cytoplasm. Individual keratinocytes are tightly bound together by intracellular junctions called desmosomes (Figure 8–2). The desmosomal junctions appear as delicate "spines" between cells in conventional microscopic sections and are most conspicuous in the epidermal spinous layer (Figure 8–3). Keratin filaments are linked intracellularly and are also attached to the desmosomes, forming a network that is vital to structural integrity.

Melanocytes and Langerhans cells are dendritic cells that are intercalated among the keratinocytes of the epidermis. Melanocytes, which are positioned in the basal layer, synthesize a reddish-brown biochrome, melanin, and dispense it to numerous adjacent keratinocytes through their dendrites (Figure 8–4). This distribution system permits melanin to provide a dispersed screen against the potentially harmful

FIGURE 8–1 Although the epidermis biologically displays a gradient of differentiation, four distinct layers are recognized on the basis of microscopic appearance. Cuboidal germinative keratinocytes serve as a foundation in the basal layer; cells with ample cytoplasm and prominent desmosomes constitute the spinous layer; cells with cytoplasmic granularity resulting from an accumulation of keratin complexes and other structural proteins are found in the granular layer; and anucleate, flattened keratinocytes compose the tough, membrane-like cornified layer. (Redrawn, with permission, from Orkin M et al, eds. *Dermatology*. Originally published by Appleton & Lange. Copyright © 1991 by The McGraw-Hill Companies, Inc.)

ultraviolet rays of the sun. Langerhans cells share a similar arborized morphology but are positioned in the midspinous layer. Langerhans cells are bone marrow–derived antigen-presenting cells (see also Chapter 3).

The epidermal–dermal junction, or basement membrane zone, is a structure that welds the epidermis to the dermis and contributes to the skin barrier. The juncture of the epidermis and dermis is arrayed in an undulating fashion to increase the

A

B

C

FIGURE 8–3 With conventional light microscopy, the numerous desmosomes of the spinous layer appear as delicate attachments ("spines") between individual keratinocytes.

FIGURE 8–2 In an ultrastructural view of a human keratinocyte (**A**), numerous desmosomes (arrows) (**B**) appear as plaques that tightly bind two cell membranes together. With very high magnification (**C**), the attachment of cytoplasmic keratin filaments (**F**) to the desmosomes can be appreciated. (Reproduced, with permission, from Junqueira LC et al. *Basic Histology*, 10th ed. McGraw-Hill, 2003.)

binding surface area between the two structures and to resist shearing forces. The downward projections of the epidermis are referred to as **rete ridges**, and the upward projections of the superficial dermis are called **dermal papillae** (Figure 8–5). Although the basement membrane comprises a thin eosinophilic (pink) band beneath the basal cells in conventional microscopic sections, it has a sophisticated multilayered structure that reaches from the hemidesmosomes of the basal keratinocytes to the collagen bundles of the superficial dermis (Figure 8–6). The lamina densa and lamina lucida are two of

FIGURE 8–4 The human melanocyte displays a branching morphology, and the dendrites of the cell maintain contact with 35–40 adjacent keratinocytes in a multicellular structure termed the epidermal melanin unit. The function of the unit is the effective dispersion of melanin pigment, packaged in organelles known as melanosomes, across a broad surface area. (Redrawn, with permission, from Junqueira LC et al. *Basic Histology*, 10th ed. McGraw-Hill, 2003.)

FIGURE 8–5 The undulating configuration of the epidermal–dermal junction consists of downward extensions of the epidermis, known as rete ridges, and upward extensions of the dermis, known as dermal papillae.

the layers of the basement membrane zone and are so named because of their electron-dense and electron-lucid appearance when viewed ultrastructurally.

The dermis consists of a connective tissue gel composed largely of proteins and mucopolysaccharides (so-called ground substance). This matrix serves as the scaffolding that supports the complex neurovascular networks, which course through the skin, and also supports the eccrine (sweat gland) and follicular (hair) adnexal structures. The vast majority of the fibrous structural proteins of the dermis are composed of collagen types I and III, and a network of elastic microfibrils is also woven throughout the full dermal thickness. Fibrocytes, the synthetic units of the structural proteins, are ubiquitous, and there are also mast cells and dendritic immune cells arrayed throughout the dermis. A discussion of the fine structure of the dermis—the dermal vascular and neural networks and the adnexal structures—is beyond the scope of this chapter.

OVERVIEW OF SKIN DISEASES

In the broadest and simplest sense, there are two types of skin diseases: growths and rashes. A skin growth is a cyst, malformation, or benign or malignant neoplasm, something that usually presents clinically as a bump on the skin. A rash is, with rare exception, a nonneoplastic skin disease; it is more precisely referred to as an inflammatory skin condition or a **dermatitis**. The pathophysiologic aspects of the huge number of described growths and rashes exceed the scope of this chapter. Therefore, our discussion in this chapter will be limited to nine prototypical rashes.

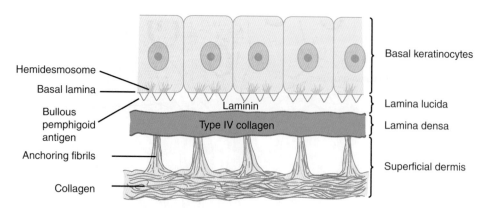

FIGURE 8–6 Schematic diagram of the basement membrane zone of human epidermis. (Redrawn, with permission, from Orkin M et al, eds. *Dermatology*. Originally published by Appleton & Lange. Copyright © 1991 by The McGraw-Hill Companies, Inc.)

TYPES OF SKIN LESIONS

Physicians interested in the skin learned decades ago that the accurate diagnosis and classification of the many patterns of dermatitis depended on a standardized nomenclature for the description and documentation of rashes. When used in association with a few well-chosen adjectives, the terms used to describe the prototypical types of inflammatory skin lesions (so-called primary lesions) permit vivid description of a rash. To illustrate the importance of terminology, imagine trying to describe a patient's condition over the telephone to another physician. Talking about a red, raised rash may truthfully describe the eruption in some sense, but the mental image evoked could be any one of dozens of skin diseases. The only way to accurately characterize an eruption is by the use of precisely defined terms.

The most important types of primary lesions include macules and patches, papules and plaques, vesicles and bullae, pustules, and nodules. The terms **macule** and **patch** denote flat areas of discoloration without any discernible change in texture. Macules are 1 cm or less in diameter, whereas patches exceed 1 cm in size. **Papules** and **plaques** are elevated, palpable skin lesions in which the breadth of the lesion exceeds its thickness. A papule is small, 1 cm or less in diameter, whereas a plaque exceeds 1 cm in size. **Vesicles** and **bullae** are fluid-filled spaces within the skin. Vesicles are less than 1 cm in diameter, whereas bullae exceed 1 cm in size. A vesicle or bulla containing purulent fluid is known as a **pustule**. A **nodule** is a solid, rounded skin lesion in which diameter and thickness are roughly equal.

TYPES OF INFLAMMATORY SKIN DISEASES

Different inflammatory processes involve different structures within the skin and display different microscopic patterns. Experience has shown that pattern analysis can serve as a useful means of diagnosis and classification. Pattern analysis depends on accurate recognition of the distribution of inflammation within the skin as well as recognition of the specific structures affected by the inflammatory reaction. There are nine distinct patterns of dermatitis (Table 8–1; Figure 8–7). All nine of these patterns and some of the diseases that produce them are discussed in detail next.

CHECKPOINT

1. What are the two most basic barrier functions of skin?
2. How is skin distinct from mucosa? Why are these terms important?
3. What are the main primary lesions? Why are these terms important?
4. What are the main patterns of inflammatory skin disease?
5. What is the value of knowing the microscopic pattern of inflammation of a skin lesion? What additional information is needed for this information to be most useful?

PATHOPHYSIOLOGY OF SELECTED SKIN DISEASES

PATTERN: PSORIASIFORM DERMATITIS

Example: Psoriasis

Overview

Psoriasis is a common chronic, persistent or relapsing, scaling skin condition. Individual lesions are distinctive in their classic form: sharply marginated and erythematous and surmounted by silvery scales (Figure 8–8). Most patients with psoriasis have a limited number of fixed plaques, but there is great variation in clinical presentation.

Epidemiology and Etiology

Psoriasis affects between 1% and 2% of individuals of both sexes in most ethnic groups. The most common age at onset is the third decade, but psoriasis can develop soon after

TABLE 8–1   Patterns of inflammatory skin disease.

Pattern	Description	Prototypes
Psoriasiform dermatitis	Inflammatory infiltrate associated with epidermal thickening as a result of elongation of rete ridges	Psoriasis
Interface dermatitis	Cytotoxic inflammatory reaction with prominent changes in the lower epidermis, characterized by vacuolization of keratinocytes	Erythema multiforme Lichen planus
Vesiculobullous dermatitis	Inflammatory reaction associated with intraepidermal or subepidermal cleavage	Bullous pemphigoid
Vasculitis	Inflammatory reaction focused on the walls of cutaneous vessels	Leukocytoclastic vasculitis
Spongiotic dermatitis	Inflammatory infiltrate associated with intercellular epidermal edema (spongiosis)	Allergic contact dermatitis (poison oak dermatitis)
Panniculitis	Inflammatory reaction involving the subcutaneous fat	Erythema nodosum
Nodular dermatitis	Inflammatory reaction with a nodular or diffuse dermal infiltrate in the absence of significant epidermal changes	Cutaneous sarcoidosis
Folliculitis	Inflammatory reaction directed against folliculosebaceous units	Acne folliculitis
Perivascular dermatitis	Perivascular inflammatory infiltrate without significant involvement of the epidermis	Urticaria (hives)

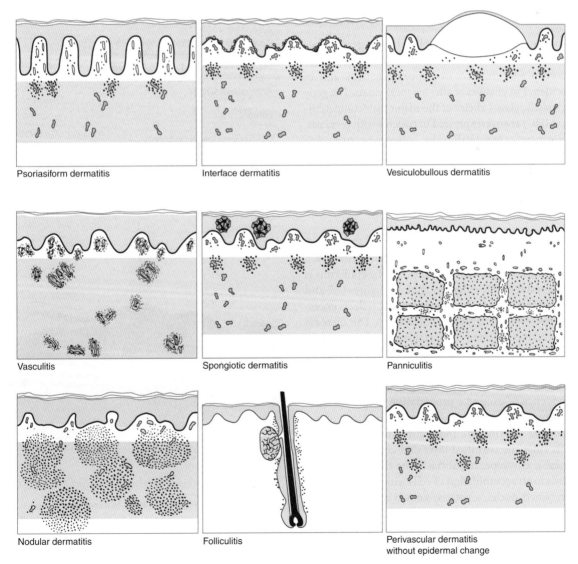

Psoriasiform dermatitis

Interface dermatitis

Vesiculobullous dermatitis

Vasculitis

Spongiotic dermatitis

Panniculitis

Nodular dermatitis

Folliculitis

Perivascular dermatitis without epidermal change

FIGURE 8–7 Nine patterns of inflammatory skin disease. (See also Table 8–1.)

FIGURE 8–8 Classic plaque-type psoriasis (psoriasis vulgaris) consisting of sharply marginated, scaling plaques. (Image used with permission from Dr. Timothy Berger.)

birth, and psoriasis of new onset has been documented in a centenarian.

Several lines of evidence have established that genetic factors contribute to the development of psoriasis. There is a high rate of concordance for psoriasis in monozygotic twins and an increased incidence in relatives of affected individuals. The gene products of specific class I alleles of the major histocompatibility complex (MHC) are overexpressed in patients with psoriasis. Psoriasis is not merely a genetic disorder, however, because some susceptible individuals never develop characteristic lesions. In other predisposed individuals, a number of environmental factors, including infection, physical injury, stress, and drugs, can serve as triggers for the development of psoriasis (Table 8–2).

Histopathology and Pathogenesis

Psoriasis is the prototypical form of psoriasiform dermatitis, a pattern of inflammatory skin disease in which the epidermis is thickened as a result of rete ridge elongation (Figures 8–7 and 8–9). In psoriatic lesions, epidermal thickening reflects excessive epidermopoiesis (epidermal proliferation). The increase in epidermopoiesis is reflected in shortening of the duration of the keratinocyte cell cycle and doubling of the proliferative cell population. Because of these alterations, lesional skin contains up to 30 times as many keratinocytes per unit area as normal skin. Evidence of excessive proliferation is also manifest microscopically as numerous intraepidermal mitotic figures.

During normal keratinocyte maturation, nuclei are eliminated as cells enter the cornified layer and condense to form a semipermeable envelope. In psoriasis, the truncation of the cell cycle leads to an accumulation of cells within the cornified layer with retained nuclei, a pattern known as parakeratosis. As parakeratotic cells accumulate, neutrophils migrate to the cornified layer. Histopathologically, the silvery scale of psoriatic plaques consists of a thick layer of parakeratotic keratinocytes with numerous intercalated neutrophils. At times, the

TABLE 8–2   Factors that induce or exacerbate psoriasis.

Physical Factors
Trauma (so-called Koebner phenomenon)
Abrasions
Contusions
Lacerations
Burns
Sunburn[1]
Bites
Surgical incisions
Cold weather
Infections
Viral bronchitis
Streptococcal pharyngitis
Human immunodeficiency virus (HIV) infection
Medications or Medication Related
Antimalarial agents
Lithium
β-Adrenergic blocking agents
Corticosteroid withdrawal

[1]Ultraviolet (UV) light in modest doses inhibits psoriasis and has been used as effective therapy for decades. UV light exacerbates psoriasis only when presented in toxic doses (sunburn).

FIGURE 8–9 Histopathologic features of psoriasis at low magnification. The rete ridges are strikingly and evenly elongated, and the overlying cornified layer contains cells with retained nuclei (parakeratosis), a pattern that reflects the increased epidermal turnover.

FIGURE 8–10 In a psoriatic plaque at high magnification, dilated capillaries are evident in an edematous portion of the superficial dermis.

number of neutrophils in the stratum corneum is so great that lesions assume a pustular appearance.

Psoriasis also induces endothelial cell hyperproliferation, which yields pronounced dilation, tortuosity, and increased capillary permeability in the superficial dermis (Figure 8–10). The vascular alterations contribute to the bright erythema seen clinically. The capillary changes are most pronounced at the advancing margins of psoriatic plaques.

After years of research, a large number of immunologic abnormalities that involve both innate and adaptive immunity have been documented in psoriatic skin. Antigenic stimuli are thought to activate the innate immune response, leading to the production of cytokines, such as interferon, tumor necrosis factor (TNF), interleukin-23 (IL-23), and IL-12, by macrophages, dendritic cells, and neutrophils. This leads to attraction, activation, and differentiation of T cells. These T cells, most importantly T-helper 1 and T-helper 17 cells, produce cytokines that lead to epidermal hyperplasia, recruitment of inflammatory cells, and ultimately a positive feedback loop that perpetuates the pathologic process. Recent studies suggest that microRNAs probably play a role in the pathogenesis of psoriasis as well.

Clinical Manifestations

The cardinal features of psoriasis plaques include sharp margination, bright erythema, and nonconfluent, whitish or silvery scales. Lesions can occur at any site, but the scalp, the extensor surfaces of the extremities, and the flexural surfaces are often involved. Psoriasis commonly affects the nail bed and matrix, yielding pitted or markedly thickened dystrophic nails. Mucosal surfaces are often spared, although the tongue can sometimes be involved (referred to as geographic tongue).

The only extracutaneous manifestation of psoriasis is psoriatic arthritis, a deforming, asymmetric, oligoarticular arthritis that can involve small or large joints. The distal interphalangeal joints of the fingers and toes are characteristically involved. Psoriatic arthritis is classified as one of the seronegative spondyloarthropathies, distinguishable from rheumatoid arthritis by a lack of circulating autoantibodies (so-called rheumatoid factors) or circulating immune complexes and by linkage with specific MHC class I alleles, including HLA-B27.

There are many variants of psoriasis, all of which are histopathologically similar but which differ greatly in clinical distribution (Table 8–3).

CHECKPOINT

6. What evidence supports a genetic role in the development of psoriasis? An environmental role?
7. Which cell types hyperproliferate in psoriasis?
8. What immunologic defects have been identified in psoriasis?

TABLE 8–3   Variants of psoriasis.

Variant	Cutaneous Findings and Distribution	Other Features
Plaque-type psoriasis (psoriasis vulgaris)	Large stationary plaques with prominent scales, commonly involving the scalp and the extensor surfaces of the extremities	
Guttate psoriasis	Scaling papules or small plaques, usually 0.5–1.5 cm in diameter, scattered on the trunk and proximal extremities	Lesions often induced or exacerbated by streptococcal pharyngitis
Erythrodermic psoriasis	Generalized erythematous plaques involving the face, trunk, and extremities, with only slight scaling	
Pustular psoriasis, generalized	Generalized eruption of sterile pustules involving erythematous skin of the trunk and extremities, often with sparing of the face	Associated with fever; may occur in pregnancy
Pustular psoriasis, localized	Scaling erythematous plaques, studded with pustules, involving the palms, soles, and nails	
Inverse psoriasis	Slightly scaling, erythematous plaques involving the axillary and inguinal regions, with sparing of areas usually involved in plaque-type disease	

PATTERN: INTERFACE DERMATITIS

Example: Lichen Planus

Overview

Lichen planus is a distinctive pruritic eruption that usually presents with numerous small papules. Individual lesions have angulated borders, flat tops, and a violaceous hue, attributes that form the basis of their alliterative description as pruritic, polygonal, purple papules (Figure 8–11). The individual papules of lichen planus sometimes coalesce to form larger plaques. Minute whitish streaks, barely visible to the naked eye and known as Wickham striae, are often found on the surfaces of lesions.

Epidemiology and Etiology

Lichen planus generally develops in adulthood and affects women slightly more commonly than men. Although the factors that trigger lichen planus remain obscure in many patients, it is clear that the rash represents a cell-mediated immune reaction that directly or indirectly damages basal keratinocytes of the epidermis. Observations that suggest a cell-mediated mechanism include the occurrence of lichen planus–like eruptions as a manifestation of graft-versus-host disease after bone marrow transplantation and the development of a lichen

FIGURE 8–11 Pruritic, polygonal, flat-topped papules of lichen planus.

TABLE 8–4   Medications that induce lichenoid (lichen planus–like) reactions.

Therapeutic gold
Antimalarial agents
Quinacrine
Quinidine
Quinine
Chloroquine
Penicillamine
Thiazide diuretics
β-Blocking agents
Antibiotics
Tetracycline
Streptomycin
Dapsone
Isoniazid
Anticonvulsants
Carbamazepine
Phenytoin
Nonsteroidal anti-inflammatory drugs

planus–like eruption in mice after injection of sensitized, autoreactive T cells. Although most lichen planus is idiopathic, drugs are one established cause of lichen planus or lichen planus–like reactions. Therapeutic gold and antimalarial agents are the medications most closely linked to the development of lichenoid eruptions, but a long list of other agents has accumulated (Table 8–4).

Histopathology and Pathogenesis

Lichen planus is a form of lichenoid interface dermatitis, a type of inflammatory skin disease in which a dense infiltrate of lymphocytes occupies the perijunctional dermis immediately subjacent to the epidermis, in association with vacuolization of the lower epidermis (Figure 8–12). The dermal infiltrate is composed largely, if not entirely, of T lymphocytes. Some of the T cells are also found within the epidermis, where adjacent vacuolated, injured keratinocytes are found. Dense eosinophilic (pink) globules, known as **colloid bodies**, are also identifiable within the epidermis and the infiltrate (Figure 8–13). Colloid bodies are condensed, anucleate keratinocytes that have succumbed to the inflammatory reaction. Although the keratinocytes bear the brunt of the lymphocyte attack, melanocytes may be coincidentally destroyed in the reaction as "innocent bystanders." Free melanin

FIGURE 8–12 Histopathologic features of lichen planus at low magnification. There is a bandlike infiltrate of lymphocytes that impinges on the epidermal–dermal junction, and some keratinocytes adjacent to the infiltrate show cytoplasmic vacuolization.

pigment is released as melanocytes are damaged, and the pigment is phagocytosed by dermal macrophages known as melanophages.

In incipient lesions of lichen planus, CD4 helper T lymphocytes predominate, and some of the cells have been found in proximity to macrophages and Langerhans cells (see also Chapter 3). In contrast, CD8 cytotoxic T cells comprise the bulk of the infiltrate in mature lesions. This shift in infiltrating T-cell composition is thought to reflect the afferent and efferent aspects of lesional development. In the afferent phase, causative antigens are processed and presented to helper T cells, probably in the context of specific HLA determinants. The stimulated CD4 lymphocytes then elaborate specific cytokines that lead to the recruitment of cytotoxic lymphocytes.

FIGURE 8–13 Necrotic keratinocytes (so-called colloid bodies) in a lesion of lichen planus appear as rounded and eosinophilic globules along the epidermal–dermal junction (arrows).

Cell-mediated cytotoxicity and cytokines such as interferon-γ and TNF are then thought to contribute to the vacuolization and necrosis of keratinocytes as a secondary event. Emerging data reveal that microRNAs may also play a role in the pathogenesis of the oral form of lichen planus.

The clinical appearance of lichen planus lesions reflects several synchronous alterations in the skin. The dense array of lymphocytes in the superficial dermis yields the elevated, flat-topped appearance of each papule or plaque. The chronic inflammatory reaction induces accentuation of the cornified layer (hyperkeratosis) of the epidermis, which contributes to the superficial whitish coloration perceived as Wickham striae. Although the many melanophages that accumulate in the papillary dermis hold a brownish-black pigment, the fact that the pigmented cells are embedded in a colloidal matrix such as the skin permits extensive scattering of light, a phenomenon known as the Tyndall effect. Thus, the human eye interprets a lesion of lichen planus as dusky or violaceous despite the fact that the pigment that serves as the basis for the coloration is melanin.

Clinical Manifestations

Lichen planus affects both skin and mucous membranes. Papules are generally distributed bilaterally and symmetrically. The sites most commonly involved include the flexor surfaces of the extremities, the genital skin, and the mucous membranes. Rarely, lichen planus may involve the mucosa of internal organs, such as the esophagus. Cutaneous lesions are virtually never seen on the palms, soles, or face.

In general, lichen planus variants can be grouped into three categories.

A. Lichen Planus Papules Arrayed in an Unusual Configuration—In these variants, typical individual papules of lichen planus are grouped in a distinctive larger pattern. In annular lichen planus, small lichenoid papules coalesce to form a larger ring. Linear and zosteriform patterns of lichen planus have also been observed. When lichen planus presents in an unusual configuration, it is prone to being underdiagnosed or misdiagnosed.

B. Lichen Planus Papules Arrayed at Distinctive Sites—Although most lichen planus is widespread, at times papules are restricted to a specific body site, such as the mouth (oral lichen planus) or genitalia. Nearly 25% of all lichen planus patients have disease limited to the mucous membranes.

C. Lichen Planus Papules with Unusual Clinical Morphology—Some examples of lichen planus defy clinical recognition because the appearance of the individual lesions is atypical. Erosive, vesiculobullous, atrophic, and hypertrophic lesions can be seen. In **erosive lichen planus**, the interface reaction directed against the epidermis is so profound that the entire epidermis becomes necrotic and ulceration ensues. The closely related entity **vesiculobullous lichen planus** is also characterized by an intense interface reaction that yields necrosis of the epidermal junctional zone across a broad front. As a result of basal layer necrosis, the epidermis becomes detached from its dermal attachments and a blister develops. In **atrophic lichen planus**, the rate of destruction of keratinocytes by the lichenoid interface reaction exceeds the rate of epidermal regeneration, and the epidermis becomes attenuated as a result. In contrast, in **hypertrophic lichen planus**, the rate of epidermal regeneration triggered by the interface reaction exceeds the rate of destruction, and thick, verrucous, hyperkeratotic lesions develop. All of these variants are histopathologically similar with the exception of the foci of ulceration seen in erosive lichen planus.

CHECKPOINT

9. Which skin cells are damaged by cell-mediated immune reactions in lichen planus?
10. Which drugs have been most commonly implicated in licheniform eruptions?
11. What synchronous alterations in the skin are reflected in the clinical appearance of lichen planus?

Example: Erythema Multiforme

Overview

Erythema multiforme is an acute cutaneous eruption that presents with a wide spectrum of clinical severity. The eruption is commonly brief and self-limited, but repetitive or generalized attacks can be disabling or even life threatening. As the name implies, variation in lesional morphology can be seen, but most patients present with a monomorphous pattern in a given bout. The prototypical lesion is a red macule or thin papule that expands centrifugally and develops a dusky or necrotic center, creating a target-like pattern (Figure 8–14).

Epidemiology and Etiology

Erythema multiforme is an uncommon but distinctive skin disease that afflicts men and women in nearly equal numbers. The peak incidence is in the second to fourth decades of life, and onset during infancy or early childhood is a rarity. Like lichen planus, erythema multiforme represents a cell-mediated immune reaction that eventuates in necrosis of epidermal keratinocytes. Herpes simplex viral infection and reactions to medications have been established as the most common causes of erythema multiforme. Other known causes include *Mycoplasma* infection, contact dermatitis, drugs, and radiation.

Histopathology and Pathogenesis

Erythema multiforme is a prototypical form of vacuolar interface dermatitis. In contrast to lichen planus, which typically presents with a dense, obscuring lichenoid infiltrate within the superficial dermis, in erythema multiforme the inflammatory infiltrate is sparse. Thus, the vacuolated keratinocytes

FIGURE 8–14 Target lesions—a characteristic pattern seen in erythema multiforme—consist of a papule or plaque with a central zone of epidermal necrosis surrounded by a rim of erythema. (Image used with permission from Dr. Timothy Berger.)

that are widely distributed within the epidermal basal layer are conspicuous in the face of a sparse infiltrate, and the damaged keratinocytes serve as the basis for the name of this pattern of inflammatory skin disease.

The dermal infiltrate in erythema multiforme is composed of a mixture of CD4 and CD8 T lymphocytes. CD8 cytotoxic cells are also found within the epidermis, in proximity to vacuolated and necrotic keratinocytes. Keratinocytes killed in the course of the inflammatory reaction become anucleate and are manifest microscopically as round, dense, eosinophilic bodies similar to the colloid bodies of lichen planus (Figure 8–15).

Although lichen planus and erythema multiforme are clinically, microscopically, and etiologically distinct, both appear to share a common pathogenetic pathway in which specific inciting agents recruit effector lymphocytes into the epidermis and papillary dermis. After this recruitment, keratinocytes are injured and killed by the combined negative influences of cytotoxicity and cytokines such as interferon-γ and TNF.

Many cases of so-called erythema multiforme minor are triggered by herpes simplex viral infection. A relationship between erythema multiforme and herpetic infection had long been suspected based on the documentation of preceding herpes simplex lesions in patients with erythema multiforme.

FIGURE 8–15 Histopathologic features of erythema multiforme, a type of vacuolar interface dermatitis. There is a modest infiltrate of lymphocytes in the vicinity of the epidermal–dermal junction where vacuolated and necrotic keratinocytes are conspicuous.

Support for this relationship was strengthened after antiherpetic drug therapy, in the form of oral acyclovir, was shown to suppress the development of erythema multiforme lesions in some individuals. Molecular studies have substantiated the relationship by confirming the presence of herpes simplex DNA within skin from erythema multiforme lesions. Herpesvirus DNA is also demonstrable within peripheral blood lymphocytes and within lesional skin after resolution but not within nonlesional skin. These findings suggest that viral DNA is disseminated from the primary infection in the peripheral blood and becomes integrated into the skin at specific target sites. The herpetic genomic fragments then contribute to the development of a cytotoxic effector response in their chosen target tissue, the skin.

The target-like clinical appearance of many erythema multiforme lesions reflects zonal differences in the intensity of the inflammatory reaction and its deleterious effects. At the periphery of an erythema multiforme lesion, only sparse inflammation, slight edema, and subtle vacuolization of the epidermis are apparent in the outer erythematous halo. In contrast, the dusky "bull's eye" often shows pronounced epidermal vacuolization, with areas of near-complete epidermal necrosis.

Clinical Manifestations

Erythema multiforme is generally limited to the skin and mucous membranes. The lesions develop rapidly in crops and are initially distributed on acral surfaces, although proximal spread to the trunk and face commonly occurs. Mucosal erosions and ulcers are seen in roughly 25% of cases, and mucositis can be the sole presenting feature of the disease. Although erythema multiforme is an epithelial disorder, nonspecific constitutional symptoms such as malaise can also occur.

Although the spectrum of erythema multiforme exists as a continuum, a given patient is usually classified as having minor or major disease. The disorder is referred to as **erythema multiforme minor** when there are scattered lesions confined to the skin or when skin lesions are observed in association with limited mucosal involvement. A diagnosis of **erythema multiforme major** is based on the presence of prominent involvement of at least two of three mucosal sites: oral, anogenital, or conjunctival. Many examples of erythema multiforme major also display severe, widespread cutaneous involvement. Although Stevens–Johnson syndrome had classically been used to describe severe cases of erythema multiforme, consensus classification has separated Stevens–Johnson syndrome from erythema multiforme and added it to the spectrum of toxic epidermal necrolysis. These two entities, Stevens–Johnson syndrome and toxic epidermal necrolysis, are now considered to represent variant dermatologic manifestations of severe idiosyncratic reactions. Most often the result of medications, these entities involve vast regions of skin and mucosal necrosis (Figure 8–16) with secondary vesiculation. Pathologically, the findings are similar to those of a severe burn in that the integrity of a patient's skin fails, resulting in an increased risk of infectious and metabolic sequelae.

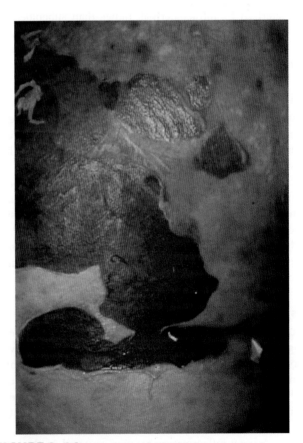

FIGURE 8–16 Toxic epidermal necrolysis. Generalized maculopapular erythema of the trunk and extremities is followed by extensive desquamation, as seen on this patient's trunk, resulting from epidermal necrosis. Patients are often admitted to a burn unit for acute care. (Image used with permission from Dr. Timothy Berger.)

PATTERN: VESICULOBULLOUS DERMATITIS

Example: Bullous Pemphigoid

Overview

Bullous pemphigoid is a blistering disease in which tense, fluid-filled spaces develop within erythematous, inflamed skin. The blisters in bullous pemphigoid develop because of detachment of the epidermis from the dermis (subepidermal vesiculation) as the result of a specific inflammatory reaction directed against structural proteins. The term "pemphigoid" reflects the clinical similarity of bullous pemphigoid to pemphigus vulgaris, another form of blistering skin disease characterized by intraepidermal, rather than subepidermal, vesiculation. The distinction between bullous pemphigoid and pemphigus vulgaris is an important one, because bullous pemphigoid has a more favorable prognosis.

Epidemiology and Etiology

Bullous pemphigoid is generally a disorder of the elderly. There are rare reports of bullous pemphigoid in children and young adults, but the vast majority of patients are older than 60 years. There is no sex predilection.

It has been known for years that immunoglobulins and complement are deposited along the epidermal–dermal junction in bullous pemphigoid. The deposited antibodies are specific for antigens within the basement membrane zone (BP180 and BP230), and bullous pemphigoid thus represents a form of autoimmune skin disease. The specific factors that induce autoantibody production have not been identified.

Histopathology and Pathogenesis

Microscopically, biopsies from fully developed bullous pemphigoid lesions show a subepidermal cleft containing lymphocytes, eosinophils, and neutrophils, as well as eosinophilic (pink) material that represents extravasated macromolecules such as fibrin (Figure 8–17). An inflammatory infiltrate of eosinophils, neutrophils, and lymphocytes is also evident in the dermis beneath the cleft. These findings represent the aftermath of an inflammatory reaction centered on the basement membrane zone.

Insights into this reaction can be obtained from direct immunofluorescence microscopy, in which fluorochrome-labeled anti-immunoglobulin G (IgG), anti-IgA, anti-IgM, and

FIGURE 8–17 Histopathologic features of bullous pemphigoid. There is a subepidermal cleft that contains numerous eosinophils and lymphocytes, and a similar infiltrate is present in the superficial dermis. Ultrastructurally, the separation is within the lamina lucida of the basement membrane zone, at the level of the bullous pemphigoid antigen (see Figure 8–6).

anticomplement antibodies are incubated with lesional skin. Using an ultraviolet microscope to localize the fluorochrome, tagged antibodies specific for IgG and complement component C3 are found in a linear distribution along the epidermal–dermal junction (Figure 8–18). Circulating IgG that binds to the basement membrane zone of human epidermis is also identifiable in bullous pemphigoid patients. These antibodies are capable of complement fixation, and pathogenicity has been confirmed by injection into laboratory animals, in whom the antibodies bind to the junctional zone and induce blisters.

FIGURE 8–18 Direct immunofluorescence findings in lesional skin from a bullous pemphigoid patient. When fluorochrome-stained sections are viewed through an ultraviolet microscope, a bright linear band, signifying deposition of immunoglobulin G, is evident along the epidermal–dermal junction. (Image used with permission from Dr. Kari Connolly.)

The autoantibodies (IgG) in bullous pemphigoid are directed against hemidesmosomal proteins, namely bullous pemphigoid antigen 180 and bullous pemphigoid antigen 230. The binding of these autoantibodies to the basement membrane zone leads to an inflammatory cascade with activation of the classic complement cascade (see Chapter 3). Complement fragments induce mast cell degranulation and attract neutrophils. The presence of eosinophils in the infiltrate of bullous pemphigoid is probably a reflection of mast cell degranulation, because mast cell granules contain eosinophil chemotactic factors. Numerous enzymes are released by granulocytes and mast cells during the reaction, and enzymatic digestion is thought to be the primary mechanism behind the separation of the epidermis from the dermis with formation of tense bullae. It is also possible that the bullous pemphigoid antigen plays a vital structural role that is compromised by autoantibody binding, leading to cleavage. Quantifiable titers of bullous pemphigoid antigen correlate to disease activity.

Clinical Manifestations

Patients with bullous pemphigoid present with large, tense blisters on an erythematous base (Figure 8–19). Lesions are most commonly distributed on the extremities and lower trunk, but blisters can develop at any site. Most patients experience considerable pruritus in association with their blisters, possibly triggered by the many eosinophils in the dermal infiltrate. Mucous membrane lesions develop in up to one-third of patients and are usually clinically innocuous.

Some patients with bullous pemphigoid present with itchy, erythematous plaques, with no blistering for an extended period of time, but blisters eventually develop in most patients. This pattern is known as pre-eruptive or urticarial bullous pemphigoid. Immunofluorescence and histopathologic examination of biopsies from such patients reveals junctional deposition of autoantibodies and complement in association with an eosinophil-rich infiltrate, implying that the inflammatory reaction is identical to that of conventional bullous pemphigoid. The explanation for the delayed blistering seen in these patients is not presently known.

Bullous pemphigoid is a disease of the skin and mucous membranes only, and systemic involvement has never been documented. Some patients with bullous pemphigoid have developed skin lesions synchronously with a diagnosis of malignancy, but careful studies with age-matched controls have not demonstrated an increased incidence of bullous pemphigoid in cancer patients.

FIGURE 8–19 Large tense bullae on erythematous bases are distributed over the lower trunk. (Image used with permission from Dr. Timothy Berger.)

CHECKPOINT

15. How do pemphigus and pemphigoid differ, and why is the distinction important?
16. How does immunoglobulin binding to the bullous pemphigoid antigen cause blistering in lesions of bullous pemphigoid?
17. Is there a connection between bullous pemphigoid and cancer?

PATTERN: VASCULITIS

Example: Leukocytoclastic Vasculitis

Overview

Leukocytoclastic vasculitis is an inflammatory disorder affecting small blood vessels of the skin that typically presents as an eruption of reddish or violaceous papules, a pattern known as **palpable purpura** (Figure 8–20). The lesions develop in crops, and individual papules persist for a few days or weeks and generally less than a month. Although each individual lesion is transient, the duration of the eruption can vary from weeks to months, and in exceptional cases crops can develop over a period of years.

Epidemiology and Etiology

Leukocytoclastic vasculitis can develop at any age, and the incidence is equal in both sexes. The most common precipitants include infections and medications. Bacterial, mycobacterial, and viral infections can all trigger bouts, but poststreptococcal and poststaphylococcal eruptions are most common.

FIGURE 8–20 Purpuric papules are scattered on the lower extremity in leukocytoclastic vasculitis. (Image used with permission from Dr. Timothy Berger.)

FIGURE 8–21 Direct immunofluorescence microscopy localizes complement component C3 within the walls of small cutaneous vessels. The complement fragments are present after activation of the complement cascade by immune complexes. Immunoglobulin deposition within vessel walls is detectable by the same method. (Image used with permission from Dr. Kari Connolly.)

A wide variety of drugs have been established as leukocytoclastic vasculitis elicitors, including antibiotics, thiazide diuretics, and nonsteroidal anti-inflammatory agents. Among antibiotics, penicillin derivatives are the foremost offenders.

Histopathology and Pathogenesis

The name of this disorder conveys its chief pathological attributes, namely an inflammatory reaction involving blood vessels in association with an accumulation of necrotic nuclear (leukocytoclastic) debris. The key steps that contribute to this pattern include the accumulation of triggering molecules within the walls of small blood vessels, subsequent stimulation of the complement cascade with the elaboration of chemoattractants, and entry of neutrophils with oxidative enzyme release, eventuating in cellular destruction and nuclear fragmentation. The molecules that trigger leukocytoclastic vasculitis are immune complexes, consisting of antibodies bound to exogenous antigens usually derived from microbial proteins or medications. Circulating immune complexes have been documented by laboratory assays of serum from patients with active leukocytoclastic vasculitis, and the presence of circulating complexes can also be deduced based on the finding of low serum complement levels during exacerbations. The exact factors that lead to preferential deposition of immune complexes within small cutaneous vessels (venules) remain unknown, but the fact that

venules exhibit relatively high permeability in the face of a relatively low flow rate is probably contributory. The deposited complexes are detectable within vessel walls by direct immunofluorescence testing (Figure 8–21).

After becoming trapped in tissue, immune complexes activate the complement cascade, and localized production of chemotactic fragments (such as C5a) and vasoactive molecules ensues (see Chapter 3). Chemoattractants draw neutrophils out of vascular lumens and into vascular walls, where release of neutrophilic enzymes results in destruction of the immune complexes, the neutrophils, and the vessel. Microscopically, this stage is characterized by an infiltrate of neutrophils, neutrophilic nuclear dust, and protein (fibrin) in the vessel wall, a pattern that has historically been called "fibrinoid necrosis" (Figure 8–22). Throughout the inflammatory reaction, the integrity of the channel is progressively compromised. As cellular interstices widen, erythrocytes and fibrin exude through the vessel wall and enter the surrounding dermis.

Leukocytoclastic vasculitis lesions are raised and papular because lesional skin is altered and expanded by an intense vasocentric infiltrate containing numerous neutrophils. The erythematous or purpuric quality of leukocytoclastic vasculitis is attributable to the numerous extravasated erythrocytes that accumulate in the dermis of fully developed lesions. In patients with repetitive or persistent leukocytoclastic vasculitis, extravasated erythrocyte debris is metabolized into hemosiderin, which accumulates within macrophages (siderophages) in the deep dermis. The dermal hemosiderin can contribute to a dusky, violaceous clinical appearance, clinically similar to, but pathologically distinct from, the pigmentary changes seen in lichen planus. After resolution of the eruption, the hyperpigmentation resolves slowly over a period of weeks to months as the hemosiderin is resorbed.

FIGURE 8–22 Histopathologic features of leukocytoclastic vasculitis, a form of small-vessel vasculitis. Neutrophils, neutrophilic nuclear debris, and amorphous protein deposits are present within the expanded wall of a cutaneous venule.

Clinical Manifestations

Lesions of leukocytoclastic vasculitis can develop at any site but are usually distributed on the lower extremities or in dependent areas. Although purpuric lesions comprise the most common clinical pattern, a variety of other morphologic patterns, including vesicopustules, necrotic papules, and ulcers, can develop. These patterns often reflect secondary ischemic changes superimposed on the primary vasculitic papule. Vesicopustules develop after ischemic necrosis of the epidermis results in subepidermal separation or after massive dermal accumulation of neutrophils secondary to immune complex deposition. Necrotic papules, eschars, and ulcers are end-stage lesions that develop after total necrosis of the epidermis and superficial dermis. In essence, these lesions represent vasculitic infarcts.

Leukocytoclastic vasculitis is not merely a dermatitis but often part of a systemic vasculitis involving small vessels. In such cases, the vascular eruption is accompanied by arthralgias, myalgias, and malaise. Arthralgias and myalgias are probably attributable to vasculitic changes in small vessels in joint capsules and soft tissue. Vasculitic involvement of the kidneys, liver, and gastrointestinal tract can also occur. Such involvement of abdominal organ systems often presents clinically as abdominal pain. Laboratory studies are important to evaluate possible renal or hepatic impairment.

CHECKPOINT

18. Why are leukocytoclastic vasculitis lesions papular?
19. What are the most common precipitants of leukocytoclastic vasculitis?
20. When leukocytoclastic vasculitis is part of a systemic vasculitis, what additional symptoms are typically observed?

PATTERN: SPONGIOTIC DERMATITIS

Example: Allergic Contact Dermatitis
Overview

Allergic contact dermatitis is an eruption, usually pruritic, caused by a specific immune-mediated reaction to a substance that has touched the skin. The acute phase is characterized by erythematous papules, vesicles, and bullae confined to the area of primary contact of the "allergen" (Figure 8–23). Often the blisters break down and result in weeping and formation of a yellowish crust.

Epidemiology and Etiology

Reliable data on the incidence of allergic contact dermatitis are impossible to gather because of the vast number of people affected, including those with mild disease who do not come to medical attention. However, the disorder has been estimated to cost millions annually in occupation-related direct medical costs and lost productivity.

The factors that determine which individuals will react to which substances are not known, although HLA types are thought to play a role. Some animal models of allergic contact dermatitis demonstrate autosomal inheritance patterns.

FIGURE 8–23 Allergic contact dermatitis, characterized by confluent, linear, eruptive vesicles with surrounding erythema. (Image used with permission from Dr. Timothy Berger.)

FIGURE 8–24 Allergic contact dermatitis. Intercellular edema has made the "spines" (desmosomes) between keratinocytes visible.

Histopathology and Pathogenesis

As the term "spongiotic dermatitis" implies, spongiosis is the pathologic hallmark of this category of skin disease. The term "spongiosis" refers to edema of the epidermis, which separates keratinocytes from one another. Microscopically, edema makes visible the normally indiscernible "spines," or desmosomes, that interconnect the keratinocytes (Figures 8–7 and 8–24). Spongiosis may be slight and barely perceptible microscopically or so massive that it is evident clinically as a blister. Spongiotic dermatitis is accompanied by a variable amount of perivascular inflammation that may be around the superficial vascular plexus or the superficial and deep vascular plexuses, or perivascular and interstitial in distribution (Figure 8–25). The infiltrate is typically composed of lymphocytes, but

FIGURE 8–25 Histopathologic features of allergic contact dermatitis, a type of acute spongiotic dermatitis. There is a perivascular and interstitial infiltrate of inflammatory cells. The paleness of the papillary dermis is a result of edema.

eosinophils are often concurrently present in significant numbers in spongiotic dermatitis.

The series of events leading to the development of allergic contact dermatitis has been and continues to be intensively studied, because the mechanism of development of contact hypersensitivity in the skin is analogous to the cell-mediated rejection of organs used for transplantation. Delayed-type (type IV) hypersensitivity reactions consist of two phases: induction (sensitization/afferent) and elicitation (efferent). In the induction phase, the allergen that has come into contact with an individual naive to that allergen binds to an endogenous protein and alters it to make it appear foreign. This protein–allergen complex is then intercepted by the immunosurveillance cells of the skin: the Langerhans cells. Langerhans cells are bone marrow–derived dendritic cells that reside in the epidermis and form a network at the interface of the immune system with the environment. They engulf the complex, partially degrade ("process") it, migrate to the lymph nodes, and present antigenic fragments on the cell surface in conjunction with an MHC-II molecule. The Langerhans cells with antigen–MHC-II complexes on the surface contact naive T cells possessing T-cell receptors that specifically recognize the MHC-II–allergen complex. The binding of the T-cell receptors to the MHC-II–allergen complex in the context of important co-stimulatory molecules on the surface of the Langerhans cells stimulates clonal expansion of reactive T cells. This process progresses over a period of days. If the allergen exposure is transient, the first exposure often does not result in a reaction at the exposure site. However, a contingent of "armed and ready" memory T cells is now policing the skin, waiting for the allergen to reappear. The individual is now said to be sensitized.

The elicitation phase begins once the sensitized individual encounters the antigen again. Memory T cells from the prior exposure have been policing the skin constantly. The Langerhans cells again process antigen and migrate to lymph nodes, but presentation and T-cell proliferation also occur at the site of contact with the allergen. Nonspecific T cells in the vicinity are recruited and stimulated by the inflammatory cytokines released by the specifically reactive T cells, and an amplification loop ensues, eventuating in clinically recognizable dermatitis. This complex series of events takes time to develop, resulting in the 24- to 48-hour delay between re-exposure and eruption. Many individuals have experienced this delay in their own experience with poison ivy or poison oak. The onset of these disorders never occurs while the yardwork is being completed or during the hike but always a day or two later.

Delayed-type hypersensitivity serves the organism's need for defense against noxious invaders such as viruses; responding T cells recognize virally infected cells and selectively kill them. The development of contact allergy represents an aberrance of this protective mechanism, and the allergen invokes a somewhat nonselective onslaught of T cells that damage the epidermis and result in spongiotic dermatitis histopathologically and a pruritic erythematous blistering eruption clinically.

Clinical Manifestations

Few skin diseases are as well embedded in the lay lexicon as poison ivy and poison oak, which are among the most common causes of allergic contact dermatitis. Although there are many causes of allergic contact dermatitis, a number of airborne allergens are frequently identifiable in occupational settings. For those who have been unfortunate enough to experience a full-blown case of poison ivy or oak (so-called *Rhus* dermatitis, after the genus of plant involved), the salient features of the eruption are well known, manifesting as an extremely pruritic erythematous eruption on areas of skin exposed directly to the allergenic plant leaves. The eruption consists of erythematous papules, papulovesicles, vesicles, or bullae, often in a linear pattern where the offending leaf was drawn across the skin. Linear streaks, although characteristic, are not always noted because the eruption will assume the pattern of the exposure: a hand covered in allergen that then touches the face may result in a rash in a nonlinear configuration.

A common misconception regarding *Rhus* dermatitis is that blister fluid from broken blisters (or even touching the blistered area) causes the eruption to spread. In fact, once the eruption has developed, the allergen has been irreversibly bound to other proteins or has been so degraded that it cannot be transferred to other sites. Apparent spread of the eruption to other sites can be accounted for by several possible scenarios. First, the *Rhus* allergen is tremendously stable and can persist on unwashed clothing and remain capable of inducing allergic contact dermatitis for up to 1 year. Inadvertent contact with contaminated clothes or other surfaces may induce new areas of dermatitis often thought to represent spread and not additional contact. (Washing the skin with soap and water soon after contact with the offending sap will usually abort development of the eruption.) Second, intense allergic contact dermatitis can induce an eruption on skin that was never contacted by allergen. This poorly understood phenomenon is termed "autosensitization." The autosensitization eruption consists of erythematous papules or papulovesicles that are often confined to the hands and feet but may be generalized. The pattern of individual lesions is not linear or geometric, as it is at the original site of allergic contact dermatitis.

Importantly, *Rhus* is but one cause of allergic contact dermatitis. The list of known antigens numbers in the thousands, and there are countless ways for these substances to come into contact with the skin. Often an unnatural geometric pattern of an eruption is the clue to an "outside-in" disease, caused by a contactant. Importantly, a contact eruption does not develop immediately on contact but only after a delay of 24–48 hours. This sometimes makes identification of the offending agent difficult, as the connection between exposure and eruption is obscured by the time delay. Patch testing is a useful clinical technique for helping to pinpoint a possible cause when an unknown contactant is suspected as the origin of a persistent or recurrent eruption. In patch testing, a panel of small amounts of standardized antigens are applied in an array to unaffected skin (typically on the back) and left in place for 48 hours. The patches are then removed and the skin is inspected for development of erythema or vesiculation; wherever a reaction is present, the substance that induced the reaction is noted. Readings are performed again at 96 hours to detect long-delayed reactions. To be useful clinically, positive patch test reactions must be correlated with the pattern of the original eruption and the overall clinical context.

CHECKPOINT

21. What is spongiosis?
22. What are the two phases of development of allergic contact dermatitis? What steps are involved in each?
23. What is the role of patch testing in patients with suspected allergic contact dermatitis?

PATTERN: PANNICULITIS

Example: Erythema Nodosum

Overview

Panniculitis is an inflammatory process that occurs in the fat of the subcutis. Erythema nodosum is the most common form of panniculitis, presenting most often with tender red nodules on the anterior lower legs (Figure 8–26). The number of

FIGURE 8–26 Erythema nodosum on the lower legs of a woman. The lesions are firm, painful, red or red-brown plaques and nodules. Lesion borders are indistinct. (Image used with permission from Dr. Timothy Berger.)

lesions is variable, but typically a dozen or more lesions may be present at onset.

Because the infiltrate in panniculitis occurs deeply in the skin, demarcation of individual lesions is often indistinct. Fever and constitutional symptoms—in particular arthralgias—may accompany the onset of erythema nodosum. The duration of the eruption is typically a few weeks to a few months.

Epidemiology and Etiology

Erythema nodosum is a common condition, although precise data regarding its prevalence are not available. Women seem especially susceptible to its development, and there is an adult female/male predominance of 3:1. This is not true in childhood cases, in which boys and girls are equally affected. Erythema nodosum represents a final common pathway of inflammation that may develop in response to any one of a number of general causes, including infection, medication, hormones (including pregnancy), and inflammatory disease. Streptococcal pharyngitis, sulfonamide-containing drugs, estrogen-containing oral contraceptives, and inflammatory bowel disease are well-known inducers of the disorder.

Histopathology and Pathogenesis

Panniculitis can be separated into two broad categories based on the distribution of inflammation: mostly lobular panniculitis and mostly septal panniculitis (see Figure 8-7). The septa are the fibrous divisions between fat compartments and contain the neurovascular bundles. The lobules are the conglomerations of adipocytes demarcated by septa. The modifier "mostly" is meant to convey that the inflammatory process is not strictly confined to a single compartment but, in fact, will frequently spill over from one to the other. An important step in making a specific histopathologic diagnosis is deciding where the majority of the inflammatory response is located.

In the case of erythema nodosum, the inflammatory response occurs in the septal compartment and consists of lymphocytes, histiocytes, and granulocytes (neutrophils and eosinophils) (Figure 8-27). Multinucleated histiocytes within the septa are a finding of considerable diagnostic value (Figure 8-28). The septa are thickened and may become fibrotic depending on the density of the infiltrate and the duration of the reaction. Even though the infiltrate is largely confined to subcutaneous septa, there is commonly an element of fat necrosis at the edges of the subcutaneous lobules in erythema nodosum. Evidence of fat necrosis may be seen in the form of an infiltrate of foamy (lipid-laden) macrophages at the periphery of subcutaneous lobules or in the form of small stellate clefts within multinucleate macrophages, indicating an element of lipomembranous fat necrosis.

The favored hypothesis regarding the mechanism of development of erythema nodosum is that of a delayed-type hypersensitivity reaction occurring in the septal fat. Immune complex deposition has not been found in the lesions. It is not yet known why systemic hypersensitivity is localized to the fat in such a microscopically distinctive fashion.

FIGURE 8-27 Histopathologic features of erythema nodosum, a form of septal panniculitis. The septa are thickened and inflamed. There is little inflammation of the fat lobules.

Clinical Manifestations

As mentioned, erythema nodosum presents as tender, deep-seated, red to red-brown nodules. As the lesions age, they evolve to more "bruise-like" patches or thin plaques. Erythema nodosum tends to occur on the anterior shins but may involve the thighs, the extensor forearms, and, rarely, the trunk. Because the lesions represent a hypersensitivity response to some inciting stimulus, they may persist or continue to develop in crops for as long as the stimulus is present. In the case of streptococci-associated erythema nodosum, the lesions will probably resolve within a few weeks after successful antibiotic treatment of the primary infection. A prolonged course of erythema nodosum should prompt a search for persistent infection and possible other causes. Erythema

FIGURE 8-28 Erythema nodosum. There are multiple large multinucleated giant cells in this septum. Note the prominent fibrous background with increased cellularity.

nodosum may also be the presenting sign of sarcoidosis (see the following discussion).

PATTERN: NODULAR DERMATITIS

Example: Cutaneous Sarcoidosis

Overview

Sarcoidosis is an enigmatic systemic disease with a hugely variable clinical spectrum ranging from mild asymptomatic skin papules to life-threatening lung disease. Lesions are often red-brown dermal papules or nodules that may occur anywhere on the cutaneous surface but have a special predilection for the face (Figure 8–29). Similar nodular granulomas can occur in the pulmonary tree and other viscera.

Epidemiology and Etiology

Sarcoidosis can affect patients of any age or ethnic background but does occur more frequently in young adults and, in the United States, is more common in people of black African descent. Among this population, estimates of disease incidence range from 35.5 to 64 cases per 100,000 compared with 10–14 cases per 100,000 in whites. In Europe, Irish and Scandinavian populations are at increased risk.

Numerous causes of sarcoidosis have been proposed, including infectious agents. Among these, *Mycobacterium* species (especially *M tuberculosis*) have been favored suspects, although investigation has yielded contradictory results. Other proposed etiologic agents include *Histoplasma*, viruses, and minute systematized foreign particles (which may incite a reactive process in susceptible individuals), although no solid evidence supporting these suspected causes exists. One report found polarizable foreign material in diseased skin of patients with sarcoidosis, but the authors emphasized that this finding probably reflects the propensity of sarcoidal lesions to develop around a nidus of foreign material in affected patients and does not imply that sarcoidosis is directly caused by foreign detritus. The extent to which genetic heritage determines the susceptibility of an individual to sarcoidosis is unclear, although a higher than expected incidence of sarcoidosis among siblings of affected patients suggests a genetic role. Although both HLA and non-HLA genes (such as the TNF gene) have been implicated in sarcoidosis, alterations in these genes and their interaction with environmental factors continue to be areas of investigation.

Histopathology and Pathogenesis

Sarcoidosis is manifest microscopically as collections of tissue macrophages (ie, histiocytes), known as granulomas, situated within the dermis (Figures 8–30 and 8–31). Unlike the tuberculoid granulomas of tuberculosis, sarcoidal granulomas are noncaseating and do not show central coagulation necrosis. Multinucleated histiocytes formed by the fusion of individual cells are a common finding (Figure 8–32). The characteristic microscopic appearance of sarcoidal granulomas is of small numbers of lymphocytes around the granulomas ("naked granulomas"). This appearance contrasts with the dense

FIGURE 8–29 Reddish-brown papule near the nose, typical of sarcoidosis. (Image used with permission from Dr. Timothy Berger.)

FIGURE 8–30 Histopathologic features of sarcoidosis, a nodular dermatitis. Note the nodular collections of histiocytes scattered throughout the dermis.

FIGURE 8–31 Sarcoidosis. Pale-staining histiocytes form nodular aggregates among the collagen of the dermis.

lymphocytic infiltrate that blankets the granulomas in many other granulomatous disorders, including tuberculosis. Sarcoidal granulomas can occupy almost the entire dermis in affected skin or may occur only in relatively small foci that are widely spaced. Histochemical stains for infectious organisms are generally negative.

Just as the cause of sarcoidosis remains unknown, the mechanisms of granuloma formation in sarcoidosis are not completely understood. In general, certain antigenic stimuli elicit a T-cell reaction (see prior discussion regarding the pathogenesis of allergic contact dermatitis). Antigens presented in the proper context induce the responding T cells to release various cytokines. The specific cytokines **monocyte chemotactic factor** and **migration inhibitory factor**, along with a host of others, recruit macrophages to the site and direct the cells to remain there. Even though lymphocytes are a small

FIGURE 8–32 Sarcoidosis. Multinucleated giant cells such as the one seen here in the center of the field are common in sarcoidal granulomas.

component of sarcoidal granulomas microscopically, they are believed to be crucial to the pathogenesis of the disease.

Studies of the organization of sarcoidal granulomas suggest a pattern of lymphocyte arrangement similar to that of tuberculoid leprosy, a condition in which a potent immune response keeps the *M leprae* organisms in relative check. In these conditions, the lymphocytes present within the centers of the granulomas are CD4 positive, whereas CD8-positive cells are arranged at the periphery. This structure may allow the CD4 helper cells to direct the immune response to center around an offending antigen while the CD8 suppressor cells limit the extent of the response. Granulomas are not organized in this fashion in lepromatous leprosy, and the lack of an effective suppressive reaction permits uncontrolled proliferation of *M leprae* bacilli.

Clinical Manifestations

The clinical picture in sarcoidosis is quite broad. The spectrum of symptoms in an individual patient depends on which tissues are involved and to what extent. There are several prototypical presentations. One consists of bilateral pulmonary hilar lymphadenopathy (resulting from sarcoidal granulomas in perihilar lymph nodes) and acute erythema nodosum, a combination known as Löfgren syndrome. Fever, arthralgias, uveitis, and lung parenchymal involvement are common in Löfgren syndrome. Another variant of sarcoidosis involves the nose, with beadlike papules at the rims of the nares (see Figure 8–29). This presentation is known as lupus pernio, a term of some antiquity that still enjoys widespread use in dermatology. More recently, the designation "nasal rim sarcoidosis" has been proposed for this variant. This cutaneous finding usually indicates significant involvement of the tracheobronchial tree or lung parenchyma.

Skin disease occurs in systemic sarcoidosis in only one-third of cases, although about 80% of patients with sarcoidosis of the skin have concurrent systemic disease. The lungs are commonly involved, and the possibility of lung involvement should always be investigated in any case of sarcoidosis. Cutaneous sarcoidosis has been termed "the great imitator," as the clinical morphology can be variable, including skin-colored to red-brown papules, plaques, and nodules; hair loss (alopecia) on the scalp or other sites; pigmentary alteration; ulcers; and numerous other patterns. New dermal papules or nodules arising within tattoos that have been present even for many years are a well-recognized phenomenon in sarcoidosis. This should not be surprising because tattoo pigment is a foreign body that is phagocytosed by tissue macrophages and probably serves as a nidus for the development of sarcoidosis lesions. New dermal papules have also been described in association with scars.

Diagnosing sarcoidosis may be difficult. It is often a diagnosis of exclusion. Only when the clinical spectrum is consistent with sarcoidosis and standard investigations have failed to uncover a clear origin (infectious or otherwise) can a diagnosis of sarcoidosis be issued with confidence. Helpful studies include chest x-ray and bone radiographs with findings suggestive of sarcoidosis or a biopsy of skin or other involved tissue showing the noncaseating granulomas characteristic of the disease.

PATTERN: FOLLICULITIS & PERIFOLLICULITIS

Example: Acne

Overview

Acne most commonly presents as follicle-based comedones, inflammatory papules, or pustules on the face, neck, chest, and back (Figure 8–33). Teenagers are stereotypically afflicted, but neonatal acne and adult acne are also common. Disfiguring nodulocystic acne with resulting severe scarring does not occur before puberty.

Epidemiology

Acne vulgaris is so common that it is said by some authors to affect practically everyone at some point in their lives. The peak incidence is at 18 years of age, although adults can also have acne. There are studies showing that 3% of men and 5% of women have acne between 40 and 49 years of age.

Histopathology and Pathogenesis

Histopathologically, comedonal acne is manifest as a widened follicle with a dense keratin plug within its infundibulum. If the follicular orifice is patulous, the acne lesion is said to be an open comedone. If the orifice is normal and the follicle is expanded below the skin surface, the lesion is termed a closed comedone. Secondary inflammatory changes occur commonly within plugged follicular units. Neutrophils may accompany the keratinous plug within the follicular canal, creating a pustular lesion. Inflammatory acne lesions are a consequence of follicles that have ruptured with resultant spillage of keratinous debris into the perifollicular dermis, evoking a dense inflammatory reaction with a mixture of neutrophils, lymphocytes, and histiocytes (Figure 8–34).

An understanding of the evolution of acne lesions has led to therapies that are effective for the vast majority of cases. There are four essential components to the development of acne lesions: (1) plugging of the folliculosebaceous unit; (2) sebum production; (3) overgrowth of the bacterium *Propionibacterium acnes* within the plugged follicle; and (4) a secondary inflammatory response. The formation of keratin plugs within follicles is a complex process thought to be genetically controlled on a cellular level. Keratinocytes become sticky and fail to slough appropriately, yielding follicular plugging. Contrary

FIGURE 8–33 Acne vulgaris. There are numerous inflamed pustules and papules with central black plugs termed open comedones or "blackheads." (Image used with permission from Dr. Timothy Berger.)

FIGURE 8–34 Histopathologic features of acne. There is a follicle with a central keratin plug. Surrounding the follicle, there is lymphocytic inflammatory infiltrate. This lesion would correspond to an erythematous papule seen in inflammatory acne (see Figure 8–33).

to a commonly held belief, being "dirty" does not cause acne, and vigorous or frequent cleansing does not improve the condition. However, some exogenous substances such as oily cosmetics or petrolatum-based hair care products may promote comedone formation and thus exacerbate acne.

Plugged follicles alone would never become more than comedones, however, if it were not for sebum production and *P acnes* overgrowth. *P acnes* is a commensal organism of the skin. However, with ample sebum as a food source within the well-protected environment of a plugged follicle, *P acnes* overgrowth occurs. The sebum is broken down to constituent lipids and free fatty acids. The failure of keratinous debris and sebum to exit the follicle freely expands the follicular canal. The bacteria release factors chemotactic for neutrophils, and their infiltration of the follicle results in pustule formation. Neutrophilic enzymes weaken the follicle wall and follicular rupture occurs, releasing large amounts of inflammatory reactants into the dermis. Lymphocytes, macrophages, and more neutrophils respond, and the comedonal lesion is transformed into an inflamed papule, pustule, or nodule of acne. Follicular rupture and an intense secondary inflammatory reaction may eventuate with profound scarring in some hosts.

Clinical Manifestations

The spectrum of acne severity is quite broad. In the neonate, maternal androgens stimulate enlargement of and sebum overproduction from sebaceous glands. The presence of sebum promotes *P acnes* overgrowth, and acne ensues until the maternal androgens have cleared and the sebaceous glands atrophy to a normal neonatal size. Significant sebum production does not begin again until puberty. Under the stimulation of androgens at puberty, sebaceous glands enlarge once again and produce sebum in the sebaceous areas of the body, namely the face, neck, chest, and back (the same areas affected most by acne). Onset may be gradual or rapid, and severity may range from primarily comedonal to inflammatory papules and pustules to highly inflammatory, painful nodules. Severe scarring variants may be explosive in onset and present with systemic symptoms of fever and arthralgias. Age at onset and family history are predictors of the severity of acne.

Acne may present as a component of a syndrome, as in polycystic ovary disease (ie, Stein–Leventhal syndrome) or so-called SAPHO syndrome (*s*ynovitis, *a*cne, *p*almoplantar pustulosis, *h*yperostosis, and *o*steitis). At least in polycystic ovary disease, there may be hormonal influences that predispose to the acne lesion development.

CHECKPOINT

30. Why do some infants develop acne? What factors explain its spontaneous resolution?

31. What is the pathophysiology of lesion development in acne?

32. What are some broad treatment categories for acne, and which aspect of acne pathogenesis does each address?

PATTERN: PERIVASCULAR DERMATITIS WITHOUT EPIDERMAL CHANGE

Example: Urticaria
Clinical Presentation

Urticaria is a common condition that manifests clinically as relatively transient papules and/or plaques, colloquially called "hives" or "wheals." In some patients, the disease is short-lived, whereas in others it persists for decades. Urticaria is at one end of a spectrum with angioedema at the other: Urticaria involves the superficial dermis, whereas angioedema involves the deep dermis and subcutaneous tissue. Both urticaria and angioedema are sometimes accompanied by anaphylaxis, a potentially life-threating condition (see Chapter 3).

Epidemiology and Etiology

Urticaria affects approximately 15–25% of the population and affects people of all ages. Urticaria is associated with angioedema in approximately 50% of patients, whereas about 40% of patients have urticaria alone and 10% have angioedema alone. Urticaria is classified as acute if it lasts less than 6 weeks and chronic if it lasts more than 6 weeks.

In some patients, a specific cause of urticaria can be identified, such as sunlight, water, medication, pressure, vibration, heat, cold, exercise, or emotional stress. In other patients, no specific trigger can be pinpointed. Cold urticaria is usually acquired, although it can be inherited in the familial cold autoinflammatory syndrome owing to a mutation in the *CIAS1* gene on chromosome 1q44.

Histopathology and Pathogenesis

Microscopically, urticaria is characterized by a sparse, mixed, perivascular infiltrate without any alterations to the epidermis. The infiltrate is composed mostly of lymphocytes and eosinophils. A few admixed neutrophils are present in some cases. The infiltrate is sparse in intensity (Figures 8–35 and 8–36). Slight dermal edema is often present, although this may be difficult to appreciate microscopically. Most changes are located in the upper dermis.

Urticaria is the result of mast cell degranulation that causes the release of histamine and other pro-inflammatory cytokines, such as prostaglandins, leukotrienes, and platelet activating factor. While the type I hypersensitivity reaction mediated by IgE is the classic cause of mast cell degranulation, there are many other mediators of mast cell degranulation, including complement activation, physical stimuli, viral infections, and autoantibodies. The release of histamine causes capillary vasodilation in the superficial dermis with subsequent extravasation of protein-rich fluid into the superficial aspects of the skin and the development of the urticarial papules and/or plaques. The lesions resolve when the fluid gets resorbed. Angioedema is a result of the same process, although it involves the deep dermis and subcutaneous tissue and typically manifests as

FIGURE 8–35 Histopathologic features of urticaria. Low-power microscopic features of urticaria include a relatively sparse perivascular and interstitial infiltrate of lymphocytes and eosinophils without epidermal change.

FIGURE 8–37 Urticaria skin lesions with typical erythematous to white pruritic papules and plaques with surrounding rims of erythema. (Used, with permission, from Richard P. Usatine, MD in Usatine RP et al, eds. *Color Atlas of Family Medicine*, 2nd ed. McGraw-Hill, 2013.)

diffuse swelling rather than as discrete papules or plaques, owing to the deeper location of the changes.

Clinical Manifestations

The primary lesion of urticaria is a papule or plaque without epidermal change, ranging in morphologic shape from round

FIGURE 8–36 Histopathologic features of urticaria. A high-power view demonstrates numerous eosinophils (arrow) within the inflammatory infiltrate.

to annular to arcuate (Figure 8–37). The lesions range from erythematous to white and can range in size from a few millimeters to many centimeters. A surrounding rim of erythema is sometimes present. There is no change to the surface of the skin since the pathology is located in the dermis. Individual urticarial lesions are often pruritic and typically last for less than 1 day. The lesions resolve without any change to the skin. Any part of the body can be affected, although the trunk and extremities are the most common sites of involvement. Urticaria that can be elicited by physical stroking or scratching of the skin is called dermotographism. Angioedema lesions present as diffuse swelling, most often of mucous membranes and/ or the hands and feet. These lesions can persist for up to 3 days. If the respiratory tract is involved, the swelling can be life-threatening.

CHECKPOINT

33. What type of cell causes urticaria upon degranulation?
34. What are some causes of mast cell degranulation?
35. What are the typical clinical and microscopic findings of urticaria and angioedema?

CASE STUDIES

Yeong Kwok, MD

(See Chapter 25, p. 758–62 for answers)

CASE 38

A 25-year-old woman presents with a complaint of rash that has developed over the past several weeks and seems to be progressing. On examination, she is noted to have several plaque-like lesions over the extensor surfaces of both upper and lower extremities as well as similar lesions on her scalp. The plaques are erythematous, with silvery scales, and are sharply marginated.

Questions

A. What is the likely diagnosis? Is this skin disease genetic, environmental, or both? Based on what evidence?

B. What are the pathophysiologic mechanisms behind the development of the plaques, scale, and erythema characteristic of this disorder?

C. What immunologic defects have been implicated in patients with this skin disease?

CASE 39

A 35-year-old woman who recently returned from Africa presents to the clinic with complaints of a rash. During her trip, she developed an itchy rash on both arms. She has an unremarkable medical history. Medications recently taken include chloroquine for malaria prophylaxis. Examination discloses multiple small violaceous papules on the flexor surfaces of the arms. The lesions have angular borders and flat tops. Some of the lesions have minute white streaks on the surface, barely visible to the naked eye.

Questions

A. What is the likely diagnosis? What is the possible underlying cause?

B. What is the pathophysiologic mechanism by which these skin lesions are formed?

C. What histopathologic changes in the skin are responsible for the appearance of these lesions as violaceous papules with minute white striae?

CASE 40

A 27-year-old woman presents to the urgent care clinic complaining of a red, itchy rash developing suddenly the day before on her arms and legs and spreading to the trunk. She denies ulcers in the mouth or genital area. Her medical history is unremarkable except for occasional episodes of genital herpes. The most recent outbreak was approximately 2 weeks ago. She generally takes oral acyclovir on such occasions, but her prescription has run out and so she did not take any with her last bout. On physical examination, she has multiple erythematous papules over the arms, legs, and trunk. Many of the papules have a central area of duskiness or clearing, such that the lesions resemble targets. There is no evidence of mucosal involvement.

Questions

A. What is the likely diagnosis?

B. What is the pathophysiologic mechanism by which these skin lesions are formed? In what ways is this disease similar to and different from lichen planus?

C. What factors may have triggered this rash? What evidence supports this link?

D. What is responsible for the target-like appearance of these lesions, and what would the histopathology show?

CASE 41

A 65-year-old man presents to the dermatology clinic with a complaint of blisters developing on his abdomen and extremities over the past week. The lesions consisted initially of red patches followed by blister formation. They are pruritic but not painful. The patient has no other complaints and denies mucous membrane involvement. Examination shows only multiple large, tense blisters with an erythematous base over the lower trunk and extremities. The clinical picture is felt to be most consistent with bullous pemphigoid.

Questions

A. Why is this condition called bullous pemphigoid?
B. What would one expect histologic examination to show?
C. What would one expect to find on direct immunofluorescence microscopy?
D. What is the presumed mechanism by which blister formation occurs in bullous pemphigoid?

CASE 42

A 60-year-old man presents to the clinic with complaints of a recurring rash. He states that for the past 2–3 months, he has had several episodes of a painless, nonpruritic rash over his distal lower extremities. The lesions are described as purple and raised. His medical history is remarkable for hepatitis C—with no history of cirrhosis—and peripheral neuropathy. The patient has recently been treated for otitis media with amoxicillin. He has taken no other medications. Physical examination is notable only for multiple reddish-purple papules over the distal lower extremities (palpable purpura). The underlying skin is hyperpigmented. Biopsy reveals neutrophils, neutrophilic debris, and amorphous protein deposits involving the small blood vessels, consistent with fibrinoid necrosis.

Questions

A. What is the likely dermatologic diagnosis? What are some possible precipitants of that disease in this patient?
B. What is the underlying pathogenetic mechanism by which the lesions are formed?
C. What histologic characteristics are responsible for the appearance of the lesions as papular and purpuric?
D. What additional symptoms should this patient be asked about? Should any laboratory tests be ordered?

CASE 43

A 30-year-old woman presents to the clinic complaining that she has "an itchy rash all over the place." She noticed that her legs became red, itchy, and blistered about 2 days after she had been hiking in a heavily wooded area. She says that scratching broke the blisters, and afterward the rash became much worse and spread all over. She is convinced that the rash could not be poison ivy because once before she was exposed to that plant and did not develop a rash. On examination, there are erythematous vesicles and bullae in linear streaks on both of her legs. Some areas are weepy, with a yellowish crust. There are ill-defined erythematous plaques studded with papulovesicles on the trunk and arms.

Questions

A. What is the likely diagnosis? What feature on the physical examination is the cardinal sign?
B. What made the eruption spread?
C. How do you explain the diagnosis to the patient in light of the fact that she did not develop a rash after known exposure to poison ivy in the past? Why didn't the rash appear until 2 days after the apparent exposure?

CASE 44

A 45-year-old woman presents to clinic with a rash on her legs for 2 months. She notes that the rash started soon after babysitting her niece, who had "strep throat." She initially had a sore throat herself, but it stopped hurting after she took 2 days' worth of antibiotics she had left over from a previous prescription. On examination, on the anterior lower legs, she has several scattered ill-defined erythematous nodules, which are tender to palpation.

Questions

A. What is the likely diagnosis? What is the probable cause? What might explain why the eruption has persisted?
B. What are some other common causes of this condition?
C. What is the pathophysiologic mechanism of skin lesion formation?
D. What are the histopathologic findings of this disease?

CASE 45

A 52-year-old African American man presents to the clinic with a rash that has been worsening for several months. Review of systems is notable for a chronic cough. Examination reveals multiple red-brown, dermis-based papules on the trunk, arms, and face. Several lesions are clustered near the nares. The examination is otherwise unremarkable.

Questions

A. What is the likely diagnosis? What information is necessary to confirm the diagnosis?
B. Which organ system (in addition to the skin) is at risk for disease involvement based on the clinical examination?
C. What are the histopathologic features of this disease?
D. How does the disease present clinically?

CASE 46

A 15-year-old girl presents to the clinic complaining of "pimples" for 6 months. She has been using an over-the-counter face wash four times a day to keep the oil and dirt off, but it has not helped. Examination reveals several dozen erythematous papules and pustules over the forehead and central face with scattered open and closed comedones. A diagnosis of moderate inflammatory acne is entertained.

Questions

A. Why has this patient's meticulous cleansing practice not helped her condition? What advice would you give her regarding facial cleansing?
B. What is the life cycle of an inflammatory acne papule?
C. What are some general categories of acne treatment, and what component of lesion development does each address?

CASE 47

A 12-year-old boy is brought to the pediatrician's office for evaluation of hives. He has no significant past medical history and no history of allergies. He has just joined the middle school cross-country team and noticed that he gets hives about 10 minutes into each training run. The hives are very itchy, irregular blotches on his legs and trunk, about 10–20 cm in size, and they persist for about 30 minutes. He does not experience swelling of the lips or oropharynx and denies any wheezing or shortness of breath. His physical examination is normal without skin lesions or oral swelling at that moment, and his lungs are clear. He does have mild dermatographism with wheals that form on the back after stroking with a tongue depressor.

Questions

A. What is the likely cause of the patient's hives (urticaria)?
B. What is the cellular mechanism of the urticaria?
C. What more serious complication is often associated with urticaria?

REFERENCES

General

Ackerman AB et al. *The Lives of Lesions: Chronology in Dermatopathology.* Masson, 1984.

Bolognia JL et al, eds. *Dermatology,* 4th ed. Elsevier, 2017.

James WD et al. *Andrews' Diseases of the Skin: Clinical Dermatology,* 12th ed. Elsevier, 2015.

Wolff K et al, eds. *Fitzpatrick's Color Atlas and Synopsis of Clinical Dermatology,* 8th ed. McGraw-Hill, 2017.

Psoriasis

Boehncke WH et al. Psoriasis. Lancet. 2015 Sep 5;386(9997):983–94. [PMID: 26025581]

Fitch E et al. Pathophysiology of psoriasis: recent advances on IL-23 and Th17 cytokines. Curr Rheumatol Rep. 2007 Dec;9(6):461–7. [PMID: 18177599]

Hawkes JE et al. MicroRNAs in psoriasis. J Invest Dermatol. 2016 Feb;136(2):365–71. [PMID: 26802234]

Lynde CW et al. Interleukin 17A: toward a new understanding of psoriasis pathogenesis. J Am Acad Dermatol. 2014 Jul;71(1):141–50. [PMID: 24655820]

Meier M et al. Clinical spectrum and severity of psoriasis. Curr Probl Dermatol. 2009;38:1–20. [PMID: 19710547]

Tonel G et al. Cutting edge: a critical functional role for IL-23 in psoriasis. J Immunol. 2010 Nov 15:185(10):5688–91. [PMID: 20956338]

Lichen Planus

Cheng S et al. Interventions for erosive lichen planus affecting mucosal sites. Cochrane Database Syst Rev. 2012 Feb 15;2:CD008092. [PMID: 22336835]

Kurago ZB. Etiology and pathogenesis of oral lichen planus: an overview. Oral Surg Oral Med Oral Pathol Oral Radiol. 2016 Jul;122(1):72–80. [PMID: 27260276]

Lage D et al. Lichen planus and lichenoid drug-induced eruption: a histological and immunohistochemical study. Int J Dermatol. 2012 Oct;51(10):1199–205. [PMID: 22416968]

Le Cleach L et al. Clinical practice. Lichen planus. N Engl J Med. 2012 Feb 23;366(8):723–32. [PMID: 22356325]

Ma H et al. MicroRNAs in oral lichen planus and potential miRNA-mRNA pathogenesis with essential cytokines: a review. Oral Surg Oral Med Oral Pathol Oral Radiol. 2016 Aug;122(2):164–73. [PMID: 27282956]

Wang H et al. Role of distinct CD4(+) T helper subset in pathogenesis of oral lichen planus. J Oral Pathol Med. 2016 Jul;45(6):385–93. [PMID: 26693958]

Erythema Multiforme

Abe R. Toxic epidermal necrolysis and Stevens-Johnson syndrome: soluble Fas ligand involvement in the pathomechanisms of these diseases. J Dermatol Sci. 2008 Dec;52(3):151–9. [PMID: 18657400]

Dodiuk-Gad RP et al. Stevens-Johnson syndrome and toxic epidermal necrolysis: an update. Am J Clin Dermatol. 2015 Dec;16(6):475–93. [PMID: 26481651]

Hoetzenecker W et al. Adverse cutaneous drug eruptions: current understanding. Semin Immunopathol. 2016 Jan;38(1):75–86. [PMID: 26553194]

Sokumbi O et al. Clinical features, diagnosis, and treatment of erythema multiforme: a review for the practicing dermatologist. Int J Dermatol. 2012 Aug;51(8):889–902. [PMID: 22788803]

Wetter DA et al. Recurrent erythema multiforme: clinical characteristics, etiologic associations, and treatment in a series of 48 patients at Mayo Clinic, 2000 to 2007. J Am Acad Dermatol. 2010 Jan;62(1):45–53. [PMID: 19665257]

White KD et al. Evolving models of the immunopathogenesis of T cell-mediated drug allergy: the role of host, pathogens, and drug response. J Allergy Clin Immunol. 2015 Aug;136(2):219–34. [PMID: 26254049]

Bullous Pemphigoid

Feng S et al. Serum levels of autoantibodies to BP180 correlate with disease activity in patients with bullous pemphigoid. Int J Dermatol. 2008 Mar;47(3):225–8. [PMID: 18289320]

Goletz S et al. Anti-p200 pemphigoid. J Am Acad Dermatol. 2014 Jul;71(1):185–91. [PMID: 24767733]

Kershenovich R et al. Diagnosis and classification of pemphigus and bullous pemphigoid. Autoimmun Rev. 2014 Apr-May;13(4-5):477–81. [PMID: 24424192]

Nishie W. Update on the pathogenesis of bullous pemphigoid: an autoantibody-mediated blistering disease targeting collagen XVII. J Dermatol Sci. 2014 Mar;73(3):179–86. [PMID: 24434029]

van Beek N et al. IgE-mediated mechanisms in bullous pemphigoid and other autoimmune bullous diseases. Expert Rev Clin Immunol. 2016;12(3):267–77. [PMID: 26588556]

Leukocytoclastic Vasculitis

Grau RG. Drug-induced vasculitis: new insights and a changing lineup of suspects. Curr Rheumatol Rep. 2015 Dec;17(12):71. [PMID: 26503355]

Micheletti RG et al. Small vessel vasculitis of the skin. Rheum Dis Clin North Am. 2015;41(1):21–32. [PMID: 25399937]

Allergic Contact Dermatitis

de Groot AC. New contact allergens: 2008 to 2015. Dermatitis. 2015 Sep-Oct;26(5):199–215. [PMID:26367204]

Friedmann PS et al. Genetic factors in susceptibility to contact sensitivity. Contact Dermatitis. 2015 May;72(5):263–74. [PMID: 25711366]

Fyhrquist N et al. New findings in allergic contact dermatitis. Curr Opin Allergy Clin Immunol. 2014 Oct;14(5):430–5. [PMID: 25054832]

Martin SF. Immunological mechanisms in allergic contact dermatitis. Curr Opin Allergy Clin Immunol. 2015 Apr;15(2):124–30. [PMID: 25611878]

McFadden JP et al. Why does allergic contact dermatitis exist? Br J Dermatol. 2013 Apr;168(4):692–9. [PMID: 23383741]

Mowad CM et al. Allergic contact dermatitis: patient diagnosis and evaluation. J Am Acad Dermatol. 2016 Jun;74(6):1029–40. [PMID: 27185421]

Peng W et al. Pathogenesis of atopic dermatitis. Clin Exp Allergy. 2015 Mar;45(3):566–74. [PMID: 25610977]

Erythema Nodosum

Blake T et al. Erythema nodosum—a review of an uncommon panniculitis. Dermatol Online J. 2014 Apr 16;20(4):22376. [PMID: 24746312]

Kisacik B et al. Multiclinical experiences in erythema nodosum: rheumatology clinics versus dermatology and infection diseases clinics. Rheumatol Int. 2013 Feb;33(2):315–8. [PMID: 22441968]

Papagrigoraki A et al. Erythema nodosum: etiological factors and relapses in a retrospective cohort study. Eur J Dermatol. 2010 Nov–Dec;20(6):773–7. [PMID: 21030339]

Thrash B et al. Cutaneous manifestations of gastrointestinal disease: part II. J Am Acad Dermatol. 2013 Feb;68(2):211.e1–33. [PMID: 23317981]

Cutaneous Sarcoidosis

Sanchez M et al. Sarcoidosis. Dermatol Clin. 2015 Jul;33(3):389–416. [PMID: 26143421]

Wanat KA et al. A practical approach to cutaneous sarcoidosis. Am J Clin Dermatol. 2014 Aug;15(4):283–97. [PMID: 24820822]

Wanat KA et al. Cutaneous sarcoidosis. Clin Chest Med. 2015 Dec;36(4):685–702. [PMID: 26593142]

Acne

Beylot C et al. *Propionibacterium acnes*: an update on its role in the pathogenesis of acne. J Eur Acad Dermatol Venereol. 2014 Mar;28(3):271–8. [PMID: 23905540]

Gollnick HP. From new findings in acne pathogenesis to new approaches in treatment. J Eur Acad Dermatol Venereol. 2015 Jun;29(Suppl 5):1–7. [PMID: 26059819]

Liu PF et al. *Propionibacterium acnes* in the pathogenesis and immunotherapy of acne vulgaris. Curr Drug Metab. 2015;16(4):245–54. [PMID: 26264195]

Suh DH et al. What's new in the physiopathology of acne? Br J Dermatol. 2015 Jul;172(Suppl 1):13–9. [PMID: 25645151]

Urticaria

Asero R et al. Chronic urticaria: a focus on pathogenesis. F1000Res. 2017 Jul 11;6:1095. [PMID: 28751972]

Fukunaga A et al. Cholinergic urticaria: epidemiology, physiopathology, new categorization, and management. Clin Auton Res. 2018 Feb;28(1):103–13. [PMID: 28382552]

Hoffman HM et al. Identification of a locus on chromosome 1q44 for familial cold urticaria. Am J Hum Genet. 2000 May;66(5):1693–8. [PMID: 10741953]

LoVerde D et al. Angioedema. Crit Care Med. 2017 Apr;45(4):725–35. [PMID: 28291095]

Pattanaik D et al. Pediatric angioedema. Curr Allergy Asthma Rep. 2017 Aug 8;17(9):60. [PMID: 28791569]

Radonjic-Hoesli S et al. Urticaria and angioedema: an update on classification and pathogenesis. Clin Rev Allergy Immunol. 2018 Feb;54(1):88–101. [PMID: 28748365]

Pulmonary Disease

9

Thomas H. Sisson, MD, Dru Claar, MD, Mark S. Chesnutt, MD, & Thomas J. Prendergast, MD

The principal physiologic role of the lungs is to make oxygen available to tissues for metabolism and to remove the main byproduct of that metabolism, carbon dioxide. The lungs perform this function by moving inspired air into close proximity to the pulmonary capillary bed to enable gas exchange by simple diffusion. This is accomplished at a minimal workload, is regulated efficiently over a wide range of metabolic demand, and takes place with close matching of ventilation to lung perfusion. The extensive surface area of the respiratory system must also be protected from a broad variety of infectious or noxious environmental insults.

Humans possess a complex and efficient respiratory system that satisfies these diverse requirements. When injury to components of the respiratory system occurs, the integrated function of the whole is disrupted. The consequences can be profound. Airway injury or dysfunction results in **obstructive lung diseases**, including asthma and chronic obstructive pulmonary disease (COPD). Injury to the pulmonary parenchyma can produce **restrictive lung diseases**, such as idiopathic pulmonary fibrosis, acute respiratory distress syndrome, and pulmonary vascular disease. To understand the clinical presentations of lung disease, it is necessary first to understand the anatomic and functional organization of the lungs that determines normal function.

CHECKPOINT

1. What are the two principal physiologic roles of the lungs?
2. What are the requirements for successful lung function?

NORMAL STRUCTURE & FUNCTION OF THE LUNGS

ANATOMY

The mature respiratory system consists of visceral pleura-covered lungs contained by the chest wall and diaphragm, the latter serving under normal conditions as the principal bellows muscle for ventilation. The lungs are divided into lobes, each demarcated by intervening visceral pleura. Each lung possesses an upper and lower lobe; the middle lobe and lingula are the third lobes in the right and left lungs, respectively. At end expiration, most of the volume of the lungs is air (Table 9–1), whereas almost half of the mass of the lungs is accounted for by blood volume. It is a testament to the delicate structure of the gas-exchanging region of the lungs that alveolar tissue has a total weight of only 250 g but a total surface area of 75 m².

Connective tissue fibers and surfactant serve to maintain the anatomic integrity of this large and complex surface area.

The connective tissue fibers are highly organized collagen and elastic structures that radiate into the interstitium. These fibers divide segments, invest airways and vessels, and support alveolar walls with a delicate, elastic fibrous network. The multidirectional elastic support provided by this network allows the lung, from alveoli to conducting airways, to support itself and retain airway patency despite large changes in volume.

Surfactant is a complex material produced by type II alveolar cells; it is composed of multiple phospholipids and specific associated proteins. The physiologic function of a subset of surfactant lipoproteins is to enhance the anatomic stability of the alveoli. The presence of surfactant covering the alveolar epithelial surface reduces surface tension, allowing expansion of alveoli with a transpulmonary distending pressure of less than 5 cm H_2O. In the absence of this surface-active layer,

TABLE 9–1   Components of a normal human lung.

Component	Volume (mL) or Mass (g)	Thickness (μm)
Gas (functional residual capacity)	2400 mL	
Tissue	900 g	
Blood	400 g	
Lung	500 g	
Support structures	225 g	
Alveolar walls	275 g	
Epithelium	60 g	0.18
Endothelium	50 g	0.10
Interstitium	110 g	0.22
Alveolar macrophages	55 g	

Reproduced, with permission, from Albertine KH. Anatomy of the lungs. In: Broaddus C et al. *Murray & Nadel's Textbook of Respiratory Medicine,* 6th ed. Elsevier Saunders, 2016. Copyright © Saunders/Elsevier.

increasing surface tension associated with a reduction of alveolar volume during expiration would result in the collapse of alveoli. The distending pressure required to re-expand these collapsed alveoli would be greater than normal ventilatory effort could produce.

Airway & Epithelial Anatomy

Further anatomic division of the lungs is based primarily on the separation of the tracheobronchial tree into **conducting airways**, which provide for movement of air from the external environment to areas of gas exchange, and **terminal respiratory units**, or **acini**, the airways and associated alveolar structures participating directly in gas exchange (Figure 9–1). The proximal conducting airways are lined with ciliated pseudostratified columnar epithelial cells, are supported by a cartilaginous skeleton in their walls, and contain secretory glands in the epithelial wall. The ciliated epithelium has a uniform orientation of cilia that beat in unison toward the pharynx. This ciliary action, together with the mucus layer produced by submucosal mucous secretory glands, provides a mechanism for the continuous transport of contaminating or excess material out of the lungs. Circumferential airway smooth muscle is also present but, as with secretory glands, is reduced and then lost as the airways branch farther into the lung and diminish in caliber. The smallest conducting airways are nonrespiratory **bronchioles**. These are characterized by a loss of smooth muscle and cartilage but a retention of a cuboidal epithelium that may be ciliated and is not a site of gas exchange. The lobes of the lung are divided into less distinct lobules, defined as collections of terminal respiratory units incompletely bounded by connective tissue septa. Terminal respiratory units are the final physiologic and anatomic unit of the lung, with walls of thin alveolar epithelial cells that provide gas exchange with the alveolar–capillary network.

The principal site of resistance to airflow in the lungs is in medium-sized bronchi (Figure 9–2). This seems

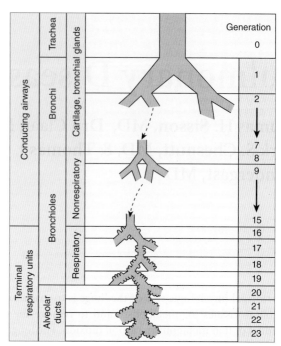

FIGURE 9–1 Subdivision of conducting airways and terminal respiratory units. This schematic illustration demonstrates the subdivisions of both the conducting airways and the respiratory airways. Successive branching produces increasing generations of airways, beginning with the trachea. Note that gas-exchanging segments of the lung are encountered only after extensive branching, with a concomitant decrease in airway caliber and an increase in total cross-sectional area (see Figures 9–2 and 9–3). (Redrawn, with permission, from Weibel ER. *Morphometry of the Human Lung.* Academic Press, 2013.)

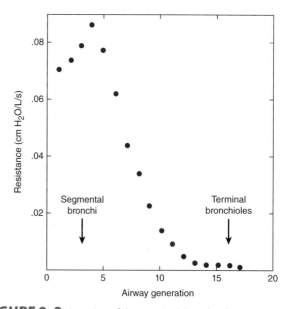

FIGURE 9–2 Location of the principal site of airflow resistance. The second- through fifth-generation airways include the segmental bronchi and larger bronchioles. They present the greatest resistance to airflow in normal individuals. The smaller airways contribute relatively little despite their smaller caliber because of the enormous number arranged in parallel. Compare with Figure 9–3. (Adapted, with permission of Elsevier, from Pedley TJ et al. The prediction of pressure drop and variation of resistance within the human bronchial airways. Respir Physiol. 1970;9(3):387.)

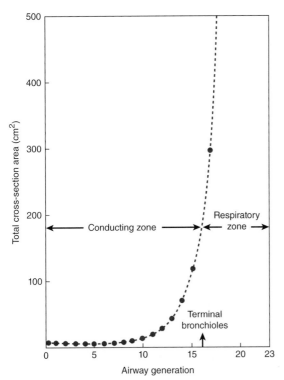

FIGURE 9–3 Airway generation and total airway cross-sectional area. Note the extremely rapid increase in total cross-sectional area in the respiratory zone (compare with Figure 9–1) and the fall in resistance as a consequence of the increase in cross-sectional area (compare with Figure 9–2). As a result, the forward velocity of gas during inspiration becomes very low at the level of the respiratory bronchioles, and gas diffusion becomes the chief mode of ventilation. (Redrawn, with permission, from West JB et al. *West's Respiratory Physiology: The Essentials*, 10th ed. Lippincott Williams & Wilkins, 2015.)

counterintuitive because one would expect smaller-caliber airways to be the major site of resistance, but repetitive branching of the small airways leads to a profound increase in cross-sectional area that does not contribute significantly to airway resistance in healthy individuals (Figure 9–3). Under pathologic conditions such as asthma, in which smaller bronchi and bronchioles become narrowed, airway resistance can increase dramatically.

The pulmonary arteries are found in close association with the branching bronchial tree in the lungs (Figure 9–4). Both arterial blood flow and bronchial airflow are actively regulated by changing vessel or airway caliber. The anatomic relationship between arteries and bronchi provides an ideal setting for the continuous matching of ventilation and perfusion to different lung segments.

Vascular & Lymphatic Anatomy

The pulmonary vascular system includes two distinct circuits that distribute blood through the lungs: the **pulmonary** and **bronchial circulations**. The right ventricle pumps its entire output of mixed venous blood through pulmonary arteries

toward alveolar capillaries. Pulmonary arteries and arterioles are smooth muscle–invested vessels located adjacent to bronchi within the pulmonary bronchovascular bundle. Pulmonary arterioles are very sensitive to alveolar PO_2, with a prominent vasoconstrictor response to hypoxia. **Hypoxic pulmonary vasoconstriction** allows matching of alveolar perfusion to ventilation (see below). Pulmonary veins arise from alveolar capillaries to form vessels that traverse the intralobular septa to return oxygenated blood to the left atrium.

Bronchial arteries that arise from the aorta and intercostal arteries deliver oxygenated blood at systemic pressures to nearly all the intrapulmonary structures proximal to the terminal bronchioles, including the bronchial tree, hilar structures, pulmonary arteries and veins, pulmonary nervous system and lymphatics, connective tissue septa, and visceral pleura. Most lung tumors receive their blood supply from the bronchial circulation. There are abundant bronchopulmonary anastomoses at the arteriolar and capillary levels that are silent in health but which may enlarge in disease to contribute to hemoptysis. Drainage of the bronchial circulation occurs both to the right atrium via the azygos vein and to the left atrium via the pulmonary veins. The latter represents an anatomic shunt of deoxygenated blood, typically representing less than 5% of cardiac output.

Pulmonary lymphatics arise in connective tissue spaces beneath the visceral pleura and in deep plexuses at the junction of the terminal bronchioles and alveoli. Lymphatics do not enter the alveolar peri-interstitial space (see Figure 9–4). As a result, fluid in the alveolar interstitium must move to the region of terminal bronchioles to gain access to draining lymphatics. Lymphatic ducts travel principally in the peribronchovascular sheath back to hilar and mediastinal lymph nodes before entering the left thoracic duct or right lymphatic duct. Lymphatic drainage of the pleural space occurs through plexuses investing the costal, diaphragmatic, and mediastinal parietal pleura that are anatomically separate from pulmonary lymphatics.

Pulmonary Nervous System

The lungs are richly innervated with neural fibers from parasympathetic (vagal), sympathetic, and the so-called nonadrenergic, noncholinergic (NANC) systems. Efferent fibers include the following: (1) parasympathetic fibers, with muscarinic cholinergic efferents that mediate bronchoconstriction, pulmonary vasodilation, and mucous gland secretion; (2) sympathetic fibers, whose stimulation produces bronchial smooth muscle relaxation, pulmonary vasoconstriction, and secretory gland activity inhibition; and (3) the NANC system, with multiple transmitters implicated, including adenosine triphosphate (ATP), nitric oxide (NO), and peptide neurotransmitters such as substance P and vasoactive intestinal peptide (VIP). The NANC system participates in inhibitory events, including bronchodilation, and may function as the

FIGURE 9–4 Airway, vascular, and lymphatic anatomy of the lung. This schematic diagram demonstrates the general anatomic relationships of the airways and terminal respiratory units with the vascular and lymphatic systems of the lung. Important points are as follows: (1) The pulmonary arterial system runs adjacent to the bronchial tree, while the draining pulmonary veins are found distant from the airways; (2) the bronchial wall blood supply is provided by bronchial arteries, branches of systemic arterial origin; (3) lymphatics are found adjacent to both the arterial and venous systems and are very abundant in the lung; and (4) lymphatics are found as far distally as the terminal respiratory bronchioles, but they do not penetrate to the alveolar wall. (A, alveolus; AD, alveolar duct; RB, respiratory bronchiole; TB, terminal bronchiole.) (Redrawn, with permission, from Staub NC. The physiology of pulmonary edema. Hum Pathol. 1970;1:419. Copyright © Elsevier.)

predominant reciprocal balance to the excitatory cholinergic system.

Pulmonary afferents consist principally of the vagal sensory fibers. These include the following:

1. Fibers from bronchopulmonary stretch receptors, located in the trachea and proximal bronchi. Stimulation of these fibers by lung inflation results in bronchodilation and an increased heart rate.
2. Fibers from irritant receptors, also found in proximal airways. Stimulation of these fibers by diverse nonspecific stimuli elicits efferent responses, including cough, bronchoconstriction, and mucus secretion.
3. C fibers, or fibers from juxtacapillary (J) receptors, which are unmyelinated fibers ending in lung parenchyma and bronchial walls and respond to mechanical and chemical stimuli. The reflex responses associated with C fiber stimulation include a rapid shallow breathing pattern, mucus secretion, cough, and heart rate slowing with inspiration.

Immune Structure & Function

Of all the body's organs, the lungs have a unique exposure to environmental insults. Nonexertional ventilation in an adult totals about 7500 L of air per day, an amount increased substantially with activity. This exposure to an open, nonsterile environment imposes an ongoing risk of toxic, infectious, and inflammatory insults. Furthermore, the pulmonary circulation contains the only capillary bed through which the entire circulating blood volume must flow in each cardiac cycle. As a consequence, the lung is an obligatory vascular sieve and functions as a principal site of defense against the hematogenous spread of infection and other noxious influences. Protecting the lungs from environmental and infectious injury involves a set of complex responses capable of providing timely and successful defense against attack via the airways or vascular bed. As outlined in Table 9–2, it is convenient for discussion purposes to separate these responses into two major categories—nonspecific physical and chemical protections and specific immune structures and actions—all functioning to prevent injury to or microbial invasion of the very large epithelial and vascular area of the lung.

LUNG VOLUMES, CAPACITIES & THE NORMAL SPIROGRAM

The volume of gas in the lungs is divided into volumes and capacities as shown by the bars at the left of the figure below. Lung volumes are primary: They do not overlap each other. **Tidal volume (V_T)** is the amount of gas inhaled and exhaled with each resting breath. A normal tidal volume in a 70 kg person is approximately 350–400 mL. **Residual volume (RV)** is the amount of gas remaining in the lungs at the end of a maximal exhalation. Lung capacities are composed of two or more lung volumes. The **vital capacity (VC)** is the total amount of gas that can be exhaled after a maximal inhalation. The vital capacity and the residual volume together constitute the **total lung capacity (TLC)**, or the total amount of gas in the lungs at the end of a maximal inhalation. The **functional residual capacity (FRC)** is the amount of gas in the lungs at the end of a resting tidal breath. (**ERV**, expiratory reserve volume; **IC**, inspiratory capacity; **IRV**, inspiratory reserve volume.)

The spirogram at the right in the figure is drawn in real time. The first tidal breath shown takes 5 seconds, indicating a respiratory rate of 12 breaths/min. The **forced vital capacity (FVC)** maneuver begins with an inhalation from FRC to TLC (lasting about 1 second) followed by a forceful exhalation from TLC to RV (lasting about 5 seconds). The amount of gas exhaled during the first second of this maneuver is the **forced expiratory volume in 1 second (FEV_1)**. Normal subjects expel approximately 80% of the FVC in the first second. The **ratio of the FEV_1 to FVC** (referred to as the **FEV_1/FVC** or **FEV_1%**) is diminished in patients with obstructive lung disease and increased in patients with restrictive lung disease.

(Redrawn, with permission, from Staub NC. *Basic Respiratory Physiology*. Churchill Livingstone, 1991. Copyright © Elsevier.)

CHECKPOINT

3. What are the roles of the connective tissue and surfactant systems in lung function?

4. What is the role of the ciliary action of the respiratory epithelium?

5. Why are medium-sized bronchi, rather than small airways, the major site of resistance to airflow in the lungs?

6. What are the physiologic functions of the efferent parasympathetic, sympathetic, and NANC neural systems of the lung?

7. What are the categories of afferent vagal sensory receptors?

8. What are the different roles of the pulmonary and bronchial arteries?

9. What sensitive mechanism do the pulmonary arteries have for matching alveolar perfusion with ventilation?

10. What are the components of the nonspecific defense system of the lungs?

11. What are the humoral and cellular components of the specific immune defense system of the lungs?

PHYSIOLOGY

At rest, the lungs take 4 L/min of air and 5 L/min of blood, direct them within 0.2 μm of each other, and then return both to their respective pools. With maximal exercise, flow may increase to 100 L/min of ventilation and 25 L/min of cardiac output. The lungs thereby perform their primary physiologic function of making oxygen available to the tissues for metabolism and removing the major byproduct of that metabolism, carbon dioxide. The lungs perform this task largely free of conscious control while maintaining $PaCO_2$ within a 5% tolerance. It is a magnificent feat of evolutionary plumbing and neurochemical control.

Static Properties: Compliance & Elastic Recoil

The lung maintains its extremely thin parenchyma over an enormous surface area by means of an intricate supporting architecture of collagen and elastin fibers. Anatomically, as well as physiologically and functionally, the lung is an elastic organ.

TABLE 9–2   Lung defenses.

I. Nonspecific defenses

  1. Clearance

    a. Cough

    b. Mucociliary escalator

  2. Secretions

    a. Tracheobronchial (mucus)

    b. Alveolar (surfactant)

    c. Cellular components (including lysozyme, complement, surfactant proteins, defensins)

  3. Cellular defenses

    a. Nonphagocytic

      Conducting airway epithelium

      Terminal respiratory epithelium

    b. Phagocytic

      Blood phagocytes (monocytes)

      Tissue phagocytes (alveolar macrophages)

  4. Biochemical defenses

    a. Proteinase inhibitors (α_1-protease inhibitor, secretory leukoprotease inhibitor)

    b. Antioxidants (eg, transferrin, lactoferrin, glutathione, albumin)

II. Specific immunologic defenses

  1. Antibody mediated (B-lymphocyte–dependent immunologic responses)

    a. Secretory immunoglobulin (IgA)

    b. Serum immunoglobulins

  2. Antigen presentation to lymphocytes

    a. Macrophages and monocytes

    b. Dendritic cells

    c. Epithelial cells

  3. Cell mediated (T-lymphocyte–dependent) immunologic responses

    a. Cytokine mediated

    b. Direct cellular cytotoxicity

  4. Nonlymphocyte cellular immune responses

    a. Mast cell dependent

    b. Eosinophil dependent

FIGURE 9–5 Interaction of the pressure–volume properties of the lungs and the chest wall. Resting lung volume (FRC) represents the equilibrium point at which the elastic recoil of the lung (tendency to collapse inward) and the chest wall (tendency to spring outward) are exactly balanced. Other lung volumes can also be defined by reference to this diagram. Total lung capacity (TLC) is the point at which the inspiratory muscles cannot generate sufficient force to overcome the elastic recoil of the lungs and chest wall. Residual volume (RV) is the point at which the expiratory muscles cannot generate sufficient force to overcome the elastic recoil of the chest wall. Compliance is calculated by taking the slope of these pressure–volume relationships at a specific volume. Note that the compliance of the lungs is greater at low lung volumes but falls considerably above two-thirds of vital capacity. (Modified, with permission, from Staub NC. *Basic Respiratory Physiology.* Churchill Livingstone, 1991. Copyright © Elsevier.)

The lungs inflate and deflate in response to changes in the volume of the semi-rigid thoracic cage in which they are suspended. An analogy is the inflation of a blacksmith's bellows by pulling the handles apart, thus increasing the volume of the bellows, lowering pressure, and causing inflow of air. Air enters the lungs when pressure in the pleural space is reduced by the expansion of the chest wall. The volume of air entering the lungs depends on the change in pleural pressure and the **compliance** of the respiratory system. Compliance is an intrinsic elastic property that relates a change in volume to a change in pressure. The compliance of both the chest wall and the lungs contributes to the compliance of the respiratory system (Figure 9–5). The compliance of the chest wall does not change significantly with thoracic volume, at least within the physiologic range. The compliance of the lungs varies inversely with lung volume. At functional residual capacity (FRC), the lungs are normally very compliant, approximately 200 mL/cm H_2O. Thus, a reduction of only 5 cm H_2O pressure in the pleural space will draw a breath of 1 L.

The tendency of a deformable body to return to its baseline shape is its **elastic recoil**. The elastic recoil of the chest wall is determined by the shape and structure of the thoracic cage. Lung elastic recoil is determined by two factors: tissue elasticity and the forces needed to change the shape of the air–liquid interface of the alveolus (Figure 9–6). Expanding the lungs requires overcoming local surface forces that are directly proportionate to alveolar **surface tension**. Surface tension is a physical property that reflects the greater attraction between

FIGURE 9–6 The effect of surface forces on lung compliance: a simple experiment demonstrating the effect of surface tension at the air–liquid interface of excised cat lungs. When inflated with saline, there are no surface forces to overcome, and the lungs are both more compliant and show no difference (hysteresis) between the inflation and deflation curves. When inflated with air, the pressure required to distend the lung is greater at every volume. The difference between the two curves represents the contribution of surface forces. There is also a pronounced hysteresis to lungs inflated with air that reflects surfactant recruited into the alveolar liquid during inflation (upward arrow), where it further reduces surface forces during deflation (downward arrow). (Reproduced, with permission, from Clements JA, Tierney DF. Alveolar instability associated with altered surface tension. In: *Handbook of Physiology, Respiration*. Sect. 3, Vol. II, Chapter 69. Washington, DC: American Physiological Society; 1965:1565–84.)

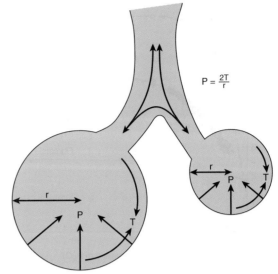

FIGURE 9–7 The importance of surface tension. If two connected alveoli have the same surface tension, then the smaller the radius, the greater the pressure tending to collapse the sphere. This could lead to alveolar instability, with smaller units emptying into larger ones. Alveoli typically do not have the same surface tension, however, because surface forces vary according to surface area as a result of the presence of surfactant: The relative concentration of surfactant in the surface layer of the sphere increases as the radius of the sphere falls, augmenting the effect of surfactant at low lung volumes. This tends to counterbalance the increase in pressure needed to keep alveoli open at diminished lung volume and adds stability to the alveoli, which might otherwise tend to collapse into one another. Surfactant thus protects against the regional collapse of lung units, a condition known as atelectasis, in addition to its other functions. (r, radius of alveolus; P, gas pressure; T, surface tension.)

molecules of a liquid than between molecules of that liquid and adjacent gas. At the air–liquid interface of the lung, molecules of water at the interface are more strongly attracted to each other than they are to the air above. This creates a net force drawing water molecules together in the plane of the interface. If the interface is stretched over a curved surface, that force acts to collapse the curve. The law of Laplace quantifies this force: The pressure needed to keep the curve open (in this case represented by a sphere) is directly proportionate to the surface tension at the interface and inversely proportionate to the radius of the sphere (Figure 9–7).

Surfactant is a mixture of phospholipid (predominantly dipalmitoylphosphatidylcholine [DPPC]) and specific surfactant proteins. These hydrophobic molecules displace water molecules from the air–liquid interface, thereby reducing surface tension. This reduction has three physiologic implications. First, it reduces the elastic recoil pressure of the lungs, thereby reducing the pressure needed to inflate them. This results in reduced work of breathing. Second, it allows surface forces to vary with alveolar surface area, thereby promoting alveolar stability and protecting against collapse and atelectasis (see Figure 9–7). Third, it limits the reduction of hydrostatic pressure in the pericapillary interstitium caused by surface tension. This reduces the forces promoting fluid transudation and the tendency to accumulate interstitial edema.

Pathologic states may result from reduced lung elastic recoil causing an increase in compliance (emphysema), increased interstitial connective tissue leading to decreased compliance (pulmonary fibrosis), or disruption of surfactant with an increase in surface forces (infant respiratory distress syndrome [IRDS]) (Figure 9–8).

Dynamic Properties: Flow & Resistance

Inflation of the lungs must overcome three opposing forces: elastic recoil, including surface forces; inertia of the respiratory system; and resistance to airflow. Since inertia is negligible, the work of breathing can be divided into work to overcome elastic forces and work to overcome flow resistance.

Increased elastic forces predominate in two common disorders: diffuse parenchymal fibrosis and obesity. The reduction in lung compliance in fibrotic lung disease, and in chest wall and respiratory system compliance in obesity, increases the work of breathing. Obese subjects also experience increased airflow resistance, largely though not entirely because of their tendency to breathe at lower lung volumes.

Flow resistance depends on the nature of the flow. Under conditions of **laminar** or **streamlined flow**, resistance is

FIGURE 9–8 Static expiratory pressure–volume curves in normal subjects and patients with emphysema and pulmonary fibrosis. The underlying physiologic abnormality in emphysema is a dramatic increase in lung compliance. Such patients tend to breathe at very high lung volumes. Patients with pulmonary fibrosis have very noncompliant lungs and breathe at low lung volumes. (Redrawn, with permission, from Pride NB et al. Lung mechanics in disease. In: Fishman AP, ed. Vol III, Part 2, of *Handbook of Physiology*. Section 3. Respiratory. American Physiological Society, 1986.)

described by the Poiseuille equation: Resistance is directly proportionate to the length of the airway and the viscosity of the gas, and inversely proportionate to the fourth power of the radius. A reduction by one-half of the airway radius leads to a 16-fold increase in airway resistance. Airway caliber is, therefore, the principal determinant of airway resistance under laminar flow conditions. Under conditions of **turbulent flow**, the driving pressure needed to achieve a given flow rate is proportionate to the square of the flow rate. Turbulent flow also depends on gas density and not on gas viscosity.

Most of the resistance to normal breathing arises in medium-sized bronchi and not in smaller bronchioles (see Figure 9–2). There are three main reasons for this counterintuitive finding. First, airflow in the normal lung is not laminar but turbulent, at least from the mouth to the small peripheral airways. Thus, where flow is highest (in segmental and subsegmental bronchi), resistance depends chiefly on flow rates. Second, in small peripheral airways, where airway caliber is the principal determinant of resistance, repetitive branching creates a very large number of small airways arranged in parallel. Their resistance is reciprocally additive, making their contribution to total airway resistance minor under normal conditions. Third, there is a transition to laminar flow approaching the terminal bronchioles as a consequence of increased cross-sectional area and decreased flow rates (see Figure 9–3). In the respiratory bronchioles and alveoli, bulk flow of gas ceases and gas movement occurs by diffusion.

Airway resistance is determined by several factors. Many disease states affect bronchial smooth muscle tone and cause

bronchoconstriction, producing an abnormal narrowing of the airways. Airways may also be narrowed by hypertrophy (chronic bronchitis) or infiltration (sarcoidosis) of the airway mucosa. Physiologically, the radial traction of the lung interstitium supports the airways and increases their caliber as lung volume increases. Conversely, as lung volume decreases, airway caliber also decreases and resistance to airflow increases. Patients with airflow obstruction often breathe at large lung volumes because higher volumes tend to increase elastic lung recoil, maximize airway caliber, and minimize flow resistance.

Analysis in terms of laminar and turbulent flow assumes that airways are rigid tubes. In fact, they are highly compressible. The compressibility of the airways underlies the important phenomenon of **effort-independent flow**; airflow rates during expiration can be increased with effort only up to a certain point. Beyond that point, further increases in effort do not increase flow rates. The explanation for this phenomenon relies on the concept of an **equal pressure point**. Pleural pressure is generally negative (sub-atmospheric) throughout quiet breathing. Peribronchiolar pressure, the pressure surrounding small, noncartilaginous conducting airways, is closely related to pleural pressure. Hence, during quiet breathing, conducting airways are surrounded by negative pressure that helps keep them open. Pleural and peribronchiolar pressure becomes positive during forced expiration, subjecting distensible conducting airways to positive pressure. The equal pressure point occurs where the surrounding peribronchiolar pressure equals or exceeds pressure inside the airway, causing **dynamic compression** of the airways, which leads to instability and potential airway collapse (Figure 9–9).

The equal pressure point is not an anatomic site but a functional result that helps clarify different mechanisms of airflow obstruction. Because the driving pressure of expiratory airflow is principally lung elastic recoil pressure, a loss of lung elasticity that reduces recoil pressure without changing pleural or peribronchiolar pressure will lead to dynamic compression at higher lung volumes. The resultant **air trapping** contributes to symptomatic dyspnea in patients with obstructive lung disease. Patients with emphysema lose lung elastic recoil and may have severely impaired expiratory flow even with airways of normal caliber. The presence of airway disease will increase the drop in driving pressure along the airways and may generate an equal pressure point at even higher lung volumes. Conversely, an increase in recoil pressure will oppose dynamic compression. Patients with pulmonary fibrosis may have abnormally high flow rates despite severely reduced lung volumes.

The Work of Breathing

A constant minute ventilation can be achieved through multiple combinations of respiratory rate and tidal volume. The two components of the work of breathing—elastic forces and resistance to airflow—are affected in opposite ways by changes in frequency and depth of breathing. Elastic resistance is minimized by frequent shallow breaths; resistive forces are minimized by fewer larger-tidal-volume breaths. Figure 9–10

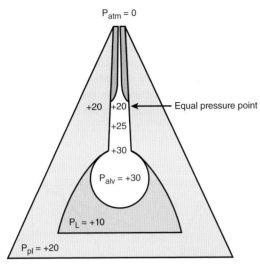

FIGURE 9–9 The concept of the equal pressure point. For air to flow through a tube, there must be a pressure difference between the two ends. In the case of forced expiration with an open glottis, this driving pressure is the difference between alveolar pressure (the sum of pleural pressure and lung elastic recoil pressure) and atmospheric pressure (assumed to be zero). Frictional resistance causes a fall in this driving pressure along the length of the conducting airways. At some point, the driving pressure may equal the surrounding peribronchial pressure; in this event, the net transmural pressure is zero. This defines the equal pressure point. Downstream (toward the mouth) from the equal pressure point, pressure outside the airway is greater than the driving pressure inside the airway. This net negative pressure tends to collapse the airway, resulting in dynamic compression. The more forcefully one expires, the more the pressure surrounding collapsible airways increases. Flow becomes effort independent. (P_{alv}, alveolar pressure; P_{atm}, atmospheric pressure; P_L, lung elastic recoil pressure; P_{pl}, pleural pressure.)

shows how these two components can be summed to provide a total work of breathing for different frequencies at a fixed minute ventilation. The set point for basal respiration is the point at which the total work of breathing is minimized.

In normal humans, this occurs at a frequency of approximately 15 breaths/min. In different diseases, this pattern is altered to compensate for the underlying physiologic abnormality.

The amount of energy needed to maintain the respiratory muscles during quiet breathing is small, approximately 2% of basal oxygen consumption. In patients with lung disease, the energy requirements are greater at rest and increase dramatically with exercise. Patients with emphysema may not be able to increase their ventilation by more than a factor of 2 because the oxygen cost of breathing exceeds the additional oxygen made available to the body.

Oxygen Transport

Oxygen is poorly soluble in blood. At a temperature of 37°C and an oxygen partial pressure of 100 mm Hg ($PaO_2 = 100$), total oxygen dissolved in 100 mL of whole blood is approximately 0.3 mL. Because basal oxygen consumption in the average adult human is approximately 250 mL/min, dissolved oxygen content would be inadequate to meet metabolic demands. Instead, the high oxygen needs of complex internal organs are met by a soluble protein that binds oxygen rapidly, reversibly, and with a high storage capacity, namely, hemoglobin.

Hemoglobin is a complex tetramer of two alpha and two beta polypeptide chains, each of which contains a heme group with an iron atom in the ferrous form (Fe^{2+}) at its center capable of binding molecular oxygen (O_2). Each molecule of hemoglobin can bind four oxygen molecules. Under physiologic conditions, 1 g of fully saturated hemoglobin can carry approximately 1.34 mL of oxygen. Therefore, 100 mL of blood containing 15 g/dL of saturated hemoglobin contains 20.1 mL of O_2, nearly 70 times the amount in solution. The conventional way to represent oxygen bound to hemoglobin is the **hemoglobin saturation (SO_2)**, the ratio of oxygen bound to hemoglobin divided by the total oxygen-binding capacity, typically expressed as a percentage. Note that SO_2 alone does not determine oxygen content. Blood oxygen content is the sum of

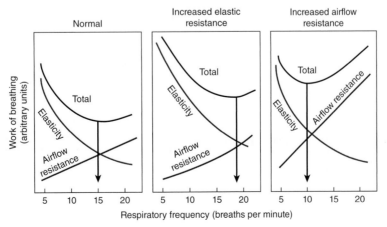

FIGURE 9–10 Minimizing the work of breathing. These diagrams divide the total work of breathing at the same minute ventilation into elastic and resistive components. In disease states that increase elastic forces (eg, pulmonary fibrosis), total work is minimized by rapid, shallow breathing; with increased airflow resistance (eg, chronic bronchitis), total work is minimized by slow, deep breathing. (Redrawn, with permission, from Lumb AB. *Nunn's Applied Respiratory Physiology*, 8th ed. Elsevier, 2016. Copyright © Elsevier.)

two terms: dissolved oxygen and oxygen bound to hemoglobin. Dissolved oxygen is a linear function of the oxygen partial pressure (PO_2) and solubility, whereas oxygen bound to hemoglobin is the product of three terms: oxygen-carrying capacity, hemoglobin concentration, and hemoglobin saturation (SO_2):

$$CO_2 = (0.003 \times PO_2) + (1.34 \times [\text{Hemoglobin}] \times SO_2)$$

This equation explains why oxygen content and tissue oxygen delivery may be low despite 100% SO_2 if hemoglobin concentration is markedly reduced.

Because of its physical chemistry, hemoglobin saturation has a complex relationship with the partial pressure of oxygen. Interactions among the four polypeptide chains in the heme molecule increase overall affinity for oxygen as each oxygen-binding site is filled. If we graph PO_2 against SO_2 to represent the **oxyhemoglobin dissociation curve**, we see that the relationship is not linear but S-shaped or sigmoidal (Figure 9–11). The curve is very steep in the physiologic range, (ie, between 10 and 70 mm Hg PO_2). Above a partial pressure of 70 mm Hg, the oxyhemoglobin dissociation curve flattens. This relationship explains the suitability of hemoglobin for its primary physiologic role: the reversible binding to oxygen with uptake in the lungs and release in the tissues. Both illness and changes in altitude can cause the PO_2 to decrease significantly, but as long as the partial pressure remains above 70 mm Hg, there will be a minimal consequence on the O_2 saturation of hemoglobin and, in turn, the oxygen content. From 70 to 40 mm Hg, a fall in PO_2 is associated with a proportionally larger increase in the release of oxygen from hemoglobin while retaining a relatively high end-capillary PO_2 to promote oxygen diffusion into tissues. Below 40 mm Hg, small changes in PO_2 continue to release oxygen to tissues, down to very low PO_2 levels encountered in some capillary beds.

Distribution of Ventilation & Perfusion

Inhaled air and pulmonary arterial blood flow are not distributed equally to all lung regions. In healthy individuals, heterogeneous distribution is due principally to two factors: the effects of gravity and the fractal geometry of repetitive branching of airways and vessels.

Pleural pressure varies from the top to the bottom of the lung by approximately 0.25 cm H_2O/cm. It is more negative at the apex and more positive at the base. The effect is shifted to an anteroposterior distribution in the supine position and is greatly diminished (although not abolished) at zero gravity. Regional ventilation depends on regional pleural pressure (Figure 9–12). More negative pleural pressure at the lung apex

FIGURE 9–12 Distribution of ventilation at different lung volumes. The effect of gravity and the weight of the lung cause pleural pressure to become more negative toward the apex of the lung. The effect of this change in pressure is to increase the expansion of apical alveoli. **A:** Total lung capacity. At high lung volumes, the compliance curve of the lung is flat; alveoli are almost equally expanded because pressure differences cause small changes in lung volume. **B:** Functional residual capacity. During quiet breathing, the lower lobes are on the steep part of the pressure–volume curve. This increased compliance at lower volumes is why ventilation at FRC is preferentially distributed to the lower lobes. **C:** Residual volume. Below functional residual capacity (FRC), there may be dependent lung units that are exposed to positive pleural pressures. These units may collapse, leading to areas of lung that are perfused but not ventilated. (Reprinted, with permission, from Hinshaw HC et al. *Diseases of the Chest*, 4th ed. WB Saunders, 1979. Copyright © Elsevier.)

PO₂ (mm Hg)	SO₂ % Hb sat	CO₂ (mL/dL) Hb-bound*	CO₂ (mL/dL) Dissolved O₂
600	100	201	1.8
200	99	199	0.6
100	98	197	0.3
90	97	195	0.27
80	96	193	0.24
70	94	188.9	0.21
60	91	182.9	0.18
50	85	170.9	0.15
40	75	150.8	0.12
30	58	116.6	0.09
27	50	100.5	0.08
20	32	64.3	0.06
10	10	20.1	0.03

*Hg = 15 g/dL

FIGURE 9–11 Oxygen–hemoglobin dissociation curve. pH 7.40, temperature 38°C. (Data from Severinghaus JW. Blood gas calculator. J Appl Physiol. 1966;21:1108.)

causes greater expansion of the apical alveoli. Because lung compliance is higher at lower lung volumes, ventilation is preferentially distributed to the lower lobes at FRC.

Pulmonary blood flow is a low-pressure system that functions in a gravitational field across 30 vertical centimeters. In the upright position, there is a nearly linear increase in blood flow from the top to the bottom of the lung. Within any horizontal (isogravitational) plane, however, there is significant heterogeneity of blood flow because of the fractal geometry of repetitive vessel branching, resulting in heterogeneous resistance. Figure 9–13 illustrates the details of this distribution.

One additional factor that regulates blood flow is **hypoxic pulmonary vasoconstriction**. The smooth muscle cells of pulmonary arterioles are sensitive to alveolar PO_2 (much more so than to arterial PO_2). As alveolar PO_2 falls, there is

arteriolar constriction, an increase in local resistance to flow, and redistribution of flow to regions of higher alveolar PO_2. When regionalized, this is an effective mechanism to diminish local blood flow without a significant increase in mean pulmonary arterial pressure. When it affects more than 20% of the pulmonary circulation, such as in the setting of global alveolar hypoxia, widespread pulmonary vasoconstriction increases mean pulmonary arterial pressure and may result in pulmonary hypertension.

Matching of Ventilation to Perfusion

The functional role of the lungs is to place ambient air in close proximity to circulating blood to permit gas exchange by simple diffusion. To accomplish this, air and blood flow must be

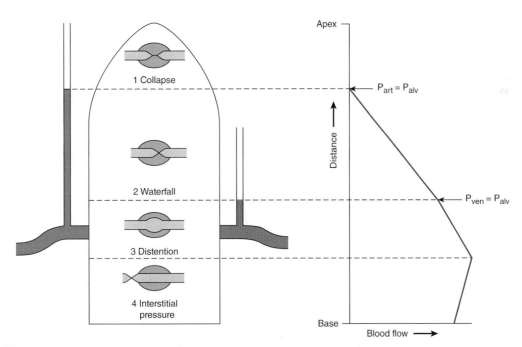

FIGURE 9–13 Effect of changing hydrostatic pressure on the distribution of pulmonary blood flow. Capillary blood flow in different regions of the lung is governed by three pressures: pulmonary arterial pressure, pulmonary venous pressure, and alveolar pressure. Pulmonary arterial pressure must be greater than pulmonary venous pressure to maintain forward perfusion; there are, therefore, three potential arrangements of these variables. **Zone 1:** $P_{alv} > P_{art} > P_{ven}$. There is no capillary perfusion in areas where alveolar pressure is greater than the capillary perfusion pressure. Because alveolar pressure is normally zero, this occurs only where mean pulmonary arterial pressure is less than the vertical distance from the pulmonary artery. **Zone 2:** $P_{art} > P_{alv} > P_{ven}$. Pulmonary arterial pressure exceeds alveolar pressure, but alveolar pressure exceeds pulmonary venous pressure. The driving pressure along the capillary is dissipated by resistance to flow until the transmural pressure is negative and compression occurs. This zone of collapse then regulates flow, which is intermittent and dependent on fluctuating pulmonary venous pressures. **Zone 3:** $P_{art} > P_{ven} > P_{alv}$. Flow is independent of alveolar pressure because the pulmonary venous pressure exceeds atmospheric pressure. **Zone 4:** Zone of extra-alveolar compression. In dependent lung regions, lung interstitial pressure may exceed pulmonary arterial pressure. In this event, capillary flow is determined by compression of extra-alveolar vessels. The right side of the diagram shows a near-continuous distribution of blood flow from the top of the lung to the bottom, demonstrating that in the normal lung there are no discrete zones. The normal human lung at FRC spans 30 vertical centimeters, half of which distance is above the pulmonary artery and left atrium, and representative pulmonary arterial pressures are 33/11 cm H_2O with a mean of 19 cm H_2O. There is, therefore, no physiologic zone 1 in upright humans except perhaps in late diastole. Left atrial pressure averages 11 cm H_2O and is sufficient to create zone 3 conditions two-thirds of the distance from the heart to the apex. However, in patients undergoing positive-pressure mechanical ventilation, or in patients with airway disease creating lung units that fail to empty during the normal respiratory cycle, alveolar pressure is no longer atmospheric. Under conditions of positive end-expiratory pressure (PEEP), P_{alv} may be as high as 15–20 cm H_2O. This potentially shifts the entire distribution of pulmonary blood flow. (Adapted and reprinted, with permission, from Hughes JM et al. Effect of lung volume on the distribution of pulmonary blood flow in man. Respir Physiol. 1968;4(1):58–72. Copyright © Elsevier.)

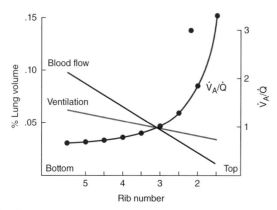

FIGURE 9–14 Changing distribution of ventilation and perfusion down the upright lung. The two straight lines reflect the progressive increases in ventilation and perfusion. The slope is steeper for perfusion. The ratio of ventilation to perfusion is, therefore, lowest at the base and highest at the apex. (Redrawn, with permission, from West JB. *Ventilation/Blood Flow and Gas Exchange*, 5th ed. Blackwell, 1990.)

directed to the same place at the same time. Optimum functioning of the respiratory system requires that ventilation be matched to perfusion.

In the normal individual, typical resting alveolar ventilation is approximately 4 L/min, whereas pulmonary artery blood flow is 5 L/min. This yields an overall ratio of ventilation to perfusion of 0.8. As noted above, ventilation and perfusion are both preferentially distributed to dependent regions at rest, although the increase in gravity-dependent flow is more marked with perfusion than with ventilation. Hence, the ratio of ventilation to perfusion is highest at the apex and lowest at the base (Figure 9–14).

Regional alterations from the **ideal** situation of matched uniform distribution of ventilation and perfusion (Figure 9–15, top left panel) are referred to as $\dot{V}/\dot{Q}$ **mismatch** and are an extremely important phenomenon underlying the functional impairment of many disease states. A distribution may favor low $\dot{V}/\dot{Q}$ ratios, with the extreme case being a shunt (perfusion without ventilation, or $\dot{V}/\dot{Q} = 0$), or it may favor high $\dot{V}/\dot{Q}$ ratios, with the extreme case being alveolar dead space (ventilation without perfusion, or $\dot{V}/\dot{Q} = \infty$). These two types of $\dot{V}/\dot{Q}$ mismatch affect respiratory function very differently. A shift toward low $\dot{V}/\dot{Q}$ ratios occurs when regional ventilation is reduced or eliminated but perfusion persists, as might happen with atelectatic lung or in areas of lung consolidation where alveoli are filled with fluid or infected debris. A **shunt** (Figure 9–15, top right panel) is the extreme case of a low $\dot{V}/\dot{Q}$ area where ventilation is absent and the ratio goes to zero. Pulmonary arterial (mixed venous) blood will then pass to the systemic arterial circulation without coming into contact with alveolar gas. The primary physiologic effect of such a right-to-left shunt is to reduce arterial PO_2. The lung is able to reflexively respond to regional hypoxemia by decreasing blood flow to these areas, thereby restoring ventilation-to-perfusion balance.

In the normal individual, approximately one-third of resting minute ventilation fills the main conducting airways. This is the anatomic dead space; it represents ventilation to areas that do not participate in gas exchange. If participating gas-exchanging regions of the lung are ventilated but not perfused, as may occur in pulmonary embolism, pulmonary vascular disease, or emphysema, these regions will also fail to function in gas exchange and are referred to as **alveolar dead space** or **wasted ventilation** (Figure 9–15, bottom left panel). Functionally, a shift toward high $\dot{V}/\dot{Q}$ ratios means that more work of breathing supports ventilation that does not participate in gas exchange, reducing the overall efficiency of ventilation and CO_2 removal. In the absence of respiratory compensation, the primary effect of increased dead space is a rise in arterial PCO_2; PaO_2 may fall as a result of increased alveolar PO_2. Because the respiratory control center is exquisitely sensitive to small changes in $PaCO_2$, however, the most common integrated response to increasing wasted ventilation is to increase total minute ventilation (which includes ventilation to perfused alveolar units), thereby maintaining $PaCO_2$ nearly constant. In this **compensated** state (Figure 9–15, bottom right panel), PaO_2 remains normal. The A–a ΔPO_2 is increased (discussed below). This adaptive response may be unconscious, but it presents a clinical problem when the individual can no longer sustain an increased minute ventilation, as in the patient with advanced emphysema.

Ventilation/perfusion mismatching commonly occurs between the limiting cases of true shunts and alveolar dead space. The effect on arterial blood gases of shifts in the distribution of $\dot{V}/\dot{Q}$ ratios can be predicted from a discussion of the limiting cases (Figure 9–16). The top panel of Figure 9–16 illustrates a respiratory unit where on one side (B), ventilation has been reduced but perfusion maintained. This defines an area of **low $\dot{V}/\dot{Q}$ ratio**. The physiologic effect of low $\dot{V}/\dot{Q}$ areas is similar to the effect of shunts: hypoxemia without hypercapnia. The difference between low $\dot{V}/\dot{Q}$ areas and true shunts can also be seen by comparing this schematic with Figure 9–15. As shown in the top right panel of Figure 9–15, shunted blood does not come into contact with inspired air; therefore, no amount of additional oxygen supplied to inspired air will reverse the fall in systemic arterial PO_2. In contrast, a low $\dot{V}/\dot{Q}$ area (Figure 9–16, top panel) does come in contact with inspired air, and the fall in systemic arterial PO_2 can be reversed with increased inspired oxygen.

The bottom panel of Figure 9–16 illustrates a respiratory unit where on one side (B), blood flow has been decreased but ventilation maintained. This defines an area of **high $\dot{V}/\dot{Q}$ ratio.** The effect on lung function can be understood by dividing the unit into an area with a normal $\dot{V}/\dot{Q}$ ratio (A) and an area of dead space or wasted ventilation (B′). The physiologic effect of high $\dot{V}/\dot{Q}$ ratios is an increase in PCO_2, typically leading to increased respiration to return $PaCO_2$ to normal.

Hyperventilation of unaffected lung regions can compensate for the increase in PCO_2 from alveolar dead space but cannot compensate for the decrease in PO_2 from areas of shunt. The reason for this is the different ways that oxygen and

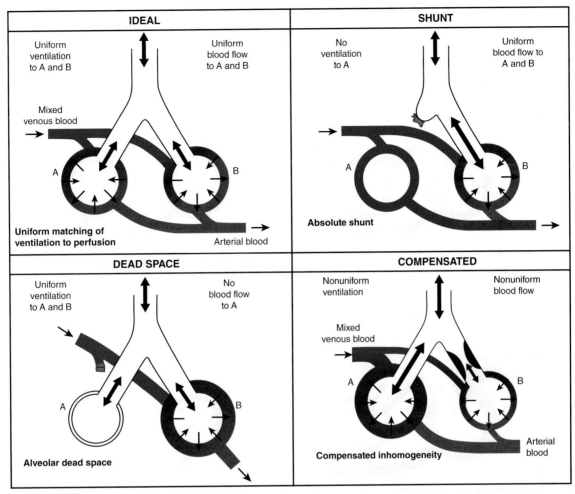

FIGURE 9–15 Four models of the relationship of ventilation to perfusion. In this schematic representation, circles represent respiratory units and tubes depict conducting airways. The colored channels represent pulmonary blood flow, which enters the capillary bed as mixed venous blood (blue) and leaves it as arterialized blood (red). Blood is depicted as purple in situations with insufficient oxygenation. Large arrows show the distribution of inspired gas; small arrows show the diffusion of O_2 and CO_2. In the **ideal** case (**top left panel**), the PaO_2 and $PaCO_2$ leaving respiratory units A and B are identical. A **shunt** (**top right panel**) is a low $\dot{V}/\dot{Q}$ area where ventilation is absent and the ratio goes to zero, reducing the arterial PO_2. If participating gas-exchanging regions of the lung are ventilated but not perfused, these regions also fail to function in gas exchange; referred to as alveolar **dead space** (**bottom left panel**), they reduce the overall efficiency of ventilation and CO_2 removal (wasted ventilation). However, one response to an increasing wasted ventilation is to increase total minute ventilation (which includes ventilation to perfused alveolar units), thereby maintaining a nearly constant $PaCO_2$ and normal PaO_2, a so-called **compensated** state (**bottom right panel**). See text for details. (Redrawn, with permission, from Comroe J. *Physiology of Respiration*, 2nd ed. Year Book, 1974. Copyright © Elsevier.)

carbon dioxide are carried in blood, and the different relationships between the content and partial pressure of these gases. Because PCO_2 and CO_2 content are linearly related within the normal physiologic range, increased ventilation to one respiratory unit will reduce the PCO_2 *and* the CO_2 content of blood leaving that unit. Overall CO_2 content will be the mean of the affected and unaffected units. Because PCO_2 is proportionate to the CO_2 content, the reduced CO_2 content of hyperventilated lung regions compensates for elevated content from areas of wasted ventilation. The PCO_2 and CO_2 content of the mixture track together.

Hyperventilation or increasing inspired oxygen to unaffected lung regions does not compensate for the decrease in PO_2 from areas of true shunt. The O_2 content of blood is not linearly related to PO_2 (see Figure 9–11). The sigmoidal shape of the oxyhemoglobin dissociation curve indicates that hemoglobin is nearly maximally saturated at a PO_2 of 60. Increasing PO_2 from 60 to 600 increases partial pressure 10-fold but O_2 content by only 10%. Increasing ventilation or increasing alveolar PO_2 to unaffected respiratory units can increase end-capillary PO_2 but will not change the O_2 content of blood leaving those units. Overall O_2 content will be the mean of normal blood oxygen content and shunted, desaturated blood. The reduced oxygen content of the mixture tends to lie on the steep portion of the oxyhemoglobin dissociation curve, with the result that modest decreases in oxygen content lead to large decreases in the PO_2.

FIGURE 9–16 Ventilation/perfusion mismatching. The top panel shows a respiratory unit where on one side (B), ventilation has been reduced but perfusion is maintained. This defines an area of **low V̇/Q̇ ratio**. The physiologic effect of low V̇/Q̇ areas appears similar to the effect of shunts: hypoxemia without hypercapnia. But since a low V̇/Q̇ area does come in contact with inspired air, the fall in PaO₂ can be reversed with increased inhaled FiO₂. The bottom panel shows a respiratory unit where on one side (B), blood flow has been decreased but ventilation is maintained. This defines an area of **high V̇/Q̇ ratio**. The effect on lung function can be understood by dividing the unit into an area with a normal V̇/Q̇ ratio (A) and an area of dead space or wasted ventilation (B′). The physiologic effect of high V̇/Q̇ ratios is to increase PCO₂, typically leading to increased respiration to return PaCO₂ to normal. (Blue, deoxygenated; red, oxygenated.) See the Figure 9–15 legend and the text for details. (Redrawn, with permission, from Comroe J. *Physiology of Respiration*, 2nd ed. Year Book, 1974. Copyright © Elsevier.)

Arterial blood gases detect major disturbances in respiratory function. One attempt to assess more subtle abnormalities of gas exchange is to calculate the difference between the alveolar and arterial PO_2. This is referred to as the A–a ΔPO_2 or A–a DO_2. The alveolar–capillary membrane permits full equilibration of alveolar and end-capillary oxygen tension under normal V̇/Q̇ matching. There is nonetheless a small A–a ΔPO_2 in normal individuals as a result of right-to-left shunting through the bronchial veins and the thebesian veins of the left heart. This accounts for approximately 2–5% of resting cardiac output and leads to an A–a ΔPO_2 of 5–8 mm Hg in healthy young adults breathing ambient air at sea level. Increasing the fractional inspired concentration of oxygen (FiO₂) increases this value: A normal A–a ΔPO_2 breathing 100% oxygen is approximately 100 mm Hg. Normal values increase with age, presumably as a result of the closure of dependent airways with a consequent shift toward low V̇/Q̇ ratios. Further increases in the A–a ΔPO_2 reflect areas of low V̇/Q̇ ratio, including shunting.

Control of Breathing

The lungs inflate and deflate passively in response to changes in pleural pressure. Therefore, control over respiration lies in control of the striated muscles—chiefly the diaphragm but also the intercostals and abdominal wall—that change pleural pressure.

These muscles are under both automatic and voluntary control. The rhythm of spontaneous breathing originates in the

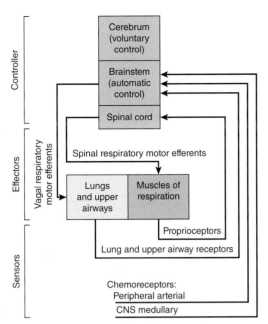

FIGURE 9–17 Schematic representation of the respiratory control system. The interrelationships among the CNS controller, effectors, and sensors are shown, as are the connections among these components. (Redrawn, with permission, from Berger AJ et al. Regulation of respiration. N Engl J Med. 1977;297:92. Copyright © 1977 Massachusetts Medical Society. Reprinted with permission from Massachusetts Medical Society.)

brainstem, specifically in several groups of interconnected neurons in the medulla. Research into the generation of the respiratory rhythm has identified that it originates in the neurons of the pre-Bötzinger complex. Respiratory neurons are either inspiratory or expiratory and may fire early, late, or in an accelerating fashion during the respiratory cycle. Their integrated output is an efferent signal via the phrenic nerve (diaphragm) and spinal nerves (intercostals and abdominal wall) to generate rhythmic contraction and relaxation of the respiratory musculature. The result is spontaneous breathing without conscious input. However, by attending to breathing, one may alter this pattern. Eating, speaking, singing, swimming, and defecating all rely on voluntary control over automatic breathing.

A. Sensory Input

The frequency, depth, and timing of spontaneous breathing are modified by information provided to the respiratory center from both chemical and mechanical sensors (Figure 9–17).

There are chemoreceptors in the peripheral vasculature and in the brainstem. The peripheral chemoreceptors are the carotid bodies, located at the bifurcation of the common carotid arteries and the aortic bodies near the arch of the aorta. The carotid bodies are particularly important in humans. They function as sensors of arterial oxygenation. There is a graded increase in firing of the carotid body in response to a fall in the PaO_2. This response is most marked below 60 mm Hg. An increase in the $PaCO_2$ or a fall in arterial pH potentiates the response of the carotid body to decreases in the PaO_2.

In humans, the carotid bodies are solely responsible for the increased ventilation seen in response to hypoxia. Bilateral carotid body resection, which has been performed to treat disabling dyspnea and may happen as an unintended consequence of carotid thromboendarterectomy, results in a complete loss of this hypoxic ventilatory drive while leaving intact the response to changes in $PaCO_2$. Central chemoreceptors mediate the response to changes in $PaCO_2$. There is growing evidence that these chemoreceptors are widely dispersed throughout the brainstem. They are separate from the neurons that generate the respiratory rhythm. The increased ventilatory response to elevation in $PaCO_2$ is mediated through changes in chemoreceptor pH. The blood–brain barrier permits free diffusion of CO_2 but not hydrogen ions. CO_2 is hydrated to carbonic acid, which ionizes and lowers brain pH. Central chemoreceptors probably respond to these changes in intracellular hydrogen ion concentration.

There are a variety of pulmonary stretch receptors located in airway smooth muscle and mucosa whose afferent fibers are carried in the vagus nerve. They discharge in response to lung distention. Increasing lung volume decreases the rate of respiration by increasing expiratory time. This is known as the Hering–Breuer reflex. There are unmyelinated C fibers located near the pulmonary capillaries (hence juxtacapillary [J] receptors). These fibers are quiet during normal breathing but can be directly stimulated by the intravenous administration of irritant chemicals such as capsaicin. They appear to stimulate the increased respiratory drive in interstitial edema and pulmonary fibrosis. Skeletal movement transmitted by proprioceptors in joints, muscles, and tendons causes an increase in respiration and may have some role in the increased ventilation of exercise. Finally, there are muscle spindle receptors in the diaphragm and intercostals that provide feedback on muscle force. They may be involved in the sensation of dyspnea when the work of breathing is disproportionate to ventilation.

B. Integrated Responses

Under normal conditions in healthy adults, the hydrogen ion concentration in the region of the central chemoreceptors determines the drive to breathe. Changes in chemoreceptor pH are largely determined by the $PaCO_2$. The PaO_2 is not an important part of the baseline respiratory drive under normal conditions.

Breathing is stimulated by a fall in the PaO_2, a rise in the $PaCO_2$, or an increase in the hydrogen ion concentration of arterial blood (fall in arterial pH).

Ventilation increases approximately 2–3 L/min for every 1 mm Hg rise in $PaCO_2$. This response (Figure 9–18) occurs first through sensitization of the carotid body receptor. The carotid body will increase its firing in response to an increased $PaCO_2$ even in the absence of changes in the PaO_2. This accounts for approximately 15% of the ventilatory response to hypercapnia. The majority of the response is mediated

FIGURE 9–18 Ventilatory response to CO_2. The curves represent changes in minute ventilation plotted against changes in inspired PCO_2 at different values of alveolar PO_2. There is a linear increase in ventilation with increasing PCO_2. The rate of increase is greater at lower PO_2 values, but the curves begin from a common point at which ventilation should cease in response to lowered PCO_2. In awake humans, arousal maintains ventilation even when the PCO_2 falls below this level; when lightly anesthetized, apnea does occur. In the case of metabolic acidosis, this x-intercept is shifted to the left, but the slope of the lines remains virtually unchanged. This indicates that the effects of metabolic acidosis are separate from and additive to the effects of respiratory acidosis. (BTPS, body temperature and pressure, saturated with water vapor.) (Redrawn, with permission, from Barrett KE et al. *Ganong's Review of Medical Physiology*, 25th ed. McGraw-Hill, 2016.)

FIGURE 9–19 Isocapnic ventilatory response to hypoxia. These curves represent changes in minute ventilation plotted against changes in alveolar PO_2 when the alveolar PCO_2 is held constant at 37, 44, or 49 mm Hg. When PCO_2 is in the normal range (37–44 mm Hg), there is little increase in ventilation until the PO_2 is reduced to between 50 and 60 mm Hg. The ventilatory response to hypoxia is augmented at elevated PCO_2 levels. The response to hypoxia is not linear, as it is in response to an increased PCO_2, but resembles a rectangular hyperbola asymptotic to infinite ventilation (at a PO_2 in the low 30s) and ventilation without tonic stimulation from the carotid bodies (which occurs above a PO_2 of 500 mm Hg). Not shown is the fall in minute ventilation that occurs with extreme hypoxia (PO_2 values below 30 mm Hg) as a result of depression of the respiratory center. (Redrawn, with permission, from Barrett KE et al. *Ganong's Review of Medical Physiology*, 25th ed. McGraw-Hill, 2016.)

through pH changes in the region of the central chemoreceptors. Changes in arterial pH are additive to changes in $PaCO_2$. CO_2 response curves under conditions of metabolic acidosis have an identical slope but are shifted to the left. The ventilatory response to an increased $PaCO_2$ falls with age, sleep, aerobic conditioning, and increased work of breathing.

The individual response to hypoxemia is extremely variable. Normally, there is little increase in ventilation until the PaO_2 falls below 50–60 mm Hg. At this point, there is a rapid increase in ventilation that reaches its maximum at approximately 32 mm Hg. Below this level, further decreases in PaO_2 lead to depression of ventilation. The response to hypoxia is affected by the $PaCO_2$. An increase in the alveolar PCO_2 will shift the isocapnic O_2 response curve upward and to the right (Figure 9–19).

A fall in arterial hydrogen ion concentration increases minute ventilation. This response results chiefly from stimulation of the carotid bodies and is independent of changes in $PaCO_2$. There is a response to severe metabolic acidosis in the absence of carotid bodies. It is assumed that this response is mediated by central chemoreceptors; it may represent a breakdown of the blood–brain barrier.

C. Special Situations

1. **Chronic hypercapnia**—In patients with chronic hypercapnia, brain pH is returned toward normal by compensatory changes in serum and tissue bicarbonate levels. As a result, central chemoreceptors become less sensitive to further changes in $PaCO_2$. In this instance, a patient's basal minute ventilation may depend on tonic stimuli from the carotid bodies. If such a patient were given high concentrations of inspired oxygen, carotid body output may be depressed, leading to a fall in minute ventilation. The change in minute ventilation does not fully account for the hypercapnia in response to supplemental oxygen, suggesting that ablation of hypoxic pulmonary vasoconstriction also plays a role.

2. **Chronic hypoxia**—Long-term residence at high altitude—or sleep apnea with repeated episodes of severe oxygen desaturation—may blunt the hypoxic ventilatory response. In such individuals, the development of lung disease and hypercapnia may attenuate all endogenous stimuli to breathing. This pattern is seen in patients with obesity-hypoventilation syndrome.

3. **Exercise**—Exercise may increase minute ventilation up to 25 times the resting level. Strenuous but submaximal exercise in a healthy individual typically causes no change or only a slight increaes in PaO_2 as a result of increased pulmonary blood flow and better matching of ventilation to perfusion, with no change or a slight fall in $PaCO_2$. Changes in arterial oxygenation are, therefore, not a factor behind the increased ventilatory response to exercise. The reason for the increased ventilatory response is not known with certainty. Two contributing factors are the increased production of carbon dioxide and increased afferent discharge from joint and muscle proprioceptors.

CHECKPOINT

12. What are the components of lung elastic recoil? What is the role of surfactant?
13. What three opposing forces must be overcome normally to inflate the lungs?
14. What are four factors affecting airway resistance?
15. What are the components of the work of breathing?
16. What factors regulate ventilation, and what factors regulate perfusion?
17. How are ventilation and perfusion normally matched?
18. What are the effects of changing CO_2 and O_2 levels on respiratory control?

PATHOPHYSIOLOGY OF SELECTED LUNG DISEASES

OBSTRUCTIVE LUNG DISEASES: ASTHMA & CHRONIC OBSTRUCTIVE PULMONARY DISEASE (COPD)

The fundamental physiologic problem in obstructive lung diseases is increased resistance to expiratory airflow as a result of caliber reduction of conducting airways. This increased resistance can be caused by processes (1) within the lumen, (2) in the airway wall, or (3) in the supporting structures surrounding the airway. Examples of luminal obstruction include the increased secretions seen in asthma and chronic bronchitis. Airway wall thickening and airway narrowing can result from inflammation, a characteristic feature of both asthma and chronic bronchitis, or from bronchial smooth muscle contraction, as occurs in asthma. Emphysema is the classic example of obstruction caused by loss of surrounding supporting structure, with expiratory airway collapse resulting from the destruction of the elastin-containing alveolar wall attachments. Although the causes and clinical presentations of these diseases are distinct, the common elements of their physiology are instructive.

1. Asthma

Clinical Presentation

Asthma is a clinical syndrome with multiple phenotypes. This diversity reflects complex interactions between genetic predisposition and environmental exposure and suggests heterogeneity in the underlying pathophysiology.

Asthma is a disease of airway inflammation and variable airflow obstruction characterized by intermittent symptoms, including wheezing, chest tightness, shortness of breath (dyspnea), and cough, together with demonstrable bronchial hyperresponsiveness. Exposure to defined allergens or to various nonspecific stimuli initiates a cascade of cellular activation events in the airways, resulting in both acute and chronic inflammatory processes mediated by a complex and integrated assortment of locally released cytokines and other mediators. Release of mediators can alter airway smooth muscle tone and responsiveness, induce mucus hypersecretion, and damage airway epithelium. These pathologic events result in chronically abnormal airway architecture and function.

Inherent in the definition of asthma is the possibility of considerable variation in the magnitude and manifestations of the disease within and between individuals over time. For example, whereas many asthmatic patients have infrequent and mild symptoms, others may have persistent or prolonged symptoms of great severity. Similarly, initiating or exacerbating stimuli may be quite different between individual patients.

Epidemiology & Risk Factors

Asthma is a common chronic pulmonary disease, affecting approximately 300 million people worldwide. Globally, asthma is estimated to be responsible for 346,000 deaths per year. Overall U.S. prevalence was 7.8% in 2015, with higher rates in males younger than 18 years (9.9%) and in females older than 18 years (9.7%). Each year, approximately 500,000 hospital admissions and 4500 deaths in the United States are attributed to asthma. Prevalence, hospitalizations, and fatal events have all increased in the United States over the past 30 years. Mortality rates reached a plateau in the late 1990s and have declined slightly over the past two decades. Hospitalization rates have been highest among blacks and children, and death rates are consistently highest among blacks aged 15–24 years.

The strongest identifiable predisposing factor for the development of asthma is atopy, or the production of immunoglobulin E (IgE) antibodies in response to allergen exposure. Fifty-six percent of asthma cases were attributable to atopy in the National Health and Nutrition Examination Survey III (NHANES III) of 12,106 Americans done between 1988 and 1994. Exposure of sensitive patients to inhaled allergens

TABLE 9–3   Asthma: Provocative factors.

Physiologic and pharmacologic mediators of normal smooth muscle contraction
Histamine
Methacholine
Adenosine triphosphate
Physicochemical agents
Exercise; hyperventilation with cold, dry air
Air pollutants
Sulfur dioxide
Nitrogen dioxide
Viral respiratory infections (eg, influenza A)
Ingestants
Propranolol
Aspirin; NSAIDs
Allergens
Low-molecular-weight chemicals (eg, penicillin, isocyanates, anhydrides, chromate)
Complex organic molecules (eg, animal danders, dust mites, enzymes, wood dusts)

increases airway inflammation, airway hyperresponsiveness, and asthma symptoms. Symptoms may develop immediately (immediate asthmatic response) or 4–6 hours after allergen exposure (late asthmatic response). Table 9–3 lists common allergens. In multiple studies, obesity is associated with an increased prevalence of asthma.

Indoor exposure to house dust mite or cockroach antigens is a strong risk factor for asthma. At the same time, it is well established that children raised on farms have *lower* prevalences of atopy and asthma, and the diversity of microbial exposure in childhood was shown in one study to be inversely related to risk of asthma. These observations, and the increased incidence of atopy, allergy, and autoimmune diseases in the developed world, have led researchers to pursue the underlying causes of atopy itself. One theory is that early childhood exposure to infections and/or organic antigens may fundamentally alter adaptive immunity. Some exposures may promote a T_H1 phenotype (differentiation of CD4+ T-helper cells toward a T_H1 response characterized by production of interferon γ), whereas the absence of these exposures may promote a T_H2 phenotype (characterized by a primary cytokine response that includes interleukin-4 [IL-4], IL-5, IL-13, and tumor necrosis factor, which together are associated with atopy, allergic diseases, and asthma). The complexity of the immune response and its interactions with the human microbiome preclude any firm conclusions at this time, but this is a rapidly expanding area of research that promises to reshape our basic understanding of the etiology of atopy and asthma.

Genetic factors are also strongly implicated in asthma risk. Twin studies have estimated that asthma is up to 60% heritable. In addition, multiple genome-wide association studies have demonstrated the genetic link between the *ORMDL3/GSDMD* locus on chromosome 17q21 and childhood asthma. The functional mechanism underlying this association remains unclear. Epigenetic changes via DNA methylation of genes involved in the T_H1 and T_H2 immune responses have also been found to be associated with asthma.

Pathogenesis

The fundamental abnormality in asthma is an increased reactivity of airways to stimuli. As outlined in Table 9–3, there are many known provocative agents (triggers) for asthma. These can be broadly categorized as follows: (1) physiologic or pharmacologic mediators of asthmatic airway responses; (2) allergens that can induce airway inflammation and reactivity in sensitized individuals; and (3) exogenous physicochemical agents or stimuli that produce airway hyperreactivity. Some of these provocative agents will produce responses in people with asthma only (eg, exercise, adenosine), whereas others produce characteristically magnified responses in people with asthma that can be used to distinguish them from people without asthma under controlled testing conditions (eg, histamine and methacholine; see later discussion). There is no single mechanism that serves to explain the occurrence of asthma in all individuals. There are, however, common events that characterize the pathologic processes that result in asthma. It is important to recognize the central role of airway inflammation in the evolution of asthma.

The earliest event in asthmatic airway responses is the activation of local inflammatory cells, principally mast cells and eosinophils. Inflammatory cell activation can occur directly by specific IgE-dependent mechanisms or indirectly via other processes (eg, osmotic stimuli or chemical irritant exposure). Acute-acting mediators, including leukotrienes, prostaglandins, and histamine, rapidly induce smooth muscle contraction, mucus hypersecretion, and vasodilation with endothelial leakage and local edema formation. Epithelial cells also appear to be involved in this process, releasing leukotrienes and prostaglandins as well as inflammatory cytokines on activation. Some of these preformed and rapidly acting mediators possess chemotactic activity that attracts additional inflammatory cells, such as eosinophils and neutrophils, to airway mucosa.

A critical process that accompanies these acute events is the recruitment, multiplication, and activation of inflammatory cells through the actions of a network of locally released cytokines and chemokines. Cytokines and chemokines participate in a complex and prolonged series of events that results in the perpetuation of local airway inflammation and hyperresponsiveness (Table 9–4). These events include the promotion of mast cell and eosinophil growth, the influx and proliferation of T lymphocytes, and the differentiation of B lymphocytes to IgE- and IgA-producing plasma cells. An important

TABLE 9–4   Asthma: Cellular inflammatory events.

Epithelial cell activation or injury
Cytokine (IL-8) and chemokine release, with neutrophil chemotaxis or activation
Antigen presentation to lymphocytes
Secretory epithelial cell hyperplasia and hypersecretion
Epithelial death; increased magnitude of airway sensory neural reflexes
Lymphocyte activation
Antigen exposure with lymphocyte proliferation
Increased cytokine and chemokine expression; activation of additional effector cells (dendritic cells, mast cells, eosinophils, macrophages)
Activation of B cells; increased IgE synthesis
Augmented lymphocyte activation by local cytokines
Mast cell and eosinophil activation
Eosinophil release of cytotoxic and acute pro-inflammatory mediators
IgE-mediated mast cell activation, with acute mediator release (eg, histamine, leukotrienes, platelets activating factor)
New expression of multiple cytokines by mast cells, with multiple effector cell activation, as with lymphocytes

component of this process now appears to be the differentiation and activation of helper T lymphocytes of the T_H2 phenotype. These T_H2 lymphocytes, through their production of cytokines, including IL-3, IL-4, IL-5, IL-6, IL-9, IL-10, and IL-13, promote the activation of mast cells, eosinophils, and other effector cells and drive IgE production by B cells, all of which are pathologic components of the asthma phenotype. Thus, through their specific mediators, these multiple cells participate in the many pro-inflammatory processes that are active in the airways of people with asthma. Among these are injury to epithelial cells and denudation of the airway, greater exposure of afferent sensory nerves, and consequent neurally mediated smooth muscle hyperresponsiveness; the upregulation of IgE-mediated mast cell and eosinophil activation, including acute and long-acting mediator release; and submucosal gland hypersecretion with increased mucus volume. Concurrently, the production of growth factors such as TGF-β, TGF-α, and fibroblast growth factor (FGF) by epithelial cells as well as macrophages and other inflammatory cells drives the process of tissue remodeling and submucosal airway fibrosis. This submucosal fibrosis can result in fixed airway obstruction that may complicate chronic airway inflammation in asthma.

Although there is a classic paradigm of allergic asthma (described above), there is an increasing recognition of alternative asthma phenotypes, reinforcing the notion of heterogeneity in the underlying pathogenesis. For example, adult onset non-allergic asthma and asthma in the obese patient are two recognized phenotypes, both of which are typically difficult to treat. The poor response to standard therapy for allergic asthma has motivated research into alternative mechanisms that underlie these phenotypes. Neutrophilic inflammation and the T_H17 immune response are areas of active investigation, but thus far, the precise mechanisms that drive these alternative phenotypes remain unclear.

Pathology

The histopathologic features of asthma reflect the cellular processes at play. Airway mucosa is thickened, edematous, and infiltrated with inflammatory cells, principally lymphocytes, eosinophils, and mast cells. Hypertrophied and contracted airway smooth muscle is also conspicuous. Bronchial and bronchiolar epithelial cells are frequently damaged, in part by secreted cytotoxic molecules from eosinophils, including major basic protein and eosinophil chemotactic protein. Epithelial cell injury and death leave portions of the airway lumen denuded, exposing autonomic and probably noncholinergic, nonadrenergic afferents that can mediate airway hyperreactivity. Secretory gland hyperplasia and mucus hypersecretion are seen, with mucus plugging of airways, a prominent finding in severe asthma. Even in mildly involved asthmatic airways, inflammatory cells are found in increased numbers in the mucosa and submucosa, and subepithelial myofibroblasts are noted to proliferate and produce increased interstitial collagen. In turn, submucosal fibrosis contributes to the relatively fixed airway obstruction that occurs in a subset of people with asthma. The pathologic findings seen in severe fatal asthma parallel the pathologic events described previously but reflect the greater magnitude of the insult. In these patients, severe airway epithelial injury and loss are noted, often with severe and complete obstruction of the airway lumen by mucus plugs.

Pathophysiology

Local cellular events in the airways have important effects on lung function. As a consequence of airway inflammation, mucus hypersecretion, and smooth muscle hyperresponsiveness leading to bronchoconstriction, the airways are narrowed, resulting in an increase in resistance (recall that Raw $\propto 1/\text{radius}^4$). The small-caliber peripheral airways do not contribute significantly to airflow resistance in healthy individuals, but as these airways narrow in patients with asthma, they contribute substantially to airflow obstruction. Bronchial neural function also appears to play a role in the evolution of asthma, although this is probably of secondary importance. Cough and reflex bronchoconstriction mediated by vagal efferents follows stimulation of bronchial irritant receptors. Peptide neurotransmitters may also play a role. The pro-inflammatory neuropeptide substance P can be released from unmyelinated afferent fibers in the airways and can induce smooth muscle contraction and mediator release from mast cells. VIP is the peptide neurotransmitter of some airway nonadrenergic, noncholinergic neurons and functions as a bronchodilator; interruption of its action by VIP cleavage can promote bronchoconstriction.

Airway obstruction occurs diffusely, although not homogeneously, throughout the lungs. As a result, ventilation of respiratory units becomes nonuniform, and the matching of ventilation to perfusion is altered. Areas of both abnormally low and abnormally high $\dot{V}/\dot{Q}$ ratios exist, with the low $\dot{V}/\dot{Q}$ ratio regions contributing to hypoxemia. Pure shunt is unusual in asthma even though mucus plugging is a common finding, particularly in severe, fatal asthma. Arterial CO_2 tension is usually normal to low, given the increased ventilation seen with asthma exacerbations. Even mild hypercapnia should be viewed as an ominous sign during a severe asthma attack, indicating progressive airway obstruction, muscle fatigue, and falling alveolar ventilation.

Clinical Manifestations

The manifestations of asthma are readily explained by the presence of airway inflammation and obstruction.

A. Symptoms & Signs—The variability of symptoms and signs is an indication of the tremendous range of disease severity, from mild and intermittent disease to chronic, severe, and sometimes fatal asthma. Importantly, symptoms of asthma do not necessarily correlate with the degree of airway obstruction.

1. **Dyspnea and chest tightness**—The sensations of dyspnea and chest tightness result from several concerted physiologic changes. The greater muscular effort required to overcome increased airway resistance is detected by spindle stretch receptors, principally of intercostal muscles and the chest wall. Hyperinflation from airway obstruction results in thoracic distention. Lung compliance falls, and the work of breathing increases, also detected by chest wall sensory nerves and manifested as chest tightness and dyspnea. As obstruction worsens, increased $\dot{V}/\dot{Q}$ mismatching produces hypoxemia. Rising arterial CO_2 tension and, later, evolving arterial hypoxemia (each alone or together as synergistic stimuli) will stimulate respiratory drive through peripheral and central chemoreceptors. This stimulus in the setting of respiratory muscle fatigue produces progressive dyspnea.

2. **Wheezing**—Smooth muscle contraction, together with mucus hypersecretion and retention, results in airway caliber reduction and prolonged turbulent airflow, producing auscultatory and audible wheezing. The intensity of wheezing does not correlate well with the severity of airway narrowing; as an example, with extreme airway obstruction, airflow may be so reduced that wheezing is barely detectable if at all.

3. **Cough**—Cough results from the combination of airway narrowing, mucus hypersecretion, and the neural afferent hyperresponsiveness seen with airway inflammation. It can also be a consequence of nonspecific inflammation after superimposed infections, particularly viral, in patients with asthma. By virtue of the compressive narrowing and high velocity of airflow in central airways, cough provides sufficient shear and propulsive force to clear collected mucus and retained particles from narrowed airways.

4. **Tachypnea and tachycardia**—Tachypnea and tachycardia may be absent in mild disease but are virtually universal in acute exacerbations.

5. **Pulsus paradoxus**—Pulsus paradoxus is a fall of more than 10 mm Hg in systolic arterial pressure during inspiration. It appears to occur as a consequence of lung hyperinflation, with compromise of left ventricular filling together with augmented venous return to the right ventricle during vigorous inspiration in severe obstruction. With increased right ventricular end-diastolic volume during inspiration, the intraventricular septum is moved to the left, compromising left ventricular filling and output. The consequence of this decreased output is a decrease in systolic pressure during inspiration, or pulsus paradoxus.

6. **Hypoxemia**—Airway narrowing reduces ventilation to affected lung units, causing $\dot{V}/\dot{Q}$ mismatching with a shift toward low $\dot{V}/\dot{Q}$ ratios, resulting in an increase in the A–a ΔPO_2 and frank hypoxemia in severe cases. True shunt is unusual except in very severe asthma.

7. **Hypercapnia and respiratory acidosis**—In mild to moderate asthma, ventilation is normal or increased, and the arterial PCO_2 is either normal or decreased. In severe attacks, airway obstruction may worsen and respiratory muscle fatigue supervenes, with the evolution of alveolar hypoventilation, hypercapnia, and respiratory acidosis. Note that this progression can occur despite continued tachypnea. An increased respiratory rate does not reverse alveolar hypoventilation because tidal volumes are reduced secondary to dynamic hyperinflation.

8. **Obstructive defects by pulmonary function testing**—Patients with mild asthma may have entirely normal pulmonary function between exacerbations. During active asthma attacks, all indices of expiratory airflow are reduced, including FEV_1, FEV_1/FVC ($FEV_1\%$), and peak expiratory flow rate (Figure 9–20). FVC is often also reduced as a result of air trapping that results from premature airway closure before full expiration. Administration of a bronchodilator improves airflow obstruction. A consequence of airflow obstruction is incomplete emptying of lung units at end expiration resulting in air trapping (increased RV) and hyperinflation (increased total lung capacity). Pulmonary diffusing capacity for carbon monoxide (DLCO) is often increased as a consequence of the increased lung (and lung capillary blood) volume.

9. **Bronchial hyperresponsiveness**—Bronchial hyperresponsiveness is defined as either (1) a 12% or greater increase in the FEV_1 in response to an inhaled bronchodilator, or (2) a 20% or greater decrease in FEV_1 in

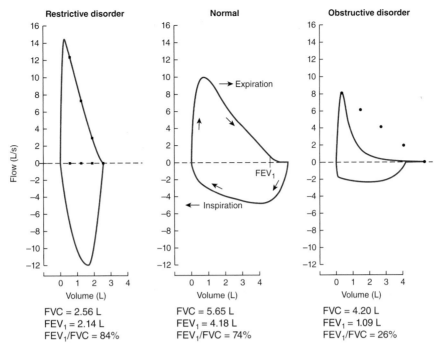

FIGURE 9–20 Flow–volume curves ("loops") from standard spirometry are shown for a normal patient (**center**), a patient with a severe obstructive ventilatory defect (**right**), and a patient with a moderate restrictive ventilatory defect (**left**).

response to a provoking factor that, at the same concentration, causes less than a 5% change in a healthy individual. Methacholine and histamine are agents for which standardized provocation testing has been established. Such testing reveals nonspecific hyperresponsiveness in virtually all people with asthma, including those with mild disease and normal spirometry findings. Other agents that have been used to establish specific exposure sensitivities include sulfur dioxide and toluene diisocyanate.

CHECKPOINT

19. What is the fundamental physiologic problem in obstructive lung disease? Give an example of each of its three principal sources.

20. What are the pathologic events that contribute to chronically abnormal airway architecture in asthma?

21. What are the three categories of provocative agents that can trigger asthma?

22. Which acute-acting mediators contribute to asthmatic airway responses?

23. What are some histopathologic features of asthma?

24. Name three reasons for increased airway resistance in asthma.

25. Why is arterial PCO_2 usually low in asthma exacerbations?

26. What are some of the common symptoms and signs of acute asthma?

2. COPD: Chronic Bronchitis & Emphysema

COPD is defined by the presence of persistent respiratory symptoms and airflow limitation secondary to airway and alveolar abnormalities resulting from exposure to noxious particles or gases. It is common, preventable, and treatable. Pathologic changes in COPD are seen throughout the respiratory tract, from the large airways to the alveoli. Therefore, in COPD, there can be a spectrum of clinical manifestations that share a common underlying etiology.

Clinical Presentation

COPD is often described as two discrete processes, chronic bronchitis and emphysema, both of which can lead to the development of fixed airway obstruction. From a physiologic perspective, it is useful to separate these two processes, as each has distinct pathologic mechanisms. However, it is important to recognize that both processes can be found within the same individual, with a varying contribution of each to the overall clinical phenotype.

A. Chronic Bronchitis—Chronic bronchitis is defined by a clinical history of productive cough for 3 months of the year for 2 consecutive years. Both dyspnea and airway obstruction, often with an element of reversibility, are intermittently to continuously present. Chronic bronchitis predominantly impacts the airways. Inflammation in the larger airways leads to mucosal thickening and to mucus hypersecretion, which contributes to the productive cough. Extension of the inflammatory changes into smaller bronchioles produces airflow obstruction.

B. Emphysema—Pulmonary emphysema is a condition marked by irreversible enlargement of the airspaces distal to the terminal bronchioles, accompanied by destruction of their walls, most often without obvious fibrosis. In contrast to chronic bronchitis, the primary pathologic defect in emphysema is not in the airways but rather in the respiratory unit walls, where the loss of elastic tissue results in a loss of the recoil tension necessary to support distal airways during expiration. Progressive dyspnea and nonreversible obstruction accompany the airspace destruction without mucus hypersecretion or productive cough. Furthermore, the loss of alveolar surface area and the accompanying capillary bed for gas exchange contribute to progressive hypoxia and dyspnea. Pathologic and etiologic distinctions can be made among various patterns of emphysema, but the clinical presentations of all are similar.

Etiology & Epidemiology

COPD is a major cause of global morbidity and mortality. It is currently the third leading cause of death worldwide. In 2012, more than 3 million people died as a result of COPD, representing 6% of all deaths globally. Furthermore, by 2030 the prevalence of the disease is projected to rise to an expected 4.5 million deaths worldwide. In the United States, COPD is also the third leading cause of death. It is estimated to have direct costs of approximately $32 billion dollars per year. The prevalence of COPD is nearly equal between men and women, but mortality rates are higher in men. Mortality also increases with age and is higher in persons of lower socioeconomic status. Despite its significant global impact, COPD is likely under-diagnosed. Cigarette smoking is the most common risk factor worldwide, representing the principal cause in up to 90% of patients. Although fewer than 50% of heavy smokers develop COPD during their lifetime, cigarette smokers have a greater mortality rate from COPD than non-smokers. Beyond tobacco smoke exposure, population-based studies suggest that chronic dust (including silica and cotton) and chemical fume exposure are significant contributing risk factors for COPD. In the developing world, indoor exposure to smoke from burning biofuels is a major cause of COPD.

The most important identified genetic risk factor for the evolution of COPD is deficiency of α_1-protease (α_1-antitrypsin) inhibitor. Reduced circulating and tissue levels can lead to the early onset of severe emphysema. Alpha$_1$-protease inhibitor is capable of inhibiting several types of proteases, including neutrophil elastase, which is implicated in the genesis of emphysema (see Pathophysiology section below). Autosomal dominant mutations, especially in northern Europeans, produce abnormally low serum and tissue levels of this inhibitor, altering the balance of connective tissue synthesis and proteolysis. A homozygous mutation (the ZZ genotype) results in inhibitor levels 10–15% of normal, and the risk of emphysema, particularly in smokers who carry this mutation, is dramatically increased.

Pathophysiology

COPD develops in response to chronic inflammation triggered by the inhalation of noxious particles or gas, such as

are found in cigarette smoke. Repeated inhalational exposure leads to persistent inflammation, producing the characteristic pathophysiologic changes seen in patients with COPD. The primary site of inflammatory involvement determines the predominant pathophysiologic process in an individual, with airway-predominant disease causing chronic bronchitis and parenchyma disease causing emphysema.

A. Chronic Bronchitis—The principal pathologic features are inflammation of airways, particularly small airways, and hypertrophy of large airway mucous glands, with increased mucus secretion and accompanying mucus obstruction of airways (Figure 9–21). The airway mucosa is variably infiltrated with inflammatory cells, including polymorphonuclear leukocytes and lymphocytes. Mucosal inflammation can substantially narrow the bronchial lumen. As a consequence of the chronic inflammation, the normal ciliated pseudostratified columnar epithelium is frequently replaced by patchy squamous metaplasia. In the absence of normal ciliated bronchial epithelium, mucociliary clearance function is severely diminished or completely abolished. Hypertrophy and hyperplasia of submucosal glands are prominent features, with the glands often making up more than 50% of the bronchial wall thickness. Mucus hypersecretion accompanies mucous gland hyperplasia, contributing to luminal narrowing. Bronchial smooth muscle hypertrophy is common, and hyperresponsiveness to nonspecific bronchoconstrictor stimuli (including histamine and methacholine) can be seen. Bronchioles are often infiltrated with inflammatory cells and are distorted, with associated peribronchial fibrosis. Mucus impaction and luminal obstruction of smaller airways are often seen. In the absence of any superimposed process, such as pneumonia, the gas-exchanging lung parenchyma, composed of terminal

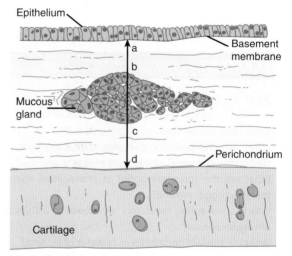

FIGURE 9–21 Bronchial wall anatomy. Structure of a normal bronchial wall. In chronic bronchitis, the thickness of the mucous glands increases and can be expressed as the ratio of (b–c)/(a–d); this is known as the Reid index. (Redrawn, with permission, from Thurlbeck WM. Chronic airflow obstruction in lung disease. In: Bennington JL, ed. *Major Problems in Pathology.* Saunders, 1976.)

respiratory units, is largely undamaged. The result of these combined changes is chronic airway obstruction and impaired clearance of airway secretions.

The nonuniform airway obstruction of chronic bronchitis has substantial effects on ventilation and gas exchange. Airway narrowing that leads to prolonged expiratory time produces hyperinflation. Ventilation/perfusion relationships are altered with increased areas of low $\dot{V}/\dot{Q}$ ratios. These low $\dot{V}/\dot{Q}$ mismatches are largely responsible for the more significant resting hypoxemia seen in chronic bronchitis, compared with that seen in emphysema. True shunt (perfusion with no ventilation) is unusual in chronic bronchitis.

B. Emphysema—The principal pathologic event in emphysema is thought to be a continuing destructive process resulting from an imbalance between lung oxidant insults and lung antioxidants and antielastases (particularly neutrophil α1-anti-protease) (Figure 9–22). Oxidants, whether endogenous (superoxide anion) or exogenous (eg, cigarette smoke), can inhibit the normal protective function of protease inhibitors (antiproteases), allowing progressive tissue destruction.

In contrast to chronic bronchitis, a disease of the airways, emphysema is a disease of the surrounding lung parenchyma. The physiologic consequences result from three important changes: (1) destruction of terminal respiratory units; (2) loss of alveolar–capillary bed; and (3) loss of the supporting structures of the lung, including elastin-containing connective tissue. This loss of connective tissue reduces the normal support of noncartilaginous airways, leading to a lung with diminished elastic recoil and increased compliance. A premature

expiratory collapse of airways ensues, with characteristic obstructive symptoms and physiologic findings.

The pathologic picture of emphysema is one of progressive destruction of terminal respiratory units or lung parenchyma distal to terminal bronchioles. Airway inflammatory changes are minimal if present, although some mucous gland hyperplasia can be seen in large conducting airways. The interstitium of respiratory units harbors some inflammatory cells, but the chief finding is a loss of alveolar walls and enlargement of airspaces. Alveolar capillaries are also lost, which can result in decreased diffusing capacity and progressive hypoxemia, particularly with exercise.

Alveolar destruction is not uniform in all cases of emphysema. Anatomic variants have been described on the basis of the pattern of destruction of the terminal respiratory unit (or acinus, as it is also known). In centriacinar emphysema, destruction is focused in the center of the terminal respiratory unit, with the respiratory bronchioles and alveolar ducts relatively spared. This pattern is most frequently associated with prolonged smoking. Panacinar emphysema involves destruction of the terminal respiratory unit globally, with diffuse airspace distention. This pattern is typically, although not uniquely, seen in α1-protease inhibitor deficiency. It is important to note that the distinction between these two patterns is largely pathologic; there is no significant difference in the clinical presentation. An additional emphysema pattern of clinical importance is bullous emphysema. Bullae are large confluent airspaces formed by greater local destruction or progressive distention of lung units. They are important because of the compressive effect they can have on surrounding lung and the large physiologic dead space associated with these structures.

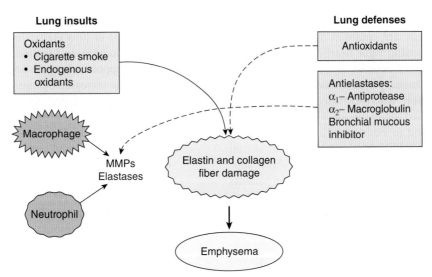

FIGURE 9–22 Schema of the elastase–antielastase hypothesis of emphysema. Activation is represented by solid lines, inhibition by dashed lines. The lung is protected from elastolytic damage by α1-protease inhibitor and α2-macroglobulin. Bronchial mucus inhibitor protects the airways. Elastase is derived primarily from neutrophils, but macrophages secrete an elastase-like metalloprotease and may ingest and later release neutrophil elastase. Oxidants derived from neutrophils and macrophages or from cigarette smoke may inactivate α1-protease inhibitor and may interfere with lung matrix repair. Endogenous antioxidants such as superoxide dismutase, glutathione, and catalase protect the lung against oxidant injury. (MMPs, matrix metalloproteinases.)

Clinical Manifestations

A. Chronic Bronchitis—The clinical manifestations of chronic bronchitis are principally the result of the obstructive and inflammatory airway process.

1. **Cough with sputum production**—Cough is productive of thick, often purulent sputum owing to the ongoing local inflammation and the high likelihood of bacterial colonization and infection. Sputum viscosity is increased largely as a result of the presence of free DNA (of high molecular weight and high viscosity) from lysed cells. With increased inflammation and mucosal injury, hemoptysis can occur but is usually scant. Cough, which is very effective in clearing normal airways, is much less effective because of the narrow airway caliber and the greater volume and viscosity of secretions.

2. **Wheezing**—Persistent airway narrowing and mucus obstruction can produce localized or more diffuse wheezing. This may be responsive to bronchodilators, representing a reversible component to the obstruction.

3. **Inspiratory and expiratory rhonchi**—Increased mucus production, together with defective mucociliary escalator function, leaves excessive secretions in the airways, despite increased coughing. Rhonchi are heard prominently in larger airways during tidal breathing or with cough.

4. **Cardiac examination**—Tachycardia is common, especially with exacerbations of bronchitis or with hypoxemia. If hypoxemia is significant and chronic, pulmonary hypertension can result; cardiac examination reveals a prominent pulmonary valve closing sound (P_2) or elevated jugular venous pressure and peripheral edema.

5. **Imaging**—Typical chest radiographic findings include increased lung volumes with relatively depressed diaphragms consistent with hyperinflation. Prominent parallel linear densities ("tram track lines") of thickened bronchial walls are common. Cardiac size may be increased, suggesting right heart volume overload. Prominent pulmonary arteries are common and are associated with pulmonary hypertension.

6. **Pulmonary function tests**—Diffuse airway obstruction is demonstrated on pulmonary function testing as a global reduction in expiratory flows and volumes. FEV_1, FVC, and the FEV_1/FVC (FEV_1%) ratio are all reduced. The expiratory flow–volume curve shows substantial flow limitation (see Figure 9–20). Some patients may respond to bronchodilators. Measurement of lung volumes reveals an increase in the RV and FRC, reflecting air trapped in the lung as a result of diffuse airway obstruction and early airway closure at higher lung volumes. DLCO is typically normal, reflecting a preserved alveolar–capillary bed.

7. **Arterial blood gases**—Ventilation/perfusion mismatching is common in chronic bronchitis. The A–a ΔPO_2 is increased and hypoxemia is common, mainly because of significant areas of low $\dot{V}/\dot{Q}$ ratios; hypoxemia at rest tends to be more profound than in emphysema. With increasing obstruction, increasing PCO_2 (hypercapnia) and respiratory acidosis, with compensatory metabolic alkalosis, are seen.

8. **Polycythemia**—Chronic hypoxemia is associated with a variable erythropoietin-mediated increase in hematocrit. With more severe and prolonged hypoxia, the hematocrit may increase to over 50%.

B. Emphysema—Emphysema presents as a noninflammatory disease manifested by dyspnea, progressive nonreversible airway obstruction, and abnormalities of gas exchange, particularly with exercise.

1. **Breath sounds**—Breath sounds in emphysema are typically decreased in intensity, reflecting decreased airflow, prolonged expiratory time, and prominent lung hyperinflation. Wheezes, when present, are of diminished intensity. Airway sounds, including crackles and rhonchi, are unusual in the absence of superimposed processes such as infection or pulmonary edema.

2. **Cardiac examination**—Tachycardia may be present as in chronic bronchitis, especially with exacerbations or hypoxemia. Pulmonary hypertension is a common consequence of pulmonary vascular obliteration. Cardiac examination may reveal prominent pulmonary valve closure (increased P_2, the pulmonary component of the second heart sound).

3. **Imaging**—Hyperinflation is common, with flattened hemidiaphragms and an increased anteroposterior chest diameter. Parenchymal destruction produces attenuated lung peripheral vascular markings, often with proximal pulmonary artery dilation as a result of secondary pulmonary hypertension. Cystic or bullous changes may also be seen.

4. **Pulmonary function tests**—Lung parenchymal destruction and loss of lung elastic recoil are the fundamental causes of pulmonary function abnormalities. The loss of elastic support in lung tissue surrounding the airways results in the increased dynamic compression of airways (see Figure 9–9), especially during forced expiration. Premature airway collapse reduces all flows, including FEV_1, FVC, and the FEV_1/FVC (FEV_1% ratio). As with chronic bronchitis and asthma, the expiratory flow–volume curve shows substantial limitation in flow (see Figure 9–20). Expiratory time prolongation and early airway closure caused by loss of elastic recoil result in air trapping (increased RV). TLC is also increased, although often a substantial amount of this increase comes from gas trapped in poorly or noncommunicating lung units, including bullae. The DLCO is generally decreased in proportion to the extent of emphysema, reflecting the progressive loss of alveoli and their capillary beds.

5. **Arterial blood gases**—Emphysema is a disease of alveolar wall destruction. The loss of alveolar capillaries creates $\dot{V}/\dot{Q}$ mismatches with areas of high ventilation relative to perfusion. Typically, patients with emphysema adapt to

high $\dot{V}/\dot{Q}$ ratios by increasing their minute ventilation. They may maintain nearly normal PO_2 and PCO_2 levels despite advanced disease. With greater disease severity and further loss of capillary perfusion, the DLCO falls, leading to exercise-related and, when severe, resting arterial hemoglobin desaturation. Hypercapnia, respiratory acidosis, and a compensatory metabolic alkalosis are common in severe disease.

6. **Polycythemia**—As in chronic bronchitis, chronic hypoxemia is frequently associated with an elevated hematocrit.

CHECKPOINT

27. What is the leading cause of COPD?
28. Describe the pathophysiologic changes in emphysema versus chronic bronchitis.
29. Mutations of which protein are strongly correlated with an increased risk of emphysema?
30. Name eight symptoms and signs of chronic bronchitis.
31. Name six symptoms and signs of emphysema.

RESTRICTIVE LUNG DISEASE: IDIOPATHIC PULMONARY FIBROSIS

Interstitial lung disease, or diffuse parenchymal lung disease, is a descriptive term that encompasses more than 180 different disorders. These disorders are grouped together because of shared pathologic, physiologic, clinical, and radiographic features. Diffuse parenchymal lung diseases are characterized by a thickened alveolar interstitium resulting from the accumulation of inflammatory cells, mesenchymal cells, and collagen-rich extracellular matrix, leading to fibrosis and capillary remodeling (Figure 9–23). Diffuse lung fibrosis leads to increased lung elastic recoil, decreased lung compliance and lung volumes, impaired oxygen diffusion, and alterations in $\dot{V}/\dot{Q}$ matching, leading to impairment in gas exchange through a pattern known as restrictive lung disease.

Diffuse parenchymal lung disease is often referred to as interstitial lung disease, but the modifier "interstitial" is an incomplete characterization of the pathologic process. The lung interstitium formally refers to the region of the alveolar wall exclusive of and separating the basement membranes of alveolar epithelial and pulmonary capillary endothelial cells. In the normal lung, this interstitium is a space that may contain a few mesenchymal cells (eg, fibroblasts), extracellular matrix molecules (eg, collagen, elastin, proteoglycans), and tissue leukocytes, including mast cells and lymphocytes. Under pathologic conditions, not only is the interstitium affected, but characteristic changes are also observed in the alveolar epithelium, including denudation and hypertrophy. In addition, the capillary endothelium can be involved with a loss or remodeling of alveolar capillaries. This extensive disruption of normal lung structure by interstitial processes profoundly influences lung function.

The known causes of diffuse parenchymal lung disease include occupational and environmental exposures to organic and inorganic dusts, collagen vascular diseases (e.g. rheumatoid arthritis, progressive systemic sclerosis, dermatomyositis/polymyositis), and medication toxicity. There are also diffuse parenchymal lung diseases of unknown etiology, such as idiopathic pulmonary fibrosis (IPF). The physiologic

FIGURE 9–23 Categories of diffuse parenchymal lung disease that often lead to restrictive lung disease. In the absence of underlying malignancy or a history of chemical or radiation therapy, diffuse parenchymal lung disease can be broadly grouped into the clinical categories shown. (IPF, idiopathic pulmonary fibrosis; IIP, idiopathic interstitial pneumonia; DIP, diffuse interstitial pneumonia; RBILD, respiratory bronchiolitis-associated interstitial lung disease; AIP, acute idiopathic pneumonia; COP, cryptogenic organizing pneumonia; NSIP, nonspecific interstitial pneumonia; LIP, lymphocytic interstitial pneumonia.)

consequences seen in IPF are typical of other causes of diffuse parenchymal lung disease, particularly in their advanced stages. For that reason, the remainder of this section focuses on IPF as a prototypical interstitial lung disease.

Clinical Presentation

IPF, previously known as interstitial pulmonary fibrosis or cryptogenic fibrosing alveolitis, is caused by progressive fibrosis leading to destruction of normal lung architecture. This process produces not only a restrictive defect, with altered ventilation and increased work of breathing, but also vascular alterations that can severely impair normal pulmonary perfusion and gas exchange.

The usual presentation of IPF is one of insidious onset. Patients present with dyspnea that has progressed over months to years and often a chronic non-productive cough. Fever and chest pain are generally absent. As the disease worsens, dyspnea may occur even at rest. Digital cyanosis, clubbing, and pulmonary hypertension are common in later stages.

The diagnosis of IPF may be made by high-resolution chest CT in the setting of an appropriate clinical history and pulmonary function tests or by surgical lung biopsy. Typical CT findings are described below. The histopathologic correlate to IPF is **usual interstitial pneumonia** (**UIP**), a temporally and spatially heterogeneous pattern of scattered clusters of mature collagen deposition and alveolar wall destruction interspersed with areas of normal alveolar architecture. These clusters of ongoing fibrosis are called fibroblastic foci and contain both fibroblasts and myofibroblasts; inflammatory cells may be present but are usually sparse.

Etiology & Epidemiology

Compared with COPD, IPF is an uncommon disorder with an estimated prevalence of 18 per 100,000 people in the United States. This disease has a male predominance and typically presents in the sixth to seventh decades of life (it is rare in individuals under 50 years of age). By definition, the term "idiopathic" indicates that none of the known causes of diffuse parenchymal lung disease are present in an individual patient. Major risk factors include tobacco smoke exposure, environmental exposures (eg, metal and wood dusts), occupational exposures (in farming and agriculture), and chronic viral infections. Beyond environmental exposures, recent studies clearly implicate both common and rare variant genetic alterations in the development of IPF. The common variants account for approximately one-third of the risk for developing IPF and include the *MUC5B* and *TOLLIP* genes. Associations with other disorders, including emphysema, gastroesophageal reflux disease, and obesity, remain undefined. The clinical, imaging, and histopathologic features of IPF can be indistinguishable from diffuse parenchymal lung diseases of known etiology. Therefore, it is critical that a thorough history and physical examination are performed on each patient, since the treatment and prognosis differ between IPF and these other interstitial disorders.

The natural history of IPF is classically one of unremitting progression, and the median survival is approximately 3 years from the time of diagnosis. The clinical course is nonetheless very heterogeneous and may reflect separate phenotypes of the disease rather than variable progression. Risk factors for accelerated progression include gender, older age at diagnosis (>70 years), cumulative tobacco smoke exposure, and severity of disease by symptoms (dyspnea score) or standardized assessment (extent of radiographic disease, severity of pulmonary restriction on pulmonary function tests, presence of pulmonary hypertension). Combining these predictive variables into scoring algorithms such as the GAP index (**G**ender, **A**ge, **P**hysiology [including FVC and DLCO]) can aid the clinician in estimating the 1-year mortality rate for a patient with IPF. Further attempts to improve such predictions have examined the utility of IPF biomarkers. One example is the serum concentration of matrix metalloproteinase 7, with increasing levels portending a worse outcome. Other less well-established prognostic biomarkers include serum levels of monomeric periostin, YKL-40, and CCL18.

A subset (5–15%) of patients with IPF will also experience an acute exacerbation of their disease characterized by an abrupt deterioration in symptoms, lung function, and radiographic abnormalities. Pathologic specimens from such patients reveal diffuse alveolar damage in addition to findings of UIP. These episodes are associated with a poor prognosis, with an associated median survival of 3–4 months.

Pathophysiology

The pathophysiology of IPF and its histopathologic correlate UIP is an active area of research with the promise that a better understanding of the basic mechanisms of this disease will translate into more effective treatments. Mounting evidence implicates repetitive microinjury to the alveolar epithelium followed by aberrant wound repair as the predominant mechanism of disease pathogenesis. Defects (both genetic and acquired) in type II alveolar epithelial cells increase the susceptibility of these cells to injury and apoptosis and also interfere with their regenerative capacity. For example, genetic mutations in type II alveolar epithelial cell-specific proteins, including surfactant proteins A and C, have been identified in individuals with familial pulmonary fibrosis. These mutations result in protein defects that induce cell stress and promote cell death. Furthermore, mutations in telomere maintenance genes (including *TERT* and *TERC*) result in telomere shortening and impair the regenerative capacity of the type II alveolar epithelium. In addition to these genetic studies, histopathologic and biomarker studies of IPF patients consistently identify abnormalities in the alveolar epithelium, including denudation and/or hyperplasia of cells in areas of active fibrosis and elevated systemic levels of surfactant proteins. Finally, animal studies confirm that a targeted injury to the type II alveolar epithelial cell is sufficient to cause fibrosis. It is currently unknown what environmental challenges are responsible for the repetitive microinjury to the susceptible type II alveolar epithelial cell (hence the idiopathic designation). It is likely that multiple different insults contribute. For example, both animal models and human studies implicate chronic herpesvirus infection as an important etiologic factor in a subset of patients. Furthermore, acute viral infections likely contribute to acute exacerbations of the disease.

Following epithelial injury, fibroblasts accumulate in the lung interstitium and typically differentiate into myofibroblasts. Myofibroblasts are highly contractile and contribute to tissue destruction. They are also responsible for the synthesis and deposition of extracellular matrix proteins such as fibronectin and collagen. In normal wound healing, fibroblasts undergo apoptosis following the successful restoration of an intact epithelium. In contrast, (myo)fibroblasts in IPF are resistant to apoptotic stimuli, favoring their persistence and ultimately contributing to the progressive nature of the disease. How epithelial injury initiates (myo)fibroblast activation is an area of ongoing study. However, current evidence suggests that the damaged type II alveolar epithelial cells secrete profibrogenic mediators, including transforming growth factor-β (TGF-β), connective tissue growth factor, and platelet-derived growth factor. Disruption of the epithelium also leads to plasma leak, activation of TGF-β, activation of the clotting cascade, and generation of thrombin, which can activate fibroblasts through cleavage of protease-activated receptors. In turn, the fibrogenic mediators, in conjunction with the development of a stiff, cross-linked, collagen-rich extracellular matrix, drive myofibroblast differentiation and apoptosis resistance.

In this working model of epithelial injury, myofibroblast activation, and failed wound repair, the inflammatory cell contribution to disease pathogenesis remains controversial. Disappointingly, a large clinical trial of the combination of an anti-inflammatory regimen of azathioprine and prednisone with N-acetylcysteine to suppress inflammation was found to *increase* the risk of death and hospitalization. And, in fact, histopathologic examination of tissue biopsies from patients with IPF typically reveals a paucity of inflammatory cells. On the other hand, it seems implausible that repetitive injury to the alveolar epithelium would not result in the activation of an immune response. Animal models implicate the interplay between recruited monocytes/macrophages and regulatory T cells in the pathogenesis of pulmonary fibrosis. In addition, many studies have demonstrated that, with fibrotic insult, activated macrophages are capable of secreting pro-fibrotic mediators such as TGF-β (Table 9–5).

Ultimately, the disruption of the alveolar epithelium with an associated perturbation in surfactant homeostasis, the accumulation of extracellular matrix proteins, and the persistence of contractile apoptosis-resistant myofibroblasts result in increased tissue stiffness, decreased lung compliance, and a reduction in lung volume. As this cycle progresses, there is continued alveolar destruction, with large areas of fibrosis and residual airspaces lined by cuboidal epithelium that originates from airway basal cells. This process, known as bronchiolization, leads to the development of honeycomb cysts that can

TABLE 9–5   Cellular events involved in lung injury and fibrosis.

Repetitive micro-injury to a susceptible type II alveolar epithelium
Injury-induced inflammatory response, including T-cell activation and monocyte/macrophage influx
Increased production/activation of profibrotic mediators, including TGF-β, CTGF, and PDGF
Accumulation and activation of apoptosis-resistant and contractile (myo)fibroblasts
Deposition of stiff cross-linked extracellular matrix with tissue destruction
Failure of type II alveolar epithelial cell reconstitution, leading to bronchiolization with the formation of honeycomb cysts
Increased pulmonary vascular resistance secondary to hypoxemia and vascular remodeling, leading to pulmonary arterial hypertension in a subset of patients

be appreciated both in pathologic specimens and on radiographic imaging. Along with alveolar destruction, pulmonary vascular changes occur. These changes can be precipitated by patchy obliteration of the accompanying vascular bed and by hypoxemic vasoconstriction. The resultant altered physiology includes increased pulmonary vascular resistance, pulmonary arterial hypertension, and right heart strain. Table 9–6 summarizes the pathophysiology of interstitial lung diseases.

Clinical Manifestations

A. Symptoms & Signs

1. **Cough**—An intermittent, irritating, nonproductive cough is often the first symptom of IPF. It may be refractory to antitussive therapy. The mechanism is likely multifactorial, with fibrotic damage to terminal respiratory units causing bronchial and bronchiolar distortion, which leads to alterations in both stimulatory and inhibitory nerve fibers involved in cough reflexes. Although epithelial cells may be injured, mucus hypersecretion and a productive cough are not typically seen in early disease.

2. **Dyspnea and tachypnea**—Multiple factors contribute to dyspnea in patients with IPF. Fibrosis of lung parenchyma decreases lung compliance; in combination with alterations in surfactant turnover, the distending pressure required to inflate the lungs increases, as does the work of breathing. Increased stimuli from C fibers in fibrotic alveolar walls or stretch receptors in the chest wall may sense the increased force necessary to inflate less compliant lungs. Tachypnea results from increased lung sensory receptor stimuli and the attempt to maintain a normal alveolar minute ventilation (and hence normal PaCO$_2$) as lung volumes decrease. A rapid, shallow breathing pattern also reduces ventilatory work

TABLE 9–6   Pathophysiology of interstitial lung diseases.

Decreased lung compliance
• Lungs are stiffer and more resistant to expansion (Figure 9–8)
• Lung compliance curve is shifted downward and to the right (Figure 9–20)
• Static recoil pressure is increased at total lung capacity (TLC) (owing to increased elastic forces)
• Work of breathing is increased

Decreased lung volumes as a consequence of decreased lung compliance
• TLC, vital capacity (VC), functional residual capacity (FRC), and residual volume (RV) are proportionally reduced
• Tidal volumes are reduced (Figure 9–10)
• Alveolar ventilation is maintained by increased respiratory rate (Figure 9–10)

Disturbances in gas exchange
• Patchy nature of fibrosis leads to severe inhomogeneity in ventilation
• Regional inhomogeneity causes mismatching of ventilation and perfusion with shift toward low $\dot{V}/\dot{Q}$ regions, including areas of absent ventilation (shunt)
• Increased A–a ΔPO_2 secondary to low regions, with hypoxemia in severe cases
• Decreased pulmonary diffusing capacity (DLCO) owing to thickened alveolar walls and loss of pulmonary capillaries, leading to a reduction in pulmonary capillary surface area
• Hypoxemia typically exacerbated by exercise (Figure 9–24)
• $PaCO_2$ typically normal or low owing to increased minute ventilation; hypercarbia in pure idiopathic pulmonary fibrosis (IPF) is indicative of very advanced disease

Pulmonary artery hypertension
• Decreased pulmonary capillary surface area
• Increased pulmonary vascular resistance from reduced FRC
• Inhomogeneity of ventilation causes regional alveolar hypoxia with consequent hypoxic pulmonary vasoconstriction
• Marked exacerbation with exercise owing to inability to recruit new vessels

in the face of increased lung elastic recoil. The diminished capillary bed and thickened alveolar–capillary membrane contribute to hypoxemia with exercise. In advanced disease, altered gas exchange with severe $\dot{V}/\dot{Q}$ mismatching can produce hypoxemia at rest.

3. **Inspiratory crackles**—Diffuse fine, dry inspiratory crackles are common and reflect the successive opening on inspiration of respiratory units that are collapsed owing to fibrosis and the loss of normal surfactant.

4. **Digital clubbing**—Clubbing of the fingers and toes is a common finding, but the cause is unknown. There is no established link with any specific physiologic variable, including hypoxemia.

5. **Cardiac examination**—As with hypoxemia from other causes, cardiac examination can reveal evidence of pulmonary hypertension with a prominent pulmonary valve closure sound (P_2). This can be accompanied by

right heart overload or decompensation, with elevated jugular venous pressure, the murmur of tricuspid regurgitation, or a right-sided third heart sound (S_3).

B. Imaging

Characteristic chest radiograph findings include reduced lung volumes with increased reticular opacities prominent in the lung periphery and loss of definition of vascular structures, diaphragms, and cardiac border. Fibrosis surrounding expanded small airspaces is seen as honeycombing. With pulmonary hypertension, central pulmonary arteries may be enlarged. Typical chest CT findings include diffuse septal thickening, increased subpleural reticular opacities, traction bronchiectasis with pleural scalloping, and subpleural, clustered, small (3–10 mm) cystic airspaces (honeycombing). Ground glass opacities are usually absent.

C. Pulmonary Function Tests

Lung fibrosis typically produces a restrictive ventilatory pattern, with reductions in TLC, FEV_1, and FVC, while maintaining a preserved or even increased ratio of FEV_1/FVC (FEV_1%) (see Figure 9–20). The increased elastic recoil produces normal to increased expiratory flow rates when adjusted for lung volume. The DLCO in lung fibrosis is progressively reduced as a function of the fibrotic obliteration of lung capillaries.

D. Arterial Blood Gases

Hypoxemia is common in advanced IPF. It results from the patchy nature of fibrosis, causing extreme variability in regional compliance and ventilation leading to prominent $\dot{V}/\dot{Q}$ mismatching shifted toward low $\dot{V}/\dot{Q}$ ratios. Cardiac output tends to be low, which reduces mixed venous PO_2 ($P_{mv}O_2$). Diffusion impairment increases with the severity of fibrosis but rarely contributes to resting hypoxemia. Diffusion impairment also contributes to abnormal oxygenation and is a significant contributor to exercise-induced desaturation when the combination of a low $P_{mv}O_2$ and reduced capillary transit time limits the oxygen loading of hemoglobin (Figure 9–24). Arterial PCO_2 is typically low because of increased ventilation owing to hypoxia and the irritant stimuli of lung fibrosis. Only in the later stages of disease, when increased lung elastic recoil and work of breathing prevent appropriate ventilation, does the $PaCO_2$ rise above normal. Hypercapnia is a grave sign, implying an inability to maintain adequate alveolar ventilation as a result of excess work of breathing.

CHECKPOINT

32. How does interstitial lung disease affect lung function?
33. Name five events in the pathophysiology of idiopathic pulmonary fibrosis.
34. Name eight symptoms and signs of idiopathic pulmonary fibrosis.

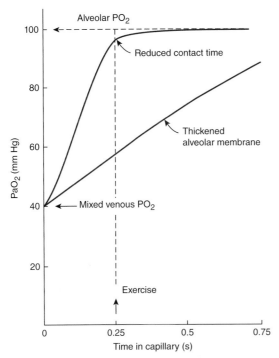

FIGURE 9–24 Change in PaO_2 along the pulmonary capillary. The typical transit time at rest for an erythrocyte through an alveolar capillary is 0.75 seconds. In the normal lung, the partial pressure difference and rate of diffusion of O_2 across the alveolar–capillary barrier assure complete saturation of hemoglobin in 0.25 seconds. Even with the shorter capillary transit time of exercise, the normal lung allows for complete saturation of hemoglobin in the alveolar capillary. If the alveolar–capillary barrier is thickened, as in lung fibrosis, and particularly if the starting point (the mixed venous PO_2) is reduced, diminished diffusion in the setting of shortened capillary transit time will cause alveolar end-capillary blood not to be fully saturated with O_2. Greater desaturation will occur with progressive exercise as peripheral extraction further decreases the mixed venous PO_2. (Redrawn, with permission, from West JB. *West's Pulmonary Pathophysiology: The Essentials*, 9th ed. Lippincott Williams & Wilkins, 2017.)

PULMONARY EDEMA

Clinical Presentation

Pulmonary edema is the accumulation of excess fluid in the extravascular compartment of the lungs, principally in the interstitium and alveolar spaces. This accumulation may occur slowly, as in a patient with occult renal failure, or emergently, as in left ventricular failure after an acute myocardial infarction. Pulmonary edema most commonly presents with dyspnea. Dyspnea is breathing perceived by a patient as both uncomfortable or anxiety-provoking and disproportionate to the level of activity. Dyspnea from pulmonary edema may be present only with exertion, or the patient may experience dyspnea at rest. In severe cases, pulmonary edema may be accompanied by edema fluid in the sputum and can cause acute respiratory failure.

Etiology

Pulmonary edema is a common problem associated with a variety of medical conditions (Table 9–7). In light of these multiple causes, it is helpful to think about pulmonary edema in terms of underlying physiologic principles.

TABLE 9–7   Causes of pulmonary edema by physiologic principle.

Increased pulmonary capillary hydrostatic pressure
Left ventricular dysfunction, acute or chronic
Myocardial ischemia or infarction
Heart failure, systolic or diastolic
Left atrial outflow obstruction
Mitral valve stenosis
Atrial myxoma
Intravascular volume overload
Iatrogenic volume expansion
Renal failure
Decreased plasma colloid osmotic pressure
Hypoalbuminemia
Nephrotic syndrome
Hepatic failure
Decreased interstitial pressure
Laryngospasm with maximal inspiratory efforts
Rapid re-expansion of collapsed lung
Increased pulmonary capillary endothelial permeability
Infectious pneumonia
Bacteremia
Sepsis
Nonthoracic trauma accompanied by hypotension ("shock lung")
Acute pancreatitis
Disseminated intravascular coagulation
Following cardiopulmonary bypass
Transfusion-related acute lung injury
Increased alveolar epithelial permeability
Aspiration of acidic gastric contents
Inhaled toxins: oxygen, phosgene, chlorine, smoke
Near-drowning and drowning
Decreased lymphatic clearance
Obstruction of intrapulmonary lymphatics by lymphangitic spread of carcinoma
Central mass or carcinoma obstructing lymphatics
Disruption of lymphatics by surgery, trauma, radiation therapy, inflammation
Multiple contributing mechanisms or uncertain
Neurogenic
High-altitude associated
Narcotic overdose
Tocolytic associated

Pathophysiology

All blood vessels leak; under normal conditions, fluid moves between blood vessels and the spaces around them while protein flux is minimal. In the adult human, the pulmonary capillaries are the major site of fluid flux from the pulmonary vasculature. The Starling equation—(Jv ≈ K ([Pc – Pi] – σ[πc – πi])—describes the movement of fluid between the pulmonary capillaries and the pulmonary extravascular compartment. The flux of fluid across a semipermeable membrane (Jv) is related to the inherent permeability of the membrane to fluid (K = fluid filtration coefficient of the capillary endothelium) and macromolecules (σ = protein reflection coefficient of the capillary endothelium), as well as the hydrostatic and colloid oncotic pressure gradients across the membrane (Pc = capillary hydrostatic pressure; Pi = interstitial hydrostatic pressure; πc and πi are the capillary and interstitial colloid oncotic pressures, respectively).

Under normal conditions, there is net flow out of the blood vessels into the interstitial space owing to the following pressure dynamics:

1. Pulmonary capillary hydrostatic pressure *exceeds* interstitial hydrostatic pressure; therefore, hydrostatic forces favor fluid movement out of the capillaries into the interstitial space.
2. Pulmonary capillary colloid oncotic pressure *exceeds* interstitial colloid oncotic pressure, favoring fluid movement out of the interstitial space into the capillaries.
3. The effect of hydrostatic forces is greater than that of colloid oncotic forces; thus, there is a net fluid movement out of the capillaries into the interstitial spaces. The net rate of fluid movement out of the pulmonary capillaries under normal conditions is approximately 15–20 mL/h, representing less than 0.01% of pulmonary blood flow.

Alveoli have homeostatic mechanisms to protect against extravascular fluid in the interstitial space. The alveolar epithelium forms a tight cellular barrier that is nearly impermeable to the passage of protein into the alveolar space. Restricting protein from the space maintains higher colloid oncotic pressure in the interstitium. In addition, alveolar epithelial cells actively transport sodium out of the alveoli. Both mechanisms create gradients that favor movement of fluid out of the alveolar space into the interstitium, maintaining alveolar function.

The pulmonary lymphatic system also helps prevent the accumulation of extravascular fluid in the interstitium under normal conditions. Fluid in the lung interstitial space is removed by pericapillary lymphatic vessels. These vessels do not enter the alveolar wall and are thus termed "juxta-alveolar." In addition, the pericapillary interstitium is contiguous with the perivascular and peribronchial interstitium. Interstitial pressure in these more central areas is negative relative to the pericapillary interstitium, so fluid tracks centrally away from the airspaces. In effect, the perivascular and peribronchiolar interstitium acts as a sump for fluid, and it can accommodate approximately 500 mL with a negligible increase in interstitial hydrostatic pressure. Because this fluid is protein-depleted relative to blood, osmotic forces favor resorption from the interstitium into blood vessels adjacent to these central areas. This is the major site of resorption of fluid from the perivascular and peribronchiolar interstitium. Edema fluid may track further into the mediastinum, where it is taken up by mediastinal lymphatics. The perivascular and peribronchiolar interstitium is also contiguous with the interlobular septa and the visceral pleura. In some patients, a significant amount of fluid transits out through the visceral pleural into the pleural space, where there is high-capacity resorption through pores on the parietal pleura into parietal pleural lymphatics. The rate of fluid resorption by the lymphatic system is usually sufficient to prevent fluid accumulation in the interstitium and the alveolar spaces.

Pulmonary edema occurs when fluid exiting the pulmonary vascular space exceeds the capacity for fluid clearance. At some undefined critical level after the perivascular and peribronchiolar interstitium has been filled, increased interstitial hydrostatic pressure causes edema fluid to enter the alveolar space (Figure 9–25). The pathway into the alveolar space remains unknown but is thought to occur by bulk flow. Pulmonary edema may occur under a number of different conditions:

1. The **hydrostatic pressure gradient** *increases* (elevated pulmonary capillary hydrostatic pressure). Pulmonary edema that occurs in this setting is termed **cardiogenic** or **hydrostatic pulmonary edema**. This is primarily a mechanical process resulting in an ultrafiltrate of plasma. Edema fluid in this setting has a relatively low protein content, generally less than 60% of a patient's plasma protein content. In normal individuals, pulmonary capillary pressure (ie, pulmonary capillary wedge pressure) must exceed approximately 20 mm Hg before the fluid leaving the vascular space exceeds the rate of resorption. Cardiogenic or hydrostatic pulmonary edema classically results from elevated pulmonary venous and left atrial pressures resulting from left ventricular systolic or diastolic failure as well as aortic or mitral valve disease.
2. **Vascular endothelial cell** and/or **alveolar epithelial cell permeability** *increases*. Pulmonary edema that occurs in this setting is termed **noncardiogenic** or **increased-permeability pulmonary edema**. The permeability of the endothelial or epithelial barrier may increase as a result of cellular injury. Local or systemic activation of inflammatory cascades typically initiates the dysfunction of both the endothelial and epithelial barriers. Following injury to these cells, both fluid and protein permeability increase, although there may be little change in hydrostatic pressure. Under conditions of increased membrane permeability, edema fluid has protein content similar to intravascular fluid, generally at least 70% of the plasma protein content. The acute respiratory distress syndrome (ARDS) epitomizes this type of pulmonary edema (detailed discussion below).
3. The **oncotic pressure gradient** *decreases* (low plasma colloid oncotic pressure). Edema fluid in this setting

Stage I
Interstitial pulmonary edema

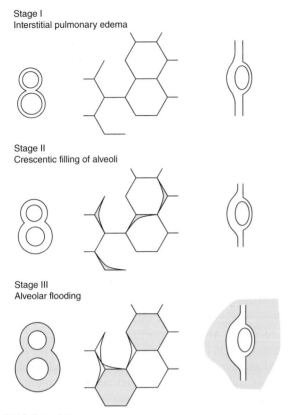

Stage II
Crescentic filling of alveoli

Stage III
Alveolar flooding

FIGURE 9–25 Stages in the accumulation of pulmonary edema fluid. The three columns represent three anatomic views of the progressive accumulation of pulmonary edema fluid. From left to right, the columns represent a cross-section of the bronchovascular bundle showing the loose connective tissue surrounding the pulmonary artery and bronchial wall, a cross-section of alveoli fixed in inflation, and the pulmonary capillary in cross-section. The first stage is an eccentric accumulation of fluid in the pericapillary interstitial space. The limitation of edema fluid to one side of the pulmonary capillary maintains gas transfer better than symmetric accumulation. When the formation of edema fluid exceeds lymphatic removal, it distends the peribronchovascular interstitium. At this stage, there is no alveolar flooding, but there is some crescentic filling of alveoli. The third stage is alveolar flooding. Note that each individual alveolus is either totally flooded or has minimal crescentic filling. This pattern probably occurs because alveolar edema interferes with surfactant, and, above some threshold, there is an increase in surface forces that greatly increases the transmural pressure and causes flooding. (Redrawn, with permission, from Lumb AB. *Nunn's Applied Respiratory Physiology*, 8th ed. Copyright Elsevier, 2016.)

has a relatively low protein content. Hypoalbuminemia owing to prolonged illness or nephrotic syndrome can cause this type of pulmonary edema.

4. **Lymphatic drainage** is *impaired*. This form of pulmonary edema is rare but may be seen with physical obstruction of the lymphatic system from malignancy (lymphoma) or infection (histoplasmosis, tuberculosis), from obliteration of lymphatics owing to radiation therapy for breast or lung cancer, or from idiopathic causes (yellow nail syndrome).

Hydrostatic and permeability pulmonary edema are not mutually exclusive and in fact may be closely linked. Pulmonary edema occurs when the hydrostatic pressure is excessive for a given capillary permeability and for a given rate of clearance of interstitial fluid. For instance, in the presence of damaged capillary endothelium, small increases in an otherwise normal hydrostatic pressure gradient may cause large increases in edema formation. Similarly, if the alveolar–epithelial barrier is damaged, even the baseline flux of fluid across an intact capillary endothelium may cause alveolar filling.

ARDS is the archetypal example of increased-permeability edema. While the underlying pathophysiology is complex, the fundamental mechanism is an inflammation-mediated disruption of the alveolar–capillary barrier. Through loss of endothelial and epithelial barrier integrity, the normal homeostatic mechanisms of fluid balance are disrupted, and protein-rich fluid accumulates in the alveolar space. This loss of integrity may result from direct injury to the alveolar epithelium following local activation of inflammation by inhaled toxins or pulmonary infection, or it may occur after primary injury to the pulmonary capillary endothelium following systemic activation of inflammation by circulating toxins, as in sepsis or pancreatitis. This is in contrast to cardiogenic pulmonary edema, in which both the alveolar epithelium and the capillary endothelium are usually intact. There are a wide range of clinical entities that can lead to ARDS, including some with increased pulmonary capillary endothelial permeability and others with increased alveolar epithelial permeability (see Table 9–7). These pathologically diverse processes can be grouped together into the syndrome of ARDS because they share a final common pathway of alveolar–capillary barrier injury, which results in characteristic changes in pulmonary mechanics and lung function.

ARDS is the byproduct of a dysregulated inflammatory response by the lung to an injurious insult. Whether the injury occurs directly or indirectly, the insult activates the innate immune response through resident immune cells such as the alveolar macrophage. These cells recognize both exogenous factors, such as those derived from microorganisms, and endogenous factors, elaborated by local or distant cellular injury, through "pattern recognition" receptors (eg, toll-like receptors). Receptor activation stimulates pro-inflammatory responses. Through the release of cytokines and chemokines, such as IL-1B, TNF, IL-6, and IL-8, circulating inflammatory cells, including neutrophils and monocytes, are recruited to the lung and undergo activation that further potentiates the pro-inflammatory signal. The propagation of this inflammatory cascade results in direct and indirect tissue injury through the release of a variety of factors, including other cytokines and chemokines, proteases, eicosanoids, and reactive oxygen species. Loss of barrier integrity as a result of injury to both the alveolar epithelium and capillary endothelium ultimately leads to the leakage of protein-rich fluid into the alveolar spaces throughout the lung. There, the edema fluid inactivates surfactant, increasing surface tension with resultant alveolar instability and atelectasis. Increased surface tension decreases the interstitial hydrostatic pressure, further favoring fluid movement into the alveolus. The loss of surfactant activity and the filling of airspaces cause the significant physiologic derangements that characterize ARDS, including decreases in lung compliance and lung volume and severe hypoxemia (secondary to low $\dot{V}/\dot{Q}$ and shunt).

The histopathology of increased-permeability pulmonary edema reflects the inflammatory disruption of the alveolar–capillary barrier. Grossly, the lungs are edematous and heavy. The surface appears violaceous, and hemorrhagic fluid exudes from the cut pleural surface. Microscopically, there is infiltration of the interalveolar septa and the interstitium by inflammatory cells and erythrocytes. Type I pneumocytes are damaged, leaving a denuded alveolar barrier. Sheets of pink-staining material, known as hyaline membranes, line the denuded basement membrane. Composed of cellular debris and plasma proteins (including fibrin), these hyaline membranes are the hallmark of the diffuse alveolar damage of ARDS. In some patients, the alveolar–capillary barrier injury progresses to fibrosis; in other, surviving patients, complete recovery with regeneration of an intact alveolar epithelium from the residual type II pneumocytes may occur.

Clinical Manifestations

Cardiogenic and noncardiogenic pulmonary edema both result in increased extravascular lung water, and both may result in respiratory failure. Given the differences in pathophysiology, it is unsurprising that the clinical manifestations are very different in the two syndromes.

A. Increased Hydrostatic Pulmonary Edema (Cardiogenic Pulmonary Edema)

Early increases in pulmonary venous pressure may be asymptomatic. The patient may notice only mild exertional dyspnea or a nonproductive cough stimulated by activation of irritant receptors coupled with C fibers. Orthopnea and paroxysmal nocturnal dyspnea occur when the patient's recumbent position allows for the redistribution of blood or edema fluid from the lower extremities into the venous circulation, thereby increasing thoracic blood volume and pulmonary venous pressures.

Clinical signs begin with the accumulation of interstitial fluid. Cardiac examination may reveal a third heart sound, but there is a paucity of lung findings in purely interstitial edema. Early evidence of interstitial edema may be appreciated on a chest radiograph as an increase in the caliber of the upper lobe vessels ("pulmonary vascular redistribution") and as fluid accumulating in the perivascular and peribronchial spaces ("cuffing"). The chest radiograph may also show Kerley B lines, which represent fluid in the interlobular septa. With increasing interstitial edema, lung compliance falls, and the patient begins to breathe more rapidly and shallowly to adapt to the increased elastic work of breathing. As alveolar flooding begins, there are further decreases in lung volume and

pulmonary compliance. With some alveoli filled with fluid, there is an increase in the fraction of the lung that is perfused but poorly ventilated. This shift toward low $\dot{V}/\dot{Q}$ ratios causes an increase in A–a ΔPO_2, if not frank hypoxemia. Supplemental oxygen corrects the hypoxemia, provided there is an absence of shunt. The $PaCO_2$ is often normal or low, reflecting the increased drive to breathe. The patient may become sweaty and cyanotic. The sputum may become pink, frothy edema fluid. It is pink from capillary hemorrhage resulting from high pulmonary venous pressures. Auscultation reveals inspiratory crackles chiefly at the bases, where the hydrostatic pressure is greatest, but potentially throughout both lungs. Rhonchi and wheezing ("cardiac asthma") may occur. On the chest radiograph, the accumulation of fluid in the interstitium and alveolar spaces results in the development of bilateral perihilar opacities.

B. Increased-Permeability Pulmonary Edema (Noncardiogenic Pulmonary Edema)

The most common form of increased-permeability pulmonary edema is ARDS. According to the consensus Berlin Definition, ARDS is characterized by acute onset (<7 days) of bilateral radiographic pulmonary infiltrates and respiratory failure not fully explained by heart failure or volume overload, with an associated impairment in oxygenation defined as a PaO_2/FiO_2 ratio of 300 or less. The severity of ARDS is defined by the severity of impairment in oxygenation. Mild, moderate, and severe ARDS are defined by PaO_2/FiO_2 ratios of 200–300 mm Hg, 100–200 mm Hg, and less than 100 mm Hg, respectively. ARDS is the final common pathway of a number of different serious medical conditions, all of which lead to increased pulmonary capillary leak. The range of clinical presentations includes all the diagnoses in the adult ICU, including sepsis, pneumonia, pancreatitis, aspiration of gastric contents, shock, lung contusion, nonthoracic trauma, toxic inhalation, near-drowning, and multiple blood transfusions. About one-third of ARDS patients initially have sepsis syndrome.

Although the mechanism of injury varies, damage to capillary endothelial cells and alveolar epithelial cells is common in ARDS regardless of cause. After the initial insult (eg, an episode of high-grade bacteremia), there is generally a period of stability, reflecting the time it takes for pro-inflammatory mediators released from stimulated inflammatory cells to cause damage. Damage to endothelial and epithelial cells causes increased vascular permeability and reduced surfactant production and activity. These abnormalities lead to interstitial and alveolar pulmonary edema, alveolar collapse, a significant increase in surface forces, markedly reduced pulmonary compliance, and hypoxemia. For the first 24–48 hours after the insult, the patient may experience increased work of breathing, manifested by dyspnea and tachypnea, but without abnormalities on the chest radiograph. At this early stage, the increased A–a ΔPO_2 reflects alveolar edema with $\dot{V}/\dot{Q}$ mismatching shifted to low $\dot{V}/\dot{Q}$ ratios that can usually be corrected by increased FiO_2 and increased minute ventilation. The clinical picture may improve, or there may be a further fall in compliance and disruption of pulmonary capillaries, leading to areas of true shunting and refractory hypoxemia. The combination of increased work of breathing and progressive hypoxemia usually requires mechanical ventilation. Because the underlying process is heterogeneous, there is normal-appearing lung adjacent to atelectatic or consolidated lung. Therefore, ventilating patients at typical tidal volumes may overdistend normal alveoli, reduce blood flow to areas of adequate ventilation, and precipitate further lung injury ("volu-trauma").

Hypoxemia can be profound in ARDS and is typically followed days later by hypercapnia owing to increasing dead space ventilation. Radiographically, there may be patchy alveolar opacities or "whiteout" of the lungs, representing diffuse confluent alveolar filling. Pathologically, diffuse alveolar damage is seen, characterized by inflammatory cell infiltration and the formation of hyaline membranes. Mortality is 20–40%. Most patients die from some complication of their presenting illness, not from refractory hypoxemia. Of those who survive, a majority will recover near-normal lung function, but their recovery may be prolonged (6–12 months). A subset of survivors will develop new pulmonary fibrosis or reactive airway disease.

CHECKPOINT

35. What four factors are involved in the production of pulmonary edema? How are they affected in cardiogenic versus noncardiogenic causes of pulmonary edema?

36. What are the common causes of noncardiogenic pulmonary edema?

37. Is lung damage from increased-permeability pulmonary edema reversible? If so, how?

38. What are the two major reasons that mechanical ventilation is often required in severe pulmonary edema?

PULMONARY EMBOLISM

Clinical Presentation

The English word "embolus" derives from a Greek word meaning "plug" or "stopper." A pulmonary embolus consists of material that gains access to the venous system and then to the pulmonary circulation. Eventually, it reaches a vessel whose caliber is too small to permit free passage where it forms a plug, occluding the lumen and obstructing perfusion. There are many types of pulmonary emboli (Table 9–8). The most common is pulmonary thromboembolism, which occurs when venous thrombi, chiefly from the lower extremities, migrate to the pulmonary circulation. Note that it is a normal function of the pulmonary microcirculation to prevent embolic material from entering the systemic arterial system. The lungs possess both excess functional capacity and a redundant vascular supply, allowing them to filter a significant number of thrombi

TABLE 9–8   Types of pulmonary emboli.

Material	Clinical Setting
Air	Cardiac surgery, neurosurgery, improper manipulation of central venous catheters
Amniotic fluid	Active labor
Fat	Long bone fracture, liposuction
Foreign body	Pieces of intravenous devices, talc
Oil	Lymphangiography
Parasite eggs	Schistosomiasis
Septic emboli	Endocarditis, thrombophlebitis
Thrombus	Deep venous thrombosis
Tumor	Renal cell carcinoma with invasion of vena cava

and platelet aggregates with minimal impact on lung function or hemodynamics. However, large thromboemboli, or a large enough accumulation of smaller ones, can cause substantial impairment of cardiac and respiratory function and death.

Pulmonary thromboemboli are common and cause significant morbidity. They are found at autopsy in 25–50% of hospitalized patients and are considered a major contributing cause of death in one-third of those. However, the diagnosis is made antemortem in only 10–20% of cases.

Etiology & Epidemiology

Pulmonary embolism (PE) and deep venous thrombosis represent a continuum of a single disease that has been coined venous thromboembolic disease (VTE). VTE is a common problem with an annual incidence of approximately 100 new cases per 100,000 persons. The risk of this disorder increases with advancing age and also differs among ethnicities (with the greatest incidence in African-Americans). Furthermore, pulmonary embolism accounts for approximately 5–10% of in-hospital deaths, making this disorder the leading cause of inpatient mortality.

The thromboemboli that cause PE almost never originate in the pulmonary circulation; they arrive there by dislodging from their site of origin and traveling through the venous circulation. More than 95% of pulmonary thromboemboli arise from thrombi in the deep veins of the lower extremity: the popliteal, femoral, and iliac veins. Venous thrombosis below the popliteal veins or occurring in the superficial veins of the leg is clinically common but not a risk factor for pulmonary thromboembolism because thrombi in these locations rarely migrate to the pulmonary circulation without first extending above the knee. Because fewer than 20% of calf thrombi will extend into the popliteal veins, isolated calf thrombi may be observed with serial tests to exclude extension into the proximal deep system. Venous thromboses occasionally occur in the

TABLE 9–9   Risk factors for venous thrombosis.

Increased venous stasis
Bed rest
Immobilization, especially after orthopedic surgery
Low cardiac output states
Pregnancy
Obesity
Hyperviscosity
Local vascular damage, especially prior thrombosis with incompetent valves
Central venous catheters
Increasing age
Increased coagulability
Tissue injury: surgery, trauma, myocardial infarction
Malignancy
Presence of a lupus anticoagulant/antiphospholipid antibody
Nephrotic syndrome
Oral contraceptive use, especially estrogen administration
Genetic coagulation disorders: resistance to activated protein C (factor V Leiden); prothrombin 20210A mutation; hyperhomocysteinemia; thermolabile variant of methylenetetrahydrofolate reductase (MTHFR); deficiency of antithrombin III, protein C, or its cofactor, protein S, or of plasminogen; dysfunctional fibrinogen
Endothelial injury
Intravenous catheter placement
Trauma
Surgery
Prior deep venous thrombosis

upper extremities or in the right side of the heart; this happens most commonly in the presence of intravenous catheters or cardiac pacing wires and may be of increasing clinical importance as the use of long-term intravenous catheters increases.

Risk factors for pulmonary thromboembolism are, therefore, the risk factors for the development of venous thrombosis in the deep veins of the legs (deep venous thrombosis) (Table 9–9). The German pathologist Rudolf Virchow described these risk factors in 1856: venous stasis, vascular wall endothelial injury, and increased activation of the clotting system. His observations remain valid today.

The most prevalent risk factor in hospitalized patients is stasis from immobilization, especially in those undergoing surgical procedures. The incidence of calf vein thrombosis in patients who do not receive appropriate anticoagulant prophylaxis after total knee replacement is reported to be as high as 84%; it is more than 50% after hip surgery or prostatectomy. The risk of fatal pulmonary thromboembolism in these patients may be as high as 5%. Physicians caring for these patients must, therefore, be aware of the magnitude of the risk and institute appropriate prophylactic therapy (Tables 9–9 and 9–10).

Malignancy and tissue damage at surgery are the two most common causes of increased activation of the coagulation system. Injury to the venous endothelium can result from stasis with local hypoxia, the insertion of intravenous catheters, or mechanical injury during surgery or trauma. Prior thrombosis can also damage venous valves and lead to venous incompetence, which promotes stasis.

Enhanced activation of the clotting cascade can result from both acquired disorders (eg, estrogen-containing medication, malignancy) and genetic predispositions (thrombophilias). Advances now permit identification of genetic disorders in up to one-third of unselected patients with venous thrombosis and in more than half of patients with familial thrombosis (see Table 9–9). It is now clear that these genetic variants may interact with other factors (eg, oral contraceptive use, dietary deficiencies) to increase thrombosis risk.

In addition to these major risk factors, recent studies implicate other risk factors for the development of VTE: specifically, inflammatory disorders such as Crohn disease, ulcerative colitis, and rheumatoid arthritis; and infections, such as urinary tract infection, respiratory tract infection, and bacteremia. The metabolic syndrome also increases the risk of VTE, especially the presence of abdominal obesity. The mechanisms by which these other risk factors increase the likelihood of VTE is unclear, but it is hypothesized that systemic inflammation upregulates procoagulant factors while concurrently inhibiting fibrinolysis. Abdominal obesity may also cause venous stasis secondary to increased abdominal pressure.

Pathophysiology

Venous thrombi are composed of a friable mass of fibrin, with many erythrocytes and a few leukocytes and platelets randomly enmeshed in the matrix. When a venous thrombus travels to the pulmonary circulation, it causes a broad array of pathophysiologic changes (Table 9–11).

A. Hemodynamic Changes

Every patient with a pulmonary embolus has some degree of mechanical obstruction of the pulmonary arterial circulation. The severity of mechanical obstruction depends on the clot burden, the neurohumoral reflexes stimulated by mediators released from the thrombus, and the presence or absence of pre-existing cardiopulmonary disease. Patients *without* pre-existing cardiopulmonary disease can accommodate occlusion of up to roughly one-third of the pulmonary circulation with a negligible increase in pulmonary vascular resistance and pulmonary arterial pressure. The normal pulmonary circulation adapts to the diverted blood flow through the recruitment and dilation of compliant pulmonary arterial vessels (see Figure 9–13). These adaptive mechanisms fail when a greater proportion of the pulmonary circulation is compromised by larger emboli and/or by the elaboration of vasoconstricting mediators, at which point pulmonary vascular resistance and pulmonary arterial pressure increase. In patients with pre-existing cardiopulmonary disease, increases in pulmonary artery pressures have not been shown to correlate with extent of embolization. The likely explanation is that normal adaptive

TABLE 9–10   Risk of postoperative deep venous thrombosis or pulmonary embolus in patients who do not receive anticoagulant prophylaxis.

Risk Category	Incidence of Calf Deep Venous Thrombosis	Incidence of Proximal Deep Venous Thrombosis	Incidence of Fatal Pulmonary Embolus
High risk	40–80%	10–20%	1–5%
1. Age >40			
2. Anesthesia >30 min			
3. At least one of the following:			
a. Orthopedic surgery			
b. Pelvic or abdominal cancer surgery			
c. History of deep venous thrombosis or pulmonary embolus			
d. Hereditary coagulopathy			
Moderate risk	10–40%	2–10%	0.1–0.7%
1. Age >40			
2. Anesthesia >30 min			
3. At least one of the following secondary risk factors:			
a. Immobilization			
b. Obesity			
c. Malignancy			
d. Estrogen use			
e. Varicose veins			
f. Paralysis			
Low risk	<10%	<1%	<0.01%
1. Any age			
2. Anesthesia <30 min			
3. No secondary risk factors			

Modified and reproduced, with permission, from Merli G. Update: deep vein thrombosis and pulmonary embolism prophylaxis in orthopedic surgery. Med Clin North Am. 1993;77:397. Copyright © Elsevier.

TABLE 9–11   Pathophysiologic changes in pulmonary embolism.

Pulmonary Physiology	Change with Pulmonary Thromboembolism	Mechanism of Observed Change
Hemodynamics	Increased pulmonary vascular resistance	Vascular obstruction
		Vasoconstriction mediated by thromboxane A2 and serotonin
Gas exchange	Decreased PO_2 (hypoxemia)	Increased perfusion of lung units with low $\dot{V}/\dot{Q}$ ratios
		Decreased cardiac output with decrease in mixed venous PO_2
		Right-to-left shunting
	Increased alveolar dead space	Vascular obstruction
		Absent perfusion $\dot{Q}$ to lung units with preserved ventilation $\dot{V}$
Work of breathing	Decreased lung compliance	Loss of surfactant causing alveolar edema and hemorrhage
	Increased airway resistance	Reflex bronchoconstriction
Ventilatory control	Increased respiratory rate (hyperventilation)	Reflex stimulation of irritant receptors

FIGURE 9–26 Arterial PO$_2$ and A–a O$_2$ difference in 74 patients with PE from the PIOPED II study. Blood gases were drawn while patients were breathing room air. (Data from Stein PD et al. Clinical characteristics of patients with acute pulmonary embolism: data from PIOPED II. Am J Med. 2007;120:871.)

mechanisms are ineffective in patients with pre-existing pulmonary hypertension, making them susceptible to significant instability with any subsequent impairment of the pulmonary vasculature.

Large emboli that do not completely occlude vessels, particularly in patients with compromised cardiac function, may cause an acute increase in pulmonary vascular resistance. This leads to acute right ventricular strain and can lead to a fatal decrease in cardiac output. The most devastating and feared complication of acute pulmonary thromboembolism is sudden occlusion of the pulmonary outflow tract ("saddle embolus"), reducing cardiac output to zero and causing immediate cardiovascular collapse and death. Such dramatic presentations occur in less than 5% of cases and are essentially untreatable. They serve to highlight the importance of primary prevention of venous thrombosis.

B. Changes in Ventilation

The immediate effect is the generation of increased "dead space" ventilation (ie, regions of the lung with preserved $\dot{V}$ but absent $\dot{Q}$). This increase in dead space impairs the elimination of carbon dioxide with minimal effect on oxygenation. However, in the setting of thromboembolism, patients typically compensate for the increase in dead space ventilation by increasing their total minute ventilation. In fact, patients classically overcompensate for the increase in dead space, exhibiting a respiratory alkalosis on their arterial blood gas analysis.

C. Changes in Oxygenation

Mild to moderate hypoxemia with a low PaCO$_2$ is the most common finding in acute pulmonary thromboembolism. Mild hypoxemia may be obscured by the tendency to rely on oximetry alone, because more than half of patients will have oxygen saturations (SaO$_2$) above 90% (Figure 9–26). Historically, the A–a ΔPO$_2$ was thought to be a more sensitive indicator of PE because it compensates for the presence of hypocapnia and the amount of inspired FiO$_2$. However, the Prospective Investigation of Pulmonary Embolism Diagnosis II (PIOPED II) study called this thinking into question. An A–a ΔPO$_2$ less than 20, which is normal or near normal depending on patient age, was

found in one-third of patients with an acute PE identified by CT scan (see Figure 9–26).

No one mechanism fully accounts for hypoxemia in acute PE. At least five mechanisms have been suggested:

1. Local hypoperfusion interfering with surfactant production by alveolar type II cells. Surfactant is subsequently depleted, resulting in alveolar edema, alveolar collapse, and areas of atelectasis creating lung units with little or no ventilation. These changes result in an increase in lung units with low $\dot{V}/\dot{Q}$ ratios, including some areas of true shunting, both of which contribute to an increased A–a ΔPO$_2$ and arterial hypoxemia.

2. The diversion of blood flow through poorly ventilated or nonventilated lung zones. Perfusion is normally reduced to hypoventilated lung regions through hypoxic pulmonary vasoconstriction. However, if pulmonary artery pressure increases after thromboembolism, perfusion may increase in areas of vasoconstriction, resulting in shifts toward low $\dot{V}/\dot{Q}$ areas causing hypoxemia.

3. True right-to-left shunts. Increased pulmonary artery, right ventricular, and right atrial pressures favor the development of shunts in a small percentage of patients with hypoxemia from acute pulmonary thromboembolism. It has been proposed that these shunts result from the opening of a foramen ovale or from pulmonary artery to pulmonary venous shunting, but their exact location is unknown.

4. Low mixed venous PO$_2$. In some patients with preexisting impaired cardiac function or with large emboli that cause acute right ventricular strain, cardiac output may fall, with a resultant fall in mixed venous oxygen concentration. This is an important cause of hypoxemia in seriously ill patients.

5. Decreased pulmonary capillary surface area resulting in decreased lung diffusion capacity.

D. Bronchoconstriction

Reflex bronchoconstriction causes wheezing and increased work of breathing in some patients.

E. Pulmonary Infarction

Obstruction of small pulmonary arterial branches that act as end arteries leads to pulmonary infarction in about 10% of cases. It is generally associated with some concomitant abnormality of the bronchial circulation such as that seen in patients with left ventricular failure and chronically elevated left atrial pressures.

Clinical Manifestations

A. Symptoms & Signs

The classic triad of a sudden onset of dyspnea, pleuritic chest pain, and hemoptysis occurs in a minority of cases. In a large study of patients with PE, dyspnea was present in 73% of cases, and pleuritic chest pain was present 44% of the time. Dyspnea probably results from reflex bronchoconstriction as well as increased pulmonary artery pressure, loss of pulmonary compliance, and stimulation of C fibers. In patients with large emboli, acute right heart strain may contribute to dyspnea. Pleuritic chest pain is more common than pulmonary infarction; one group has suggested that the pain is caused by areas of pulmonary hemorrhage. Hemoptysis is seen with pulmonary infarction but may also result from transmission of systemic arterial pressures to the microvasculature via bronchopulmonary anastomoses, with subsequent capillary disruption. It may reflect hemorrhagic pulmonary edema from surfactant depletion or neutrophil-associated capillary injury. Syncope may signal a massive embolus.

The most predictive physical finding for pulmonary embolism is not in the chest but the leg: a swollen, tender, warm, and reddened calf that provides evidence for deep venous thrombosis. The absence of such evidence does not exclude the diagnosis, because the clinical examination is insensitive and the absence of signs may indicate that the entire thrombus has embolized. Auscultatory chest findings are common but nonspecific. Atelectasis may lead to inspiratory crackles; infarction may cause a focal pleural friction rub; and the release of mediators may cause bronchoconstriction and wheezing. In large embolization, one may find signs of acute right ventricular strain such as a right ventricular lift and accentuation of the pulmonary component of the second heart sound.

Difficulty in recognizing patients with pulmonary embolism results from the lack of sensitivity and specificity of symptoms and signs. This challenge has motivated the development of clinical probability scoring systems. The Wells and Geneva scores are examples of two well-validated diagnostic aids that allow the clinician to assign disease likelihoods to individual patients. In both scoring systems, points are tabulated based on the presence of specific clinical features that are readily assessed. Patients can then be categorized into different tiers of disease probability to facilitate clinical decisions on the performance and interpretation of diagnostic tests and the initiation of treatments.

B. Electrocardiography

The electrocardiogram is abnormal in 70% of patients with acute PE. However, the most common abnormalities are sinus tachycardia and nonspecific ST and T wave changes, each seen in approximately 40% of patients. The classic finding of an acute right ventricular strain pattern on ECG—a deep S wave in lead I and both a Q wave and an inverted T wave in lead III ($S_1Q_3T_3$)—was observed in 11% of patients in the Urokinase Pulmonary Embolism Trial.

C. Laboratory Findings

An increase in the A–a ΔPO_2 is seen in more than two-thirds of cases, and hypoxemia is a common yet nonspecific finding. Measurement of the degradation product of cross-linked fibrin, D-dimers, can be used to exclude the diagnosis of acute PE in symptomatic outpatients deemed to have a low pretest probability of PE based on clinical criteria. Depending on the specific assay and patient population, the D-dimer has a high sensitivity (85–99%) and moderate to high specificity (40–93%). Most studies suggest that D-dimer cannot be used to exclude PE in a patient with an intermediate or a high pretest probability for PE.

Brain natriuretic peptide (BNP), an indicator of ventricular stretch, and cardiac troponins, which indicate cardiac myocyte injury, are commonly measured in patients with PE. Because of low sensitivity and specificity, these markers cannot be used to diagnose PE. However, an elevation of BNP or troponins in the setting of known PE has been shown to correlate with the presence of right ventricular overload and a greater risk of adverse outcomes, including respiratory failure and death.

D. Chest Radiography

The chest radiograph was normal in only 12% of patients with confirmed pulmonary thromboembolism in the PIOPED study. The most common findings were atelectasis, parenchymal opacities, and small pleural effusions. However, the prevalence of these findings was the same in hospitalized patients without suspected pulmonary thromboembolism. Local oligemia (Westermark sign) or pleura-based areas of increased opacity that represent intraparenchymal hemorrhage (Hampton hump) are rare. The chest radiograph is necessary to exclude other common lung diseases and to permit interpretation of the ventilation/perfusion scan, but it does not itself establish the diagnosis. Paradoxically, it may be most helpful when normal in the setting of acute severe hypoxemia.

E. Ventilation/Perfusion Scanning

A perfusion scan is obtained by injecting microaggregated radiolabeled albumin with a particle size of 50–100 μm into the venous system and allowing the particles to embolize to the pulmonary capillary bed (approximate diameter 10 μm). The substance is labeled with a gamma-emitting isotope of technetium (Tc-99m pertechnetate) that permits imaging of the distribution of pulmonary blood flow. A ventilation scan is performed by having the patient breathe xenon (Xe-133) or a radioactive aerosol and doing sequential scans during inhalation and exhalation. A normal perfusion scan excludes clinically significant pulmonary thromboembolism. A segmental or larger perfusion defect in a radiographically normal area that shows normal ventilation is diagnostic. This is referred to as a "mismatched" defect and is highly specific (97%) for pulmonary thromboembolism.

Only a minority of ventilation/perfusion scans reveal clearly diagnostic findings, however. The PIOPED study demonstrated that nondiagnostic ventilation/perfusion scans can stratify a patient's risk of pulmonary thromboembolism. Furthermore, within the categories of high-, medium-, and low-probability studies, the clinician's pretest assessment of the probability of pulmonary thromboembolism can further stratify patients. When clinical probabilities and scan interpretations are discordant, additional evaluation for VTE should be performed.

F. Computed Tomography and Pulmonary Angiography

Computed tomography scanning with intravenous contrast (CT pulmonary angiography) has widely supplanted ventilation/perfusion scanning as the initial test of choice to diagnose PE. The diagnostic strength of this imaging modality lies in its high negative predictive value and its ability to identify other conditions that cause dyspnea and chest pain (eg, pneumonia, aortic dissection). Multiple trials have shown a high sensitivity and specificity of this imaging technique, although the diagnostic test characteristics depend on patient selection, expertise of the technician performing the contrast injection, and the experience of the interpreting radiologist. The PIOPED II trial evaluated CT angiography for the diagnosis of PE and found a sensitivity of 83% and a specificity of 96% (Table 9–12). Several other studies indicate that the risk of PE after a negative CT scan in patients with a low or intermediate clinical probability of PE is less than 2%. Consistent with the first PIOPED trial comparing ventilation/perfusion scanning and traditional pulmonary angiography, pretest probability based on clinical risk scores must be taken into account when interpreting CT pulmonary

angiography. As is true with the ventilation/perfusion scan, if test results and clinical probabilities are discordant, further testing, such as ventilation/perfusion scanning, lower extremity Doppler ultrasonography, or pulmonary angiography, must be considered.

Pulmonary angiography is a safe but invasive procedure with well-defined morbidity and mortality data. Minor complications occur in approximately 5% of patients. Most are allergic contrast reactions or transient kidney injury or are related to percutaneous catheter insertion; cardiac perforation and arrhythmias are reported but rare. Among the PIOPED I patients who underwent angiography, five deaths (0.7%) were directly related to the procedure. Pulmonary angiography remains the reference standard for the diagnosis of PE, but its role compared with CT angiography is a subject of ongoing debate. There is general agreement that angiography is indicated when the diagnosis is in doubt but there is a high clinical pretest probability of PE, or when the diagnosis of PE must be established with certainty, as when anticoagulation is contraindicated or placement of an inferior vena cava filter is contemplated. An intraluminal filling defect in more than one projection establishes a definitive diagnosis. Secondary findings highly suggestive of PE include an abrupt arterial cutoff, asymmetry of blood flow (especially segmental oligemia), and a prolonged arterial phase with slow filling. Pulmonary angiography was performed in 755 patients in the PIOPED I study. A definitive diagnosis was established in 97%; in 3%, the studies were nondiagnostic. Four patients (0.8%) with negative angiograms subsequently had pulmonary thromboemboli at autopsy. Serial angiography has demonstrated minimal resolution of thrombus prior to day 7 following presentation. Thus, negative angiography within 7 days of presentation excludes the diagnosis.

G. Resolution

The variability among patients is so great that generalizations are difficult. The largest number of patients monitored serially

TABLE 9–12 Positive and negative predictive values of CT angiography for acute pulmonary embolism (PE).

| CT Scan Results | Clinical Probability[1] (%) | | | | | |
| | High | | Intermediate | | Low | |
	PE+/No. of Patients	%	PE+/No. of Patients	%	PE+/No. of Patients	%
CT+ (likelihood PE present)	22/23	96	93/101	92	22/38	58
CT– (likelihood PE absent)	9/15	60	121/136	89	158/164	96

[1]Clinical probability based on the Wells score: less than 2.0, low probability; 2.0–6.0, moderate probability; more than 6.0, high probability.

Data from Stein PD et al. Multidetector computed tomography for acute pulmonary embolism. N Engl J Med. 2006;354(12):2317–27.

with quantitative assessments was in the Urokinase Pulmonary Embolism Trial. In that study, serial perfusion scans showed a resolution of 35–56% of perfusion defects at 9–14 days. More recent studies, some involving quantitative angiography, have tended to support the time course of these findings.

In a few patients, pulmonary emboli do not resolve completely but become organized and incorporated into the pulmonary arterial wall as an epithelialized fibrous mass, producing what is termed chronic pulmonary thromboembolism. This entity presents with stenosis of the central pulmonary arteries, with associated pulmonary hypertension and right ventricular failure (cor pulmonale). Treatment is surgical.

CHECKPOINT

39. Where do 95% of pulmonary thromboemboli originate?
40. What are the risk factors for pulmonary thromboemboli?
41. What hemodynamic changes are brought about by significant pulmonary thromboemboli?
42. What changes in ventilation/perfusion relationships are brought about by significant pulmonary thromboemboli?
43. Suggest some possible explanations for hypoxemia in pulmonary thromboembolism.
44. What are the clinical manifestations of pulmonary thromboembolism?

CASE STUDIES

Yeong Kwok, MD

(See Chapter 25, p. 762–65 for answers)

CASE 48

A 25-year-old previously well woman presents to your office with complaints of episodic shortness of breath and chest tightness. She has had the symptoms on and off for about 2 years but states that they have worsened lately, occurring two or three times a month. She notes that the symptoms are worse during the spring months. She has no exercise-induced or nocturnal symptoms. The family history is notable for a father with asthma. She is single and works as an administrative assistant in a high-tech firm. She lives with a roommate, who moved in approximately 2 months ago. The roommate has a cat. The patient smokes occasionally when out with friends and drinks socially, but has no history of illicit drug use. Examination is notable for mild end-expiratory wheezing. The history and physical examination are consistent with a diagnosis of asthma. Pulmonary function tests are ordered to confirm the diagnosis.

Questions

A. What are the three categories of provocative agents that can trigger asthma? What are some possible triggers in this patient?
B. Describe the early events responsible for the pathogenesis of asthma. How does this result in chronic airway inflammation and airway hyperresponsiveness?
C. What pathogenetic mechanisms are responsible for this patient's symptoms of wheezing, shortness of breath, and chest tightness?
D. What might you expect the results of her pulmonary function tests to be? Why?

CASE 49

A 67-year-old man presents to your office with worsening cough, sputum production, and shortness of breath. He has been a cigarette smoker for the past 50 years, smoking approximately 1 pack a day. He has a chronic AM cough productive of some yellow sputum but generally feels okay during the day. He was in his usual state of health until two weeks ago when he developed a cold. Since then, he has had a hacking cough and increased thick sputum production. He also has had difficulty walking more than a block without stopping due to shortness of breath. Physical examination reveals prolonged expiration, audible wheezing, and diffuse rhonchi throughout both lung fields. Chest x-ray shows hyperinflation of both lungs with a flattened diaphragm.

Questions

A. What are the two major clinical syndromes classified as chronic obstructive pulmonary disease? How do they differ?

B. Of the two syndromes above, which is predominant in this patient? What are the epidemiology and predisposing factors for this condition?

C. What might the pulmonary function tests show in this patient?

D. How do arterial blood gases differ in chronic bronchitis and emphysema?

CASE 50

A 68-year-old man presents to the clinic with a complaint of shortness of breath. He states that he has become progressively more short of breath over the last 2 months, such that he is now short of breath with walking one block. In addition, he has noted a nonproductive cough. He denies fever, chills, night sweats, chest pain, orthopnea, and paroxysmal nocturnal dyspnea. He has noted no lower extremity edema. The medical history is unremarkable. Physical examination reveals a respiratory rate of 19/min and fine, dry inspiratory crackles heard throughout both lung fields. Digital clubbing is present. A diagnosis of idiopathic pulmonary fibrosis is made.

Questions

A. What are the cellular events involved in lung injury and fibrosis in idiopathic pulmonary fibrosis?

B. What pathophysiologic mechanisms are responsible for this patient's symptoms of dyspnea and cough? What pathogenetic mechanisms are responsible for his physical findings of tachypnea, inspiratory crackles, and digital clubbing?

C. What might you expect the chest x-ray film and pulmonary function tests to show?

CASE 51

A 72-year-old man presents to the emergency department complaining of severe shortness of breath. He has long-standing poorly controlled hypertension and a history of coronary artery disease and two myocardial infarctions. About 1 week before admission, he had an episode of sub-sternal chest pain lasting approximately 30 minutes. Since then he has noted progressive shortness of breath to the point that he is now dyspneic on minimal exertion such as walking across the room. He notes a new onset of shortness of breath while lying down. He is only comfortable when propped up by three pillows. He is occasionally awakened from sleep acutely short of breath. On examination he is afebrile, with a blood pressure of 160/100 mm Hg, heart rate of 108/min, respiratory rate of 22/min, and oxygen saturation of 88% on room air. He is pale, cool, and diaphoretic. Jugular venous pressure is 10 cm H_2O. Chest auscultation reveals rales in both lungs to the mid-lung fields. Cardiac examination reveals tachycardia, with an audible S_3 and S_4. No murmurs or rubs are heard. Extremities are without edema. The ECG shows left ventricular hypertrophy and Q waves in the anterior and lateral leads, consistent with this patient's history of hypertension and myocardial infarction. Chest x-ray film reveals bilateral fluffy infiltrates consistent with pulmonary edema. He is admitted to the ICU with a diagnosis of heart failure and possible myocardial infarction.

Questions

A. What are the four factors that account for almost all cases of pulmonary edema? Which are probably responsible for this patient's pulmonary edema?

B. How does poor cardiac function cause pulmonary edema?

CASE 52

A 57-year-old man undergoes total knee replacement for severe degenerative joint disease. Four days after surgery, he develops an acute onset of shortness of breath and right-sided pleuritic chest pain. He is now in moderate respiratory distress with a respiratory rate of 28/min, heart rate of 120 bpm, and blood pressure of 110/70 mm Hg. Oxygen saturation is 90% on room air. Lung examination is normal. Cardiac examination reveals tachycardia but is otherwise unremarkable. The right lower extremity is postsurgical, healing well, with 2+ pitting edema, calf tenderness, erythema, and warmth; the left leg is normal. He has a positive Homan sign on the right. Acute pulmonary embolism is suspected.

Questions

A. Where did the pulmonary embolism probably arise from?

B. What are this patient's risk factors for thromboembolism?

C. What are the hemodynamic changes seen in acute pulmonary embolism?

D. What changes might be expected in ventilation/perfusion relationships and why?

CASE 53

A 46-year-old man presents to the hospital with a 5-day history of worsening cough, high fever, and shortness of breath. On physical examination, he is noted to be tachypneic (respiratory rate of 30 breaths/min), hypoxic with a low oxygen saturation (89%), and febrile (39°C). Chest x-ray film reveals infiltrates in both lower lobes. A complete blood count reveals a high white blood cell count. He is admitted to the hospital. Despite treatment with oxygen and antibiotics, he becomes more hypoxic and requires endotracheal intubation and mechanical ventilation. Blood cultures grow *Streptococcus pneumoniae*. Despite mechanical ventilation using high oxygen concentrations, his arterial blood oxygen level remains low. His chest x-ray film shows progression of infiltrates throughout both lung fields. He is diagnosed with acute respiratory distress syndrome (ARDS).

Questions

A. What are the main pathophysiologic factors in ARDS that cause an accumulation of extravascular fluid in the lungs?
B. What are the common causes of ARDS?
C. What accounts for the severe hypoxia often found in ARDS, despite the use of mechanical ventilation and high concentrations of oxygen?

REFERENCES

General

Broaddus VC et al. *Murray & Nadel's Textbook of Respiratory Medicine*, 6th ed. Elsevier, 2015.

Lumb AB. *Nunn's Applied Respiratory Physiology*, 8th ed. Elsevier, 2016.

West JB. *Pulmonary Pathophysiology: The Essentials*, 8th ed. Lippincott Williams & Wilkins, 2012.

West JB et al. *West's Respiratory Physiology: The Essentials*, 10th ed. Lippincott Williams & Wilkins, 2015.

Physiology & Pathophysiology

Akulian J et al. The evaluation and clinical application of pleural physiology. Clin Chest Med. 2013 Mar;34(1):11–9. [PMID: 23411052]

Brusasco V et al. Chronic obstructive pulmonary disease. Compr Physiol. 2014 Jan;4(1):1–31. [PMID: 24692133]

Chan ED et al. Pulse oximetry: understanding its basic principles facilitates appreciation of its limitations. Respir Med. 2013 Jun;107(6):789–99. [PMID: 23490227]

Nici L et al. Pulmonary rehabilitation: definition, concept, and history. Clin Chest Med. 2014 Jun;35(2):279–82. [PMID: 24874123]

Piper AJ et al. Hypoventilation syndromes. Compr Physiol. 2014 Oct;4(4):1639–76. [PMID: 25428856]

Prabhakar NR et al. Oxygen sensing and homeostasis. Physiology (Bethesda). 2015 Sep;30(5):340–8. [PMID: 26328879]

Wagner PD. The physiological basis of pulmonary gas exchange: implications for clinical interpretation of arterial blood gases. Eur Respir J. 2015 Jan;45(1):227–43. [PMID: 25323225]

Obstructive Lung Diseases

Berg K et al. The pathology of chronic obstructive pulmonary disease: progress in the 20th and 21st centuries. Arch Pathol Lab Med. 2016 Dec;140(12):1423–28. [PMID: 27922768]

Decramer M et al. Chronic obstructive pulmonary disease. Lancet. 2012;379(9823):1341–51. [PMID: 22314182]

Gauthier M et al. Evolving concepts of asthma. Am J Respir Crit Care Med. 2015 Sep 15;192(6):660–8. [PMID: 26161792]

Global Initiative for Asthma. 2018 Global Strategy for Asthma Management and Prevention. 2018. Available from: http://ginasthma.org/gina-reports/

Global Initiative for Chronic Obstructive Lung Disease (GOLD). GOLD 2017 Global Strategy for the Diagnosis, Management and Prevention of COPD. 2017. Available from: http://goldcopd.org/gold-2017-global-strategy-diagnosis-management-prevention-copd/

Hogg JC et al. The contribution of small airway obstruction to the pathogenesis of chronic obstructive pulmonary disease. Physiol Rev. 2017 Apr;97(2):529–52. [PMID: 28151425]

Holt PG et al. Defective respiratory tract immune surveillance in asthma: a primary causal factor in disease onset and progression. Chest. 2014 Feb;145(2):370–8. [PMID: 24493508]

Kent BD et al. Hypoxemia in patients with COPD: cause, effects and disease progression. Int J Chron Obstruct Pulmon Dis. 2011;6:199–208. [PMID: 21660297]

Kim V et al. Chronic bronchitis and chronic obstructive pulmonary disease. Am J Respir Crit Care Med. 2013 Feb 1;187(3):228–37. [PMID: 23204254]

Olin JT et al. Asthma: pathogenesis and novel drugs for treatment. BMJ. 2014 Nov 24;349:g5517. [PMID: 25420994]

Postma DS et al. The asthma-COPD overlap syndrome. N Engl J Med. 2015 Sep 24;373(13):1241–9. [PMID: 26398072]

Wenzel SE. Asthma phenotypes: the evolution from molecular approaches. Nat Med. 2012 May 4;18(5):716–25. [PMID: 22561835]

Zhang Z et al. Molecular pathogenesis in chronic obstructive pulmonary disease and therapeutic potential by targeting AMP-activated protein kinase. J Cell Physiol. 2018 Mar;233(3):1999–2006. [PMID: 28160496]

Interstitial Lung Diseases

Ahluwalia N et al. New therapeutic targets in idiopathic pulmonary fibrosis. Aiming to rein in runaway wound-healing responses. Am J Respir Crit Care Med. 2014 Oct 15;190(8):867–78. [PMID: 25090037]

Collard HR et al. Acute exacerbation of idiopathic pulmonary fibrosis. An International Working Group Report. Am J Respir Crit Care Med. 2016 Aug 1;194(3):265–75. [PMID: 27299520]

Goodwin A et al. Molecular endotyping of pulmonary fibrosis. Chest 2016 Jan;149(1):228–37. [PMID: 26356594]

Guiot J et al. Blood biomarkers in idiopathic pulmonary fibrosis. Lung. 2017 Jun;195(3):273–80. [PMID: 28353114]

Hambly N et al. Molecular classification of idiopathic pulmonary fibrosis: personalized medicine, genetics and biomarkers. Respirol 2015 Oct;20(7):1010–22. [PMID: 26109466]

Jankowich MD et al. Combined pulmonary fibrosis and emphysema syndrome: a review. Chest. 2012 Jan 14;141(1):222–31. [PMID: 22215830]

Johannson KA et al. Air pollution exposure: a novel environmental risk factor for interstitial lung disease? Chest. 2015 Apr;147(4):1161–7. [PMID: 25846532]

King TE Jr et al. Idiopathic pulmonary fibrosis. Lancet. 2011 Dec 3;378(9807):1949–61. [PMID: 21719092]

Larsen BT et al. Update for pathologists on idiopathic interstitial pneumonias. Arch Pathol Lab Med. 2012 Oct;136(10):1234–41. [PMID: 23020729]

Ley B et al. A multidimensional index and staging system for idiopathic pulmonary fibrosis. Ann Intern Med. 2012 May 15;156(10):684–91. [PMID: 22586007]

Luppi F et al. Acute exacerbation of idiopathic pulmonary fibrosis: a clinical review. Intern Emerg Med. 2015 Jun;10(4):401–11. [PMID: 25672832]

Mathai SK et al. Pulmonary fibrosis in the era of stratified medicine. Thorax. 2016 Dec;71(12):1154–60. [PMID: 27799632]

Noble PW et al. Pulmonary fibrosis: patterns and perpetrators. J Clin Invest. 2012 Aug 1;122(8):2756–62. [PMID: 22850886]

Ohta S et al; Consortium for Development of Diagnostics for Pulmonary Fibrosis Patients (CoDD-PF). The usefulness of monomeric periostin as a biomarker for idiopathic pulmonary fibrosis. PLoS One. 2017 Mar 29;12(3):e0174547. [PMID: 28355256]

Panagiotou M et al. Pulmonary vascular and cardiac impairment in interstitial lung disease. Eur Respir Rev. 2017 Jan 17;26(143). p111:160053. [Epub ahead of print] [PMID: 28096284]

Putman RK et al. Genetics and early detection in idiopathic pulmonary fibrosis. Am J Respir Crit Care Med. 2014 Apr 1;189(7):770–8. [PMID: 24547893]

Richeldi L et al. Idiopathic pulmonary fibrosis. Lancet 2017 May 13;389(10082):1941–52. [PMID: 28365056]

Ryu JH. Idiopathic pulmonary fibrosis: evolving concepts. Mayo Clin Proc. 2014 Aug;89(8):1130–42. [PMID: 24867394]

Solomon JJ et al. Connective tissue disease-associated interstitial lung disease: a focused review. J Intensive Care Med. 2015 Oct;30(7):392–400. [PMID: 24371251]

Pulmonary Edema

Birukov KG et al. Barrier enhancing signals in pulmonary edema. Compr Physiol. 2013 Jan;3(1):429–84. [PMID: 23720293]

Busl KM et al. Neurogenic pulmonary edema. Crit Care Med. 2015 Aug;43(8):1710–5. [PMID: 26066018]

MacIver DH et al. The vital role of the right ventricle in the pathogenesis of acute pulmonary edema. Am J Cardiol. 2015 Apr 1;115(7):992–1000. [PMID: 25697920]

O'Connor ME et al. Fluid overload. Crit Care Clin. 2015 Oct;31(4):803–21. [PMID: 26410146]

Platz E et al. Assessment and prevalence of pulmonary oedema in contemporary acute heart failure trials: a systematic review. Eur J Heart Fail. 2015 Sep;17(9):906–16. [PMID: 26230356]

Siddall E et al. Capillary leak syndrome: etiologies, pathophysiology, and management. Kidney Int. 2017 Jul;92(1):37–46 [PMID: 28318633]

Acute Respiratory Failure & ARDS

ARDS Definition Task Force; Ranieri VM et al. Acute respiratory distress syndrome: the Berlin Definition. JAMA. 2012 Jun 20;307(23):2526–33. [PMID: 22797452]

Burnham EL et al. The fibroproliferative response in acute respiratory distress syndrome: mechanisms and clinical significance. Eur Respir J. 2014 Jan;43(1):276–85. [PMID: 23520315]

Fujishima S. Pathophysiology and biomarkers of acute respiratory distress syndrome. J Intensive Care. 2014 May 7;2(1):32. [PMID: 25520844]

Han S et al. The acute respiratory distress syndrome: from mechanism to translation. J Immunol. 2015 Feb 1;194(3):855–60. Erratum in: J Immunol. 2015 Jun 1;194(11):5569. [PMID: 25596299]

Huppert LA et al. Alveolar fluid clearance in pathologically relevant conditions: in vitro and in vivo models of acute respiratory distress syndrome. Front Immunol. 2017 Apr 7;8:371. [PMID: 28439268]

Mac Sweeney RM et al. Acute respiratory distress syndrome. Lancet. 2016 Nov 12;388(10058): 2416–30. [PMID: 27133972]

Matthay MA et al. The acute respiratory distress syndrome. J Clin Invest. 2012 Aug 1;122(8):2731–40. [PMID: 22850883]

Millar FR et al. The pulmonary endothelium in acute respiratory distress syndrome: insights and therapeutic opportunities. Thorax. 2016 May;71(5):462–73. [PMID: 26968969]

Monahan LJ. Acute respiratory distress syndrome. Curr Probl Pediatr Adolesc Health Care. 2013 Nov-Dec;43(10):278–84. [PMID: 24295609]

Sharp C et al. Advances in understanding of the pathogenesis of acute respiratory distress syndrome. Respiration. 2015;89(5):420–34. [PMID: 25925331]

Pulmonary Embolism

Becattini C et al. Risk stratification of patients with acute symptomatic pulmonary embolism based on presence or absence of lower extremity DVT: systematic review and meta-analysis. Chest. 2016 Jan;149(1):192–200. [PMID: 26204122]

Cutts S et al. Adult respiratory distress syndrome. Ann R Coll Surg Engl. 2017 Jan;99(1):12–6. [PMID: 27513791]

Jiménez D et al. Risk stratification of patients with acute symptomatic pulmonary embolism. Intern Emerg Med. 2016 Feb;11(1):11–8. [PMID: 26768476]

Moorjani N et al. Massive pulmonary embolism. Cardiol Clin. 2013 Nov;31(4):503–18. [PMID: 24188217]

Piovella F et al. Acute pulmonary embolism: risk assessment, risk stratification and treatment options. Clin Respir J. 2016 Sep;10(5):545–54. [PMID: 25619266]

Riva N et al. Epidemiology and pathophysiology of venous thromboembolism: similarities with atherothrombosis and the role of inflammation. Thromb Haemost. 2015 Jun;113(6):1176–83. [PMID: 25472800]

Yan C et al. Recent progress in research on the pathogenesis of pulmonary thromboembolism: an old story with new perspectives. Biomed Res Int. 2017;2017:6516791. [PMID: 28484717]

Zhou XY et al. The prognostic value of pulmonary embolism severity index in acute pulmonary embolism: a meta-analysis. Respir Res. 2012 Dec 4;13:111. [PMID: 23210843]

Cardiovascular Disorders: Heart Disease

Fred M. Kusumoto, MD, FACC

Diseases of the cardiovascular system frequently confront the physician involved in the day-to-day care of patients. Knowledge of the underlying pathophysiologic processes associated with diseases of the heart and blood vessels provides a critical framework for patient management. This chapter deals with diseases of the heart, with the following chapter focusing on diseases of the blood vessels. Normal cardiac structure and function are summarized here, and pathophysiologic mechanisms for commonly encountered cardiac problems are then discussed, with emphasis on arrhythmias, heart failure, valvular heart disease, coronary artery disease, and pericardial disease.

NORMAL STRUCTURE & FUNCTION OF THE HEART

ANATOMY

The heart is a complex organ whose primary function is to pump blood through the pulmonary and systemic circulations. It is composed of four muscular chambers: the main pumping chambers, the left and right ventricles, and the left and right atria, which act like "priming pumps" responsible for the final 20–30% of ventricular filling (Figure 10–1A). Peripheral venous return from the inferior and superior venae cavae fills the right atrium and ventricle (through the open tricuspid valve) (Figure 10–1B). With atrial contraction, additional blood flows through the tricuspid valve and completes the filling of the right ventricle. Unoxygenated blood is then pumped to the pulmonary artery and lung by the right ventricle through the pulmonary valve (Figure 10–1C). Oxygenated blood returns from the lung to the left atrium via four pulmonary veins (Figure 10–1D). Sequential left atrial and ventricular contraction pumps blood back to the peripheral tissues. The mitral valve separates the left atrium and ventricle, and the aortic valve separates the left ventricle from the aorta (Figures 10–1D and 10–1E).

The heart lies free in the pericardial sac, attached to mediastinal structures only at the great vessels. During embryologic development, the heart invaginates into the pericardial sac like a fist pushing into a partially inflated balloon. The pericardial sac is composed of a serous inner layer (visceral pericardium) directly apposed to the myocardium and a fibrous outer layer called the parietal pericardium. Under normal conditions, approximately 40–50 mL of clear fluid, which probably is an ultrafiltrate of plasma, fills the space between the layers of the pericardial sac.

The left main and right coronary arteries arise from the root of the aorta and provide the principal blood supply to the heart (Figure 10–2). The large left main coronary artery usually branches into the left anterior descending artery and the circumflex coronary artery. The left anterior descending coronary artery gives off diagonal and septal branches that supply blood to the anterior wall and septum of the heart, respectively. The circumflex coronary artery continues around the heart in the left atrioventricular groove and gives off large obtuse marginal arteries that supply blood to the left ventricular free wall. The right coronary artery travels in the right atrioventricular groove and supplies blood to the right ventricle via acute marginal branches. The posterior descending artery, which supplies blood to the posterior and inferior walls of the left ventricle, arises from the right coronary artery in 80% of people (right-dominant circulation) and from the circumflex artery in the remainder (left-dominant circulation).

Contraction of the heart chambers is coordinated by several regions in the heart composed of myocytes with specialized

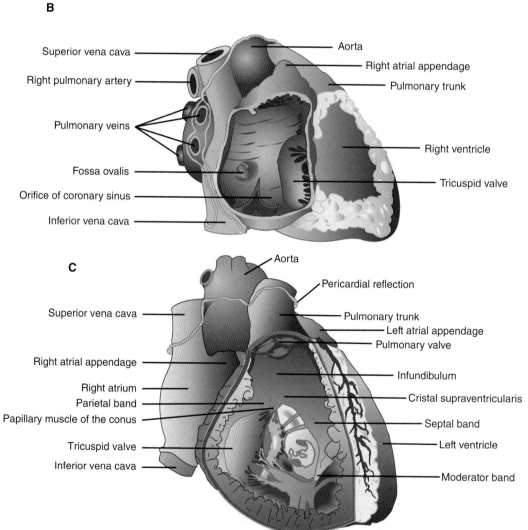

FIGURE 10–1 Anatomy of the heart. **A:** Anterior view of the heart. **B:** View of the right heart with the right atrial wall reflected to show the right atrium. **C:** Anterior view of the heart with the anterior wall removed to show the right ventricular cavity. (Redrawn, with permission, from Cheitlin MD et al, eds. *Clinical Cardiology*, 6th ed. Originally published by Appleton & Lange. Copyright © 1993 by The McGraw-Hill Companies, Inc.)

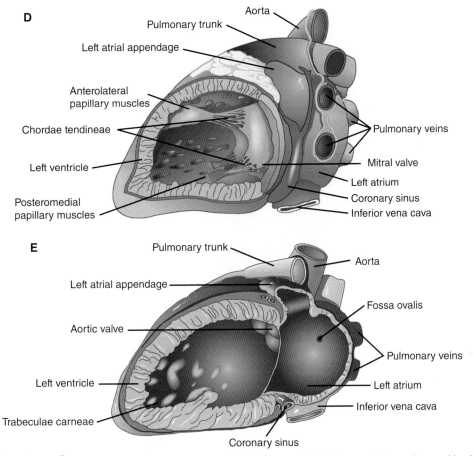

FIGURE 10–1 (Continued) Anatomy of the heart. **D:** View of the left heart with the left ventricular wall turned back to show the mitral valve. **E:** View of the left heart from the left side with the left ventricular free wall and mitral valve cut away to reveal the aortic valve. (Redrawn, with permission, from Cheitlin MD et al, eds. *Clinical Cardiology*, 6th ed. Originally published by Appleton & Lange. Copyright © 1993 by The McGraw-Hill Companies, Inc.)

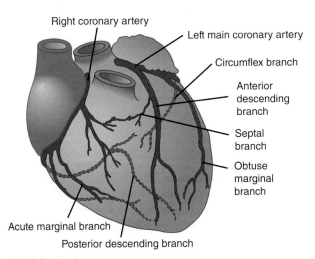

FIGURE 10–2 Coronary arteries and their principal branches in humans. (Redrawn, with permission, from Ross G. The cardiovascular system. In: Ross G, ed. *Essentials of Human Physiology*. Copyright © 1978 by Year Book Medical Publishers, Inc., Chicago. Copyright © Elsevier.)

automaticity (pacemaker) and conduction properties (Figure 10–3). Cells in the sinoatrial (SA) node and the atrioventricular (AV) node have fast pacemaker rates (SA node: 60–100 bpm; AV node: 40–70 bpm), and the His bundle and Purkinje fibers are characterized by rapid rates of conduction. Because it has the fastest intrinsic pacemaker rhythm, the SA node is usually the site of initiation of the cardiac electrical impulse during a normal heartbeat. The impulse then rapidly depolarizes both the left and right atria as it travels to the AV node. Conduction velocity slows from 1 m/s in atrial tissue to 0.05 m/s in nodal tissue. After the delay in the AV node, the impulse moves rapidly down the His bundle (1 m/s) and Purkinje fibers (4 m/s) to simultaneously depolarize the right and left ventricles. The atria and ventricles are separated by a fibrous framework that is electrically inert, so under normal conditions the AV node and the contiguous His bundle form the only electrical connection between the atria and ventricles. This arrangement allows the atria and ventricles to beat in a synchronized fashion and minimizes the chance of electrical feedback between the chambers.

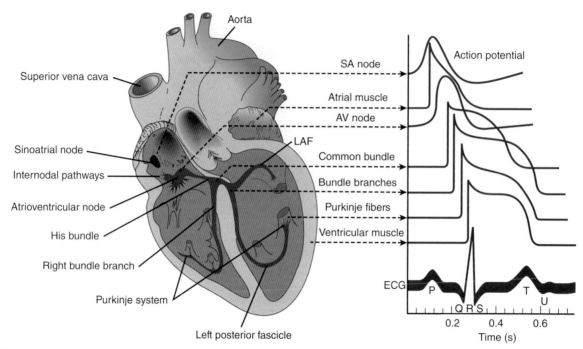

FIGURE 10–3 Conducting system of the heart. Typical transmembrane action potentials for the SA and AV nodes, other parts of the conduction system, and the atrial and ventricular muscles are shown along with the correlation to the extracellularly recorded electrical activity (ie, the electrocardiogram [ECG]). The action potentials and ECG are plotted on the same time axis but with different zero points on the vertical scale. The PR interval is measured from the beginning of the P wave to the beginning of the QRS. (LAF, left anterior fascicle.) (Redrawn, with permission, from Barrett KE et al, eds. *Ganong's Review of Medical Physiology,* 25th ed. McGraw-Hill, 2016.)

The electrical activity of the heart can be measured from the body surface at standardized positions by electrocardiography. On the electrocardiogram (ECG), the P wave represents depolarization of atrial tissue; the electrocardiographic wave (QRS) interval, ventricular depolarization; and the T wave, ventricular repolarization (see Figure 10–3). Because normal ventricular depolarization occurs almost simultaneously in the right and left ventricles—usually within 60–100 ms—the QRS complex is narrow. Although the electrical activity of the small specialized conduction tissues cannot be measured directly from the surface, the interval between the P wave and the start of the QRS complex (PR interval) primarily represents the conduction time of the AV node and His bundle.

HISTOLOGY

Ventricular myocytes are normally 50–100 mm long and 10–25 mm wide. Atrial and nodal myocytes are smaller, whereas myocytes of the Purkinje system are larger in both dimensions. Myocytes are filled with hundreds of parallel striated bundles termed myofibrils. Myofibrils are composed of repeating units, termed sarcomeres, that form the major contractile unit of the myocyte (Figure 10–4). Sarcomeres are complex structures composed of contractile proteins, myosin and actin, which are connected by cross-bridges, and a regulatory protein complex, tropomyosin. (See Cellular Physiology section later.)

PHYSIOLOGY

Physiology of the Whole Heart

Because the ventricles are the primary physiologic pumps of the heart, analysis has focused on these chambers, particularly the left ventricle. The function of intact ventricles is traditionally studied by evaluating pressure–time and pressure–volume relationships.

In **pressure–time analysis** (Figure 10–5), pressures in the heart chambers and great vessels are measured during the cardiac cycle and plotted as a function of time. At the beginning of the cardiac cycle, the left atrium contracts, forcing additional blood into the left ventricle and giving rise to an *a* wave on the left atrial pressure tracing. At end diastole, the mitral valve closes, producing the first heart sound (S_1), and a brief period of isovolumic contraction follows, during which both the aortic and mitral valves are closed but the left ventricle is actively contracting. When intraventricular pressure rises to the level of aortic pressure, the aortic valve opens and blood flows into the aorta. Beyond this point, the aorta and left ventricle form a contiguous chamber with equal pressures, but left ventricular volume decreases as blood is expelled. Left ventricular contraction stops and ventricular relaxation begins, and end systole is reached when intraventricular pressure falls below aortic pressure. The aortic valve then closes, producing the second heart sound (S_2). Throughout systole, blood has slowly accumulated in the left atrium (because the mitral valve is closed),

FIGURE 10–4 **A:** Electron photomicrograph of cardiac muscle. The fuzzy thick lines are intercalated disks (×12,000). (Reproduced, with permission, from Bloom W et al. *A Textbook of Histology*, 10th ed. Saunders, 1975. Copyright © Elsevier.) **B:** Diagram of cardiac muscle as seen under the light microscope (**top**) and the electron microscope (**bottom**). (N, nucleus.) (Redrawn, with permission, from Braunwald E et al. Mechanisms of contraction of the normal and failing heart. N Engl J Med. 1967;277:794. Copyright © 1967 Massachusetts Medical Society. Reprinted with permission from Massachusetts Medical Society.)

giving rise to the *v* wave on the left atrial pressure tracing. During the first phase of diastole—isovolumic relaxation—no change in ventricular volume occurs, but continued relaxation of the ventricle leads to an exponential fall in left ventricular pressure. Left ventricular filling begins when left ventricular pressure falls below left atrial pressure and the mitral valve opens. Ventricular relaxation is a relatively long process that begins before the aortic valve closes and extends past the mitral valve opening. The rate and extent of ventricular

relaxation depend on multiple factors: heart rate, wall thickness, chamber volume and shape, aortic pressure, sympathetic tone, and presence or absence of myocardial ischemia. Once the mitral valve opens, there is an initial period of rapid filling of the ventricle that contributes 70–80% of blood volume to the ventricle and occurs largely because of the atrioventricular pressure gradient. By mid-diastole, flow into the left ventricle has slowed, and the cardiac cycle begins again with the next atrial contraction. Right ventricular pressure–time analysis

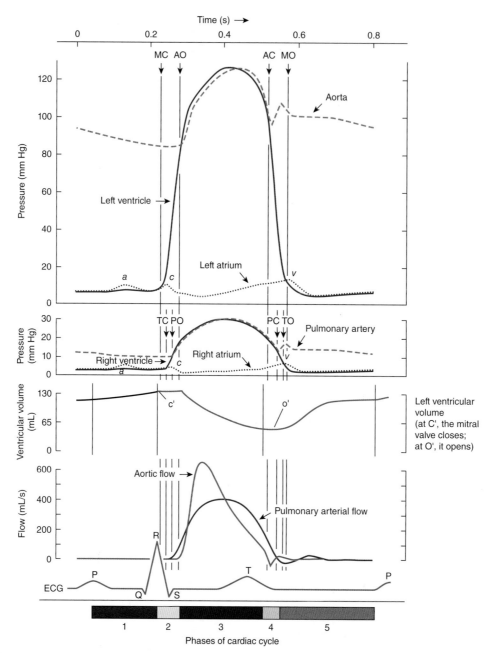

FIGURE 10–5 Diagram of events in the cardiac cycle. From top downward: pressure (mm Hg) in aorta, left ventricle, left atrium, pulmonary artery, right ventricle, right atrium; blood flow (mL/s) in ascending aorta and pulmonary artery; ECG. Abscissa, time in seconds. (Valvular opening and closing are indicated by AO and AC, respectively, for the aortic valve; MO and MC for the mitral valve; PO and PC for the pulmonary valve; TO and TC for the tricuspid valve.) Events of the cardiac cycle at a heart rate of 75 bpm. The phases of the cardiac cycle identified by the numbers at the bottom are as follows: 1, atrial systole; 2, isovolumetric ventricular contraction; 3, ventricular ejection; 4, isovolumetric ventricular relaxation; 5, ventricular filling. Note that late in systole, aortic pressure actually exceeds left ventricular pressure. However, the momentum of the blood keeps it flowing out of the ventricle for a short period. The pressure relationships in the right ventricle and pulmonary artery are similar. (Redrawn, with permission, from Milnor WR. The circulation. In: Mountcastle VB, ed. *Medical Physiology*, 2 vols. Mosby, 1980. Copyright © Elsevier.)

is similar but with lower pressures because the impedance to flow in the pulmonary vascular system is much lower than in the systemic circulation.

In **pressure–volume analysis** (Figure 10–6), pressure during the cardiac cycle is plotted as a function of volume rather than time. During diastole, as ventricular volume increases

during both the initial rapid filling period and atrial contraction, ventricular pressure increases (curve **da**). The shape and position of this curve, the **diastolic pressure–volume relationship**, depend on relaxation properties of the ventricle, the elastic recoil of the ventricle, and the distensibility of the ventricle. The curve shifts to the left (higher pressure for a given

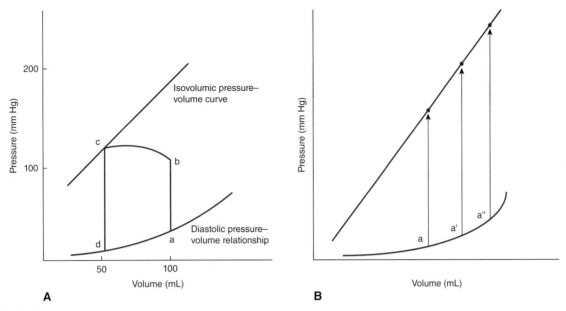

FIGURE 10–6 **A:** Pressure–volume loop for the left ventricle. During diastole, the left ventricle fills and pressure increases along the diastolic pressure–volume curve from **d** to **a**. Line **ab** represents isometric contraction, and **bc** the ejection phase of systole. The aortic valve closes at point **c**, and pressure drops along **cd** (isovolumic relaxation), until the mitral valve opens at point **d** and the cycle repeats. The distance from **b** to **c** represents the stroke volume ejected by that beat. Point **a** represents end-diastole, and point **c** represent end-systole. **B:** If the left ventricle is filled by varying amounts (**a**, **a'**, **a''**) and allowed to undergo isovolumic contraction, a relatively linear relationship, the isovolumic pressure–volume relation, can be defined.

volume) if relaxation of the ventricle is decreased, the ventricle loses elastic recoil, or the ventricle becomes stiffer. At the beginning of systole, active ventricular contraction begins and volume remains unchanged (isovolumic contraction period) (**ab**). When left ventricular pressure reaches aortic pressure, the aortic valve opens, and ventricular volume decreases as the ventricle expels its blood (curve **bc**). At end systole (**c**), the aortic valve closes and isovolumic relaxation begins (**cd**). When the mitral valve opens, the ventricle begins filling for the next cardiac cycle, repeating the entire process. The area encompassed by this loop represents the amount of work done by the ventricle during a cardiac cycle. The position of point **c** depends on the **isovolumic systolic pressure–volume curve**. If the ventricle is filled with variable amounts of blood (preloads) and allowed to contract, but the aortic valve is prevented from opening, a relatively linear relationship exists, termed the isovolumic systolic pressure–volume curve (Figure 10–6B). The slope and position of this line describe the inherent contractile state of the ventricle. If contractility is increased by catecholamines or other positive inotropes, the line will shift to the left.

Pressure–volume relationships help illustrate the effects of different stresses on cardiac output. Cardiac output of the ventricle is the product of the **heart rate** and the volume of blood pumped with each beat (**stroke volume**). The width of the pressure–volume loop is the difference between end-diastolic volume and end-systolic volume, or the stroke volume (see Figure 10–6). The stroke volume depends on three parameters: contractility, afterload, and preload (Figure 10–7).

Changing the contractile state of the heart will change the width of the pressure–volume loop by changing the position of the isovolumic systolic pressure curve. The impedance against which the heart must work (aortic pressure for the left ventricle) is termed **afterload**; increased afterload will cause a decrease in stroke volume. **Preload** is the amount of filling of the ventricle at end-diastole. Up to a point, the more a myocyte or ventricular chamber is stretched, the more it will contract (**Frank–Starling relationship**), so that increased preload will lead to an increase in stroke volume.

Pressure–time and pressure–volume relationships are critical for understanding the pathophysiologic mechanisms of diseases that affect the entire ventricular chamber function, such as heart failure and valvular abnormalities.

Cellular Physiology

A. Ventricular and Atrial Myocytes

The cellular mechanism of myocyte contraction after electrical stimulation is too complex to fully address in this section, but excellent discussions of electromechanical coupling can be found. Briefly, when the myocyte is stimulated, sodium channels on the cell surface membrane (sarcolemma) open, and sodium ions (Na^+) flow down their electrochemical gradient into the cell. This sudden inward surge of ions is responsible for the sharp upstroke of the myocyte action potential (phase 0) (Figure 10–8). A plateau phase follows, during which the cell membrane potential remains relatively unchanged owing to the inward flow of calcium ions (Ca^{2+}) and the outward flow of

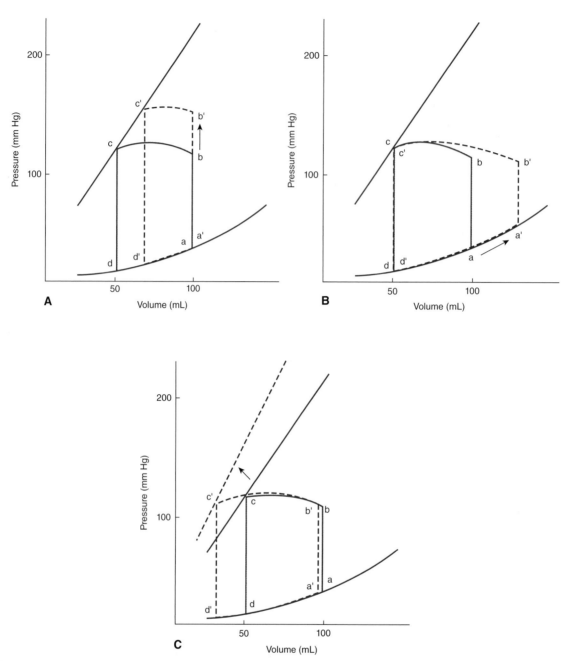

FIGURE 10–7 **A:** Increasing afterload from **b** to **b'** decreases stroke volume from **bc** to **b'c'**. **B:** Increasing preload from **a** to **a'** increases stroke volume from **bc** to **b'c'**, but at the expense of increased end-diastolic pressure. **C:** An increasingly contractile state shifts the isovolumic pressure–volume relationship leftward, increasing stroke volume from **bc** to **b'c'**.

potassium ions (K⁺) through several different specialized potassium channels. Repolarization occurs because of the continued outward flow of K⁺ after the inward flux of Ca²⁺ has stopped.

Within the cell, the change in membrane potential from the sudden influx of Na⁺ and the subsequent increase in intracellular Ca²⁺ causes the sarcoplasmic reticulum to release large numbers of calcium ions via specialized Ca²⁺ release channels, although the exact signaling mechanism is unknown. Once in the cytoplasm, however, Ca²⁺ released from the sarcoplasmic

reticulum binds with the regulatory proteins troponin and tropomyosin. Myosin and actin are then allowed to interact and the cross-bridges between them bend, giving rise to contraction (Figure 10–9). The process of relaxation is also poorly understood but appears to involve return of Ca²⁺ to the sarcoplasmic reticulum via two transmembrane sarcoplasmic reticulum-embedded proteins: Ca²⁺-ATPase and phospholamban. Reuptake of Ca²⁺ is an active process that requires adenosine triphosphate (ATP).

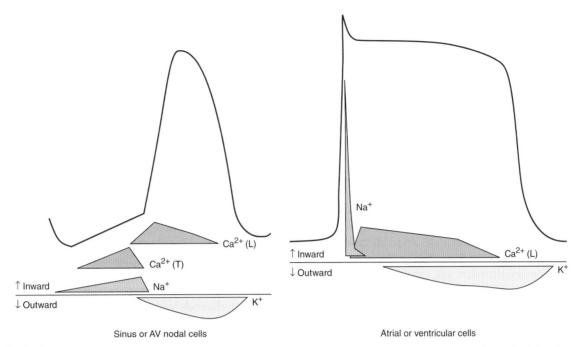

FIGURE 10–8 Changes in ionic conductances responsible for generating action potentials for ventricular or atrial tissue (right) and a sinus or AV node cell (left). In nodal cells, rapid Na^+ channels are absent, so that the action potential upstroke is much slower. Diastolic depolarization observed in nodal cells is a result of decreased K^+ efflux and slow Na^+ and Ca^{2+} influx. Ca^{2+} (T): influx via Ca^{2+} (T) channels; Ca^{2+} (L): influx via Ca^{2+} (L) channels.

B. Pacemaker Cells

The action potential of pacemaker cells is different from that described for ventricular and atrial myocytes (see Figure 10–8). Fast sodium channels are absent, so that a rapid phase 0 depolarization is not observed in SA nodal and AV nodal cells. In addition, these cells are characterized by increased automaticity from a relatively rapid spontaneous phase 4 depolarization. A combination of a reduced outward flow of K^+ and an inward flow of Na^+ and Ca^{2+} via specialized channels appears to be responsible for this dynamic change in membrane potential. Myofibrils are sparse, although present, in the specialized pacemaker cells.

CHECKPOINT

1. What are the differences in pacemaker and conduction properties in different regions of the heart, and why do these differences explain the observation that cardiac electrical impulses normally arise in the SA node?
2. Describe pressure–time analysis through the cardiac cycle.
3. Describe pressure–volume analysis through the cardiac cycle.
4. What are preload and afterload?
5. Briefly describe the molecular mechanism of electromechanical coupling in cardiac myocyte contraction.

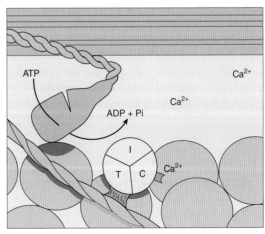

FIGURE 10–9 Initiation of muscle contraction by Ca^{2+}. When Ca^{2+} binds to troponin C, tropomyosin is displaced laterally, exposing the binding site for myosin on actin (dark area). ATP hydrolysis then changes the conformation of the myosin head and fosters its binding to the exposed site. For simplicity, only one of the two heads of the myosin-II molecule is shown. (Redrawn, with permission, from Ganong WF. *Review of Medical Physiology*, 22nd ed. McGraw-Hill, 2005.)

PATHOPHYSIOLOGY OF SELECTED CARDIOVASCULAR DISORDERS

ARRHYTHMIAS

At rest, the heart is normally activated at a rate of 50–100 bpm. Abnormal rhythms of the heart (arrhythmias) can be classified as either too slow (bradycardias) or too fast (tachycardias).

Bradycardia

Bradycardia can arise from two basic mechanisms. First, reduced automaticity of the sinus node can result in slow heart rates or pauses. As shown in Figure 10–10, if sinus node pacemaker activity ceases, the heart will usually be activated at a slower rate by other cardiac tissues with pacemaker activity. Reduced sinus node automaticity can occur during periods of increased vagal tone (sleep, carotid sinus massage, "common faint"), with increasing age, and secondary to drugs (beta blockers, calcium channel blockers).

Second, slow heart rates can occur if the cardiac impulse is prevented from activating the ventricles normally because of blocked conduction (Figure 10–11). Because the fibrous valvular annulus is electrically inert, the AV node and His bundle normally form the only electrically active connection between the atria and the ventricles. Although this arrangement is useful for preventing feedback between the two chambers, it also makes the AV node and His bundle vulnerable sites for blocked conduction between the atria and ventricles. Although block can be observed in either the left or right bundle branches, bradycardia does not necessarily occur, because the ventricles can still be activated by the contralateral bundle. Atrioventricular block has been classified as first degree when there is an abnormally long atrioventricular conduction time (PR interval >0.22 s) but activation of the atria and ventricles still demonstrates a 1:1 association. In second-degree atrioventricular block, some but not all atrial impulses are conducted to the ventricles. Finally, in third-degree block, there is no association between atrial and ventricular activity. Atrioventricular block can occur with increasing age, with increased vagal input, and as a side effect of certain drugs. Atrioventricular block can sometimes also be observed in congenital disorders, such as muscular dystrophy, tuberous sclerosis, and maternal systemic lupus erythematosus, and in acquired disorders, such as sarcoidosis, gout, Lyme disease, systemic lupus erythematosus, ankylosing spondylitis, and coronary artery disease.

Bradycardia resulting from either decreased automaticity or blocked conduction requires evaluation to search for reversible causes. However, implantation of a permanent pacemaker is often required.

Tachycardia

Tachycardias can arise from three basic cellular mechanisms (Figure 10–12). First, increased automaticity resulting from more rapid phase 4 depolarization can cause rapid heart rate. Second, if repolarization is delayed (longer plateau period), spontaneous depolarizations (caused by reactivation of sodium or calcium channels) can sometimes occur in phase 3 or phase 4 of the action potential. These depolarizations are called triggered activity because they depend on the existence of a preceding action potential. If these depolarizations reach threshold, tachycardia can occur in certain pathologic conditions. Third, and most commonly, tachycardias can arise from a re-entrant circuit. Any condition that gives rise to parallel but electrically separate regions with different conduction velocities (such as the border zone of a myocardial infarction or an accessory atrioventricular connection) can serve as the substrate for a re-entrant circuit.

The best studied example of re-entrant tachyarrhythmias is Wolff–Parkinson–White syndrome (Figure 10–13). As mentioned, the AV node normally forms the only electrical connection between the atria and the ventricles. Perhaps because of incomplete formation of the annulus, an accessory atrioventricular connection is found in approximately 1 in 1000 persons. This accessory pathway is usually composed of normal atrial or ventricular tissue. Because part of the ventricle is "pre-excited" over the accessory pathway rather than via the AV node, the surface ECG shows a short PR interval and a relatively wide QRS with a slurred upstroke, termed a **delta wave**. Because the atria and ventricles are linked by two parallel connections, re-entrant tachycardias are readily initiated. For example, a premature atrial contraction could be blocked in the accessory pathway but still conduct to the ventricles via the AV node. If enough time has elapsed so that the accessory pathway has recovered excitability, the cardiac impulse can travel in retrograde fashion to the atria over the accessory pathway and initiate a re-entrant tachycardia.

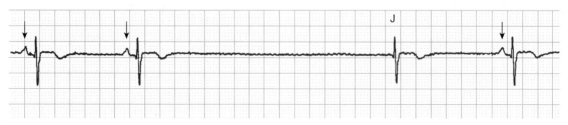

FIGURE 10–10   Rhythm strip showing bradycardia resulting from sinus node pause. Atrial activity (**arrows**) suddenly ceases, and after approximately 3 s a junctional escape beat is observed (J).

FIGURE 10–11 Rhythm strip demonstrating third-degree (complete) heart block with no association between atrial activity (**arrows**) and ventricular activity (**dots**).

FIGURE 10–12 Tachyarrhythmias can arise from three different mechanisms. First, increased automaticity from more rapid phase 4 depolarization can cause arrhythmias. Second, in certain conditions, spontaneous depolarizations during phase 3 (early after-depolarizations [EAD]) or phase 4 (delayed after-depolarizations [DAD]) can repetitively reach threshold and cause tachycardia. This appears to be the mechanism of the polymorphic ventricular tachycardia (torsades de pointes) observed in some patients taking procainamide or quinidine and the arrhythmias associated with digoxin toxicity. Third, the most common mechanism for tachyarrhythmia is re-entry. In re-entry, two parallel pathways with different conduction properties exist (perhaps at the border zone of a myocardial infarction or a region of myocardial ischemia). The electrical impulse normally travels down the fast pathway and the slow pathway (shaded region), but at the point where the two pathways converge, the impulse traveling down the slow pathway is blocked since the tissue is refractory from the recent depolarization via the fast pathway (**a**). However, when a premature beat reaches the circuit, block can occur in the fast pathway, and the impulse will travel down the slow pathway (shaded region) (**b**). After traveling through the slow pathway, the impulse can then enter the fast pathway in retrograde fashion (which, because of the delay, has recovered excitability) and then re-enter the slow pathway to start a continuous loop of activation, or re-entrant circuit (**c**).

The best example of tachycardias from triggered activity is long QT syndrome. More than 40 years ago, investigators described several clusters of patients with a congenital syndrome associated with a long QT interval and ventricular arrhythmias. Data have shown that the long QT interval can be a result of several specific ion channel defects. For example, a reduction in potassium channel function leads to a prolonged plateau period (Figure 10–14). The prolonged plateau phase in ventricular tissue leads to a prolonged QT interval. These patients are prone to triggered activity because of the reactivation of sodium and calcium channels (early after depolarizations). Triggered activity in the ventricles can lead to life-threatening ventricular arrhythmias.

Regardless of the mechanism, the approach to the immediate clinical management of tachycardias depends on whether the QRS complex is narrow or wide. If the QRS complex is narrow, ventricular depolarization must be occurring normally over the specialized conduction tissues of the heart, and the arrhythmia must be originating at or above the AV node (supraventricular) (Figure 10–15).

A wide QRS complex suggests that ventricular activation is not occurring normally over the specialized conduction tissues of the heart. The tachycardia is arising from ventricular tissue or is a supraventricular tachycardia with aberrant conduction over the His–Purkinje system or an accessory pathway. Criteria have been developed to distinguish between ventricular and supraventricular tachycardia with aberrance.

HEART FAILURE

Inadequate pump function of the heart, which leads to congestion resulting from fluid in the lungs and peripheral tissues, is a common end result of many cardiac disease processes. Heart failure (HF) is present in approximately 3 million people in the United States; more than 400,000 new cases are reported annually. The clinical presentation is highly variable; for an individual patient, symptoms and signs depend on how quickly heart failure develops and whether it involves the left, right, or both ventricles.

1. Left Ventricular Failure

Clinical Presentation

Patients with left ventricular failure most commonly present with a sensation of breathlessness (dyspnea), particularly

FIGURE 10–13 Re-entrant tachyarrhythmia resulting from Wolff–Parkinson–White syndrome. **A:** The first two beats demonstrate sinus rhythm with pre-excitation of the ventricles over an accessory pathway. The large arrows show the delta wave. An atrial premature contraction (APC) blocks in the accessory pathway, which leads to normalization of the QRS, and the atria are activated in retrograde fashion via the accessory pathway (small arrows), and supraventricular tachycardia ensues. **B:** The left panel schematically depicts the first two beats of the rhythm strip. The QRS is wide owing to activation of the ventricles over both the AV node and the accessory pathway. The middle panel depicts the atrial premature contraction, which is blocked in the accessory pathway but conducts over the AV node. In the right panel, the atria are activated in retrograde fashion over the accessory pathway, and a re-entrant circuit is initiated.

when lying down (orthopnea) or at night (paroxysmal nocturnal dyspnea). In addition, the patient may complain of blood-tinged sputum (hemoptysis) and occasionally chest pain. Fatigue, nocturia, and confusion can also be caused by heart failure.

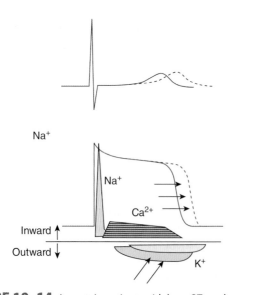

FIGURE 10–14 In certain patients with long QT syndrome, potassium channel function is reduced (diagonal arrows), which leads to prolongation of the action potential of ventricular myocytes and prolongation of the QT interval. In some cases, reactivation of sodium and calcium channels can lead to triggered activity that can initiate life-threatening ventricular arrhythmias.

On physical examination, the patient usually has elevated respiratory and heart rates. The skin may be pale, cold, and sweaty. In severe heart failure, palpation of the peripheral pulse may reveal alternating strong and weak beats (pulsus alternans). Auscultation of the lungs reveals abnormal sounds, called rales, that have been described as "crackling leaves." In addition, the bases of the lung fields may be dull to percussion. On cardiac examination, the apical impulse is often displaced laterally and sustained. Third and fourth heart sounds can be heard on auscultation of the heart. Because many patients with left ventricular failure also have accompanying failure of the right ventricle, signs of right ventricular failure may also be present (see next section).

Etiology

Heart failure is a pathophysiologic complex associated with dysfunction of the heart and is a common end point for many diseases of the cardiovascular system. There are many possible causes (Table 10–1), and the specific reason for heart failure in a given patient must always be sought. In general, heart failure can be caused by (1) inappropriate workloads placed on the heart, such as volume overload or pressure overload; (2) restricted filling of the heart; (3) myocyte loss; or (4) decreased myocyte contractility. Any one of these causes can initiate an evolving sequence of events that are described next. Each of these four causes can have several possible underlying mechanisms. For example, in developed countries, the most common cause of myocyte loss is cell death owing to an

Atrial fibrillation   Atrial flutter

AV nodal   Atrioventricular
re-entrant tachycardia   re-entrant tachycardia

Atrial tachycardia

FIGURE 10–15 In supraventricular tachycardia, the QRS is narrow because the ventricles are depolarized over the normal specialized conduction tissues (light blue region). Five possible arrhythmias are commonly encountered. First, in atrial fibrillation, multiple microreentrant circuits can lead to chaotic activation of the atrium. Because impulses are reaching the AV node at irregular intervals, ventricular depolarization is irregular. Second, in atrial flutter, a macroreentrant circuit, traveling up the interatrial septum and down the lateral walls, can activate the atria in a regular fashion at approximately 300 bpm. The AV node can conduct only every other or every third beat, so that the ventricles are depolarized at 150 or 100 bpm. In AV nodal re-entrant tachycardia, slow and fast pathways exist in the region of the AV node and a microreentrant circuit can be formed. Fourth, in atrioventricular re-entry, an abnormal connection between the atrium and ventricle exists so that a macroreentrant circuit can be formed with the AV node forming the slow pathway, and the abnormal atrioventricular connection forming the fast pathway. Finally, in atrial tachycardia, an abnormal focus of atrial activity as a result of either re-entry, triggered activity, or abnormal automaticity can activate the atria in a regular fashion.

obstructed artery (see the discussions of atherosclerosis and myocardial infarction later in the chapter). However, myocyte loss can also arise from genetic disorders (often of the intracellular proteins responsible for myocyte architecture; eg, dystrophin) or as an inflammatory response (eg, after a viral infection or other insult).

TABLE 10–1   Causes of left ventricular failure.

Volume overload
Regurgitant valves (mitral or aortic) High-output states: anemia, hyperthyroidism
Pressure overload
Systemic hypertension Outflow obstruction: aortic stenosis, asymmetric septal hypertrophy
Loss of muscle
Myocardial infarction from coronary artery disease Connective tissue disease: systemic lupus erythematosus
Loss of contractility
Poisons: alcohol, cobalt, doxorubicin Infections: viral, bacterial Genetic mutations of cellular architecture or sarcomere proteins
Restricted filling
Mitral stenosis Pericardial disease: constrictive pericarditis, pericardial tamponade Infiltrative diseases: amyloidosis

Pathophysiology

The pathophysiology of heart failure is complex and must be understood at multiple levels. Traditionally, research has focused on the hemodynamic changes of the failing heart, considering the heart as an isolated organ. However, studies of the failing heart have emphasized the importance of understanding changes at the cellular level and the neuro-hormonal interactions between the heart and other organs of the body (Table 10–2).

TABLE 10–2   Pathophysiologic changes associated with heart failure.

Hemodynamic changes
Decreased output (systolic dysfunction) Decreased filling (diastolic dysfunction)
Neuro-hormonal changes
Sympathetic system activation Renin–angiotensin system activation Vasopressin release Cytokine release
Cellular changes
Inefficient intracellular Ca^{2+} handling Adrenergic desensitization Myocyte hypertrophy Re-expression of fetal phenotype proteins Cell death (apoptosis) Fibrosis

A. Hemodynamic Changes—From a hemodynamic standpoint, heart failure can arise from worsening systolic or diastolic function or, more frequently, a combination of both. In **systolic dysfunction**, the isovolumic systolic pressure curve of the pressure–volume relationship is shifted downward (Figure 10–16A). This reduces the stroke volume of the heart with a concomitant decrease in cardiac output. To maintain cardiac output, the heart can respond with three compensatory mechanisms: First, increased return of blood to the heart (preload) can lead to increased sarcomere contraction (Frank–Starling relationship). In the pressure–volume relationship, the heart operates at **a′** instead of **a**, and stroke volume increases, but

at the cost of increased end-diastolic pressure (Figure 10–16D). Second, an increase in catecholamine release can increase cardiac output both by increasing the heart rate and shifting the systolic isovolumetric curve to the left (Figure 10–16C). Finally, the cardiac muscle can hypertrophy and ventricular volume can increase, which shifts the diastolic curve to the right (Figure 10–16B). Although each of these compensatory mechanisms can temporarily maintain cardiac output, each is limited in its ability to do so, and if the underlying reason for systolic dysfunction remains untreated, the heart ultimately fails.

In **diastolic dysfunction**, the position of the systolic isovolumic curve remains unchanged (myocyte contractility is

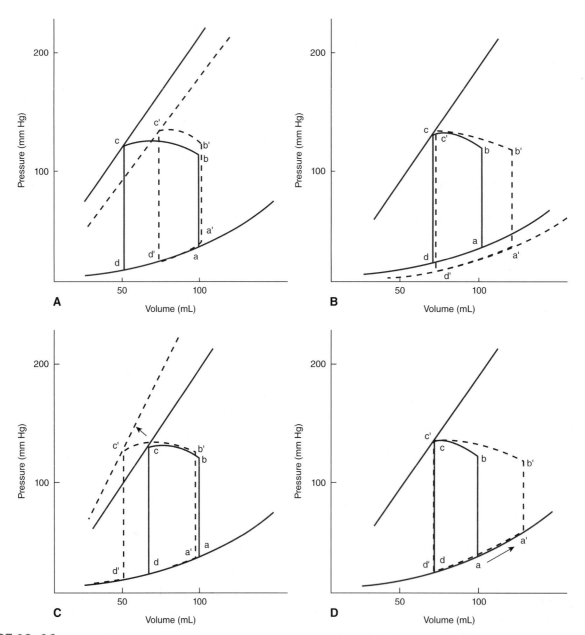

FIGURE 10–16 **A:** Systolic dysfunction is represented by a shift of the isovolumic pressure–volume curve to the right (dashed line), thus decreasing stroke volume. The ventricle can compensate by (**B**) shifting the diastolic pressure–volume relationship rightward (dashed line) by increasing left ventricular volume or elasticity, (**C**) increasing contractile state (dashed line) by activating circulating catecholamines, and (**D**) increasing filling or preload (**a** to **a′**).

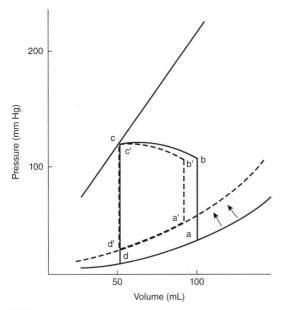

FIGURE 10–17 In diastolic dysfunction, the diastolic pressure–volume relation is shifted upward and to the left (dashed line), which leads to an elevated left ventricular end-diastolic pressure (**a′**) and reduced stroke volume.

preserved). However, the diastolic pressure–volume curve is shifted to the left, with an accompanying increase in left ventricular end-diastolic pressure and symptoms of heart failure (Figure 10–17). Diastolic dysfunction can be present in any disease that causes decreased relaxation, decreased elastic recoil, or increased ventricle stiffness. Hypertension often leads to compensatory increases in left ventricular wall thickness that can cause diastolic dysfunction by changing all three parameters. Lack of sufficient blood to the myocytes (ischemia) can also cause diastolic dysfunction by decreasing relaxation. If ischemia is severe, as in myocardial infarction, irreversible damage to the myocytes can occur, with replacement of contractile cells by fibrosis, which will lead to systolic dysfunction. In most patients, a combination of systolic and diastolic dysfunction is responsible for the symptoms of heart failure.

B. Neuro-hormonal Changes—After an injury to the heart (see Table 10–1), an increased secretion of endogenous neurohormones and cytokines is observed. Initially, an increase in the activity of the adrenergic and renin–angiotensin systems provides a compensatory response that maintains perfusion of vital organs. However, over time these changes can lead to a progressive deterioration of cardiac function.

Increased sympathetic activity occurs early in the development of heart failure. Elevated plasma norepinephrine levels cause increased cardiac contractility and an increased heart rate that initially help maintain cardiac output. However, continued increases lead to increased preload (as a result of venous vasoconstriction) and afterload (from arterial vasoconstriction), which can worsen heart failure. In addition, sympathetic hyperactivity causes deleterious cellular changes, discussed in the next section.

Reduced renal blood pressure stimulates the release of renin and increases the production of angiotensin II. Both angiotensin II and sympathetic activation cause efferent glomerular arteriolar vasoconstriction, which helps maintain the glomerular filtration rate despite a reduced cardiac output. Angiotensin II stimulates aldosterone synthesis, which leads to sodium resorption and potassium excretion by the kidneys. However, a vicious circle is initiated as the continued hyperactivity of the renin–angiotensin system leads to severe vasoconstriction, increased afterload, and a further reduction in cardiac output and the glomerular filtration rate.

Heart failure is associated with an increase in the release of vasopressin from the posterior pituitary gland. Vasopressin is another powerful vasoconstrictor that also promotes reabsorption of water in the renal tubules.

Heart failure is associated with the release of cytokines and other circulating peptides. Cytokines are a heterogeneous family of proteins that are secreted by macrophages, lymphocytes, monocytes, and endothelial cells in response to injury. The **interleukins (ILs)** and **tumor necrosis factor (TNF)** are the two major groups of cytokines that may have an important pathophysiologic role in heart failure. Upregulation of the gene responsible for TNF with an accompanying increase in circulating TNF plasma levels has been found in patients with heart failure. TNF appears to have an important role in the cycle of myocyte hypertrophy and cell death (apoptosis), described in the next section. Preliminary in vitro data suggest that IL-1 may accelerate myocyte hypertrophy. Another peptide important for mediating some of the pathophysiologic effects observed in heart failure is the potent vasoconstrictor **endothelin**, which is released from endothelial cells. Preliminary data have suggested that excessive endothelin release may be responsible for hypertension in the pulmonary arteries observed in patients with left ventricular heart failure. Endothelin is also associated with myocyte growth and collagen deposition in the interstitial matrix.

C. Cellular Changes—Pathophysiologic changes at the cellular level are very complex and include changes in Ca^{2+} handling, adrenergic receptors, the contractile apparatus, and myocyte structure.

In heart failure, both delivery of Ca^{2+} to the contractile apparatus and reuptake of Ca^{2+} by the sarcoplasmic reticulum are slowed. Decreased levels of messenger ribonucleic acid (mRNA) for the specialized Ca^{2+} release channels have been reported by some investigators. Similarly, myocytes from failing hearts have reduced levels of mRNA for the two sarcoplasmic reticulum proteins, phospholamban and Ca^{2+}-ATPase.

Two major classes of adrenergic receptor are found in the human heart. Alpha$_1$-adrenergic receptors are important for inducing myocardial hypertrophy; levels of α1 receptors are slightly increased in heart failure. Heart failure is associated with significant β-adrenergic receptor desensitization as a result of chronic sympathetic activation. This effect is mediated by downregulation of $β_1$-adrenergic receptors, downstream uncoupling of the signal transduction pathway, and upregulation of inhibitory G proteins. All these changes lead to a further reduction in myocyte contractility.

Cardiac myocytes cannot proliferate once they have matured to their adult form. However, there is a constant turnover of the contractile proteins that make up the sarcomere. In response to the hemodynamic stresses associated with heart failure, angiotensin II, TNF, norepinephrine, and other molecules induce protein synthesis via intranuclear mediators of gene activity such as c-*fos*, c-*jun*, and c-*myc*. This causes myocyte hypertrophy with an increase in sarcomere numbers and a re-expression of fetal and neonatal forms of myosin and troponin. Activation of this primitive program results in the development of large myocytes that do not contract normally and have decreased ATPase activity.

The heart enlarges in response to continued hemodynamic stress. Changes in myocardial size and shape associated with heart failure are collectively referred to as left ventricular remodeling. Several tissue changes appear to mediate this process. First, heart failure is associated with myocyte loss via a process called apoptosis (programmed cell death). Unlike the process of necrosis, apoptotic cells initially demonstrate decreased cell volume without disruption of the cell membrane. However, as the apoptotic process continues, the myocyte ultimately dies, and "holes" are left in the myocardium. Loss of myocytes places increased stress on the remaining myocytes. The process of apoptosis is accelerated by the proliferative signals that stimulate myocyte hypertrophy such as TNF. Although apoptosis is a normal process essential in organs made up of proliferating cells, in the heart apoptosis initiates a vicious circle whereby cell death causes increased stress that leads to hypertrophy and the further acceleration of apoptosis.

A second tissue change observed in heart failure is an increased amount of fibrous tissue in the interstitial spaces of the heart. Collagen deposition results from fibroblast activation and myocyte death. Endothelin release leads to interstitial collagen deposition. The increase in connective tissue increases chamber stiffness and shifts the diastolic pressure–volume curve to the left.

Finally, heart failure is associated with gradual ventricle dilation. Myocyte "slippage" as a result of the activation of collagenases that disrupt the collagen network may be responsible for this process.

Clinical Manifestations

A. Symptoms

1. **Shortness of breath, orthopnea, paroxysmal nocturnal dyspnea**—Although many details of the physiologic mechanisms for the sensation of breathlessness are unclear, the inciting event is probably increasing pulmonary capillary pressure as a consequence of elevated left ventricular and atrial pressures. The rise in pulmonary capillary pressure relative to plasma oncotic pressure causes fluid to move into the interstitial spaces

FIGURE 10–18 Posteroanterior chest x-ray film in a man with acute pulmonary edema resulting from left ventricular failure. Note the bat's-wing density, cardiac enlargement, increased size of upper lobe vessels, and pulmonary venous congestion. (Reproduced, with permission, from Cheitlin MD et al, eds. *Clinical Cardiology*, 6th ed. Originally published by Appleton & Lange. Copyright © 1993 by The McGraw-Hill Companies, Inc.)

of the lung (pulmonary edema), which can be seen on chest x-ray film (Figure 10–18). Interstitial edema probably stimulates juxtacapillary J receptors, which in turn causes reflex shallow, rapid breathing. Replacement of air in the lungs by blood or interstitial fluid can cause a reduction of vital capacity, restrictive physiology, and air trapping as a result of closure of small airways. The work of breathing increases as the patient tries to distend stiff lungs, which can lead to respiratory muscle fatigue and the sensation of dyspnea. Alterations in the distribution of ventilation and perfusion result in relative ventilation–perfusion mismatch, with consequent widening of the alveolar–arterial O_2 gradient, hypoxemia, and increased dead space. Edema of the bronchial walls can lead to small airway obstruction and produce wheezing ("cardiac asthma"). Shortness of breath occurs in the recumbent position (orthopnea) because of reduced blood pooling in the extremities and abdomen, and, because the patient is operating on the steep portion of the diastolic pressure–volume curve, any increase in blood return leads to marked elevations in ventricular pressures. Patients usually learn to minimize orthopnea by sleeping with the upper body propped up by two or more pillows. Sudden onset of severe respiratory distress at night—paroxysmal nocturnal dyspnea—probably occurs because of the reduced adrenergic support of ventricular function that occurs with sleep, the increase in blood return as described previously, and normal nocturnal depression of the respiratory center.

2. **Fatigue, confusion**—Fatigue probably arises because of the inability of the heart to supply appropriate amounts of blood to skeletal muscles. Confusion may arise in advanced heart failure because of under-perfusion of the cerebrum.

3. **Nocturia**—Heart failure can lead to reduced renal perfusion during the day while the patient is upright, which normalizes only at night while the patient is supine, with consequent diuresis.

4. **Chest pain**—If the cause of failure is coronary artery disease, patients may have chest pain secondary to ischemia (angina pectoris). In addition, even without ischemia, acute heart failure can cause chest pain by unknown mechanisms.

B. Physical Examination

1. **Rales, pleural effusion**—Increased fluid in the alveolar spaces from the mechanisms described previously can be heard as rales. Increased capillary pressures can also cause fluid accumulation in the pleural spaces.

2. **Displaced and sustained apical impulse**—In most people, contraction of the heart can be appreciated by careful palpation of the chest wall (apical impulse). The normal apical impulse is felt in the midclavicular line in the fourth or fifth intercostal space and is palpable only during the first part of systole. When the apical impulse can be felt during the latter part of systole, it is sustained. Sustained impulses suggest that increases in left ventricular volume or mass are present. In addition, when left ventricular volume is increased as a compensatory mechanism of heart failure, the apical impulse is displaced laterally.

3. **Third heart sound (S_3)**—The third heart sound is a low-pitched sound heard during rapid filling of the ventricle in early diastole (Figure 10–19A). The exact mechanism responsible for the genesis of the third heart sound is unknown, but the sound appears to result either from the sudden deceleration of blood as the elastic limits of the ventricular chamber are reached or from the actual impact of the ventricular wall against the chest wall. Although a third heart sound is normal in children and young adults, it is rarely heard in healthy adults older than 40 years. In these individuals, the presence of a third heart sound is almost pathognomonic of ventricular failure. The increased end-systolic volumes and pressures characteristic of the failing heart are probably responsible for the prominent third heart sound. When it arises because of left ventricular failure, the third heart sound is usually heard best at the apex. It can be present in patients with either diastolic or systolic dysfunction.

4. **Fourth heart sound (S_4)**—Normally, sounds arising from atrial contraction are not heard. However, if there is increased ventricle stiffness, a low-pitched sound at end-diastole that occurs concomitantly with atrial contraction can sometimes be heard (Figure 10–19B). As with the third heart sound, the exact mechanism for the genesis of the fourth heart sound is unknown. However, it probably arises from the sudden deceleration of blood in a non-compliant ventricle or from the sudden impact of a stiff ventricle against the chest wall. It is best heard laterally over the apex at the point of maximal impulse, particularly when the patient is partially rolled over onto the left side. The fourth heart sound is commonly heard in any patient with heart failure resulting from diastolic dysfunction.

5. **Pale, cold, and sweaty skin**—Patients with severe heart failure often have peripheral vasoconstriction, which maintains blood flow to the central organs and head. In some cases, the skin appears dusky because of reduced oxygen content in venous blood as a result of increased oxygen extraction from peripheral tissues that are receiving low blood flow. Sweating occurs because body heat cannot be dissipated through the constricted vascular bed of the skin.

FIGURE 10–19 **A:** Phonocardiogram showing typical third heart sound (S_3). It follows the second sound (S_2) by 0.16 s. **B:** Phonocardiogram showing a fourth heart sound (S_4) and its relation to first sound (S_1).

2. Right Ventricular Failure

Clinical Presentation

Symptoms of right ventricular failure include shortness of breath, pedal edema, and abdominal pain.

The findings on physical examination are similar to those of left ventricular failure but in different positions, because the right ventricle is anatomically anterior and to the right of the left ventricle (see Figure 10–1). Patients with right ventricular failure may have a third heart sound heard best at the sternal border or a sustained systolic heave of the sternum. Inspection of the neck reveals elevated jugular venous pressures. Because the most common cause of right ventricular failure is left ventricular failure, signs of left ventricular failure are often also present.

Etiology

Right ventricular failure can have several causes. As mentioned, left ventricular failure can cause right ventricular failure because of the increased afterload placed on the right ventricle. Increased afterload can also be present from abnormalities of the pulmonary arteries or capillaries. For example, increased flow from a congenital shunt can cause reactive pulmonary artery constriction, increased right ventricular afterload, and, ultimately, right ventricular failure. Right ventricular failure can occur as a sequela of pulmonary disease (cor pulmonale) because of destruction of the pulmonary capillary bed or hypoxia-induced vasoconstriction of the pulmonary arterioles. Right ventricular failure can also be caused by right ventricular ischemia, usually in the setting of an inferior wall myocardial infarction (Table 10–3).

Pathophysiology

The pathophysiology of right ventricular failure is similar to that described for the left ventricle. Both systolic and diastolic abnormalities of the right ventricle can be present and usually occur because of inappropriate loads placed on the ventricle or primary loss of myocyte contractility.

TABLE 10–3   Causes of right ventricular failure.

Left-sided failure
Precapillary obstruction
Congenital (shunts, obstruction)   Idiopathic pulmonary hypertension
Primary right ventricular failure
Right ventricular infarction
Cor pulmonale
Hypoxia-induced vasoconstriction   Pulmonary embolism   Chronic obstructive pulmonary disease

Patients with isolated right ventricular failure (pulmonary hypertension, cor pulmonale) can have a mechanical reason for left ventricular failure. The interventricular septum is usually bowed toward the thinner-walled and lower-pressure right ventricle. When right ventricular pressure increases relative to the left, the interventricular septum can bow to the left and prevent efficient filling of the left ventricle, which may lead to pulmonary congestion. Rarely, the bowing can be so severe that left ventricular outflow is partially obstructed.

Clinical Manifestations

A. Shortness of Breath—In left ventricular failure, patients may be short of breath because of pulmonary edema, as discussed previously. In patients with right-sided failure resulting from pulmonary disease, shortness of breath may be a manifestation of the underlying disease (eg, pulmonary embolus, chronic obstructive pulmonary disease). In some patients with right ventricular failure, congestion of the hepatic veins with formation of ascites can impinge on normal diaphragmatic function and contribute to the sensation of dyspnea. In addition, reduced right-sided cardiac output alone can cause acidosis, hypoxia, and air hunger. If the cause of right-sided failure is a left-sided defect such as mitral stenosis, the onset of right heart failure can sometimes lessen the symptoms of pulmonary edema because of the decreased load placed on the left ventricle.

B. Elevated Jugular Venous Pressure—The position of venous pulsations of the internal jugular vein can be observed during examination of the neck (Figure 10–20A). The vertical distance above the heart at which venous pulsations are observed is an estimate of the right atrial or central venous pressure. Because the position of the right atrium cannot be precisely determined, the height of the jugular venous pulsation is measured relative to the angle of Louis on the sternum. Right atrial pressure can then be approximated by adding 5 cm to the height of the venous column (because the right atrium is approximately 5 cm inferior to the angle). Jugular venous pulsations are usually observed less than 7 cm above the right atrium. Elevated atrial pressures are present any time this distance is greater than 10 cm. Elevated atrial pressures indicate that the preload of the ventricle is adequate but ventricular function is decreased and fluid is accumulating in the venous system. Other causes of elevated jugular pressures besides heart failure include pericardial tamponade, constrictive pericarditis, and massive pulmonary embolism.

In addition to relative position, individual waveforms of the jugular venous pulse can be assessed. Three positive waves (*a*, *c*, and *v*) and two negative waves (*x* and *y*) can be recognized (Figure 10–20B). The *a* wave is caused by transmitted right atrial pressure from atrial contraction. The *c* wave is usually not present on bedside examination; it is thought to arise from bulging of the tricuspid valve during isovolumic

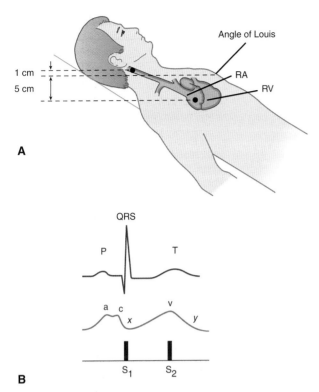

FIGURE 10–20 **A:** Examination of jugular venous pulse and estimation of venous pressure. (RA, right atrium; RV, right ventricle.) **B:** Jugular venous pressure waveforms in relation to the electrocardiogram (P wave, QRS, and T wave) and the first and second heart sounds (S_1 and S_2). The bottom of the *x* descent occurs coincident with the first heart sound (S_1). The *v* wave occurs just after the apical impulse is felt at the same time the second heart sound (S_2) is heard. See text for further explanation of jugular venous waveforms.

contraction of the right ventricle. The *x* descent is thought to result from atrial relaxation and downward displacement of the tricuspid annulus during systole. The *v* wave arises from continued filling of the right atrium during the latter part of systole. Once the tricuspid valve opens, blood flows into the right ventricle and the *y* descent begins. Evaluation of the individual waveforms will become particularly important when pericardial disease is discussed.

C. Anasarca, Ascites, Pedal Edema, Hepatojugular Reflux & Abdominal Pain—Elevated right-sided pressure leads to fluid accumulation in the systemic venous circulation. Venous congestion can be manifested by generalized edema (anasarca), ascites (collection of fluid in the peritoneal space), and dependent edema (swelling of the feet and legs). Pressing on the liver for approximately 5 seconds can lead to displacement of blood into the vena cava; when the right ventricle cannot accommodate this additional volume, an increase in jugular venous pressure ("hepatojugular reflux") can be observed. Expansion of the liver from fluid accumulation can cause distention of the liver capsule with accompanying right upper quadrant abdominal pain.

CHECKPOINT

6. What are the clinical presentations of left ventricular heart failure (HF) and right ventricular failure?
7. What are the four general categories that account for almost all causes of HF?
8. Explain the differences between the pathophysiology of HF resulting from systolic versus diastolic dysfunction.
9. What are the major clinical manifestations and complications of left- versus right-sided heart failure?

VALVULAR HEART DISEASE

Dysfunctional cardiac valves can be classified as either narrow (stenosis) or leaky (regurgitation). Although the tricuspid and pulmonary valves can become dysfunctional in patients with endocarditis, congenital lesions, or carcinoid syndrome, primary right-sided valvular abnormalities are relatively rare and are not discussed further here. In this section, the pathophysiologic mechanisms of stenotic and regurgitant aortic and mitral valves are addressed.

Figure 10–21 provides a general classification of heart murmurs. Any disease process that creates turbulent flow in the heart or great vessels can cause a murmur. For instance, ventricular septal defect is associated with a systolic murmur because of the abnormal interventricular connection and the pressure difference between the left and right ventricles; patent ductus arteriosus is associated with a continuous murmur because of a persistent connection between the pulmonary artery and the aorta. However, valvular lesions are the principal cause of heart murmurs. Thus, an understanding of heart murmurs gives insight into the underlying pathophysiologic processes of specific valvular lesions.

Heart murmurs can be either systolic or diastolic. During systole, while the left ventricle is contracting, the aortic valve is open and the mitral valve is closed. Turbulent flow can occur either because of an incompetent mitral valve, leading to regurgitation of blood back into the atrium, or from a narrowed aortic valve. In diastole, the situation is reversed, with filling of the left ventricle through an open mitral valve while the aortic valve is closed. Turbulent flow occurs when there is mitral valve narrowing or aortic valve incompetence. Valve stenosis usually develops slowly over time; lesions that cause valvular regurgitation can be either chronic or acute.

1. Aortic Stenosis

Clinical Presentation

For all causes of aortic stenosis, there is usually a long latent period of slowly increasing obstruction before symptoms appear. In descending order of frequency, the three characteristic symptoms of aortic stenosis are chest pain (angina pectoris), syncope, and heart failure (see prior discussion). Once symptoms occur, the prognosis is poor if the obstruction is

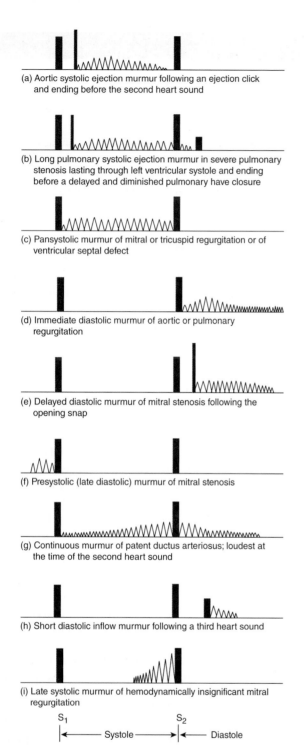

(a) Aortic systolic ejection murmur following an ejection click and ending before the second heart sound

(b) Long pulmonary systolic ejection murmur in severe pulmonary stenosis lasting through left ventricular systole and ending before a delayed and diminished pulmonary have closure

(c) Pansystolic murmur of mitral or tricuspid regurgitation or of ventricular septal defect

(d) Immediate diastolic murmur of aortic or pulmonary regurgitation

(e) Delayed diastolic murmur of mitral stenosis following the opening snap

(f) Presystolic (late diastolic) murmur of mitral stenosis

(g) Continuous murmur of patent ductus arteriosus; loudest at the time of the second heart sound

(h) Short diastolic inflow murmur following a third heart sound

(i) Late systolic murmur of hemodynamically insignificant mitral regurgitation

S_1 S_2

|← Systole →|← Diastole

FIGURE 10–21 The timing of the principal cardiac murmurs.

TABLE 10–4   Causes of aortic stenosis.

Type	Pathology	Clinical Presentation
Congenital	The valve can be unicuspid, bicuspid, or tricuspid with partially fused leaflets. Abnormal flow can lead to fibrosis and calcification of the leaflets.	Patient usually develops symptoms before age 30 years.
Rheumatic	Tissue inflammation results in adhesion and fusing of the commissures. Fibrosis and calcification of the leaflet tips can occur because of continued turbulent flow.	Patient usually develops symptoms between ages 30 and 70 years. Often the valve will also be regurgitant. Accompanying mitral valve disease is frequently present.
Degenerative	Leaflets become inflexible because of calcium deposition at the bases. The leaflet tips remain relatively normal.	The most likely cause of aortic stenosis in patients older than 70 years. Particularly prevalent in patients with diabetes or hypercholesterolemia.

the sternal notch and the neck. Depending on the cause of the aortic stenosis, a crisp, relatively high-pitched aortic ejection sound can be heard just after the first heart sound. Finally, a fourth heart sound (S_4) is often present.

Etiology

Table 10–4 lists and describes various causes of aortic stenosis.

Pathophysiology

The normal aortic valve area is approximately 3.5–4.0 cm². Critical aortic stenosis is usually present when the area is less than 0.8 cm². At this point, the systolic gradient between the left ventricle and the aorta can exceed 150 mm Hg, and most patients are symptomatic (Figure 10–22A). The fixed outflow obstruction places a large afterload on the ventricle. The compensatory mechanisms of the heart can be understood by examining the Laplace law for a sphere, where wall stress (T) is proportionate to the product of the transmural pressure (P) and cavitary radius (r) and inversely proportionate to wall thickness (W):

$$T \propto P \times \frac{r}{W}$$

In response to the pressure overload (increased P), left ventricular wall thickness markedly increases—while the cavitary radius remains relatively unchanged—by parallel sarcomere replication. These compensatory changes, termed "concentric hypertrophy," reduce the increase in

untreated, with average life expectancies of 2, 3, and 5 years for angina pectoris, syncope, and heart failure, respectively.

On physical examination, palpation of the carotid upstroke reveals a pulsation (pulsus) that is both decreased (parvus) and late (tardus) relative to the apical impulse. Palpation of the chest reveals an apical impulse that is laterally displaced and sustained. On auscultation, a midsystolic murmur is heard, loudest at the base of the heart, and often with radiation to

FIGURE 10–22 Aortic stenosis. **A:** Drawing of the left heart in left anterior oblique view showing anatomic features of aortic stenosis. Note structures enlarged: left ventricle (thickened); poststenotic dilation of the aorta. **B:** Drawing showing auscultatory and hemodynamic features of predominant aortic stenosis. Cardinal features include left ventricular hypertrophy and systolic ejection murmur. (A, aortic valve; EC, ejection click; P, pulmonary valve; SM, systolic murmur.) (Redrawn, with permission, from Cheitlin MD et al, eds. *Clinical Cardiology*, 6th ed. Originally published by Appleton & Lange. Copyright © 1993 by The McGraw-Hill Companies, Inc.) **C:** Pressure–volume loop in aortic stenosis. The left ventricle becomes thickened and less compliant, forcing the diastolic pressure–volume curve upward, which results in elevated left ventricular end-diastolic pressure (**a′**). Because the left ventricle must pump against a fixed gradient (increased afterload), **b** increases to **b′**. Finally, the hypertrophy of the ventricle results in increased inotropic force, which shifts the isovolumic pressure curve leftward.

wall tension observed in aortic stenosis (see Aortic Regurgitation). Analysis of pressure–volume loops reveals that, to maintain stroke volume and because of decreases in ventricular compliance, left ventricular end-diastolic pressure increases significantly (Figure 10–22C). The thick ventricle leads to a prominent *a* wave on left atrial pressure tracings as the ventricle becomes more dependent on atrial contraction to fill the ventricle.

Clinical Manifestations

A. Symptoms

1. **Angina pectoris**—Angina can occur because of several mechanisms. First, approximately half of all patients with aortic stenosis have significant concomitant coronary artery disease. Even without significant coronary artery disease, the combination of increased oxygen demands because of ventricular hypertrophy and decreased supply as a result of excessive compression of the vessels can lead to relative ischemia of the myocytes. Finally, coronary artery obstruction from calcium emboli arising from a calcified stenotic aortic valve has been reported, although it is an uncommon cause of angina.

2. **Syncope**—Syncope in aortic stenosis usually results from decreased cerebral perfusion from the fixed obstruction but may also occur because of transient atrial arrhythmias with loss of effective atrial contribution to ventricular filling. In addition, arrhythmias arising from ventricular tissues are more common in patients with aortic stenosis and can cause syncope.

3. **Heart failure**—(See Heart Failure.) The progressive increase in left ventricular end-diastolic pressure can cause elevated pulmonary venous pressure and pulmonary edema.

B. Physical Examination—Because there is a fixed obstruction to flow, the carotid upstroke is decreased and late. Left ventricular hypertrophy causes the apical impulse to be displaced laterally and to become sustained. The increased dependence on atrial contraction is responsible for the prominent S_4. Flow through the restricted orifice gives rise to a midsystolic murmur. The murmur is usually heard best at the base of the heart but often radiates to the neck and apex. It usually presents as a crescendo–decrescendo murmur, and, in contrast to mitral regurgitation, the first and second heart sounds are easily heard. As aortic valve narrowing worsens, the murmur peaks later in systole. When calcified leaflets are present, the murmur tends to have a harsher quality. An aortic ejection sound, caused by the sudden checking of the leaflets as they open, is heard only when the leaflets remain fairly mobile, as in congenitally malformed valves.

Although obstruction of blood flow from the left ventricle usually results from valvular disease, obstruction can also occur above or below the valve and can present in somewhat the same way as valvular aortic stenosis. A membranous shelf that partially obstructs flow just above the valve in the aorta can sometimes be present from birth. In this condition, the systolic murmur is usually heard best at the first intercostal space at the right sternal border. Subvalvular stenosis can occur in some patients who develop severe hypertrophy of the heart (Figure 10–23). Hypertrophic cardiomyopathy is a genetic disorder that often involves a mutation of one of the sarcomere proteins such as myosin or actin. This well-recognized clinical entity—hypertrophic cardiomyopathy—can also be manifested by a crescendo–decrescendo systolic murmur noted on physical examination. However, obstruction of the outflow tract in hypertrophic cardiomyopathy is dynamic, with greater obstruction when preload is decreased from decreased intra-ventricular volume. For this reason, having the patient stand or perform the Valsalva maneuver (expiratory effort against a closed glottis), both of which decrease venous return, causes the murmur to increase. Both maneuvers cause a decrease in murmurs caused by valvular stenosis, because less absolute blood volume flows across the stenotic aortic valve.

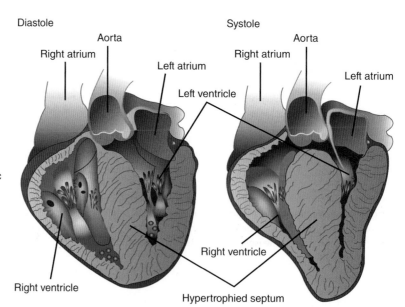

Cardinal features:
Left ventricular (especially septal) hypertrophy, diastolic dysfunction; systolic outflow obstruction, systolic anterior motion of mitral valve; excessive left ventricular emptying.

Variable factors:
Severity; level of peripheral resistance; low resistance and low blood volume lead to obstruction.

FIGURE 10–23 Hypertrophic cardiomyopathy (left lateral view). The cardinal features are displayed. (Redrawn, with permission, from Cheitlin MD et al, eds. *Clinical Cardiology*, 6th ed. Originally published by Appleton & Lange. Copyright © 1993 by The McGraw-Hill Companies, Inc.)

2. Aortic Regurgitation

Clinical Presentation

Aortic regurgitation can be either chronic or acute. In chronic aortic regurgitation, there is a long latent period during which the patient remains asymptomatic as the heart responds to the volume load. When the compensatory mechanisms fail, symptoms of left-sided failure become manifest. In acute aortic regurgitation, compensatory mechanisms have no time to be activated, so shortness of breath, pulmonary edema, and hypotension—often with cardiovascular collapse—occur suddenly.

Physical examination of patients with chronic aortic regurgitation reveals hyperdynamic (pounding) pulses. The apical impulse is hyperdynamic and displaced laterally. On auscultation, three murmurs may be heard: a high-pitched early diastolic murmur, a diastolic rumble called the Austin Flint murmur, and a systolic murmur. A third heart sound is often present. However, in acute aortic regurgitation, the peripheral signs are often absent, and in many cases the left ventricular impulse is normal. On auscultation, the diastolic murmur is much softer, and the Austin Flint murmur, if present, is short. The first heart sound will be soft and sometimes absent.

Etiology

Chronic and acute aortic regurgitation can result either from valvular or aortic root abnormalities (Table 10–5).

Pathophysiology

Aortic regurgitation places a volume load on the left ventricle because during diastole, blood enters the ventricle both from the left atrium and from the aorta. If the regurgitation develops slowly, the heart responds to the increased diastolic pressure by fiber elongation and replication of sarcomeres in series, which leads to increased ventricular volumes. Because systolic pressure remains relatively unchanged, increased wall stress—by the Laplace law—can be compensated for by an additional increase in wall thickness. This response, "eccentric hypertrophy"—so named because the ventricular cavity enlarges laterally in the chest and becomes eccentric to its normal position—explains the different ventricular geometry observed in patients with aortic regurgitation versus those with aortic stenosis (concentric hypertrophy caused by the systolic pressure overload). Ultimately, chronic aortic regurgitation leads to huge ventricular volumes as demonstrated in the pressure–volume loops (Figure 10–24). The left ventricle operates as a low-compliance pump, handling large end-diastolic and stroke volumes, often with little increase in end-diastolic pressure. In addition, no truly isovolumic period of relaxation or contraction exists because of the persistent flow into the ventricle from the systemic circulation. Aortic pulse pressure is widened. Diastolic pressure decreases because of regurgitant flow back into the left ventricle and increased compliance of the large central vessels (in response to increased stroke volume); elevated stroke volume leads to increased systolic pressures (Figure 10–24C).

TABLE 10–5   Causes of aortic regurgitation.

Site	Pathology	Causes	Time Course
Valvular	Cusp abnormalities	Endocarditis	Acute or chronic
		Rheumatic disease	Acute or chronic
		Ankylosing spondylitis	Usually chronic
		Congenital	Chronic
Aortic root	Dilation	Aortic aneurysm	Acute or chronic
		Heritable disorders of connective tissue	Usually chronic
		Marfan syndrome	
		Ehlers–Danlos syndrome	
		Osteogenesis imperfecta	
	Inflammation	Aortitis (Takayasu arteritis)	Usually chronic
		Syphilis	Usually chronic
		Arthritic diseases	Usually chronic
		Ankylosing spondylitis	
		Reiter syndrome	
		Rheumatoid arthritis	
		Systemic lupus erythematosus	Acute or chronic
		Cystic medial necrosis	
	Tears with loss of commissural support	Trauma	Usually acute
		Dissection, often from hypertension	Usually acute

FIGURE 10–24   Aortic insufficiency (regurgitation). **A:** Drawing of the left heart in left anterior oblique view showing the anatomic features of aortic insufficiency. Note structures enlarged: left ventricle, aorta. **B:** Drawing showing the auscultatory and hemodynamic features of predominant aortic insufficiency. Cardinal features include large hypertrophied left ventricle, large aorta, increased stroke volume, wide pulse pressure, and diastolic murmur. (A, aortic valve; DM, diastolic murmur; P, pulmonary valve; SM, systolic murmur.) (Redrawn, with permission, from Cheitlin MD et al, eds. *Clinical Cardiology*, 6th ed. Originally published by Appleton & Lange. Copyright © 1993 by The McGraw-Hill Companies, Inc.) **C:** Pressure–volume loop in chronic aortic insufficiency. A marked enlargement in left ventricular volume shifts the diastolic pressure–volume curve rightward. Hypertrophy of the ventricle shifts the isovolumic pressure–volume curve leftward (not shown), but ultimately the ventricle dilates, contractility decreases, and the isovolumic pressure–volume curve shifts to the right. Stroke volume is enormous, although effective stroke volume may be minimally changed because much of the increase in stroke volume leaks back into the ventricle. Because the ventricle is constantly being filled from the mitral valve or the incompetent aortic valve, no isovolumic periods exist.

Clinical Manifestations

A. Shortness of Breath—Pulmonary edema can develop, particularly if the aortic regurgitation is acute and the ventricle does not have time to compensate for the sudden increase in volume. In chronic aortic regurgitation, compensatory mechanisms eventually fail and the heart begins to operate on the steeper portion of the diastolic pressure–volume curve.

B. Physical Examination

1. **Hyperdynamic pulses**—In chronic aortic regurgitation, a widened pulse pressure is responsible for several characteristic peripheral signs. Palpation of the peripheral pulse reveals a sudden rise and then drop in pressure (water-hammer or Corrigan pulse). Head bobbing (DeMusset sign), rhythmic pulsation of the uvula (Müller sign), and arterial pulsation seen in the nail bed (Quincke pulse) have been described in patients with chronic aortic regurgitation.

2. **Murmurs**—Three heart murmurs can be heard in patients with aortic regurgitation: First, flow from the regurgitant volume back into the left ventricle can be heard as a high-pitched, blowing, early diastolic murmur usually perceived best along the left sternal border. Second, the rumbling murmur described by Austin Flint can be heard at the apex during any part of diastole. The Austin Flint murmur is thought to result from regurgitant flow from the aortic valve impinging on the anterior leaflet of the mitral valve, producing functional mitral stenosis. Finally, a crescendo–decrescendo systolic murmur, thought to arise from the increased stroke volume flowing across the aortic valve, can be heard at the left sternal border.

   In acute, severe aortic regurgitation, the early diastolic murmur may be softer because of rapid diastolic equalization of ventricular and aortic pressures. The first heart sound is soft because of early mitral valve closure from aortic regurgitation and elevated ventricular pressures.

3. **Third heart sound**—A third heart sound can be heard because of concomitant heart failure or because of the exaggerated early diastolic filling of the left ventricle.

4. **Apical impulse**—The apical impulse is displaced laterally because of the increased volume of the left ventricle.

3. Mitral Stenosis

Clinical Presentation

The symptoms of mitral stenosis include dyspnea, fatigue, and hemoptysis. Occasionally, the patient complains of palpitations or a rapid heartbeat. Finally, the patient with mitral stenosis may present with neurologic symptoms such as transient numbness or weakness of the extremities, sudden loss of vision, or difficulty with coordination.

The characteristic murmur of mitral stenosis is a late low-pitched diastolic rumble. In addition, an opening snap may be heard in the first portion of diastole (Figure 10–25). Auscultation of the lungs may reveal rales.

Etiology

Mitral stenosis is most commonly a sequela of rheumatic heart disease (Table 10–6). Infrequently, it may be caused by congenital lesions or calcium deposition. Atrial masses (myxomas) can cause intermittent mitral valve obstruction.

Pathophysiology

The mitral valve is normally bicuspid, with the anterior cusp approximately twice the area of the posterior cusp. The mitral valve area is usually 5–6 cm^2; clinically relevant mitral stenosis usually occurs when the valve area decreases to less than 1 cm^2. Because obstruction of flow protects the ventricle from pressure and volume loads, the left ventricular pressure–volume relationship shows relatively little abnormality other than decreased volumes. However, analysis of hemodynamic tracings shows the characteristic elevation in left atrial pressures (Figure 10–25B). For this reason, the main pathophysiologic abnormalities in mitral stenosis are elevated pulmonary venous pressure and elevated right-sided pressures (pulmonary artery, right ventricle, and right atrium). Dilation and reduced systolic function of the right ventricle are commonly observed in patients with advanced mitral stenosis.

Clinical Manifestations

A. Symptoms

1. **Shortness of breath, hemoptysis, and orthopnea**—All these symptoms occur because of elevated left atrial, pulmonary venous, and pulmonary capillary pressures (the actual mechanisms are described in the section on heart failure).

2. **Palpitations**—Increased left atrial size predisposes patients with mitral stenosis to atrial arrhythmias. Chaotic atrial activity (ie, atrial fibrillation) is commonly observed. Because ventricular filling is particularly dependent on atrial contraction in patients with mitral stenosis, acute hemodynamic decompensation may occur when organized contraction of the atrium is lost.

3. **Neurologic symptoms**—Reduced outflow leads to dilation of the left atrium and stasis of blood flow. A thrombus in the left atrium is observed on echocardiography in approximately 20% of patients with mitral stenosis, and the prevalence increases with age, the presence of atrial fibrillation, the severity of stenosis, and any reduction in cardiac output. Embolic events that lead to neurologic symptoms occur in 8% of patients in sinus rhythm and in 32% of patients with chronic or paroxysmal atrial fibrillation. In addition, left atrial enlargement can sometimes impinge on the recurrent laryngeal nerve and lead to hoarseness (Ortner syndrome).

FIGURE 10–25 Mitral stenosis. **A:** Drawing of the left heart in left anterior oblique view showing the anatomic features of mitral stenosis. Note the enlarged left atrium and small left ventricle. **B:** Drawing showing the auscultatory and hemodynamic features of mitral stenosis. Cardinal features include thickening and fusion of mitral valve cusps, elevated left atrial pressure, left atrial enlargement, opening snap, and diastolic murmur. (A, aortic; DM, diastolic murmur; M, mitral; OS, opening snap; P, pulmonary; PSM, presystolic murmur; T, tricuspid.) **C:** Pressure–volume loop in mitral stenosis. Filling of the left ventricle is restricted from **a** to **a′**, decreasing stroke volume to **b′c′**.

B. Physical Examination—On auscultation of the heart, the diastolic rumble occurs because of turbulent flow across the narrowed mitral valve orifice. An opening snap, analogous to the ejection click described for aortic stenosis, may be heard in early diastole. The opening snap is heard only when the patient has relatively mobile leaflets.

Rales occur because elevated pulmonary capillary pressures lead to an accumulation of intra-alveolar fluid.

4. Mitral Regurgitation

Clinical Presentation

The presentation of mitral regurgitation depends on how quickly valvular incompetence develops. Patients with chronic mitral regurgitation develop symptoms gradually over time. Common complaints include dyspnea, easy fatigability, and palpitations. Patients with acute mitral

TABLE 10–6   **Causes of mitral stenosis.**

Type	Comments
Rheumatic	Most common. Narrowing results from fusion and thickening of the commissures, cusps, and chordae tendineae. Symptoms usually develop 20 years after acute rheumatic fever.
Calcific	Usually causes mitral regurgitation but can cause mitral stenosis in some cases.
Congenital	Usually presents during infancy or childhood.
Collagen–vascular disease	Systemic lupus erythematosus and rheumatoid arthritis (rare).

TABLE 10–7   **Causes of mitral regurgitation.**

Type	Causes
Acute	
Ruptured chordae tendineae	Infective endocarditis
	Trauma
	Acute rheumatic fever
	"Spontaneous"
Ruptured or dysfunctional papillary muscles	Ischemia
	Myocardial infarction
	Trauma
	Myocardial abscess
Perforated leaflet	Infective endocarditis
	Trauma
Chronic	
Inflammatory	Rheumatic heart disease
	Collagen–vascular disease
Infection	Infective endocarditis
Degenerative	Myxomatous degeneration of the valve leaflets
	Calcification of the mitral annulus
Rupture or dysfunction of the chordae tendineae or papillary muscles	Infective endocarditis
	Trauma
	Acute rheumatic fever
	"Spontaneous"
	Ischemia
	Myocardial infarction
	Myocardial abscess
Congenital	
	Developmental anomalies

regurgitation present with symptoms of left heart failure: shortness of breath, orthopnea, and shock. Chest pain may be present in patients whose mitral regurgitation is due to coronary artery disease.

On physical examination, patients have a pansystolic regurgitant murmur that is heard best at the apex and often radiates to the axilla. This murmur often obscures the first and second heart sounds. When mitral valve incompetence is severe, a third heart sound is often present. In chronic mitral regurgitation, the apical impulse is often hyperdynamic and displaced laterally.

Etiology

In the past, rheumatic heart disease accounted for most cases of mitral regurgitation. Mitral valve prolapse is now probably the most common cause, followed by coronary artery disease. The tips of the anterior and posterior mitral valve leaflets are held in place during ventricular contraction by the anterolateral and posteromedial papillary muscles. The valves are connected to the papillary muscles via thin fibrous structures called chordae tendineae. In patients with mitral valve prolapse, extra tissue present on the valvular apparatus can undergo myxomatous degeneration by the fifth or sixth decade. Mitral regurgitation follows as a result of either poor coaptation of the valve leaflets or sudden rupture of the chordae tendineae. In coronary artery disease, obstruction of the circumflex coronary artery can lead to ischemia or rupture of the papillary muscles (Table 10–7).

Pathophysiology

When the mitral valve fails to close properly, regurgitation of blood into the left atrium from the ventricle occurs during systole. In chronic mitral regurgitation, the compensatory mechanism to this volume load is similar to the changes seen in aortic regurgitation. The left ventricle and atrium dilate, and to normalize wall stress in the ventricle there is also concomitant hypertrophy of the ventricular wall (see prior discussion of the Laplace law). Diastolic filling of the ventricle

increases because it is now the sum of right ventricular output and the regurgitant volume from the previous beat. In acute mitral regurgitation, the sudden volume load on the atrium and ventricle is not compensated for by chamber enlargement and hypertrophy. The sudden increase in atrial volume leads to prominent atrial *v* waves with transmission of this elevated pressure to the pulmonary capillaries and the development of pulmonary edema (Figure 10–26).

Clinical Manifestations

A. Symptoms

1. **Pulmonary edema**—Rapid elevation of pulmonary capillary pressure in acute mitral regurgitation leads to the sudden onset of pulmonary edema, manifested by shortness of breath, orthopnea, and paroxysmal nocturnal dyspnea. In chronic mitral regurgitation, the symptoms

FIGURE 10–26 Mitral insufficiency (regurgitation). **A:** Drawing of the left heart in left lateral view showing the anatomic features of mitral insufficiency. Note the structures enlarged: left atrium and left ventricle. **B:** Drawing showing the auscultatory and hemodynamic features of mitral insufficiency. Cardinal features include systolic backflow into left atrium, left atrial enlargement, left ventricular enlargement (hypertrophy in acute lesions), prominent *v* wave caused by filling from both the pulmonary veins and the regurgitant jet, and holosystolic murmur. (3, third heart sound; A, aortic; P, pulmonary; SM, systolic murmur.) (Redrawn, with permission, from Cheitlin MD et al, eds. *Clinical Cardiology*, 6th ed. Originally published by Appleton & Lange. Copyright © 1993 by The McGraw-Hill Companies, Inc.) **C:** Pressure–volume loop in mitral insufficiency. Increased ventricular volumes shift the diastolic pressure–volume curve rightward. Stroke volume is increased because the ventricle can now eject blood into the low-pressure left atrium. With chronic volume loads, the isovolumic pressure–volume curve eventually shifts to the right.

develop gradually, but at some point, the compensatory mechanisms fail and pulmonary edema develops, particularly with exercise.

2. **Fatigue**—Fatigue can develop because of decreased forward blood flow to the peripheral tissues.

3. **Palpitations**—Left atrial enlargement may lead to the development of atrial fibrillation and accompanying palpitations. Patients with atrial fibrillation and mitral regurgitation have a 20% incidence of cardioembolic events.

B. Physical Examination

1. **Holosystolic murmur**—Regurgitant flow into the atrium produces a high-pitched murmur heard throughout systole. The murmur begins with the first heart sound, continues to the second heart sound, and is of constant intensity throughout systole. It finally ends when left ventricular pressure drops to equal left atrial pressure during isovolumic relaxation. Unlike with the murmur of aortic stenosis, there is little variation in the intensity of the murmur as the heart rate changes. In addition, the murmur does not change in intensity with respiration. It is usually heard best at the apex and often radiates to the axilla. If anterior leaflet rupture has occurred, the mitral regurgitation murmur will sometimes radiate to the back.

2. **Third heart sound**—A third heart sound is heard if heart failure is present. Because of increased and rapid filling of the ventricle during diastole, it may also be heard in the absence of overt failure in patients with severe mitral regurgitation.

3. **Displaced and hyperdynamic apical impulse**—The compensatory increase in left ventricular volume and wall thickness in patients with chronic mitral regurgitation is manifested by a laterally displaced apical impulse. Because the ventricle now has a low-pressure chamber (the left atrium) into which to eject blood, the apical impulse is often hyperdynamic. When mitral regurgitation develops suddenly, the apical impulse is not displaced or hyperdynamic, because the left ventricle has not had enough time for compensatory volume increases to occur.

CHECKPOINT

10. What are the clinical presentations of each of the four major categories of valvular heart disease?

11. What are the most common causes of each category of valvular heart disease?

12. What is the pathogenesis of each category of valvular heart disease?

13. What are the major clinical manifestations and complications of each category of valvular heart disease?

CORONARY ARTERY DISEASE

Clinical Presentation

Chest pain is the most common symptom associated with coronary artery disease. It is usually described as dull and can often radiate down the arm or to the jaw. It does not worsen with a deep breath and can be associated with shortness of breath, diaphoresis, nausea, and vomiting. This entire symptom complex has been termed **angina pectoris**, or "pain in the chest"; this phrase was first used by Heberden in 1744.

Clinically, angina is classified according to the precipitant and the duration of symptoms. If the pain occurs only with exertion and has been stable over a long period of time, it is termed **stable angina**. If the pain occurs at rest, it is termed **unstable angina**. Finally, regardless of the precipitant, if the chest pain persists without interruption for prolonged periods and irreversible myocyte damage has occurred, it is termed **myocardial infarction**.

On physical examination, the patient with coronary artery disease may have a fourth heart sound or signs of heart failure and shock. However, more than any other cardiovascular problem, the initial diagnosis relies on patient history.

Etiology

Atherosclerotic obstruction of the large epicardial vessels is by far the most common cause of coronary artery disease. Spasm of the coronary arteries from various mediators such as serotonin and histamine has been well described and is more common in Japanese individuals. Rarely, congenital abnormalities can cause coronary artery diseases (Table 10–8).

Pathophysiology

Coronary blood flow brings oxygen to myocytes and removes waste products such as carbon dioxide, lactic acid, and hydrogen ions. The heart has a tremendously high metabolic requirement; although it accounts for only 0.3% of body weight, it is responsible for 7% of the body's resting oxygen consumption. Cellular ischemia occurs when there is either an increased demand for oxygen relative to maximal arterial supply or an absolute reduction in oxygen supply. Although situations of increased demand such as thyrotoxicosis and aortic stenosis can cause myocardial ischemia, most clinical cases result

TABLE 10–8 Causes of coronary artery disease.

Type	Comments
Atherosclerosis	Most common cause. Risk factors include hypertension, hypercholesterolemia, diabetes mellitus, smoking, and a family history of atherosclerosis.
Spasm	Coronary artery vasospasm can occur in any population but is most prevalent in Japanese. Vasoconstriction appears to be mediated by histamine, serotonin, catecholamines, and endothelium-derived factors. Because spasm can occur at any time, the chest pain is often not exertion related.
Emboli	Rare cause of coronary artery disease. Can occur from vegetations in patients with endocarditis.
Congenital	Congenital coronary artery abnormalities are present in 1–2% of the population. However, only a small fraction of these abnormalities causes symptomatic ischemia.

from decreased oxygen supply. Rarely, reduced oxygen supply can arise from decreased oxygen content in blood—such as occurs in carbon monoxide poisoning and anemia—but more commonly stems from coronary artery abnormalities (see Table 10–8), particularly atherosclerotic disease. Myocardial ischemia may arise from a combination of increased demand and decreased supply; for example, cocaine abuse increases oxygen demand (by inhibiting reuptake of norepinephrine at adrenergic nerve endings in the heart) and can reduce oxygen supply by causing vasospasm.

Atherosclerosis of large coronary arteries remains the predominant cause of angina and myocardial infarction. Raised fatty streaks, which appear as yellow spots or streaks in the vessel walls, are seen in coronary arteries in almost all members of any population by 20 years of age (see Chapter 11). They are found mainly in areas exposed to increased shear stresses, such as bending points and bifurcations, and are thought to arise from isolated macrophage foam cell migration into areas of minimal chronic intimal injury. In many people, this process progresses with additional foam cell migration, smooth muscle cell proliferation, and extracellular fat and collagen deposition (Figure 10–27). The extent and incidence of these advanced lesions vary among persons in different geographic regions and ethnic groups.

The underlying pathophysiologic processes differ for each clinical presentation of coronary artery disease. In patients with stable angina, fixed narrowing of one or several coronary arteries is usually present. Because the large coronary arteries usually function as conduits and do not offer resistance to flow, the arterial lumen must be decreased by 90% to produce cellular ischemia when the patient is at rest. However, with exercise, a 50% reduction in lumen size can lead to symptoms. In patients with unstable angina, fissuring of the atherosclerotic plaque can lead to platelet accumulation and transient episodes of thrombotic occlusion, usually lasting 10–20 minutes.

In addition, platelet release of vasoconstrictive factors, such as thromboxane A_2 or serotonin, and endothelial dysfunction may cause vasoconstriction and contribute to decreased flow. In myocardial infarction, deep arterial injury from plaque rupture may cause the formation of a relatively fixed and persistent thrombus. Recent research has emphasized that plaque composition mediated by inflammation has an important role in clinical presentation. Loss of the extracellular matrix and cellular necrosis owing to the inflammatory response appear to be the key mediators of plaque rupture.

The heart receives its energy primarily from ATP generated by the oxidative phosphorylation of free fatty acids, although glucose and other carbohydrates can be used. Within 60 seconds after coronary artery occlusion, myocardial oxygen tension in the affected cells falls essentially to zero. Cardiac stores of high-energy phosphates are rapidly depleted, and the cells shift rapidly to anaerobic metabolism with consequent lactic acid production. A dysfunction of myocardial relaxation and contraction occurs within seconds, even before the depletion of high-energy phosphates occurs. The biochemical basis for this abnormality is not well understood. If perfusion is not restored within 40–60 minutes, an irreversible stage of injury characterized by diffuse mitochondrial swelling, damage to the cell membrane, and marked depletion of glycogen begins. The exact mechanism by which irreversible damage occurs is multifactorial, and severe ATP depletion, increased extracellular calcium concentrations, lactic acidosis, and free radicals are all likely mediators of this process.

In experimental preparations, if ischemic myocardium is perfused within 5 minutes, systolic function returns promptly, whereas diastolic abnormalities may take up to 40 minutes to normalize. With prolonged episodes of ischemia—up to 1 hour—it may take up to 1 month to restore ventricular function. When the heart demonstrates this prolonged period of decreased function despite normal perfusion, the myocardium

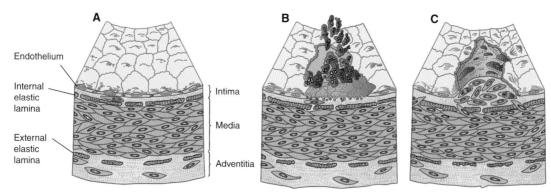

FIGURE 10–27 Mechanisms of atheroma production. **A:** Structure of the normal muscular artery. The adventitia, or outermost layer of the artery, consists principally of recognizable fibroblasts intermixed with smooth muscle cells loosely arranged between bundles of collagen and surrounded by proteoglycans. It is usually separated from the media by a discontinuous sheet of elastic tissue, the external elastic lamina. **B:** Platelet aggregates, or microthrombi, form as a result of platelet adherence to the exposed subendothelial connective tissue. Platelets that adhere to the connective tissue release granules whose constituents may gain entry into the arterial wall. Platelet factors thus interact with plasma constituents in the artery wall and may stimulate events shown in the next illustration. **C:** Smooth muscle cells migrate from the media into the intima through fenestrae in the internal elastic lamina and actively multiply within the intima. Endothelial cells regenerate in an attempt to re-cover the exposed intima, which thickens rapidly owing to smooth muscle proliferation and the formation of new connective tissue. (Redrawn, with permission, from Ross R et al. The pathogenesis of atherosclerosis. [Part 1.] N Engl J Med. 1976;295:369. Copyright © 1976 Massachusetts Medical Society. Reprinted with permission from Massachusetts Medical Society.)

is said to be "stunned." The biochemical basis for stunning is poorly understood. If reperfusion occurs later or not at all, systolic function often will not return to the affected area.

Clinical Manifestations

A. Chest Pain

Chest pain has traditionally been ascribed to ischemia. However, more recent evidence suggests that, in patients with coronary artery disease, 70–80% of episodes of ischemia are actually asymptomatic. When present, the chest pain is thought to be mediated by sympathetic afferent fibers that richly innervate the atrium and ventricle. From the heart, the fibers traverse the upper thoracic sympathetic ganglia and the five upper thoracic dorsal roots of the spinal cord. In the spinal cord, the impulses probably converge with impulses from other structures. This convergence is probably the mechanism for the chest wall, back, and arm pain that sometimes accompanies angina pectoris. The importance of these fibers can be demonstrated in patients who have had a heart transplant. When these patients develop atherosclerosis, they remain completely asymptomatic, without development of angina.

Evidence suggests that the actual trigger for nerve stimulation is adenosine. Adenosine infusion into the coronary arteries can produce the characteristic symptoms of angina without evidence of ischemia. In addition, blocking the adenosine receptor (P_1) with aminophylline leads to reduced anginal symptoms despite similar degrees of ischemia.

Three factors probably account for the large proportion of asymptomatic episodes: dysfunction of afferent nerves, transient reduced perfusion, and differing pain thresholds among patients. Dysfunction of afferent nerves may cause silent ischemia. Patients with transplanted hearts do not sense cardiac pain despite significant atherosclerosis. Peripheral neuropathy in patients with diabetes may explain the increased episodes of silent ischemia described in this patient population. Transient reduced perfusion may also be an important mechanism for silent ischemia. Within a few seconds after cessation of perfusion, systolic and diastolic abnormalities can be observed. Angina is a relatively late event, occurring after at least 30 seconds of ischemia. Finally, differing pain thresholds among patients may explain the high prevalence of silent ischemia. The presence of angina is moderately correlated with a decreased pain tolerance. The mechanism for different pain thresholds is unknown but may result from differences in plasma endorphins.

B. Fourth Heart Sound and Shortness of Breath

Both these findings may occur because of diastolic and systolic dysfunction of the ischemic myocardium. (See Heart Failure.)

C. Shock

The site of coronary artery occlusion determines the clinical presentation of myocardial ischemia or infarction. As a general rule, the more myocardium that is supplied by the occluded vessel, the more significant and severe are the symptoms. For example, obstruction of the left main coronary artery or the proximal left anterior descending coronary artery will usually present as severe cardiac failure, often with associated hypotension (shock). In addition, shock may be associated with coronary artery disease in several special situations. If septum necrosis occurs from left anterior descending artery occlusion, myocardial rupture with the formation of an interventricular septal defect can occur. Rupture of the anterior or lateral free walls from occlusion of the left anterior descending or circumflex coronary arteries, respectively, can lead to the formation of pericardial effusion and tamponade. Rupture of myocardial tissue usually occurs 4–7 days after the acute ischemic event, when the myocardial wall has thinned and is in the process of healing. Sudden hemodynamic decompensation during this period should arouse suspicion of these complications. Finally, circumflex artery occlusion may result in ischemia and dysfunction or overt rupture of the papillary muscles, which can produce severe mitral regurgitation and shock.

D. Bradycardia

Inferior wall myocardial infarctions usually arise from occlusion of the right coronary artery. Because the area of left ventricular tissue supplied by this artery is small, patients usually do not present with heart failure. However, the artery that provides blood supply to the AV node branches off the posterior descending artery, so that inferior wall myocardial infarctions are sometimes associated with slowed or absent conduction in the AV node. Besides ischemia, AV nodal conduction abnormalities can occur because of reflex activation of the vagus nerve, which richly innervates the AV node.

Dysfunction of the sinus node is rarely seen in coronary artery disease, because this area receives blood from both the right and the left coronary arteries.

E. Nausea and Vomiting

Nausea and vomiting may arise from activation of the vagus nerve in the setting of an inferior wall myocardial infarction.

F. Tachycardia

Levels of catecholamines are usually raised in patients with myocardial infarction. This helps maintain stroke volume but leads to an increased heart rate.

CHECKPOINT

14. What is the clinical presentation of coronary artery disease along the continuum from stable angina to unstable angina to myocardial infarction?

15. What are the most common causes of coronary artery disease?

16. How do the pathophysiologies of stable angina, unstable angina, and myocardial infarction differ?

17. What are the major clinical manifestations and complications of coronary artery disease?

PERICARDIAL DISEASE

Pericardial disease may include inflammation of the pericardium (pericarditis) or abnormal amounts of fluid in the space between the visceral and parietal pericardia (pericardial effusion).

Pericarditis

Clinical Presentation

The patient presents with severe chest pain. Descriptions of the pain are variable, but the usual picture is of a sharp retrosternal onset with radiation to the back and worse with deep breathing or coughing. The pain is often position dependent: worse when lying flat and improved while sitting up and leaning forward.

On physical examination, the pericardial rub is pathognomonic of pericarditis. It is a high-pitched squeaking sound, often with two or more components.

Occasionally, continual inflammation of the pericardium leads to fibrosis and the development of constrictive pericarditis (Figure 10–28). Examination of the jugular venous pulsation is critical in the patient who may have constrictive pericarditis. The jugular venous pressure is elevated, and the individual waveforms are often quite prominent. In addition, there can be an inappropriate increase in the jugular venous pulsation level with inspiration (Kussmaul sign). Hepatomegaly and ascites may be noted on physical examination. On auscultation of the heart, a high-pitched sound called a pericardial knock can be heard just after the second heart sound, often mimicking a third heart sound.

Etiology

Table 10–9 lists the causes of acute pericarditis. Viruses, particularly the coxsackieviruses, are the most common cause of acute pericarditis. Viruses are also probably responsible for "idiopathic" pericarditis.

FIGURE 10–28 Magnetic resonance image of a cross-section of thorax showing pericardial thickening (**arrows**) in a patient with constrictive pericarditis. (Used, with permission, from Charles Higgins, MD in Cheitlin MD et al, eds. *Clinical Cardiology*, 6th ed. Appleton & Lange, 1993.)

TABLE 10–9   Causes of pericarditis.

Infections
Viral: coxsackievirus
Bacterial
Tuberculosis
Purulent: staphylococcal, pneumococcal
Protozoal: amebiasis
Mycotic: actinomycosis, coccidioidomycosis
Collagen–vascular disease
Systemic lupus erythematosus
Scleroderma
Rheumatoid arthritis
Neoplasm
Metabolic
Renal failure
Injury
Myocardial infarction
Postinfarction
Postthoracotomy
Trauma
Radiation
Idiopathic

Pathophysiology

In pericarditis, microscopic examination of pericardial specimens obtained at surgery (eg, stripping or window) or autopsy shows signs of acute inflammation, with increased numbers of polymorphonuclear leukocytes, increased vascularity, and fibrin deposition. If the inflammation is of long duration, the pericardium can become fibrotic and scarred, with calcium deposition.

The heavily fibrotic pericardium can inhibit the filling of the ventricles. At this point, signs of constrictive pericarditis appear (see following discussion).

Clinical Manifestations

A. Chest Pain—Chest pain is probably a result of pericardium inflammation. Inflammation of adjacent pleura may account for the characteristic worsening of pain with deep breathing and coughing.

B. Physical Examination

1. **Friction rub**—The pericardial friction rub is thought to arise from friction between the visceral and parietal pericardial surfaces. The rub is traditionally described as having three components, each associated with rapid movement of a cardiac chamber: The systolic component, which is probably related to ventricular contraction, is the most common and most easily heard. During

FIGURE 10–29 Phonocardiogram of the typical sharp, early diastolic pericardial knock (K). (Reproduced, with permission, from Cheitlin MD et al, eds. *Clinical Cardiology*, 6th ed. Originally published by Appleton & Lange. Copyright © 1993 by The McGraw-Hill Companies, Inc.)

diastole, there are two components: one during early diastole, resulting from rapid filling of the ventricle, and another quieter component that occurs in late diastole, thought to be due to atrial contraction. The diastolic components often merge so that a two-component or "to-and-fro" rub is most commonly heard.

2. **Signs of constriction**—In the patient with constrictive pericarditis, early diastolic filling of the ventricle occurs normally, but the filling is suddenly stopped by the nonelastic thickened pericardium. This cessation of filling can be observed on the pressure–time curve of the ventricle and is probably responsible for the diastolic knock (Figure 10–29). In addition, the rapid emptying of the atrium leads to a prominent *y* descent that makes the *v* wave more noticeable on the atrial pressure tracing (Figure 10–30). Systemic venous pressure is elevated, because flow entering the heart is limited. Usually with inspiration, the decrease in intrathoracic pressure is transmitted to the heart, and filling of the right side of the heart increases with an accompanying fall in systemic venous pressure. In patients with constrictive pericarditis, this normal response is prevented and the patient develops Kussmaul sign (Figure 10–31). Elevated

systemic venous pressure can cause fluid accumulation in the liver and intraperitoneal space, leading to hepatomegaly and ascites.

PERICARDIAL EFFUSION & TAMPONADE

Clinical Presentation

Pericardial effusion may occur in response to any cause of pericarditis, so the patient may develop chest pain or pericardial rub, as described previously. In addition, pericardial effusion may develop slowly and may be asymptomatic. However, sudden filling of the pericardial space with fluid can have catastrophic consequences by limiting ventricular filling (pericardial tamponade). Patients with pericardial tamponade often complain of shortness of breath, but the diagnosis is most commonly made by noting the characteristic physical examination findings associated with pericardial tamponade.

These characteristic physical signs arise from the limited filling of the ventricle. The three classic signs of pericardial tamponade are called the Beck triad after the surgeon who described them in 1935: (1) hypotension, (2) elevated jugular venous pressure, and (3) muffled heart sounds. In addition, the patient may have a decrease in systemic pressure with inspiration (paradoxical pulse).

Etiology

Almost any cause of pericarditis can cause pericardial effusion.

Pathophysiology

The pericardium is normally filled with a small amount of fluid (30–50 mL) with an intrapericardial pressure that is usually about the same as the intrapleural pressure. With the sudden addition

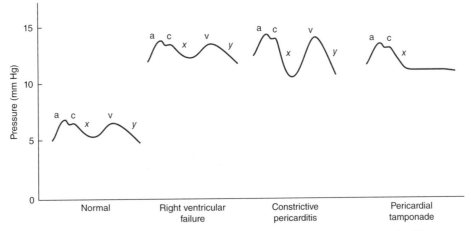

FIGURE 10–30 Jugular venous pressure waveforms in various kinds of heart disease. In right ventricular failure, mean jugular venous pressure is elevated, but the waveforms remain relatively unchanged. If right ventricular failure is accompanied by tricuspid regurgitation, the *v* wave may become more prominent (because the right atrium is receiving blood from both systemic venous return and the right ventricle). In constrictive pericarditis, the *y* descent becomes prominent because the right ventricle rapidly fills in early diastole. In contrast, in pericardial tamponade, the right ventricle fills only during early systole, so that only an *x* descent is observed. In both constrictive pericarditis and pericardial tamponade, mean jugular venous pressure is elevated.

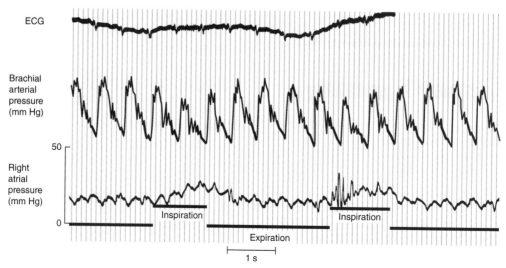

FIGURE 10–31 Brachial arterial and right atrial pressures showing pulsus paradoxus in a patient with constrictive pericarditis and an increase in right atrial pressure on inspiration (Kussmaul sign). Both the systolic and diastolic atrial pressures rise with inspiration. (Redrawn, with permission, from Cheitlin MD et al, eds. *Clinical Cardiology*, 6th ed. Originally published by Appleton & Lange. Copyright © 1993 by The McGraw-Hill Companies, Inc.)

of fluid, the pericardial pressure can increase, at times to the level of the right atrial and right ventricular pressures. The transmural distending pressure of the ventricle decreases and the chamber collapses, preventing appropriate filling of the heart from systemic venous return. The four chambers of the heart occupy a relatively fixed volume in the pericardial sac, and hemodynamic evaluation reveals equilibration of ventricular and pulmonary artery diastolic pressures with right atrial and left atrial pressures, all at approximately intrapericardial pressure.

Clinical Manifestations

Because the clinical manifestations of pericardial effusion without tamponade are similar to those of pericarditis, they are not described here. Instead, the pathophysiologic mechanisms for the symptoms and signs of pericardial tamponade are described.

A. Shortness of Breath

Dyspnea is the most common symptom of pericardial tamponade. The pathogenesis probably relates to a reduction in cardiac output and, in some patients, the presence of pulmonary edema.

B. Elevated Jugular Venous Pressure

Jugular venous pressure is elevated (see Figure 10–30). In addition, cardiac tamponade alters the dynamics of atrial filling. Normally, atrial filling occurs first during ventricular ejection (*y* descent) and then later when the tricuspid valve opens (*x* descent). In cardiac tamponade, the atrium can fill during ventricular contraction so that the *x* descent can still be seen. However, when the tricuspid valve opens, further filling of the right atrium is prevented because chamber size is limited by the surrounding pericardial fluid. For this reason, the *y* descent is not seen in the patient with pericardial tamponade. Loss of

the *y* descent in the setting of elevated jugular venous pressure should always arouse suspicion of pericardial tamponade.

C. Hypotension

Hypotension occurs because of reduced cardiac output.

D. Paradoxical Pulse

Arterial systolic blood pressure normally drops 10–12 mm Hg with inspiration. Marked inspiratory drop in systolic blood pressure (>20 mm Hg) is an important physical finding in the diagnosis of cardiac tamponade but can also be seen in severe pulmonary disease and, less commonly, in constrictive pericarditis (see Figure 10–31). Marked inspiratory decline in left ventricular stroke volume occurs because of decreased left ventricular end-diastolic volume. With inspiration, increased blood return augments filling of the right ventricle, which causes the interventricular septum to bow to the left and reduce left ventricular end-diastolic volume (reverse Bernheim effect). Also during inspiration, flow into the left atrium from the pulmonary veins is reduced, further reducing left ventricular preload.

E. Muffled Heart Sounds

Pericardial fluid can cause the heart sounds to become muffled or indistinct.

CHECKPOINT

18. What are the clinical presentations of each form of pericardial disease discussed?

19. What are the most common causes of pericarditis and pericardial effusion?

20. What are the major clinical manifestations and complications of pericarditis and pericardial effusion with tamponade?

CASE STUDIES

Yeong Kwok, MD

(See Chapter 25, p. 765–68 for answers)

CASE 54

A 25-year-old man presents to the hospital with light-headedness and palpitations for the past 2 hours. He had four or five previous episodes of palpitations in the past, but they had lasted only a few minutes and went away on their own. These episodes were not associated with any specific activity or diet. He denies any chest pain. On physical examination, he is noted to be tachycardic with a heart rate of 180 bpm and a blood pressure of 105/70 mm Hg. An ECG shows a narrow complex tachycardia at 180 bpm. The tachycardia terminates suddenly, and the patient's heart rate drops to 90 bpm. A repeat ECG shows sinus rhythm with a short PR interval and a wide QRS with a slurred upstroke (delta wave). The patient is diagnosed as having Wolff–Parkinson–White syndrome.

Questions

A. What is the significance of the delta wave on this patient's ECG?
B. How are re-entrant tachycardias initiated in this condition?
C. What are two other mechanisms that give rise to tachycardias?

CASE 55

A 66-year-old woman presents to the clinic with shortness of breath, leg swelling, and fatigue. She has a long history of type 2 diabetes and hypertension but until recently had been able to go for daily walks with her friends. In the past month, the walks have become more difficult owing to shortness of breath and fatigue. She also sometimes awakens in the middle of the night owing to shortness of breath and has to prop herself up on three pillows. On physical examination, she is noted to be tachycardic with a heart rate of 110 bpm and a blood pressure of 105/70 mm Hg. Her lung exam is notable for fine crackles on inspiration at both bases. Her cardiac exam is notable for the presence of a third and fourth heart sound and jugular venous distension. She has 2+ pitting edema to the knees bilaterally. An ECG shows sinus rhythm at 110 bpm with Q waves in the anterior leads. An echocardiogram shows decreased wall motion of the anterior wall of the heart and an estimated ejection fraction of 25%. She is diagnosed with systolic heart failure, likely secondary to a silent myocardial infarction.

Questions

A. What are the four broad mechanisms that can lead to heart failure? Which of these are at work in this case?
B. What are the differences between systolic and diastolic dysfunction?
C. What are the causes of this patient's shortness of breath, awakening in the middle of the night, and need to prop herself up on three pillows?

CASE 56

A 59-year-old man is brought to the emergency department by ambulance after experiencing a syncopal episode. He states that he was running in the park when he suddenly lost consciousness. He denies any symptoms preceding the event, and he had no deficits or symptoms upon arousing. On review of systems, he does say that he has had substernal chest pressure associated with exercise for the past several weeks. Each episode was relieved with rest. He denies shortness of breath, dyspnea on exertion, orthopnea, and paroxysmal nocturnal dyspnea. His medical history is notable for multiple episodes of pharyngitis as a child. He is otherwise well. He has no significant family history. He was born in Mexico and moved to the United States at age 10 years. He does not smoke, drink alcohol, or use illicit drugs. On examination, his blood pressure is 110/90 mm Hg, heart rate 95 bpm, respiratory rate 15/min, and oxygen saturation 98%. Neck examination reveals both pulsus parvus and pulsus tardus. Cardiac examination reveals a laterally displaced and sustained apical impulse. He has a grade 3/6 midsystolic murmur, loudest at the base of the heart, radiating to the neck, and a grade 1/6 high-pitched, blowing, early diastolic murmur along the left sternal border. An S_4 is audible. Lungs are clear to auscultation. Abdominal examination is benign. He has no lower extremity edema. Aortic stenosis is suspected.

Questions

A. What are the most common causes of aortic stenosis? Which is most likely in this patient? Why?
B. How does aortic stenosis cause syncope?
C. What is the pathophysiologic mechanism by which aortic stenosis causes angina pectoris?
D. How does aortic stenosis result in the physical findings described?
E. Based on the way this patient presented, what is his life expectancy if left untreated?

CASE 57

A 64-year-old man presents to the clinic with a 3-month history of worsening shortness of breath. He finds that he becomes short of breath after walking one block or one flight of stairs. He awakens at night, gasping for breath, and has to prop himself up with pillows in order to sleep. On physical examination, his blood pressure is 190/60 mm Hg and his pulses are hyperdynamic. His apical impulse is displaced to the left and downward. On physical examination, there are rales over both lower lung fields. On cardiac examination, there are three distinct murmurs: a high-pitched, early diastolic murmur loudest at the left lower sternal border, a diastolic rumble heard at the apex, and a crescendo–decrescendo systolic murmur heard at the left upper sternal border. Chest x-ray film shows cardiomegaly and pulmonary edema, and an echocardiogram shows severe aortic regurgitation with a dilated and hypertrophied left ventricle.

Questions

A. What accounts for the dilation and hypertrophy of the left ventricle in aortic regurgitation?
B. What is the pathophysiology of the wide pulse pressure (difference between the systolic and diastolic blood pressure) and the hyperdynamic pulses?
C. What explains the murmurs heard in this patient?
D. What are the underlying mechanisms responsible for the patient's shortness of breath with exertion and at night?

CASE 58

A 45-year-old man presents with a history of shortness of breath, irregular heartbeat, and hemoptysis. He notes that over the past 2 weeks, he has become easily "winded" with minor activities. Also, he has coughed up some flecks of blood on a few occasions. He has noted a fast heartbeat and, on occasion, a pounding sensation in his chest. He gives a history of being ill for several weeks after a severe sore throat in childhood. On physical examination, his pulse rate is noted to be 120–130 bpm and his rhythm is irregularly irregular. He has distended jugular venous pulses and rales at the bases of both lung fields. On cardiac examination, there is an irregular heartbeat as well as a soft diastolic decrescendo murmur, loudest at the apex. An ECG shows atrial fibrillation as well as evidence of left atrial enlargement.

Questions

A. What is the likely diagnosis in this patient, and what are the elements in the history, physical examination, and ECG that support the diagnosis?

B. What is the main pathophysiologic mechanism in this condition, and how does it explain the irregular heartbeat, shortness of breath, and hemoptysis?

C. What neurologic complication might this patient develop?

CASE 59

A 59-year-old man presents to the emergency department with a 4-hour history of "crushing" chest pain. His cardiac examination is normal with no murmurs and normal heart sounds. An ECG reveals ST segment elevation in the lateral precordial leads, and cardiac enzymes show evidence of myocardial injury. He undergoes emergent cardiac catheterization that shows a thrombus in the left circumflex artery. He undergoes successful angioplasty, and a stent is placed. He is monitored in the cardiac intensive care unit. He does well until the next day, when he develops sudden shortness of breath and decreasing oxygen saturations. Physical examination now reveals jugular venous distention, rales at both lung bases, and a blowing holosystolic murmur loudest at the apex, radiating into the axilla.

Questions

A. What likely accounts for this patient's sudden decompensation?

B. What is the main pathophysiologic derangement in this condition?

C. What changes in the heart take place if this condition develops slowly rather than suddenly?

CASE 60

A 55-year-old man presents to the clinic with complaints of chest pain. He states that for the past 5 months he has noted intermittent substernal chest pressure radiating to the left arm. The pain occurs primarily when exercising vigorously and is relieved with rest. He denies associated shortness of breath, nausea, vomiting, or diaphoresis. He has a medical history significant for hypertension and hyperlipidemia. He is taking atenolol for his high blood pressure and is eating a low-cholesterol diet. His family history is notable for a father who died of myocardial infarction at age 56 years. He has a 50-pack-year smoking history and is currently trying to quit. His physical examination is within normal limits with the exception of his blood pressure, which is 145/95 mm Hg, with a heart rate of 75 bpm.

Questions

A. What is the likely diagnosis? How would you classify his diagnosis clinically?

B. What are the most common causes of this disease? Which is the most likely in this patient?

C. What are this patient's risk factors for coronary artery disease?

D. What is the hypothesized mechanism by which atherosclerotic plaques form?

E. What is the pathogenetic mechanism by which plaque formation results in the symptoms mentioned?

CASE 61

A 35-year-old man presents to the emergency department with complaints of chest pain. The pain is described as 8 on a scale ranging from 1 to 10, retrosternal, and sharp in nature. It radiates to the back, is worse with taking a deep breath, and is improved by leaning forward. On review of systems, he has noted a "flu-like illness" over the past several days, including fever, rhinorrhea, and cough. He has no medical history and is taking no medications. He denies tobacco, alcohol, or drug use. On physical examination, he appears in moderate distress from pain, with a blood pressure of 125/85 mm Hg, heart rate 105 bpm, respiratory rate 18/min, and oxygen saturation of 98% on room air. He is currently afebrile. His head-and-neck examination is notable for clear mucus in the nasal passages and a mildly erythematous oropharynx. The neck is supple, with shotty anterior cervical lymphadenopathy. The chest is clear to auscultation. Jugular veins are not distended. Cardiac examination is tachycardic with a three-component high-pitched squeaking sound. Abdominal and extremity examinations are normal.

Questions

A. What is the likely diagnosis?
B. What are the most common causes of this disease, and which is most likely in this patient?
C. What is the pathophysiologic mechanism for his chest pain?
D. What is the sound heard on cardiac examination? What is its cause?
E. What are two possible complications of this disease? What might you look for on physical examination to make certain these complications are not present?

CASE 62

A 65-year-old woman is hospitalized with a large anterior myocardial infarction. After 4 days in the hospital, she is doing well and plans are being made for discharge to a rehabilitation facility to help her regain her strength and recover her cardiac function. While going to the bathroom, she passes out suddenly. On examination, her blood pressure is ~60/40 mm Hg, her heart rate is 120, and she has distant heart sounds. An emergent echocardiogram shows rupture of the anterior wall and pericardial tamponade.

Questions

A. What are the three classic signs of pericardial tamponade (Beck triad)?
B. What is the pathophysiology of pericardial tamponade?
C. What is the mechanism of paradoxica pulse?

REFERENCES

General

Fuster V et al. *Hurst's The Heart*, 14th ed. McGraw-Hill, 2017.
Kusumoto FM. *Cardiovascular Pathophysiology*. Hayes Barton, 2004.
Mohrman DE et al. *Cardiovascular Physiology*, 8th ed. McGraw-Hill, 2014.

Arrhythmias

Benson DW et al. Wolff-Parkinson-White syndrome: lessons learnt and lessons remaining. Cardiol Young. 2017 Jan;27(S1):S62–S67. [PMID: 28084962]

Guasch E et al. Diagnosis, pathophysiology, and management of exercise-induced arrhythmias. Nat Rev Cardiol. 2017 Feb;14(2):88–101. [PMID: 27830772]

Jacobson JT et al. Management of ventricular arrhythmias in structural heart disease. Postgrad Med. 2015 Jun;127(5):549–59. [PMID: 25971427]

Pedersen CT et al. EHRA/HRS/APHRS expert consensus on ventricular arrhythmias. Heart Rhythm. 2014 Oct;11(10):e166–96. [PMID: 25179489]

Prystowsky EN et al. Treatment of atrial fibrillation. JAMA. 2015 Jul 21;314(3):278–88. [PMID: 26197188]

Wung SF. Bradyarrhythmias: clinical presentation, diagnosis, and management. Crit Care Nurs Clin North Am. 2016 Sep;28(3):297–308. [PMID: 27484658]

Heart Failure

Arany Z et al. Peripartum cardiomyopathy. Circulation. 2016 Apr 5;133(14):1397–409. [PMID: 27045128]

Argulian E et al. Misconceptions and facts about 'diastolic' heart failure. Am J Med. 2014 Dec;127(12):1144–7. [PMID: 24937156]

Brown DA et al. Expert consensus document: mitochondrial function as a therapeutic target in heart failure. Nat Rev Cardiol. 2017 Apr;14(4):238–50. [PMID: 28004807]

Callan PD et al. Heart failure – what's new and what's changed? Clin Med (Lond). 2016 Dec;16(Suppl 6):S37–S42. [PMID: 27956439]

Dharmarajan K et al. Epidemiology, pathophysiology, and prognosis of heart failure in older adults. Heart Fail Clin. 2017 Jul;13(3):417–26. [PMID: 28602363]

Oren O et al. Heart failure with preserved ejection fraction: diagnosis and management. Am J Med. 2017 May;130(5):510–6. [PMID: 28163048]

Pfeffer MA. Heart failure and hypertension: importance of prevention. Med Clin North Am. 2017 Jan;101(1):19–28. [PMID: 27884228]

Reddy S et al. Molecular mechanisms of right ventricular failure. Circulation. 2015 Nov 3;132(18):1734–42. [PMID: 26527692]

Viau DM et al. The pathophysiology of hypertensive acute heart failure. Heart. 2015 Dec;101(23):1861–7. [PMID: 26123135]

Valvular Heart Disease

Abramowitz Y et al. Mitral annulus calcification. J Am Coll Cardiol. 2015 Oct 27;66(17):1934–41. [PMID: 26493666]

Argulian E et al. Misconceptions and facts about mitral regurgitation. Am J Med. 2016 Sep;129(9):919–23. [PMID: 27059381]

Asgar AW et al. Secondary mitral regurgitation in heart failure: pathophysiology, prognosis, and therapeutic considerations. J Am Coll Cardiol. 2015 Mar 31;65(12):1231–48. Erratum in: J Am Coll Cardiol. 2015 May 26;65(20):2265. [PMID: 25814231]

Carabello B. How to follow patients with mitral and aortic valve disease. Med Clin North Am. 2015 Jul;99(4):739–57. [PMID: 26042880]

Coffey S et al. The prevalence, incidence, progression, and risks of aortic valve sclerosis: a systematic review and meta-analysis. J Am Coll Cardiol. 2014 Jul 1;63(25 Pt A):2852–61. [PMID: 24814496]

Joseph J et al. Aortic stenosis: pathophysiology, diagnosis, and therapy. Am J Med. 2017 Mar;130(3):253–63. [PMID: 27810479]

Nappi F et al. Ischemic mitral valve prolapse. J Thorac Dis. 2016 Dec;8(12):3752–61. [PMID: 28149574]

Rader F et al. Left ventricular hypertrophy in valvular aortic stenosis: mechanisms and clinical implications. Am J Med. 2015 Apr;128(4):344–52. [PMID: 25460869]

Small A et al. Biomarkers of calcific aortic valve disease. Arterioscler Thromb Vasc Biol. 2017 Apr;37(4):623–32. [PMID: 28153876]

Sritharen Y et al. Pathophysiology of aortic valve stenosis: is it both fibrocalcific and sex specific? Physiology (Bethesda). 2017 May;32(3):182–96. [PMID: 28404735]

Coronary Artery Disease

Boudoulas KD et al. Coronary atherosclerosis: pathophysiologic basis for diagnosis and management. Prog Cardiovasc Dis. 2016 May-Jun;58(6):676–92. [PMID: 27091673]

Brown RA et al. Current understanding of atherogenesis. Am J Med. 2017 Mar;130(3):268–82. [PMID: 27888053].

Dalen JE et al. The epidemic of the 20(th) century: coronary heart disease. Am J Med. 2014 Sep;127(9):807–12. [PMID: 24811552]

Fanaroff AC et al. Does this patient with chest pain have acute coronary syndrome? The rational clinical examination systematic review. JAMA. 2015 Nov 10;314(18):1955–65. [PMID: 26547467].

Khera AV et al. Genetics of coronary artery disease: discovery, biology and clinical translation. Nat Rev Genet. 2017 Jun;18(6):331–44. [PMID: 28286336]

Tweet MS et al. What clinicians should know about spontaneous coronary artery dissection. Mayo Clin Proc. 2015 Aug;90(8):1125–30. [PMID: 26250728]

Pericardial Disease

Dad T et al. Pericarditis and pericardial effusions in end-stage renal disease. Semin Dial. 2016 Sep;29(5):366–73. [PMID: 27228946]

Fardman A et al. European guidelines on pericardial diseases: a focused review of novel aspects. Curr Cardiol Rep. 2016 May;18(5):46. [PMID: 27007597]

González-Moreno J et al. Serosal involvement in IgG4-related disease: report of two cases and review of the literature. Rheumatol Int. 2016 Jul;36(7):1033–41. [PMID: 27207156]

Hoit BD. Pathophysiology of the pericardium. Prog Cardiovasc Dis. 2017 Jan-Feb;59(4):341–8. [PMID: 27916673]

Imazio M et al. Evaluation and treatment of pericarditis: a systematic review. JAMA. 2015 Oct 13;314(14):1498–506. Erratum in: JAMA. 2015 Nov 10;314(18):1978. JAMA. 2016 Jan 5;315(1):90. [PMID: 26461998]

Lestuzzi C et al. 2015 update on the diagnosis and management of neoplastic pericardial disease. Expert Rev Cardiovasc Ther. 2015 Apr;13(4):377–89. [PMID: 25797903]

Miranda WR et al. Constrictive pericarditis: a practical clinical approach. Prog Cardiovasc Dis. 2017 Jan-Feb;59(4):369–79. [PMID: 28062267]

Vakamudi S et al. Pericardial effusions: causes, diagnosis, and management. Prog Cardiovasc Dis. 2017 Jan-Feb;59(4):380–8. [PMID: 28062268]

Yusuf SW et al. Pericardial disease: a clinical review. Expert Rev Cardiovasc Ther. 2016;14(4):525–39. [PMID: 26691443]

Cardiovascular Disorders: Vascular Disease

Igor Mitrovic, MD

This chapter reviews the normal structure and function of the vascular component of the cardiovascular system and then considers the pathophysiology of three common conditions frequently seen by practicing physicians: atherosclerosis, hypertension, and shock.

NORMAL VASCULAR STRUCTURE & FUNCTION

ANATOMY & HISTOLOGY

The blood vessels are a closed system of conduits that carry blood from the heart to the tissues and back to the heart. All of the blood flows through the lungs, but the systemic circulation is made up of many different circuits in parallel (Figure 11–1). This permits wide variation in regional systemic blood flow without changing the total systemic flow.

Figure 11–2 summarizes the characteristics of the various types of blood vessels in humans. Note that as the diameter of the vessels decreases, their number in the body increases so that the total cross-sectional area increases.

All blood vessels are lined by a single layer of endothelial cells. Collectively, the endothelial cells constitute a remarkable organ that secretes substances that affect the diameter of the vessels and provide for their growth, their repair when injured, and the formation of new vessels that carry blood to growing tissues.

Arterial Vessels

The aorta, the large arteries, and the arterioles are made up of an outer layer of connective tissue, the **adventitia**; a middle layer of smooth muscle, the **media**; and an inner layer, the **intima**, containing the layer of endothelial cells and some subendothelial connective tissue. The walls of the aorta and the large arteries contain abundant elastic tissue, much of it concentrated in the **internal elastic lamina**, a prominent band between the intima and the media, and another band, the **external elastic lamina**, between the media and the adventitia

(Figure 11–3). The vessels are stretched by the force of cardiac ejection during systole, and the elastic tissue permits them to recoil during diastole. This maintains diastolic pressure and aids the forward motion of the blood. The walls of the arterioles contain less elastic tissue than the arteries but proportionately more smooth muscle (see Figure 11–2). The muscle is extensively innervated by noradrenergic nerve fibers, which are constrictor in function. In some instances, there is a cholinergic innervation, which is vasodilator in function. The arteries and the arterioles offer considerable resistance to the flow of blood and are known as the **resistance vessels**.

Capillaries

The terminal portions of the arterioles, sometimes called metarterioles, drain into the **capillaries**. On the upstream side, the openings of the capillaries are surrounded by smooth muscle **precapillary sphincters**. There is debate about whether the metarterioles and sphincters are innervated. The capillaries themselves are made up of a single layer of endothelial cells. Outside these cells are occasional pericytes that serve numerous functions, including the mechanical support, signaling (eg, regulation of endothelial cell proliferation and migration), and regulation of protein diffusion, as well as cell extravasation across the capillary walls). Pericytes have also been shown to possess a variety of stem cell properties (Figure 11–4). The capillaries anastomose extensively, and although each capillary is only 5–9 μm in diameter, there are so many of them that the total cross-sectional area of all the capillaries is about 4500 cm^2.

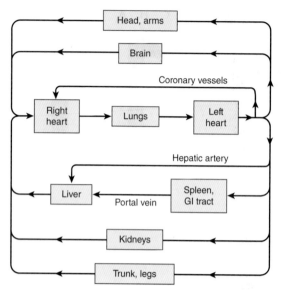

FIGURE 11-1 Diagram of circulation in the adult. (GI, gastrointestinal.) (Redrawn, with permission, from Barrett KE et al, eds. *Ganong's Review of Medical Physiology*, 25th ed. McGraw-Hill, 2016.)

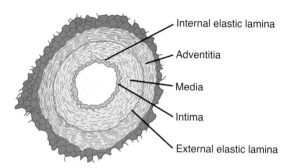

FIGURE 11-3 Cross-section of a small artery. (Redrawn, with permission, from Ganong WF. *Review of Medical Physiology*, 22nd ed. McGraw-Hill, 2005.)

(Chapter 14). In endocrine tissues, the small intestine, and the kidneys, tissues in which there is bulk flow of material across capillary walls, the cytoplasm of the endothelial cells is attenuated to form gaps called fenestrations. These gaps appear to be closed by a discontinuous membrane, which permits the passage of substances up to approximately 600 nm in diameter. In skeletal muscle, cardiac muscle, and many other tissues, there are no fenestrations, but the junctions between endothelial cells permit the passage of substances up to 10 nm in diameter. Finally, in brain capillaries, there are tight junctions between the endothelial cells. These tight junctions permit very little passive transport and are a key component of the blood–brain barrier. Water and carbon dioxide enter the brain with ease, but movement of most other substances in and out of brain tissue is mainly via transport proteins in the endothelial cells.

Some substances cross capillary walls by vesicular transport, a process that involves plasma endocytosis, movement of the vesicles formed in this way across the endothelial cell cytoplasm, and exocytosis on the tissue side. However, relatively little material is moved in this fashion, and most fluid and solute exchange occurs at the junctions between endothelial cells. In the liver, there are large gaps between endothelial cells

* In systemic vessels. There is an additional 12% in the heart and 18% in the pulmonary circulation.

FIGURE 11-2 Characteristics of systemic blood vessels. Cross-sections of the vessels are not drawn to scale because of the huge range in size from aorta and vena cava to capillaries. (Redrawn from Burton AC. Relation of structure to function of the tissues of the wall of blood vessels. Physiol Rev. 1954;34:619.)

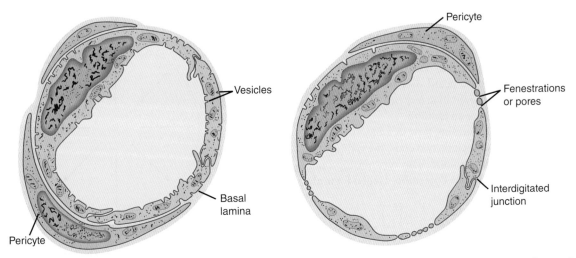

FIGURE 11–4 Cross-sections of capillaries. **Left:** Continuous type of capillary found in skeletal muscle. **Right:** Fenestrated type of capillary. (Adapted from Fawcett DW. Comparative observations on the fine structure of blood capillaries. In: Orbison JL et al, eds. *The Peripheral Blood Vessels*. Williams & Wilkins, 1962.)

Venules & Veins

The venules are very similar to capillaries; they are about 20 μm in diameter, and their approximate total cross-sectional area is 4000 cm². They drain into veins that have modest amounts of smooth muscle and elastic tissue in their relatively thin walls and average 5 mm in diameter. The veins drain into the superior and inferior vena cavae, which in turn drain into the right atrium of the heart. The walls of the veins, unlike those of the arteries and arterioles, are easily distended and can expand to hold more blood without much increase in intravascular pressure. Therefore, they are known as **capacitance vessels**. They are innervated, and their smooth muscle can contract in response to noradrenergic stimulation, pushing blood into the heart and the arterial side of the circulation. The intima of the limb veins is folded at intervals to form the venous valves that prevent retrograde flow.

Lymphatics

The smallest lymphatic vessels are made up of endothelial tubes. Fluid appears to enter them through loose junctions between the endothelial cells. They drain into larger endothelial tubes that have valves and contractile walls containing smooth muscle, so that the fluid they contain moves centrally. The central lymphatics drain into the right and left subclavian veins. Thus, the lymphatic system drains excess fluid from the tissues back into the vascular system.

CHECKPOINT

1. How does the composition of the wall of an arteriole differ from that of an artery?
2. What are the modes of transport across the capillary wall? In which organ is transport greatest?
3. Why are veins termed capacitance vessels?

PHYSIOLOGY

Biophysical Considerations

In any system made up of a pump and a closed system of pipes such as the heart and the blood vessels, the flow of fluid between the two ends of the system depends on the pressure difference generated by the pump and the resistance to flow in the pipes:

$$Q = \frac{\Delta P}{R}$$

In the cardiovascular system, this translates into:

$$CO = \frac{MAP - Pra}{R}$$

where CO is cardiac output, MAP is mean arterial pressure, and Pra is the pressure in the right atrium. Since Pra is normally close to 0 mm Hg, this expression has the following corollary:

$$MAP = CO \times R$$

Thus, mean arterial pressure increases when there is an increase in cardiac output or when the diameter of the blood vessels (principally the arterioles, the main resistance vessels) is decreased.

Flow in blood vessels is laminar (ie, an infinitely thin layer of blood next to the vessel wall does not move, the next layer moves slowly, and the next layer moves more rapidly, with the fastest flow in the center). Usually the flow is smooth, and no sound is generated. However, if flow is accelerated, it becomes turbulent when a **critical velocity** is reached. Constriction of a blood vessel or a heart valve causes faster flow in the constricted region because the kinetic energy of flow is increased and the potential energy is decreased (the **Bernoulli principle**). Therefore, critical velocity is more often reached. The turbulence causes noise. The examining physician hears this noise through the stethoscope as a **bruit** or **murmur**. The two terms are often used interchangeably, although the term "murmur" is more commonly applied to noise heard over the heart and the term "bruit" to noise heard over blood vessels. The sounds of Korotkoff heard over an artery below a blood pressure cuff (discussed later) are an example.

The main factors that determine flow in a blood vessel are the pressure difference between its two ends, the radius of the vessel, and the viscosity of the blood. This relationship can be expressed mathematically by the **Poiseuille–Hagen formula**:

$$F = (P_A - P_B) \times \left(\frac{\pi}{8}\right) \times \left(\frac{1}{\eta}\right) \times \left(\frac{r^4}{L}\right)$$

where

F = flow

$P_A - P_B$ = pressure difference between the two ends of the tube

η = viscosity

r = radius of tube

L = length of tube

Because flow is equal to pressure difference divided by resistance (R),

$$R = \frac{8\eta L}{\pi r^4}$$

Note that flow varies directly and pressure inversely with the fourth power of the radius of the vessel. This is why small changes in the diameter of the arterioles, the principal resistance vessels, cause large changes in pressure. For example, when the radius of a vessel is doubled, resistance is decreased to 6% of its previous value. Conversely, a small decrease in arterial diameter produces a relatively marked increase in blood pressure. Viscosity also has an effect, but, except at very high or very low values, the effect is small. Viscosity is high in polycythemia and low in anemia.

Figure 11–5 illustrates the relationship between distending pressure and wall tension. This relationship is called the **law of Laplace**. It states that the wall tension (T) in a hollow viscus is equal to the product of the **transmural pressure** (P) and the radius (r) divided by the thickness of the wall (W):

$$T = \frac{Pr}{W}$$

In thin-walled structures, wall thickness is negligible, but in structures such as arteries it becomes a significant factor. The transmural pressure is the pressure inside the viscus minus the pressure outside the viscus, but in the body the latter is negligible. Therefore, in a distensible hollow viscus, transmural pressure at equilibrium is equal to wall tension divided by the two principal radii of curvature of the object (r_1 and r_2):

$$P = T\left(\frac{1}{r_1} + \frac{1}{r_2}\right)$$

FIGURE 11–5 Law of Laplace. In a hollow object (eg, viscus, blood vessel), the distending pressure (P) equals the wall tension (T). (Redrawn, with permission, from Barrett KE et al, eds. *Ganong's Review of Medical Physiology*, 24th ed. McGraw-Hill, 2012.)

The operation of this law in the lungs is discussed in Chapter 9. In a cylinder such as a blood vessel, one radius is infinite, so

$$P = \frac{T}{r}$$

Thus, the smaller the radius of a vessel, the lower the wall tension necessary to balance the distending pressure. For example, the wall tension in the aorta is about 170,000 dynes/cm, whereas in capillaries it is about 16 dynes/cm. This is why the thin-walled, delicate capillaries do not collapse. The law of Laplace also applies to the heart. When the heart is dilated, it must develop more wall tension to function. Consequently, its work increases.

With these principles and Figure 11–2 in mind, plus the fact that the major sites of vascular resistance are the arterioles, it is possible to understand the pressures in the various parts of the vascular system (Figure 11–6) and the velocity of flow in them. Systolic and diastolic pressures in the aorta and large arteries are stable, and there is a large pulse pressure. Normal pressure is about 120/80 mm Hg in healthy young adults. In the arterioles, there is a sharp drop, so that pressure at the entrances to the capillaries is about 37 mm Hg and pulse pressure has disappeared. At the ends of the capillaries, it is about 17 mm Hg and falls steadily in the venous system to about 5 mm Hg at the entrance of the vena cavae into the right atrium. Velocity falls in the arterioles, is low in the capillaries because of the large total cross-sectional area, and increases again in the large veins.

The pressures mentioned previously are, of course, those recorded with patients in the supine position.

Because of the weight of the blood, there is a pressure increase in the standing position in both arteries and veins of 0.77 mm Hg for each centimeter below the heart it is measured and a corresponding decrease of 0.77 mm Hg for

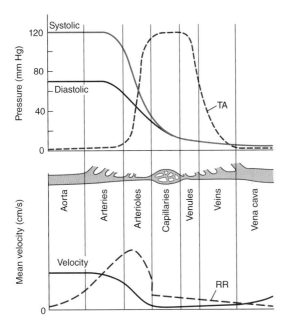

FIGURE 11–6 Diagram of the changes in pressure and velocity as blood flows through the systemic circulation. (RR, relative resistance, which is highest in the arterioles; TA, total cross-sectional area of the vessels, which increases from 4.5 cm² in the aorta to 4500 cm² in the capillaries [Figure 11–2].) (Redrawn, with permission, from Barrett KE et al, eds. *Ganong's Review of Medical Physiology*, 25th ed. McGraw-Hill, 2016.)

each centimeter above the heart. Thus, when the mean arterial pressure at the level of the heart is 100 mm Hg, the mean arterial pressure in a large artery in the foot of a standing averaged-sized adult is about 180 mm Hg; in the head, it is about 62 mm Hg.

Measurement of Arterial Pressure

Arterial pressure can be measured directly by inserting a needle into an artery. Alternatively, it can be measured by the auscultatory method. The familiar inflatable cuff attached to a manometer is placed around the upper arm at the level of the heart and a stethoscope is placed over the brachial artery below the cuff. The cuff is inflated to well above the suspected systolic pressure and then deflated slowly. At the systolic pressure, a faint tapping sound is heard as blood first begins to pass beyond the cuff. With further lowering of the pressure, the sound becomes louder and then dull and muffled before finally disappearing. These are the **sounds of Korotkoff**, which are produced by turbulent flow in the brachial artery. The change from staccato to muffled sound occurs when blood first passes under the cuff continuously, even though the artery is still partially constricted. Continuous flow has a different auditory quality than interrupted flow. Finally, at the diastolic pressure, the sound disappears. Although diastolic pressure measured directly with a catheter in the brachial artery correlates best with the disappearance of sound in normal adults, in children and after exercise it correlates better with the change to a muffled sound.

Normal Arterial Pressure

Normal blood pressure in the brachial artery at heart level in healthy young adults is about 120/80 mm Hg. It is affected by many factors, including emotion and anxiety, and in some individuals, blood pressure is higher when taken by a physician in the clinic than it is during normal activities at home ("**white-coat hypertension**"). Systolic and diastolic pressures normally fall by as much as 20 mm Hg during sleep. Therefore, normal subjects are called "dippers." In individuals with hypertension, the fall during sleep is reduced or absent (ie, hypertensives are "nondippers").

There is general agreement that blood pressure rises with advancing age, but there has been uncertainty about the magnitude of this rise because hypertension is a common disease whose incidence increases with advancing age. However, individuals who have systolic blood pressures <120 mm Hg at age 50–60 years and never develop clinical hypertension still have systolic pressures that rise throughout life (Figure 11–7). This rise may be the closest approximation to the rise in normal individuals. Individuals with mild hypertension that is untreated show a significantly more rapid rise in systolic pressure. In both groups, diastolic pressure also rises but then starts to fall in middle age as the stiffness of arteries increases. Consequently, pulse pressure rises with advancing age.

It is interesting that systolic and diastolic blood pressures are lower in young women than in young men until the age of 55–65 years, after which they become comparable. Because there is a positive correlation between blood pressure and the incidence of heart attacks and strokes (discussed later), the lower blood pressure before menopause in women may be one reason why, on average, women live longer than men.

Capillary Circulation

In the capillaries, the velocity of blood flow is decreased because, although single-vessel diameter is small, there is a large total cross-sectional area. It is in the capillary bed that nutrients leave and wastes enter the circulation. The forces producing movement of solute and solvent across capillary walls are called **Starling forces** after the physiologist who first described them and analyzed their function. They are the hydrostatic pressure difference across the capillary wall (capillary pressure minus tissue pressure) and the osmotic pressure gradient across the capillary wall (capillary oncotic pressure minus tissue oncotic pressure). The hydrostatic pressure gradient is outward because tissue pressure is low, and the oncotic pressure gradient is inward because large molecules in the blood do not cross the capillary wall. Obviously, most of the net movement of substances out of a typical capillary occurs at its arteriolar end, where the net pressure gradient is outward primarily because hydrostatic pressure in the capillary (about 37 mm Hg; Figure 11–8) is greater than the oncotic pressure. As the capillary resistance and the filtration progressively cause a decrease in the hydrostatic pressure along the length of the vessel, the inwardly directed oncotic pressure gradient

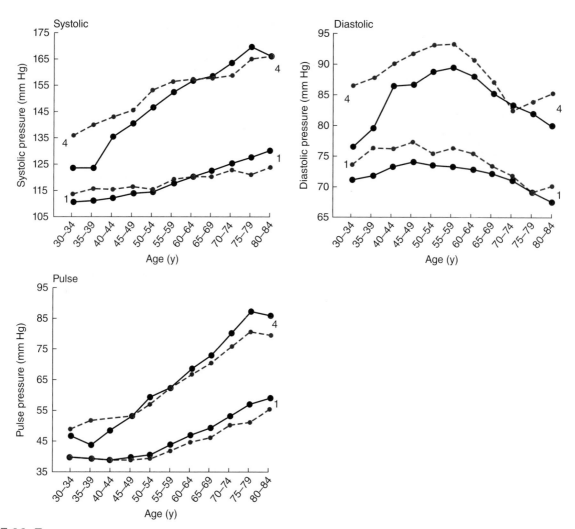

FIGURE 11–7 Effects of age and sex on systolic, diastolic, and pulse pressure in humans. Data are from a large group of individuals who were studied every 2 years throughout their adult lives. Group 1: individuals who had systolic blood pressures <120 mm Hg at age 50–60 years. Group 4: Individuals who had systolic blood pressure ≥160 mm Hg at age 50–60 years and had not received treatment for hypertension (ie, individuals with mild, untreated hypertension). Values for females are shown by the solid black lines, and those for males are shown by the dashed red lines. (Redrawn, with permission, from Franklin SS et al. Hemodynamic patterns of age-related changes in blood pressure: the Framingham Heart Study. Circulation. 1997;96:308.)

becomes greater than the hydrostatic pressure gradient so that, at the venular end, fluid is reabsorbed. Thus, net flow is out of the capillary at the arteriolar end and into the capillary at the venular end. Any excess solute and solvent in the tissues is picked up by the lymph vessels and moved to the venous circulation by the main lymphatic ducts. Flow in the small lymphatics is passive, but in the larger lymphatic ducts there are valves and the walls contract.

REGULATION OF THE CARDIOVASCULAR SYSTEM

Given the vital nature of the cardiovascular system in maintaining blood flow to vital organs and adjusting flow so that it is increased in active tissues and decreased in inactive tissues, it is not surprising that multiple cardiovascular regulatory mechanisms have evolved. Cardiovascular adjustments are effected by altering the output of the pump (the heart), changing the diameter of the resistance vessels (chiefly the arterioles), and altering the amount of blood pooled in the capacitance vessels (the veins).

The regulation of cardiac output is discussed in Chapter 10. The caliber of the arterioles is regulated by vasodilator metabolites produced in metabolically active tissues, by the process of autoregulation, by a variety of vasoregulatory substances produced by endothelial cells, by circulating vasoactive hormones, and by a system of vasomotor nerves to the blood vessels and the heart. Discharge in the vasomotor nerves is regulated in feedback fashion by carotid sinus and aortic arch baroreceptors that monitor pressure in the arteries (the high-pressure baroreceptor system) and baroreceptors in the cardiac atria and great veins (the low-pressure baroreceptor system).

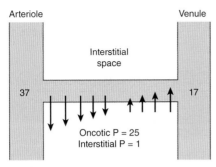

FIGURE 11–8 Schematic representation of pressure (P) gradients across the wall of a muscle capillary. The numbers at the arteriolar and venular ends of the capillary are the hydrostatic pressures in millimeters of mercury at these locations. The arrows indicate the approximate magnitude and direction of fluid movement. In this example, the pressure differential at the arteriolar end of the capillary is 11 mm Hg ([37 − 1] − 25) outward; at the opposite end, it is 9 mm Hg (25 − [17 − 1]) inward. (Redrawn, with permission, from Barrett KE et al, eds. *Ganong's Review of Medical Physiology*, 25th ed. McGraw-Hill, 2016.)

Vasodilator Metabolites

Various metabolic changes occurring in active tissues produce substances that dilate vessels supplying the tissues. This helps ensure the increased blood flow necessary to support the increased tissue activity. One important vasodilator is CO_2. Another is K^+, and adenosine dilates blood vessels in some tissues. In addition, the rise in temperature and the fall in pH that occur in some metabolically active tissues have a vasodilator effect.

Autoregulation

Many tissues have the ability to maintain a relatively constant blood flow during changes in perfusion pressure; this process is called **autoregulation**. The physiologic basis of autoregulation is unsettled. One factor is the myogenic response to stretch of the smooth muscle in arterioles; as pressure inside a vessel rises, its smooth muscle is stretched, and its response is to contract. Smooth muscle contracts in the absence of extrinsic innervation. Another factor may be the accumulation of vasodilator metabolites; when flow to a tissue is reduced, the metabolites are not washed away, and they accumulate even in the absence of increased activity.

Substances Secreted by the Endothelium

The blood vessels are lined by a continuous layer of endothelial cells, and these cells play a vital role in the regulation of vascular function. They respond to flow changes (shear stress), stretch, a variety of circulating substances, and inflammatory mediators. In response to these stimuli, they secrete growth regulators and vasoactive substances. The growth factors regulate vascular development and are important in a number of diseases. The vasoactive substances produced by the endothelium generally act in a paracrine fashion to regulate local vascular tone. They include prostaglandins, such as prostacyclin, and also thromboxanes, nitric oxide, and endothelins.

A. Prostaglandins & Thromboxanes

Prostacyclin is produced by endothelial cells and thromboxane A_2 by platelets from their common precursor, arachidonic acid. Thromboxane A_2 causes platelet aggregation and vasoconstriction, whereas prostacyclin promotes vasodilation. The balance between the two is one of the mechanisms favoring local vasoconstriction and clot formation at sites of vascular injury while keeping the clot from extending, thereby maintaining normal flow in neighboring uninjured areas. The balance between platelet thromboxane A_2 and endothelial prostacyclin can be shifted by the administration of low doses of aspirin. Thromboxane A_2 and prostacyclin are both produced from arachidonic acid by the cyclooxygenase pathway. Aspirin produces an irreversible inhibition of cyclooxygenase. However, endothelial cells make more cyclooxygenase within a few hours, whereas circulating platelets do not, and new platelet cyclooxygenase appears only as new platelets enter the circulation over a period of days. Therefore, the chronic administration of small doses of aspirin reduces intravascular clotting for prolonged periods and is of value in preventing myocardial infarctions, unstable angina, transient ischemic attacks, and stroke.

B. Nitric Oxide

The production of a potent vasodilator by endothelial cells was first suspected when it was noted that removal of the endothelium from rings of arterial tissue converted the normal dilator response to acetylcholine into a constrictor response. The responsible agent was first called **endothelium-derived relaxing factor**, but it is now known to be **nitric oxide (NO)**. NO is produced from arginine (Figure 11–9) in a reaction catalyzed by **nitric oxide synthase (NOS)**. Three forms of NOS have been cloned: NOS1, found in the nervous system; NOS2, found in macrophages and related immune cells; and NOS3, found in endothelial cells. NOS1 and NOS3 are activated by agents that increase intracellular Ca^{2+}, including the vasodilators acetylcholine and bradykinin, whereas NOS2 is activated by cytokines. The NO formed in endothelial cells diffuses to adjacent vascular smooth muscle cells, where it activates soluble guanylyl cyclase, producing cyclic guanosine monophosphate (cGMP; see Figure 11–9). The cGMP mediates the relaxation of vascular smooth muscle.

The vasodilators that act by way of NO in vivo include not only acetylcholine and bradykinin but vasoactive intestinal polypeptide (VIP), substance P, and some other polypeptides. In addition, various substances that produce vasoconstriction in vivo would have a much greater constrictor effect if they did not simultaneously release NO. Consequently, NO is a major local regulator of blood flow. Its widespread role in regulation of the vascular system is indicated by the fact that an infusion of amino acid analogs of arginine that inhibit NOS causes blood pressure to rise. Thus, it appears that NOS is acting in a chronic fashion to keep the vascular system dilated.

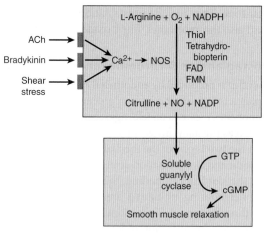

FIGURE 11–9 Synthesis of nitric oxide (NO) from arginine in endothelial cells and its action via stimulation of soluble guanylyl cyclase and generation of cyclic guanosine monophosphate (cGMP) to produce relaxation in vascular smooth muscle cells. The endothelial form of nitric oxide synthase (NOS) is activated by increased intracellular Ca^{2+}, and an increase in Ca^{2+} is produced by acetylcholine (ACh), bradykinin, or shear stress acting on the cell membrane. Thiol, tetrahydrobiopterin, flavin adenine dinucleotide (FAD), and flavin mononucleotide (FMN) are requisite cofactors. (GTP, guanosine triphosphate; NAD, nicotinamide adenine dinucleotide; NADP, nicotinamide adenine dinucleotide phosphate.) (Redrawn, with permission, from Barrett KE et al, eds. *Ganong's Review of Medical Physiology,* 24th ed. McGraw-Hill, 2012.)

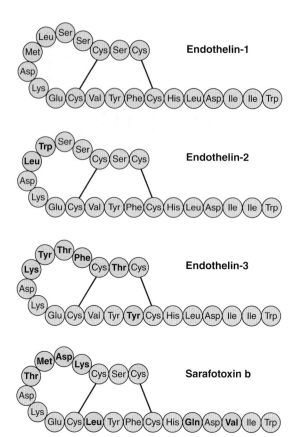

FIGURE 11–10 Structure of human endothelins and one of the snake venom sarafotoxins. The amino acid residues that differ from endothelin-1 are indicated in blue. (Redrawn, with permission, from Ganong WF. *Review of Medical Physiology,* 22nd ed. McGraw-Hill, 2005.)

NO is responsible in large part for reactive hyperemia, the vasodilation and increased blood flow that occur in tissues and organs after a transient obstruction of their blood supply is removed. It can be seen in the forearm after occlusion of the blood supply above the elbow, and it can be quantitated by measuring the increase in forearm volume by plethysmography. NO-dependent vasodilation can also be measured clinically by determining the dilator response to graded doses of acetylcholine injected intra-arterially.

Recent advances in the field of NO research have led to the identification of asymmetric-dimethylarginine (ADMA), an endogenous inhibitor of NOS enzymes. ADMA has been shown to be associated with endothelial dysfunction, cardiovascular mortality, and chronic kidney disease. The plasma ADMA level can serve as a component of a diagnostic tool for assessing cardiovascular health. Experimental evidence indicates that ADMA can be therapeutic target.

NO is present in many tissues in addition to the vascular system. Its function in some of these tissues is discussed in other chapters of this book.

C. Endothelins

Endothelial cells also produce endothelin-1 (ET-1), the most potent vasoconstrictor agent yet discovered. Three closely related endothelins have been identified in mammals: ET-1, endothelin-2 (ET-2), and endothelin-3 (ET-3). All are polypeptides related to the sarafotoxins, polypeptides found in snake venoms. They contain 21 amino acid residues and two disulfide bonds (Figure 11–10). All are cleaved from larger prohormones (big endothelins) by endothelin-converting enzymes. The most widely expressed endothelin, ET-1, is found in vascular endothelial cells, vascular smooth muscle cells, macrophages, fibroblasts, myocardiocytes, brain neurons, and pancreatic and intestinal epithelial cells, among others. Alternatively, ET-2 expression is restricted to intestinal epithelial cells and ovarian cells, whereas ET-3 expression is observed only in vascular endothelial cells and intestinal epithelial cells.

Over the past several years, our understanding of endothelin physiology and pathophysiology (particularly related to ET-1) has increased tremendously. Two G protein–coupled receptors—A and B—that mediate endothelin effects have been identified. Endothelin A receptor has the greatest affinity for ET-1, whereas endothelin B receptor has the same affinity for all three polypeptide isoforms. Interestingly, vascular smooth muscle cells express both endothelin receptors, and their activation leads to vasoconstriction. Endothelial cells, however, express only endothelin B receptor, which stimulates endothelial NOS, leading to NO-dependent smooth muscle relaxation. Recent animal data suggest that the activation of the endothelin B receptor in collecting ducts leads to a similar NO-dependent increase in sodium excretion. Moreover, there are indications that ET-1 may contribute to the extracellular matrix remodeling in vascular, cardiac, and kidney disease, and endothelin receptor antagonists are emerging as important agents in the treatment of pulmonary hypertension.

Circulating Hormones That Affect Vascular Smooth Muscle

Hormones in the circulation that have general effects on the vascular system include vasoconstrictors and vasodilators. The principal vasoconstrictors are norepinephrine and epinephrine (Chapter 12), vasopressin (Chapter 19), and angiotensin II (Chapter 21). The principal vasodilators are vasoactive intestinal peptide (VIP; Chapter 13), kinins, and natriuretic peptides.

A. Kinins

The kinins are two related vasodilator polypeptides called **bradykinin** and **lysyl-bradykinin** (Figure 11–11). The decapeptide lysyl-bradykinin can be converted to the nonapeptide bradykinin by aminopeptidase. Both are metabolized to inactive fragments by the carboxypeptidase kininase I or the dipeptidylcarboxypeptidase kininase II. Kininase II and angiotensin-converting enzyme are the same enzyme, so inhibition of angiotensin-converting enzyme for the treatment of hypertension or heart failure increases plasma and tissue kinins.

Kinins are formed from two **kininogens**: high-molecular-weight (HMW) kininogen and low-molecular-weight (LMW) kininogen. These kinin precursor proteins are products of a single gene produced by alternative splicing. The proteases responsible for the cleavage of kininogens are the **kallikreins**, a family of enzymes encoded in humans by three genes situated on chromosome 19.

Lysyl-bradykinin and bradykinin are primarily tissue hormones produced, for example, by the kidneys and actively secreting glands, but small amounts are also found in the circulating blood. They act on two receptors, B_1 and B_2, both coupled to G proteins. Kinins increase blood flow to actively secreting glands by producing vasodilation, and, when injected systemically, they are relatively potent vasodilators.

B. Natriuretic Hormones

Atrial natriuretic peptide (**ANP**), a polypeptide containing 28 amino acid residues, is secreted from the atria when atrial

FIGURE 11–11 Kinins. Lysyl-bradykinin (top) can be converted to bradykinin (bottom) by aminopeptidase. The peptides are inactivated by kininase I (KI) or kininase II (KII) at the sites indicated by the short arrows. (Redrawn, with permission, from Barrett KE et al, eds. *Ganong's Review of Medical Physiology*, 24th ed. McGraw-Hill, 2012.)

myocytes are stretched. **Brain natriuretic peptide** (**BNP**) was originally isolated from the brains of experimental animals, but in humans it is secreted by the ventricular myocytes and is also known as **β-type natriuretic peptide**. **CNP**, a third type of natriuretic peptide, is also found in humans. These peptides cause natriuresis through at least two mechanisms: (1) direct inhibition of epithelial sodium channels (ENaC) in the renal collecting ducts; and (2) inhibition of renin release from the renal juxtaglomerular cells, which ultimately leads to decreased aldosterone production. This leads to the urinary excretion of sodium and water, a reduction of intravascular volume, and a decreased stretch of the atrial myocytes. The natriuretic peptides also antagonize the pressor effects of angiotensin II and other pressor hormones by increasing intracellular cGMP. All three have vasodilatory activity, but CNP uniquely induces a greater effect on veins than arterioles. While circulating levels of these peptides are increased in heart failure, the elevations are presumed to be a compensatory response to the detrimental changes of volume overload secondary to a decrease in cardiac output. Nevertheless, measurement of the circulating BNP level is used in the differential diagnosis and evaluation of heart failure. As all three natriuretic peptides have cardio- and reno-protective properties, their therapeutic potential in chronic heart failure treatment is currently under study.

An additional uncharacterized natriuretic hormone that acts by inhibiting Na^+-K^+ adenosine triphosphatase (ATPase) is present in the circulation, but it raises rather than lowers blood pressure (see sections below concerning hypertension and salt sensitivity). There is substantial evidence that this hormone is actually ouabain and that it is secreted by the adrenal glands in response to increased dietary sodium intake.

Neural Control Via the Sympathetic Vasomotor System

Table 11–1 summarizes the factors affecting the caliber of the arterioles in the body, and hence peripheral resistance and tissue blood flow. This list includes the factors discussed previously plus a few additional polypeptides that have minor or special effects. It also includes the control of blood pressure by noradrenergic and, in some instances, cholinergic sympathetic vasomotor nerves to the arterioles. In addition to the extensive nerve supply to these resistance vessels, there is a moderate innervation of the capacitance vessels.

Discharge of the noradrenergic vasomotor nerves causes constriction of the arterioles innervated by the nerves, and if the discharge is general rather than local, there is an increase in blood pressure. In addition, the discharge of sympathetic noradrenergic nerves innervating the heart increases blood pressure by increasing the force and rate of cardiac contraction (inotropic and chronotropic effects), increasing stroke volume and cardiac output. Noradrenergic stimulation also inhibits the effect of vagal stimulation, which normally slows the heart and decreases cardiac output.

TABLE 11–1   Summary of factors affecting the caliber of the arterioles.

Constriction
Local factors
Decreased local temperature
Autoregulation
Locally released platelet serotonin
Endothelial cell products
Endothelin-1
Hormones
Norepinephrine
Epinephrine (except in skeletal muscle and liver)
Arginine vasopressin
Angiotensin II
Circulating Na^+-K^+ ATPase inhibitor
Neuropeptide Y
Neural control
Increased discharge of noradrenergic vasomotor nerves
Dilation
Local factors
Increased CO_2, K^+, adenosine, lactate
Decreased O_2
Decreased local pH
Increased local temperature
Endothelial cell products
Nitric oxide
Hormones
Vasoactive intestinal peptide
CGRPα (calcitonin gene-related peptide, α form)
Substance P
Histamine
Kinins
Natriuretic peptides (ANP, BNP, CNP)
Epinephrine in skeletal muscle and liver
Neural control
Activation of cholinergic dilator fibers to skeletal muscle
Decreased discharge of noradrenergic vasomotor nerves

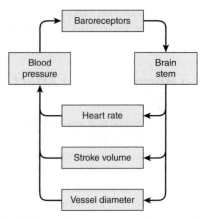

FIGURE 11–12 Feedback regulation of systemic blood pressure by baroreceptors. (Redrawn, with permission, from Barrett KE et al, eds. *Ganong's Review of Medical Physiology*, 25th ed. McGraw-Hill, 2016.)

The main control of vasomotor discharge is feedback regulation via the baroreceptors in the high-pressure and low-pressure portions of the circulatory system (Figure 11–12). The baroreceptors are stretch-sensitive nerve endings located in the carotid sinuses and aortic arch on the arterial side and in the walls of the great veins and the cardiac atria on the venous side. The nerve fibers relay impulses in cranial nerves IX and X to the medulla oblongata, where the fibers end in the nucleus tractus solitarius (Figure 11–13). From the nucleus, second-order neurons pass to the caudal portion of the ventrolateral medulla and environs. From there, third-order inhibitory neurons pass to the rostral ventrolateral medulla, the location of the cell bodies of the neurons that control blood pressure. The axons of these neurons descend into the spinal cord and innervate the cell bodies of the blood pressure–regulating preganglionic sympathetic neurons in the intermediolateral gray column of the spinal cord. The axons of the preganglionic neurons leave the spinal cord and synapse on the postganglionic neurons in the ganglionic chain and collateral ganglia, as well as on the catecholamine-secreting cells in the adrenal medulla. The axons of the postganglionic noradrenergic neurons innervate the blood vessels and the heart. Figure 11–13 illustrates these pathways and the probable synaptic mediator at each synapse in the chain. Note in particular that the increased activity in the baroreceptor afferents produced by increases in blood pressure inhibits sympathetic vasomotor outflow, whereas a decreased baroreceptor afferent discharge stimulates sympathetic vasomotor outflow. This is brought about by the inhibitory γ-aminobutyric acid–secreting neuron link between the caudal portion of the ventrolateral medulla and the rostral ventrolateral medulla. In addition, an increased baroreceptor discharge stimulates afferents from the nucleus tractus solitarius to the dorsal motor nucleus of the vagus and the nucleus ambiguus. This increases the vagal discharge to the heart, slowing the cardiac rate and decreasing cardiac output.

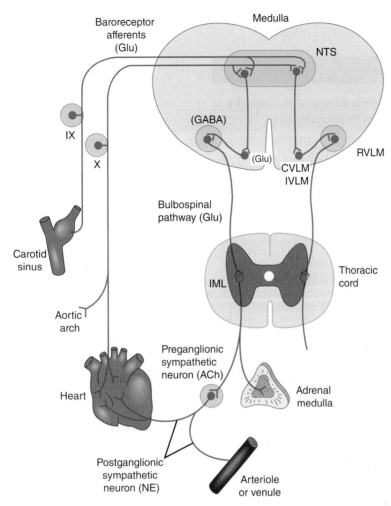

FIGURE 11–13 Basic pathways involved in the medullary control of blood pressure. The vagal efferent pathways to the heart are not shown. The probable neurotransmitters in the pathways are indicated in parentheses. (ACh, acetylcholine; CVLM, IVLM, and RVLM, caudal, intermediate, and rostral ventrolateral medulla, respectively; GABA, γ-aminobutyric acid; Glu, glutamate; IML, intermediolateral gray column; IX, glossopharyngeal nerve; NE, norepinephrine; NTS, nucleus tractus solitarius; X, vagus nerve.) (Reproduced, with permission, from Reis DJ et al. Role of adrenaline neurons of the ventrolateral medulla [the C1 group] in the tonic and phasic control of arterial pressure. Clin Exp Hypertens [A]. 1984;6:221. By permission of the publisher Taylor & Francis Ltd, http://www.informaworld.com)

There are ancillary reciprocal circuits between the nucleus tractus solitarius and the more dorsal portions of the brainstem and the hypothalamus that smooth and adjust the response of the baroreceptor pathway, but the primary neural regulation of blood pressure is mediated by the baroreceptor pathway in the medulla oblongata.

In addition to direct effects on vasomotor discharge, the baroreceptor pathway causes changes in endocrine function that augment the homeostatic value of baroreceptor responses. Adrenal medullary secretion is increased by the discharge of the sympathetic nervous system, although the contributions of circulating catecholamines to the increase in blood pressure are relatively small. An increased sympathetic discharge also increases renin secretion from the kidneys. The resultant increase in circulating angiotensin II not only acts directly on vascular smooth muscle to cause constriction but also increases aldosterone secretion, which in turn increases Na$^+$ retention, expanding intravascular volume. Associated with an increased vasomotor discharge, there is also an increase in antidiuretic hormone (ADH; also referred to as vasopressin) secretion from the posterior pituitary. ADH expands total body water by increasing free water retention in the kidney (acting through the V$_2$ vasopressin receptor). Although the primary role of ADH is to facilitate the lowering of osmolality, ADH also facilitates the expansion of intravascular volume. Although the volume expansion resulting from ADH is relatively small, ADH release increases with the severity of the effective circulating volume loss. Moreover, activation of the lower affinity V$_1$ vasopressin receptor on vascular smooth muscle results in a marked increase in vascular tone.

Baroreceptor function can be tested in experimental animals and judiciously in humans by infusing the pressor drug phenylephrine at different doses and at each dose measuring the slowing of the heart rate by determining the interval between the R waves (RR interval) of the ECG. Figure 11–14 provides an example of results of this type of testing.

FIGURE 11–14 Baroreflex-mediated lowering of the heart rate during phenylephrine infusion in a human subject. Note that the values for the RR interval of the ECG, which are plotted on the vertical axis, are inversely proportionate to the heart rate. (Redrawn, with permission, from Kotrly K et al. Effects of fentanyl-diazepam-nitrous oxide anaesthesia on arterial baroreflex control of heart rate in man. Br J Anaesth. 1986;58:406.)

PATHOPHYSIOLOGY OF SELECTED VASCULAR DISORDERS

ATHEROSCLEROSIS

Prevalence & Significance

A condition that afflicts the large and medium-sized arteries of almost every human, at least in societies in which cholesterol-rich foodstuffs are abundant and cheap, is **atherosclerosis**. This condition begins in childhood and, in the absence of accelerating factors, develops slowly until it is widespread in old age. However, it is accelerated by a wide variety of genetic and environmental factors (see later discussion). It is characterized by localized fibrous thickenings of the arterial wall associated with lipid-infiltrated plaques that may eventually calcify. Old plaques are also prone to ulceration and rupture, triggering the formation of thrombi that obstruct flow. Therefore, atherosclerosis leads to vascular insufficiency in the limbs, abnormalities of the renal circulation, and dilations (aneurysms) and even rupture of the aorta and other large arteries. It also leads to common severe and life-threatening diseases of the heart and brain because of the formation of intravascular clots at the site of the plaques.

In the United States and most other developed countries, it has been calculated that atherosclerosis is the underlying cause of about 50% of all deaths. Almost all patients with myocardial infarction—and most of those with stroke resulting from cerebral thrombosis—have atherosclerosis. The incidence of ischemic heart disease and strokes has been declining in the United States since 1963, but atherosclerosis is still very common. Thus, atherosclerosis underlies and is fundamentally responsible for a large portion of the clinical problems seen by physicians caring for adult patients.

Pathogenesis

The initial event in atherosclerosis is the infiltration of low-density lipoproteins (LDLs) into the subendothelial region. The endothelium is subject to **shear stress**, the tendency to be pulled along or deformed by flowing blood. This is most marked at points where the arteries branch, which is also where the lipids accumulate to the greatest degree.

The LDLs are oxidized or altered in other ways. Thus, altered LDLs activate various components of the innate immune system, including macrophages, natural antibodies, and innate effector proteins such as C-reactive protein and complement. Altered LDLs are recognized by a family of **scavenger receptors** expressed on macrophages that cooperate with toll-like receptors to stimulate inflammation and drive atherogenesis. The scavenger receptors mediate uptake of the oxidized LDL into macrophages and the formation of **foam cells** (Figure 11–15). The foam cells form **fatty streaks**. The streaks appear in the aorta in the first decade of life, in the coronary arteries in the second decade, and in the cerebral arteries in the third and fourth decades.

Oxidized LDLs have a number of deleterious effects, including stimulating the release of pro-inflammatory cytokines (such as macrophage migration inhibitory factor and type I interferon) and inhibiting NO production. Vascular smooth muscle cells in the vicinity of foam cells are stimulated and move from the media to the intima, where they proliferate, lay down collagen and other matrix molecules, and contribute to the bulk of the lesion. Smooth muscle cells also take up oxidized LDL and become foam cells. Lipids accumulate both intracellularly and extracellularly.

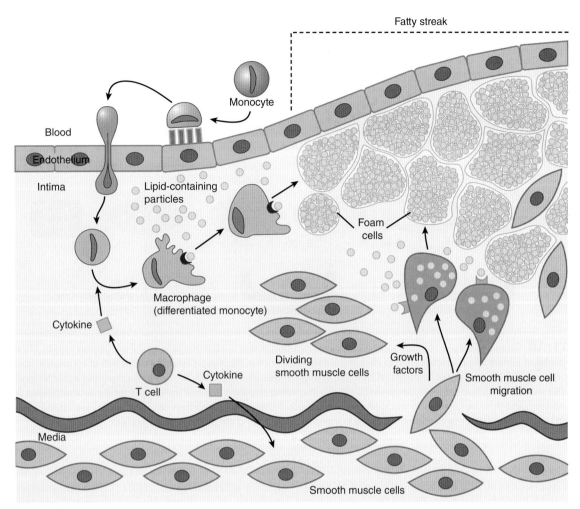

FIGURE 11–15 Formation of a fatty streak in an artery. After vascular injury, monocytes bind to the endothelium, then cross it to the subendothelial space, and become activated tissue microphages. The macrophages take up oxidized low-density lipoproteins (LDLs), becoming foam cells. T cells release cytokines, which also activate macrophages. In addition, the cytokines cause smooth muscle cells to proliferate. Under the influence of growth factors, the smooth muscle cells then move to the subendothelial space, where they produce collagen and take up LDL, adding to the population of foam cells. (Redrawn, with permission, from Hajjar DP et al. Atherosclerosis. Am Scientist. 1995;83:460.)

Although an elevated serum LDL level is a major risk factor for, and oxidized LDL is a critical participant in, the development of atherosclerotic plaques, not all circulating LDLs are the same. Small, dense LDL particles are more atherogenic than large LDL particles. The small, dense LDL particles appear to be more rapidly oxidized and may more easily invade the subendothelial layer of arterial walls. Moreover, evidence suggests that the level of small, dense LDL particles also correlates with other atherogenic metabolic abnormalities.

The intercellular "soup" in the plaques contains a variety of cell-damaging substances, including ozone. In addition, the "loading" of macrophages with cholesterol can be lipotoxic to the endoplasmic reticulum, resulting in macrophage apoptosis and plaque necrosis. Cholesterol crystals associated with necrotized macrophages further stimulate inflammation and lead to the recruitment of neutrophils. As the atherosclerotic lesions age, immune system T cells and monocytes are attracted to them, creating a vicious cycle of necrosis and inflammation.

As plaques mature, a fibrous cap forms over them. The plaques with defective or broken caps are most prone to rupture. The lesions alone may distort vessels to the point that they are occluded, but it is usually the rupture or ulceration of plaques that triggers thrombosis, blocking blood flow.

Atherosclerotic lesions have been shown to have many of the characteristics of a low-grade infection. A substantial number of studies support an association of various infections, including *Chlamydophila pneumoniae* (an organism usually associated with respiratory infection), with the development of atherosclerosis. However, only *C pneumoniae* (and no other bacteria) has actually been isolated in the atherosclerotic plaque. Clinical trials have been conducted to assess the effects of antibiotics in the secondary prevention of composite cardiovascular events, but results have been disappointing. Although these studies have yet to establish a definitive causal link between infection and atherosclerosis, it is clear that infections, by increasing an organism's inflammatory state, can at least promote atherosclerosis. A characteristic

FIGURE 11–16 Simplified diagram of the lipoprotein systems for transporting lipids in humans. In the exogenous system, chylomicrons rich in triglycerides of dietary origin are converted to chylomicron remnants rich in cholesteryl esters by the action of lipoprotein lipase. In the endogenous system, very-low-density lipoproteins (VLDLs) rich in triglycerides are secreted by the liver and converted into intermediate-density lipoproteins (IDLs) and then to low-density lipoproteins (LDLs) rich in cholesteryl esters. Some of the LDLs enter the subendothelial space of arteries, are oxidized, and then are taken up by macrophages, which become foam cells. The letters on the chylomicrons, chylomicron remnants, VLDL, IDL, and LDL, identify the primary apoproteins found in them. (LCAT, lecithin-cholesterol acyltransferase.)

of atherosclerosis that is currently receiving considerable attention is its association with a deficient release of NO and defective vasodilation. As noted, oxidized LDLs inhibit NO production. If acetylcholine is infused via catheter into normal coronary arteries, the vessels dilate; however, if it is infused when atherosclerosis is present, the vessels constrict. This indicates that the endothelial secretion of NO is defective.

Interestingly, recent experimental evidence indicates that the activation of the vasculature endothelial receptor for endothelin B both stimulates eNOS and exerts antiprolif-erative effects on vascular smooth muscle cells. It has been speculated that the disrupted signaling via this receptor can be an additional contributing factor in the pathophysiology of atherosclerosis.

Relation to Dietary Cholesterol & Other Lipids

Transforming a monocyte into a lipid-ingesting macrophage involves the appearance on its surface of a unique type of oxi-dized LDL receptor, the **scavenger receptor**. Monocytes are stimulated to produce these receptors by the action of **mac-rophage colony-stimulating factor** secreted by endothelial cells and vascular smooth muscle cells. When oxidized LDL-receptor complexes are formed, they are internalized and the receptors recycle to the membrane while the lipid is stored.

Obviously, lipid accumulation in foam cells is a key event in the progression of atherosclerotic lesions, and it is well established that lowering plasma cholesterol slows the prog-ress of atherosclerosis. Figure 11–16 summarizes the main pathways of the metabolism of ingested lipids. Because lipids are relatively insoluble, they are transported as special lipopro-tein particles that increase their solubility. Dietary cholesterol and triglycerides are packaged in the protein-coated **chylo-microns** in intestinal epithelial cells. Under the influence of lipoprotein lipase, these particles release triglycerides to fat depots and muscles, and the resulting **chylomicron remnants** are taken up by the liver. The liver also synthesizes choles-terol and packages it with specific proteins to form **very-low-density lipoproteins (VLDLs)**. These lipoprotein particles enter the circulation, and, under the influence of lipoprotein lipase, donate triglycerides to tissues. In this way, they become cholesterol-rich **intermediate-density lipoproteins (IDLs)** and **low-density lipoproteins (LDLs)**. The LDLs supply cho-lesterol to the tissues. They provide all cells with cholesterol for the production of cell membranes and other uses. They also provide most of the cholesterol that is the precursor for all ste-roid hormones. As noted, oxidized LDLs are taken up by mac-rophages and smooth muscle cells in atherosclerotic lesions. On the other hand, **high-density lipoproteins (HDLs)** take cholesterol from peripheral cells and transport it to the liver where it is metabolized, keeping plasma and tissue cholesterol low. For this reason, it is referred to as "good cholesterol" as opposed to LDL cholesterol, which is "bad cholesterol." Efforts are being made to increase HDL levels by pharmaceutical means in the treatment of atherosclerosis.

Clinical Manifestations

Because atherosclerosis is an abnormality of arterial blood vessels, it can affect almost any organ in the body. Calcified atherosclerotic plaques are occasionally detected on x-ray film, and angiographic visualization of deformed arterial walls is possible. In general, however, atherosclerosis is asymptomatic until one of its complications develops.

In coronary arteries, atherosclerotic narrowing that reduces the lumen of a coronary artery more than 75% causes **angina pectoris**, the chest pain that results when pain-producing substances accumulate in the myocardium. Typically, the pain comes on during exertion and disappears with rest, as the substances are washed out by the blood. When atherosclerotic lesions cause clotting and occlusion of a coronary artery, the myocardium supplied by the artery dies (**myocardial infarction**). (Myocardial infarction is also discussed in Chapter 10.)

In the cerebral circulation, arterial blockage at the site of atherosclerotic plaques causes **thrombotic strokes**. (Strokes are discussed in Chapter 7.) In the abdominal aorta, extensive atherosclerosis can lead to aneurysmal dilation and rupture of the vessel. In the renal vessels, the localized constriction of one or both renal arteries causes **renovascular hypertension** (see later discussion). In the circulation to the legs, vascular insufficiency causes **intermittent claudication** (fatigue and usually pain on walking that is relieved by rest). If the circulation of a limb is severely compromised, the skin can ulcerate, producing lesions that are slow to heal. Frank **gangrene** of the extremities may also occur. Less frequently, clot formation and obstruction may occur in vessels supplying the intestines or other parts of the body.

Risk Factors

As noted, the progression of atherosclerosis is accelerated by a wide variety of genetic and environmental factors (risk factors), which are summarized in Table 11–2. Obviously, treating the accelerating conditions that are treatable and avoiding those that are avoidable should reduce the incidence of myocardial infarctions, strokes, and other complications of atherosclerosis.

Estrogen increases cholesterol removal by the liver, and the progression of atherosclerosis is less rapid in premenopausal women than in men. In addition, epidemiologic evidence suggests that estrogen replacement therapy may protect the cardiovascular system in postmenopausal women. On the other hand, large doses of estrogens increase the incidence of blood clots, and even small doses produce a slight increase in clotting. In addition, in several studies, estrogen treatment of postmenopausal women failed to prevent second heart attacks. The reason for the discrepancies between the epidemiologic and experimental data is currently unsettled.

The effect of increased plasma levels of homocysteine and related molecules, such as homocystine and homocysteine

TABLE 11–2 Conditions that accelerate the progression of atherosclerosis and the mechanisms responsible.

Condition	Mechanism
Male gender (and females after menopause)	Lack of LDL-lowering effect of estrogens; estrogens probably act by increasing the number of LDL receptors in the liver.
Family history of ischemic heart disease, stroke	Probably multiple genetic mechanisms.
Primary hyperlipidemia	Inherited disorders causing lipoprotein lipase deficiency (type I), defective LDL receptors (type IIa), abnormal apoprotein E (type III), deficiency of apoprotein C (type V), or unknown cause (types IIb and IV).
Secondary hyperlipidemia[1]	Increased circulating triglycerides produced by diuretics, β-adrenergic blocking drugs, excess alcohol intake.
Cigarette smoking	Probably carbon monoxide–induced hypoxic injury to endothelial cells.
Hypertension	Increased shear stress, with damage to endothelium.
Diabetes mellitus (types 1 and 2)	Decreased hepatic removal of LDL from the circulation; increased glycosylation of collagen, which increases LDL binding to blood vessel walls.
Obesity, particularly abdominal obesity	Fat tissue (including perivascular fat) is very active in releasing a number of endocrine and paracrine factors (including TNF) that can alter endothelial function and increase the inflammatory state of an individual.
Nephrotic syndrome	Increased hepatic production of lipids and lipoprotein(a).
Hypothyroidism	Decreased formation of LDL receptors in the liver.
High lipoprotein(a)	Unsettled.
Elevated plasma homocysteine	Unsettled. Probably increased homocysteine provides more H_2O_2 and other reactive oxygen molecules that foster the formation of oxidized LDL.

[1]Hypercholesterolemia and hypertriglyceridemia are both risk factors.

thiolactone, a condition sometimes called hyperhomocystinemia, deserves emphasis. These increases are associated with accelerated atherosclerosis, and the magnitude of the plasma elevation is positively correlated with the severity of the atherosclerosis. Markedly elevated levels resulting from documented mutations of relevant genes are rare, but mild elevations occur in 7% of the general population. The mechanism responsible for the accelerated vascular damage is unsettled, but homocysteine is a significant source of H_2O_2 and other reactive forms of oxygen, and this may accelerate LDL oxidation.

Homocysteine is an intermediate in the synthesis of methionine. It is metabolized by enzymes dependent on vitamin B_6, vitamin B_{12}, and folic acid. Supplementing the diet with these vitamins reduces plasma homocysteine, usually to normal. Determining whether such supplements also reduce the incidence of accelerated atherosclerosis will require prolonged, careful clinical trials, and the results of such studies to date are inconclusive.

Evidence is now overwhelming that lowering plasma cholesterol and triglyceride levels and increasing plasma HDL levels slows, and in some cases reverses, the atherosclerotic process. The desired decrease in lipids can sometimes be achieved with the dietary restriction of cholesterol and saturated and trans fat alone, even though dietary restriction initiates a compensatory increase in cholesterol synthesis in the body. When dietary treatment is not adequate, reducing the conversion of mevalonate to cholesterol with statins, drugs that inhibit hepatic 3-methylglutaryl coenzyme A (HMG-CoA) reductase, the enzyme that catalyzes this reaction, is beneficial. The currently available HMG-CoA reductase inhibitors include atorvastatin, lovastatin, pitavastatin, pravastatin, simvastatin, fluvastatin, and rosuvastatin.

Despite promising preliminary experimental results using gene therapy for severe hypercholesterolemia in animals with congenitally defective LDL receptors, this approach has proven challenging in humans owing to the lack of efficient gene targeting. The development of the CRISPR/Cas9 system, a more precise and efficient gene editing technique, is anticipated to ameliorate this problem. Other molecular biologic approaches to slowing or preventing the development of atherosclerosis are under development.

Antioxidant treatment with agents such as α-tocopherol, vitamin E, and β-carotene has been used to inhibit LDL oxidation, which reduces the incidence of atherosclerotic changes in experimental animals. However, the results of antioxidant treatment in humans have generally been disappointing or negative.

Men who smoke a pack of cigarettes a day have a 70% increase in death rate from ischemic heart disease compared with nonsmokers, and there is also an increase in women. Smoking cessation lessens the risk of death and of myocardial infarction. The deleterious effects of smoking include endothelial damage caused by carbon monoxide–induced hypoxia. Other factors may also be involved. Thus, stopping smoking is a major way to slow the progress of atherosclerosis.

Because of the increased shear stress imposed on the endothelium by an elevated blood pressure, hypertension is another important modifiable risk factor for atherosclerosis. Lowering blood pressure has its greatest effect in reducing the incidence of stroke, but there are beneficial effects on ischemic heart disease as well. With modern methods of treatment, blood pressure in people with hypertension can generally be reduced to normal or near-normal values, and the decrease in strokes, myocardial infarctions, and renal failure produced by such treatment is clear testimony to the value of reducing or eliminating this risk factor.

In people with diabetes, there are both microvascular and macrovascular complications (see Table 18–6). The latter are primarily related to atherosclerosis. People with diabetes face a twofold increase in the incidence of myocardial infarction compared with those without diabetes; severe circulatory deficiency in the legs with gangrene is relatively common; people with diabetes experience more thrombotic strokes; and renal failure is a serious problem (Chapter 18). While chronic hyperglycemia itself can induce vascular damage, it is becoming more apparent that insulin resistance, such as occurs in type 2 diabetes mellitus, contributes markedly to the development of atherosclerosis. Insulin activation of the PI3K/Akt pathway leads to the increased expression of endothelin B receptor, the consequent activation of nitric oxide synthase in endothelial cells, and a resultant enhancement of local vasodilation and decrease in local inflammation. Insulin resistance downregulates the P13K/Akt pathway, leading to the selective activation of the p-ERK pathway, facilitating the proliferation and migration of vascular smooth muscle cells that contribute to the development of atherosclerosis. Importantly, however, the rigorous control of blood pressure in people with diabetes is more efficacious in reducing cardiovascular complications than is the rigorous control of blood glucose.

Obesity has long been appreciated as an independent risk factor for atherosclerosis. However, the mechanism(s) through which obesity promotes atherosclerosis has remained enigmatic until recently. Despite the overproduction of the satiety-inducing adipose-derived adipokines (eg, leptin and adiponectin) in obese subjects, they exhibit marked resistance to the effects of these adipokines. Moreover, obesity induces a low-grade inflammation of adipose tissue by producing pro-inflammatory cytokines such as TNFα and interleukin 6, as well as by recruiting inflammatory cells. In addition to the enhanced production of adipokines, perivascular fat also produces pro-inflammatory molecules. Taken together, these findings indicate that perivascular adipose tissue may be a major contributor to obesity-induced atherosclerosis.

Nephrotic syndrome and hypothyroidism also accelerate the progression of atherosclerosis and are treatable conditions.

Although local inflammation clearly plays a direct role in the pathogenesis of atherosclerosis, the possibility that indirect mechanisms associated with autoimmune diseases, infections (including gum disease and gastric infections), or exposure to various pollutants contribute to (or even initiate) atherosclerosis remains controversial.

CHECKPOINT

10. What is the most common cause of death in the United States among individuals older than 45 years?
11. What is the hypothesized mechanism of atherosclerotic plaque formation?
12. What are some ways in which atherosclerotic plaques can cause cardiovascular disease?
13. Name five treatable risk factors that accelerate the progression of atherosclerosis.

HYPERTENSION

Hypertension is not a single disease but rather a syndrome with multiple causes. In most instances, the cause remains unknown, and the cases are lumped together under the term **essential hypertension** (Table 11–3). However, mechanisms are continuously being discovered that explain hypertension in new subsets of the formerly monolithic category of essential hypertension, and the percentage of cases in the essential category continues to decline. Essential hypertension is often called **primary hypertension**, and hypertension in which the cause is known is called **secondary hypertension**, although this separation seems somewhat artificial. This chapter discusses the pathogenesis of hypertension and its complications in general terms and then discusses the specific causes of the currently defined subgroups and the unique features, if any, that each adds to the general findings in patients with high blood pressure.

Pathogenesis

Current guidelines of the Joint National Committee on Prevention, Detection, Evaluation, and Treatment of High Blood Pressure define normal blood pressure as a systolic pressure of less than 120 mm Hg and a diastolic pressure of less than 80 mm Hg. Hypertension is defined as an arterial pressure greater than 140/90 mm Hg in adults on at least three consecutive visits to the doctor's office. People whose blood pressure is between normal and 140/90 mm Hg are considered to have pre-hypertension, and people whose blood pressure falls in this category should appropriately modify their lifestyle to lower their blood pressure to below 120/80 mm Hg. As noted (see Figure 11–7), systolic pressure normally rises throughout life, and diastolic pressure rises until age 50–60 years but then falls, so that pulse pressure continues to increase. In the past, emphasis has been on treating individuals with elevated diastolic pressure. However, it now appears that, particularly in elderly individuals, treating systolic hypertension is equally important or even more so in reducing the cardiovascular complications of hypertension. Moreover, some studies indicate that overly aggressive treatment (particularly of diastolic hypertension) may be associated with adverse cardiac events (primarily myocardial infarctions) in patients with coronary

TABLE 11–3 Primary and secondary causes of hypertension.

Primary
Essential (idiopathic) hypertension

Secondary
Renal hypertension
Renovascular (atherosclerosis, fibromuscular dysplasia)
Parenchymal (chronic kidney disease, polycystic kidney disease, obstructive uropathy)
Endocrine–metabolic hypertension
Primary aldosteronism
Cushing syndrome
Pheochromocytoma
Other adrenal enzyme deficiencies
(11β-hydroxylase deficiency, 17α-hydroxylase deficiency, 11-hydroxysteroid deficiency [licorice])
Hyperthyroidism
Hyperparathyroidism
Acromegaly
Obesity and metabolic syndrome
Drug-induced or drug-related
Estrogen treatment ("pill hypertension")
Exogenous corticosteroids, androgens
Nonsteroidal anti-inflammatory drugs
Cocaine, amphetamine, or alcohol use
Decongestants
Appetite suppressants
Cyclosporine, tacrolimus
Antidepressants (some; eg, venlafaxine)
Miscellaneous
Pre-eclampsia and eclampsia
Liddle syndrome
Coarctation of the aorta
Sleep apnea
Polycythemia, erythropoietin
Increased intracranial pressure

artery disease or chronic heart failure. The explanation for this may be that because the coronary arteries fill during diastole, in individuals with coronary artery disease or heart failure, adequate cardiac muscle perfusion depends a somewhat higher diastolic blood pressure.

The most common cause of hypertension is increased peripheral vascular resistance. However, because blood pressure equals total peripheral resistance times cardiac output, prolonged increases in cardiac output can also cause hypertension. These are seen, for example, in hyperthyroidism and beriberi. In addition, increased blood volume causes hypertension, especially in individuals with mineralocorticoid excess or renal failure (see later discussion); and increased blood viscosity, if marked, can increase arterial pressure.

Clinical Presentation

Hypertension by itself does not cause symptoms. Headaches, fatigue, and dizziness are sometimes ascribed to hypertension, but nonspecific symptoms such as these are no more common in people with hypertension than they are in normotensive controls. Instead, the condition is discovered during routine screening or when patients seek medical advice for its complications. These complications are serious and potentially fatal. They include myocardial infarction, heart failure, thrombotic and hemorrhagic strokes, hypertensive encephalopathy, and renal failure (Figure 11–17). This is why hypertension is called "the silent killer."

Physical findings are also absent in early hypertension, and observable changes are generally found only in advanced severe cases. These may include **hypertensive retinopathy**

(ie, narrowed arterioles seen on funduscopic examination) and, in more severe cases, retinal hemorrhages and exudates, along with swelling of the optic nerve head (papilledema). Prolonged pumping against an elevated peripheral resistance causes left ventricular hypertrophy, which can be detected by echocardiography, and cardiac enlargement, which can be detected on physical examination. It is important to listen with the stethoscope over the kidneys because in renal hypertension (see later discussion), narrowing of the renal arteries may cause bruits. These bruits are usually continuous throughout the cardiac cycle. It has been recommended that the blood pressure response to rising from the sitting to the standing position be determined. A blood pressure rise on standing sometimes occurs in essential hypertension, presumably because of a hyperactive sympathetic response to the erect posture. This rise is usually absent in other forms of hypertension.

In many patients with hypertension, the condition is benign and progresses slowly; in others, it progresses rapidly. Actuarial data indicate that, on average, untreated hypertension reduces life expectancy by 10–20 years. Atherosclerosis is accelerated, and this in turn leads to ischemic heart disease with angina pectoris and myocardial infarctions (Chapter 10), thrombotic strokes and cerebral hemorrhages (Chapter 7), and renal failure (Chapter 16). Another complication of severe hypertension is **hypertensive encephalopathy**, in which there is confusion, disordered consciousness, and seizures. This condition, which requires vigorous treatment, is probably due to arteriolar spasm and cerebral edema.

In all forms of hypertension regardless of cause, the condition can suddenly accelerate and enter the malignant phase. In **malignant hypertension**, there is widespread fibrinoid

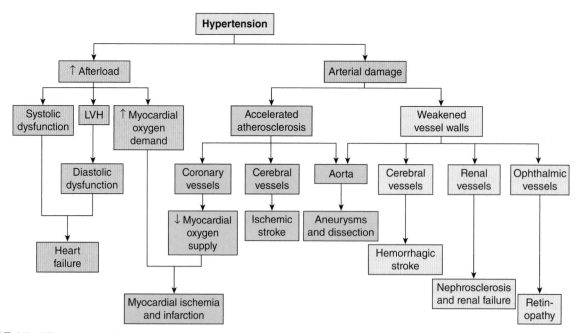

FIGURE 11–17 Pathogenesis of the complications produced by arterial hypertension. (LVH, left ventricular hypertrophy.) (Redrawn, with permission, from Drago J et al. Hypertension. Chapter 13 in Lilly LS et al, eds. *Pathophysiology of Heart Disease: A Collaborative Project of Medical Students and Faculty*, 6th ed. Wolters Kluwer, 2016.)

necrosis of the media with intimal fibrosis in the arterioles, narrowing them and leading to progressive severe retinopathy, heart failure, and renal failure. If untreated, malignant hypertension is usually fatal in 1 year.

MANAGEMENT

A discussion of disease treatment is beyond the scope of this book. However, it should be noted that in all forms of hypertension, modern treatment with β-adrenergic blocking drugs, inhibitors of the renin–angiotensin system, Ca^{2+} channel inhibitors, and diuretics reduce blood pressure, usually to normal levels. Though these drugs use different signaling and effector cascades, they all lower blood pressure either by decreasing arterial vascular tone and/or by decreasing intravascular volume. In addition, these treatments delay or prevent complications and lengthen life expectancy. Moreover, evidence indicates that aggressive blood pressure lowering in high-risk individuals (including those with a systolic blood pressure below 140 mm Hg) has substantial benefits in preventing major cardiovascular events.

In the case of essential hypertension, these therapies are not curative and must be continued indefinitely. Unfortunately, a significant number of patients with essential hypertension do not achieve adequate blood pressure control despite treatment. Recent evidence suggests that management approaches could be both improved and simplified if plasma renin measurement was added to current diagnostic algorithms. Patients with high and normal plasma renin would be treated primarily with renin-angiotensin-aldosterone inhibitors (such as ACE inhibitors or ARBs), and patients with low renin would be treated primarily with volume-depleting agents. The principle behind this approach lies in the assumption that hypertension arises as a consequence of either abnormally high activity of endogenous vasoconstrictors or abnormally elevated total body salt and subsequent expanded blood volume. While these two variables are not completely independent, renin measurement can facilitate the identification of the prevailing mechanism: If a patient has an elevated (or even normal) level of renin in the face of hypertension, the renin-angiotensin-aldosterone system (RAAS) is inappropriately reacting in the face of high blood pressure. If renin is low and pressure is high, the RAAS response is appropriate, so the likely culprit is the elevated body fluid volume. In the first situation, a preferred treatment approach is RAAS inhibition. In the second scenario, a therapy that decreases intravascular volume is preferred. While this approach can be effective in the long-term treatment of essential hypertension, if a cause of hypertension can be identified (so-called secondary hypertension), its treatment may result in a cure. Consequently, it is important to identify such cases. For example, an important exception to the above algorithm is the case of primary aldosteronism (autonomous excessive aldosterone secretion) in which pathologic aldosterone-mediated intravascular volume expansion is the cause of the hypertension. In this disease, renin is appropriately physiologically suppressed owing to the pathologic aldosterone excess. Treatment focuses on removing an inciting aldosterone-secreting adrenal tumor or medically treating the aldosterone excess, most often with a mineralocorticoid receptor antagonist.

Etiology

A. Coarctation of the Aorta

Congenital narrowing of the aorta usually occurs just distal to the origin of the left subclavian artery. Peripheral resistance is increased above the constriction. Therefore, blood pressure is elevated in the arms, head, and chest but lowered in the legs. However, because the constriction is proximal to the renal arteries, renin secretion is increased in most cases of coarctation as a result of the reduction in arterial pressure in the renal arteries. This tends to increase blood pressure throughout the body. Elimination of the constriction by resecting the narrowed segment of the aorta usually cures the condition.

B. Salt Sensitivity

Although salt intake has been recognized as a factor in the pathophysiology of hypertension, not all hypertension is salt sensitive. As shown in Table 11–4, about 30% of whites with normal renal function and normal blood pressure are salt sensitive compared with 55% of whites with essential hypertension. For unknown reasons, a much larger percentage of black people with hypertension are salt sensitive (73%). These figures have obvious significance in terms of recommendations about salt intake in hypertension.

It should be emphasized that the figures just cited refer to individuals with normal renal function and normal (or reduced) secretion of mineralocorticoid hormones. When renal function is reduced, mineralocorticoid secretion is increased (or the effects of mineralocorticoids are enhanced), there is an abnormal retention of salt and water, and hypertension is produced on this basis (see later discussion).

TABLE 11–4   Salt sensitivity in humans.

	Percentage of Individuals	
	Normal	Hypertensive
White		
Salt-sensitive[1]	30	55
Salt-resistant	70	45
Black		
Salt-sensitive[1]	32	73
Salt-resistant	68	27

Used, with permission, from MH Weinberger. Data from Luft FC et al. Salt sensitivity and resistance of blood pressure. Hypertension. 1991;17(Suppl I):1102.

[1]Mean blood pressure decrease of more than 10 mm Hg with furosemide and low-salt diet.

The genetic mechanisms responsible for the differences in salt sensitivity are still debated. One leading hypothesis posits that salt-mediated hypertension stems from salt-induced vascular dysfunction leading to increased total peripheral resistance. Salt can activate three pathways that may lead to vascular smooth muscle contraction: (1) salt stimulates a subset of G proteins (G_{12-13}) responsible for the activation of myosin light chain kinase, which phosphorylates myosin to initiate contraction; (2) salt stimulates the Rho/Rho kinase pathway, which inhibits myosin light chain phosphatase to prevent smooth muscle relaxation; and (3) short-term increases in dietary salt intake stimulate the release of endogenous ouabain (whose effect on the vascular smooth muscle parallels the effects of the cardiac glycoside) to inhibit Na^+-K^+ ATPase with a consequent decrease in Na^+–Ca^+ exchanger activity, ultimately elevating intracellular calcium levels and increasing smooth muscle tone. Experimental evidence suggests that individual differences in these signaling pathways may indeed contribute to salt-related hypertension.

A second hypothesis proposes that the kidney of salt-sensitive individuals cannot effectively excrete a salt load, leading to an inappropriate increase in intravascular volume and resultant hypertension. Supporting data include the frequent finding that kidney transplantation often ameliorates hypertension in salt-sensitive patients. Also, animal studies that have defined an aldosterone-independent activation of mineralocorticoid receptors and a sympathetically mediated activation of sodium reabsorption in the distal renal tubule both support the contribution of renal defects in sodium handling to salt-sensitive hypertension. Regardless of the mechanism, however, the salt sensitivity of blood pressure is an influential risk factor of prognostic importance in cardiovascular disease.

C. Renal Abnormalities

Goldblatt's observation that **renal artery constriction** increased blood pressure in experimental animals was rapidly followed by demonstration of the same event in humans. However, disappointment followed when it was found that **renal hypertension** resulting from constriction of one or both renal arteries accounted for only a very small percentage of cases of clinical hypertension. The narrowing can result from atherosclerosis, the fibroelastic overgrowth of the renal artery wall, or external pressure on the vessel. The initial constriction decreases renal arteriolar pressure, which leads to increased renin secretion. (The renin–angiotensin system is discussed in Chapters 16 and 21.) However, in many cases, some other mechanism takes over chronically to maintain the hypertension. The nature of this other mechanism is unknown.

Ureteral obstruction can cause hypertension in animals and probably in humans by increasing renal interstitial pressure, thus decreasing the pressure gradient across the renin-secreting juxtaglomerular cells.

Acute and chronic glomerulonephritis and other forms of diffuse kidney disease can cause hypertension when the loss of the ability to excrete salt is severe enough that Na^+ and water are retained and blood volume is expanded.

D. Hormonal Disorders (Chapters 12 & 21)

A remarkable number of adrenal abnormalities cause hypertension. These mainly include conditions in which mineralocorticoids are secreted in excess, but **excess cortisol secretion** can also cause hypertension (albeit, through mineralocorticoid receptor activation), as does **excess catecholamine secretion** by adrenal medulla tumors. (These disorders are covered in detail in Chapters 12 and 21.)

One particular contributing factor to hypertension in women is **estrogen**. Secretion of angiotensinogen from the liver is under endocrine control and is uniquely stimulated by estrogens. Consequently, it is increased in women taking contraceptive pills containing large amounts of estrogens. When circulating angiotensinogen is increased, more angiotensin II is formed and blood pressure rises. The normal compensation for this response is decreased renin secretion because angiotensin II feeds back directly on the juxtaglomerular cells to reduce renin secretion. However, in some women, the compensation is incomplete and the estrogens cause a significant increase in blood pressure. Some women with this condition have underlying essential hypertension, which is triggered by the estrogens, but in others, the hypertension is cured by stopping estrogen treatment.

In view of the fact that Na^+ retention resulting from mineralocorticoid excess causes hypertension, it may seem surprising that a natriuretic hormone is also a suspected cause of hypertension. ANP and other natriuretic peptides of cardiac origin cause sodium loss in the urine and generally lower blood pressure. However, there is also a digitalis-like natriuretic substance in the circulation. Its source seems to be the adrenals, although it has also been claimed that it is secreted by the hypothalamus. This substance, which may be naturally occurring ouabain, inhibits Na^+-K^+ ATPase. This results in a loss of Na^+ in the urine, but an accumulation of Ca^{2+} in cells because of the Na^+ gradient decrease across the cell membrane. The increase in intracellular Ca^{2+} causes vascular smooth muscle to contract. Consequently, blood pressure is increased. However, the physiologic and pathophysiologic significance of this natriuretic hormone remains unsettled, and its hypersecretion cannot yet be considered a proved cause of clinical hypertension.

E. Neurologic Disorders

The nervous system plays a key role in maintaining blood pressure in normal individuals (see prior discussion). Clonidine and other drugs lower blood pressure by acting on the brain to decrease sympathetic discharge, and several of the most effective treatments for chronic hypertension act peripherally to reduce the effect of vasomotor sympathetic discharge to the blood vessels and heart. These and other observations suggest that clinical hypertension could be caused by central nervous system (CNS) abnormalities. Interruption of the afferent input from the baroreceptors to the CNS in experimental animals causes increased blood pressure. However, emphasis has been placed on the variability of the blood pressure in such animals rather than on any consistent elevation of mean arterial pressure. There is some evidence that chronic pressure on the rostral ventrolateral medulla (see Figure 11–13) caused by minor anatomic abnormalities can cause hypertension in humans. However, this evidence is controversial, and as yet it cannot be said that this is an established cause of hypertension.

F. Nitric Oxide

An intriguing observation in experimental animals is that the administration of drugs that inhibit the production of NO increase blood pressure. Furthermore, there is a sustained elevation in blood pressure in knockout mice in which the genetic expression of the endothelial form of NOS has been disrupted. These observations suggest that NO has a chronic blood pressure–lowering effect and raise the possibility that inhibiting the production (or the effects) of NO may contribute to the development of hypertension in humans. The corollary of this conclusion is that therapies targeting vascular NO production or responsiveness could be successful in treating hypertension.

G. Facilitation of Na⁺–H⁺ Exchange

In approximately 50% of patients with essential hypertension, the function of a ubiquitous pH-regulating Na^+–H^+ exchanger in cell membranes is enhanced. Evidence indicates that this is associated with a polymorphism in the gene for one of the β subunits of a G protein that facilitates the function of the G protein. However, the overall significance of this abnormality remains to be determined.

H. Obesity

An association between body weight and hypertension has been appreciated for some time now. Moreover, insulin resistance and hyperlipidemia (along with obesity) are more prevalent in patients with essential hypertension and in their normotensive relatives than in the general population (or in patients with hypertension from known causes). This has led to a speculation that insulin resistance (via the hyperinsulinemia-mediated stimulation of the sympathetic nervous system) contributes to hypertension. However, experimental evidence is limited. It is more likely that the hypertension seen in obesity stems from a number of metabolic, hormonal, and humoral perturbations triggered by the accumulation of visceral (and perivascular) fat tissue. Increased fat tissue either directly (through local synthesis) or indirectly leads to an increase in the number of signaling molecules (eg, leptin, TNFα, VEGF, angiotensin II, and other molecules) that trigger an increased activation of the RAAS and sympathetic systems, endothelial dysfunction, and sodium retention. These changes can lead to an increase in peripheral vascular resistance and/or an increase in fluid retention, resulting in elevated blood pressure.

CHECKPOINT

14. Describe five physical findings in long-standing or severe hypertension.
15. Name 10 known causes of hypertension and a means by which each could be identified as the cause of hypertension in a patient.
16. What is the effect on blood pressure of disrupting the gene for the endothelial cell form of NOS in mice?

SHOCK

The term "shock" is used to denote various conditions, including the response to the passage of electric current through the body, the state that follows immediately after interruption of the spinal cord, and the stunned reaction to bad news. In the current context, it refers to an abnormality of the circulatory system in which there is inadequate tissue perfusion because of a relatively or absolutely inadequate cardiac output. The causes are divided into four groups: **hypovolemic shock**, an inadequate volume of blood to fill the vascular system; **distributive, vasogenic,** or **low-resistance shock**, an increase in the size of the vascular system produced by vasodilation in the presence of a normal blood volume; **cardiogenic shock**, inadequate heart output as a result of myocardial abnormalities; and **obstructive shock**, inadequate cardiac output as a result of blood flow obstruction in the lungs or heart. Table 11–5 provides examples of the conditions or diseases that can cause each type of shock.

Hypovolemic Shock

Hypovolemic shock is characterized by hypotension; a rapid, thready pulse; cold, pale, clammy skin; intense thirst; rapid respiration; and restlessness or, alternatively, torpor. Urine volume is markedly decreased. However, none of these findings is invariably present. Hypovolemic shock is commonly subdivided into categories on the basis of cause. The use of terms such as "hemorrhagic shock," "traumatic shock," "surgical shock," and "burn shock" is of some benefit because although there are similarities among these various forms of shock, there are important features that are unique to each.

In hypovolemic and other forms of shock, inadequate tissue perfusion leads to increased anaerobic glycolysis, with the production of large amounts of lactic acid. In severe cases, the blood lactate level rises from a normal value of about 1 mmol/L to 9 mmol/L or more. The resulting lactic acidosis depresses the myocardium, decreases peripheral vascular responsiveness to catecholamines, and may be severe enough to cause coma.

Multiple compensatory reactions come into play to defend extracellular fluid volume (Table 11–6). The large number of reactions that have evolved indicates the importance of maintaining blood volume for survival.

TABLE 11–5   Types of shock, with examples of conditions or diseases that can cause each type.

Hypovolemic shock (decreased blood volume)
Hemorrhage
Trauma
Surgery
Burns
Fluid loss associated with vomiting or diarrhea
Distributive shock (marked vasodilation; also called vasogenic or low-resistance shock)
Fainting (neurogenic shock)
Anaphylaxis
Sepsis (also causes hypovolemia owing to increased capillary permeability with loss of fluid into tissues)
Cardiogenic shock (inadequate output by a diseased heart)
Myocardial infarction
Heart failure
Arrhythmias
Obstructive shock (obstruction of blood flow)
Tension pneumothorax
Pulmonary embolism
Cardiac tumor
Pericardial tamponade

TABLE 11–6   Compensatory reactions activated by hypovolemia.

Vasoconstriction
Tachycardia
Venoconstriction
Tachypnea → Increased thoracic pumping
Restlessness → Increased skeletal muscle pumping (in some cases)
Increased movement of interstitial fluid into capillaries
Increased secretion of vasopressin
Increased secretion of glucocorticoids
Increased secretion of renin and aldosterone
Increased secretion of erythropoietin
Increased plasma protein synthesis

A decrease in pulse pressure or mean arterial pressure decreases the number of impulses ascending to the brain from the arterial baroreceptors, resulting in an increased vasomotor discharge. The resulting vasoconstriction is generalized, sparing only the vessels of the brain and the heart. The coronary vessels are dilated because of the increased myocardial metabolism secondary to an increase in heart rate. Vasoconstriction in the skin accounts for the coolness and pallor, and vasoconstriction in the kidneys accounts for the shutdown in renal function.

The immediate cardiac response to hypovolemia is tachycardia. With more extensive loss of volume, tachycardia can be replaced by bradycardia. With very severe hypovolemia, tachycardia reappears. Bradycardia may be due to the unmasking of a vagally mediated depressor reflex, perhaps related to limiting blood loss.

Vasoconstriction in the kidney reduces glomerular filtration. This reduces water loss, but it reaches a point at which nitrogenous products of metabolism accumulate in the blood (**prerenal azotemia**). If hypotension is prolonged, there may be severe renal tubular damage, leading to acute kidney injury.

The fall in blood pressure and the decreased O_2-carrying power of the blood caused by the loss of red cells results in the stimulation of the carotid and aortic chemoreceptors. This not only stimulates respiration but increases vasoconstrictor discharge. In severe hypovolemia, the pressure is so low that there is no longer any discharge from the carotid and aortic baroreceptors. This occurs when the mean blood pressure is about 70 mm Hg. Under these circumstances, if the afferent discharge from the chemoreceptors via the carotid sinus and vagus nerves is stopped, there is a paradoxic further fall in blood pressure rather than a rise.

Hypovolemia causes a marked increase in the circulating levels of the pressor hormones angiotensin II, epinephrine, norepinephrine, and vasopressin. ACTH secretion is also increased, and angiotensin II and ACTH both cause an acute increase in aldosterone secretion. The resulting retention of Na^+ and water helps re-expand blood volume.

Forms of Hypovolemic Shock

Hemorrhagic shock is probably the most carefully studied form of shock because it is easily produced in experimental animals. With moderate hemorrhage (5–15 mL/kg body weight), pulse pressure is reduced but mean arterial pressure may remain normal. With more severe hemorrhage, blood pressure always falls.

After hemorrhage, the plasma protein lost in shed blood is gradually replaced by hepatic synthesis, and the concentration of plasma proteins returns to normal in 3–4 days. The increase in circulating erythropoietin increases red blood cell formation, but it takes 4–8 weeks to restore red cell counts to normal.

Traumatic shock develops when there is severe damage to muscle and bone. This is the type of shock seen in battle casualties and automobile accident victims. Bleeding into the injured areas is the principal cause of such shock. The amount of blood that can be lost into a site of injury that appears relatively minor is remarkable; the thigh muscles can accommodate 1 L of extravasated blood, for example, with an increase in the diameter of the thigh of only 1 cm.

Breakdown of skeletal muscle is a serious additional problem when shock is accompanied by extensive muscle crushing (**crush syndrome**). When pressure on tissues is relieved and they are once again perfused with blood, free radicals are generated, which cause further tissue destruction (**reperfusion-induced injury**). Increased Ca^{2+} in damaged cells can reach toxic levels. Large amounts of K^+ enter the circulation. Myoglobin and other products from reperfused tissue can accumulate in the kidneys, where glomerular filtration is already reduced by hypotension, and the tubules can become clogged, causing anuria.

Surgical shock is a result of combinations, in various proportions, of external hemorrhage, bleeding into injured tissues, and dehydration.

In **burn shock**, there is a loss of plasma from burn surfaces, and the hematocrit rises rather than falls, producing severe hemoconcentration. In addition, there are complex metabolic changes. For these reasons, as well as the ease of infection in burned areas and kidney damage, the mortality rate when third-degree burns cover more than 75% of the body is close to 100%.

Distributive Shock

In distributive shock, most of the symptoms and signs described previously are present. However, vasodilation causes the skin to be warm rather than cold and clammy. **Anaphylactic shock** is a good example of distributive shock. In this condition, an accelerated allergic reaction causes the release of large amounts of histamine, producing marked vasodilation. Blood pressure falls because the size of the vascular system exceeds the amount of blood in it even though blood volume is normal.

A second type of distributive shock is **neurogenic shock**, in which a sudden loss of sympathetic autonomic activity (as seen in head and spinal cord injuries) results in vasodilation and blood pooling in the veins. The resulting decrease in venous return reduces cardiac output and frequently produces fainting, or **syncope**, a sudden transient loss of consciousness. A more benign and much more common form is **postural syncope**, which occurs on rising from a sitting or lying position. This is common in patients taking drugs that block sympathetic discharge or its effects on the blood vessels. Falling to the horizontal position restores blood flow to the brain, and consciousness is regained. Pressure on the carotid sinus produced, for example, by a tight collar can cause sufficient bradycardia and hypotension to cause fainting (**carotid sinus syncope**). Fainting caused by a variety of activities has been given appropriate names, such as **micturition syncope**, **cough syncope**, **deglutition syncope**, and **effort syncope**.

Syncope resulting from neurogenic shock is usually benign. However, it must be distinguished from syncope resulting from other causes and, therefore, merits investigation.

Another form of distributive shock is **septic shock**. (This condition is discussed in detail in Chapter 4.) It is now the most common cause of death in ICUs in the United States. It is a complex condition that includes elements of hypovolemic shock resulting from loss of plasma into the tissues ("third spacing") and cardiogenic shock resulting from toxins that depress the myocardium. It is associated with excess NO production, and therapy with drugs that scavenge NO may be beneficial.

Streptococcal toxic shock syndrome is a particularly severe form of septic shock in which group A streptococci infect deep tissues; the M protein on the surface of those bacteria has an antiphagocytic effect. This M protein is also released into the circulation, where it aggregates with fibrinogen.

Cardiogenic Shock

About 25% of syncopal episodes are of cardiac origin and are due either to the transient obstruction of blood flow through the heart or to sudden decreases in cardiac output caused by various cardiac arrhythmias. In addition, fainting is the presenting symptom in 7% of patients with myocardial infarctions.

Cardiogenic shock results whenever the pumping function of the heart is impaired to the point that blood flow to tissues is no longer adequate to meet resting metabolic demands; most commonly, it is due to extensive infarction of the left ventricle. The incidence of shock in patients with myocardial infarction is about 10%, and the mortality rate is 60–90%.

However, cardiogenic shock can also be caused by other diseases (eg, heart failure, arrhythmias) that severely compromise normal ventricular function. The symptoms are those of hypovolemic shock plus congestion of the lungs and viscera resulting from failure of the heart to put out all the venous blood returned to it. Consequently, the condition is sometimes called "congested shock."

Obstructive Shock

The picture of congested shock is also seen in **obstructive shock**. Causes include massive pulmonary emboli, tension pneumothorax with kinking of the great veins, and bleeding into the pericardium with external pressure on the heart (**cardiac tamponade**). In the latter two conditions, prompt surgery is required to prevent death. Pulsus paradoxus occurs in cardiac tamponade. Normally, blood pressure falls about 5 mm Hg during inspiration. In pulsus paradoxus, this response is exaggerated, and blood pressure falls 10 mm Hg or more as a result of increased fluid pressure in the pericardial sac on the external surface of the heart. However, pulsus paradoxus also occurs with labored respiration in severe asthma, emphysema, and upper airway obstruction.

Refractory Shock

Some patients with hypovolemia or septic shock die soon after the onset of the condition, whereas others recover as compensatory mechanisms gradually restore the circulation to normal. In an intermediate group of patients, shock persists for hours and gradually progresses. It eventually reaches a state in which there is no longer any response to vasopressor drugs and in which, even if the blood volume is returned to normal, cardiac output remains depressed. This condition, once known as **irreversible shock**, is now known as **refractory shock**. Patients often die despite vigorous treatment; however, more and more are now saved as our understanding of the pathophysiologic mechanisms has increased and treatment has improved. Therefore, "refractory shock" seems to be a more appropriate term than "irreversible shock."

Various factors appear to make shock refractory. Precapillary sphincters are constricted for several hours but then relax, whereas postcapillary venules remain constricted. Therefore, blood flows into the capillaries and remains there. Various positive feedback mechanisms contribute to the refractory state. For example, cerebral ischemia depresses vasomotor and cardiac discharge, causing blood pressure to fall and making the shock worse. This, in turn, causes a further reduction in cerebral blood flow. In addition, myocardial blood flow is reduced in severe shock. Myocardial failure makes the pumping action of the heart less effective and consequently makes the shock worse and further lowers myocardial blood flow.

A complication of shock that has a very high mortality rate is pulmonary damage with the production of acute respiratory distress syndrome. The cause appears to be capillary endothelial cell damage and damage to alveolar epithelial cells with the release of cytokines (Chapter 9).

CHECKPOINT

17. What are the four major pathophysiologic forms of shock?
18. Name three pathophysiologic consequences of lactic acidosis in shock.
19. Describe five specific forms of hypovolemic shock.
20. Name three specific forms of distributive shock, and distinguish them from hypovolemic shock.
21. Name three factors that tend to make shock refractory.

CASE STUDIES

Yeong Kwok, MD

(See Chapter 25, p. 769–70 for answers)

CASE 63

A 65-year-old woman presents to the clinic to establish care. Her past medical history is notable for type 2 diabetes and hypertension. She has a 45-pack-year smoking history. A few weeks ago, she was shovelling her driveway when she had to stop owing to tightness in her chest. She does not get any regular exercise because her calves become very painful after walking one block.

Questions

A. What is the likely diagnosis?
B. What is the pathogenesis of this condition?
C. What are this patient's rick factors, and how do they contribute to the development of atherosclerosis?

CASE 64

A 56-year-old black man presents to the clinic for a routine physical examination. He has not seen a physician for 10 years. On arrival, he is noted to have a blood pressure of 160/90 mm Hg.

Questions

A. Does this man have hypertension? Why or why not?
B. What physical findings might be present if he has had long-standing hypertension?
C. What are some of the important complications of hypertension?
D. What are some causes of hypertension?

CASE 65

A young woman is brought to the emergency department by ambulance after a severe motor vehicle accident. She is unconscious. Her blood pressure is 64/40 mm Hg, and her heart rate is 150 bpm. She is intubated and hand-ventilated. There is no evidence of head trauma. The pupils are 2 mm and reactive. She withdraws to pain. Cardiac examination reveals no murmurs, gallops, or rubs. The lungs are clear to auscultation. The abdomen is tense, with decreased bowel sounds. The extremities are cool and clammy, with thready pulses. Despite aggressive blood and fluid resuscitation, the patient dies.

Questions

A. What are the four major pathophysiologic causes of shock? Which was likely in this patient?

B. What pathogenetic mechanism accounts for this patient's unresponsiveness? For the cool, pale extremities?

C. What forms of hypovolemic shock may have been present in this patient? Why?

REFERENCES

General

Madonna R et al. Pathways and drugs in pulmonary arterial hypertension—focus on the role of endothelin receptor antagonists. Cardiovasc Drugs Ther. 2015;29(5):469–79. [PMID: 26145170]

Németh B et al. The issue of plasma asymmetric dimethylarginine reference range—a systematic review and meta-analysis. PLoS One. 2017 May 11;12(5):e0177493. [PMID: 28494019]

Thomas H et al. The importance of pericytes in healing: wounds and other pathologies. Int J Mol Sci. 2017 Jun;18(6):1129. [PMID: 28538706]

Atherosclerosis

Boudoulas KD et al. Coronary atherosclerosis: pathophysiologic basis for diagnosis and management. Prog Cardiovasc Dis. 2016 May-Jun;58(6):676–92. [PMID: 27091673]

Dahal U et al. An unsettled debate about the potential role of infection in pathogenesis of atherosclerosis. J Clin Med Res. 2017 Jul;9(7):547–54. [PMID: 28611853]

Engin A. Endothelial dysfunction in obesity. Adv Exp Med Biol. 2017;960:345–79. [PMID: 28585207]

Feingold KR et al, eds. The effect of inflammation and infection on lipids and lipoproteins. Endotext [Internet]. South Dartmouth (MA): MDText.com, Inc.; 2015 Jun. [PMID: 26561701] http://www.ncbi.nlm.nih.gov/books/NBK326741/

Huang Cao ZF et al. Role of perivascular adipose tissue in vascular physiology and pathology. Hypertension. 2017 May;69(5):770–7. [PMID: 28320849]

Janus A et al. Insulin resistance and endothelial dysfunction constitute a common therapeutic target in cardiometabolic disorders. Mediators Inflamm. 2016;2016:3634948. [PMID: 27413253]

Low Wang CC et al. Clinical update: cardiovascular disease in diabetes mellitus: atherosclerotic cardiovascular disease and heart failure in type 2 diabetes mellitus—mechanisms, management, and clinical considerations. Circulation. 2016 Jun 14;133(24):2459–502. [PMID: 27297342]

Ruscica M et al. Translating the biology of adipokines in atherosclerosis and cardiovascular diseases: gaps and open questions. Nutr Metab Cardiovasc Dis. 2017 May;27(5):379–95. [PMID: 28237179]

Savić N et al. Advances in therapeutic CRISPR/Cas9 genome editing. Transl Res. 2016 Feb;168:15–21. [PMID: 26470680]

Hypertension

Ettehad D et al. Blood pressure lowering for prevention of cardiovascular disease and death: a systematic review and meta-analysis. Lancet. 2016 Mar 5;387(10022):957–67. [PMID: 26724178]

Funder JW. Aldosterone and mineralocorticoid receptors—physiology and pathophysiology. Int J Mol Sci. 2017 May 11; 18(5):1032. [PMID: 28492512]

Furberg CD et al. Unsuccessfully treated hypertension: a major public health problem with a potential solution. Am J Hypertens. 2017 Sep 1;30(9):857–60. [PMID: 28482060]

Hall JE. Renal dysfunction, rather than nonrenal vascular dysfunction, mediates salt-induced hypertension. Circulation. 2016 Mar 1;133(9):894–906. [PMID: 26927007]

Hwang AY et al. Resistant hypertension: mechanisms and treatment. Curr Hypertens Rep. 2017 Jul;19(7):56. [PMID: 28597403]

Kurtz TW et al. An alternative hypothesis to the widely held view that renal excretion of sodium accounts for resistance to salt-induced hypertension. Kidney Int. 2016 Nov;90(5):965–73. [PMID: 27546606]

Kusche-Vihrog K et al. Salt controls endothelial and vascular phenotype. Pflugers Arch. 2015 Mar;467(3):499–512. [PMID: 25420527]

Seravalle G et al. Obesity and hypertension. Pharmacol Res. 2017 May 19;122:1–7. [PMID: 28532816]

Stowasser M. Update in primary aldosteronism. J Clin Endocrinol Metab. 2015 Jan;100(1):1–10. [PMID: 25365316]

Xie X et al. Effects of intensive blood pressure lowering on cardiovascular and renal outcomes: updated systematic review and meta-analysis. Lancet. 2016 Jan 30;387(10017):435–43. [PMID: 26559744]

Shock

Furer A et al. Hemodynamics of cardiogenic shock. Interv Cardiol Clin. 2017 Jul;6(3):359–71. [PMID: 28600090]

Gotts JE et al. Sepsis: pathophysiology and clinical management. BMJ. 2016 May 23;353:i1585. [PMID: 27217054]

Lord JM et al. The systemic immune response to trauma: an overview of pathophysiology and treatment. Lancet. 2014 Oct 18;384(9952):1455–65. [PMID: 25390327]

Mohsenin V. Assessment of preload and fluid responsiveness in intensive care unit. How good are we? J Crit Care. 2015 Jun;30(3):567–73. [PMID: 25682347]

Reyentovich A et al. Management of refractory cardiogenic shock. Nat Rev Cardiol. 2016 Aug;13(8):481–92. [PMID: 27356877]

Singer M et al. The third international consensus definitions for sepsis and septic shock (Sepsis-3). 2. JAMA. 2016 Feb 23;315(8):801–10. [PMID: 26903338]

Vincent JL et al. Optimum treatment of vasopressor-dependent distributive shock. Expert Rev Anti Infect Ther. 2017 Jan;15(1):5–10. [PMID: 27774825]

Disorders of the Adrenal Medulla

12

Lauren Fishbein, MD, PhD, &
Tobias Else, MD

The **adrenal medulla** secretes catecholamines (epinephrine, norepinephrine, dopamine). The catecholamines help prepare the body to deal with emergency situations. The major disorder of the adrenal medulla is **pheochromocytoma**, a neoplasm characterized by excessive catecholamine secretion.

NORMAL STRUCTURE & FUNCTION OF THE ADRENAL MEDULLA

ANATOMY

The adrenal medulla is the reddish-brown central portion of the adrenal gland. Accessory medullary tissue is sometimes located in the retroperitoneum near the sympathetic ganglia or along the abdominal aorta (paraganglia) (Figure 12–1).

HISTOLOGY

The adrenal medulla is made up of polyhedral cells arranged in cords or clumps. Embryologically, the adrenal medullary cells derive from neural crest cells. Medullary cells are innervated by cholinergic preganglionic nerve fibers that reach the gland via the splanchnic nerves. The adrenal medulla can be regarded as a specialized sympathetic ganglion, in which preganglionic sympathetic nerve fibers (using acetylcholine as a neurotransmitter) directly make contact with postganglionic cells, which secrete catecholamines (mainly epinephrine) directly into the circulation. This relationship is analogous to the other sympathetic ganglia, which connect preganglionic cholinergic sympathetic nerve fibers with postganglionic fibers using catecholamines (mainly norepinephrine) as neurotransmitters. Medullary parenchymal cells accumulate and store their hormone products in prominent, dense secretory granules, 150–350 nm in diameter. Histologically, these cells and granules have a high affinity for chromium salts (**chromaffin reaction**) and thus are called **chromaffin cells** and contain **chromaffin granules**. The granules contain the catecholamines epinephrine and norepinephrine. Morphologically, two types of medullary cells can be distinguished: epinephrine-secreting cells, which have larger, less dense granules, and norepinephrine-secreting cells, which have smaller, very dense granules. Separate dopamine-secreting cells have not been identified. Ninety percent of medullary cells are the epinephrine-secreting type, and 10% are the norepinephrine-secreting type.

PHYSIOLOGY

The catecholamines help to regulate metabolism, the contractility of cardiac and smooth muscle, and neurotransmission.

Formation, Secretion & Metabolism of Catecholamines

The adrenal medulla secretes three catecholamines: epinephrine, norepinephrine, and dopamine. Secretion occurs after the release of acetylcholine from the preganglionic neurons that innervate the medullary cells. Figure 12–2 illustrates the major biosynthetic pathways and hormonal intermediates for the catecholamines. In humans, most (80%) of the catecholamine output of the adrenal medulla is epinephrine. This epinephrine predominance occurs because the enzyme phenylethanolamine *N*-methyltransferase (PMNT), which converts norepinephrine to epinephrine, is upregulated by cortisol, which is found in high concentration locally from

FIGURE 12–1 Anatomic distribution of extra-adrenal chromaffin tissue in the newborn. (Redrawn, with permission, from Coupland R. *The Natural History of the Chromaffin Cell*. Longman, Green, 1965.)

the surrounding adrenal cortex. Norepinephrine is principally found in paraganglial cells associated with the sympathetic nervous system and in the central nervous system, where it functions as a major neurotransmitter.

Approximately 70% of the epinephrine and norepinephrine and 95% of the dopamine found in plasma are conjugated to sulfate and are inactive. In the supine state, the normal plasma level of free epinephrine is about 30 pg/mL (0.16 nmol/L); there is a 50–100% increase on standing. The normal plasma level of free norepinephrine is about 300 pg/mL (1.8 nmol/L), and the plasma free dopamine level is about 35 pg/mL (0.23 nmol/L).

Most catecholamine metabolism takes place within the same cells in which they are synthesized, mainly because of catecholamines leaking from the vesicular stores into the cytoplasm. These vesicular stores exist in a dynamic equilibrium, with outward passive leakage counterbalanced by an inward active transport controlled by vesicular monoamine transporters. Typically, the catechol–O–methyltransferase (COMT) enzyme methylates norepinephrine and epinephrine to form normetanephrine and metanephrine, respectively. These are then deaminated by monoamine oxidase.

In catecholaminergic neurons, the presence of monoamine oxidase in the cytoplasm leads to the formation of reactive catecholaldehydes. Production of these toxic aldehydes depends on the dynamics of the vesicular–axoplasmic monoamine exchange and an enzyme-catalyzed conversion to nontoxic acids or alcohols. In sympathetic nerves, the aldehyde produced from norepinephrine is converted to 3,4-dihydroxyphenylglycol. Subsequent extraneuronal O-methylation leads to the production of 3-methoxy-4-hydroxyphenylglycol, and its oxidation in the liver, catalyzed by alcohol and aldehyde

dehydrogenases, leads to the formation of vanillylmandelic acid (VMA). Compared with intraneuronal deamination, the extraneuronal O-methylation of norepinephrine and epinephrine represents a minor pathway of metabolism.

The single largest source of epinephrine is the adrenal medulla. In the circulation, the catecholamines have a short half-life of about 2 minutes. Normally, only very small quantities of free epinephrine (about 6 μg/day) and norepinephrine (about 30 μg/day) are excreted, but about 700 μg of VMA is excreted daily.

Regulation of Catecholamine Secretion

Physiologic stimuli affect medullary secretion through the nervous system. Medullary cells secrete catecholamines after the release of acetylcholine from the preganglionic neurons that innervate them. Catecholamine secretion is low in the basal state and is reduced even further during sleep. Emergency situations cause an increase in adrenal catecholamine secretion as part of a generalized sympathetic discharge that serves to prepare the individual for stress ("fight-or-flight") response). Physiological stress such as psychological, physical (eg, mechanical, thermal), metabolic (eg, hypoglycemia, exercise), or pathologic (eg, obstructive sleep apnea) stress leads to catecholamine secretion.

Mechanism of Action of Catecholamines

The effects of epinephrine and norepinephrine are mediated by their actions on two classes of receptors: α- and β-adrenergic receptors (Table 12–1). Alpha receptors are subdivided into α_1 and α_2 receptors, and β receptors are subdivided into β_1, β_2, and β_3 receptors. Alpha$_1$ receptors mediate smooth muscle contraction in blood vessels and the genitourinary (GU) tract and increase glycogenolysis. Alpha$_2$ receptors mediate smooth muscle relaxation in the gastrointestinal (GI) tract and the vasoconstriction of some blood vessels. Alpha$_2$ receptors also decrease insulin secretion. Beta$_1$ receptors mediate an increased rate and force of myocardial contraction and stimulate lipolysis and renin release. Beta$_2$ receptors mediate smooth muscle relaxation in the bronchi, blood vessels, GU tract, and GI tract and increase hepatic gluconeogenesis and glycogenolysis, muscle glycogenolysis, and the release of insulin and glucagon.

Intracellular post-receptor signaling is different for each subclass of adrenergic receptor. Stimulation of α_1-adrenergic receptors results in an increase in intracellular Ca^{2+} concentrations. First, phospholipase C is activated by the guanine nucleotide binding stimulatory protein, G_s. Phospholipase C hydrolyzes the membrane-bound phospholipid, phosphatidylinositol-4,5-bisphosphate, to generate two second messengers: diacylglycerol and inositol-1,4,5-trisphosphate. Diacylglycerol in turn activates protein kinase C, which phosphorylates various cellular substrates. Inositol-1,4,5-trisphosphate stimulates the release of intracellular Ca^{2+}, which then initiates various cellular responses.

FIGURE 12-2 Biosynthesis and catabolism of catecholamines. The catecholamines are synthesized from tyrosine (TYR). The enzyme catechol-O-methyltransferase (COMT) generates metanephrine (MN) from epinephrine (E) and normetanephrine (NM) from norepinephrine (NE). COMT is constitutively active in pheochromocytomas and paragangliomas, and the release of these substances is constant rather than episodic. (3MT, 3-methoxytyramine; AADC, aromatic L-amino acid decarboxylase; DA, dopamine; DBH, dopamine beta-hydroxylase; DOPAC, dihydroxyphenylacetic acid; HVA, homovanillic acid; MAO, monoamine oxidase; PNMT, phenylethanolamine N-methyltransferase; VMA, vanillylmandelic acid.)

Activation of α_2-adrenergic receptors results in a decrease in intracellular cyclic adenosine 3′,5′-monophosphate (cAMP). The mechanism involves receptor interaction with an inhibitory G protein, G_i, leading to inhibition of the adenylyl cyclase enzyme and, therefore, a decrease in cAMP. The fall in cAMP level leads to a decrease in activity of the cAMP-dependent protein kinase A. The G_i protein also stimulates K$^+$ channels and inhibits voltage-sensitive Ca^{2+} channels.

On the other hand, β-adrenergic receptors stimulate adenylyl cyclase through the mediation of G_s. Activation of β-adrenergic receptors thus leads to an increase in cAMP, activation of the cAMP-dependent protein kinase A, and the consequent phosphorylation of various cellular proteins. The G_s protein can also directly activate voltage-sensitive Ca^{2+} channels in the plasma membrane of cardiac and skeletal muscle.

The α_1- and β_1-adrenergic receptors are generally found in organs and tissues (eg, heart and gut) heavily innervated by—and situated so as to be readily activated by the stimulation of—the sympathetic nerves. The α_1- and β_1-adrenergic receptors are preferentially stimulated by norepinephrine, especially that released by nerve endings. In contrast, the α_2- and β_2-adrenergic receptors are generally situated in post-junctional sites in organs and tissues (eg, uterine and bronchial skeletal muscle) remote from sites of norepinephrine release. The α_2- and β_2-adrenergic receptors are preferentially stimulated by circulating catecholamines, especially epinephrine.

Differences in tissue distribution, accessibility by nerve fibers, preferences for epinephrine versus norepinephrine, and differences in post-receptor signaling are thus responsible for the diverse effects of catecholamines in an organ- and cell-specific manner.

TABLE 12–1   Physiologic effects of catecholamines on the adrenergic receptors of selected tissues.

Organ or Tissue	Adrenergic Receptor	Effect
Heart (myocardium)	β_1	Increased force of contraction (inotropic)
	α_1, β_1	Increased rate of contraction (chronotropic)
	β_1	Increased excitability (predisposes to arrhythmia)
	β_1	Increased AV nodal conduction velocity
Blood vessels (vascular smooth muscle)	α_1, α_2	Vasoconstriction, hypertension
	β_2	Vasodilation
Kidney (juxtaglomerular cells)	β_1	Increased renin release
	β_2	Increased peripheral conversion of T_4 to T_3
Gut (intestinal smooth muscle)	α_1, β_2	Increased sphincter tone (hyperpolarization); decreased motility (relaxation)
	β_3	Increased motility
Pancreas (B cells)	α_2	Decreased insulin release
		Decreased glucagon release
	β_2	Increased insulin release
		Increased glucagon release
Liver	α_1, β_2	Increased gluconeogenesis
		Increased glycogenolysis
		Increased peripheral conversion of T_4 to T_3
Adipose tissue	α_2	Decreased lipolysis
	β_1, β_3	Increased lipolysis
Skin (eg, apocrine glands on hands, axillas; hair)	α_1	Increased sweating
		Increased piloerection
Lung (bronchial smooth muscle)	β_2	Dilation of bronchi and bronchioles
Uterus (genitourinary smooth muscle)	α_1	Increased contraction of gravid uterus; decreased contraction of nongravid uterus (relaxation)
	β_2	Relaxation
Bladder (genitourinary smooth muscle)	α_1	Contraction
	β_2	Relaxation
Prostate	α_1	Increased contraction and ejaculation
Skeletal muscle	β_2	Increased muscle contraction speed
		Increased glycogenolysis
		Increased release of lactic acid
Platelets	α_2	Aggregation
Central nervous system	α	Increased alertness, anxiety, fear
Eye	α_1	Increased ciliary muscle contraction (pupillary dilation)
Peripheral nerves	β_2	Increased conduction velocity
Most tissues	β_1, β_3	Increased calorigenesis
		Increased metabolic rate

Modified and reproduced, with permission, from Fitzgerald P. Adrenal medulla and paraganglia. In: Gardner DG et al, eds. *Greenspan's Basic & Clinical Endocrinology*, 10th ed. McGraw-Hill, 2017.

Effects of Catecholamines

The catecholamines have been termed fight-or-flight hormones because their effects on the heart, blood vessels, smooth muscle, and metabolism assist organisms in responding to stress. Table 12–1 presents the principal physiologic effects of the catecholamines.

In the peripheral circulation, norepinephrine produces vasoconstriction in most organs (via α_1 receptors). Epinephrine produces vasodilation via β_2 receptors in skeletal muscle and the liver and vasoconstriction elsewhere. The former usually outweighs the latter, and for that reason epinephrine usually lowers total peripheral resistance.

Norepinephrine causes both systolic and diastolic blood pressures to rise. The rise in blood pressure stimulates the carotid and aortic baroreceptors, resulting in reflex bradycardia and a fall in cardiac output. Epinephrine causes a widening of pulse pressure but does not stimulate the baroreceptors to the same degree, so the pulse rises and cardiac output increases. Hence, pheochromocytomas and other tumors of the adrenal medulla, which usually secrete norepinephrine, lead to vasoconstriction and an increase in blood pressure.

The effects of catecholamines on metabolism include effects on glycogenolysis, lipolysis, and insulin secretion, mediated by both α- and β-adrenergic receptors. These metabolic effects result primarily from the action of epinephrine on four target tissues: liver, muscle, pancreas, and adipose tissue (see Table 12–1). The result is an increase in the levels of circulating glucose and free fatty acids. The increased levels of these two substances help provide an adequate supply of metabolic fuel to the nervous system and muscle during physiologic stress.

The amount of circulating plasma epinephrine and norepinephrine needed to produce these various physiologic and metabolic effects has been determined by infusing catecholamines into resting subjects. For norepinephrine, the threshold for cardiovascular and metabolic effects is a plasma level of about 1500 pg/mL, or about five times the basal level. In normal individuals, the plasma norepinephrine level rarely exceeds this threshold. However, for epinephrine, the threshold for tachycardia occurs at a plasma level of about 50 pg/mL, or about twice the basal level. The threshold for increasing systolic blood pressure and lipolysis is about 75 pg/mL of epinephrine; for increasing glucose and lactate, about 150 pg/mL; and for increasing insulin secretion, about 40 pg/mL. In healthy individuals, plasma epinephrine levels often exceed these thresholds.

The physiologic effect of circulating dopamine is unknown. Centrally, dopamine acts to inhibit prolactin secretion. Peripherally, in small doses, injected dopamine produces renal vasodilation, probably by binding to a specific dopaminergic receptor. In moderate doses, it also produces vasodilation of the mesenteric and coronary circulation and vasoconstriction peripherally. It has a positive inotropic effect on the heart, mediated by action on the β_1-adrenergic receptors. Moderate to large doses of dopamine increase the systolic blood pressure without affecting diastolic pressure.

Overview of Adrenal Medullary Disorders

Pheochromocytoma is an uncommon tumor of adrenal medullary tissue that causes the production of excessive amounts of catecholamines. Patients typically present with sustained or episodic hypertension or with a syndrome characterized by episodic palpitations, tachycardia, chest pain, headache, anxiety, pallor, excessive sweating, and hyperglycemia. Pheochromocytomas can usually be cured if diagnosed and treated properly. Pheochromocytomas are closely related to paragangliomas, which sometimes are termed extra-adrenal pheochromocytomas. Paragangliomas arise from paraganglia, which are cell conglomerates found in close proximity to the sympathetic and parasympathetic ganglia. Most parasympathetic paragangliomas are found in the head and neck area (eg, carotid body, vagal nerve) and often do not secrete any catecholamines. Most sympathetic paragangliomas arise in the abdomen and often secrete norepinephrine.

CHECKPOINT

1. What is the embryologic origin of the cells of the adrenal medulla?
2. Which nerve fibers innervate the adrenal medulla?
3. Which catecholamines are secreted by the human adrenal medulla? Of these, which is the major product?
4. What are the major physiologic stimuli of catecholamine secretion?
5. What are the subtypes and distribution of catecholamine receptors?
6. What physiologic processes do each subtype of catecholamine receptor control, and how do catecholamines bring about each of these physiologic processes?

PATHOPHYSIOLOGY OF SELECTED DISORDERS OF THE ADRENAL MEDULLA

Pheochromocytomas are the main pathological entity of the adrenal medulla. Other tumors of the adrenal medulla or its embryonic precursors include neuroblastomas and ganglioneuromas. Neuroblastomas are one of the most common tumors of early childhood. In response to therapy (or even spontaneously), neuroblastomas can differentiate into ganglioneuromas. Both of these tumors secrete catecholamines, but symptoms due to catecholamine excess are usually absent because catecholamine levels do not reach those observed with pheochromocytomas. The absence of the adrenal medulla (eg, after bilateral adrenalectomy) is usually well tolerated, though sometimes symptoms such as orthostatic hypotension may be observed.

PHEOCHROMOCYTOMA AND PARAGANGLIOMA

Pheochromocytomas are neoplasms of the chromaffin cells of the adrenal medulla or paraganglial cells of extramedullary sites (and hence termed paragangliomas). These tumors secrete excessive amounts of epinephrine, norepinephrine, or both; dopamine is rarely secreted. Most pheochromocytomas and paragangliomas secrete norepinephrine and cause sustained or episodic hypertension. Tumors that secrete epinephrine cause hypertension less often; more frequently, they produce episodic hyperglycemia, glucosuria, and other metabolic effects.

Table 12–2 summarizes the clinical features of pheochromocytomas. Pheochromocytomas and paragangliomas are uncommon, probably found in about 0.1% of all patients with hypertension and in approximately two to eight individuals per million in the population. They occur in both sexes and in all age groups but are most often diagnosed in the fourth or fifth decade of life. Children with pheochromocytomas are more likely to have a familial cancer syndrome and to present with multifocal and/or extra-adrenal tumors.

The diagnosis is important because a sudden release of catecholamines from these tumors during anesthesia, surgery, or obstetric delivery may prove fatal. Pheochromocytoma was classically referred to as the "tumor of tens" because it was previously believed that 10% are extra-adrenal, 10% are outside the abdomen, 10% are multiple, 10% are bilateral, 10% are asymptomatic, 10% are hereditary, and 10% are malignant. Recent research has proved this designation to be untrue. It is now appreciated that about 23% occur at extra-adrenal sites, that multifocal pheochromocytomas or paragangliomas can be found in roughly one-third of pediatric cases, that about 30–40% of cases are hereditary, and that up to 20% of cases are malignant.

Etiology

Several genetic syndromes, all transmitted in an autosomal dominant fashion, are associated with an increased risk of pheochromocytoma and sympathetic or parasympathetic nervous system paragangliomas. Most familial cases are caused by one of four syndromes: neurofibromatosis type 1 (NF1; also known as von Recklinghausen disease), von Hippel–Lindau syndrome, multiple endocrine neoplasia type 2 (MEN 2), and hereditary paraganglioma syndrome (Table 12–3). The genetic basis of these syndromes is now well defined.

Although not part of the diagnostic criteria, patients with NF1 have an increased incidence of pheochromocytoma caused by mutation of the *NF1* gene. Pheochromocytomas associated with NF1 often secrete both epinephrine and norepinephrine.

Pheochromocytoma is a frequent occurrence in patients with von Hippel–Lindau syndrome, a multiple-cancer predisposition syndrome caused by mutations of the *VHL* tumor suppressor gene. VHL-associated pheochromocytomas often secrete norepinephrine.

MEN 2 has two subtypes. In MEN 2A, patients develop pheochromocytomas as well as calcitonin-producing medullary thyroid carcinoma or C-cell hyperplasia of the thyroid and parathyroid hormone (PTH)–producing adenomas of the parathyroid (primary hyperparathyroidism). In MEN 2B, patients develop pheochromocytomas in association with medullary carcinoma of the thyroid and numerous oral mucosal neuromas, but no parathyroid adenomas. About 50% of patients with MEN 2A and MEN 2B have pheochromocytomas, often bilaterally. MEN 2–associated pheochromocytomas often predominately secrete epinephrine. A mutated *RET* proto-oncogene localized to chromosome 10q11.2 is responsible for MEN 2A and MEN 2B. The codon position of the *RET* mutation is related to disease phenotype. For example, mutations in *RET* at the specific codon 634 are associated with MEN 2A, and mutations at the specific codon 918 are associated with MEN 2B. These germline mutations of the *RET* proto-oncogene were the first examples of a dominantly acting oncogenic point mutation found to cause a heritable neoplasm in humans. Missense mutations in *RET* can be detected by DNA analysis, allowing for the identification of patients predisposed to MEN 2 to be screened for early detection and treatment of the associated neoplasms.

TABLE 12–2   Clinical features of pheochromocytoma and paraganglioma.

Epidemiology	Adults; both sexes; all ages, especially 30–50 years
Biologic behavior	80% benign; 20% malignant
Secretion	High levels of catecholamines; most secrete norepinephrine
Clinical presentation	Sustained or episodic hypertension, headaches, sweating, palpitations, hyperglycemia, glycosuria
	Occasionally asymptomatic (found incidentally on CT scan or MRI)
Macroscopic features	Mass, often hemorrhagic; 10% bilateral, ~23% extra-adrenal
Microscopic features	Nests of large cells, vascular stroma

Adapted, with permission, from Chandrasoma P et al, eds. *Concise Pathology*, 2nd ed. Originally published by Appleton & Lange. Copyright © 1994 by The McGraw-Hill Companies, Inc.

TABLE 12–3   Major genetic syndromes associated with pheochromocytoma and paraganglioma.

Syndrome	Clinical Features	Pheochromocytomas/Paragangliomas	Gene	Locus
MEN 2A	Medullary thyroid carcinoma	50% develop pheochromocytoma	RET	10q11.2
	Primary hyperparathyroidism	Bilateral, asynchronous pheochromocytoma		
	Pheochromocytoma			
MEN 2B	Medullary thyroid carcinoma		RET	10q11.2
	Pheochromocytoma			
	Ganglioneuromas			
	Oral mucosal neuromas			
	Marfanoid habitus			
NF1	Neurofibromas	0.1–5.0% develop pheochromocytoma (20–50% of hypertensive patients)	NF1	17q11.2
	Café-au-lait spots	12% malignant		
	Lisch nodules	Often bilateral		
	Plexiform neurofibromas			
	Sphenoid dysplasia			
	Optic gliomas			
	Axillary and inguinal freckling			
	Pheochromocytoma			
VHL	Hemangioblastomas (brain, spine, retina)	30% develop pheochromocytoma	VHL	3p26-25
	Clear-cell renal cell carcinoma			
	Pancreatic cysts and neuroendocrine tumors			
	Pheochromocytoma			
Hereditary PGL	Paraganglioma (parasympathetic or sympathetic)	25% of SDHB pheochromocytoma/paraganglioma cases are malignant	SDHD	3p26-25
	Pheochromocytoma	SDHD and SDHAF2 are paternally inherited	SDHAF2	11q12.2
	Clear-cell renal cell carcinoma		SDHC	1q21
	Gastrointestinal stromal tumor		SDHB	1q35-36
			SDHA	3q29
Hereditary PGL	Paraganglioma		TMEM127	2q11
	Pheochromocytoma			
	Clear-cell renal cell carcinoma			
Familial PGL	Pheochromocytoma	Often bilateral, sometimes multifocal	MAX	14q23
Hereditary leiomyomatosis and renal cell carcinoma syndrome	Uterine leiomyoma	Increased risk of malignant paraganglioma	FH	1q43
	Renal cell carcinoma (type 2 papillary)			
	Pheochromocytoma (rare)			
	Paraganglioma (rare)			
Polycythemia PGL syndrome	Polycythemia	Germline or somatic mosaic mutations	EPAS1	2p21
	Pheochromocytoma			
	Paraganglioma			
	Somatostatinoma			

MEN, multiple endocrine neoplasia; NF1, neurofibromatosis type 1; PGL, paraganglioma; SDH, succinate dehydrogenase; VHL, von Hippel–Lindau syndrome.

The most prevalent mutation in *RET* involves a cysteine residue at amino acid position 634. *RET* encodes a plasma membrane–associated tyrosine kinase that associates with a number of different related receptors. When these receptors are activated, they dimerize and bring two molecules of the RET tyrosine kinase close together, which initiates the cellular transmission of the signal. The 634-cysteine residue is part of an intramolecular sulfide bridge between associated cysteine residues. When one cysteine is absent, two RET molecules form intermolecular bridges, resulting in the initiation of intracellular signaling even in the absence of receptor association or ligand activation.

Hereditary paraganglioma syndromes are transmitted in an autosomal dominant fashion and most often are caused by germline mutations in genes coding for subcomponents of the succinate–dehydrogenase complex (*SDHD, SDHB, SDHC,* and rarely *SDHA* and *SDHAF2*) that serves as complex II of the mitochondrial respiratory chain. Extra-adrenal paragangliomas of the abdomen (*SDHB*) and head and neck area (*SDHD* and *SDHC*) are more common in patients with hereditary paraganglioma. *SDHD* (and *SDHAF2*) mutations are influenced by a "parent-of-origin effect." Affected patients always inherit the defective allele from their father. Individuals who inherit a mutant maternal allele do not exhibit an increased risk for a paraganglioma, but such carriers of a maternally inherited allele can transmit the defect to offspring. Patients with *SDHx* mutations are at risk for multiple primary paragangliomas in various locations, including adrenal pheochromocytoma, as well as other tumor types such as renal carcinomas and gastrointestinal stromal tumors. Recently, mutations have been identified in other genes, including *TMEM127, MAX, FH,* and *EPAS1,* which can more rarely cause hereditary pheochromocytomas and/or paragangliomas.

SDHx and *VHL* mutations cause perturbations in the same intracellular signaling cascade typically induced by hypoxia, thereby leading to a "pseudo-hypoxia" state. *SDHx* mutations lead to an accumulation of succinate, which in turn inhibits an enzyme that hydroxylates the transcription factor hypoxia-inducible factor α (HIF1α.) Normally, the hydroxylated HIF1α is recognized by the VHL protein and marked for destruction by the proteosome. Therefore, *SDHx* mutations and *VHL* mutations essentially protect HIF1α from degradation. This protection leads to an increase in HIF1α-induced transcription of downstream genes in the hypoxia pathway, which is in part responsible for the neoplastic phenotype.

Germline mutations in *NF1, RET, VHL, SDHx,* and others account for up to 30–40% of cases of pheochromocytomas and paragangliomas. Given the high frequency of germline mutations, genetic counseling and genetic testing are recommended for all patients with pheochromocytomas or paragangliomas, particularly those with a positive family history, multifocal disease, or a diagnosis before age 50 years. If a patient tests positive for a susceptibility gene mutation, their blood relatives should be offered genetic counseling and testing, and if positive for a gene mutation, those relatives can be screened for early detection of disease. Almost all pheochromocytomas and

FIGURE 12–3 Cross-section of adrenal, showing a pheochromocytoma and hyperplasia of the medulla in a patient with multiple endocrine neoplasia type 2a. The patient also had a medullary carcinoma of the thyroid and a large pheochromocytoma in the contralateral adrenal. (Reproduced, with permission, from Chandrasoma P et al, eds. *Concise Pathology,* 3rd ed. Originally published by Appleton & Lange. Copyright © 1998 by The McGraw-Hill Companies, Inc.)

paragangliomas (at least 80%) occur in the abdomen, and most of these are in the adrenal medulla. Extra-adrenal paragangliomas (including sympathetic and parasympathetic paragangliomas) are found in the para-aortic and perirenal area, the organ of Zuckerkandl, the urinary bladder, the heart, the neck, and the posterior mediastinum (see Figure 12–1). Some of these tumors can lead to very specific symptoms (eg, urinary bladder paraganglioma can cause a hypertensive crisis with voiding). Grossly, pheochromocytomas and paragangliomas are generally well circumscribed but vary in size, with weights ranging from less than 1 g to several kilograms (Figure 12–3). They are highly vascular tumors and frequently have cystic, necrotic, or hemorrhagic areas. Microscopically, the tumor consists of large pleomorphic cells arranged in sheets separated by a highly vascular stroma. In the cytoplasm, there are catecholamine-containing storage granules similar to those in normal adrenal medullary cells. Mitoses are rare, but tumor invasion of the adrenal capsule and blood vessels is common even in benign pheochromocytomas and paragangliomas. About 20% of pheochromocytomas and paragangliomas are malignant. Malignancy is established only when a metastasis occurs in a site where chromaffin cells are not usually found (eg, liver, lung, bone, brain). Unfavorable prognostic factors suggesting a malignant course include large tumor size, extra-adrenal location, younger age, dopamine secretion, and *SDHB* mutation.

Pathogenesis

Most pheochromocytomas and paragangliomas predominantly release norepinephrine, and many also release epinephrine (Table 12–4). Rarely, a pheochromocytoma releases predominantly or only epinephrine; even more rarely, paragangliomas can predominantly secrete dopamine.

In about half of patients with a pheochromocytoma or a paraganglioma, clinical manifestations vary in intensity and occur in an episodic or paroxysmal fashion. The paroxysms are related to sudden catecholamine discharge from the tumor. The sudden catecholamine excess causes hypertension,

TABLE 12–4 Pathophysiologic and clinical manifestations of catecholamine excess.

Target Tissue	Physiologic Effect	Catecholamine Excess	
		Pathophysiologic Manifestations	Clinical Manifestations
Heart	Increased heart rate	Tachycardia	Palpitations
		Tachyarrhythmia	Angina pectoris
	Increased contractility	Increased myocardial O_2 consumption	Angina pectoris
		Myocarditis	Heart failure
		Cardiomyopathy	
Blood vessels	Arteriolar constriction	Hypertension	Headache
			Heart failure
			Angina pectoris
	Venoconstriction	Decreased plasma volume	Dizziness
			Orthostatic hypotension
			Circulatory collapse
Gut	Intestinal relaxation	Impaired intestinal motility	Ileus
			Obstipation
Pancreas (B cells)	Suppression of insulin release	Carbohydrate intolerance	Hyperglycemia
			Glucosuria
Liver	Increased glucose output	Carbohydrate intolerance	Hyperglycemia
			Glucosuria
Adipose	Lipolysis	Increased free fatty acids	Weight loss
Skin (apocrine glands)	Stimulation	Sweating	Diaphoresis
Bladder neck	Contraction	Elevated urethral pressures	Urinary retention
Most tissues	Increased basal metabolic rate	Increased heat production	Heat intolerance
			Sweating
			Weight loss

Data from Werbel SS et al. Pheochromocytoma: update on diagnosis, localization, and management. Med Clin North Am. 1995;79:131.

palpitations, tachycardia, chest pain, headache, anxiety, blanching, and excessive sweating. Such paroxysms usually occur several times a week but may occur only once every few months or up to 25 times daily. Paroxysms typically last for 15 minutes or less but may last for days. As time passes, the paroxysms usually become more frequent but generally do not change in character. A typical paroxysm may be produced by activities that compress the tumor (eg, bending, lifting, exercise, defecation, eating, deep palpation of the abdomen) and by emotional distress or anxiety.

Other patients have persistently secreting tumors and more chronic symptoms, including sustained hypertension. However, such patients also usually experience paroxysms related to transient increases in catecholamine release. The long-term exposure to high levels of circulating catecholamines seems not to produce the classic hemodynamic responses observed after the acute administration of catecholamines. This may be due in part to desensitization of the cardiovascular system to catecholamines and may explain why some patients with a pheochromocytoma or a paraganglioma are entirely asymptomatic.

Clinical Manifestations

The clinical manifestations of pheochromocytoma and paraganglioma result from the increased secretion of epinephrine and norepinephrine. Table 12–5 lists commonly reported manifestations.

TABLE 12–5   Clinical findings in pheochromocytoma.

Symptoms	Frequency (%)
Spells	67
Headache	59
Palpitations	50
Diaphoresis	50
Fainting episode	40
Bone pain	35
Weight loss	30
Anxiety	19
Nausea, vomiting	19
Dizziness	18
Flushing	14
Weakness, fatigue	14
Abdominal pain	14
Dyspnea	13
Paresthesias	13
Chest pain	12
Constipation	11
Flank pain	7
Visual symptoms	7
Diarrhea	6
Signs	
Hypertension	92
Sustained	48
Paroxysmal	44
Fever	28
Tachycardia	15
Orthostatic hypotension	12
Palpable mass	8
Shock	4
Laboratory findings	
Hyperglycemia	42
Hypercalcemia	4
Polycythemia	3

Data from Werbel SS et al. Pheochromocytoma: update on diagnosis, localization, and management. Med Clin North Am. 1995;79:131.

The classical pentad of symptoms in patients with a pheochromocytoma or a paraganglioma consists of headache, palpitation, perspiration, pallor, and orthostasis. The most common presenting feature is hypertension. In about half of cases, hypertension is sustained but the blood pressure shows marked fluctuations, with peak pressures during symptomatic paroxysms. During a hypertensive episode, the systolic blood pressure can rise to as high as 300 mm Hg. In about one-third of cases, hypertension is truly intermittent. In some individuals, hypertension is absent. The blood pressure elevation caused by the catecholamine excess results from two mechanisms: α-adrenergic receptor–mediated arteriolar vasoconstriction, leading to an increase in peripheral resistance; and β_1 receptor–mediated increases in cardiac output and in renin release, leading to increased circulating levels of angiotensin II. The increased total peripheral vascular resistance is probably primarily responsible for the maintenance of high arterial pressures.

Hypertensive crisis may be precipitated by a variety of drugs, including tricyclic antidepressants, antidopaminergic agents, metoclopramide, and naloxone. Beta blockers should not be administered until alpha blockade has been established. Otherwise, blockade of β_2-adrenergic receptors, which promote vasodilation, will allow unopposed α-adrenergic receptor activation and produce marked vasoconstriction and hypertension.

Peripheral vasoconstriction, mediated by α receptors, causes both facial pallor and cool, moist hands and feet. Chronic vasoconstriction of the arterial and venous beds leads to a reduction in plasma volume and predisposes to postural hypotension. In others, orthostatic hypotension is associated with decreased cardiac stroke volume and an impaired response of total peripheral vascular resistance to changes in posture, perhaps indicative of diminished arteriolar and venous responsiveness. The reduced responsiveness of the vasculature to norepinephrine in patients with a pheochromocytoma or a paraganglioma is probably related to the downregulation of α-adrenergic receptors resulting from persistently elevated norepinephrine levels.

Table 12–6 summarizes the complications of pheochromocytoma and paraganglioma. If unrecognized and untreated, pheochromocytoma and paraganglioma may be complicated by hypertensive retinopathy (retinal hemorrhages or papilledema); nephropathy; myocardial infarction, resulting from either myocarditis or coronary artery vasospasm; pulmonary edema, secondary either to left-sided heart failure or noncardiogenic causes; and stroke from cerebral infarction, intracranial hemorrhage, or embolism. Cerebral infarction results from hypercoagulability, vasospasm, or both. Hemorrhage occurs secondary to severe arterial hypertension. Emboli can originate in mural thrombi in patients with dilated cardiomyopathy. Cardiomyopathy during a catecholamine surge often resembles takotsubo (stress/catecholamine-induced) cardiomyopathy (the so-called "broken heart" syndrome). Takotsubo cardiomyopathy may be a presenting sign in patients with undiagnosed pheochromocytoma or paraganglioma. In

TABLE 12-6   Complications of pheochromocytoma and paraganglioma.

Cardiovascular	Renal
Arrhythmias	Renal artery stenosis (resulting from kinking by adrenal mass)
Ventricular tachycardia	Renal infarction
Torsades de pointes	**Endocrine and metabolic**
Wolff–Parkinson–White syndrome	Hyperglycemia, glucose intolerance, diabetic ketoacidosis
Ventricular fibrillation	Hypoglycemia
ECG changes	Thyrotoxicosis (transient)
ST segment elevations or depressions	Reactivation of Graves disease
Inverted or flattened T waves	Hypercalcemia
Prolonged QT intervals	Lactic acidosis
High or peaked P waves	Fever
Cardiomyopathy	**Skeletal**
Dilated	Osseous microthrombi (from hemoconcentration)
Hypertrophic	Brachydactyly
Left ventricular hypertrophy	**Skin**
Myocarditis	Leukocytoclastic vasculitis
Subendocardial, intramyocardial hemorrhages	**Crisis**
Acute myocardial infarction	Obtundation, shock, disseminated intravascular coagulation, seizures, rhabdomyolysis, acute renal failure, death
Pulmonary	
Pulmonary edema (noncardiogenic)	
Gastrointestinal	
Ileus	
Obstipation	
Megacolon	
Acute abdominal pain	

pregnancy, pheochromocytoma may lead to significant maternal morbidity and fetal demise.

The metabolic effects of excessive levels of circulating catecholamines increase both blood glucose and free fatty acid levels. Increased glycolysis and glycogenolysis, combined with an α-adrenergic receptor–mediated inhibition of insulin release, cause an increase in blood sugar levels. In addition, epinephrine stimulates glucose production by gluconeogenesis and decreases insulin-mediated glucose uptake by peripheral tissues such as skeletal muscle. In pheochromocytoma, impaired glucose homeostasis may also result from β-adrenergic receptor desensitization, which produces relative insulin resistance. Glucose intolerance is common, and diabetes mellitus may occur.

Epinephrine raises blood lactate concentrations by stimulating glycogenolysis and glycolysis. An increase in oxygen consumption from the catecholamine stimulation of metabolism occurs in combination with a decrease in oxygen delivery to tissues from vasoconstriction, leading to lactate accumulation.

Occasionally, pheochromocytomas may also produce peptide hormones leading to specific paraneoplastic phenomena. For example, hypercalcemia may occur, related to an excessive production of PTH-related peptide (PTHrP) in cases of malignant pheochromocytomas (similar to some other malignancies). Hypercalcemia may also occur as a result of the excessive production of PTH itself in cases of MEN 2A in which pheochromocytoma occurs in conjunction with primary hyperparathyroidism. Very rarely, the ectopic production of adrenocorticotropic hormone (ACTH) by pheochromocytoma may lead to "ectopic" Cushing syndrome. Rare cases have been described in which a pheochromocytoma produces vasoactive intestinal peptide (VIP) (causing severe diarrhea), growth hormone–releasing hormone (GHRH) (causing acromegaly), corticotropin-releasing hormone (CRH) (causing Cushing syndrome), insulin (causing hypoglycemia), or other peptide hormones.

An increase in metabolic rate may cause weight loss (or, in children, lack of weight gain), and impaired heat loss from peripheral vasoconstriction may cause a mild elevation of basal body temperature, heat intolerance, flushing, or increased sweating.

During paroxysms, patients may experience marked anxiety, and when episodes are prolonged or severe, there may be visual disturbances, paresthesias, or seizures. A feeling of fatigue or exhaustion usually follows these episodes. Some patients present with psychosis or confusion.

There may be abdominal discomfort resulting from a large adrenal or extra-adrenal mass. Remarkably, some patients with pheochromocytomas or paragangliomas are entirely asymptomatic.

Somewhat different clinical manifestations occur with predominantly epinephrine-releasing pheochromocytomas. Symptoms and signs include hypotension, prominent tachycardia, widened pulse pressure, cardiac arrhythmias, and noncardiogenic pulmonary edema. Acute hemorrhagic necrosis of the tumor may present initially as acute abdominal pain with marked hypertension, followed by hypotension, shock, and sudden death as a consequence of the sudden cessation of catecholamine production ("fulminant pheochromocytoma crisis"). Death may also result from cardiovascular collapse secondary to prolonged vasoconstriction and loss of blood volume into the interstitium.

Patients with pure epinephrine-producing pheochromocytomas may be hypotensive because of epinephrine-induced peripheral vasodilation. Other patients with severe arterial vasoconstriction may appear to be in shock. In still others, the prolonged vasoconstriction of a hypertensive crisis may lead to shock.

Diagnosis

Pheochromocytoma and paraganglioma are diagnosed by demonstrating abnormally high concentrations of catecholamines or their breakdown products in the plasma or urine. Increases in plasma metanephrine and normetanephrine concentrations are greater and more consistent than increases in plasma catecholamines. Pheochromocytoma tumor cells produce large amounts of metanephrines from catecholamines leaking into the cytoplasm from vesicular stores and metabolized by catechol-O-methyltransferase (COMT) present in pheochromocytoma cells. Thus, the elevated plasma levels of free metanephrine and normetanephrine in patients with pheochromocytoma are probably due mostly to metabolism

before, and not after, the release of catecholamines into the circulation. These metabolites are particularly useful for detecting pheochromocytomas. There is a long list of medications and drugs that can lead to false positive tests, and patients, especially those with indeterminate levels of metanephrines and catecholamines, should be taken off these if possible and retested before the diagnosis of a pheochromocytoma or a paraganglioma is made.

In addition to these catecholamine metabolites, plasma levels of chromogranin A (a substance found in chromaffin granules) are significantly higher in patients with pheochromocytomas, especially those with malignant tumors. For malignant pheochromocytomas, serum chromogranin A levels can also be monitored during chemotherapy of malignant pheochromocytomas to gauge tumor response and to detect relapse. However, chromogranin A is a nonspecific marker for a pheochromocytoma and a paraganglioma and several medications, including proton pump inhibitors, can increase chromogranin A levels.

Administration of the antihypertensive agent clonidine can be used to differentiate essential hypertension from hypertension caused by pheochromocytoma or paraganglioma. This is especially useful in cases in which plasma or urine metanephrine/catecholamine levels are indeterminate. Clonidine is a potent α_2 agonist that stimulates α_2 receptors in the brain, reducing sympathetic outflow and blood pressure. A dose of 0.3 mg of clonidine is given orally, and blood pressure and plasma catecholamine levels are determined periodically over the next 3 hours. Essential hypertension depends partly on centrally mediated catecholamine release. Normally, administering clonidine suppresses sympathetic nervous system activity and substantially lowers plasma norepinephrine levels, reducing blood pressure. However, in patients with a pheochromocytoma or a paraganglioma, the drug has little or no effect on plasma catecholamine levels because the tumor behaves autonomously. Thus, blood pressure remains unchanged.

Once a diagnosis of a pheochromocytoma or paraganglioma is made, the next step is to localize the neoplasm or neoplasms radiographically to permit surgical removal. Computed tomography (CT) or magnetic resonance imaging (MRI) can be used in tumor localization. CT and MRI have good sensitivity but poor specificity for detecting pheochromocytomas. Nuclear imaging studies such as iodine-123–metaiodobenzylguanidine (^{123}I-MIBG) scintigraphy have limited sensitivity but better specificity in diagnosis. For example, the specificity of ^{123}I-MIBG scintigraphy is very good for confirming that a tumor is a pheochromocytoma or a paraganglioma and for ruling out metastases, but not all tumors are MIBG avid, limiting the test's sensitivity. In addition, 6-[fluorine-18]-fluorodopamine positron emission tomography (PET) can aid in both tumor diagnosis and localization in patients with positive biochemical test results. Some pheochromocytomas and paragangliomas also express somatostatin receptors and can be imaged with an octreotide scan or a Gallium-68-DOTATATE-PET scan, which uses radiolabeled somatostatin receptor agonists.

Treatment

Surgical resection is the main treatment for a pheochromocytoma and a paraganglioma. Nevertheless, any surgery in patients with pheochromocytoma or paraganglioma, including resection of the tumor itself, involves the risk of significant complications, including stroke and death. Operative and postoperative complications are directly associated with preoperative systolic blood pressure, tumor size, excretion of urinary catecholamines and their metabolites, duration of anesthesia, and number of previous surgeries. Patients with a pheochromocytoma or paraganglioma must be treated with the proper adrenergic blockade with medication prior to any surgical or interventional procedure. Understanding the pathophysiology of the hormonal secretion is critically important in preparing the patient for surgery. For example, as noted previously, it is important that hypertension not be treated with β blockers, which could cause a paradoxical worsening of hypertension by allowing unopposed α stimulation. Instead, an α receptor blocker, such as phenoxybenzamine, a noncompetitive antagonist, should be used as treatment of catecholamine-induced hypertension. Other medications that can be used impair catecholamine production, such as methyltyrosine, which blocks the enzyme tyrosine hydroxylase.

CHECKPOINT

7. What genetic mutations are found in patients with pheochromocytoma?
8. What are the symptoms and signs of pheochromocytoma?
9. What are some complications of untreated pheochromocytoma?
10. What are the metabolic and neurologic effects of pheochromocytoma?
11. How is the diagnosis of pheochromocytoma made?

CASE STUDIES

Yeong Kwok, MD

(See Chapter 25, p. 770 for answers)

CASE 66

A 39-year-old woman comes to the office complaining of episodic anxiety, headache, and palpitations. She states that without dieting, she has lost 15 pounds over the past 6 months. The physical examination is normal except for a blood pressure of 200/100 mm Hg and a resting pulse rate of 110 bpm. The chart review shows that prior blood pressures have always been normal, including one 6 months ago. A diagnosis of pheochromocytoma is entertained.

Questions

A. What other features of the history should be elicited? Why is family history important?
B. What laboratory tests should be ordered, and what results should be anticipated? If the laboratory tests are nondiagnostic but suspicion is high, what other test can be done?
C. What is the pathogenesis of the symptoms of anxiety, headache, palpitations, and weight loss in pheochromocytomas?

REFERENCES

General

Fitzgerald PA. Adrenal medulla and paraganglia. In: Gardner DG et al, eds. *Greenspan's Basic & Clinical Endocrinology*, 10th ed. McGraw-Hill, 2017.

Kwatampora L et al. Endocrine malignancies. In: Kantarjian HM et al, eds. *The MD Anderson Manual of Medical Oncology*, 3rd ed. McGraw-Hill, 2016.

Pheochromocytoma & Paraganglioma

Barron J. Phaeochromocytoma: diagnostic challenges for biochemical screening and diagnosis. J Clin Pathol. 2010 Aug;63(8):669–74. [PMID: 20547690]

Chen Y et al. Accuracy of plasma free metanephrines in the diagnosis of pheochromocytoma and paraganglioma: a systematic review and meta-analysis. Endocr Pract. 2017 Oct;23(10):1178–92. [PMID: 28704094]

Eisenhofer G et al. Diagnostic tests and biomarkers for pheochromocytoma and extra-adrenal paraganglioma: from routine laboratory methods to disease stratification. Endocr Pathol. 2012 Mar;23(1):4–14. [PMID: 22180288]

Eisenhofer G et al. Supine or sitting? Economic and other considerations for the use of plasma metanephrines for diagnosis of pheochromocytoma. Clin Endocrinol. 2015 Mar; 82(3):463–4. [PMID: 25186957]

Else T. 15 years of paraganglioma: pheochromocytoma, paraganglioma and genetic syndromes: a historical perspective. Endocr Relat Cancer. 2015 Aug:22(4):T147–59. [PMID: 26273101]

Favier J et al. Paraganglioma and pheochromocytoma: from genetics to personalized medicine. Nat Rev Endocrinol. 2015 Feb;11(2):101–11. [PMID: 25385035]

Fishbein L. Pheochromocytoma and paraganglioma: genetics, diagnosis and treatment. Hematol Oncol Clin North Am. 2016 Feb;30(1):135–50. [PMID: 26614373]

Gagnon N et al. Takotsubo-like cardiomyopathy in a large cohort of patients with pheochromocytoma and paraganglioma. Endocr Pract. 2017 Oct;23(10):1178–92. [PMID: 28704094]

Galetta F et al. Cardiovascular complications in patients with pheochromocytoma: a mini-review. Biomed Pharmacother. 2010 Sep; 64(7):505–9. [PMID: 20580187]

Gimm O et al. Malignant pheochromocytomas and paragangliomas: a diagnostic challenge. Langenbecks Arch Surg. 2012 Feb;397(2):155–77. [PMID: 22124609]

Harari A et al. Malignant pheochromocytoma: a review. Am J Surg. 2011 May;201(5):700–8. [PMID: 20870212]

Lenders J et al. Pheochromocytoma and paraganglioma: an Endocrine Society Clinical Practice Guideline. J Clin Endocrinol Metab. 2014 Jun;99(6):1915–42. [PMID: 24893135]

Prejbisz A et al. Cardiovascular manifestations of phaeochromocytoma. J Hypertens. 2011 Nov;29(11):2049–60. [PMID: 21826022]

Roman-Gonzalez A et al. Malignant pheochromocytoma-paraganglioma: pathogenesis and TNM staging and current clinical trials. Curr Opin Endocrinol Diabetes Obes. 2017 Jun:24(3):174–83. [PMID: 28234804]

Sarathi V. Characteristics of pediatric pheochromocytoma/paraganglioma. Indian J Endocrinol Metab. 2017 May-Jun;21(3):470–4. [PMID: 28553607]

Tischler AS et al. 15 years of paraganglioma: pathology of pheochromocytoma and paraganglioma. Endocr Relat Cancer. 2015 Aug;22(4):T123–33. [PMID: 26136457]

Gastrointestinal Disease

Jason C. Mills, MD, PhD, AGAF, & Matthew A. Ciorba, MD

Gastrointestinal (GI) diseases most often present with one or more of four common classes of symptoms and signs: (1) abdominal or chest pain; (2) altered ingestion of food (eg, resulting from nausea, vomiting, **dysphagia** [difficulty swallowing], **odynophagia** [painful swallowing], or **anorexia** [lack of appetite]); (3) altered bowel movements (ie, diarrhea or constipation); and (4) GI tract bleeding, either occurring without warning or preceded by one or more of the foregoing (Table 13–1). However, not all cases of a particular GI disease present in the same way. For example, peptic ulcer disease, although typically accompanied by abdominal pain, may be painless.

GI disease may be limited to the GI tract (eg, reflux esophagitis, peptic ulcer, diverticular disease), be a manifestation of a systemic disorder (eg, inflammatory bowel disease), or present as a systemic disease resulting from a primary GI pathologic process (eg, vitamin deficiencies resulting from malabsorption). Because different parts of the GI tract are specialized for certain functions, the most prominent causes, consequences, and manifestations of disease differ from one anatomic site to another.

Acutely, GI disease can be complicated by dehydration, sepsis, or bleeding or by their consequences, such as shock. **Dehydration** can occur as a consequence of even subtle alterations in fluid input or outflow because the volume of fluid traversing the GI tract daily is enormous (see later discussion). **Sepsis** can result from disruption of the barrier function against pathogens in the environment, including bacteria resident in the colon. The tendency for **bleeding** is a reflection of the tremendous vascularity of the GI tract and the difficulty of applying pressure at the site of bleeding.

Chronically, GI disease can be complicated by malnutrition and deficiency states. These occur because many primary GI diseases result in **malabsorption** (failure to absorb one or more necessary nutrients in ingested food).

GI tract disease can present as partial or complete **obstruction** (blockage of movement of contents down the GI tract) caused by **adhesions** and **stenosis** resulting from the proliferation of connective tissue in response to inflammation. The symptoms and signs of obstruction can range from mild nausea, abdominal pain, and anorexia to projectile vomiting and rebound tenderness. In severe cases, obstruction can result in perforation, infarction and bleeding, hypotension, shock, sepsis, and death. The severity of symptoms depends on the extent of obstruction, the degree to which the obstruction compromises blood flow to the affected region, and the stage in the natural history of the process at which the patient presents for medical attention.

CHECKPOINT

1. What are the cardinal symptoms and signs of GI disease?
2. What are some acute systemic complications of primary GI disease?
3. What additional systemic manifestations can occur as a result of chronic GI disease?

STRUCTURE, FUNCTION & CONTROL OF THE GI TRACT

STRUCTURE OF THE GI TRACT

The GI tract is one of the most complex and important organ systems. It comprises the alimentary canal, a hollow structure extending from the mouth to the anus, and associated glandular organs that empty their contents into the canal (Figure 13–1). The alimentary canal is 7–9 m in the adult and includes the mouth, esophagus (23–25 cm), stomach, small

TABLE 13–1   Common presentations of GI disease.

Cardinal GI Symptom or Sign	Esophagus	Stomach	Intestines	Gallbladder
Pain	Achalasia, reflux	Gastric ulcer	Duodenal ulcer	Cholelithiasis
		Gastric cancer	Irritable bowel syndrome	
			Diverticular disease	
Altered ingestion				
Dysphagia	Achalasia, reflux			
Nausea, vomiting	Achalasia, reflux	Gastroparesis	Acute gastroenteritis	Cholelithiasis
	Esophageal cancer		Obstruction	
Altered bowel movements				
Constipation			Diverticular disease	
			Diabetic autonomic neuropathy	
Diarrhea (including steatorrhea)		Gastric surgery, dumping syndrome	Gastroenteritis	Cholelithiasis
			Irritable bowel syndrome	
			Inflammatory bowel disease	
			Diabetic autonomic neuropathy	
Bleeding				
Hematemesis	Varices resulting from portal hypertension	Gastric ulcer	Duodenal ulcer	
		Mucosal laceration (eg, after violent retching)		
Bloody stools (including melena, frank blood, and occult blood)	Varices	Gastric ulcer	Inflammatory bowel disease	
			Duodenal ulcer	
			Diverticular disease	
			Colon cancer	
			Gastroenteritis	
			Infarction	

intestine (duodenum, jejunum, ileum; 6–7 m), large intestine (cecum and colon; 1.0–1.5 m), rectum, and anus. The canal is connected to the salivary glands, the pancreas, and the gallbladder, the sources of **exocrine** secretions that play an essential role in digestion.

The wall of the GI tract is composed of four main layers. From the lumen outward, these include the **mucosa, submucosa, muscularis externa,** and **serosa** (Figure 13–2). The precise structure of some of these layers, most notably the mucosa, varies from one region of the GI tract to the next. The **mucosa** has three components: specialized epithelial cells that line the lumen; the underlying **lamina propria,** a layer of connective tissue that contains small blood and lymphatic vessels, immune cells, and nerve fibers; and the **muscularis**

mucosa, a thin layer of muscle cells. The muscularis mucosa is an important boundary in determining whether cancer of the GI tract is still localized to its site of origin or is likely to have metastasized (ie, spread to distant regions of the body). The **submucosa** is a layer of loose connective tissue directly beneath the mucosa containing larger blood and lymphatic vessels and a nerve plexus of the intrinsic or **enteric nervous system,** termed the **submucosal nerve (Meissner) plexus.** This nerve plexus is particularly important for secretion control in the GI tract. In some areas, the submucosa also contains glands and lymphoid tissue. The **muscularis externa** is composed of an inner circular and an outer longitudinal layer of smooth muscle and is responsible for the motility of the GI tract. Between these muscle layers lies the **myenteric nerve (Auerbach) plexus,** a

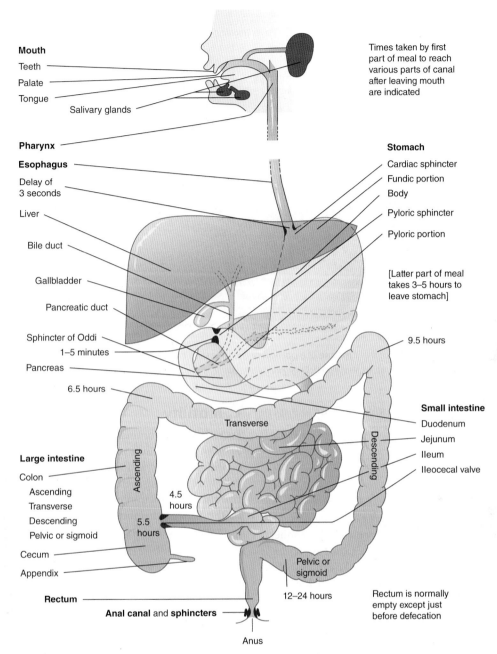

FIGURE 13–1 Progress of food along the alimentary canal. Food undergoes both mechanical and chemical changes to render it suitable for absorption and assimilation. (Redrawn, with permission, from Mackenna BR et al, eds. *Illustrated Physiology*, 6th ed. Churchill Livingstone, 1997. Copyright © Elsevier.)

division of the enteric nervous system that regulates motility. The **serosa** is an outer sheath of squamous mesothelial cells and connective tissues, where larger nerves and blood vessels travel in a bed of connective and adipose tissue.

FUNCTIONS OF THE GI TRACT

The overall function of the GI tract is to take in nutrients and process them into a form that can be used by the body and to eliminate wastes. The major physiological processes that occur in the GI tract are **digestion**, **secretion**, **motility**, and **absorption**.

A. Digestion

Food is taken into the mouth as large particles containing macromolecules that are not immediately absorbable into the body. **Digestion** is the process that converts nutrients in food to products that can be **absorbed** by cells of the mucosa. Digestion includes **physical processes** (eg, chewing, GI contractions) that break up the food, mix it with digestive secretions, and propel it along the alimentary canal, and **chemical processes** (involving digestive enzymes) that degrade food components (proteins, fats, polysaccharides) to products that can be absorbed (amino acids, fatty acids, monosaccharides). Digestive enzymes arise from exocrine glands (salivary gland, pancreas, gallbladder, and

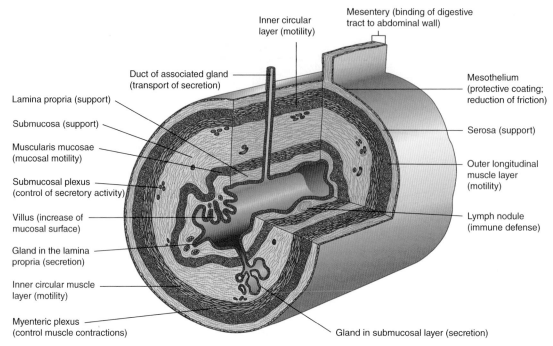

FIGURE 13–2 Schematic illustration of the structure of a portion of the digestive tract with various possible components. (Redrawn, with permission, from Bevelander G. *Outline of Histology*, 7th ed. Mosby, 1971. Copyright © Elsevier.)

liver) and from cells and glands in the mucosa or are found on the apical surface of certain epithelial cells.

B. Secretion

During the process of digestion, large volumes of fluid are **secreted** into the lumen of the GI tract. Secretions arise from exocrine glands (salivary glands, pancreas, gallbladder) and from epithelial cells lining the GI lumen (or glands that connect to the lumen). The daily fluid load in the GI tract is approximately 2 L of oral intake and 7 L of secretions (1.5 L saliva, 2.5 L gastric juice, 0.5 L bile, 1.5 L pancreatic juice, and 1 L intestinal secretions). From this total of 9 L, approximately 100 mL ends up in stool daily; the balance is recycled (Figure 13–3).

Flow rate mL/d	\multicolumn{4}{c}{Ion concentrations mEq/L}	Osmolality mOsm/kg
	Na^+	K^+	Cl^-	HCO_3^-	
9000	60	15	60	15	Variable
3000	140	6	100	30	Isotonic
1000	140	8	60	70	Isotonic
100	40	90	15	30	Isotonic

Colon absorption capacity (3–4 L/d)

FIGURE 13–3 Approximate flow rates per day and ionic constituents of fluid passing through different levels of the intestine. (Redrawn, with permission, from Schiller et al. Diarrhea. In: Feldman M et al, eds. *Sleisenger and Fordtran's Gastrointestinal and Liver Disease*, 10th ed. Elsevier, 2016.)

C. Motility

Secretions and luminal contents are moved from mouth to anus and mixed by a process termed **motility** because of the coordinated contractions of smooth muscle. Smooth muscle cells have a resting membrane potential (small excess of negative charge) in their interior as a result of the activity of pumps in the plasma membrane. When a cell is depolarized, this potential difference is transiently abolished, generating a signal that (1) causes contraction of actin and myosin filaments and (2) is propagated to neighboring cells, resulting in the coordinated response of muscle contraction. Depolarization of a cell can occur spontaneously or in response to a neural or hormonal stimulus depending on the specific characteristics of different cells. GI smooth muscle displays differences in contractile properties in different regions of the tract. "Slow-wave" oscillating depolarizations occur in some areas, and rapid "spike" depolarizations occur in other areas. Each type occurs with a characteristic intrinsic frequency, but each can also be triggered by specific stimuli such as stretch, neuronal input, or hormones. Short bursts of spikes cause phasic motor activity; longer bursts cause tonic muscle contraction. Tonic contraction occurs at **sphincters** ("gates" that allow further movement down the GI tract only during relaxation). Phasic electrical activity occurs at the intervening regions of the GI tract (between sphincters).

D. Absorption

The products of digestion (amino acids, small peptides, monosaccharides, fatty acids) are taken into the body by the process of **absorption**. Absorbed molecules can pass across (**transcellular route**) or between (**paracellular route**) the epithelial cells lining the intestine to enter the blood or lymphatic systems. In general, this transport can occur by either a **passive**, energy-independent mechanism that occurs down an **electrochemical gradient** (of charge or concentration) or by an **active**, energy-requiring process that occurs against an electrochemical gradient. **Passive transport** can occur by simple **diffusion** (random molecular motion) of uncharged molecules that readily pass the lipid layer plasma membrane. In this manner, short-chain fatty acids are absorbed in the small intestine. Charged molecules that cannot cross the plasma membrane diffuse through specialized **channels** (transmembrane proteins) within the apical and basolateral membrane of epithelial cells. For instance, water is absorbed by diffusion through aquaporins (proteins that form water channels) in the small intestine. Some molecules that are absorbed by diffusion bind to transporter proteins in the plasma membrane that facilitate their transfer into the cell (**facilitated diffusion**). For example, fructose is absorbed into epithelial cells of the small intestine by facilitated diffusion through the apical membrane GLUT-5 transporter.

Active transport requires metabolic energy. There are two classes of active transport. In **primary active transport**, the transport molecule itself hydrolyzes adenosine triphosphate (ATP). An example of primary active transport is the Na^+-K^+ ATPase found in the basolateral membrane of intestinal epithelial cells, which expels three Na^+ ions from cells in exchange for two K^+ ions that are pumped into the cell. This unequal transport of ions generates a transmembrane potential (negative inside; ie, transport is **electrogenic**). In **secondary active transport**, the transporter itself does not hydrolyze ATP, but transport depends on an electrochemical gradient that has been established by primary active transport. The Na^+-K^+ ATPase maintains a low intracellular Na^+ concentration and an inside negative potential in epithelial cells, thereby providing the electrochemical gradient for the secondary active transport of many absorbed molecules. For example, glucose is absorbed against a concentration gradient across the apical membrane of epithelial cells in the small intestine by secondary active transport with Na^+ ions by the SGLT1 transporter. Two Na^+ ions are transported down their electrochemical gradient (generated by the Na^+-K^+ ATPase), dragging with them one glucose molecule. For large molecules such as proteins, transport occurs by pinching off from, and fusion of membrane vesicles with, the plasma membrane. These processes are termed **endocytosis** (uptake into epithelial cells) and **exocytosis** (export out of epithelial cells).

In addition to the major roles of the GI tract related to digestion and absorption, the digestive tract has other functions essential for the maintenance of health and homeostasis.

E. Defense

The mucosa of the GI tract is the largest surface of the body exposed to the environment, and the gut, like the skin, must protect the body from the external environment. Defense involves protection against ingested toxins, bacteria, and viruses, as well as the bacteria and toxins that normally exist in the large intestine (Table 13–2). The magnitude of the problem is illustrated by the observation that there are more bacterial cells in the human colon than cells in the entire body. Defense involves two mechanisms:

1. **Adaptive immune defense**—The mucosal immune system or gut-associated lymphoid tissue (GALT) surveys the contents of the intestinal lumen through a variety of mechanisms that use cells of both myeloid and lymphoid lineages. Myeloid-derived cells (specific populations of dendritic cells and macrophages) extend processes that interact with the intestinal epithelial barrier to sense the luminal environment. Aggregates of lymphoid cells include Peyer patches (larger aggregates in the distal small intestine) and isolated lymphoid follicles located throughout the intestine. These lymphoid aggregates also play important roles in immune surveillance (Figure 13–4). GALT protects against pathogenic bacteria, viruses, and toxins and enables tolerance of potentially immunogenic dietary substances and bacteria.

2. **Innate immune defense**—These mechanisms include the secretion of fluid (eg, abundant acid secreted by the stomach), electrolytes, and mucus, as well as the tight junctions between epithelial cells. The secretions neutralize and flush away potentially damaging bacteria and macromolecules, and the tight junctions of the gut epithelium prevent their ingress into tissues.

In the intestine, mucus is secreted by specialized goblet cells. The mucus forms a protective layer over the epithelial cells. A group of antimicrobial peptides are secreted into the intestinal lumen. The specialized cells in the small intestine that perform this function are the Paneth cells that produce and secrete lysozyme and alpha-defensins that contribute to defense and healing. Alpha-defensins have broad-spectrum activity and are thought to create holes in bacterial cell walls and prevent them from colonizing the small intestine. **Trefoil peptides** are secreted into the lumen of the GI tract with mucus. Among their many effects, they promote the healing of mucosal lesions.

F. Regulation of Fluid & Electrolyte Balance

The small intestine receives 8–9 L of fluid with electrolytes per day and secretes a further 1 L with electrolytes per day. Most of the fluid is absorbed. Thus, secretion and absorption must be regulated to maintain balance. Increased secretion or diminished absorption causes diarrhea, which can be fatal because of fluid and electrolyte loss.

G. Excretion

Undigested food products, bacteria, and certain heavy metals (eg, copper and iron excreted in bile) are excreted in feces.

TABLE 13–2   **Mechanisms of defense of the GI tract (and features of structure and function involved).**

Form of Defense	Structural Adaptation	Functional Adaptation	Mechanism of Defense
Defense from acid			
Mucus production	Large numbers of mucus-secreting stomach surface cells	Mucin gene expression	Prevents direct contact of acid with epithelium
Bicarbonate production (alkaline tide)	Duodenal Brunner glands	Ion channel gene expression	Neutralizes any acid that breaches epithelium
Prostaglandin production	Specialized prostaglandin-producing cells in lamina propria	Cyclo-oxygenase 1 and 2 (*Ptgs1/2*) gene expression	Attenuates acid production
Tight junctions	Tight junction formation	Tight junction gene expression	Prevents breach of epithelium
Bicarbonate from pancreas	Pancreatic duct opening into duodenum	Secretin release in response to gastric acid	Neutralizes acid leaving stomach
Defense from infection			
Secretory immune system	Mucosa-associated lymphoid tissue and transcytotic epithelial cells	Machinery for transcytosis of immunoglobulin (*PIGR* gene expression)	Extends the protective umbrella of blood-borne immunity to the GI tract lumen
Rapid epithelial cell turnover	Cell proliferation in glands/crypts; cell release into lumen	Actively proliferating stem cells	Limits the consequences of enterocyte infection
Normal colonic microbiota		Induce expression of specific antimicrobial proteins (angiogenin4, Reg3γ)	
Stomach acid	Gastric glands containing parietal cells	Multiple humoral controls on acid secretion (histamine, acetylcholine, and gastrin)	Kills pathogenic organisms on ingestion

CHECKPOINT

4. What are the major functions of the GI tract?
5. Describe the four major layers of a cross-section through the GI tract.
6. What volumes of fluid are transferred into and out of the GI tract each day?
7. Describe the general mechanism of electrolyte transport across epithelial cells.
8. Describe how the GI tract defends itself.

REGULATION MECHANISMS OF THE GI TRACT

The processes of motility, secretion, digestion, and absorption are under close physiologic regulation by nerves, hormones, and paracrine substance (Figure 13–5).

A. Neural Control

There are two components of GI innervation:

1. **Intrinsic innervation by the enteric nervous system—** The enteric nervous system is the third division of the autonomic nervous system (Figure 13–6). An enteric neuron has its cell body within the wall of the GI tract and is thus intrinsic to the gut. The enteric nervous system comprises a series of ganglionated nerve plexuses that extend from the esophagus to the rectum and are organized into two principal components: (1) the myenteric, or Auerbach, plexus, which is sandwiched between the layers of the muscularis externa; and (2) the submucosal or Meissner plexus, which lies in the submucosa. The enteric nervous system is extensive, containing as many neurons as are present in the spinal cord. It contains sensory or afferent neurons (sometimes called **intrinsic primary afferent neurons [IPANs]**) that sense the environment (eg, intestinal pH, osmolality, wall stretch), **interneurons** (the connectors), and **secretomotor** or **efferent neurons** that control many cell types to stimulate or inhibit the motility, secretion, absorption, and immune functions of the GI tract. In this manner, the enteric nervous system can regulate the GI tract in a reflex manner without input from the central nervous system (CNS). For this reason, it is often called the "little brain." Enteric neurons use many neurotransmitters, most notably **neuropeptides**.

2. The degree to which the CNS regulates the enteric nervous system varies by region. The characteristic

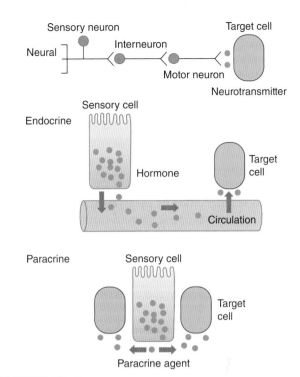

FIGURE 13–5 Neural, endocrine, and paracrine mechanisms of control in the GI tract.

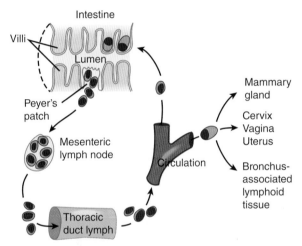

FIGURE 13–4 Systemic and local features of gut immunology. (Redrawn, with permission, from Dotan I et al. Mucosal immunology and inflammation. In: Feldman M et al, eds. *Sleisenger and Fordtran's Gastrointestinal and Liver Disease*, 10th ed. Elsevier, 2016. Copyright © Elsevier.)

functions of structures derived from the embryonic foregut (eg, esophageal peristalsis, relaxation of the lower esophageal sphincter, gastric accommodation and peristalsis, pyloric sphincter function) depend more on CNS control. However, functions of structures derived from the embryonic midgut and hindgut (eg, intestinal peristalsis, mucosal secretion) can continue without input from the CNS.

3. The clinical importance of the enteric nervous system is seen in clinical syndromes in which its function is lost;

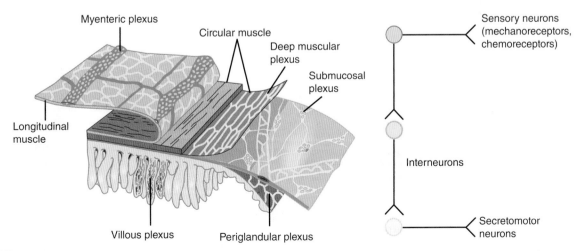

FIGURE 13–6 The enteric nervous system. **Left:** Enteric nervous system of the small intestine. Enteric neurons are organized in two nerve plexuses, the submucosal plexus and myenteric plexus. Additional plexuses, including the deep muscular, periglandular, and villous plexuses are discussed in the text. (Redrawn with permission from Brookes SJH et al. Functional histoanatomy of the enteric nervous system. In: Johnson LR, ed. *Physiology of the Gastrointestinal Tract*, 4th ed. Elsevier, 2006.) **Right:** The enteric nervous system includes sensory neurons, interneurons, and motor neurons. Complete reflex arcs exist within the enteric nervous system.

this can occur at several levels. In esophageal achalasia, for example, as a result of enteric nervous system defects, the body of the esophagus is quiet and the lower sphincter is tonically contracted, making ingestion of food difficult or impossible. More distally, failure of the enteric nerves to migrate into the colon during development (as in Hirschsprung disease) or the loss of enteric nervous system function (as in pseudo-obstruction of the small bowel) has severe clinical consequences, including abdominal pain, distension, and a risk of catastrophic intestinal perforation.

4. **Extrinsic innervation by parasympathetic and sympathetic nerves**—Extrinsic neurons that innervate the GI tract have cell bodies outside the gut wall and allow a bidirectional communication between the brain and the gut (**the brain–gut axis**) (Figure 13–7). This communication can regulate the function of the enteric nervous system or directly control the activity of other cell types.

In **parasympathetic innervation**, the vagus nerve (cranial nerve X) innervates the esophagus, stomach, gallbladder, pancreas, and the first part of intestine, cecum, and proximal colon. The pelvic nerve from the sacral spinal cord innervates the distal colon and the rectum. Preganglionic cell bodies in the medulla (vagus) or sacral spinal cord (pelvic nerve) project fibers to some enteric neurons in the gut wall, which are thus in a sense postganglionic parasympathetic nerves. The preganglionic nerves use acetylcholine as a neurotransmitter, which activates **nicotinic receptors** on enteric neurons. The postganglionic enteric nerves use acetylcholine (acting on **muscarinic receptors**) and neuropeptides as neurotransmitters. Parasympathetic stimulation can stimulate and inhibit GI functions.

In **sympathetic innervation**, preganglionic sympathetic nerves arise from cell bodies in the thoracic spinal cord and project fibers to prevertebral ganglia (celiac, cranial, and caudal mesenteric ganglion). They release acetylcholine as a neurotransmitter that interacts with **nicotinic** receptors on the postganglionic nerves. Postganglionic fibers innervate some enteric neurons or directly innervate effector cells in the GI tract, such as vascular smooth muscle cells. Norepinephrine is the major postganglionic neurotransmitter. Sympathetic innervation is often inhibitory to GI functions.

Regarding **extrinsic sensory nerves**, parasympathetic and sympathetic nerve tracts also carry sensory fibers from the gut to cell bodies located in nodose ganglia and the dorsal root

FIGURE 13–7 The extrinsic innervation of the GI tract by the parasympathetic and sympathetic nerves. Preganglionic parasympathetic nerves from the medulla and the sacral spinal cord project fibers in the vagal and pelvic nerves, respectively, to the wall of the GI tract and innervate enteric neurons that serve as postganglionic parasympathetic nerves. Preganglionic sympathetic nerves project fibers from the thoracolumbar regions of the spinal cord to the prevertebral ganglia, where they innervate postganglionic sympathetic nerves that project to the GI tract. Both the parasympathetic and sympathetic preganglionic nerves release acetylcholine (ACh), which activates nicotinic receptors on postganglionic nerves. Postganglionic parasympathetic nerves release acetylcholine and peptides, whereas postganglionic sympathetic nerves release norepinephrine (NE).

ganglia, respectively. Cell bodies in the nodose and dorsal root ganglia then project fibers to the brainstem (from nodose ganglia) or spinal cord (from dorsal route ganglia). Sensory nerve fibers in the wall of the GI tract detect mucosal pH and osmolality and can respond to amino acids or glucose, temperature, tension, and touch. In this manner, the extrinsic sensory nerves sense changes in the environment of the intestine and trigger central reflexes that initiate secretomotor changes to maintain normal homeostasis. Extrinsic sensory nerves also contribute to GI inflammation and pain. Sensory nerve endings in the wall of the gut detect noxious chemical and mechanical stimuli, including acid, inflammatory agents, and distension. These stimuli trigger the release of the neuropeptides, substance P, and calcitonin gene-related peptide from the endings of sensory nerves within the gut wall, where they induce plasma protein extravasation, granulocyte infiltration, and arteriolar vasodilatation to cause neurogenic inflammation. The same stimuli induce the release of neuropeptides from the central projections of these neurons, where they participate in pain transmission. Additional research is required to define the mechanisms of neurogenic inflammation and GI pain.

B. Hormonal Control

Hormones are blood-borne messengers released from endocrine cells or glands into the circulation, which carries them to distant target cells (see Figure 13–5). This mechanism of endocrine regulation was discovered in the GI tract in 1902, when Bayliss and Starling discovered the hormone **secretin** in the small intestine and showed that it stimulates secretion from the exocrine pancreas. Since then, a large number of hormones have been identified in all regions of the GI tract. In this respect, the GI tract is the largest endocrine organ.

GI hormones have several characteristics in common. They are secreted from endocrine cells scattered throughout the mucosa of the stomach and intestine, rather than being concentrated in specialized glands. GI hormones are invariably peptides, and many of these peptides are present not only in endocrine cells but also in the nerves of the enteric system and CNS (Table 13–3). Thus, they have dual functions as hormones and neurotransmitters. After feeding, there are elevated levels of many GI hormones in the circulation. These hormones have multiple biological effects, ranging from the stimulation of gastric acid secretion to the suppression of appetite. The physiologic role of some GI hormones has been clearly established by demonstrating that antagonists of hormone receptors block certain physiologic processes. However, in many cases, such antagonists are not available, and the physiologic relevance of hormones that cannot be antagonized remains to be determined.

C. Paracrine Control

Many substances used for intercellular signaling are rapidly removed from the extracellular fluid by uptake into nearby cells or by enzymatic degradation. Such substances have a short half-life in the extracellular fluid and are consequently capable of regulating only neighboring cells. Paracrine substances are released from non-neuronal sensory cells and neurons and regulate the function of neighboring cells, rather than influencing distant organs by passage through the circulation (see Figure 13–5 and Table 13–3). Examples include **histamine** and **somatostatin**, which are released from cells in the stomach to control acid secretion, and **serotonin** (**5-hydroxytryptamine** [**5-HT**]), which is released in the small intestine to control vagus nerve activity.

CHECKPOINT

9. What are the three general mechanisms of control observed in the GI tract?
10. What are the two components of the enteric nervous system?
11. What are the three general types of enteric neuron?
12. Describe the parasympathetic and sympathetic innervation of the GI tract.
13. What is the relationship between the enteric and central nervous systems?

GI SMOOTH MUSCLE

A. Structure of GI Smooth Muscle

The two principal muscle layers that control the motility of the GI tract are the inner circular layer and the outer longitudinal layer of the muscularis externa. They vary in thickness in different regions of the GI tract. For example, the muscles are thickened in the gastric antrum, where strong contractions break up food before it enters the small intestine, and muscle layers are thickened to form sphincters. Most of the GI muscle is **smooth muscle**, except the pharynx, parts of the esophagus, and the external anal sphincter, which are made up of **striated** (skeletal) muscle. GI smooth muscle is similar to smooth muscle in other organs: Fusiform cells are packed together in bundles by connective tissue sheaths. **Gap junctions** between cells allow signals to readily pass from cell to cell so that the contraction of bundles occurs synchronously. **Interstitial cells of Cajal** form an extensive network of stellate cells in the muscle layers of the stomach and intestine that are intimately associated with smooth muscle cells and enteric neurons (Figure 13–8). They may have two functions. First, they transmit information from enteric neurons to the smooth muscle cells. Second, they are the **pacemaker cells**, which have the capacity to generate the basic electrical rhythm or slow waves that are a consistent feature of GI smooth muscle. Animals lacking interstitial cells of Cajal show markedly abnormal GI motility, including defective gastric emptying and intestinal stasis or ileus. Defects in interstitial cells of Cajal may be associated with motility disturbances in patients, and this is an area of active investigation.

TABLE 13–3   Secretory products of the GI tract.

Product	Physiologic Actions	Site of Release	Stimulus for Release	Disease Association
True hormones				
Gastrin	Stimulates acid secretion and growth of gastric oxyntic gland mucosa	Gastric antrum (and duodenum)	Peptides, amino acids, distension, vagal stimulation	Zollinger–Ellison syndrome, peptic ulcer disease
CCK	Stimulates gallbladder contraction, pancreatic enzyme and bicarbonate secretion, and growth of exocrine pancreas	Duodenum and jejunum	Peptides, amino acids, long-chain fatty acids, (acid)	
Secretin	Stimulates pancreatic bicarbonate secretion, biliary bicarbonate secretion, growth of exocrine pancreas, pepsin secretion; inhibits gastric acid secretion, trophic effects of gastrin	Duodenum	Acid (fat)	
GIP	Stimulates insulin release (inhibits gastric acid secretion)	Duodenum and jejunum	Glucose, amino acids, fatty acids	
Other polypeptides with hormone function				
Motilin	Stimulates gastric and duodenal motility	Duodenum and jejunum	Unknown	Irritable bowel syndrome; diabetic gastroparesis
Pancreatic polypeptide	Inhibits pancreatic bicarbonate and enzyme secretion	Pancreatic islets of Langerhans	Protein (fat and glucose)	
Glucagon-like peptide-1 (GLP-1)	Stimulates insulin secretion, thereby lowering blood glucose	Ileum and colon	Glucose and fat	Inflammatory conditions and diabetes mellitus
Paracrine factors				
Somatostatin	Inhibits release of most other peptide hormones (eg, acid stimulates somatostatin to block gastrin)	GI tract mucosa, pancreatic islets of Langerhans	Acid stimulates, vagus nerve inhibits release	Gallstones
Prostaglandins	Promote blood flow, increase mucus and bicarbonate secretion from gastric mucosa	Multiple	Various	NSAID-induced gastritis and ulcer disease
Histamine	Stimulates gastric acid secretion	Oxyntic gland mucosa	Gastrin and unknown others	
Neurocrines				
VIP	Relaxes sphincters and gut circular muscle; stimulates intestinal and pancreatic secretion	Mucosa and smooth muscle of GI tract	Enteric nervous system	Secretory diarrhea
Bombesin	Stimulates gastrin release	Gastric mucosa	Enteric nervous system	
Enkephalins	Stimulate smooth muscle contraction; inhibit intestinal secretion	Mucosa and smooth muscle of GI tract	Enteric nervous system	
Other products				
Intrinsic factor	Binds vitamin B_{12} to facilitate its absorption	Parietal cells of the stomach	Constitutive secretion	Autoimmune destruction of parietal cells causes pernicious anemia
Mucin	Lubrication and protection	Goblet cells along entire intestinal mucosa and surface cells in stomach	GI tract irritation	Viscid mucus in cystic fibrosis, attenuation in some cases of peptic ulcer
Acid	Prevents infection; initiates digestion	Parietal cells of the stomach	Gastrin, histamine, acetylcholine, NSAIDs (indirectly)	Acid-peptic disease

CCK, cholecystokinin; GI, gastrointestinal; GIP, gastric inhibitory polypeptide; NSAID, nonsteroidal anti-inflammatory drug; VIP, vasoactive intestinal peptide.

Note: Parentheses indicate minor components and effects.

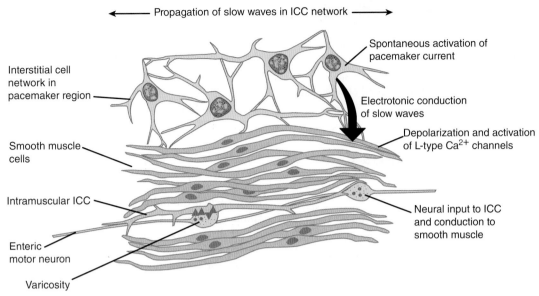

FIGURE 13–8 Diagrammatic view of interstitial cells of Cajal (ICC) in the intestine, showing their interaction with enteric nerves and smooth muscle cells.

B. Electrophysiology of GI Smooth Muscle

GI smooth muscle cells have a resting membrane potential of −40 to −80 mV as a result of the relative conductances of K^+, Na^+, and Cl^- ions. An electrogenic Na^+-K^+ ATPase contributes significantly to the resting membrane potential. Less is known about the electrophysiological properties of interstitial cells of Cajal, in part because of difficulties in isolating these cells for study. The resting membrane potential of smooth muscle cells varies characteristically with time and is called a slow wave or basic electrical rhythm. Slow waves occur at a rate of 3–5/min in the stomach and at a rate of 12–20/min in the intestine. Interstitial cells of Cajal set the frequency of the slow waves, and slow waves are transmitted between cells through gap junctions. Nerves and hormones modulate the amplitude of slow waves. Depending on the amplitude of the slow waves and the excitability of the smooth muscle, slow waves can give rise to action potentials. If the slow-wave depolarization reaches a threshold, a train of action potentials will fire. Action potentials depolarize the membrane of the smooth muscle cells and induce an influx of Ca^{2+} ions into the cytoplasm through voltage-sensitive Ca^{2+} channels in the plasma membrane and from intracellular stores, causing contraction. What causes an action potential to occur? The presence of neurotransmitters or hormones released close to the smooth muscle cells alters the resting membrane potentials of the cells, which makes the oscillations in membrane potential (the slow waves) more or less likely to reach threshold and initiate an action potential. However, because inhibitory motor neurons of the GI tract are highly active and can prevent the generation of action potentials, not all slow waves result in active contractions. Action potentials and contractions can only occur when these inhibitory motor neurons are switched off by input from interneurons. Thus, the tonic inhibition serves to control the inherent excitability of the pacemaker cells.

C. Mechanical Properties of GI Smooth Muscle

Several characteristic patterns of contraction can be observed in GI smooth muscle. **Tonic contractions** are best represented by sphincters that act as one-way valves to prevent the retrograde movement of material from distal to more proximal regions and thus to facilitate flow in an aboral direction. The proximal parts of the stomach and the gallbladder also exhibit tonic contractions. **Peristaltic contractions** are moving waves of contraction that propel digesta along the GI tract. Peristalsis involves the neurally mediated contraction of smooth muscle on the oral side of a bolus of digesta and a neurally mediated relaxation of muscle on the anal side of the digesta. Peristalsis occurs in the pharynx, esophagus, gastric antrum, and small and large intestine. **Segmental contractions** produce narrow contracted segments between relaxed segments. These movements allow mixing of the luminal contents with GI tract secretions and increase exposure to mucosal surfaces where absorption occurs. Segmentation occurs in the stomach and intestine. **Pathologic patterns of motility** include **spasms**, which are very strong and often painful contractions that occur continuously in a dysregulated manner, and **ileus**, in which contractile activity is markedly decreased or absent. Ileus often results from irritation of the peritoneum that may occur with surgery, peritonitis, and pancreatitis. Further research is required to understand the mechanisms of these abnormal contractions, which may lead to improved therapies.

CHECKPOINT

CHECKPOINT

14. What are the positive and negative regulators of smooth muscle cell action potentials?

15. What are the functions of interstitial cells of Cajal?

16. What are the general types of contractions observed in the GI tract after feeding?

OROPHARYNX & ESOPHAGUS

Anatomy & Histology

The oropharynx provides entry to the GI tract during swallowing and to the respiratory tract during breathing. It includes the vocal cords, which separate the two tracts and provide the structural basis for speech. Much of the oropharynx is lined with a respiratory-type ciliated pseudocolumnar epithelium.

The esophagus is a hollow tube (25–30 cm long, 2–3 cm wide). The wall of the esophagus consists of a stratified squamous epithelial cell layer, an inner layer of circular muscle, a myenteric nerve plexus, and an outer layer of longitudinal muscle. The first third of the esophagus is composed of striated muscle, the middle third is mixed striated and smooth muscle, and the lower third is purely smooth muscle. The esophagus is delimited by an **upper esophageal sphincter** (a distinct thickening of striated circular muscle) and a **lower esophageal sphincter** (a tonically contracted 3–4 cm ring of smooth muscle). The two sphincters generate small luminal zones of high pressure, whereas the rest of the esophageal lumen is at a pressure equal to that of the surrounding body cavities. Between swallows, the two sphincters are closed, preventing entry of air and gastric acid into the esophagus. Regulation of the lower esophageal sphincter is especially important because it controls the passage of digesta into the stomach and prevents the reflux of gastric contents into the esophagus, where they can damage the mucosa. Between swallows, the lower esophageal sphincter is contracted, in large part by vagal cholinergic mechanisms. During swallowing, vagal inhibitory fibers allow the lower esophageal sphincter to relax, possibly because of a release of inhibitory neurotransmitters from enteric nerves, including nitric oxide and vasoactive intestinal peptide (VIP).

Swallowing Reflex

Swallowing begins as a voluntary process that rapidly becomes an involuntary reflex mechanism. During the voluntary oral phase, the tongue pushes a bolus of food to the back of the mouth and into the oropharynx. From there on, the process is involuntary. In the **pharyngeal phase**, the food bolus stimulates touch receptors in the pharynx. Sensory signals pass by the glossopharyngeal, vagal, and trigeminal nerves to the swallowing center in the medulla and pons. Motor impulses pass through cranial nerves to control an involuntary process that directs food into the esophagus and away from the airway. Breathing is interrupted and the soft palate is elevated,

closing the pharyngeal opening of the nasopharynx and preventing food from entering the internal openings of the nostrils. The tongue is pressed against the hard palate, closing the oral opening of the pharynx. The glottis is pulled under the epiglottis, which blocks the laryngeal opening. Cartilages around the larynx are pulled together, further restricting food from entering the respiratory tract. When all openings to the pharynx are closed, a wave of muscular contraction pushes the bolus of food toward the opening of the esophagus. As the food reaches the esophagus, the upper esophageal sphincter relaxes to accept the material and then closes after the bolus has moved through. The **esophageal phase** of swallowing begins when the bolus passes through the upper esophageal sphincter. Vagal stretch receptors in the wall of the esophagus detect distension by the bolus and induce a **vagovagal** reflex, during which vagal motor nerves induce a wave of contraction that spreads along the esophagus at 3–5 cm/s. This is termed **primary peristalsis** (Figure 13–9). As the wave of primary peristalsis reaches the lower esophageal sphincter, the sphincter relaxes to allow the bolus to enter the stomach. Distension of the esophagus by the bolus can initiate another wave of contraction called **secondary peristalsis**. Often, repetitive waves of secondary peristalsis are required to clear the esophagus of food. Various hormones and neurotransmitters, foods, and drugs can affect the tone of the lower esophageal sphincter pressure.

The importance of oropharyngeal motility and its control is seen in patients who have had strokes or have dementia. The inability to swallow properly often makes them unable to manage their own oral secretions, resulting in the aspiration of oral contents into the lungs with the development of pneumonia. This is a common cause of death in individuals with these kinds of CNS disorders. Disordered lower esophageal sphincter tone can cause gastroesophageal reflux disease (GERD), presenting as heartburn and potentially increasing the risk for adenocarcinoma of the esophagus.

CHECKPOINT

17. What is the histologic difference between the proximal one-third and the distal two-thirds of the esophagus?

18. What are the functions of the upper and lower esophageal sphincters, and how are they regulated?

19. Describe the three phases of the swallowing reflex.

STOMACH

Anatomy & Histology

The stomach is a complex glandular organ guarded by two sphincters: the lower esophageal sphincter and the **pyloric sphincter** (Figure 13–10). The mucosa is formed by a single layer of epithelial cells that line the lumen of the stomach and descend into funnel-shaped invaginations (ie, broad at the top

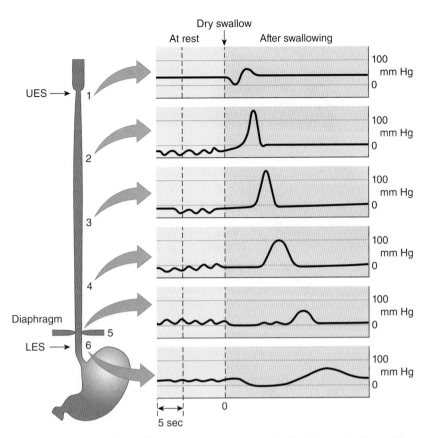

FIGURE 13–9 Primary peristalsis of the esophagus. The tracings show pressures in the indicated regions of the esophagus at rest and at various times after swallowing. (LES, lower esophageal sphincter; UES, upper esophageal sphincter.) (Redrawn from data in Conklin JL et al. Motor functions of the pharynx and esophagus. In: Johnson LR, ed. *Physiology of the Gastrointestinal Tract*, 4th ed. Elsevier, 2006.)

near the surface and then narrow as they descend deeper). The broad upper portion is called the pit zone. The middle portion, where the invaginations narrow into glands, is the neck, and the deepest zone is the base. The stomach can be divided anatomically into several regions on the basis of structure and function. The **cardia** is a small region of variable size just distal to the lower esophageal sphincter where the gastric glands are almost entirely composed of mucus-secreting cells. The **corpus**, or **body**, is the major part of the stomach and includes the **fundus**, which is the portion of the body superior to the insertion of the esophagus. Gastric glands in the corpus contain **parietal cells** (mostly in the neck zone), which secrete **hydrochloric acid** and **intrinsic factor**, and **chief cells** (mostly in the base zone), which secrete the digestive enzyme precursor **pepsinogen**. The corpus is the principal site of gastric digestion. The **pyloric antrum** is the distal region of the stomach that secretes the hormone **gastrin** from G cells. Glands of the antrum, like those of the cardia, secrete mostly mucus. The antrum, a highly muscular portion of the stomach, grinds food and regulates gastric emptying.

Gastric Acid Secretion

A number of products are secreted from the stomach. Of these, hydrochloric acid (HCl) is perhaps the most important

from a pathophysiologic standpoint. Secretion of acid by the parietal cells of the gastric glands occurs in a basal diurnal pattern but can be stimulated by such diverse factors as the thought of food, distension of the stomach, and protein ingestion. Gastric secretions were the subject of some of the first GI experimentalists. The Italian Lazzaro Spallanzani fed and retrieved from animal stomachs tubes filled with various substances to examine digestion. And Pavlov received his Nobel prize for studying digestive organ secretion long before his work was appreciated for its psychological implications.

A. Molecular Mechanisms of HCl Secretion

The mechanisms by which parietal cells secrete HCl into the stomach have been intensively studied because of the importance of acid secretion to digestion and in disease states. Parietal cells are roughly pyramidal in shape. Their membranes express a **H⁺-K⁺ ATPase**, a primary active transporter responsible for the secretion of HCl. Parietal cells undergo a remarkable change in appearance when stimulated to secrete HCl (Figure 13–11). In the unstimulated state, they harbor an intracellular tubulovesicular network studded with H⁺-K⁺ ATPase molecules. On activation, the tubulovesicular membranes fuse with the plasma membrane to form a canalicular membrane with microvilli. The result is an increase in the area

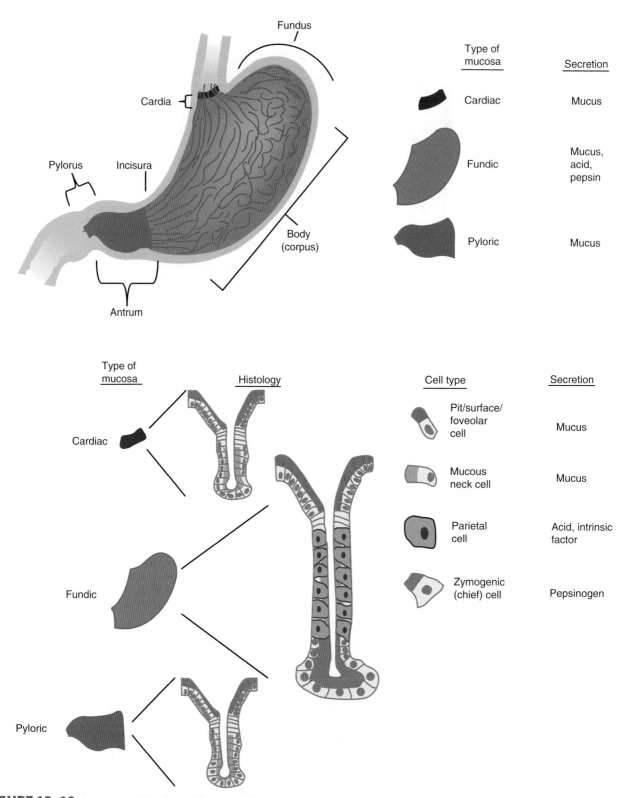

FIGURE 13–10 Anatomy and histology of the stomach. (Redrawn, with permission, from Boron WF et al, eds. *Medical Physiology*, 2nd ed. Saunders Elsevier, 2009.)

of the apical membrane by 50- to 100-fold that allows a markedly increased secretion of HCl by the H⁺-K⁺ ATPase pumps directly into the glandular lumen, which in turn squirts the acid into the lumen of the stomach.

The H⁺-K⁺ ATPase is a heterodimer of an α-subunit (the catalytically active unit) and a β-subunit (involved in fixing the intracellular location). The H⁺-K⁺ ATPase pumps H⁺ ions from the cell across the apical membrane in exchange for K⁺

FIGURE 13–11 Acid secretion by parietal cells. **Top:** Upon stimulation, the tubulovesicular network in the parietal cell fuses to form an extensive canalicular membrane with microvilli, which increases the surface area. **Bottom:** The mechanisms of HCl secretion by parietal cells, stimulated by histamine, acetylcholine, and gastrin, are demonstrated. For abbreviations, see the legend for Figure 13–12.

ions (see Figure 13–11). This is an example of primary active transport driven by ATP, which pumps H^+ ions against an enormous concentration gradient (1,000,000:1). Tight junctions between cells prevent the re-entry of H^+ ions into the mucosa. The K^+ ions that have entered the cells then recycle to the lumen or enter interstitial fluid by K^+ channels. To maintain electroneutrality, Cl^- ions are secreted passively across the apical membrane into the lumen through Cl^- channels, forming HCl. The secreted H^+ ions are provided by H_2O and CO_2, which form H_2CO_3. Carbonic anhydrase generates H^+ ions for secretion and HCO_3^- ions, which enter the interstitial fluid by exchange for Cl^- ions. Cl^- ions enter against their electrochemical gradient, driven by the efflux of HCO_3^- down an electrochemical gradient. The secretion of HCO_3^- into the blood forms the "**alkaline tide**," which can lead to alkalosis when H^+ ion secretion is excessive. Water movement maintains the osmotic balance in all regions.

An understanding of the mechanisms of HCl secretion by parietal cells permitted the development of **proton pump inhibitors** (**PPIs**), a class of drugs that inhibit the H^+-K^+ ATPase. Drugs such as omeprazole, a benzimidazole, are inactive at neutral pH levels but, when acidified (in the stomach), bind to sulfhydryl groups of cysteine residues on the external surface of the H^+-K^+ ATPase, irreversibly inhibiting activity and blocking the hypersecretion of gastric acid. Other experimental drugs, termed **acid pump antagonists**, competitively interfere with K^+ ion binding to block acid secretion. These drugs can be used to inhibit the hypersecretion of gastric acid that causes GERD.

B. Stimulants and Inhibitors of HCl Secretion

The three main stimulants of H^+ ion secretion are acetylcholine, gastrin, and histamine, all of which stimulate HCl secretion and induce characteristic shape changes in the stimulated parietal cell. **Acetylcholine** is released from vagal postganglionic or enteric neurons during feeding. It binds to muscarinic M3-type muscarinic receptors on parietal cells to stimulate H^+ ion secretion. **Gastrin** is a peptide hormone of 17 or 34 amino acids secreted from G cells in the gastric antrum during feeding. Gastrin binds to cholecystokinin (CCK) type B receptors on parietal cells, which also stimulates H^+ ion secretion.

Both acetylcholine and gastrin receptors activate the same signal transduction pathways: activation of phospholipase Cβ, leading to the generation of inositol trisphosphate, which mobilizes Ca^{2+} from intracellular stores, and diacylglycerol, which activates protein kinase C. Because both acetylcholine and gastrin act through similar intracellular pathways, the combined effects of gastrin and acetylcholine are additive.

Histamine is a paracrine substance secreted by enterochromaffin-like (ECL) and mast cells in the corpus mucosa during feeding. Histamine binds to H_2 receptors on parietal cells to activate adenylyl cyclase and increase cAMP. The cAMP activates protein kinase A to stimulate H^+ ion secretion. The combination of histamine and acetylcholine or gastrin can increase the rate of acid production by up to 10-fold over basal levels, a much greater effect than simple addition of the effects of the agonists would predict. This effect is known as **potentiation**. Potentiation requires that two different signal molecules bind to receptors that act through different intracellular mechanisms. Increased intracellular Ca^{2+} and cAMP activate K^+ channels on the apical membrane of parietal cells, thereby promoting K^+ ion efflux from the cell. This hyperpolarizes the cell (more negative inside) to promote Cl^- ion secretion across the apical membrane. Ca^{2+} and cAMP also increase insertion of Cl^- channels and H^+-K^+ ATPase into the apical membrane. The combined effects are to stimulate HCl secretion.

Gastrin also regulates growth of the gastric epithelium. Excess gastrin aberrantly produced by certain tumors causes the hyperproliferation of gastric glands and parietal cells and an excess secretion of gastric acid. The excess acid in the small intestine can lead to ulceration of the mucosa, steatorrhea as a result of the inactivation of pancreatic lipases (which are inhibited by low pH), and diarrhea. This condition is termed **Zollinger–Ellison syndrome**. The excessive administration of PPIs can result in prolonged high luminal pH, which stimulates the hypersecretion of gastrin, which can increase mucosal growth and, in particular, stimulate the hyperplasia (overproliferation) of histamine-secreting ECL cells. Termination of drug treatment then results in an acid production rebound because of the increased content of parietal cells and gastrin-secreting G cells.

In addition to the direct mechanisms by which acetylcholine, gastrin, and histamine stimulate HCl secretion from parietal cells, acetylcholine and gastrin also indirectly stimulate secretion by acting on enterochromaffin-like cells to promote the release of histamine, which in turn stimulates parietal cells. The importance of histamine to H^+ ion secretion is illustrated by studies with **histamine H_2 receptor antagonists**, such as cimetidine. These drugs not only inhibit histamine-stimulated H^+ ion secretion but also block the effects of acetylcholine and gastrin. By preventing such potentiation, these agents can be used to effectively treat the hypersecretion of gastric acid.

Somatostatin, a peptide of 14 or 28 amino acids, is an important inhibitor of gastric acid secretion. Somatostatin directly inhibits proton secretion by activating receptors on parietal cells, which couple to inhibit cAMP. Somatostatin also inhibits gastrin and histamine secretion, which indirectly inhibits proton secretion. Somatostatin is secreted by **D cells** in the gastric antrum and corpus. D cells in the gastric antrum have direct contact with the stomach lumen (open endocrine cells), allowing them to sense the luminal contents. Protons in the antrum stimulate somatostatin secretion, which acts as a paracrine agent to inhibit gastrin secretion from neighboring G cells and to thereby indirectly reduce gastric acid secretion. This is an example of **negative-feedback regulation**. D cells in the corpus do not have contact with the lumen (closed cells) and thus cannot sense luminal protons. Instead, multiple neurohumoral factors (eg, noradrenalin, CCK, VIP) increase the release of corpus somatostatin, which in turn inhibits acid production indirectly by decreasing histamine release from ECL cells and directly by inhibiting parietal cells. Vagal ACh and the T_H1 cytokine interferon-γ inhibit somatostatin release and promote acid secretion. Recent studies indicate that the endocrine cells in the stomach sense luminal nutrient and acid via primary cilia on their apical surfaces.

C. Integrated Regulation of Gastric Acid Secretion

The secretion of gastric acid between meals is low. Three phases of acid secretion occur during feeding (Figure 13–12). **The cephalic phase** (~30% of response) of secretion, first illustrated by Pavlov's elegant experiments, is initiated by the sight, smell, taste, and swallowing of food. These stimuli activate the dorsal motor nucleus of the vagal nerve in the medulla, resulting in activation/discharge of the vagus nerve and tributary parasympathetic motor nerves. Stimulation has several consequences. In the corpus, postganglionic nerves release acetylcholine, which directly activates parietal cells by M3 receptors. Acetylcholine also induces histamine release from enterochromaffin cells, which stimulates H^+ ion secretion by parietal cells. In the antrum, vagal stimulation induces the release of **gastrin-releasing peptide** from postganglionic fibers, which stimulates gastrin release and thus indirectly stimulates H^+ ion secretion. Acetylcholine also inhibits somatostatin release from D cells in the corpus and pylorus to stimulate H^+ ion secretion.

The **gastric phase** (~70% of response) of secretion is induced by stimuli within the stomach. Vagal sensory nerves detect gastric distension with food and trigger a vagovagal reflex during which vagal motor nerves release acetylcholine in the stomach to promote acid secretion. Partially digested proteins and amino acids stimulate gastrin release from G cells in the pylorus. G cells, like D cells, are open-type endocrine cells that directly sense the contents of the stomach. Gastrin then further stimulates acid secretion. Acidification of the pylorus stimulates the release of somatostatin, which inhibits acid secretion by a negative-feedback loop as described.

During the **intestinal phase**, the products of protein digestion, on entering the small intestine, can stimulate gastrin release from G cells in the duodenum. Many substances, most notably fat and acid, stimulate the secretion of hormones from the small intestine that inhibit gastric acid secretion. Examples include secretin and cholecystokinin.

Helicobacter pylori is a bacterium that lives in the mucous layer of the stomach where the enzyme urease is active, converting urea to CO_2 and ammonia. Ammonia buffers luminal acid and protects the organism. *H pylori* also secretes proteins, such as CagA and VacA, that modulate immune responses and directly alter mucosal cell signaling pathways. More than half the world's population is infected with *H pylori*. In most cases, the infection, though chronic, is mild and does not cause symptoms. In some individuals, however, the infection remains confined to the antrum but leads to increased acid secretion and symptomatic inflammation that causes ulceration of the stomach or duodenum. Almost all duodenal peptic (ie, acid-associated) ulcers and about half of gastric peptic

FIGURE 13–12 Regulation of gastric acid secretion by nerves and hormones. During the cephalic phase of digestion, vagal cholinergic nerves directly stimulate parietal cells and induce the release of histamine from enterochromaffin-like (ECL) cells, which also stimulate parietal cells. Vagal fibers also release gastrin-releasing peptide (GRP) in the antrum to induce gastrin secretion, which is carried in the bloodstream to induce the release of histamine and stimulate parietal cells. During the gastric phase of digestion, food in the stomach triggers vagovagal reflexes and stimulates gastrin secretion. Acidification of the gastric antrum stimulates the release of somatostatin, which inhibits gastrin release and thus acid secretion; vagal acetylcholine (Ach) inhibits somatostatin release. (CCKB-R, cholecystokinin B receptor; G, gastrin; GRP, gastrin-releasing peptide; GRP-R, GRP receptor; H2-R, histamine 2 receptor; M3-R, muscarinic 3 receptor; S-R, somatostatin receptor.)

ulcers have *H pylori* infection as a root cause; the remaining gastric ulcers are caused by medications (eg, aspirin, nonsteroidal anti-inflammatory drugs). In some patients, chronic *H pylori* infection can spread to the corpus and lead to chronic inflammation that triggers the death (atrophy) of parietal cells and altered mucosal differentiation patterns (metaplasias) that increase the risk of progression to gastric cancer. In certain geographical regions (eg, East Asia and parts of Central and South America), owing to environmental and/or lifestyle factors that have not been fully elucidated, the risk for progression to gastric cancer is much higher than in other regions (eg, United States, Canada).

Other Gastric Secretions

Chief cells in the glands of the gastric corpus secrete **pepsinogen**, an inactive precursor (zymogen) of the active protease pepsin. Acetylcholine is the main stimulant of pepsinogen secretion, although other factors (eg, gastrin) also stimulate secretion. Once released into the lumen of the stomach, gastric acid and pre-existing pepsin convert pepsinogen to pepsin. Pepsin has a pH optimum of 3.0 and is thus active in the stomach. It is an endopeptidase that begins the degradation of dietary proteins into peptides. However, pepsin accounts for only 10% of the total protein digestion.

Mucins are high-molecular-weight glycoproteins secreted by mucous cells of gastric glands in the corpus and antrum. The peptide backbone of mucins is densely populated with carbohydrate side chains enriched with sulfate groups. Mucins combine with phospholipids, bicarbonate, and water to form the mucous gel layer that adheres to the surface of stomach epithelial cells. This layer acts as physical protection for epithelial cells from damage by contractile food grinding as well as noxious substances such as acid, pepsin, and bile acids. Acetylcholine and mucosal irritation stimulate mucin secretion.

Epithelial cells of the corpus and antrum secrete HCO_3^- ions. Although the secretion of HCO_3^- is minor compared with H^+ ion secretion, HCO_3^- plays a major role in epithelial defense. HCO_3^- ions are trapped in the mucous gel to form an "unstirred layer" in proximity to the epithelium, where the pH is 7.0 compared with 1.0–3.0 in the lumen. Acetylcholine and intraluminal acid stimulate HCO_3^- secretion.

Intrinsic factor is a glycoprotein secreted by parietal cells required for vitamin B_{12} absorption. Vitamin B_{12} (cobalamin) is not made in mammalian cells, and the only source is the diet: meat, fish, and dairy products, but not vegetables or fruit. In the stomach, acid and pepsin release B_{12} from dietary carrier proteins. The acidic environment permits the binding of B_{12} to **haptocorrin** (R factor), a glycoprotein produced by salivary and gastric glands. The B_{12}–haptocorrin complex enters the duodenum, where pancreatic proteases digest the haptocorrin. Free intrinsic factor also enters the duodenum. Intrinsic factor combines with B_{12} in the less acidic environment of the small intestine, forming a degradation-resistant complex for transport to the ileum. Specific receptors on epithelial cells lining the ileum bind the vitamin B_{12}–intrinsic factor complex, which is taken into cells by endocytosis. The absorbed complex dissociates within the epithelial cells, and then vitamin B_{12} binds to transcobalamin II, a protein required for exocytosis and transport to the liver. In autoimmune gastritis, parietal cells are destroyed, leading to a loss of intrinsic factor secretion, which can result in vitamin B_{12} deficiency and **pernicious anemia**. This anemia is caused by the impaired synthesis of purines and thymine for which vitamin B_{12} is required. The only reliable therapy is regular intramuscular injections of vitamin B_{12}.

GASTRIC MOTILITY

A. Patterns of Gastric Motility

In terms of motility, the proximal and distal regions of the stomach are distinct. The gastric corpus is a reservoir for gastric digestion. During each swallow, the stretch of the esophagus induces a vagovagal reflex that causes the gastric corpus to relax in preparation to receive the food, a phenomenon known as **receptive relaxation**. When food enters the stomach, it relaxes further to accommodate a meal of 1.5 L without any increase in pressure, a phenomenon called **accommodation**, which involves vagovagal and local enteric reflexes. Thus, the stomach is a reservoir for ingested food. The antrum of the stomach is highly muscular, and here contractions serve to break food into smaller pieces, thereby facilitating digestion. The pyloric sphincter controls the rate at which the antral contractions propel partially digested food, or **chyme**, into the duodenum. During fasting, the antrum is relatively quiescent, with occasional forceful contractions occurring every 75–90 min. These intense

contractions, of 5–10 min in duration, are part of a general wave of contractions that sweep the entire length of the GI tract during fasting: the **migrating myoelectric complex**. Feeding disrupts the migrating myoelectric complex, and now the antrum contracts frequently at a rate of about three contractions per minute. These slow waves of peristaltic contraction originate from spontaneously active interstitial cells of Cajal in the pacemaker zone in the middle of the body of the stomach, and they sweep toward the antrum. When the membrane potential of muscle cells depolarizes to reach threshold, action potentials fire. Contractions occur during the plateau phase of the action potential. Gastrin and acetylcholine stimulate contraction by increasing the magnitude and duration of the action potentials.

B. Gastric Emptying

Immediately after a meal, the stomach may contain up to 1 L of material, which empties slowly into the small intestine. Regulation of gastric emptying occurs by alterations in the motility of the proximal and distal stomach, pylorus, and duodenum. Gastric emptying is brought about by an increase in tone (intraluminal pressure) in the proximal stomach, an increase in the strength of antral contractions, the opening of the pylorus, and the inhibition of duodenal segmental contractions.

The rate of gastric emptying depends on the chemical and physical composition of chyme that enters the duodenum through the stimulation of both neural and hormonal pathways. Solids and liquids empty at different rates: Liquids empty rapidly, and solids empty only after a lag phase. Acid, fat, and hyperosmolar solutions entering the duodenum slow gastric emptying through the stimulation of neuronal and hormonal mechanisms. Sensory neurons in the duodenum, both vagal and spinal, respond to nutrients, H^+ ions, and the hyperosmolar content of chyme. Vagal motor nerves decrease antral contractions, contract the pylorus, and decrease proximal gastric motility. This results in the **intestinal feedback inhibition (slowing) of gastric emptying**. The main vagal mediator that stimulates contraction is acetylcholine. VIP and nitric oxide are neuronal mediators that inhibit contraction. Many hormones released by endocrine cells in the small intestine have been implicated in the feedback inhibition of gastric emptying. **Secretin**, the release of which is stimulated by acid, inhibits antral contractions and stimulates pyloric sphincter contraction to slow emptying. **Cholecystokinin**, the release of which is stimulated by fat, acts on vagal sensory nerve receptors to produce a vagovagal reflex that decreases gastric emptying.

The importance of nervous system control over gastric motility is reflected in the high incidence of **dumping syndrome** (nausea, bloating, flushing, and explosive diarrhea) that occurs as a consequence of stomach dysmotility in some patients who have undergone surgical procedures such as partial gastrectomy or nonselective vagotomy.

CHECKPOINT

20. Describe the cell types found in the mucosa of the gastric corpus and antrum, and indicate the products of each cell type.

21. What are the roles of the proximal and distal stomach?

22. Describe the ionic basis of HCl secretion from the gastric parietal cells.

23. Name a neurotransmitter, hormone, and paracrine agent that stimulates acid secretion from parietal cells.

24. Name a peptide that inhibits acid secretion from the parietal cells.

25. Describe the mechanisms of the cephalic, gastric, and intestinal phases of gastric acid secretion.

26. Name two types of drug with distinct mechanisms of action that can be used to treat the hypersecretion of gastric acid.

27. What is the role of the parietal cell in the absorption of vitamin B_{12}?

28. Describe two processes by which the gastric mucosa is protected from acid in the lumen.

29. What are the patterns of motility in the corpus and the antrum?

30. How does the composition of the digesta in the lumen of the small intestine affect the rate of gastric emptying?

GALLBLADDER

Anatomy & Histology

The gallbladder is a muscular sac with a resting volume of about 50 mL that lies on the inferior surface of the liver. It is connected to the hepatic biliary system by the cystic duct, which leads to the common bile duct whose opening into the proximal duodenum is controlled by the sphincter of Oddi. The common bile duct and the pancreatic duct usually join just proximal to this sphincter.

Physiology

A. Bile Secretion

Bile, which is produced by the liver, flows down the hepatic duct and into the gallbladder through the cystic duct. It is stored there until gallbladder contraction is stimulated to expel the contents of the gallbladder back through the cystic duct into the common bile duct and through the sphincter of Oddi into the duodenum. Stimuli for gallbladder contraction and sphincter of Oddi relaxation necessary for proper bile flow include both hormones and neural inputs. Fat in the intestine stimulates secretion of the hormone CCK from I-cells. CCK causes the gallbladder to contract and the sphincter of Oddi to relax. Depending on how long it remains in the gallbladder, bile becomes concentrated. Bile composition is further modified by mucin production under the control of prostaglandins and by the saturation of bile cholesterol controlled in part by

estrogens. The most prominent disorders of the gallbladder involve gallstone formation (see later discussion).

SMALL INTESTINE

Anatomy & Histology

Three regions can be distinguished along the approximately 6–7 m length of the small intestine. The pyloric sphincter marks the beginning of the **duodenum**, which is largely retroperitoneal, fixed in its location, and 20–25 cm in length. Because of this sphincter, stomach contents normally enter the duodenum in small spurts containing tiny suspended particles. In the duodenum, gastric contents are mixed with the secretions of the common bile duct and pancreatic duct. Beyond the duodenum, the small intestine is mobile and suspended in the peritoneal cavity by a mesentery. The proximal two-fifths is called the **jejunum**. The distal three-fifths is called the **ileum**, which ends at the ileocecal valve at the start of the large intestine.

The most striking gross structural features of the small intestine are the numerous **villi** (projections of the mucosa into the lumen of the intestine that measure approximately 1 mm in height) (Figure 13–13). Each villus contains a single terminal branch of the arterial, venous, and lymphatic trees. Villi increase the absorptive capacity 5-fold and allow efficient transfer to the circulatory system of substances absorbed from the gut lumen by **enterocytes** (surface epithelial cells). By electron microscopy, each enterocyte contains 3000–5000 **microvilli**, plasma membrane evaginations on the apical side of the cell that further increase the absorptive surface area by 200-fold. Many digestive enzymes expressed by intestinal epithelial cells are located at the tips of these microvilli. As a group, these densely packed microvilli make up a "brush border" facing the intestinal lumen.

Invaginations of the intestinal epithelium into the wall, called the crypts of Lieberkühn, surround the villi. These structures are the location of epithelial intestinal stem cells and their proliferative daughters that together constantly produce new differentiated epithelial cells that form the epithelial lining of the intestine. Each small intestinal crypt contains tetrapotential stem cells at or near the crypt base that produces the four mature epithelial cell types: absorptive enterocytes, mucus-secreting goblet cells, hormone-secreting enteroendocrine cells, and antimicrobial peptides and growth factor–secreting Paneth cells. Enterocytes, goblet cells, and enteroendocrine cells migrate out of crypts and onto adjacent villi. These cells then die by apoptosis at the tips of villi and are extruded into the lumen of the intestine; the average life span of these cells is about 4–6 days. On the other hand, Paneth cells are much longer lived (~60 days), and they migrate to the crypt base where they are in close contact with epithelial stem cells.

It has been increasingly appreciated that the external and internal surfaces of the human body are inhabited by commensal microbes that are not mere passengers but actually

FIGURE 13–13 Anatomy and histology of the small and large intestine. (Redrawn, with permission, from Boron WF et al, eds. *Medical Physiology*, 2nd ed. Saunders Elsevier, 2009. Copyright © Elsevier.)

perform critical functions. In the adult small intestine, a large and diverse population of commensal microbes inhabits the lumen. Most of these microbes are bacteria, and the major phyla represented are *Bacteroides* and *Firmicutes*. Most of these microbes are anaerobes (able to live in the absence of oxygen). The density increases dramatically in the lumen of the intestine (from hundreds per milliliter in the duodenum to trillions per milliliter in the colon). These bacteria function to aid in the digestion of complex carbohydrates. Based on studies in germ-free organisms, it is estimated that these

intestinal microbiota increase our ability to extract nutrients from food by as much as 30%. The microbiota also play key roles in training the mucosal immune system and developing blood vessels in the intestine. The microbial populations most closely associated with the mucosa appear to be quite distinct from those associated with the lumen and include many members of the Lachnospiraceae and Ruminococcaceae families. Functioning cooperatively, these microbes form a critical barrier to pathogens. Furthermore, bacteria are not the only commensal microorganisms in the intestine: *Archaea* (single-cell microorganisms without nuclei), fungi, and viruses are normally present in the lumen of the intestine. In most cases, their roles are still undefined.

Digestion & Absorption in the Small Intestine

The small intestine is the main site of digestion and the principal site of nutrient absorption. Thus, it is appropriate to review all steps of digestion in the GI tract and then to consider the mechanisms by which nutrients are absorbed.

A. Carbohydrates

Carbohydrates, which are mainly present in the diet as polysaccharides and disaccharides, must be digested to monosaccharides for absorption. Intestinal microbes (in particular, *Bacteroides* spp) contain a large repertoire of glycoside hydrolases that aid in the breakdown of complex plant polysaccharides. This is an important beneficial function of commensal intestinal microbes. Alpha-amylases in salivary and pancreatic secretions cleave interior **α**-1,4 glucose linkages in large polymers of starch to form fragments (disaccharides, trisaccharides, and oligosaccharides). Oligosaccharidases and disaccharidases in the brush border of enterocytes digest small fragments to monosaccharides, glucose, galactose, and fructose. Glucose and galactose, along with two Na^+ ions, are absorbed across the apical membrane of enterocytes by the same transporter, SGLT1. The passive uptake of water also occurs, maintaining osmolality on both sides of the cell membrane. The extrusion of Na^+ out of the basolateral membrane by Na^+-K^+ ATPase provides an electrochemical Na^+ gradient that drives the absorption of glucose and galactose against their concentration gradients. Fructose is absorbed into the cell by facilitated diffusion through the apical membrane by a different transporter, GLUT-5. All three hexoses leave the cell by facilitated diffusion through a common transporter, GLUT-2, located in the basolateral membrane.

Lactose intolerance is the most common problem of carbohydrate digestion. It results mainly from the reduction of lactase activity in adults. Lactase is expressed normally at high levels in the jejunum of neonatal and infant humans. In many parts of the world, lactase levels are gradually reduced after weaning. However, lactase levels do not decrease significantly in populations in which milk products are an important part of the adult diet. Lactase activity is rate limiting for lactose digestion in most adults throughout other regions of the world. If lactase is deficient, nondigested lactose is not absorbed. The nonabsorbed lactose retains water in the lumen to maintain the osmolality of chyme equivalent to that of plasma. This fluid retention causes abdominal pain (cramps), nausea, and diarrhea. Bacterial fermentation of lactose in the distal small intestine and colon further exacerbates these symptoms.

Mutations of the gene encoding SGLT1 impair glucose and galactose absorption in some patients. Affected individuals develop diarrhea when they consume sugars normally absorbed by SGLT1, because of defects in the absorption of Na^+, monosaccharides, and water. In contrast, fructose, which is absorbed by GLUT-5, does not cause diarrhea.

B. Proteins

Proteins entering the intestine derive from the diet and also from cells shed from the mucosa. Protein digestion begins in the stomach by the action of pepsin, but most protein digestion occurs in the lumen of the duodenum and the jejunum by the action of pancreatic proteases (**trypsin, chymotrypsin, carboxypeptidases**), yielding small oligopeptides and free amino acids. Peptidases on the surfaces of intestinal epithelial cells are required for the digestion of larger oligopeptides to yield smaller peptides and additional amino acids. Dipeptides and tripeptides are absorbed into enterocytes by secondary active cotransport with H^+ ions by the oligopeptide cotransporter, PepT1. The H^+ ions in the lumen are provided by a Na^+-K^+ transporter in the apical membrane. Amino acid uptake from the lumen occurs through several different transporters. Each transporter is specific for various side chain groups: acidic, basic, neutral, and imino. The uptake of most amino acids into enterocytes is coupled to cotransport with Na^+ ions driven by the Na^+-K^+ ATPase in the basolateral membrane. Absorbed dipeptides and tripeptides are hydrolyzed to amino acids within the enterocytes by independent cytosolic peptidases. Amino acids exit the cell through the basolateral membrane by cation-independent amino acid transporters. Infants can absorb proteins by endocytosis, providing a mechanism for the transfer of immunoglobulins, and thus passive immunity, from mother to child.

C. Lipids

Triglycerides constitute about 90% of dietary lipid; cholesterol, phospholipids, sphingolipids, fatty acids, and fat-soluble vitamins make up the balance. Dietary lipids are first emulsified by mechanical digestion (chewing, antral contractions, segmentation), which produces fine droplets suspended in aqueous fluid. Lipid digestion begins in the stomach by the combined action of swallowed **lingual lipase** from salivary glands and **gastric lipase** secreted by gastric gland chief cells in the fundus. These lipases convert triglycerides to fatty acids and diglycerides. Most lipid digestion occurs in the duodenum and jejunum. Lipids in the lumen form micelles as a result of the emulsifying properties of bile salts, phospholipids, and mixing contractions of the stomach and intestine. The most important enzyme in lipid digestion is **pancreatic lipase**. Lipase is secreted as an active enzyme, but full activity requires an alkaline pH and binding to a cofactor called **colipase**. Procolipase is also secreted in pancreatic juice and is converted to colipase by trypsin in the intestinal lumen. Lipase is only active at the oil–water interface of the triglyceride droplets. Colipase promotes the binding of lipase to the surface of micelles and thereby facilitates digestion. Lipase cleaves the fatty acid ester linkages at the 1 and 3 positions of the glycerol backbone of triglycerides to yield free fatty acids and a 2-monoglyceride.

The major barrier to lipid absorption is an **unstirred layer** on the surface of the enterocytes that is not readily mixed with the bulk fluid in the intestinal lumen because of the highly convoluted surface of the epithelium. The short- and medium-chain fatty acids that are water soluble and the long-chain fatty acids, monoglycerides, lysophospholipids, and cholesterol in the micelles diffuse through the unstirred layer to the surface of the enterocytes. Proton secretion creates an acidic micro-environment at the surface of enterocytes and promotes the protonation of fatty acids. Protonated (uncharged) fatty acids, monoglycerides, lysophospholipids, and cholesterol leave the micelles. Being protonated and thus lipid soluble, they readily diffuse into the cell. Fatty acids of less than 10 carbon atoms in length can pass through cells and enter the blood directly. The uptake of long-chain fatty acids (and some phospholipids) appears to be mediated by a specialized fatty acid transporter protein: microvillous membrane **fatty acid–binding protein**. Within the enterocyte, long-chain fatty acids bind to fatty acid–binding proteins that transport the newly absorbed long-chain fatty acids to the smooth endoplasmic reticulum for reassembly into triglycerides with absorbed 2-monoglycerides. The triglycerides, cholesterol esters, and phospholipids are combined with specific proteins in the Golgi apparatus of enterocytes and assembled into **chylomicrons**, which are exported from the basolateral membrane of the cell. They enter the lymphatic system through the large intraendothelial channels and subsequently are delivered to the bloodstream. During a relatively brief circulation, they are partially lipolyzed by cell-surface lipases and acquire more protein components. The liver is the main destination for chylomicron remnants. Note that chylomicrons serve as the primary transporters of fat-soluble vitamins in the circulation.

D. Fluid and Electrolytes

The small intestine is the major site of water absorption. Water moves into and out of the lumen of the intestine to keep its contents iso-osmotic with plasma. Water transport in either direction is thus passive, being secondary and proportional to the movement of ions (especially Na^+ and Cl^- ions) and nutrients. In the small intestine, water absorption is greatest in mature epithelial cells at villous tips. Water secretion is greatest in immature cells at villous crypts. Most passage of water (and ions) occurs by transcellular transport through aquaporins, a family of water channels. There is also some paracellular transport of water and ions. Epithelial cells lining the GI tract are interconnected by tight junctions. Junctions are somewhat leaky, allowing some water and small ions to move between the lumen and the mucosa via paracellular transport. The resistance of tight junctions is an important determinant of the relative degree that transcellular transport occurs, and this resistance varies throughout the intestines. Tight junctions are most leaky in the duodenum and jejunum, becoming progressively less leaky (tighter) in the ileum and colon. Larger ions and organic solutes are more restricted in their movement across tight junctions.

The jejunum is the main site of absorption of Na^+ ions. Na^+ absorption is mainly transcellular, either by **cotransport** with nutrients (sugars, amino acids) or by **Na^+–K^+ exchange**. There is also **parallel Na^+ and Cl^- absorption** by a paracellular route. HCO_3^- ions are secreted in the proximal duodenum, but in the jejunum, HCO_3^- and Cl^- ions are absorbed in large amounts. In the ileum, HCO_3^- is secreted and Cl^- is absorbed. K^+ ion absorption from the lumen of the small intestine occurs mainly by passive paracellular transport. The Na^+-coupled glucose transporter (SGLT1) in the apical membrane of the small intestine takes up two Na^+ ions with each glucose molecule. This property is central to the development of effective therapeutic oral rehydration solutions that contain glucose, Na^+, Cl^-, and HCO_3^- to enhance water and electrolyte uptake during severe diarrhea (eg, cholera).

The absorption of electrolytes and water is regulated by hormones and neurotransmitters. For example, angiotensin II and aldosterone, which are generated and released during dehydration, promote the absorption of NaCl in the intestine.

Secretion in the Small Intestine

The cells of the crypts of Lieberkühn are important sites of electrolyte and water secretion. The Na^+-K^+ ATPase in the basolateral membrane of epithelial cells provides the electrochemical gradients for secondary active transport and the diffusion of other ions. An Na-K-$2Cl^-$ transporter in the basolateral membrane mediates the uptake of Na^+, Cl^-, and K^+ ions into the cell (Figure 13–14). This is an example of secondary active transport: With the entry of Na^+ ions, an electrochemical gradient drives the uptake of K^+ and Cl^- ions against electrochemical gradients. Excess K^+ ions leave the cell by basolateral K^+ channels that can be regulated by Ca^{2+} and cAMP. Cl^- ions diffuse across the apical membrane of the enterocytes and into the intestinal lumen through a Cl^- channel that is regulated by cAMP. This electrogenic secretion of Cl^- ions provides a small negative charge to the lumen relative to the interstitial fluid, which drives the secretion of Na^+ ions by a paracellular route. Water follows by transcellular and paracellular routes to maintain iso-osmolality with plasma. The net result is thus the secretion of NaCl and water.

Fluid and electrolyte secretion flushes bacterial products and toxins away from the surface of the epithelium and thus plays a role in mucosal defense. Numerous substances, termed **secretagogues**, stimulate fluid and electrolyte secretion in both health and diseases (see Figure 13–14). **Neurotransmitter secretagogues** from the submucosal plexus include VIP and acetylcholine. **Paracrine secretagogues** include bradykinin, serotonin, histamine, and prostaglandins. Some products from immune cells indirectly stimulate secretion by acting on submucosal neurons to induce the release of acetylcholine or VIP, which then acts on enterocytes to stimulate secretion. **Luminal secretagogues** include bacterial toxins. A toxin from **cholera** modifies G proteins and thereby permanently activates adenylyl cyclase and increases intracellular levels of cAMP. Strong activation of the apical Cl^- channels of crypt cells results in a massive

FIGURE 13–14 Mechanisms of fluid and electrolyte secretion by epithelial cells of the intestinal crypts. **Top:** Ionic basis of secretion of Cl⁻ and Na⁺ ions. **Bottom:** Regulation of fluid and electrolyte secretion by submucosal neurons and mast cells of the lamina propria. Activated mast cells release histamine, which either directly acts on epithelial cells or acts on submucosal neurons to stimulate the release of acetylcholine, which then acts on epithelial cells.

secretion of Cl⁻ ions and, in consequence, of water and Na⁺ ions. Patients with cholera may excrete up to 20 L of diarrhea per day, leading to rapid dehydration and death. An inexpensive and effective treatment is oral rehydration with glucose-containing solutions. The glucose drives the sodium–glucose cotransporter to transport both molecules into enterocytes, and with them chloride and water, thereby offsetting the fluid efflux mediated by the bacterial toxin. Because these cotransporters are lacking in the colon, its maximum absorptive capacity (5 L/d) is considerably less than that of the small intestine (12 L/d).

One type of Cl⁻ ion channel in the apical membrane is encoded by the gene for cystic fibrosis and is termed the **cystic fibrosis conductance regulator** (**CFTR**). The CFTR is expressed in many epithelial cells throughout the body. Mutations in the channel result in improper folding and premature degradation of the channel protein. The secretion of Cl⁻ ions and, in consequence, of Na⁺ ions and water, is diminished. In the airway, this results in the production of thick secretions that impair ventilation.

Motility of the Small Intestine

A. Electrical Activity of Small Intestinal Muscle

In the human duodenum, slow waves occur at a frequency of 11–13/min. The slow-wave frequency declines to the ileum.

The slow waves may or may not be associated with action potentials. In the intestine, slow waves alone do not cause contractions. However, when action potentials fire, they give rise to strong but highly localized contractions, the magnitude of which depends on the frequency of the action potentials. The slow waves are entirely intrinsic: They are generated within the intestine and probably depend on the unstable membrane potentials of the interstitial cells of Cajal. The frequency with which action potentials fire depends on the excitability of the muscle cells, which is influenced by circulating hormones, extrinsic nerves, and the enteric nervous system.

B. Mechanical Activity of Small Intestinal Muscle

During periods of fasting, the intestine is quiescent. However, every 90–120 min, there are bursts of action potentials in the muscle that induce waves of contraction lasting about 5 min. These **migrating myoelectric complexes** take 90 min to traverse the small intestine. By the time the migrating myoelectric complex reaches the ileum, another begins in the stomach. These waves of contraction clear the small intestine of its contents, acting as a "housekeeper" to keep the lumen relatively clean, thereby minimizing bacterial overgrowth (Figure 13–15). The migrating myoelectric complex is associated with cycling levels of **motilin**, a 22–amino acid peptide hormone secreted by endocrine cells in the duodenum.

FIGURE 13–15 Mechanical activity of the small intestine during fasting and after feeding. The recordings are of intraluminal pressures measured at indicated regions of the intestine of a conscious dog. The migrating myoelectric complexes in the fasting state are disrupted by feeding, which induces segmentation and peristaltic contractions. (Redrawn, with permission, from Boron WF et al, eds. *Medical Physiology*, 2nd ed. Saunders Elsevier, 2009. Copyright © Elsevier.)

Motilin may act on the enteric nervous system to regulate the migrating myoelectric complex. Its release appears to be under neural control, although luminal contents can also stimulate motilin release. The effect of motilin is to stimulate the contraction of gastric and intestinal smooth muscle during the interdigestive period between meals.

During feeding, the migrating myoelectric complexes cease, probably because of the action of the vagus and gut hormones such as gastrin and cholecystokinin (see Figure 13–15). The migrating myoelectric complexes are replaced by **phasic contractions** that are brief (a few seconds at each site) and restricted to short lengths of intestine (a few centimeters). Phasic contractions serve both to mix and propel food through the small intestine. **Rhythmic segmented contractions** provide the major local mixing activity in the small intestine. In this process, a short segment contracts while adjacent segments are relaxed. Then, the contracted segment relaxes while previously relaxed adjacent segments contract. As these contractions alternate, chyme is forced in both directions, mixed with cell secretions, and brought into contact with cells lining the lumen. Short waves of **peristalsis** propel chyme distally, mixing chyme in successive segments and propelling it through the intestine.

C. Peristaltic Reflex

Localized chemical or mechanical stimulation of the small intestine results in a contraction on the oral side of the stimulus and relaxation on the anal side. These responses are controlled by the enteric nervous system. Sensory neurons that respond to chemicals (eg, acids) or mechanical stimuli (stroking the mucosa or stretching the muscle with a bolus of digesta) activate excitatory ascending interneurons, which then innervate excitatory motor neurons (Figure 13–16). These neurons release excitatory neurotransmitters, acetylcholine, and the neuropeptide substance P, which activates receptors on circular muscle cells to trigger contraction. The sensory neurons also excite descending interneurons that innervate inhibitory motor neurons. They, in turn, release inhibitory neurotransmitters, VIP, and nitric oxide, which relax circular muscle.

Opioid drugs such as morphine, which are highly effective for the relief of chronic pain (eg, cancer pain), have the detrimental side effect of inhibiting the motility of the small intestine. Opioids act on enteric nerves to inhibit the secretion of excitatory neurotransmitters to thereby inhibit peristalsis. The inhibition of motility slows down intestinal transit, allowing for more complete absorption, so the volume entering the colon is diminished and constipation results.

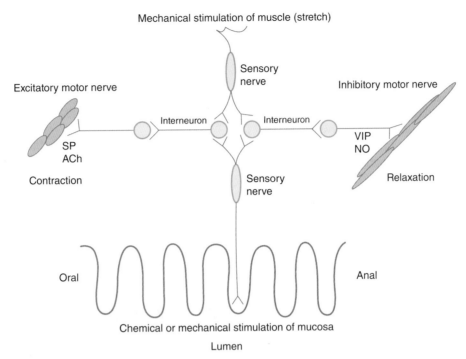

FIGURE 13–16 The peristaltic reflex of the small intestine. Enteric sensory nerves detect chemical or mechanical stimulation of the mucosa or stretch of the muscle layer. Signals are transmitted in an oral or anal direction by interneurons. Excitatory motor nerves release acetylcholine (ACh) and substance P (SP), which cause muscle contraction on the oral side of the stimulus. Inhibitory motor nerves release vasoactive intestinal peptide (VIP) and nitric oxide (NO), which cause muscle relaxation on the anal side of the stimulus.

CHECKPOINT

31. Describe the hormonal reflex by which fat in the intestine stimulates the secretion of bile.

32. Describe the mechanism by which glucose is absorbed across the apical and basolateral membranes of an enterocyte.

33. What is the mechanism of absorption of tripeptides across an intestinal epithelial cell?

34. What is the role of bile in lipid absorption in the intestine?

35. List three general mechanisms of Na+ ion absorption in the small intestine.

36. Describe the mechanism of fluid and electrolyte secretion in the crypts of Lieberkühn.

37. Name two neurotransmitters that are secretagogues.

38. How do certain bacterial toxins stimulate fluid and electrolyte secretion in the crypts of Lieberkühn?

39. Describe the pattern of intestinal motility during fasting and after feeding.

40. Name one hormone that maintains the fasting pattern of motility and one that induces the fed pattern of motility in the small intestine.

41. Name the neurotransmitters that mediate the ascending and descending limbs of the peristaltic reflex.

COLON

Anatomy & Histology

The adult colon is 1.0–1.5 m in length. Its various segments (cecum; ascending, transverse, descending, and sigmoid colon; and rectum) are involved in absorbing water and electrolytes; secreting mucus; and forming, propelling, and storing unabsorbed material (feces). The colon is also the home of the majority of the intestinal microbes.

The surface of the colon consists of a columnar epithelium with no villi and few folds except in the distal rectum (see Figure 13–13). The epithelial cells include absorptive cells and contain microvilli on their surface as well as mucus-secreting goblet cells. Colonic crypts contain goblet cells, endocrine cells, absorptive cells, and epithelial stem cells. As in the small intestine, the stem cells and their daughter progenitor cells serve to replenish the differentiated cells of the epithelium that continually turn over throughout life.

Digestion & Absorption in the Colon

Digestion in the colon occurs as a consequence of the action of the colonic microbiota. Short-chain fatty acids released by microbial action on dietary fiber are an important source of energy for the colon. More importantly, these short-chain fatty acids promote survival of healthy colonic epithelium while inducing apoptosis (programmed cell death) in epithelial cells that are progressing toward malignant transformation.

Fluid and electrolyte absorption has been well studied and is a major function of the colon. Up to 5 L of water can be absorbed per day across the colonic epithelium. Furthermore, the colonic epithelium can also take up sodium against a considerable concentration gradient. Aldosterone, a hormone involved in fluid and electrolyte homeostasis, increases colonic sodium conductance in response to volume depletion, thus playing an important role in maintaining fluid and electrolyte balance.

Secretion in the Colon

The major secretory products of the colon are the mucin proteins produced and secreted by goblet cells that reside in the epithelial layer. Mucins are very-high-molecular-weight proteins (mostly due to the extensive glycosylation). In the lumen of the colon, they are hydrated and form a layer overlying the epithelial cells. They serve to lubricate and prevent the opposing sides of the intestinal tube from sticking together (thus collapsing the tube). In addition, mucins participate in innate immunity. As antimicrobial peptides bound by immunoglobulins that are secreted into the lumen, mucins form a barrier to intestinal microbes and pathogens.

Motility of the Colon

Unlike the stomach and small intestine, the colon is rarely inactive, although its activity is less easily characterized than that of the stomach, which has the pattern known as receptive relaxation, or than that of the small intestine, which displays the pattern known as the migrating motor complex and segmental to-and-fro action. Some patterns are discernible, however, such as the gastrocolic reflex (colonic mass peristalsis after a meal). Disorders of colonic motility are common complications of autonomic neuropathy in patients with diabetes mellitus and can cause severe GI complaints. Stool continence requires contraction of the puborectalis muscle and the anal sphincter. Defecation involves relaxation of the puborectalis by the sacral parasympathetic nerves, resulting in a straightening of the anorectal angle. Rectal distension results in reflex sympathetic-mediated internal and external sphincter relaxation.

CHECKPOINT

42. How does colonic motility differ from small intestine motility?
43. What is the major secretory product of the colon?
44. What volume of water is the colon capable of absorbing per day?

OVERVIEW OF GI DISORDERS

DISORDERS OF MOTILITY

Disorders of motility affect all major regions of the GI tract. Because GI tract motility is a complex result of smooth muscle contraction under neural and hormonal control, abnormal motility of the GI tract can occur through damage to GI smooth muscle or to the neural and hormonal mechanisms by which it is controlled, or both. An example of muscle damage leading to abnormal motility is seen in esophageal stricture as a result of caustic ingestion or acid reflux. Abnormal neural control of motility is seen in esophageal achalasia. Esophageal motility disorders are typically characterized by dysphagia and odynophagia. An example of a neural defect that affects motility is Hirschsprung disease. These patients are typically younger than 2 years and either present after birth with the inability to pass meconium or later with severe constipation. The structural defect is a lack of myenteric neurons in the distal colon owing to a congenital defect whereby the migration of neural crest precursor cells does not occur properly.

Motility disorders of the stomach include gastroparesis as a complication of diabetes mellitus, and dysmotility as a consequence of stomach surgery, from either resection of part of the stomach or **vagotomy**. Vagotomy entails the surgical transection of the vagus nerve trunks, which prevents vagus-stimulated acid secretion and regulation of gastric motility. Before the availability of histamine H$_2$ receptor antagonists and PPIs, selective vagotomy of the stomach was used as a treatment for the hypersecretion of gastric acid. Vagotomy is still sometimes performed as a treatment for Zollinger–Ellison syndrome (ie, acid hypersecretion and severe peptic ulcer disease caused by a gastrin-secreting tumor). In **hypertrophic pyloric stenosis**, food cannot pass freely out of the stomach owing to spasmodic narrowing of the pyloric outlet caused by hypertrophy of the pyloric musculature. It is more common in boys and presents shortly after birth with nonbilious vomiting. It is readily managed surgically.

The symptoms and signs of motility disorders in the stomach depend on their cause. Because vagotomy cuts fibers influencing the enteric nervous system as well as the intended fibers that influence acid secretion, a classic complication of vagotomy is disordered gastric motility. This may present clinically as either partial outlet obstruction or as too-rapid emptying of gastric contents into the duodenum, with resulting fluid shifts and vasomotor symptoms (“**dumping syndrome**”). Sometimes, however, patients may develop symptoms of stomach distension, nausea, early satiety, and vomiting suggestive of partial gastric outlet obstruction. To ameliorate the latter symptoms, **pyloroplasty** (severing the fibers of the pyloric sphincter) is done to render the sphincter less competent, so that food can pass more easily into the duodenum. Intrinsic neuropathy (eg, in diabetes mellitus) results in delayed gastric emptying, nausea, vomiting, and constipation rather than the classic dumping syndrome. The pathophysiologic basis for these differences is unknown.

In the small intestine and colon, disordered motility occurs in **irritable bowel syndrome**. Irritable bowel syndrome is characterized by recurrent episodes of abdominal pain, bloating, and diarrhea alternating with constipation in the absence of detectable organic disease and structural abnormalities. The cause of this condition is still unclear.

DISORDERS OF SECRETION

Clinically recognized disorders of secretion involve the production of acid, intrinsic factor, or mucus by the stomach; digestive enzymes and bicarbonate by the pancreas; bile by the liver; and water and electrolytes by the small intestine in response to secretagogues.

Either elevated gastric acid secretion or diminished mucosal defense can predispose to the development of **peptic ulcers**. Ulcers represent discrete regions of erosion through the entire mucosa. Acid-induced damage may occur in the form of an ulcer either in the stomach (**gastric ulcer**) or in the first part of the small intestine (**duodenal ulcer**). Acid-induced injury may also occur in the form of more diffuse and less clearly demarcated inflammation anywhere along the GI tract from the lower esophagus through the duodenum. It appears that elevated acid secretion, almost always in the setting of *H pylori* infection, is relatively more important in the development of duodenal ulcer, whereas diminished mucosal defense (eg, from diminished mucus secretion in some cases) is a more crucial factor in the development of gastric ulcer, with *H pylori* underlying only about half the cases. Disorders of secretion involving the liver and pancreas are discussed in Chapters 14

and 15, respectively. Diarrhea, the major secretory disorder of the small intestine, is discussed later.

DISORDERS OF DIGESTION & ABSORPTION

Physiologically significant digestion and absorption can occur throughout the GI tract. Indeed, the effectiveness of sublingual nitroglycerin therapy for patients with angina is a testimonial to the efficacy of sublingual absorption. Nevertheless, the clinically prominent disorders of digestion and absorption focus on the small intestine and colon and the accessory organs (pancreas and liver) whose secretions (digestive enzymes, bicarbonate, and bile) are necessary for digestion and absorption in the small intestine.

GI MANIFESTATIONS OF SYSTEMIC DISEASE

A wide range of systemic conditions and diseases may produce symptoms and signs in the GI tract. These include endocrine disorders that alter control of GI tract functions or that predispose to pancreatitis or peptic ulcer disease; complications of diabetes mellitus, including autonomic neuropathy and ketoacidosis; pregnancy, deficiency disorders, including deficiency of zinc, and niacin; and neoplastic, hematologic, and rheumatologic conditions (Table 13–4).

CHECKPOINT

45. What are some common symptoms of esophageal dysmotility?
46. Why does vagotomy often create motor disorders in the stomach?

PATHOPHYSIOLOGY OF DISORDERS OF THE ESOPHAGUS

The major disorders of the esophagus are related to motor functions: Disordered peristalsis and increased lower esophageal sphincter tone are seen in esophageal achalasia, whereas inappropriate lower esophageal sphincter relaxation results in reflux esophagitis.

ESOPHAGEAL ACHALASIA

Clinical Presentation

Esophageal achalasia is a motor disorder in which the lower esophageal sphincter fails to relax properly. As a result, a **functional obstruction** (ie, obstruction as a result

of abnormal function in the absence of a visible mass or lesion) is created that is manifested as dysphagia (inability to swallow), regurgitation, and chest pain. It is a progressive disease in which severe radiographic distortion of the esophagus develops.

Etiology

The underlying cause of esophageal achalasia, which occurs with an incidence of 0.5–1.0 per 100,000 population per year, is unknown. Degeneration of the myenteric plexus and loss of inhibitory neurons that release VIP and nitric oxide, which dilate the lower esophageal sphincter, may contribute.

TABLE 13–4   GI manifestations of systemic diseases and their pathophysiologic mechanisms.

Disease or Condition	Commonly Associated GI Manifestations	Mechanism
Thyroid disease		
Autoimmune thyroiditis	Achlorhydria and pernicious anemia	Autoimmune destruction of parietal cells
Hypothyroidism	Esophageal reflux	Lower esophageal sphincter dysfunction
	Bezoars	Gastric dysmotility
	Constipation	Intestinal dysmotility
	Malabsorption	Villous atrophy and pancreatic insufficiency
Hyperthyroidism	Diarrhea and weight loss	Intestinal hypermotility with rapid transit and malabsorption
Adrenal disease		
Adrenal insufficiency	Abdominal pain	Unknown
	Diarrhea	Malabsorption resulting from loss of trophic effect of corticosteroids on enterocyte brush border
Parathyroid disease		
Primary hyperparathyroidism	Nausea and vomiting	Hypercalcemia-induced alteration in signal transduction resulting in gastric atony and dysmotility
	Pancreatitis	Hypercalcemia-induced premature activation of pancreatic enzymes
	Acid-peptic disease	Hypercalcemia-induced increased acid secretion
Diabetes mellitus		
	Esophageal, gastric, small and large intestinal, and rectal dysfunction	Autonomic neuropathy
	Nausea, vomiting, abdominal pain	Ketoacidosis with gastric atony
Pregnancy		
	Esophageal reflux, nausea and vomiting, hematemesis, constipation, hemorrhoids	Pressure effects of gravid uterus on lower esophageal sphincter, gastric emptying, intestinal transit time, and venous return
Deficiency states		
Zinc, niacin	Malabsorption syndrome	Altered enterocyte brush border
Cancer		
	Pain, fever, bleeding, ascites, obstruction, perforation	Metastases (most commonly breast cancer, melanoma, bronchogenic lung carcinoma)
	Paraneoplastic syndromes, hypercalcemia	Tumor-produced peptides
Hematologic conditions		
Bleeding disorders	Intramural hematoma	Hemorrhage
Hypercoagulable states	Bowel infarction	Intestinal ischemia
Dysproteinemias	Hemorrhage, obstruction, amyloidosis	Infiltration
Rheumatologic disorders		
Scleroderma	Dysphagia, esophageal reflux, obstruction, bleeding, perforation, pseudo-obstruction, pancreatitis, malabsorption	Inflammation, vasculitis, vascular obliteration, villous atrophy
Systemic lupus erythematosus	Nausea, vomiting, mucosal ulceration	Inflammation, vasculitis, vascular obstruction, villous atrophy
Rheumatoid arthritis	Gastric ulcers, gastritis	Aspirin or NSAID use

(continued)

TABLE 13-4   GI manifestations of systemic diseases and their pathophysiologic mechanisms. (Continued)

Disease or Condition	Commonly Associated GI Manifestations	Mechanism
Metabolic and infiltrative disorders		
Dyslipidemias; sarcoidosis, amyloidosis	Malabsorption	Infiltration, muscle atrophy, dysmotility
	Infarction	Infiltration, mucosal ischemia
Renal disorders		
Chronic renal failure and renal transplantation	Abdominal pain, GI bleeding, intestinal perforation	Gastritis, duodenitis, pancreatitis
Neurologic disorders		
Spinal cord injury, myotonic dystrophy, CNS disease	Impaired gut motility with nausea, vomiting, chronic constipation	Disordered central and enteric nervous system communication
	Gastroduodenal (Cushing) ulcers	Hemodynamic changes and/or increased vagal activity
Pulmonary disorders		
Asthma	Esophageal reflux	Nocturnal aspiration
Cystic fibrosis	Diarrhea, malabsorption, weight loss	Pancreatic exocrine insufficiency

CNS, central nervous system; GI, gastrointestinal; NSAID, nonsteroidal anti-inflammatory drug.

Reproduced, with permission, from Hunter TB et al. Gastrointestinal complications of leukemia and its treatment. AJR Am J Roentgenol. 1984;143:513; Riley SA et al. Maldigestion and malabsorption. In: Sleisenger MH et al, eds. *Gastrointestinal Disease,* 4th ed. Saunders, 1989; and Sack TL et al. Effects of systemic and extraintestinal disease on the gut. In: Sleisenger MH et al, eds. *Gastrointestinal Disease,* 4th ed. Saunders, 1989. Copyright © Elsevier.

Esophageal involvement in Chagas disease, resulting from damage of the neural plexuses of the esophagus by the parasite *Trypanosoma cruzi*, bears a striking resemblance to esophageal achalasia. A number of other disorders, including malignancies, may present with manometric pressure characteristics or radiographic features similar to those observed in idiopathic esophageal achalasia.

Pathology & Pathogenesis

Although achalasia is manifested as a motor disorder of esophageal smooth muscle, it is actually a result of defective innervation of smooth muscle in the esophageal body and lower esophageal sphincter. Lower esophageal sphincter tone is normally characterized by tonic contraction with intermittent relaxation resulting from a neural reflex arc (see earlier discussion). In achalasia, the lower esophageal sphincter is even more tightly contracted and does not relax properly in response to swallowing because of a partial loss of neurons in the wall of the esophagus. Thus, achalasia can be thought of as a disorder caused by defective inhibitory pathways of the esophageal enteric nervous system. Interestingly, injecting botulinum toxin into the lower esophageal sphincter diminishes the activity of the excitatory pathways, thereby ameliorating symptoms. In addition to dysfunction of the lower esophageal sphincter, loss of normal peristalsis in the esophageal body is often seen in achalasia, consistent with the hypothesis of myenteric plexus degeneration. Variations of achalasia also exist in which normal peristalsis is replaced by simultaneous contractions of large or small amplitude.

Clinical Manifestations

Over months and years, lower esophageal sphincter dysfunction results in tremendous enlargement of the esophagus. Normally intended as a direct conduit to the stomach, the esophagus in advanced cases of achalasia can hold as much as 1 L of putrid, infected material, imposing a high risk of aspiration pneumonia. Without treatment, patients display progressive, severe weight loss with worsening chest pain, mucosal ulceration, lung infection, and occasional esophageal rupture, culminating in death.

REFLUX ESOPHAGITIS

Clinical Presentation

The predominant presenting symptom of reflux is burning chest pain (heartburn) resulting from recurrent mucosal injury. Patients also frequently report the sensation of burning in the back of their throat and a sour (acidic) taste from the reflux. Symptoms are often worse at night, when lying supine, or after consuming foods or drugs that diminish lower esophageal sphincter tone, such as caffeinated beverages.

Etiology

Common causes of reflux esophagitis are those conditions that result in persistent or repetitive acid exposure to the esophageal mucosa. These include disorders that increase the rate of spontaneous transient lower esophageal sphincter relaxations (Table 13–5) or impair reflexes that normally follow transient

TABLE 13–5   Modulators of lower esophageal sphincter pressure.

Factors	Increase Pressure	Decrease Pressure
Hormones	Gastrin	Secretin
	Motilin	Cholecystokinin
	Substance P	Somatostatin
		Vasoactive intestinal peptide (VIP)
		Progesterone
Neural agents	α-adrenergic agonists	β-adrenergic agonists
	β-adrenergic antagonists	α-adrenergic antagonists
	Cholinergic agonists	Anticholinergic agents
Foods	Protein meals	Fat
		Chocolate
		Peppermint
Other	Histamine	Theophylline
	Antacids	Prostaglandins E_2, I_2
	Metoclopramide	Serotonin
	Domperidone	Meperidine
	Cisapride[1]	Morphine
	Prostaglandin F_2	Dopamine
	Baclofen	Calcium channel–blocking agents
		Diazepam
		Barbiturates

[1]Drug withdrawn from U.S. market.

Reproduced, with permission, from Richter JE et al. Gastroesophageal reflux disease. In: Feldman M et al, eds. *Sleisenger and Fordtran's Gastrointestinal and Liver Disease*, 9th ed. Saunders, 2010. Copyright © Elsevier.

lower esophageal sphincter relaxations with a secondary wave of esophageal peristalsis. Conditions that increase gastric volume or pressure (eg, partial or complete gastric outlet obstruction) and conditions that increase acid production also contribute. Occasionally, reflux esophagitis can be caused by alkaline injury (eg, pancreatic juice or bile refluxing through both an incompetent pyloric sphincter and a relaxed lower esophageal sphincter). Hiatal hernia, a disorder in which a portion of the proximal stomach slides into the chest cavity with upward displacement of the lower esophageal sphincter, can also contribute to the development of reflux.

Pathology & Pathogenesis

Normally, the tonically contracted lower esophageal sphincter provides an effective barrier to reflux of acid from the stomach back into the esophagus. This is reinforced by secondary esophageal peristaltic waves in response to transient lower esophageal sphincter relaxation. Loss of lower esophageal sphincter tone (ie, the opposite of achalasia), increased frequency of transient relaxations, loss of secondary peristalsis after a transient relaxation, increased stomach volume or pressure, or increased acid production, can all make the reflux of acidic stomach contents more likely, causing pain or erosion. Recurrent reflux can damage the mucosa, resulting in inflammation, hence the term "reflux esophagitis." Recurrent reflux itself predisposes to further reflux because the scarring that occurs with healing of the inflamed epithelium renders the lower esophageal sphincter progressively less competent as a barrier.

Pepsin and bile can be refluxed in addition to acid to cause esophagitis. In most cases of esophageal reflux disease, a common pathophysiologic thread can be identified (Figure 13–17). Recurrent mucosal damage results in the infiltration of granulocytes and eosinophils, basal cell hyperplasia, and eventually the development of friable, bleeding ulcers and exudates over the mucosal surface. These pathologic changes set the stage for scar formation and sphincter incompetence, predisposing to recurrent cycles of inflammation.

An increased frequency of transient lower esophageal sphincter relaxations may be partly in response to increased gastric distension. Normally, transient lower esophageal sphincter relaxations are accompanied by increased esophageal peristalsis. Individuals with defects in excitatory pathways that promote peristalsis may, therefore, be at increased risk for the development of esophageal reflux. Changes in the types of prostaglandin produced by the esophagus have been noted in reflux esophagitis, perhaps contributing to impairment of healing and predisposing to recurrences. In contrast to other forms of acid-mediated injury, *H pylori* infection does not appear to contribute to the development of reflux or esophagitis.

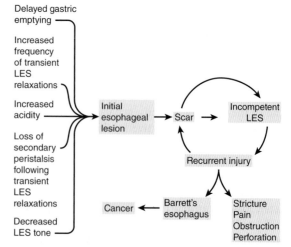

FIGURE 13–17 Pathophysiology of esophageal reflux disease. (LES, lower esophageal sphincter.)

Clinical Manifestations

Heartburn is the usual symptom of reflux esophagitis, typically worsening on lying prone. With recurrent reflux, a range of complications may develop. The most common complication is the development of stricture in the distal esophagus. Progressive obstruction, initially to solid food and later to liquid, presents as dysphagia. Other complications of recurrent reflux include hemorrhage or perforation; hoarseness, coughing, or wheezing; and pneumonia as a result of aspiration of gastric contents into the lungs, particularly during sleep. Chronic recurrent reflux can also result in a change in the esophageal epithelium from squamous to columnar histology (resembling that of the stomach and/or intestine). Termed **Barrett esophagus**, the disorder is more common in men and in smokers, and it leads to a greatly increased risk of adenocarcinoma. Adenocarcinomas in the distal esophagus and proximal (cardiac) stomach related to Barrett esophagus are among the most rapidly increasing types of cancer in young male patients in the United States.

CHECKPOINT

47. What are the roles of the lower esophageal sphincter structure in achalasia and in reflux esophagitis?
48. What are possible causes of achalasia?
49. What is the relationship of esophageal reflux to Barrett esophagus and cancer?

PATHOPHYSIOLOGY OF DISORDERS OF THE STOMACH

Common disorders involving the stomach reflect the importance of its role as a secretory organ, in particular of acid and intrinsic factor. Disorders of acid secretion result in **acid-peptic disease**, whereas loss of intrinsic factor secretion results in the inability to absorb vitamin B_{12}, manifesting as **pernicious anemia**. The major motility disorder of the stomach is gastroparesis.

ACID-PEPTIC DISEASE

Clinical Presentation

Patients with acid-peptic disease typically present with chronic, mild, gnawing or burning abdominal or chest pain resulting from superficial or deep erosion of the GI mucosa. Sudden complications include GI tract bleeding, resulting in hematemesis (vomiting of blood) or melena (tarry stools from the effect of acid on blood), and perforation and infection, resulting in severe abdominal pain and signs of acute abdomen (absence of bowel sounds, guarding, rebound tenderness). The latter presentation reflects the fact that in some cases, acid-peptic disease can be painless in the early stages and detected only when it leads to an intra-abdominal catastrophe.

Classically, duodenal ulcer presents as gnawing or burning epigastric pain occurring 1–3 hours after meals, often waking the patient at night, with antacids or food producing relief. However, many patients later documented to have duodenal ulcer do not fit this symptom profile. Elderly patients in particular often present with a complication of duodenal ulcer but no history of pain.

Etiology

Various causes of absolute or relative increased acid production (see Figure 13–12) or decreased mucosal defenses (see Table 13–2) predispose to acid-peptic disease. As mentioned, the bacterium *H pylori* is the root cause of a number of forms of acid-peptic disease, including duodenal ulcer, gastric ulcer, and gastritis (Figure 13–18).

Pathology & Pathogenesis

Corrosive agents (acid and pepsin) secreted by the stomach play a key role in gastric ulcer, duodenal ulcer, and acute erosive gastritis. These diseases have distinctive but overlapping pathogeneses with the common themes of either excessive acid secretion or diminished mucosal defense. Exactly why one but not another form of acid-peptic disease should develop in a given individual remains unclear. *H pylori* infection can cause acid-peptic disease by multiple mechanisms, including direct alteration of signal transduction in mucosal and immune cells, which in turn can increase acid secretion and diminish mucosal defenses. Figure 13–19 illustrates the complex interactions of *H pylori* infection and its location and virulence, along with its clinical consequences (eg, inflammation, increased or decreased acid secretion).

H pylori is an extremely common pathogen; rates of infection are highest in the world's poorest countries, where sanitation facilities and standards of personal hygiene are low. The most likely route of spread from person to person is fecal–oral. As many as 90% of infected individuals show signs of inflammation (gastritis or duodenitis) on endoscopy, although many, if not most, of these individuals are clinically asymptomatic. Despite this high rate of association of inflammation with *H pylori* infection, the important role of other factors is indicated by the fact that only about 15% of infected individuals ever develop a clinically significant ulcer. These other factors (both genetic and environmental, such as cigarette smoking) must account for the individual variations and are pathophysiologically important. Nevertheless, the role of *H pylori* is of particular clinical importance because, of patients who do develop acid-peptic disease, especially among those with

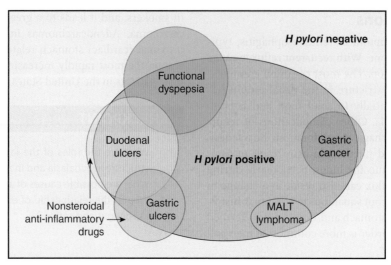

FIGURE 13–18 Relation of *H pylori* infection to upper GI tract conditions. The figure shows that most patients with gastroduodenal ulcers, gastric lymphoma, or adenocarcinoma have also been infected with *H pylori*. Note, however, that the circles are not to scale, because gastric cancer occurs in less than 1% of those infected with *H pylori*. Note, too, that relationships among the different conditions are more complex than depicted. Despite the fact that patients with cancer often have a prior history of ulcers, as shown in Figure 13–19, patients with a history of *H pylori* infection (which causes ulcers) are less likely to develop cancer. (MALT, mucosa-associated lymphoid tissue.) (Redrawn, with permission, from Calam J et al. Pathophysiology of duodenal and gastric ulcer and gastric cancer. BMJ. 2001;323:980. With permission from BMJ Publishing Group Ltd.)

duodenal ulcers, the vast majority have *H pylori* infection. Furthermore, treatment that does not eradicate *H pylori* is associated with the rapid recurrence of acid-peptic disease in most patients. There are numerous strains of *H pylori* that vary in their production of toxins such as CagA and VacA that directly alter cellular signaling pathways. Variations in bacterial strains, natural variation in the balance of inflammatory mediators (eg, T_H1 vs. T_H2 vs. T_H17 cytokines) triggered by infection, and a variety of environmental and lifestyle factors may explain why *H pylori* infection is asymptomatic in most patients, causes peptic ulcers in some, and increases the risk of developing lymphoma and adenocarcinoma in a few.

1. Gastric Ulcer

Gastric ulcer is distinguished from erosive gastritis by the depth of the lesion, with gastric ulcers penetrating through the mucosa. The actual ulcer crater is often surrounded by an area of intact but inflamed mucosa, suggesting that gastritis is a lesion that predisposes to the development of gastric ulcer. Most gastric ulcers occur on the lesser curvature of the stomach. It is likely that gastric ulcer represents the outcome of a number of different abnormalities summarized next.

Some gastric ulcers are believed to be related to impaired mucosal defenses, because the acid and pepsin secretory capacity of some affected patients is normal or even below normal.

Motility defects have been proposed to contribute to the development of gastric ulcer in at least three ways. First, they may contribute because of a tendency of duodenal contents to reflux back through an incompetent pyloric sphincter. Bile acids in the duodenal reflux material act as an irritant and may be an important contributor to a diminished mucosal barrier

against acid and pepsin. Second, they may contribute as a result of delayed emptying of gastric contents, including reflux material, into the duodenum. Third, they may contribute as a result of delayed gastric emptying and hence food retention, causing increased gastrin secretion and gastric acid production. It is not known whether these motility defects are a cause or a consequence of gastric ulcer formation.

Mucosal ischemia may play a role in the development of gastric ulcer. Prostaglandins are known to increase mucosal blood flow as well as bicarbonate and mucus secretion and to stimulate mucosal cell repair and renewal. Thus, their deficiency, resulting from nonsteroidal anti-inflammatory drug (NSAID) ingestion or other insults, may predispose to gastritis and gastric ulcer, as might diminish bicarbonate or mucus secretion resulting from other causes. Subsets of gastric ulcer patients with each of these defects have been identified. Thus, the risk factors (NSAID ingestion, smoking, psychologic stress, *H pylori* infection) that have been associated with gastric ulcer probably act by diminishing one or more mucosal defense mechanisms.

Gastritis (inflammation of the gastric mucosa) as a result of aspirin or other NSAID use, bile salts, alcohol use, or other insults may predispose to ulcer formation by (1) attenuating the barrier created by the epithelial cells or the mucus and bicarbonate they secrete; or (2) reducing the quantity of prostaglandins produced by epithelial cells that might otherwise diminish acid secretion.

2. Acute Erosive Gastritis

Acute erosive gastritis includes inflammation resulting from superficial mucosal injury, mucosal erosion, or shallow ulcers caused by a wide variety of insults, most notably alcohol use,

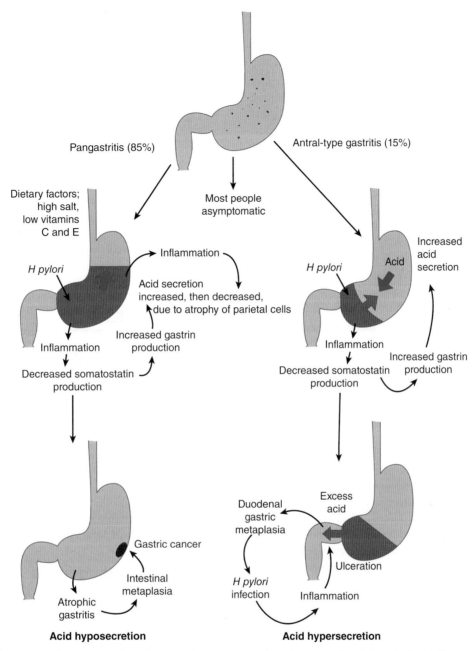

FIGURE 13–19 Patterns of chronic *H pylori* infection with respect to acid production and pathology. **Left:** Acid hyposecretion. *H pylori* infection spreads into the stomach body and causes the suppression of parietal cells, low acid secretion, atrophic gastritis, intestinal metaplasia, and predisposition to gastric cancer. **Right:** Acid hypersecretion. *H pylori* infection primarily of the stomach antrum causes decreased somatostatin and increased gastrin secretion, increasing acid secretion and predisposition to duodenal ulceration. (Redrawn from Calam J et al. Pathophysiology of duodenal and gastric ulcer and gastric cancer. BMJ. 2001;323:980. With permission from BMJ Publishing Group Ltd.)

drug use, and stress. Ethanol ingestion predisposes to gastritis but not to gastric ulcer. Unlike gastric or duodenal ulcers, in erosive gastritis the submucosa and muscularis mucosa are not penetrated. Acid hypersecretion, gastric anoxia or ischemia (eg, in shock), altered natural defenses (especially diminished mucus secretion), altered epithelial renewal, changes in tissue mediators (eg, prostaglandins), reduced intramucosal pH, and intramucosal energy deficits have been suggested as factors in the development of superficial gastric mucosal injury.

3. Chronic Atrophic Gastritis

Chronic atrophic gastritis is a heterogeneous group of conditions characterized by inflammatory cell infiltration into the corpus of the stomach with gastric mucosal atrophy that leads to the death of parietal cells and, ultimately, the dropout of gastric glands. In chronic disease, unlike in acute erosive gastritis, endoscopic abnormalities may not be grossly apparent. The capacity to secrete gastric acid is progressively reduced, and the serum levels of gastrin are elevated in an attempt to restore parietal cell activity. Atrophic gastritis can be a purely autoimmune disease associated with the production of auto-antibodies to parietal cells, intrinsic factor, and gastrin, but it can also be the result of *H pylori* infection. Traditionally, it has been thought that autoimmune gastritis is more likely to cause pernicious anemia, whereas atrophic gastritis in the setting of *H pylori* infection is more associated with the risk of progression to gastric adenocarcinoma. More recent epidemiological studies have disputed this supposition. Specifically, any condition with chronic loss of parietal cell mass or activity can lead to compensatory GI endocrine hyperplasia of reactive G cells. Progression to an autonomous gastrin-producing neuroendocrine tumor of the GI tract (gastrinoma) is a rare cause of ulcer disease. Alternatively, *H pylori*–mediated atrophic gastritis greatly increases the risk of the inflammatory infiltrate progressing to a lymphoma of mucosa-associated lymphoid tissue type (called a MALToma).

4. Duodenal Ulcer

Even more commonly than gastric ulcers, duodenal ulcers are sequelae of *H pylori* infection, caused by altered mucosal inflammatory responses and excessive acid secretion. Various other risk factors, including diet, smoking, and excessive alcohol consumption, may influence the development of duodenal ulcers, although specific associations (eg, between coffee or spicy foods and the development of ulcers) have not been demonstrated. Genetic factors also play a role; studies support the existence of a heritable component in duodenal ulcers distinct from that involved in gastric ulcer. Likewise, psychologic stress has been implicated in duodenal ulcer disease, perhaps by an autonomic-mediated influence on acid secretion (see Figure 13–12). Interestingly, duodenal ulcers are associated with a decreased risk of developing gastric adenocarcinoma, perhaps because chronic *H pylori* infection predisposes to cancer in the setting of atrophic gastritis, in which parietal cells are lost, whereas duodenal ulcers are caused by acid secretion; thus, patients with duodenal ulcers are not likely to have pronounced parietal cell atrophy (see Figure 13–19).

Clinical Manifestations

Those forms of acid-peptic disease characterized by exclusively superficial mucosal lesions (eg, acute erosive gastritis) can result in either acute or chronic GI tract bleeding, accompanied by a significant drop in hematocrit and related complications (eg, precipitating angina in a patient with coronary artery disease). Patients with acute massive bleeding present with hematemesis, rectal bleeding, or melena, depending on the site of origin, the rate of transit of blood through the GI tract, and the extent of hemorrhage. Acute massive hemorrhage (>10% of blood volume over minutes to hours) is manifested by hypotension, tachycardia, and orthostatic blood pressure and heart rate changes on standing, often with dizziness.

In addition to hemorrhage, complications of duodenal ulcer and gastric ulcer include life-threatening perforation and obstruction.

CHECKPOINT

50. How does pernicious anemia result from a secretory disorder of the stomach?
51. What is the typical acid secretion status of patients with pernicious anemia?
52. In which acid-peptic disorder are diminished mucosal defenses more important than acid hypersecretion?
53. How might motility defects contribute to gastric ulcer?
54. What factors may predispose a patient to duodenal ulcer disease?
55. How do NSAIDs contribute to acid-peptic disease?
56. What is the importance of *H pylori* infection in acid-peptic disease?
57. What other factors besides *H pylori* infection contribute to acid-peptic disease?

GASTROPARESIS

Clinical Presentation

A common complication of stomach disorders is delayed gastric emptying (Table 13–6). Known as gastroparesis, it is manifested by nausea, bloating, vomiting, and either constipation or diarrhea. The condition can also occur silently, producing metabolic derangements (eg, of blood glucose in patients with diabetes mellitus) in the absence of somatic symptoms.

Etiology

Gastroparesis is a common complication of poorly controlled diabetes mellitus, with consequent autonomic neuropathy.

Pathology & Pathogenesis

Disorders of gastric motility result from alterations in a number of normal gastric functions. These include (1) serving as a reservoir for ingested solids and liquids (eg, alteration caused by resection of the stomach); (2) mixing and homogenizing ingested food; and (3) functioning as a barrier that allows only small spurts of well-mixed chyme beyond the pyloric sphincter. The resulting disorders span the range from partial or complete gastric outlet obstruction to excessively rapid emptying and typically result from interference with the normal mechanisms by which these functions are controlled. These include the intrinsic contractility of gastric smooth muscle, the enteric nervous system, the autonomic nervous system's control over enteric nervous system function, and gut hormones.

Because the pyloric sphincter, like all sphincters, displays tonic contraction with intermittent transient relaxation, loss of vagal control results in excessive tonic contraction and symptoms of various degrees of gastric outlet obstruction. Disorders that affect the enteric nervous system, such as the neuropathy of diabetes mellitus and surgical cutting of the stomach wall or vagal trunk, typically cause delayed emptying. However, it

TABLE 13–6 Conditions producing symptomatic gastric motor dysfunction.

Acute Conditions	Chronic Conditions	
Abdominal pain, trauma, inflammation	Mechanical	Pseudo-obstruction
Postoperative state	Gastric ulcer	Idiopathic, hollow visceral myopathy
Acute infections, gastroenteritis	Duodenal ulcer	Secondary (eg, amyloidosis, Chagas disease,
Acute metabolic disorders:	Idiopathic hypertrophic pyloric stenosis	muscular dystrophies, paraneoplastic
Acidosis, hypokalemia, hypercalcemia	Superior mesenteric artery syndrome	syndrome)
or hypocalcemia, hepatic coma,	Acid-peptic disease	Postgastric surgery
myxedema	Gastroesophageal reflux	Postvagotomy or postgastric resections
Immobilization	Gastric ulcer disease, nonulcer dyspepsia	Medications
Hyperglycemia (glucose >200 mg/dL)	Gastritis	Anticholinergics, opioid analgesics, levodopa,
Pharmaceutical agents and hormones	Atrophic gastritis with or without pernicious	tricyclic antidepressants
Opioids, including endorphins and	anemia	Hormones (pharmacologic studies)
pharmacologic agents (eg, morphine)	Viral gastroenteritis (acute or chronic gastritis)	Gastrin, cholecystokinin, somatostatin
Anticholinergics	Metabolic and endocrine	Anorexia nervosa: bulimia
Tricyclic antidepressants	Diabetic ketoacidosis (acute)	Idiopathic
Beta-adrenergic agonists	Diabetic gastroparesis (chronic)	Gastric dysrhythmias: tachygastria
Levodopa	Addison disease	Gastroduodenal dyssynchrony
Aluminum hydroxide antacids	Hypothyroidism	Central nervous system: tabes dorsalis,
Gastrin	Pregnancy?	depression
Cholecystokinin	Uremia?	
Somatostatin	Collagen–vascular diseases	
	Scleroderma	
	Dermatomyositis	
	Polymyositis	
	Systemic lupus erythematosus?	

Reproduced, with permission, from McCallum RW. Motor function of the stomach in health and disease. In: Sleisenger MH et al, eds. *Gastrointestinal Disease*, 4th ed. Saunders, 1989. Copyright © Elsevier.

is important to remember that, in some cases, delayed emptying can result in symptoms expected from excessively rapid emptying. For example, an excessively contracted pylorus that can open completely but does so infrequently can result in entry into the duodenum of too large a bolus of chyme from the excessively distended stomach. Such a bolus may not be efficiently handled by the small intestine, resulting in poor absorption and diarrheal symptoms characteristic of dumping syndrome.

Hormones play an ill-defined but important role in regulating GI motility in health and disease. For example, the antibiotic erythromycin is recognized by the receptor for the GI hormone motilin, affecting GI motility. Some patients with gastroparesis are observed to experience substantial improvement with erythromycin analogs, especially when complaints related to partial gastric outlet obstruction, such as bloating, nausea, and constipation, are prominent.

Because different patients have different relative contributions of the intrinsic nervous system, enteric nervous system, autonomic nervous system, higher centers of the CNS, and hormones over control of their GI tract motility, not all treatments for gastroparesis are effective for a majority of patients even with the same initial complaints.

Clinical Manifestations

Complications of gastroparesis include the development of bezoars from retained gastric contents, bacterial overgrowth, erratic blood glucose control, and, when nausea and vomiting are profound, weight loss. Elevated blood glucose can be either a cause or a consequence of delayed gastric emptying. Bacterial overgrowth itself can result in both malabsorption and diarrhea. For unknown reasons, the symptoms of gastroparesis are variable from patient to patient as well as over time in a given patient and often correlated poorly with delayed gastric emptying. In some cases, serotonin antagonists that decrease visceral perception may be more helpful than prokinetic agents in alleviating symptoms.

CHECKPOINT

58. What are the symptoms of delayed versus rapid gastric emptying?
59. What are the complications of gastroparesis?
60. Why might erythromycin improve diabetic gastroparesis?

DISORDERS OF THE GALLBLADDER

Gallbladder disease is most commonly due to gallstones (cholelithiasis).

1. Cholelithiasis

Clinical Presentation

Gallstones are most often asymptomatic, discovered incidentally at autopsy or during surgery for an unrelated condition. Of patients who do have symptoms referable to cholelithiasis, presentations range from mild nausea or abdominal discomfort after eating fatty or fried foods to severe right upper quadrant or midepigastric abdominal pain and jaundice. A history of chronic mild symptoms with dietary association typically predates an acute episode of abdominal pain. The typical patient with gallstones is female, has a history of high dietary fat intake, has had prior pregnancies (reflecting the role of estrogens in gallstone pathogenesis), and is in her 40s (reflecting the time necessary for progression to symptomatic disease).

Etiology

Gallstones come in several varieties. Most are composed largely of cholesterol with or without calcium deposits. Occasionally, especially in patients with a chronic hemolytic disease, bilirubin stones may form. Depending on the cause and the pathophysiologic mechanism involved, patients can have one or more of the following: a few large individual stones; many smaller stones; or "sludge," a thickened viscous gel resulting from a concentration of bile believed to be highly prone to stone formation.

Pathology and Pathogenesis

Cholelithiasis is of multifactorial origin. However, the formation of cholesterol gallstones usually requires the formation of bile whose cholesterol concentration is greater than its percentage solubility. The normal processes that prevent gallstone formation probably include the fact that bile does not normally stay in the gallbladder long enough to become lithogenic (prone to stone formation). Thus, the loss of gallbladder muscular wall motility (resulting from intrinsic disease of the muscle wall, altered levels of hormones such as CCK, or altered neural control) and excessive sphincteric contraction, which impair emptying, are important predisposing factors. One consequence of decreased gallbladder emptying is excessive bile concentration, leading to heightened lithogenicity. This can occur from decreased water absorption or altered

FIGURE 13–20 Pathophysiology of cholelithiasis.

bile composition resulting from increased cholesterol content or saturation. Other factors can cause an increased tendency to form stones at any given degree of concentration and saturation, including the presence of nucleating versus antinucleating factors in bile and the size and composition of the bile acid pool. Figure 13–20 summarizes the factors that predispose to gallstone formation, including estrogens, prostaglandins, increased mucus and glycoprotein production by the gallbladder epithelium, and chronic bacterial colonization or infection. Estrogens may play multiple roles, first affecting bile composition (increasing cholesterol and its saturation in bile) but also diminishing gallbladder motility (hence predisposing to stasis, sludge formation, and lithogenicity). Prostaglandins, which are protective in the stomach by increasing mucus production, may actually contribute to lithogenicity by the same mechanism. Thus, NSAIDs that block prostaglandin production are often beneficial for the prevention of gallstones in patients so predisposed, probably by decreasing mucus production.

Clinical Manifestations

The major clinical presentation of gallstones is inflammation of the gallbladder, or **cholecystitis**. Cholecystitis can be acute, chronic, or acute against a background of chronic disease. An episode of acute cholecystitis can progress to acute pancreatitis if a stone travels down the common bile duct but fails to clear the sphincter of Oddi, thereby blocking the pancreatic duct. Likewise, an inflamed gallbladder can become infected or can undergo infarction and necrosis, setting the stage for systemic sepsis if the patient does not receive systemic broad-spectrum antibiotics and undergo emergency cholecystectomy (Figure 13–21).

PATHOPHYSIOLOGY OF DISORDERS OF THE SMALL INTESTINE & COLON

Diseases of the small and large intestine include diarrhea, inflammatory bowel disease, and diverticular disease. **Diarrhea** is a symptom that has many causes and diverse

pathogenetic mechanisms, including altered motility, secretion, digestion, and absorption. Although intestinal disorders are particularly prominent causes, disease of the stomach,

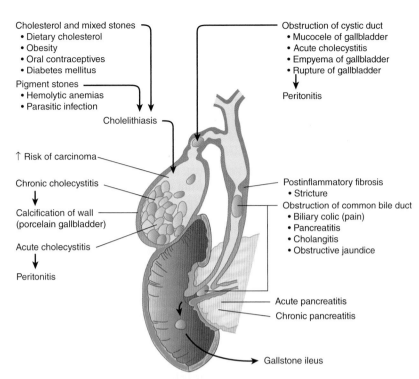

FIGURE 13–21 Clinical and pathologic effects of cholelithiasis. (Redrawn, with permission, from Chandrasoma P et al, eds. *Concise Pathology*, 3rd ed. Originally published by Appleton & Lange. Copyright © 1998 by The McGraw-Hill Companies, Inc.)

pancreas, and biliary tract can also cause diarrhea. **Inflammatory bowel diseases** (IBDs) are poorly understood chronic autoimmune processes in the small intestine, colon, or both. Diarrhea, abdominal pain, and malabsorption are prominent features. Important systemic manifestations may complicate IBDs. **Diverticular disease** occurs most prominently in the colon, in part as a direct or indirect consequence of altered motor function. **Irritable bowel syndrome** (IBS) is not a disease per se but a functional disorder manifested by abdominal pain with diarrhea or constipation in the absence of organic disease or gross structural changes of the intestine.

DIARRHEA

Clinical Presentation

The symptoms of diarrhea are an increased stool frequency, increased stool volume, and a decrease in stool consistency. Any process that increases the frequency of defecation or volume of stool makes it looser, because time-dependent water absorption is responsible for the normal soft but formed consistency of stool. Infectious diarrheas are discussed in Chapter 4. This chapter focuses on general aspects of diarrhea and diarrheas from other causes.

Patients' subjective assessments of bowel movements are colored by their baseline bowel habits. An individual with chronic constipation, with bowel movements once every 3 days or so, may regard three soft stools in a day as diarrhea. In contrast, an individual on a high-fiber diet may normally have bowel movements twice or even three times a day.

Diarrhea can be acute (<2 weeks' duration) or chronic (>4 weeks). Acute diarrhea is usually due to an infectious cause. The most common noninfectious causes are medication side effects.

The simplest idea is that diarrhea is caused by too much secretion or not enough absorption. **Osmotic (malabsorptive) diarrhea** is caused by malabsorbed nutrients or poorly absorbed electrolytes that retain water in the lumen. Malabsorption occurs when the ability to digest or absorb a particular nutrient is defective and may result from disordered mixing (altered motility), pancreatic insufficiency (altered digestion), or damage to enterocytes or their surface transporters (altered absorption). This type of diarrhea stops when the patient fasts. **Secretory diarrhea** results when secretagogues maintain elevated rates of fluid transport out of epithelial cells into the GI tract lumen. This type of diarrhea does not stop when the patient fasts. These physiologic distinctions are useful in both the diagnosis and therapy of diarrheal disorders. In terms of transport capacity, the small intestine far exceeds the colon (owing to the enormous surface area of the brush border). Thus, infectious, toxic, or other causes of heightened secretion in the small intestine can overwhelm absorptive mechanisms in the colon, resulting in diarrhea.

Etiology

Flow in the GI tract is a steady state involving massive fluid secretion into and absorption from the GI lumen. Each process is controlled by both extrinsic and intrinsic factors. Subtle aberrations in input or output at any of several levels can result

TABLE 13–7   Mechanisms of diarrhea and major specific causes.

Mechanisms of Diarrhea	Specific Causes
Osmotic/malabsorption	Disaccharidase deficiencies (eg, lactase deficiency)
	Glucose-galactose or fructose malabsorption
	Mannitol, sorbitol ingestion
	Lactulose therapy
	Some salts (eg, magnesium sulfate)
	Some antacids (eg, calcium carbonate)
	Generalized malabsorption
	Pancreatic enzyme inactivation (eg, by excess acid)
	Defective fat solubilization (disrupted enterohepatic circulation or defective bile formation)
	Ingestion of nutrient-binding substances
	Bacterial overgrowth
	Loss of enterocytes (eg, radiation, infection, ischemia)
	Lymphatic obstruction (eg, lymphoma, tuberculosis)
	Pancreatic enzyme deficiency
Secretory	Enterotoxins
	Tumor products (eg, VIP, serotonin)
	Laxatives
	Bile acids
	Fatty acids
	Congenital defects
Motility disorder	Diabetes mellitus
	Postsurgical
Inflammatory exudation	Inflammatory bowel disease
	Infection (eg, shigellosis)

VIP, vasoactive intestinal peptide.

Data from Fine KD et al. Diarrhea. In: Sleisenger MH et al, eds. *Gastrointestinal Disease*, 4th ed. Saunders, 1989.

in diarrhea with or without nutrient malabsorption. Thus, an excessive osmotic load, increased secretion, or diminished fluid resorption may result in diarrhea (Table 13–7).

An excessive osmotic load in the GI tract may come about in three different ways: by direct oral ingestion of excessive osmoles, by ingestion of a substrate that may be converted into excessive osmoles (eg, when bacterial action on the nondigestible carbohydrate lactulose generates a diarrhea-causing osmotic load in the colon), and as a manifestation of a genetic disease such as an enzyme deficiency in the setting of a particular diet (eg, milk consumption by a lactase-deficient individual).

Secretion is increased by either blood-borne or intraluminal secretagogues. These include endogenous endocrine products (eg, overproduction of VIP by a tumor), exotoxins resulting from direct ingestion (eg, acute food poisoning) or infection (eg, cholera), or GI luminal substances (eg, bile acids) that stimulate secretion.

Absorption of fluid, electrolytes, and nutrients can be diminished by many factors, including the toxic effects of alcohol and mucosal damage from infectious agents and from cytokines and prokinetic agents. Cytokines are released by immune and other cells (eg, in response to infection). Prokinetic agents speed up GI motility, thereby diminishing the time available for the absorption of any given nutrient, fluid, or electrolyte load. Finally, inflammatory and other disorders resulting in loss of mucus, blood, or protein from the GI tract may be manifested as diarrhea. Table 13–8 lists symptoms and signs suggesting specific causes of diarrhea.

Pathology & Pathogenesis

Recognizing the pathophysiologic subtypes of secretory (Tables 13–9 and 13–10) and osmotic diarrheas provides a means of approaching the diagnosis and therapy of diarrheal disorders. For example, nonbloody diarrhea that continues in the absence of oral intake must be due to a secretory mechanism, whereas diarrhea that diminishes as oral intake is curtailed (eg, in a patient receiving intravenous hydration) suggests an osmotic/malabsorptive cause. Likewise, the presence of white blood cells in the stool suggests an infectious or inflammatory origin of diarrhea, although their absence does not rule out such causes.

Of the many causes of diarrhea (Table 13–11), infectious agents are among the most important because they cause acute, sometimes life-threatening diseases whose pathogenesis is relatively well understood and because they are usually treatable. The symptoms of diarrhea caused by infectious agents are due either to toxins that alter small bowel secretion and absorption or direct mucosal invasion. The noninvasive toxin-producing bacteria are generally small bowel pathogens, whereas the invasive organisms are typically localized to the colon. Diarrheas caused by infectious agents are discussed in Chapter 4.

Evidence suggests that infectious causes of diarrhea can interface more intimately with normal mechanisms of secretory control than had been previously realized. Thus, in addition to its direct effect on the G protein controlling Cl^- ion secretion in the crypts of the small intestinal epithelium, cholera activates the enteric nervous system to cause fluid and electrolyte secretion in the colon.

TABLE 13–8 Clues to diagnosis of diarrhea from other symptoms and signs.

Symptom or Sign Associated with Diarrhea	Diagnoses to be Considered
Arthritis	Ulcerative colitis, Crohn disease, Whipple disease, enteritis resulting from *Yersinia enterocolitica*, gonococcal proctitis
Liver disease	Ulcerative colitis, Crohn disease, colon cancer with metastases to liver
Fever	Ulcerative colitis, Crohn disease, amebiasis, lymphoma, tuberculosis, Whipple disease, other enteric infections (especially viral or toxin-producing bacterial)
Marked weight loss	Malabsorption, inflammatory bowel disease, colon cancer, thyrotoxicosis
Eosinophilia	Eosinophilic gastroenteritis, parasitic disease (particularly *Strongyloides*)
Lymphadenopathy	Lymphoma, Whipple disease, AIDS
Neuropathy	Diabetic diarrhea, amyloidosis
Postural hypotension	GI bleeding, diabetic diarrhea, Addison disease, idiopathic orthostatic hypotension
Flushing	Malignant carcinoid syndrome, pancreatic cholera syndrome
Erythema	Systemic mastocytosis, glucagonoma syndrome
Proteinuria	Amyloidosis
Collagen–vascular disease	Mesenteric vasculitis
Peptic ulcers	Zollinger–Ellison syndrome
Chronic lung disease	Cystic fibrosis
Systemic arteriosclerosis	Ischemic injury to gut
Frequent infections	Immunoglobulin deficiency
Hyperpigmentation	Whipple disease, celiac disease, Addison disease
Good response to corticosteroids	Ulcerative colitis, Crohn disease, Whipple disease, Addison disease, eosinophilic gastroenteritis
Good response to antibiotics	Blind loop syndrome, tropical sprue, Whipple disease
Good response to elimination diet	Celiac disease (gluten), lactase deficiency (milk products)

Reproduced and modified, with permission, from Fine KD et al. Diarrhea. In: Sleisenger MH et al, eds. *Gastrointestinal Disease*, 4th ed. Saunders, 1989. Copyright © Elsevier.

Clinical Manifestations

Dehydration, malnutrition, weight loss, and specific vitamin deficiency syndromes (eg, glossitis, cheilosis, and stomatitis) are common signs in diarrhea depending on its cause, severity, and chronicity (see Tables 13–8 and 13–10). In certain circumstances (eg, in young children), viral gastroenteritis is associated with a high mortality rate from dehydration when supportive measures (ie, oral or intravenous rehydration) are not promptly provided. Some individuals with diarrhea from parasitic infections remain relatively asymptomatic, whereas others may develop more severe symptoms and complications, including intestinal perforation.

CHECKPOINT

61. By what mechanisms do infectious agents cause diarrhea?
62. Name three ways in which an excessive osmotic load can occur in the GI tract.

INFLAMMATORY BOWEL DISEASE

Clinical Presentation

Inflammatory bowel disease is distinguished from infectious entities by exclusion and by chronicity (months; not days or weeks). Patients often experience recurrent episodes of mucopurulent (ie, containing mucus and white cells), bloody diarrhea characterized by lack of positive cultures for known microbial pathogens and failure to respond to antibiotics alone. Because inflammatory bowel disease is characterized by exacerbations and remissions, favorable responses to therapy may be difficult to distinguish from spontaneous remissions occurring as part of the natural history of the disease.

Etiology

Triggers for the development of IBD remain elusive. However, epidemiologic studies suggest that smoking and gastrointestinal infections are possible contributory factors. There are two forms of chronic inflammatory bowel disease: **Crohn disease**, which is transmural and granulomatous in character, occurring anywhere along the GI tract; and **ulcerative colitis**, which is superficial and limited to the colonic mucosa. The exact causes of inflammatory bowel disease are unknown despite progress in understanding its pathogenesis.

Pathology & Pathogenesis

Genetic risk and environmental factors are recognized as two key elements in the pathogenesis of inflammatory bowel disease. An explosion of newly recognized susceptibility genes for both Crohn disease and ulcerative colitis have been discovered through genome-wide associations. These studies evaluated

TABLE 13-9 Histologic features of small intestinal diseases causing malabsorption.

Disease	Pathologic Features	Pattern of Distribution
Celiac (nontropical) disease (gluten enteropathy)	Villus flattening, crypt hyperplasia, increased lymphocytes and plasma cells in lamina propria	Diffuse in proximal jejunum
Tropical sprue	Shortened villi, increased lymphocytes and plasma cells in lamina propria	Diffuse in proximal jejunum
Crohn disease	Noncaseating granulomas with or without giant cells	Patchy lesions throughout GI tract but particularly affecting terminal ileum
Collagenous sprue	Subepithelial collagen deposits	Diffuse
Primary lymphoma	Malignant lymphocytes or histiocytes in lamina propria, variable villus flattening	Patchy
Whipple disease	Lamina propria laden with periodic acid-Schiff (PAS)–staining foamy macrophages, bacilli in macrophages	Diffuse
Amyloidosis	Amyloid deposition in blood vessels, muscle layers	Diffuse in muscularis mucosae, mucosal sparing
Abetalipoproteinemia	Lipid-laden, vacuolated epithelial cells, normal villi	Diffuse
Radiation enteritis	Flattened villi, mucosal inflammation, fibrosis, ulceration	Patchy
Lymphangiectasia	Dilated lymphatics in lamina propria	Patchy
Eosinophilic gastroenteritis	Eosinophilic infiltrate in the intestinal wall	Patchy
Hypogammaglobulinemia	Villus flattening, *Giardia* trophozoites often present, few plasma cells	Patchy
Giardiasis	Trophozoites may be present, variable villus flattening	Patchy
Opportunistic infections	Organisms may be seen (*Isospora belli*, cryptosporidia, Microsporida), PAS-staining macrophages (*Mycobacterium avium* complex)	Patchy

thousands of single nucleotide polymorphisms (SNPs) in thousands of patients with inflammatory bowel disease and compared them with SNPs from thousands of people without the disease (controls). These studies found abnormalities in several categories of susceptibility genes in patients with inflammatory bowel disease. These included modulators of immune function, autophagy, and epithelial function that participate in the interaction of host and microorganism. Importantly, the relative risk of most of these susceptibility genes is low (most have a 20–30% increase in relative risk of developing disease). Therefore, most people who harbor risk alleles for inflammatory bowel disease do not develop disease.

Genetic factors are clearly not the sole contributor to inflammatory bowel disease. Many environmental factors have been found to contribute to the development of Crohn disease, including pathogenic microorganisms (bacteria and viruses), the repertoire of indigenous intestinal microbes (the microbiota), dietary factors, smoking, defective immune responses, and psychosocial factors. Moreover, recent studies suggest that patterning the activity of certain aspects of the immune system during the neonatal period strongly influences immune responses in the adult. Because the composition of the intestinal microbiota is in large part transmitted by the mother, maternal effects are thought to be a contributing factor to GI disease as well. Specifically, early exposure to

intestinal microbiota may be an important component of the pathogenesis of inflammatory bowel disease.

The normal intestine is able to modulate frank inflammatory responses to its constant bombardment with dietary and microbial antigens in the lumen. This process may be defective in Crohn disease, resulting in uncontrolled inflammation. There has been considerable interest in the role of cytokines, such as interleukins and tumor necrosis factor, in Crohn disease. Cytokine profiles of T_H1 and T_H17 categories have been implicated in Crohn disease. Mice lacking the T_H1-inhibiting cytokine interleukin-10 have a T_H1 cytokine profile and develop spontaneous intestinal inflammation. Monoclonal antibodies to tumor necrosis factor alpha (TNFα) reduce inflammation in these animals and patients. Similar factors may contribute to the pathogenesis of ulcerative colitis, including infections, allergies to dietary components, immune responses to bacteria and self-antigens, and psychosocial factors. In mice, targeted disruption of the genes for the T-cell receptor and the cytokine IL-2 results in GI tract disease resembling ulcerative colitis.

The two forms of inflammatory bowel disease have characteristic differences and in many cases considerable overlap in presentation (Table 13–12). The features common to all forms of inflammatory bowel disease are mucosal ulceration and GI tract inflammation, indistinguishable, in fact, from that which can occur acutely during invasive infectious diarrhea. Other factors

TABLE 13–10 **Symptoms and signs of malabsorption and relevant pathophysiology.**

Symptom or Sign	Pathophysiologic Explanation
Gastrointestinal	
Diarrhea	Osmotic activity of carbohydrates or short-chain fatty acids
	Secretory effects of bile acids and fatty acids
	Decreased absorptive surface
	Intestinal loss of conjugated bile acids
	Ileal resection
	Severe ileal mucosal disease
	Congenital defects of the ileal sodium–bile acid cotransporter
Abdominal distension, flatulence	Bacterial gas production from carbohydrates in colon, small intestinal bacterial overgrowth
Foul-smelling flatulence or stool	Malabsorption of proteins or intestinal protein loss
Pain	Gaseous distension of intestine
Ascites	Protein loss or malabsorption
Musculoskeletal	
Tetany, muscle weakness, paresthesias	Malabsorption of vitamin D, calcium, magnesium, and phosphate
Bone pain, osteomalacia, fractures	Protein, calcium, or vitamin D deficiency; secondary hyperparathyroidism
Cutaneous and mucosal	
Easy bruisability, ecchymoses, petechiae	Vitamin K deficiency and vitamin C deficiency (scurvy)
Glossitis, cheilosis, stomatitis	Vitamin B complex, vitamin B_{12}, folate, or iron deficiency
Edema	Protein loss or malabsorption
Acrodermatitis, scaly dermatitis	Zinc and essential fatty acid deficiency
Follicular hyperkeratosis	Vitamin A deficiency
Hyperpigmented dermatitis	Niacin deficiency (pellagra)
Thin nails with spoon-shaped deformity	Iron deficiency
Perifollicular hemorrhage	Malabsorption of vitamin C (scurvy)
Spiral or curly hair	Malabsorption of vitamin C (scurvy)
Other	
Weight loss, hyperphagia	Nutrient malabsorption
Growth and weight retardation, infantilism	Nutrient malabsorption in childhood, adolescence
Anemia	Iron, folate, or vitamin B_{12} deficiency
Kidney stones	Increased colonic oxalate absorption
Amenorrhea, erectile dysfunction, infertility	Multifactorial (including protein malabsorption, secondary hypopituitarism, anemia)
Night blindness, xerophthalmia	Vitamin A deficiency
Peripheral neuropathy	Vitamin B_{12} or thiamine deficiency
Fatigue, weakness	Calorie depletion, iron and folate deficiency, anemia
Neurologic symptoms, ataxia	Vitamin B_{12}, vitamin E, or folate deficiency

TABLE 13–11   Most likely causes of diarrhea in seven different clinical categories.

1. Acute diarrhea (<2–3 weeks' duration)	**5. Chronic and recurrent diarrhea**
Viral, bacterial, parasitic, and fungal infections	Irritable bowel syndrome
Food poisoning	Inflammatory bowel disease
Drugs[1] and food additives	Parasitic and fungal infections
Fecal impaction	Malabsorption syndromes
Pelvic inflammation	Drugs,[1] food additives, sorbitol
Heavy metal poisoning (acute or chronic)	Colon cancer
2. Traveler's diarrhea	Diverticulitis
Bacterial infections	Fecal impaction
Mediated by enterotoxins produced by *Escherichia coli*	Heavy metal poisoning (acute or chronic)
Mediated mainly by invasion of mucosa and inflammation (eg, invasive *E coli, Shigella*)	Raw milk–related diarrhea
Mediated by combinations of invasion and enterotoxins (eg, *Salmonella*)	**6. Chronic diarrhea of unknown origin (previous workup failed to reveal diagnosis)**
Viral and parasitic infections	Surreptitious laxative abuse
3. Diarrhea in men who have sex with men, without AIDS	Defective anal sphincter competence masquerading as diarrhea
Amebiasis	Microscopic colitis syndrome
Giardiasis	Previously unrecognized malabsorption
Shigellosis	Pseudopancreatic cholera syndrome
Campylobacter	Idiopathic fluid malabsorption
Rectal syphilis	Hypermotility-induced diarrhea
Rectal spirochetosis other than syphilis	Neuroendocrine tumor
Rectal gonorrhea	**7. Incontinence**
Chlamydia trachomatis infection (lymphogranuloma venereum and non-LGV serotypes D–K)	Causes of sphincter dysfunction:
Herpes simplex	Anal surgery for fissures, fistulas, or hemorrhoids
4. Diarrhea in people with AIDS	Episiotomy or tear during childbirth
Cryptosporidium	Anal Crohn disease
Amebiasis	Diabetic neuropathy
Giardiasis	Causes of diarrhea: same as under 5 and 6 above
Isospora belli	
Herpes simplex, cytomegalovirus	
Mycobacterium avium-intracellulare complex	
Salmonella typhimurium	
Cryptococcus	
Candida	
AIDS enteropathy	

[1]Digitalis, propranolol, quinidine, diuretics, colchicine, antibiotics, lactulose, antacids, laxatives, chemotherapeutic agents, bile acids, meclofenamate, and many others. (See drug compendiums for adverse effects of drugs the patient has been taking.)

Reproduced and modified, with permission, from Fine KD et al. Diarrhea. In: Sleisenger MH et al, eds. *Gastrointestinal Disease*, 5th ed. Saunders, 1993. Copyright © Elsevier.

TABLE 13–12 **Similarities and differences between ulcerative colitis and Crohn disease.**

	Ulcerative Colitis	Crohn Disease
Clinical features		
Rectal bleeding	>90%	<50%
Diarrhea	90%	>70%
Abdominal mass	Rare	Common
Perianal abscesses, sinuses, and fistulas	2%	30%
Bowel perforation (free)	2–3%	<1%
Toxic megacolon	5–10%	<5%
Cancer of colon	Increased	Increased with colon involvement
Pyoderma gangrenosum	<5%	1%
Erythema nodosum	5%	15%
Renal stones	<5% (uric acid stones)	10% (oxalate stones)
Stomatitis	10%	10%
Aphthous ulceration	4%	4%
Uveitis	45%	5–10%
Spondylitis	<5%	15–20%
Peripheral arthritis	10%	20%
Thromboembolism with increased platelets and increased coagulant activity	Occurs	Occurs
Radiologic, endoscopic, and pathologic findings		
Rectal involvement	Almost 100%	<50%
Ulcers	Superficial, multiple	Solitary ulcers in the rectum
	Irregular	Linear, serpiginous, and aphthoid ulcers
Crypt abscesses, pseudopolyps, diminished goblet cells	Frequent	Common
Lymphoid aggregates and noncaseating granulomas	<10%	60–70%
Extent of disease	Mucosal and continuous	Transmural and discontinuous with "skip lesions"
Ileal involvement	Nonspecific with mild inflammation and dilation (backwash ileitis)	Ulcers, fissures, and stenosis
Fatty liver	Frequent	Frequent
Pericholangitis	30%	20%
Sclerosing cholangitis	30%	20–30%
Cirrhosis	Rare	<1%
Gallstones	Rare	10–15%
Treatment		
General	Supportive and symptomatic	Supportive and symptomatic
Definitive (drugs)	Sulfasalazine, mesalamine, corticosteroids, TNFα inhibitors, anti-integrin therapies and immunomodulators such as azathioprine	Sulfasalazine, mesalamine, corticosteroids, TNFα inhibitors, anti-integrin therapies, IL12-23 inhibitors and immunomodulators such as azathioprine

besides the presence of key gene products, including infectious agents, altered host immune responses, immune-mediated intestinal damage, psychologic factors, and dietary and environmental factors, may contribute to a final common pathway of disordered immune response.

Clinical Manifestations

A. Crohn Disease

Crohn disease most typically occurs in the distal ileum. However, the distribution of the disease can also involve the colon or less commonly any other region of the GI tract (including the oral cavity, esophagus, stomach, and proximal small intestine). A characteristic feature is that areas of ulceration and inflammation occur in a discontinuous fashion and involve the entire thickness of the bowel wall. Recurrence of disease can occur in previously uninvolved regions of the intestine and can even involve adjacent mesentery and lymph nodes. The combination of deep mucosal ulceration and submucosal thickening gives the involved mucosa a characteristic "cobblestone" appearance.

Perforation, fistula formation, abscess formation, and small intestinal obstruction are frequent complications of Crohn disease, although an indolent course occurs in most patients. The full-thickness involvement of the bowel wall may predispose to these complications. Frank bleeding from the mucosal ulcerations can be either insidious or massive, as can **protein-losing enteropathy**. Another important complication is an increased incidence of intestinal and colon cancer.

Patients with Crohn disease often manifest symptoms outside the GI tract. Most commonly, inflammatory disorders of the joints (arthritis), skin (erythema nodosum), eye (uveitis, iritis), mucous membranes (aphthous ulcers of the buccal mucosa), bile ducts (sclerosing cholangitis), and liver (autoimmune chronic active hepatitis) are also observed in these patients. Renal disorders, especially nephrolithiasis, are observed in one-third of patients with Crohn disease, probably related to increased oxalate absorption associated with steatorrhea. Amyloidosis is a serious complication of Crohn disease, as is thromboembolic disease. Both complications are probably reflections of the systemic character of the inflammatory process. Patients are often malnourished and show evidence of nutrient deficiency states.

B. Ulcerative Colitis

In contrast to Crohn disease, inflammation in ulcerative colitis is restricted to the mucosa of the colon and rectum. It typically begins at the anorectal junction and extends proximally. Ulcerative colitis and Crohn disease are similar in presentation (eg, bloody diarrhea and malabsorption) and in at least some of the complications (eg, protein-losing enteropathy and malnutrition), reflecting the widespread involvement of the mucosa in both entities. In both conditions, acute inflammatory cells (neutrophils) are located within the crypt epithelium (cryptitis) and crypt lumens (crypt abscesses). There is

also a robust infiltration of chronic inflammatory cells in the mucosa. However, because ulcerative colitis generally is limited to the mucosa, obstruction, perforation, and fistula formation are not typical complications. Most patients have mild disease, and, as with Crohn disease, some patients will have only one or two episodes during their lifetimes. As with Crohn disease, there is an increased risk of colonic adenocarcinoma that increases with the duration of the disease. Chronic disease can also lead to damage of the muscularis propria, leading to toxic megacolon, a thin-walled, dilated, poorly motile area of the colon susceptible to rupture. In the mucosa, chronic damage and ulceration can lead to excess granulation tissue that protrudes into the lumen of the intestine (pseudopolyps).

Both ulcerative colitis and Crohn disease can go into remission after treatment with first-line anti-inflammatory agents such as sulfasalazine and glucocorticoids. Crohn disease and ulcerative colitis also respond to therapy with monoclonal antibodies against the inflammatory cytokine TNFα. These anti-TNFα therapies are now commonly used to treat patients with moderate to severe disease as the benefit-to-risk profile of these agents is superior to that of corticosteroids. Moreover, these steroid-sparing agents can be used long term to maintain clinical remission. Newer and developing therapies for IBD include those that target cytokines (interleukin-23), inflammatory signaling kinases (Janus kinase [JAK]), and cell trafficking (integrins and adhesions molecules).

The natural history of both diseases is of periods of remission interrupted by active disease; medical therapy during exacerbations is directed toward supportive measures and attempts to induce remission. Because these diseases can recur after resecting involved regions of the GI tract, operative management is generally limited to relief of persistently symptomatic intestinal obstruction or bleeding.

CHECKPOINT

63. How is inflammatory bowel disease distinguished from infectious diarrhea?
64. What are the differences between ulcerative colitis and Crohn disease?
65. What are the complications of inflammatory bowel disease?

DIVERTICULAR DISEASE

Clinical Presentation

Nearly 80% of patients with diverticula are asymptomatic except for chronic constipation. Of those who develop other symptoms, the most common presentation is an intermittent and unpredictable griping lower abdominal pain (diverticulitis). Additional features of the presentation depend on which of the two major complications of diverticula the patient develops.

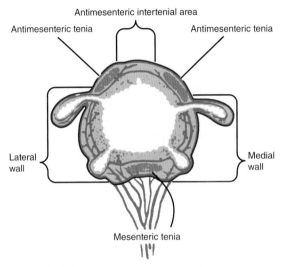

FIGURE 13–22 **Top:** Pathophysiology of diverticular disease. **Bottom:** Cross-sectional drawing of the colon, showing principal points of diverticula formation between mesenteric and antimesenteric teniae. (Redrawn, with permission, from Goligher JC. *Surgery of the Anus, Rectum and Colon*, 5th ed. Baillière Tyndall, 1984.)

A patient who develops diverticulitis (see later discussion) may present with fever and with symptoms and signs of peritoneal irritation (guarding, rebound tenderness, absence of bowel sounds). A patient who develops diverticular bleeding may present with stools that are either frankly bloody or positive for occult blood.

Etiology

Diverticulosis results from an acquired deformity of the colon in which the mucosa and submucosa herniate through the underlying muscularis (Figure 13–22). The incidence of this disease is increased with affluent, Westernized lifestyles. A rarity at the turn of the century, today it afflicts 30% of adults in the U.S. population. Its incidence increases with age, starting from about 40 years. Epidemiologic studies suggest that the consumption of highly refined foods and less fiber, with a resulting increased prevalence of chronic constipation, may be responsible for the increased prevalence of diverticular disease.

Pathology & Pathogenesis

A. Diverticulosis

Most acquired diverticula occur in the colon; the descending colon and sigmoid (left side) are involved in more than 90% of cases. Both structural and functional factors are believed to contribute to the development of diverticulosis. Acquired abnormalities in colonic wall connective tissue are believed to be the structural basis of diminished resistance to mucosal and submucosal herniation (see Figure 13–22). The functional abnormality is believed to be related to chronic constipation and the development of a transmural pressure gradient from the colonic lumen to the peritoneal space as a result of vigorous muscle contraction in the colonic wall. This functional abnormality is most likely related to changes in dietary habits; decreased dietary fiber makes the forward propulsion of feces at normal transmural pressures more difficult. This increased muscle contraction, which contributes to the development of diverticular disease, is also believed to cause the abdominal pain that is the cardinal symptom of uncomplicated diverticular disease. The pain may last hours to days, with sudden relief on passing flatus or feces. Constipation or diarrhea and flatulence are common findings during such episodes, leading to the suggestion that there is a relationship between irritable bowel syndrome and the development of diverticulosis. Treatment of the pain of diverticular disease with opioids is contraindicated because opioids directly raise intraluminal pressure and hence may increase the risk of perforation.

B. Diverticular Bleeding

Diverticula are a source of bleeding in 3–5% of patients with diverticulosis. Branches of the colonic intramural arteries (vasa recta) are closely associated with the diverticular sac, presumably leading to occasional rupture and bleeding. This is the most common cause of massive lower GI bleeding in the elderly. Diverticular bleeding is typically painless and not believed to be associated with a focus of inflammation.

The differential diagnosis of painless bleeding per rectum also includes internal hemorrhoids (dilated venous channels in the anal canal) and angiodysplasia. The latter consists of small, focal proliferations of dilated blood vessels in the mucosa, typically found in elderly patients.

C. Diverticulitis

This most common complication of diverticulosis develops when a focal area of inflammation occurs in the wall of a diverticulum in response to irritation by fecal material. The patient develops symptoms of abdominal pain and fever with a risk of progression to abscess with or without perforation. These symptoms mimic acute appendicitis; however, pain localizes typically to the left (rather than the right) lower abdominal quadrant. Perforations usually are self-contained, but the potential for subsequent fistula formation and intestinal obstruction is high. Approximately 15–25% of patients who develop diverticulitis will require surgery.

Clinical Manifestations

About one-fifth of all individuals with diverticular disease develop one of the two major complications: diverticular bleeding or diverticulitis. These disorders must be distinguished from carcinoma, inflammatory bowel disease, infection, and ischemic injury. Ischemia can arise from a variety of conditions, including atherosclerosis, vasculitis, hypercoagulable states, heart failure, and shock. Definitive diagnosis is typically made by colonoscopy.

CHECKPOINT

66. Where in the GI tract do most diverticula occur?
67. What predisposing factors contribute to the development of diverticular disease?
68. What are the major complications of diverticular disease?

IRRITABLE BOWEL SYNDROME

Irritable bowel syndrome is the most common cause of referral to gastroenterologists. It is characterized by altered bowel habits with abdominal pain in the absence of any detectable organic pathological process or specific motility or structural abnormalities.

A change in bowel habits with increasing diarrhea, constipation, or alternating diarrhea and constipation, is the principal symptom of irritable bowel syndrome. Abdominal pain, which may be caused by intestinal spasms, is also common to all patients with irritable bowel syndrome. Bloating or perceived abdominal distension is another common feature. Intraluminal gas can result from swallowing air, diminished gas absorption, and bacterial fermentation, although the cause of irritable bowel syndrome is unknown. Stress appears to have a considerable influence on these symptoms. Symptoms of irritable bowel syndrome frequently occur during or after a stressful event, and stressful events in early life may predispose to the development of irritable bowel syndrome.

Much of our understanding of the pathophysiology of irritable bowel syndrome derives from the study of motility. In normal persons, high-amplitude peristaltic contractions occur 6–8 times per day. In constipated patients with irritable bowel syndrome, the frequency of high-amplitude peristaltic contractions of the intestine is diminished compared with normal subjects, suggesting that the constipation may be due to diminished motility. Visceral hyperalgesia may also occur in patients with irritable bowel syndrome. In patients with irritable bowel syndrome, distension of the colon with a balloon, to a degree that is not painful in normal individuals, can induce pain, indicative of visceral hyperalgesia.

Irritable bowel syndrome is a complex disorder, and its cause is poorly understood. Several theories have been proposed to explain the disorder, including alterations in sensitivity of the extrinsic and intrinsic nervous systems of the intestine, which may contribute to exaggerated sensations of pain and to abnormal control of intestinal motility and secretion. An alteration in the balance of secretion and absorption is also a potential cause. Microbial dysbiosis is another important potential etiology. This etiology is supported by the response of the symptoms of some patients to either antibiotic or probiotic therapy. Although there is no gross inflammation of the intestine, there are reports of an increased influx of inflammatory cells (lymphocytes) into the colon of affected individuals as well as of the destruction of enteric neurons. One proposed theory is that irritable bowel syndrome develops as a result of an earlier and resolved bout of interstitial inflammation. In experimental animals, induction of intestinal inflammation induces visceral hyperalgesia and altered intestinal motility and secretion that persists many months after the inflammation is resolved. A similar mechanism may occur in a subset of patients who develop irritable bowel syndrome after an infection causes intestinal inflammation.

CHECKPOINT

69. List three characteristics of irritable bowel syndrome.
70. What are possible factors in the pathogenesis of irritable bowel syndrome?

CASE STUDIES

Yeong Kwok, MD

(See Chapter 25, p. 770–73 for answers)

CASE 67

A 60-year-old man presents to the clinic with a 3-month history of gradually worsening dysphagia (difficulty swallowing). He first noticed the problem when eating solid food such as steak, but now it happens even with drinking water. He has a sensation that whatever he swallows becomes stuck in his chest and does not go into the stomach. He has also developed worsening heartburn, especially upon lying down, and has had to prop himself up at night to lessen the heartburn. He has lost 10 kg as a result of his swallowing difficulties. His physical examination is unremarkable. A barium swallow x-ray reveals a decrease in peristalsis of the body of the esophagus along with dilatation of the lower esophagus and tight closure of the lower esophageal sphincter. The distal esophagus and lower esophageal sphincter have a beaked appearance. There is very little passage of barium into the stomach.

Questions

A. What is the likely diagnosis in this patient, and what is the underlying pathophysiology of this condition?
B. Botulinum toxin can be used to treat this disorder. How does it help ameliorate the symptoms?
C. What are the possible complications of this disorder, and how do they arise?

CASE 68

A 32-year-old woman presents to her primary care provider complaining of a persistent burning sensation in her chest and upper abdomen. The symptoms are worse at night while she is lying down and after meals. She has tried drinking hot cocoa to help her sleep. She is a smoker and frequently relies on benzodiazepines for insomnia. She notes a sour taste in her mouth every morning. Her physical examination is normal.

Questions

A. What is the pathogenetic mechanism of this patient's GI disorder?
B. How may her lifestyle impact her symptoms?
C. What are some complications of chronic esophageal reflux disease?

CASE 69

A 74-year-old man with severe osteoarthritis presents to the emergency department reporting two episodes of melena (black stools) without hematochezia (bright red blood in the stools) or hematemesis (bloody vomitus). He takes 600 mg of ibuprofen three times a day to control his arthritis pain. He denies alcohol use. On examination, his blood pressure is 150/70 mm Hg, and his resting pulse is 96/min. His epigastrium is minimally tender to palpation. Rectal examination reveals black tarry stool in the vault, grossly positive for occult blood. Endoscopy demonstrates a 3 cm gastric ulcer. *Helicobacter pylori* is identified on biopsies of the ulcer site.

Questions

A. What are some of the proposed mechanisms for acid-peptic disease and specifically gastric ulcer disease?
B. How may this patient's analgesic use predispose him to acid-peptic disease?
C. What role does *H pylori* infection play in the pathogenesis of ulcer disease? How should this be taken into account when treating this patient?

CASE 70

A 67-year-old man with type 2 diabetes is seen by his primary care provider for frequent nausea, vomiting, bloating, and intermittent diarrhea over the preceding 2 weeks. The vomiting typically occurs approximately 1–2 hours after eating. He states that over the past year, he has become increasingly depressed after the death of his wife and has been less adherent to his oral hypoglycemic regimen and evening insulin. He also reports 6 months of worsening neuropathic pain in his feet. His fasting fingerstick blood glucose level is 253 mg/dL.

Questions

A. How may diabetes contribute to the development of gastroparesis? Is this patient's poor glucose control a cause or consequence of gastroparesis?
B. How can delayed gastric emptying cause diarrhea?

CASE 71

A 40-year-old woman presents to the emergency department with a history of worsening right upper quadrant pain. The pain started after she had pizza for dinner 2 days ago and is described as a sharp, stabbing sensation under her right ribs. She has also felt ill, developed slight nausea, and had a low-grade fever. There has been no vomiting or diarrhea. The physical examination reveals an obese woman with a low-grade fever and tenderness to palpation of the right upper quadrant of her abdomen. An abdominal ultrasound reveals a 2 cm gallstone lodged in the cystic duct with swelling of the gallbladder and thickening of the gallbladder wall.

Questions

A. What are the mechanisms involved in gallstone formation?
B. What factors in the pathogenesis of gallstones may be responsible for the fact that it is more common in premenopausal women?
C. What local complications can ensue from gallstone disease?

CASE 72

A 45-year-old man comes to clinic with a history of excessive bloating, foul-smelling flatus, and loose stools for the past several months. He notes that about 30–60 minutes after breakfast each morning, he experiences cramping, bloating, passage of smelly flatus, and a very loose, watery bowel movement. He has not seen any blood or mucus in the stool and also denies any weight loss. This does not happen with lunch or dinner. Every day for breakfast, he eats a big bowl of cereal with milk and a yogurt smoothie. The physical exam is unremarkable with normal bowel sounds, no organomegaly, and no abdominal tenderness. He was advised to do a dietary trial of stopping dairy intake for 1 week. All his symptoms resolve, and he is diagnosed with lactose intolerance.

Questions

A. Why do people develop lactose intolerance?
B. Why does the inability to digest lactose lead to diarrhea?

CASE 73

A 42-year-old man with long-standing Crohn disease presents to the emergency department with a 1-day history of increasing abdominal distension, pain, and obstipation. He is nauseated and has vomited bilious material. He has no history of abdominal surgery and has had two exacerbations of his disease this year. He is febrile with a temperature of 38.5°C. Examination reveals multiple oral aphthous ulcers, hyperactive bowel sounds, and a grossly distended, diffusely tender abdomen without an appreciable mass. Abdominal radiographs reveal multiple air–fluid levels in the small bowel with minimal colonic gas, findings consistent with a small bowel obstruction.

Questions

A. Describe the significance of the oral aphthous ulcers in the distribution of Crohn disease.
B. What factors are thought to be involved in the pathogenesis of Crohn disease? What is the evidence to support the role of cytokines in the pathogenesis of Crohn disease?
C. What are the GI complications of Crohn disease?
D. Describe some of the extraintestinal manifestations of Crohn disease.

CASE 74

A 56-year-old man presents to his doctor with an 8-week history of gradually worsening diarrhea. He has had as many as eight loose watery bowel movements per day, occasionally mixed with blood. He has felt fatigued and has some left lower quadrant discomfort. He denies any travel, recent infections, or recent use of antibiotics. A colonoscopy shows chronic colitis of the entire rectum and sigmoid colon. Stool cultures and other studies for enteric pathogens are negative.

Questions

A. What is the likely diagnosis, and why?
B. Anti-inflammatory agents such as sulfasalazine and glucocorticoids have traditionally been used in the treatment of this condition. What are some of the newer agents that can also be used?
C. Why do patients with this condition often get frequent surveillance colonoscopies? What is another feared complication of this condition?

CASE 75

A 76-year-old woman with chronic constipation reports a 4-day history of "achy" left lower quadrant abdominal pain, graded 7/10, accompanied by low-grade fever and nausea. A colonoscopy performed 2 years ago revealed sigmoid diverticular disease. On examination, she has a temperature of 38.6°C. Her abdomen has a tender 3 × 2 cm mass in the left lower quadrant. Bowel sounds are normal. Her stool is positive for occult blood. An abdominal series shows a bowel gas pattern consistent with ileus and no evidence of free peritoneal air. A CT scan with contrast of the abdomen and pelvis shows pericolonic fat stranding with no evidence of an abscess. She is started on antibiotics and intravenous fluids with significant improvement in her symptoms.

Questions

A. Describe the pathogenesis of diverticular disease.
B. Why should opioids be avoided in the treatment of her abdominal pain?
C. What are the complications of diverticular disease?

CASE 76

A 32-year-old woman comes to the clinic complaining of a 3-month history of abdominal bloating, crampy abdominal pain, and a change in her bowel habits. Previously she had regular bowel movements, but 4 months ago, she developed gastroenteritis with nausea and vomiting after a cruise. The constant diarrhea and vomiting went away after a week, but since then she has had periods of constipation, lasting up to 3 days, alternating with periods of diarrhea. During the diarrheal episodes, she can have three to four loose bowel movements per day, though without blood or mucus in the stool. She describes diffuse abdominal cramping and bloating that are somewhat relieved by bowel movements. Her symptoms worsen during periods of stress. There has been no weight loss or fever. There is no association with particular foods (eg, wheat or dairy products). Her physical examination is unremarkable except for mild abdominal tenderness with no rebound or guarding. Serologic tests for celiac disease are negative. Stool cultures and examinations are negative for bacterial or parasitic infections. A colonoscopy is unremarkable.

Questions

A. What is the likely diagnosis?
B. What are the theories about the pathophysiology of this condition?

REFERENCES

General

Beumer J et al. Regulation and plasticity of intestinal stem cells during homeostasis and regeneration. Development. 2016 Oct 15;143(20):3639–49. [PMID: 27802133]

Bridwell-Rabb J et al. Vitamin B$_{12}$ in the spotlight again. Curr Opin Chem Biol. 2017 Apr;37:63–70. [PMID: 28167430]

Browning KN et al. The vagus nerve in appetite regulation, mood, and intestinal inflammation. Gastroenterology. 2017 Mar;152(4):730–44. [PMID: 27988382]

Lechuga S et al. Disruption of the epithelial barrier during intestinal inflammation: quest for new molecules and mechanisms. Biochim Biophys Acta. 2017 Jul;1864(7):1183–94. [PMID: 28322932]

Martini E et al. Mend your fences: the epithelial barrier and its relationship with mucosal immunity in inflammatory bowel disease. Cell Mol Gastroenterol Hepatol. 2017 Mar 23;4(1):33–46. [PMID: 28560287]

Powell N et al. The mucosal immune system: master regulator of bidirectional gut-brain communications. Nat Rev Gastroenterol Hepatol. 2017 Mar;14(3):143–59. [PMID: 28096541]

Singh V et al. Translating molecular physiology of intestinal transport into pharmacologic treatment of diarrhea: stimulation of Na$^+$ absorption. Clin Gastroenterol Hepatol. 2014 Jan;12(1):27–31. [PMID: 24184676]

Smith JP et al. Gastrin and gastric cancer. Cell Mol Gastroenterol Hepatol. 2017 Mar 14;4(1):75–83. [PMID: 28560291]

Willet SG et al. Stomach organ and cell lineage differentiation: from embryogenesis to adult homeostasis. Cell Mol Gastroenterol Hepatol. 2016 Sep;2(5):546–59. [PMID: 27642625]

GI Disease

Buckley A et al. Cell biology of tight junction barrier regulation and mucosal disease. Cold Spring Harb Perspect Biol. 2018 Jan 2;10(1):a029314. [PMID: 28507021]

Coati I et al. Autoimmune gastritis: pathologist's viewpoint. World J Gastroenterol. 2015 Nov 14;21(42):12179–89. [PMID: 26576102]

Hunt RH et al. The stomach in health and disease. Gut. 2015 Oct;64(10):1650–68. [PMID: 26342014]

Mills JC et al. Reserve stem cells: differentiated cells reprogram to fuel repair, metaplasia, and neoplasia in the adult gastrointestinal tract. Sci Signal. 2015 Jul 14;8(385):re8. [PMID: 26175494]

Postler TS et al. Understanding the holobiont: how microbial metabolites affect human health and shape the Immune System. Cell Metab. 2017 Jul 5;26(1):110–30. [PMID: 28625867]

Rokkas T et al. A systematic review and meta-analysis of the role of *Helicobacter pylori* eradication in preventing gastric cancer. Ann Gastroenterol. 2017;30(4):414–23. [PMID: 28655977]

Udager AM et al. Proper development of the outer longitudinal smooth muscle of the mouse pylorus requires Nkx2-5 and Gata3. Gastroenterology. 2014 Jan;146(1):157–65. [PMID: 24120474]

Achalasia & Esophageal Reflux

Boeckxstaens GE et al. Achalasia. Lancet. 2014 Jan 4;383(9911):83–93. [PMID: 23871090]

Elias PS et al. The role of acid suppression in Barrett's esophagus. Am J Med. 2017 May;130(5):525–9. [PMID: 28159599]

Furuzawa-Carballeda J et al. New insights into the pathophysiology of achalasia and implications for future treatment. World J Gastroenterol. 2016 Sep 21;22(35):7892–907. [PMID: 27672286]

Kalatskaya I. Overview of major molecular alterations during progression from Barrett's esophagus to esophageal adenocarcinoma. Ann N Y Acad Sci. 2016 Oct;1381(1):74–91. [PMID: 27415609]

Mikami DJ et al. Physiology and pathogenesis of gastroesophageal reflux disease. Surg Clin North Am. 2015 Jun;95(3):515–25. [PMID: 25965127]

Nadaleto BF et al. Gastroesophageal reflux disease in the obese: pathophysiology and treatment. Surgery. 2016 Feb;159(2):475–86. [PMID: 26054318]

Pandolfino JE et al. Achalasia: a systematic review. JAMA. 2015 May 12;313(18):1841–52. [PMID: 25965233]

Pressman A et al. Etiology and pathogenesis of idiopathic achalasia. J Clin Gastroenterol. 2017 Mar;51(3):195–202. [PMID: 28009686]

Spechler SJ et al. A Summary of the 2016 James W. Freston Conference of the American Gastroenterological Association: Intestinal metaplasia in the esophagus and stomach: origins, differences, similarities and significance. Gastroenterology. 2017 Jul;153(1):e6–e13. [PMID: 28583825]

Stavropoulos SN et al. Diagnosis and management of esophageal achalasia. BMJ. 2016 Sep 13;354:i2785. [PMID: 27625387]

Tuason J et al. Current status of achalasia management: a review on diagnosis and treatment. J Gastroenterol. 2017 Apr;52(4):401–6. [PMID: 28188367]

Wang DH et al. Transcommitment: paving the way to Barrett's metaplasia. Adv Exp Med Biol. 2016;908:183–212. [PMID: 27573773]

Acid-Peptic Disease

Backert S et al. Pathogenesis of *Helicobacter pylori* infection. Helicobacter. 2016 Sep;21(Suppl 1):19–25. [PMID: 27531534]

Freedberg DE et al. The risks and benefits of long-term use of proton pump inhibitors: expert review and best practice advice from the American Gastroenterological Association. Gastroenterology. 2017 Mar;152(4):706–15. [PMID: 28257716]

Lanas A et al. Peptic ulcer disease. Lancet. 2017 Aug 5;390(10094):613–24. [PMID: 28242110]

Potamitis GS et al. *Helicobacter pylori* and nonmalignant diseases. Helicobacter. 2015 Sep;20(Suppl 1):26–9. [PMID: 26372821]

Schubert ML. Gastric acid secretion. Curr Opin Gastroenterol. 2016 Nov;32(6):452–60. [PMID: 27607343]

Gastroparesis & Other Gastrointestinal Motility Disorders

Bragg D et al. Postoperative ileus: recent developments in pathophysiology and management. Clin Nutr. 2015 Jun;34(3):367–76. [PMID: 25819420]

Camilleri M. Functional dyspepsia and gastroparesis. Dig Dis. 2016;34(5):491–9. [PMID: 27332558]

Chen JD et al. Electrical therapies for gastrointestinal motility disorders. Expert Rev Gastroenterol Hepatol. 2017 May;11(5):407–18. [PMID: 28277856]

Koch KL et al. Diabetic gastroparesis. Gastroenterol Clin North Am. 2015 Mar;44(1):39–57. [PMID: 25667022]

Liu N et al. Gastroparesis updates on pathogenesis and management. Gut Liver. 2017 Sep 15;11(5):579–89. [PMID: 28535580]

Nguyen LA et al. Clinical presentation and pathophysiology of gastroparesis. Gastroenterol Clin North Am. 2015 Mar;44(1):21–30. [PMID: 25667020]

Parkman HP. Idiopathic gastroparesis. Gastroenterol Clin North Am. 2015 Mar;44(1):59–68. [PMID: 25667023]

Stein B et al. Gastroparesis: a review of current diagnosis and treatment options. J Clin Gastroenterol. 2015 Aug;49(7):550–8. [PMID: 25874755]

Tack J et al. Gastroparesis. Curr Opin Gastroenterol. 2015 Nov;31(6):499–505. [PMID: 26406565]

Taylor RW. Gut motility issues in critical illness. Crit Care Clin. 2016 Apr;32(2):191–201. [PMID: 27016161]

Westfal ML et al. Pediatric enteric neuropathies: diagnosis and current management. Curr Opin Pediatr. 2017 Jun;29(3):347–53. [PMID: 28319561]

Gallstone Disease

Gomes CA et al. Acute calculous cholecystitis: review of current best practices. World J Gastrointest Surg. 2017 May 27;9(5):118–26. [PMID: 28603584]

Shabanzadeh DM et al. Determinants for gallstone formation—a new data cohort study and a systematic review with meta-analysis. Scand J Gastroenterol. 2016 Oct;51(10):1239–48. [PMID: 27232657]

Tazuma S et al. Evidence-based clinical practice guidelines for cholelithiasis 2016. J Gastroenterol. 2017 Mar;52(3):276–300. [PMID: 27942871]

Diarrhea

Camilleri M et al. Pathophysiology, evaluation, and management of chronic watery diarrhea. Gastroenterology. 2017 Feb;152(3):515–32. [PMID: 27773805]

DuPont HL. Persistent diarrhea: a clinical review. JAMA. 2016 Jun 28;315(24):2712–23. [PMID: 27357241]

Giddings SL et al. Traveler's diarrhea. Med Clin North Am. 2016 Mar;100(2):317–30. [PMID: 26900116]

Odenwald MA et al. The intestinal epithelial barrier: a therapeutic target? Nat Rev Gastroenterol Hepatol. 2017 Jan;14(1):9–21. [PMID: 27848962]

Thiagarajah JR et al. Secretory diarrhoea: mechanisms and emerging therapies. Nat Rev Gastroenterol Hepatol. 2015 Aug;12(8):446–57. [PMID: 26122478]

Inflammatory Bowel Disease

Abraham C et al. Lessons learned from trials targeting cytokine pathways in patients with inflammatory bowel diseases. Gastroenterology. 2017 Feb;152(2):374–88. [PMID: 27780712]

Dalal SR et al. The microbial basis of inflammatory bowel diseases. J Clin Invest. 2014 Oct;124(10):4190–6. [PMID: 25083986]

Kaplan GG et al. Understanding and preventing the global increase of inflammatory bowel disease. Gastroenterology. 2017 Feb;152(2):313–21. [PMID: 27793607]

McGovern DP et al. Genetics of inflammatory bowel diseases. Gastroenterology. 2015 Oct;149(5):1163–76. [PMID: 26255561]

Park JR et al. Primary care of the patient with inflammatory bowel disease. Med Clin North Am. 2015 Sep;99(5):969–87. [PMID: 26320042]

Rosen MJ et al. Inflammatory bowel disease in children and adolescents. JAMA Pediatr. 2015 Nov;169(11):1053–60. [PMID: 26414706]

Sartor RB et al. Roles for intestinal bacteria, viruses, and fungi in pathogenesis of inflammatory bowel diseases and therapeutic approaches. Gastroenterology. 2017 Feb;152(2):327–39. [PMID: 27769810]

Diverticular Disease

Feuerstein JD et al. Diverticulosis and diverticulitis. Mayo Clin Proc. 2016 Aug;91(8):1094–104. [PMID: 27156370]

Scaioli E et al. Pathophysiology and therapeutic strategies for symptomatic uncomplicated diverticular disease of the colon. Dig Dis Sci. 2016 Mar;61(3):673–83. [PMID: 26458921]

Irritable Bowel Syndrome

Chey WD et al. Irritable bowel syndrome: a clinical review. JAMA. 2015 Mar 3;313(9):949–58. [PMID: 25734736]

Deiteren A et al. Irritable bowel syndrome and visceral hypersensitivity: risk factors and pathophysiological mechanisms. Acta Gastroenterol Belg. 2016 Mar;79(1):29–38. [PMID: 26852761]

Martin-Viñas JJ et al. Immune response in irritable bowel syndrome: a systematic review of systemic and mucosal inflammatory mediators. J Dig Dis. 2016 Sep;17(9):572–81. [PMID: 27426409]

Sayuk GS et al. Irritable bowel syndrome: modern concepts and management options. Am J Med. 2015 Aug;128(8):817–27. [PMID: 25731138]

Liver Disease

Nizar A. Mukhtar, MD, &
Mandana Khalili, MD, MAS

CHAPTER

14

Although many different pathogenic agents and processes can affect the liver (Table 14–1), they are generally manifested in individual patients in a limited number of ways that can be assessed by evaluating some key parameters. Liver disease can be acute or chronic, focal or diffuse, mild or severe, and reversible or irreversible. Most cases of **acute liver disease** (eg, caused by viral hepatitis) are so mild that they never come to medical attention. Transient symptoms of fatigue, loss of appetite, and nausea are often ascribed to other causes (eg, flu), and minor biochemical abnormalities referable to the liver that would be identified in blood studies are not discovered. The patient recovers without any lasting medical consequences. In other cases of acute liver injury, symptoms and signs are severe enough to call for medical attention. The entire range of liver functions may be affected or only a few, as is the case with liver injury resulting from certain drugs that cause isolated impairment of the liver's role in bile formation (**cholestasis**). Occasionally, viral, drug-induced, and other acute liver injury occurs in an overwhelming manner, resulting in massive liver cell death and progressive multi-organ failure. This syndrome of **acute liver failure** (also referred to as fulminant hepatic failure) carries a high mortality rate; however, in recent years, use of emergency liver transplantation has significantly improved survival.

Liver injury may continue beyond the initial acute episode or may be recurrent (chronic hepatitis). In some cases of chronic hepatitis, liver function remains stable or the disease process ultimately resolves altogether. In other cases, there is progressive and irreversible deterioration of liver function.

Cirrhosis is the ultimate consequence of progressive liver injury. Cirrhosis can occur in a subset of cases of chronic hepatitis that do not resolve spontaneously or after repeated episodes of acute liver injury, as in the case of chronic alcoholism. In cirrhosis, the liver becomes hard, shrunken, and nodular and displays impaired function and diminished reserve because of a decreased amount of functioning liver tissue. More importantly, the physics of blood flow is altered such

that the pressure in the portal vein is elevated. As a result, the blood is *diverted around* the liver rather than *filtered through* the liver. This phenomenon, termed **portal-to-systemic** (or **portosystemic**) **shunting**, has profound effects on the function of various organ systems and sets the stage for certain devastating complications of liver disease (described later).

Although liver disease resulting from many different causes may present in common ways, the reverse is also true (ie, liver disease from specific causes may have distinctly different presentations in different patients). For example, consider two patients with acute viral hepatitis: One may present with yellow eyes and skin—a manifestation of impaired liver function—complaining of nothing more than itching, fatigue, and loss of appetite, whereas the other may be brought to the emergency department moribund, with massive gastrointestinal (GI) bleeding and encephalopathy. Such variations in the severity of liver disease are probably due to genetic, immunologic, and environmental (including perhaps nutritional) factors that are currently poorly understood.

The consequences of liver disease can be either reversible or irreversible. Those arising directly from acute damage to the functional cells of the liver, most notably **hepatocytes**, without destruction of the liver's capacity for regeneration, are generally reversible. Like many organs of the body, the liver normally has both a huge reserve capacity for the various biochemical reactions it carries out and the ability to regenerate fully differentiated cells and thereby recover completely from acute injury. Thus, only in the most fulminant cases or in end-stage disease are there insufficient residual hepatocytes to maintain minimal essential liver functions. More commonly, patients display transient signs of liver cell necrosis and disordered function followed by full recovery. The symptoms and signs of this sort of acute liver injury can best be understood as an impairment of the normal biochemical functions of the liver.

Other consequences of liver disease are irreversible, typically seen in the patient with cirrhosis. These are best understood as

TABLE 14–1   Liver diseases.

Inherited hyperbilirubinemia	Acute fatty liver of pregnancy
Gilbert syndrome	**Liver involvement in systemic diseases**
Crigler–Najjar syndrome, types I and II	Sarcoidosis
Dubin–Johnson syndrome	Amyloidosis
Rotor syndrome	Glycogen storage diseases
Viral hepatitis	Celiac disease
Hepatitis A	Tuberculosis
Hepatitis B	*Mycobacterium avium–intracellulare* infection
Hepatitis C	**Cholestatic syndromes**
Hepatitis D	Benign postoperative cholestasis
Hepatitis E	Jaundice of sepsis
Others (Epstein–Barr [mononucleosis] virus, herpesvirus, adenovirus hepatitis)	Total parenteral nutrition (TPN)–induced jaundice
Cryptogenic hepatitis	Cholestasis of pregnancy
Immune and autoimmune liver diseases	Cholangitis and cholecystitis
Primary biliary cirrhosis	Extrahepatic biliary obstruction (stone, stricture, cancer)
Autoimmune hepatitis	Biliary atresia
Sclerosing cholangitis	Caroli disease
Overlap syndromes	Cryptosporidiosis
Graft-versus-host disease	**Drug-induced liver disease**
Allograft rejection	Hepatocellular patterns (isoniazid, acetaminophen)
Genetic liver diseases	Cholestatic patterns (methyltestosterone)
Alpha-1-antitrypsin deficiency	Mixed patterns (sulfonamides, phenytoin)
Hemochromatosis	Microvesicular and macrovesicular steatosis (methotrexate)
Wilson disease	**Vascular injury**
Benign recurrent intrahepatic cholestasis	Venoocclusive disease
Progressive familial intrahepatic cholestasis, types 1–3	Budd–Chiari syndrome
Others (galactosemia, tyrosinemia, cystic fibrosis, Neiman–Pick disease, Gaucher disease)	Ischemic hepatitis
Alcoholic liver disease	Passive congestion
Acute fatty liver	Portal vein thrombosis
Acute alcoholic hepatitis	Nodular regenerative hyperplasia
Laennec cirrhosis	**Mass lesions**
Nonalcoholic fatty liver	Hepatocellular carcinoma
Steatosis	Cholangiocarcinoma
Steatohepatitis	Adenoma
	Focal nodular hyperplasia
	Metastatic tumors
	Abscess
	Cysts
	Hemangioma

Reproduced, with permission, from Ghany M et al. Approach to the patient with liver disease. In: Kasper D et al, eds. *Harrison's Principles of Internal Medicine,* 19th ed. McGraw-Hill, 2015.

a result of portosystemic shunting of blood flow. They include a heightened sensitivity to noxious substances absorbed from the GI tract (encephalopathy), an increased risk of massive GI bleeding (development of varices and coagulopathy), and malabsorption of fat in the stool (as a result of decreased bile flow). Nevertheless, some of these consequences are treatable. Commonly, patients with cirrhosis present with superimposed acute liver injury (eg, caused by an alcoholic binge or other drug exposure). Because they have a decreased hepatocyte mass and much less functional reserve, they are more sensitive to acute liver injury than patients with a normal liver.

STRUCTURE & FUNCTION OF THE LIVER

ANATOMY, HISTOLOGY & CELL BIOLOGY

The liver is located in the right upper quadrant of the abdomen in the peritoneal space just below the right side of the diaphragm and under the rib cage (Figure 14–1). It is anatomically separated into two predominant lobes: right and left. The right lobe has two lesser segments: the posterior caudate lobe and the inferior quadrate lobe. The liver can also be differentiated functionally via the portal blood flow into four sectors, which are further subdivided into eight segments. The liver weighs approximately 1400 g in the adult and is covered by a fibrous capsule. It receives nearly 25% of the cardiac output, approximately 1500 mL of blood flow per minute, via two sources: venous flow from the **portal vein**, which is crucial to the performance of the liver's roles in bodily functions, and arterial flow from the **hepatic artery**, which is important for liver oxygenation and which supplies the biliary system via the cystic artery. These vessels converge within the liver, and the combined blood flow exits via the so-called **central veins** (also

called terminal veins or hepatic venules) that drain into the hepatic vein and ultimately the inferior vena cava.

The portal vein carries venous blood from the small intestine, rich in freshly absorbed nutrients—as well as drugs and poisons—directly to the liver. Also flowing into the portal vein before its entry into the liver is the pancreatic venous drainage, rich in pancreatic hormones (insulin, glucagon, somatostatin, and pancreatic polypeptide). The portal vein forms a specialized capillary bed that allows individual hepatocytes to be bathed directly in portal blood. In part because of this system of blood supply, the liver is a prime site for the metastatic spread of cancer, especially from the GI tract, breast, and lung.

Concepts of Liver Organization

The substance (**parenchyma**) of the liver is organized into plates of hepatocytes lying in a cage of supporting cells termed **reticuloendothelial cells** (Figure 14–2A). The plates of hepatocytes are generally only one cell thick, and individual plates are separated from each other by vascular spaces called **sinusoids**. It is in these sinusoids that blood from the hepatic artery is mixed with blood from the portal vein on the way to the central vein. The reticuloendothelial cell meshwork in which the hepatocytes reside includes diverse cell types, most importantly the **endothelial cells** that make up the walls of the sinusoids; specialized macrophages, termed **Kupffer cells**, which are anchored in the sinusoidal space; and stellate cells or **lipocytes**, fat-storing cells involved in vitamin A metabolism, which lie between the hepatocytes and the endothelial cells. Approximately 30% of all cells in the liver are reticuloendothelial cells, and about 33% of these are Kupffer cells. Yet, because reticuloendothelial cells are smaller than hepatocytes, the reticuloendothelial system accounts for only 2–10% of the total protein in the liver. The reticuloendothelial cells are much more than just a cage for hepatocytes. They perform specific functions, including phagocytosis and cytokine secretion, and communicate with each other as well as with hepatocytes. Their dysfunction contributes both to hepatocyte necrosis in acute liver disease and to hepatic fibrosis in chronic liver disease.

FIGURE 14–1 Location of the liver. (Redrawn, with permission, from Wolf DC. Evaluation of the size, shape and consistency of the liver. In: Walker HK et al, eds. *Clinical Methods*, 3rd ed. Butterworth, 1990.)

FIGURE 14–2   **A:** Detailed structure of the liver lobule. (Redrawn, with permission, from Chandrasoma P et al. *Concise Pathology,* 3rd ed. Originally published by Appleton & Lange. Copyright © 1998 by The McGraw-Hill Companies, Inc.) **B:** Relationship of lobule to acinus. (CV, central vein; PS, portal space [or triad].) (Redrawn, with permission, from Leeson CR. *Histology,* 2nd ed. Saunders, 1970. Copyright © Elsevier.) **C:** Hepatic acinus. (HV, hepatic venule.) (Reproduced, with permission, from Gumucio JJ. Hepatic transport. In: Kelley WN (ed): *Textbook of Internal Medicine.* Lippincott, 1989.)

A. Lobules

Under the microscope at low-power magnification, liver architecture has been traditionally described in terms of the **lobule** (Figure 14–2B). Neat arrays of hepatocyte plates are organized around individual central veins to form hexagons with **portal triads** or **tracts** (sheath-like structures containing a portal venule, hepatic arteriole, and bile canaliculus) at their corners. The hepatocytes adjacent to the portal triad are termed the **limiting plate**. Disruption of the limiting plate is a significant diagnostic marker of some forms of immune-mediated liver

disease. This may be seen in liver biopsies from patients with liver disease of unknown cause.

B. Functional Zonation

Physiologically, it is more useful to think of liver architecture in terms of the portal-to-central direction of blood flow: Blood entering the sinusoids from a terminal portal venule or hepatic arteriole flows past hepatocytes closest to those vessels first (termed zone 1 hepatocytes) and then percolates past zone 2 hepatocytes (so called because they are not the first hepatocytes reached by blood entering the hepatic parenchyma). The last hepatocytes reached by the blood before it enters the central vein are termed zone 3 hepatocytes. Thus, the microscopic organization of the liver can be viewed in terms of functional zones. A liver **acinus** is defined as the unit of liver tissue centered around the portal venule and hepatic arteriole whose hepatocytes can be imagined to form concentric rings of cells in the order in which they come into contact with portal blood, first to last (Figure 14–2C). Hepatocytes at either extreme of the acinus (zones 1 and 3) appear to differ in both enzymatic activity and physiologic functions. Zone 1 hepatocytes, exposed to the highest oxygen concentrations, are particularly active in gluconeogenesis and oxidative energy metabolism. They are also the major site of urea synthesis (because freely diffusible substances such as ammonia absorbed from protein breakdown in the gut are largely extracted in zone 1). Conversely, zone 3 hepatocytes are more active in glycolysis and lipogenesis (processes requiring less oxygen). Zone 2 hepatocytes display attributes of both zone 1 and zone 3 cells.

C. Receptor-Mediated Uptake

Functional zonation applies only to processes driven by the presence of diffusible substances. The liver, however, is also involved in many pathways participating in receptor-mediated uptake and active transport of substances unable to diffuse freely into cells. These substances enter whichever hepatocytes have the appropriate transporters regardless of their zone. Similarly, substances tightly bound to carrier proteins for which the liver does *not* have receptors are cleared equally poorly by hepatocytes in all three zones.

Hepatocytes: Polarized Cells with Functional Segregation

All surfaces of a hepatocyte are not the same. Hepatocytes have three sides. One side, the **apical surface**, forms the wall of the bile canaliculus. The second side, the **basolateral surface**, is in contact with the bloodstream via the sinusoids. The last side, the **lateral domain**, is bordered by the two other surfaces. Very different activities go forward at these regions of the hepatocyte plasma membrane; **tight junctions** between hepatocytes serve to maintain segregation of apical and basolateral plasma membrane domains. Processes related to bile transport and excretion act at the apical plasma membrane (Figure 14–3A). Uptake from and secretion into the bloodstream are activities that occur across the basolateral membrane (Figure 14–3B).

FIGURE 14–3 A: Mechanism of bile acid secretion. About 90% of these compounds derive from bile acids absorbed in the intestinal epithelium and recirculated to the liver. The remainder are synthesized in the liver by conjugating cholic acid with the amino acids glycine and taurine. This process occurs in the smooth endoplasmic reticulum (SER). **B:** Protein synthesis and carbohydrate storage in the liver. Protein synthesis occurs in the rough endoplasmic reticulum, which explains why liver cell lesions or starvation leads to a decrease in the amounts of albumin, fibrinogen, and prothrombin in a patient's blood. In several diseases, glycogen degradation is depressed, with an abnormal intracellular accumulation of this compound. (RER, rough endoplasmic reticulum; SER, smooth endoplasmic reticulum.) (Redrawn, with permission, from Junqueira LC et al. *Basic Histology*, 10th ed. McGraw-Hill, 2003.)

Effects of Hepatocyte Dysfunction

In view of this organization, it is perhaps not surprising that hepatocyte dysfunction can sometimes involve disruption of bile flow (cholestasis) with relative preservation of other functions. There is, however, no clear line between the consequences of disturbed apical and basolateral functions: Cholestasis, although initially a disorder of apical bile flow, is ultimately manifested at the basolateral surface. This is because it is at the basolateral surface that bilirubin and other substances to be excreted across the apical plasma membrane into the bile must first be taken up from the bloodstream. Similarly, disruption of energy metabolism or protein synthesis, although initially impinging on the secretory and metabolic processes of the hepatocyte, will ultimately affect the bile transport machinery in the apical plasma membrane as well.

Capacity for Regeneration

Although the normal liver contains very few cells in mitosis, when hepatocytes are lost, poorly understood mechanisms stimulate proliferation of the remaining hepatocytes. This is why in most cases of fulminant hepatic failure with massive hepatocellular death, if the patient survives the acute period of hepatic dysfunction (usually with medical therapy in the hospital), recovery will be complete. Similarly, surgical resection of liver tissue is followed by proliferation of the remaining hepatocytes (**hyperplasia**). Numerous growth factors (eg, HGF, TGF-α) and cytokines (eg, TNF, IL-1, IL-6) are involved in positioning the liver on a continuum between cell proliferation and cell death.

CHECKPOINT

4. From which vascular beds do the hepatic central veins derive their blood flow?

5. Why is the liver a major site for metastasis of malignant neoplasms from other parts of the body?

6. What cell types make up the liver, and what are their distinguishing characteristics?

7. What is the difference between the lobule concept and the acinus concept of liver subarchitecture?

8. What are some physiologic consequences of functional zonation in the liver?

9. What activities are found in zone 1 hepatocytes? In zone 3 hepatocytes?

10. Which structures normally maintain the separation of the apical and basolateral plasma membrane domains of the hepatocyte?

11. What happens to the remaining hepatocytes when part of the liver is surgically resected?

LIVER BLOOD FLOW & ITS CELLULAR BASIS

The portal blood flow, being venous in nature, is normally under low hydrostatic pressure (about 10 mm Hg). Accordingly, there must be little resistance to its flow within the liver, allowing the blood to percolate through the sinusoids and achieve maximal contact—for exchange of substances—with hepatocytes. Two unique features—fenestrations in the endothelial cells and lack of a typical basement membrane between endothelial cells and hepatocytes—aid in making the liver a low-pressure circuit for the flow of portal blood. These features are altered in cirrhosis, resulting in increased portal pressure and profound changes in liver blood flow, with devastating clinical consequences.

Fenestrations are spaces between the endothelial cells that make up the walls of the portal capillary system that allow plasma and its proteins, but not red blood cells, free and direct access to the surface of the hepatocytes. This feature is crucial to the liver's function of uptake from and secretion into the bloodstream. This feature also contributes to the efficiency of the liver as a filter of portal blood. Most of the capillary beds in the body lack such fenestrations.

PHYSIOLOGY

Table 14–2 lists the diverse functions of the liver grouped into four broad categories. Although there is considerable overlap between them, systematically considering each category is a useful way to approach the patient with liver disease.

Energy Generation & Substrate Interconversion

Much of the body's carbohydrate, protein, and lipid is synthesized, metabolized, and interconverted in the liver; products are removed from or released into the bloodstream in response to the energy and substrate needs of the body.

A. Carbohydrate Metabolism

After a meal, the liver achieves net glucose consumption (eg, to synthesize glycogen and generate metabolic intermediates via glycolysis and the tricarboxylic acid cycle). This occurs as a result of a confluence of several effects. First, the levels of substrates such as glucose increase. Second, the levels of hormones that affect the amount and activity of metabolic enzymes change. Thus, when blood glucose levels increase, the ratio of insulin to glucagon in the bloodstream also increases. The net effect is increased glucose use by the liver. In times of fasting (low blood glucose) or stress (when higher blood glucose is needed), hormone and substrate levels in the bloodstream drive the liver's metabolic pathways responsible for net glucose production (eg, the pathways of glycogenolysis and gluconeogenesis). As a result, blood glucose levels are raised to, or maintained in, the normal range in spite of wide and sudden changes in the rate of glucose input (eg, ingestion

TABLE 14–2   Functions of the normal liver.

Energy metabolism and substrate interconversion
Glucose production through gluconeogenesis and glycogenolysis
Glucose consumption by pathways of glycogen synthesis, fatty acid synthesis, glycolysis, and the tricarboxylic acid cycle
Cholesterol synthesis from acetate, triglyceride synthesis from fatty acids, and secretion of both in VLDL particles
Cholesterol and triglyceride uptake by endocytosis of HDL and LDL particles with excretion of cholesterol in bile, β-oxidation of fatty acids, and conversion of excess acetyl-CoA to ketones
Deamination of amino acids and conversion of ammonia to urea via the urea cycle
Transamination and de novo synthesis of nonessential amino acids
Protein synthetic functions
Synthesis of various plasma proteins, including albumin, clotting factors, binding proteins, apolipoproteins, angiotensinogen, and insulin-like growth factor I
Solubilization, transport, and storage functions
Drug and poison detoxification through phase I and phase II biotransformation reactions and excretion in bile
Solubilization of fats and fat-soluble vitamins in bile for uptake by enterocytes
Synthesis and secretion of VLDL and pre-HDL lipoprotein particles and clearance of HDL, LDL, and chylomicron remnants
Synthesis and secretion of various binding proteins, including transferrin, steroid hormone–binding globulin, thyroid hormone–binding globulin, ceruloplasmin, and metallothionein
Uptake and storage of vitamins A, D, and B_{12} and folate
Protective and clearance functions
Detoxification of ammonia through the urea cycle
Detoxification of drugs through microsomal oxidases and conjugation systems
Synthesis and export of glutathione
Clearance of damaged cells and proteins, hormones, drugs, and activated clotting factors from the portal circulation
Clearance of bacteria and antigens from the portal circulation

HDL, high-density lipoprotein; LDL, low-density lipoprotein; VLDL, very-low-density lipoprotein.

and absorption) and output (eg, use by tissues) from the bloodstream (Figure 14–4).

B. Protein Metabolism

Related to its important role in protein metabolism, the liver is a major site for processes of oxidative deamination and transamination (Figure 14–5). These reactions allow amino groups to be shuffled among molecules to generate substrates for both carbohydrate metabolism and amino acid synthesis. Likewise, the urea cycle allows nitrogen to be excreted in the form of urea, which is much less toxic than free amino groups in the form of ammonium ions. Impairment of this function in liver disease is discussed in greater detail later.

C. Lipid Metabolism

The liver is the center of lipid metabolism. The liver manufactures nearly 80% of the cholesterol synthesized in the body from acetyl-CoA via a pathway that connects the metabolism of carbohydrates with that of lipids (see Figure 14–4). Moreover, the liver can synthesize, store, and export triglycerides (see Figure 14–4). The liver is also the site of keto acid production via the pathway of fatty acid oxidation that connects lipid catabolism with activity of the tricarboxylic acid cycle.

In the process of controlling the body's cholesterol and triglyceride levels, the liver assembles, secretes, and takes up various lipoprotein particles (Figure 14–6). Dietary fat is first absorbed into the small intestine, then packaged into chylomicrons. Following the removal of triglycerides, the chylomicron remnant is taken up by the liver via **low-density lipoprotein** (**LDL**) receptor–mediated endocytosis. To distribute lipids systemically, **very-low-density lipoproteins** (**VLDLs**) are secreted by the liver and transport triglycerides and cholesterol to adipose tissue for storage or to other tissues for immediate use. As triglycerides are removed, the structure of VLDL particles is modified by the loss of lipid and protein components rendering intermediate-density lipoprotein (IDL) and further downstream LDL. LDL particles are then returned to the liver via the **LDL receptor**. On the other hand, **high-density lipoproteins** (**HDLs**), lipoproteins synthesized and secreted from the liver, scavenge excess cholesterol and triglycerides from other tissues and from the bloodstream, returning them to the liver, where they are excreted. Thus, HDL secretion and LDL removal are both mechanisms by which cholesterol in excess of that needed by various tissues is removed from the circulation (Figures 14–6B and 14–6C).

Synthesis & Secretion of Plasma Proteins

The liver manufactures and secretes many of the proteins found in plasma, including albumin, several clotting factors, a number of binding proteins, and even certain hormones and hormone precursors. By virtue of the actions of these proteins, the liver has important roles in maintaining plasma oncotic pressure (serum albumin), coagulation (clotting factor synthesis and modification), blood pressure (angiotensinogen), growth (insulin-like growth factor-1), and metabolism (steroid and thyroid hormone–binding proteins).

Solubilizing, Transport & Storage Functions

The liver plays an important role in solubilizing, transporting, and storing a variety of very different substances that would

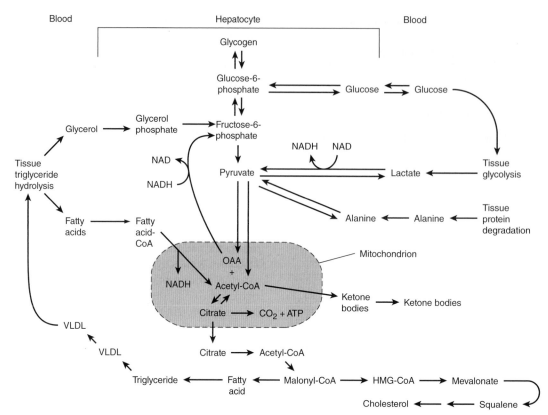

FIGURE 14–4 Pathways of hepatic carbohydrate and lipid metabolism. (ATP, adenosine triphosphate; CoA, co-enzyme A; HMG, hepatic 3-methylglutaryl; NAD, nicotinamide adenine dinucleotide (oxidized form); NADH, nicotinamide adenine dinucleotide hydride (reduced form); OAA, oxaloacetic acid; VLDL, very-low-density lipoprotein.) (Redrawn, with permission, from Schwartz CC. Hepatic metabolism. In: Kelley WN, ed. *Textbook of Internal Medicine.* Lippincott, 1989.)

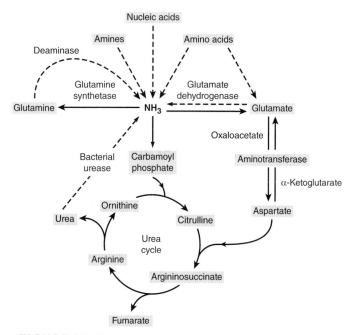

FIGURE 14–5 Urea cycle. Dashed lines signify pathways whose extent of involvement varies from patient to patient depending on genetic, dietary, and other factors. (Redrawn, with permission, from Powers-Lee SG et al. Urea synthesis and ammonia metabolism. In: Arias IM et al, eds. *The Liver: Biology and Pathology*, 3rd ed. Raven Press, 1994.)

otherwise be difficult for tissues to obtain or move in and out of cells. Specific cells in the liver perform these functions by manufacturing specialized proteins that serve as receptors, binding proteins, or enzymes.

A. Enterohepatic Circulation of Bile Acids

Bile is a detergent-like substance synthesized by the liver that permits a variety of otherwise insoluble substances to be dissolved in an aqueous environment for transport into or out of the body. Bile acids are a major component of bile and are recycled via the so-called **enterohepatic circulation** between the liver and the intestines. After synthesis and active transport from hepatocyte cytoplasm into the bile canaliculus (across the apical plasma membrane of the hepatocyte), bile is collected in the biliary tract (and sometimes stored in the gallbladder) and excreted via the common bile duct into the duodenum. While still in the cytoplasm of the hepatocyte, many bile acids are conjugated to sugars, which increases their water solubility. Once in the duodenum, bile acids serve to solubilize lipids, facilitating the digestion and absorption of fats. In the terminal ileum, both conjugated and deconjugated bile acids are taken up and transported from enterocytes to portal blood flow. Portal blood returns them to the liver, where specialized bile acid transporters (predominantly sodium taurocholate cotransporter [Ntcp]) return them to the hepatocyte cytosol via the basolateral plasma membrane facing the space of Disse.

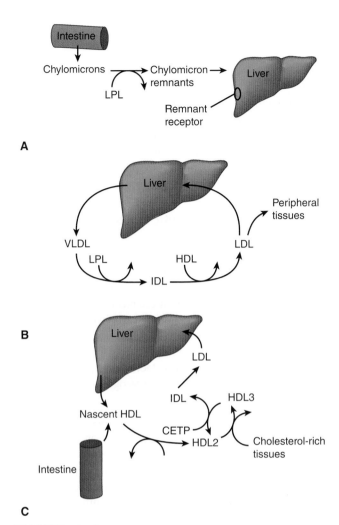

FIGURE 14–6 Lipoprotein metabolism in the liver. **A:** Exogenous fat transport pathway. **B:** Endogenous fat transport pathway. **C:** Pathway of reverse cholesterol transport. In each pathway, lipoprotein particles are used to solubilize cholesteryl esters (and triglyceride), either for the purpose of import from the GI tract (**A**), distribution to various tissues (**B**), or transport to the liver for excretion in bile (**C**). During their circulation, specific lipoprotein particles are transformed by the addition and removal of apoproteins and by the action of enzymes in plasma or in tissues (eg, lipoprotein lipase [LPL], cholesteryl ester transfer protein [CETP]). Intermediate-density lipoproteins (IDLs) are intermediates in the conversion of very-low-density lipoproteins (VLDLs) to low-density lipoproteins (LDLs). (HDL, high-density lipoprotein.) (Redrawn from Breslow JL. Genetic basis of lipoprotein disorders. J Clin Invest. 1989;84:373.)

There they are subject to reconjugation and secretion across the apical membrane along with other components (eg, pigment, cholesterol) to form new bile. Thereafter, they engage in another cycle of enterohepatic transport.

B. Drug Metabolism and Excretion

Most of the enzymes that catalyze metabolic processes needed to detoxify and excrete drugs and other substances are located in the smooth endoplasmic reticulum of hepatocytes. These pathways are used to metabolize not only exogenous drugs, but also many endogenous substances that would otherwise be difficult for cells to excrete (eg, bilirubin and cholesterol). In most cases, this metabolism involves the conversion of **hydrophobic** (lipophilic) substances (which are difficult to excrete from cells because they tend to partition into cellular membranes) into more **hydrophilic** (polar) substances. This process involves the catalysis of covalent modifications to make the substance more charged, so that it will partition more readily into an aqueous medium or at least be solubilized sufficiently in bile. As a result of these processes, collectively termed biotransformations, some substances that would otherwise be retained in cellular membranes can be excreted directly in the urine or transported into the bile for excretion in feces.

C. Phases of Biotransformation

Biotransformation generally occurs in two phases. **Phase I reactions** involve oxidation reductions in which an oxygen-containing functional group is added to the substance to be excreted. While oxidation itself does not necessarily have a major effect on water solubility, it usually introduces into the drug a reactive "handle" that makes possible other reactions that do render the modified substance water soluble. These **phase II reactions** usually involve covalent attachment of the drug to a water-soluble carrier molecule, such as the sugar glucuronic acid or the peptide glutathione. Unfortunately, by making substances more chemically reactive, phase I oxidation reactions often convert mildly toxic drugs into more toxic reactive intermediates. If conjugation by phase II enzymes is impaired for some other reason, the reactive intermediate can sometimes react with and damage other cellular structures. This feature of drug detoxification has important clinical implications.

D. The Role of Apolipoprotein in the Solubilization and Transport of Lipids

The detoxification and bile transport pathways allow hepatocytes to convert a wide range of hydrophobic low-molecular-weight substances (eg, drugs and bilirubin) into more hydrophilic and hence water-soluble forms in which they can be excreted (eg, in bile or by the kidney). However, these are not the only solubilization challenges facing the body. The body also needs a mechanism that makes lipids available to various tissues (eg, to synthesize membranes) and one that removes any excess lipid the tissues do not use. For these processes to occur, lipid must be solubilized in a dispersed form that can be carried through the bloodstream. For this purpose, hepatocytes synthesize a class of specialized **apolipoproteins**. Apolipoproteins assemble into a variety of lipoprotein particles that transport lipids to and from various tissues by receptor-mediated endocytosis (see prior discussion of lipid metabolism).

E. The Liver's Role in Producing Binding Proteins

Various cells in the liver synthesize proteins that bind certain substances very tightly (eg, some vitamins, minerals, and hormones). In some cases, this allows their transport in the bloodstream, where they would otherwise not be soluble (eg, steroids bound to steroid-binding globulin, which is synthesized and secreted by hepatocytes). In other cases, binding proteins made by the liver (eg, thyroid hormone–binding globulin) allow transport of specific substances (eg, thyroxine) in a form not fully accessible to tissues. In this way, the effective concentration of the substance is limited to its free concentration at equilibrium, and the tightly bound fraction forms a reservoir of the substance that is made available slowly as the free fraction is metabolized, thereby prolonging its half-life.

In some cases, binding proteins allow the liver to accumulate specific substances in relatively high concentrations and store them in a nontoxic form. Consider iron, for example, an essential nutrient. Free iron can be quite toxic to cells both directly as an oxidant and indirectly as an essential nutrient needed by infectious agents. Control of body iron occurs at the level of the enterocyte in the duodenum (see Chapter 13). Thus, the primary defect in the iron overload disorder hemochromatosis probably involves the enterocyte. Nevertheless, the liver is responsible for making a variety of proteins crucial for iron binding and metabolism. Through the actions of these proteins, the body gets the iron it needs without allowing excess free iron to cause damage or support pathogens.

Transferrin is an iron-binding protein synthesized and secreted into the bloodstream by the liver. On binding of free iron at normal pH, transferrin undergoes a conformational change that gives it high affinity for a specific membrane receptor of the hepatocyte (**transferrin receptor**). On receptor binding, the transferrin–transferrin receptor complex is internalized into the endocytic pathway, a progressively more acidic environment. There, at low pH, iron no longer remains bound to transferrin. However, conformational changes that occur at low pH allow transferrin to maintain high-affinity binding to its receptor even in the absence of bound iron. Thus, when the receptor recycles back to the surface, it brings the "empty" transferrin with it. On presentation to the pH 7.4 environment of the bloodstream, transferrin lacking bound iron is released from the receptor, and the cycle can start over again. In this way, transferrin and its receptor keep the bloodstream free of unbound iron. Meanwhile, the free iron released from transferrin in the acidic environment of the endosome is transported into the cytoplasm of the hepatocyte, where it binds to **ferritin**, a cytoplasmic iron storage protein. This provides a reservoir that can be mobilized in response to the body's needs but makes iron inaccessible to pathogens and keeps it from causing direct toxic effects. Similar dynamics of plasma-binding proteins, receptors, or cytosolic storage proteins occur for many other substances, including fat-soluble vitamins and steroid hormones.

Whereas most solubilization functions are performed in hepatocytes, some of the binding and storage functions involve accessory cells. Thus, vitamin A storage occurs in fat droplets seen in the **lipocytes** of the reticuloendothelial system. Lipocytes have been implicated in the pathogenesis of chronic liver injury and cirrhosis. Injury to other cells releases cytokines, which activate the lipocytes. The lipocytes respond by proliferating and by synthesizing collagen and other basement membrane components, leading to an increase in the extracellular matrix and contributing to hepatic fibrosis.

Protective & Clearance Functions

Many of the functions of the liver already discussed (eg, drug detoxification and excretion of excess cholesterol by conversion to and solubilization in bile) can also be considered protective. Nevertheless, it is useful to conceptualize the protective function as a separate category because of its clinical importance in ameliorating the consequences of liver disease.

A. Phagocytic and Endocytic Functions of Kupffer Cells

The liver helps remove bacteria and antigens that breach the defenses of the gut to enter the portal blood and also participates in clearing the circulation of endogenously generated cellular debris. It appears that specialized receptors on the Kupffer cell surface bind to glycoproteins (via carbohydrate receptors), to material coated with immunoglobulin (via the Fc receptor), or to complement (via the C3 receptor), thus allowing damaged plasma proteins, activated clotting factors, immune complexes, senescent blood cells, and so on to be recognized and removed.

B. Endocytic Functions of Hepatocytes

Hepatocytes have a number of specific receptors for damaged plasma proteins distinct from the receptors present on Kupffer cells (eg, the asialoglycoprotein receptor that specifically binds glycoproteins whose terminal sialic acid sugar residues have been removed). The precise physiologic significance of this metabolic action remains unclear.

C. Ammonia Metabolism

Ammonia generated from the deamination of amino acids is metabolized within hepatocytes into the much less toxic substance urea. Loss of this function results in altered mental status, a common manifestation of severe or end-stage liver disease.

D. Hepatocyte Synthesis of Glutathione

Glutathione is the major intracellular (cytoplasmic) reducing reagent and thus is crucial for preventing oxidative damage to cellular proteins. This molecule is a nonribosomally synthesized tripeptide (γ-glutamyl-cystinyl-glycine) that is also a substrate for many phase II drug detoxification conjugation reactions. The liver may also export glutathione for use by other tissues.

Some additional indirect liver functions (eg, its role in maintaining normal sodium and water balance) are inferred from the derangements observed in patients with liver disease, as discussed in the following section.

Tests to Assess Liver Function

A number of blood tests are commonly used to assess liver injury. Serum aspartate aminotransferase (AST) and alanine aminotransferase (ALT) are measurements of levels of enzymes normally situated within hepatocytes. Their presence in the serum is thus actually a sign of liver cell necrosis rather than an indication of liver function.

To assess liver function more directly, a number of other tests can be used. The levels of albumin, clotting factors, and bilirubin can be measured in blood samples. Each of these tests has advantages and disadvantages, and no one of them serves as an ideal sole indicator of liver function. For example, albumin has a relatively long half-life (18–20 days); its synthesis can be stimulated in excess of need, and it can be lost via the kidneys in renal disease. Furthermore, about two-thirds of body albumin is located in the extravascular, extracellular space, so changes in fluid distribution can alter serum albumin concentration. Likewise, the simplest measure of clotting factor levels, the prothrombin time (PT), is a relatively insensitive measure because it does not become abnormal until more than 80% of hepatic synthetic capacity is lost. Furthermore, vitamin K deficiency, occurring in patients with nutritional deprivation, chronic cholestasis, or fat malabsorption, can prolong the PT. Serum bilirubin is a good measure of cholestasis, and determining conjugated (direct) versus unconjugated (indirect) bilirubin provides a good assessment of whether cholestasis is intrinsic to the liver or due solely to obstruction (eg, by a stone in the common bile duct). Furthermore, cholestasis, even when caused by liver disease, often does not reflect the degree to which other hepatic functions are lost, and unconjugated hyperbilirubinemia can occur for other reasons (eg, hemolysis).

For these reasons, an accurate assessment of liver function requires several blood tests (eg, AST, ALT, albumin, PT, bilirubin), as well as a clinical assessment of the patient.

The two most common schemes for grading liver function are the modified Child–Pugh score (Table 14–3) and the Model for End-Stage Liver Disease (MELD) score (MELD score = 3.78[Ln serum bilirubin (mg/dL)] + 11.2[Ln INR] + 9.57[Ln serum creatinine (mg/dL)] + 6.43). The Child–Pugh score predicts 1- and 2-year survival, whereas the MELD score predicts short-term (3-month) survival. In the United States, the MELD score is currently used to prioritize patients for donor allocation and liver transplantation. However, the patient's serum sodium has been found to predict waitlist mortality independent of the MELD score, and its incorporation into the MELD score to generate the MELD-Na score has been shown to improve its accuracy with respect to predicting waitlist mortality (MELD-Na = MELD + 1.32 × (137-Na) − [0.033 ×

TABLE 14–3 Grading liver function using the modified Child–Pugh score.

Parameter	Points		
	1	2	3
Ascites	None	Slight	Moderate to severe
Encephalopathy	None	Slight to moderate	Moderate to severe
Bilirubin	<2.0 mg/dL	2.0–3.0 mg/dL	>3.0 mg/dL
Albumin	>3.5 g/dL	2.8–3.5 g/dL	<2.8 g/dL
Prothrombin time prolongation	1–3 s	4–6 s	>6.0 s

Modified Child–Pugh classification of the severity of liver disease according to the degree of ascites, the degree of encephalopathy, the plasma concentrations of serum bilirubin and albumin, and the prothrombin time. A total score of 5–6 is considered grade A (well-compensated disease); a score of 7–9 is grade B (significant functional compromise); and a score of 10–15 is grade C (decompensated disease). These grades correlate with 1- and 2-year patient survival: grade A, 100–85%; grade B, 80–60%; and grade C, 45–35%.

Reproduced, with permission, from Papadaakis MA et al, eds. *Current Medical Diagnosis & Treatment*, 57th ed. McGraw-Hill, 2018.

MELD × (137-Na)]). Accordingly, to improve the allocation of donor livers in the United States, the Organ Procurement and Transplantation Network has changed its policy to adopt the newer MELD-Na score instead of the older MELD score for determining priority for liver transplantation.

CHECKPOINT

12. What are the roles of the liver in carbohydrate, protein, and lipid metabolism?

13. What are two physiologic mechanisms by which the body transports cholesterol?

14. Explain phase I and phase II reactions in drug detoxification.

15. Name and explain four of the liver's clearance or protective functions.

16. What specializations allow the liver normally to be a low-pressure conduit for blood flow?

OVERVIEW OF LIVER DISEASE

TYPES OF LIVER DYSFUNCTION

Most of the clinical consequences of liver disease can be understood either as a failure of one of the liver's four broad functions (summarized in Table 14–2) or as a consequence of portal hypertension, the altered hepatic blood flow of cirrhosis.

Hepatocyte Dysfunction

One mechanism of liver disease, particularly in acute liver injury, is dysfunction of the individual hepatocytes that make up the liver parenchyma. The pathway and extent of hepatocellular dysfunction determine the specific manifestations of liver disease. The outcomes to anticipate when normal hepatic functions fail are described later.

Portal Hypertension

Some consequences of liver disease, particularly of cirrhosis, are best understood in terms of what we know about hepatic blood flow. Of greatest clinical importance are the existence under normal circumstances of a low-pressure portal venous capillary bed throughout the liver parenchyma and the functional zonation of portal blood flow.

When pathologic processes (eg, fibrosis) result in an elevation of the normally low intrahepatic venous pressure, blood backs up and a substantial fraction of it finds alternative routes back to the systemic circulation, bypassing the liver. Thus, blood from the GI tract is, in effect, filtered less efficiently by the liver before entering the systemic circulation. The consequences of this portal-to-systemic shunting are loss of the protective and clearance functions of the liver, functional abnormalities in renal salt and water homeostasis, and a greatly increased risk of GI hemorrhage from the development of engorged blood vessels carrying venous blood bypassing the liver (eg, **esophageal**, **gastric**, and **umbilical varices**).

Even in the absence of any intrinsic parenchymal liver disease, portal-to-systemic blood shunting can produce or contribute to **encephalopathy** (altered mental status resulting from failure to clear poisons absorbed from the GI tract), GI bleeding (resulting from esophageal varices), and the malabsorption of fats and fat-soluble vitamins (caused by the loss of the enterohepatic recirculation of bile), with associated coagulopathy. Table 14–4 categorizes the syndromes observed in liver disease as being a consequence of hepatocyte dysfunction, portal-to-systemic shunting, or both.

Pathophysiology of Functional Zonation

The fact that hepatocytes in the different zones of the acinus "see" blood in a particular sequence has great pathophysiologic significance. Because zone 1 hepatocytes receive blood that has just left the portal venule or hepatic arteriole, they have access to the highest concentrations of various substances, both good (eg, oxygen, nutrients) and bad (eg, drugs and toxins absorbed from the GI tract). Zone 2 hepatocytes receive blood containing less of these substances, and zone 3 hepatocytes are bathed in blood largely depleted of them. However, zone 3 hepatocytes see the highest concentrations of products (eg, drug metabolites) released into the bloodstream by the hepatocytes of zones 1 and 2. Thus, direct poisons have their most severe impact on zone 1 hepatocytes, whereas poisons generated as a result of hepatic metabolism cause more damage to zone 3 hepatocytes. Similarly, because sinusoidal blood around zone 3 has the lowest oxygen concentration, hepatocytes of this zone are at the greatest risk of injury under conditions of hypoxia.

TABLE 14–4 Pathophysiology of syndromes of aberrant function in liver disease.

Syndrome of Aberrant Function in Liver Disease	Hepatocellular Dysfunction	Portal-to-Systemic Shunting
Energy metabolism and substrate conversion		
Alcoholic hypoglycemia	✓	
Alcoholic ketoacidosis	✓	
Hyperglycemia		✓
Familial hypercholesterolemia	✓	
Hepatic encephalopathy	✓	✓
Fatty liver	✓	
Solubilization, transport, and storage function		
Drug reactions	✓	
Drug sensitivity	✓	✓
Steatorrhea	✓	✓
Fat-soluble vitamin deficiency	✓	✓
Coagulopathy	✓	✓
Protein synthetic function		
Edema due to hypoalbuminemia	✓	
Protective and clearance functions		
Hypergammaglobulinemia		✓
Hypogonadism and hyperestrogenism	✓	✓
Renal dysfunction		
Sodium retention		✓
Impaired water excretion		✓
Impaired renal concentrating ability		✓
Deranged potassium metabolism		✓
Prerenal azotemia		✓
Acute kidney injury		✓
Glomerulopathies		✓
Impaired renal acidification		✓
Hepatorenal syndrome		✓
Pulmonary complications		
Hepatic hydrothorax		✓
Hepatopulmonary syndrome		✓
Portopulmonary hypertension		✓

MANIFESTATIONS OF LIVER DYSFUNCTION

Whether as a result of hepatocyte dysfunction or portal-to-systemic shunting, failure of normal hepatic function underlies the clinical manifestations of liver disease. An understanding of these mechanisms offers insight into the probable causes of illness in a patient with acute or chronic liver disease.

Diminished Energy Generation & Substrate Interconversion

A first category of altered liver function involves the intermediary metabolism of carbohydrates, fats, and proteins.

A. Carbohydrate Metabolism

Severe liver disease can result in either hypoglycemia or hyperglycemia. Hypoglycemia results largely from a decrease in functional hepatocyte mass, whereas hyperglycemia is a result of portal-to-systemic shunting, which decreases the efficiency of postprandial glucose extraction from portal blood by hepatocytes, thus elevating the systemic blood glucose concentration.

B. Lipid Metabolism

Disturbance of lipid metabolism in the liver can result in syndromes of fat accumulation within the liver early in the course of liver injury. Perhaps this is because the complex steps involved in assembling lipoprotein particles for the export of cholesterol and triglycerides from the liver are more sensitive to disruption than are the pathways of lipid synthesis. Such disruption results in a buildup of fat that cannot be exported in the form of VLDL.

In certain chronic liver diseases such as primary biliary cirrhosis, bile flow decreases as a result of the destruction of bile ducts. The decrease in bile flow results in decreased lipid clearance via bile, with consequent hyperlipidemia. These patients often develop subcutaneous accumulations of cholesterol termed **xanthomas**.

C. Protein Metabolism

Any disturbance of protein metabolism in the liver can result in a syndrome of altered mental status and confusion known as **hepatic encephalopathy**. As with carbohydrate metabolism, altered protein metabolism can result from either hepatocyte failure or portal-to-systemic shunting, with the net effect of elevated blood concentrations of centrally acting toxins, including ammonia generated by amino acid metabolism.

Loss of Solubilization & Storage Functions

A. Disordered Bile Secretion

The clinical significance of bile synthesis can be seen in the prominence of cholestasis—failure to secrete bile—in many forms of liver disease. Cholestasis can occur as a result of extrahepatic obstruction (eg, from a gallstone in the common bile duct) or selective dysfunction of the bile synthetic and secretory machinery within the hepatocytes themselves (eg, from a reaction to certain drugs). The mechanisms responsible for cholestatic drug reactions are not well understood. Regardless of the mechanism, however, the clinical consequences of severe cholestasis may be profound: A failure to secrete bile results in a failure to solubilize substances such as dietary lipids and fat-soluble vitamins, resulting in **malabsorption** and **deficiency** states, respectively. Retained bile salts are also cytotoxic, but in the setting of cholestasis, hepatocytes adapt to the decrease in bile salt uptake by downregulating Na$^+$–bile acid cotransporter while maintaining bile salt excretion. As a result, hepatic necrosis is minimized in predominantly cholestatic syndromes, with the typical laboratory findings of minimally elevated levels of AST and ALT in the presence of marked jaundice and high levels of bilirubin. However, prolonged exposure to bile salts in chronic cholestatic diseases, such as primary biliary cirrhosis, leads to portal tract cytotoxic injury and inflammation, leading eventually to fibrosis and cirrhosis.

The solubilization function of bile works both to excrete and absorb substances. Thus, in cholestasis, endogenous substances normally excreted via the biliary tract can accumulate to high levels. One such substance is bilirubin, a product of heme degradation (Figure 14–7). The buildup of bilirubin results in **jaundice** (**icterus**), which is a yellow discoloration of the sclera and skin. In the adult, the most significant feature of jaundice is that it serves as a readily monitored index of cholestasis, which may occur alone or with other abnormalities in hepatocyte function (ie, as part of the presentation of acute hepatitis). In the neonate, however, elevated bilirubin concentrations can be toxic to the developing nervous system, producing a syndrome termed **kernicterus**.

Similarly, cholesterol is normally excreted either by conversion into bile acids or by forming complexes, termed micelles, with pre-existing (recycled) bile acids. In cholestasis, the resultant buildup of bile acids can lead to their deposition in the skin. This is believed to cause intense itching, or **pruritus**. Data suggest that, in at least some patients, cholestasis results in altered levels of endogenous opioids. Instead of skin deposition of bile acids, altered endogenous opioid-mediated neurotransmission may be responsible for pruritus. Disorders of bile production are a basis for the formation of cholesterol gallstones. Nevertheless, as mentioned, other hepatocyte functions are often relatively well preserved in the face of significant cholestasis. Table 14–5 summarizes the syndromes that produce jaundice.

Hemolysis causes an unconjugated hyperbilirubinemia because the hepatic capacity to take up and conjugate bilirubin is exceeded. Gilbert syndrome reflects a genetic defect in bilirubin conjugation. Thus, the findings in blood and urine are different from what is observed in hemolytic jaundice even though the pathway of bilirubin metabolism is backed up at a similar initial point. Extrahepatic biliary tract

FIGURE 14–7 Bilirubin secretion. This water-insoluble compound is derived from the metabolism of hemoglobin in macrophages of the mononuclear phagocyte system. Glucuronyl transferase activity in the hepatocytes causes bilirubin to be conjugated with glucuronide in the smooth endoplasmic reticulum, forming a water-soluble compound. An accumulation of bilirubin and bilirubin glucuronide in the tissues produces jaundice. Several defective processes in the hepatocytes can cause diseases that produce jaundice: a defect in the capacity of the cell to trap and absorb bilirubin (rectangle 1), the inability of the cell to conjugate bilirubin because of a deficiency in glucuronyl transferase (rectangle 2), or problems in the transfer and excretion of bilirubin glucuronide into the biliary canaliculi (rectangle 3). One of the most frequent causes of jaundice, however—unrelated to hepatocyte activity—is the obstruction of bile flow as a result of gallstones or tumors of the pancreas. This causes jaundice primarily as a result of the accumulation of bilirubin glucuronide in the tissues. (Redrawn, with permission, from Junqueira LC et al, eds. *Basic Histology*, 10th ed. McGraw-Hill, 2003.)

obstruction presents the other extreme, in which the actual pathway of bile formation is entirely intact, at least initially. In obstruction, the bilirubin level in the urine is high because the backed-up metabolite is conjugated and hence much more water soluble than unconjugated bilirubin, which accumulates in hemolysis. Most forms of jaundice that result from liver dysfunction caused by hepatocellular damage reflect variable degrees of overlap between unconjugated and conjugated hyperbilirubinemia.

B. Impaired Drug Detoxification

Two features of the mechanisms of drug detoxification are of particular clinical importance. One is the phenomenon of **enzyme induction**. It is observed that the presence in the bloodstream of any of the large class of drugs inactivated by phase I enzymes increases the amount and activity of these enzymes in the liver. This property of enzyme induction makes physiologic sense (as a response to the body's need for increased biotransformation) but can have undesired effects as well: A patient who chronically consumes large amounts of a substance metabolized by phase I enzymes (eg, ethanol) will induce the formation of these enzymes and thus speed up the metabolism of other substances metabolized by the same detoxifying enzymes (eg, antiseizure or anticoagulant medications, resulting in subtherapeutic blood levels of the drugs).

A second clinically important phenomenon in drug metabolism is that phase I reactions often convert relatively benign compounds into more reactive and hence more toxic ones. Normally, this heightened reactivity of phase I reaction products serves to facilitate phase II reactions, making detoxification more efficient. However, under certain conditions in which phase II reactions are impaired (eg, during glutathione deficiency from inadequate nutrition), continued phase I enzyme activity can cause increased liver injury. This is

TABLE 14–5   Laboratory findings in the differential diagnosis of jaundice.

Type of Jaundice	Blood Tests					
	Hct	Unconjugated Bilirubin (Indirect)	Conjugated Bilirubin (Direct)	Alkaline Phosphatase	Aminotransferases	Cholesterol
Hemolytic	↓	↑	N	N	N	N
Hepatocellular						
Gilbert syndrome	N	↑	N	N	N	N
Abnormal conjugation	N	↑↑	N	N	N	N
Hepatocellular damage	N	↑	↑	N or ↑	↑↑	N
Obstructive						
Defective excretion	N	N	N	N	N	N
Intrahepatic cholestasis	N	N	↑	N	N	N or ↑
Extrahepatic biliary obstruction	N	N	↑↑	↑↑	N or ↑	↑

N, normal; ↑, increased compared with normal; ↓, decreased compared with normal.

Data obtained from Sanyal AJ et al, eds. *Zakim and Boyer's Hepatology: A Textbook of Liver Disease*, 7th ed. Elsevier, 2017.

because the products of many phase I reactions, in the absence of glutathione, react with and damage cellular components. Such damage rapidly kills the hepatocytes.

Thus, the combined effects of certain common conditions can make the individual abnormally sensitive to the toxic effects of drugs. For example, the combination of induced phase I activity (eg, caused by alcoholism) with low phase II activity (eg, caused by low glutathione levels from nutritional deprivation) can result in the heightened generation of reactive intermediates with an inadequate capacity to conjugate and detoxify them. A classic example of this phenomenon is acetaminophen toxicity. As little as 2.5 g of acetaminophen can produce significant liver damage in such susceptible individuals, whereas normal individuals have the capacity to detoxify 10 g/d or more. Table 14–6 lists common drugs and chemicals that cause morphologically distinctive changes in the liver.

C. Lipoprotein Dynamics and Dyslipidemias

The liver's role in lipid metabolism is illustrated by the genetic defect causing familial hypercholesterolemia. Lack of a functional LDL receptor in such cases renders the liver unable to clear LDL cholesterol from the bloodstream, resulting in markedly elevated serum cholesterol and accelerated atherosclerosis and coronary artery disease. Heterozygotes with one normal LDL receptor allele can be treated with drugs (eg, HMG-CoA reductase inhibitors) that inhibit endogenous cholesterol synthesis and thus upregulate LDL receptor levels. However, there is no effective drug therapy for homozygotes because they have no normal LDL receptors. Hepatic transplantation is an effective therapy for homozygous familial hypercholesterolemia because it provides a genetically different liver with normal LDL receptors.

In acquired liver diseases, the serum cholesterol is elevated in biliary tract obstruction as a result of a blockage of cholesterol excretion in bile, and it is diminished in severe alcoholic cirrhosis, in which fat malabsorption prevents cholesterol intake.

D. Altered Hepatic Binding and Storage Functions

Liver disease influences the liver's ability to store various substances. As a result, patients with liver disease are at high risk for certain deficiency states such as folic acid and vitamin B_{12} deficiency. Because these vitamins are needed for DNA synthesis, their deficiency results in **macrocytic anemia** (low red blood cell count with large red cells reflecting abnormal nuclear maturation), a common finding in patients with liver disease.

Diminished Synthesis & Secretion of Plasma Proteins

The clinical significance of liver protein synthesis and secretion derives from the wide range of functions carried out by these proteins. For example, because albumin is the major contributor to plasma oncotic pressure, hypoalbuminemia as a consequence of liver disease or nutritional deficiency presents with marked edema formation. Other important proteins synthesized and secreted by the liver include clotting factors and hormone-binding proteins.

Loss of Protective & Clearance Functions

A crucial protective function of the liver is its role as a filter of blood from the GI tract, by which various substances are

TABLE 14–6   Principal alterations of hepatic morphology produced by some commonly used drugs and chemicals.[1]

Principal Morphologic Change	Class of Agent	Example
Cholestasis	Anabolic steroid	Methyltestosterone
	Antibiotic	Erythromycin estolate, nitrofurantoin, rifampin, amoxicillin-clavulanic acid, oxacillin
	Anticonvulsant	Carbamazepine
	Antidepressant	Duloxetine, mirtazapine, tricyclic antidepressants
	Anti-inflammatory	Sulindac
	Antiplatelet	Clopidogrel
	Antihypertensive	Irbesartan, fosinopril
	Antithyroid	Methimazole
	Calcium channel blocker	Nifedipine, verapamil
	Immunosuppressive	Cyclosporine
	Lipid-lowering	Ezetimibe
	Onco-therapeutic	Anabolic steroids, busulfan, tamoxifen, irinotecan, cytarabine, temozolomide
	Oral contraceptive	Norethynodrel with mestranol
	Oral hypoglycemic	Chlorpropamide
	Tranquilizer	Chlorpromazine[2]
Fatty liver	Antiarrhythmic	Amiodarone
	Antibiotic	Tetracycline (high-dose, intravenous)
	Anticonvulsant	Valproic acid
	Antiretroviral	Dideoxynucleosides (zidovudine), protease inhibitors (indinavir, ritonavir)
	Onco-therapeutic	Asparaginase, methotrexate, tamoxifen
Hepatitis	Anesthetic	Halothane
	Antiandrogen	Flutamide
	Antibiotic	Isoniazid,[3] rifampin, nitrofurantoin, telithromycin, minocycline,[4] pyrazinamide, trovafloxcin[5]
	Anticonvulsant	Phenytoin, carbamazepine, valproic acid, phenobarbital
	Antidepressant	Amitriptyline, trazodone, venlafaxine, fluoxetine, paroxetine, duloxetine, sertraline, nefazodone[5]
	Antifungal	Ketoconazole, fluconazole, itraconazole
	Antihypertensive	Methyldopa,[3] captopril, enalapril, lisinopril, losartan
	Anti-inflammatory	Ibuprofen, indomethacin, diclofenac, sulindac, bromfenac
	Antipsychotic	Risperidone
	Antiretroviral	Zidovudine, didanosine, stavudine, nevirapine, ritonavir, indinavir, tipranavir, zalcitabine
	Calcium channel blocker	Nifedipine, verapamil, diltiazem
	Cholinesterase inhibitor	Tacrine
	Diuretic	Chlorothiazide
	Laxative	Oxyphenisatin
	Norepinephrine reuptake inhibitor	Atomoxetine
	Oral hypoglycemic	Acarbose, troglitazone[5]

(continued)

TABLE 14–6 Principal alterations of hepatic morphology produced by some commonly used drugs and chemicals.[1] (Continued)

Principal Morphologic Change	Class of Agent	Example
Mixed hepatic/cholestatic	Antibiotic	Amoxicillin-clavulanic acid, trimethoprim-sulfamethoxazole
	Antibacterial	Clindamycin
	Antifungal	Terbinafine
	Antihistamine	Cyproheptadine
	Immunosuppressive	Azathioprine
	Lipid-lowering	Nicotinic acid, lovastatin, ezetimibe
Toxic (necrosis)	Analgesic	Acetaminophen
	Hydrocarbon	Carbon tetrachloride
	Metal	Yellow phosphorus
	Mushroom	*Amanita phalloides*
	Solvent	Dimethylformamide
Granulomas	Antiarrhythmic	Quinidine, diltiazem
	Antibiotic	Sulfonamides
	Anticonvulsant	Carbamazepine
	Anti-inflammatory	Phenylbutazone
	Xanthine oxidase inhibitor	Allopurinol
Vascular injury	Chemotherapeutic	Oxaliplatin, melphalan

[1]Several agents cause more than one type of liver lesion and appear in more than one category.

[2]Rarely associated with primary biliary cirrhosis-like lesion.

[3]Occasionally associated with chronic hepatitis or bridging hepatic necrosis or cirrhosis.

[4]Associated with an autoimmune hepatitis-like syndrome.

[5]Withdrawn from use because of severe hepatotoxicity.

Reproduced, with permission, from Lee WM. Toxic and drug-induced hepatitis. In: Kasper D et al, eds. *Harrison's Principles of Internal Medicine*, 19th ed. McGraw-Hill, 2015.

removed from portal blood before it re-enters the systemic circulation.

A. Clearance of Bacteria and Endotoxins

The clearance of bacteria by the liver's Kupffer cells is the final line of defense in keeping gut-derived bacteria and their endotoxins out of the systemic circulation. Loss of this capacity in liver disease as a result of portal-to-systemic shunting may help to explain why, in patients with severe liver disease, infections can rapidly become systemic and result in sepsis and the effects of endotoxins.

B. Altered Metabolism of Ammonia

Impairment of the liver's ability to detoxify ammonia to urea leads to hepatic encephalopathy that manifests as an altered mental status. While several overlapping mechanisms have been implicated in the pathogenesis of hepatic encephalopathy, ammonia is the most well-characterized neurotoxin that precipitates encephalopathy. Ammonia is primarily produced from deamination of glutamine by glutaminase in the enterocytes of the small bowel and colon but is also produced from urea hydrolysis via the bacterial catabolism of nitrogenous sources, including dietary protein and urea. The intact liver clears nearly all the ammonia that arrives via the portal vein by converting it to glutamine, which prevents ammonia from entering into the systemic circulation. Increased ammonia in the bloodstream can be the direct consequence of impaired liver function (either acute hepatocellular dysfunction or progressive chronic disease) and/or significant shunting of blood around the liver (portal-to-systemic shunting) with consequent bypass of its clearance mechanisms.

Precipitants of increased ammonia levels in the bloodstream and consequent altered mental status include the following: (1) increased protein intake (urea hydrolysis via bacterial catabolism of nitrogenous sources); (2) GI bleeding (increased levels of ammonia and other nitrogenous substances are produced by the breakdown of blood proteins by GI tract microbes); and (3) the systemic inflammatory response to infection (stimulation of proinflammatory cytokine release and endogenous protein catabolism, leading to elevated ammonia production). Thus, once increased protein intake has been excluded, the development of encephalopathy in a patient with chronic liver disease calls for an investigation of possible acute GI bleeding, as well as a search for a potentially catastrophic infection. Pending the outcome of diagnostic studies (eg, serial hemoglobin and hematocrit measurements and cultures of blood, urine, and ascitic fluid), therapy is aimed at diminishing the absorption of ammonia and other noxious substances from the GI tract. When the patient is given the nonabsorbable carbohydrate **lactulose**, its metabolism by microbes creates an acidic environment. Ammonia is trapped as charged NH_4^+ species in the gut lumen and excreted by the resultant osmotic diarrhea. In this way, the toxin is prevented from ever entering the portal circulation, and the patient's mental status gradually improves. Lactulose also selects for a gut bacterial flora that produces less ammonia. Antibiotics, and in particular rifaximin, have been used in conjunction with lactulose to treat hepatic encephalopathy. Antibiotics are thought to act by decreasing the intestinal production and absorption of ammonia by modulating the intestinal microbiota and preventing bacterial translocation across the gut mucosal surface.

Furthermore, the resulting elevations in blood ammonia and other nitrogen-containing compounds can upregulate peripheral receptors for endogenous benzodiazepine-like products. These effects may also contribute to altered systemic hemodynamics in liver disease.

C. Altered Hormone Clearance in Liver Disease

Normally, the liver removes from the bloodstream the fraction of steroid hormones not bound to steroid hormone–binding globulin. On uptake by hepatocytes, these steroids are oxidized, conjugated, and excreted into bile, where a fraction undergoes enterohepatic circulation. In liver disease accompanied by significant portal-to-systemic shunting, steroid hormone clearance is diminished, extraction of the circulated enterohepatic fraction is impaired, and enzymatic conversion of androgens to estrogens (peripheral aromatization) is increased. The net effect is an elevation of blood estrogens, which in turn alters hepatocyte protein synthesis and secretion, together with the activation of the metabolizing P450 enzymes. The synthesis of some hepatic proteins increases, whereas the synthesis of others is diminished. Enzymatic P450 activity increases as the liver attempts to partially compensate for the higher blood estrogen levels by increased metabolism. Thus, male patients with liver disease display both gonadal and pituitary suppression as well as feminization.

Sodium & Water Balance

Patients with liver disease often display renal abnormalities and complications, most commonly sodium retention and difficulty excreting water. An intrinsic renal lesion is apparently not involved, because the kidneys of patients with liver

TABLE 14–7   Factors influencing renal sodium retention in liver disease.

Hemodynamic
Arterial (systemic and splanchnic vasodilation)
Alterations to intrarenal blood flow
Portal-to-systemic shunting
Hypoalbuminemia
Neurohumoral
Elevated renal endothelin production
Activation of renin–angiotensin system
Increased sympathetic nervous system activity
Elevated peripheral nitric oxide production
Diminished angiotensinogen synthesis by the liver
Diminished renin and angiotensin clearance by the liver
Altered kallikrein–kinin system

Data obtained from Kasper D et al, eds. *Harrison's Principles of Internal Medicine*, 19th ed. McGraw-Hill, 2015; and from Sanyal AJ et al, eds. *Zakim and Boyer's Hepatology: A Textbook of Liver Disease*, 7th ed. Elsevier, 2017.

disease typically function normally when transplanted into patients whose liver is normal. Instead, renal abnormalities associated with liver disease are functional, occurring because liver disease induces altered intravascular pressures and perhaps because of elevated nitric oxide levels or the loss of as yet poorly understood factors secreted from the liver or the endothelium. By whatever homeostatic mechanisms, intravascular volume is perceived as being inadequate when it is actually only maldistributed. Renal mechanisms of salt and water retention are then stimulated to correct what has been sensed as volume depletion. Table 14–7 summarizes some factors that influence renal sodium retention in liver disease. Patients with severe liver disease are at risk for renal failure related to these hemodynamic and neurohumoral alterations.

CHECKPOINT

17. Under what circumstances is hypoglycemia seen in liver disease?
18. Name three clinical consequences of cholestasis.
19. The development of hepatic encephalopathy in a patient with chronic liver disease should lead you to investigate what possible precipitating factors?
20. By what mechanisms can coagulation defects be a consequence of liver disease?
21. What is an explanation for hypogonadism in male patients with liver disease?

PATHOPHYSIOLOGY OF SELECTED LIVER DISEASES

ACUTE HEPATITIS

Acute hepatitis is an inflammatory process causing liver cell death either by necrosis or by triggering apoptosis (programmed cell death). A wide range of clinical entities can cause global hepatocyte injury of sudden onset. Worldwide, acute hepatitis is most commonly caused by infection with one of several types of virus. Although these viral agents can be distinguished by serologic laboratory tests based on their antigenic properties, all produce clinically similar illnesses. Other less common infectious agents can also cause liver injury (see Table 14–1). Acute hepatitis is also sometimes caused by exposure to drugs (eg, isoniazid) or poisons (eg, ethanol).

Clinical Presentation

The severity of illness in acute hepatitis ranges from asymptomatic and clinically unapparent to fulminant and potentially fatal. The clinical presentation of acute hepatitis can also be quite variable. Some patients are relatively asymptomatic, with abnormalities noted only by laboratory studies. Others may have a range of symptoms and signs, including anorexia, fatigue, weight loss, nausea, vomiting, right upper quadrant abdominal pain, jaundice, fever, splenomegaly, and ascites. The extent of hepatic dysfunction can also vary tremendously, correlating roughly with the severity of liver injury. The relative extent of cholestasis versus hepatocyte necrosis is also highly variable. Figure 14–8 illustrates the potential interrelationship of acute hepatitis, chronic hepatitis, and cirrhosis.

Etiology

A. Acute Viral Hepatitis

Acute viral hepatitis is commonly caused by one of five major viruses: hepatitis A virus (HAV), hepatitis B virus (HBV), hepatitis C virus (HCV), hepatitis D virus (HDV), and hepatitis E virus (HEV). Table 14–8 summarizes important characteristics of these viral agents. Other viral agents that can cause acute hepatitis, though less commonly, include the Epstein–Barr virus (cause of infectious mononucleosis), cytomegalovirus, varicella virus, measles virus, herpes simplex virus, rubella virus, and yellow fever virus. A newly discovered DNA virus, SEN virus, may be associated with transfusion-associated acute hepatitis not attributable to other viruses.

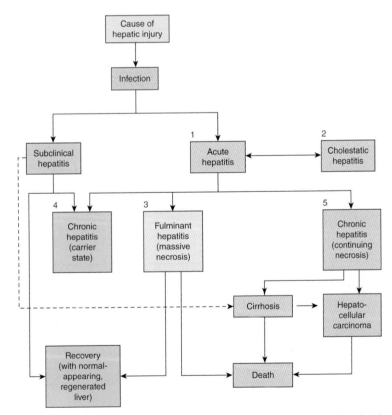

FIGURE 14–8 Clinical syndromes associated with hepatitis: acute hepatitis (1) is sometimes associated with intrahepatic cholestasis (and thus termed "cholestatic hepatitis") (2). Fulminant hepatitis (3) is associated with massive necrosis and has a high mortality rate. Chronic viral hepatitis may lead to a carrier state without (4) or with (5) continuing hepatocyte necrosis. Chronic hepatitis associated with continuing necrosis often progresses to cirrhosis, whereas chronic hepatitis associated simply with a carrier state does not. (Redrawn, with permission, from Chandrasoma P et al, eds. *Concise Pathology*, 3rd ed. Originally published by Appleton & Lange. Copyright © 1998 by The McGraw-Hill Companies, Inc.)

TABLE 14-8   **Characteristics of various types of viral hepatitis.**

	Hepatitis A	Hepatitis B	Hepatitis C	Hepatitis D	Hepatitis E
Clinical presentation					
Onset	Abrupt	Insidious	Insidious	Insidious	Abrupt
Incubation period					
Range (days)	15–50	28–160	14–160	30–180	15–60
Mean (days)	30	80	50		40
Symptoms					
Arthralgia, rash	Uncommon	Common	Uncommon	Uncommon	Common
Fever	Uncommon	Uncommon	Uncommon	Common	Common
Nausea, vomiting	Common	Common	Common	Common	Common
Jaundice	Uncommon in children	Less common than hepatitis A	Uncommon	Common	Common
Laboratory data					
Duration of enzyme elevation	Short	Prolonged	Prolonged	Like hepatitis B	Short
Virus type	RNA	DNA	RNA	RNA	RNA
Family	Picornavirus	Hepadnavirus	Flavivirus	Delta Viridae	Caliciviridae
Serologic tests					
Antigen	Yes	Yes	No	No	Yes
Antibody	Yes	Yes	Yes	Yes	Yes
Outcome					
Severity of acute disease	Mild	Moderate	Mild	Can be severe	Severe in pregnant woman
Mortality rate	Low (<0.5%)	Low (<0.5%)	Low	High (5%)	Moderate to high (0.2–1% in general population but as high as 15–20% in pregnant women)
Chronic hepatitis	No	Yes	Yes	Yes	Yes, but almost exclusively among immunocompromised persons
Associated with malignancy	No	Yes	Yes	Yes	No
Transmission					
Oral	+	±	–	–	+
Percutaneous	Rare	+	+	+	+
Sexual	+	+	+	+	–
Perinatal	–	+	+	Rare	+
Vaccine	Yes	Yes	No	No (vaccinate against HBV)	Yes (but only in certain countries)

Data obtained from Sanyal AJ et al, eds. *Zakim and Boyer's Hepatology: A Textbook of Liver Disease*, 7th ed. Elsevier, 2017.

HAV, a small RNA virus, causes liver disease both by directly killing hepatocytes and by stimulating the host's immune response to infected hepatocytes. It is spread by the fecal–oral route from infected individuals. Although most cases are mild, hepatitis A occasionally causes fulminant liver failure and massive hepatocellular necrosis, resulting in death. Regardless of the severity, patients who recover do so completely, show no evidence of residual liver disease, and have antibodies that protect them from reinfection.

HBV is a DNA virus transmitted through sexual contact or contact with infected blood or other body fluids. Perinatal and early childhood transmission is the most common mode of HBV acquisition worldwide, whereas sexual transmission is most common among adults in the United States. This virus does not kill the cells it infects. Rather, the infected hepatocytes die almost exclusively as a consequence of attack by the immune system after recognition of viral antigens on the hepatocyte surface. Although most cases of hepatitis B infection are asymptomatic or produce only mild disease, an excessive immune response can result in acute liver injury and even liver failure. In a minority of those infected as adults but a majority of individuals infected at birth, the immune response is inadequate to clear the virus and chronic hepatitis B develops. The incidence of infection has significantly declined in the era of HBV vaccination, although prevalence remains high, in part because of the immigration of infected patients from endemic countries. Although the true burden of chronic hepatitis B infection in the United States is unknown, it is estimated that 1.25 million Americans are infected with HBV, with a likely higher prevalence among those who are foreign born. Indeed, data suggest that the number of foreign-born individuals with chronic HBV living in the United States may be greater than previously reported, and the actual prevalence of chronic HBV infection may be as high as 2.2 million persons. Additionally, complications of HBV-induced liver disease result in 3000–5000 deaths each year in the United States.

HCV is an RNA virus, also transmitted by blood and body fluids; it causes a form of hepatitis similar to HBV infection but with a far greater proportion of cases (60–85%) progressing to chronic hepatitis. Acute infection is characterized by mild to moderate illness but is usually asymptomatic. However, chronic HCV can lead to life-threatening complications, including cirrhosis and hepatocellular carcinoma (HCC), usually after decades of infection. It is estimated that between 2.7 and 3.9 million Americans are infected with HCV, many unaware of their infection, and the rate of attributable mortality is rising, currently at approximately 12,000 deaths each year. The Centers for Disease Control and Prevention (CDC) estimates that persons born during 1945–1965 account for approximately three-fourths of all HCV infections in the United States; this cohort thus represents a high-prevalence group that warrants universal screening. Based on joint guidelines from the American Association for the Study of Liver Diseases (AASLD) and the Infectious Diseases Society of America (IDSA), additional high-prevalence groups that warrant HCV screening include the following: (1) people with a history of high-risk behaviors, such as injection drug or intranasal drug use; (2) people exposed to risks, such as children born to HCV-infected women; (3) people who have been exposed to HCV-infected blood via long-term hemodialysis, tattoos, or needlestick or mucosal exposure; (4) people who received blood products or organ transplants prior to 1992; (5) people who received clotting factor concentrates prior to 1987; (6) people who have been incarcerated; (7) people with human immunodeficiency virus (HIV) infection; and (8) people with unexplained chronic hepatitis or liver disease.

HDV, also known as delta agent, is a defective RNA virus that requires HBV helper functions to cause infection. Thus, individuals chronically infected with HBV are at high risk for HDV infection, whereas those who have been vaccinated against HBV are at no risk. HDV infection occurs either as coinfection with HBV or superinfection in the setting of chronic HBV. HDV infection causes a much more severe form of hepatitis, both in terms of the proportion of fulminant cases of hepatitis B and in the percentage of cases that progress to chronic hepatitis B. In North America, HDV coinfection primarily occurs in high-risk groups, such as injection drug users and those with hemophilia, and in up to 9% of those high-risk patients who have chronic HBV infection. In the United States, the prevalence of HDV coinfection in the general HBV-infected population is not well known.

HEV is an unclassified RNA virus, and like HAV, it is spread primarily via the fecal–oral route. Worldwide, HEV causes approximately 20 million infections and 70,000 deaths annually. Epidemics and acute illnesses predominantly occur in areas of high endemicity, including Asia, Africa, and Mexico, where transmission is propagated by poor sanitation and hygienic practices. In industrialized countries, the incidence of HEV infections has increased over the past decade, with seroprevalence estimated to range between 6% and 26% in the United States, in part owing to travel to endemic areas, to close environmental contact with farm animals, and to consumption of contaminated produce, as well as to increasing clinical recognition. Acute HEV infection is generally benign and self-limited, but can progress to chronic hepatitis, especially in immunocompromised patients, including organ transplant recipients and HIV-infected individuals. Many (up to 70%) pregnant women infected with HEV during their third trimester progress to acute liver failure. Individuals with chronic liver disease are also at increased risk for hepatic decompensation and mortality upon acquiring acute HEV. HEV remains an under-recognized clinical entity because the laboratory test for HEV viral load is not routinely available in clinical practice. Indeed, it is suspected that many cases of acute HEV infection are misdiagnosed as cases of drug-induced liver injury.

B. Toxic Hepatitis

Most cases of drug-induced liver injury present as acute hepatitis, although some present as cholestasis or with other patterns (see Table 14–6). The incidence of drug-induced hepatitis has been rising. Although fewer than 10% of drug-induced liver injury cases progress to acute liver failure, acetaminophen is

TABLE 14–9   Idiosyncratic drug reactions and the affected cells.

Type of Reaction	Effect on Cells	Examples of Drugs
Hepatocellular	Direct effect or production by enzyme–drug adduct leads to cell dysfunction, membrane dysfunction, cytotoxic T-cell response	Isoniazid, trazodone, diclofenac, nefazodone, venlafaxine, lovastatin
Cholestasis	Injury to canalicular membrane and transporters	Chlorpromazine, estrogen, erythromycin and its derivatives
Immunoallergic	Enzyme–drug adducts on cell surface induce IgE response	Halothane, phenytoin, sulfamethoxazole
Granulomatous	Macrophages, lymphocytes infiltrate hepatic lobule	Diltiazem, sulfa drugs, quinidine
Microvesicular fat	Altered mitochondrial respiration, oxidation leads to lactic acidosis and triglyceride accumulation	Didanosine, tetracycline, acetylsalicylic acid, valproic acid
Steatohepatitis	Multifactorial	Amiodarone, tamoxifen
Autoimmune	Cytotoxic lymphocyte response directed at hepatocyte membrane components	Nitrofurantoin, methyldopa, lovastatin, minocycline
Fibrosis	Activates stellate cells	Methotrexate, excess vitamin A
Vascular collapse	Causes ischemic or hypoxic injury	Nicotinic acid, cocaine, methylene-dioxymethamphetamine
Oncogenesis	Encourages tumor formation	Oral contraceptives, androgens
Mixed	Cytoplasmic and canalicular injury, direct damage to bile ducts	Amoxicillin-clavulanate, carbamazepine, herbs, cyclosporine, methimazole, troglitazone

Modified and reproduced, with permission, from Lee WM. Drug-induced hepatotoxicity. N Engl J Med. 2003;349:474. Copyright © 2003 Massachusetts Medical Society. Reprinted, with permission, from Massachusetts Medical Society.

now the most common cause of acute liver failure in the United States and the United Kingdom. Hepatic toxins can be further subdivided into those for which hepatic toxicity is predictable and dose dependent for most individuals (eg, acetaminophen) and those that cause unpredictable (idiosyncratic) reactions without relationship to dose (Table 14–9).

C. Alcoholic Hepatitis

Alcohol consumption is the major cause of the burden of liver disease burden in Western countries. Alcoholic liver disease comprises a spectrum of injury, including simple steatosis, acute alcoholic hepatitis, and cirrhosis, and many patients with advanced liver disease present with "acute-on-chronic" liver injury as a result of ongoing alcohol consumption. Acute alcoholic hepatitis can vary in severity from mild and self-limited to severe and life-threatening. Alcoholic hepatitis is associated with female sex, prolonged heavy alcohol consumption, and binge drinking. There is considerable variation among individuals in the amount of ethanol required to cause acute liver injury; this reflects the complex interplay of genetic, nutritional, and environmental factors that contribute to alcoholic liver disease.

Pathogenesis

A. Viral Hepatitis

The viral agents responsible for acute hepatitis first infect the hepatocyte. During the incubation period, intense viral replication in the liver cell leads to the appearance of viral components (first antigens, later antibodies) in urine, stool, and body fluids. Liver cell death and an associated inflammatory response then ensue, followed by changes in laboratory tests of liver function and the appearance of various symptoms and signs of liver disease.

1. **Liver damage**—Host immunologic response plays an important though incompletely understood role in the pathogenesis of liver damage. In hepatitis B, for example, the virus is probably not directly cytopathic. Indeed, there are asymptomatic HBV carriers who have normal liver function and histologic features. Instead, the host's cellular immune response has an important role in causing liver cell injury. Patients with defects in cell-mediated immunity are more likely to remain chronically infected with HBV than to clear the infection. Histologic specimens from patients with HBV-related liver injury demonstrate lymphocytes next to necrotic liver cells. It is thought that cytolytic T lymphocytes become sensitized to recognize hepatitis B viral antigens (eg, small quantities of hepatitis B surface antigen [HBsAg]) and host antigens on the surfaces of HBV-infected liver cells.

2. **Extrahepatic manifestations**—Immune factors may also be important in the pathogenesis of the extrahepatic manifestations of acute viral hepatitis. For example, in hepatitis B, a serum sickness–like prodrome characterized by fever, urticarial rash and angioedema, and arthralgias and arthritis appears to be related to immune complex–mediated tissue damage. During the early

prodrome, circulating immune complexes are composed of HBsAg in high titer in association with small quantities of anti-HBs. These circulating immune complexes are deposited in blood vessel walls, leading to activation of the complement cascade. In patients with arthritis, serum complement levels are depressed, and complement can be detected in circulating immune complexes containing HBsAg, anti-HBs, immunoglobulin (Ig) G, IgM, IgA, and fibrin.

Cryoglobulinemia is a common finding in chronic hepatitis C infection. Diabetes mellitus also occurs frequently and is now considered an extrahepatic manifestation of HCV. Although the mechanism is not fully understood, it is thought to be predominantly related to an increase in insulin resistance. Insulin resistance appears to diminish following HCV therapy.

Immune factors are thought to be important in the pathogenesis of some clinical manifestations in patients who become chronic HBsAg carriers after acute hepatitis. For example, in patients developing glomerulonephritis with nephrotic syndrome, histopathologic investigation demonstrates deposition of HBsAg, immunoglobulin, and complement in the glomerular basement membrane. In patients developing polyarteritis nodosa, similar deposits have been demonstrated in affected small and medium-sized arteries.

Other rarer extrahepatic manifestations include papular acrodermatitis and Guillain–Barré syndrome for HBV, and idiopathic thrombocytopenic purpura, lichen planus, Sjögren syndrome, lymphoproliferative diseases, membranoproliferative glomerulonephritis, and porphyria cutanea tarda for HCV.

B. Toxic Hepatitis

The pathogenesis of drug-induced liver injury is not well understood. Table 14–9 and Figure 14–9 summarize speculations on the mechanisms of idiosyncratic and dose-related drug-induced liver injury. Idiosyncratic drug reactions may be due to genetic predisposition in susceptible individuals to certain pathways of drug metabolism that generate toxic intermediates.

Prominent examples of drugs causing acute liver failure that have been withdrawn from the U.S. market include bromfenac, a nonsteroidal anti-inflammatory drug (NSAID), and troglitazone sulfate, a thiazolidinedione used as an insulin-sensitizing agent in diabetes mellitus. Other thiazolidinediones such as rosiglitazone and pioglitazone do not seem to have the same complication, although routine testing of transaminases has been recommended for those taking the drugs. HMG-CoA reductase inhibitors (eg, "statins") are associated with elevated levels of transaminases in fewer than 3% of individuals but very rarely result in clinical acute liver failure.

Drug- and toxin-induced hepatitis typically occurs at any time during or shortly after exposure and resolves with discontinuation of the offending agent. This is usually the case for both idiosyncratic and dose-dependent reactions.

C. Alcoholic Hepatitis

Ethanol has both direct and indirect toxic effects on the liver, as well as effects on many other organ systems. Table 14–10 lists the mechanisms thought to be responsible for ethanol-induced liver injury. Its direct effects may result from increasing the fluidity of biologic membranes and thereby disrupting cellular functions. Its indirect effects on the liver are in part a consequence of its metabolism. Ethanol is sequentially oxidized to acetaldehyde and then to acetate, with the generation of nicotinamide adenine dinucleotide hydride (NADH) and adenosine triphosphate (ATP). As a result of the high ratio of reduced to oxidized NAD generated, the pathways of fatty acid oxidation and gluconeogenesis are inhibited, whereas fatty acid synthesis is promoted.

Ethanol can also quantitatively and qualitatively alter the pattern of gene expression in various tissues but especially in the liver, resulting in impaired homeostasis and greater sensitivity to other toxins. These and other biochemical mechanisms may contribute to the common observation of fat accumulation in the liver and the tendency of hypoglycemia to develop in individuals with alcoholism whose liver glycogen has been depleted by fasting. Ethanol metabolism also affects the liver by generating acetaldehyde, which reacts with primary amino groups to inactivate enzymes, resulting in direct toxicity to the hepatocyte in which it is generated. Proteins so modified may activate the immune system against antigens that were previously tolerated as "self." Alcohol metabolism results in oxidative stress and hepatocyte death, and damaged hepatocytes release endogenous damage-associated molecular patterns (DAMPs) that recruit innate and adaptive immune cells, propagating further liver injury. Additional molecular mechanisms triggered by ethanol that have been implicated in the development of alcoholic liver disease include the induction of oxidative stress with resultant mitochondrial damage, activation of programmed hepatocyte necrosis, development of pericentral hypoxia, disruption of the gut microbiome, and alteration of intestinal epithelia resulting in increased permeability and influx of lipopolysaccharides into the liver that can cause systemic inflammation and trigger apoptotic pathways (Figure 14–10).

The histopathologic findings of alcoholic hepatitis differ from those of viral hepatitis and include the accumulation of Mallory's hyaline within hepatocytes and the infiltration of polymorphonuclear leukocytes.

Pathology

In uncomplicated acute hepatitis, the typical histologic findings consist of (1) focal liver cell degeneration and necrosis, with cell dropout, ballooning, and acidophilic degeneration (shrunken cells with eosinophilic cytoplasm and pyknotic nuclei); (2) the inflammation of portal areas, with infiltration by mononuclear cells (small lymphocytes, plasma cells, eosinophils); (3) a prominence of Kupffer cells and bile ducts; and (4) cholestasis (arrested bile flow) with bile plugs. Characteristically, although the regular pattern of hepatocyte cords is disrupted, the reticulin framework is preserved. This reticular

Six Mechanisms of Liver Injury

A. Rupture of cell membrane.
B. Injury of bile canaliculus (disruption of transport pumps).
C. P-450-drug covalent binding (drug adducts).

D. Drug adducts targeted by CTLs/cytokines.
E. Activation of apoptotic pathway by TNF/Fas.
F. Inhibition of mitochondrial function.

FIGURE 14–9 Potential mechanisms of drug-induced liver injury. The normal hepatocyte may be affected adversely by drugs through (**A**) disruption of intracellular calcium homeostasis that leads to the disassembly of actin fibrils at the surface of the hepatocyte, resulting in blebbing of the cell membrane, rupture, and cell lysis; (**B**) disruption of actin filaments next to the canaliculus (the specialized portion of the cell responsible for bile excretion), leading to a loss of villous processes and the interruption of transport pumps such as multidrug resistance–associated protein 3 (MRP3), which in turn prevents the excretion of bilirubin and other organic compounds; (**C**) covalent binding of heme-containing cytochrome P450–metabolizing enzymes to the drug, thus creating nonfunctioning adducts; (**D**) migration of these enzyme–drug adducts to the cell surface in vesicles to serve as target immunogens for cytolytic attack by T cells, stimulating an immune response involving cytolytic T cells and cytokines; (**E**) activation of apoptotic pathways by tumor necrosis factor (TNF) receptor or Fas ("DD" denotes "death domain"), triggering the cascade of intercellular caspases, resulting in programmed cell death; or (**F**) inhibition of mitochondrial function by a dual effect on both β-oxidation and the respiratory-chain enzymes, leading to failure of free fatty acid metabolism, a lack of aerobic respiration, and an accumulation of lactate and reactive oxygen species (which may disrupt mitochondrial DNA). Toxic metabolites excreted in bile may damage bile-duct epithelium (not shown). (CTLs, cytolytic T lymphocytes.) (Reproduced, with permission, from Lee WM. Drug-induced hepatotoxicity. N Engl J Med. 2003;349:474. Copyright © 2003 Massachusetts Medical Society. Reprinted, with permission, from Massachusetts Medical Society.)

TABLE 14–10 Mechanisms of hepatocyte injury by ethanol.

Disorganizes the lipid portion of cell membranes, leading to adaptive changes in their composition
Increased membrane fluidity and permeability
Impaired assembly of glycoproteins into membranes
Impaired glycoprotein secretion
Impaired binding and internalization of large ligands
Formation of abnormal mitochondria
Impairment of transport of small ligands
Impairment of membrane-bound enzymes
Adaptive changes in lipid composition, leading to increased lipid peroxidation
Abnormal display of antigens on the plasma membrane
Alters the capacity of liver cells to cope with environmental toxins
Induces xenobiotic metabolizing enzymes
Directly inhibits xenobiotic metabolizing enzymes
Induces deficiency in mechanisms protecting against injury from reactive metabolites
Enhances O_2 toxicity
Oxidation of ethanol produces acetaldehyde, a toxic and reactive intermediate
Inhibits export of proteins from the liver
Modifies hepatic protein synthesis in fasted animals
Alters the metabolism of cofactors essential for enzymatic activity: pyridoxine, folate, choline, zinc, vitamin E
Alters the oxidation–reduction potential of the liver cell
Induces malnutrition

Reproduced, with permission, from Zakim D et al. Alcoholic liver disease. In: Zakim D et al, eds. *Hepatology: A Textbook of Liver Disease*, 2nd ed. Saunders, 1990.

framework provides scaffolding for liver cells when the hepatocytes regenerate.

Recovery from acute hepatitis from any cause is characterized histologically by hepatocyte regeneration, with numerous mitotic figures and multinucleated cells, and by an almost complete restoration of normal lobular architecture.

Less commonly in acute hepatitis (1–5% of patients), there is a more severe histologic lesion called **bridging hepatic necrosis** (also called subacute, submassive, or confluent necrosis). Bridging is said to occur between lobules because necrosis involves contiguous groups of hepatocytes, resulting in large areas of hepatic cell loss and a collapse of the reticulin framework. Necrotic zones ("bridges"), consisting of condensed reticulin, inflammatory debris, and degenerating liver cells, link adjacent portal or central areas or may involve entire lobules.

Rarely, in massive hepatic necrosis or fulminant hepatitis (<1% of patients), the liver becomes small, shrunken, and soft (acute yellow atrophy). Histologic examination reveals massive hepatocyte necrosis in most lobules, leading to extensive collapse and condensation of the reticulin framework and portal structures (bile ducts and vessels).

Clinical Manifestations

A. Acute viral hepatitis

Usually there are three phases to acute viral hepatitis: the pre-icteric phase (prodrome), the icteric phase, and the convalescent phase (Figure 14–11).

1. **Pre-icteric phase (prodrome)**—The pre-icteric phase (prodrome), typically lasting 3 or 4 days, is characterized by three sets of symptoms and signs: (1) nonspecific constitutional symptoms and signs: malaise, fatigue, and mild fever; (2) gastrointestinal symptoms and signs: anorexia, nausea, vomiting, altered senses of olfaction and taste (loss of taste for coffee or cigarettes), and right upper quadrant abdominal discomfort (reflecting the enlarged liver); and (3) extrahepatic symptoms and signs: headache, photophobia, cough, coryza, myalgias, urticarial skin rash, arthralgias or arthritis (10–15% of patients with HBV), and, rarely, hematuria and proteinuria (see Figure 14–11).

2. **Icteric phase**—The icteric phase typically lasts 1–4 weeks. The constitutional symptoms usually improve, although mild weight loss may occur. Pruritus occurs if cholestasis is severe. Right upper quadrant abdominal pain as a result of the enlarged and tender liver, which was present in the prodromal phase, continues. Splenomegaly is noted in 10–20% of patients.

Jaundice may be observed as a yellowing of the scleras, skin, or mucous membranes. Jaundice is generally not appreciated on physical examination before the serum bilirubin rises above 2.5 mg/dL (41.75 μmol/L). **Direct hyperbilirubinemia** is an elevated level of conjugated bilirubin in the bloodstream. Its occurrence indicates an unimpaired ability of the hepatocytes to conjugate bilirubin but a defect in the excretion of bilirubin into the bile as a result of intrahepatic cholestasis or posthepatic obstructive biliary tract disease, with overflow of conjugated bilirubin out of hepatocytes into the bloodstream.

Changes in stool color (lightening) and urine color (darkening) often precede clinically evident jaundice. This reflects a loss of bilirubin metabolites from the stool as a consequence of disrupted bile flow. Water-soluble (conjugated) bilirubin metabolites are excreted in the urine, whereas water-insoluble metabolites accumulate in tissues, giving rise to jaundice. Note that in most cases of acute viral hepatitis, the degree of liver impairment is sufficiently mild that jaundice does not develop.

Ecchymoses suggest coagulopathy, which may be due to a loss of vitamin K absorptive capacity from the intestine

FIGURE 14–10 Alcohol consumption leads to hepatocyte apoptosis and necrosis. Increased intestinal permeability following alcohol use results in a lipopolysaccharide (LPS) influx into the liver. LPS induces inflammation, necroptosis, and apoptosis pathways via tumor necrosis factor-alpha (TNFα) and its receptor, tumor necrosis factor receptor-1 (TNFR1). (TRADD, TNFR-associated death domain; cIAP1/2, cellular inhibitor of apoptosis proteins 1 and 2; LUBAC, linear ubiquitin chain assembly complex; NF-Bκ, nuclear factor κB; TAB2/3, transforming growth factor beta-activated kinase 1/MAP3K7 binding proteins 2 and 3; TAK1, transforming growth factor beta-activated kinase 1; IKK, I-κB kinase; CYLD, CYLD lysine 63 deubiquitinase; RIP1/3, receptor-interacting proteins 1 and 3; FADD, fas-associated protein with a death domain; CFLAR, CASP8 and FADD-like apoptosis regulator; RHIM, RIP homotypic interaction motif; MLKL, mixed lineage kinase domain-like protein.) (Redrawn, with permission, from Nagy LE et al. Linking pathogenic mechanisms of alcoholic liver disease with clinical phenotypes. Gastroenterology. 2016 Jun;150(8):1756–68. Copyright © Elsevier.)

(caused by cholestasis) or decreased coagulation factor synthesis. Rarely, loss of clearance of activated clotting factors triggers disseminated intravascular coagulation. A coagulopathy in which the prothrombin time can be corrected by parenteral vitamin K but not by oral vitamin K suggests cholestatic disease, because vitamin K uptake from the gut depends on bile flow. If the prothrombin time cannot be corrected with either oral or parenteral vitamin K, an inability to synthesize clotting factor polypeptides (eg, as a result of massive hepatocellular dysfunction) should be suspected. Correction of prothrombin time with oral vitamin K alone suggests a nutritional deficiency rather than liver disease as the basis for the coagulopathy.

Tests for serum levels of various enzymes normally localized primarily within hepatocytes provide an indication of the extent of liver cell necrosis. For unclear reasons, perhaps related to liver cell polarity, certain forms of liver disease typically result in disproportionate elevations in some parameters. Thus, in alcoholic hepatitis but not in viral hepatitis, AST is often disproportionately elevated relative to ALT (AST:ALT ratio >2.0). One hypothesis is that this is due to a pyridoxine deficiency in alcoholism. Likewise, in cholestasis, alkaline

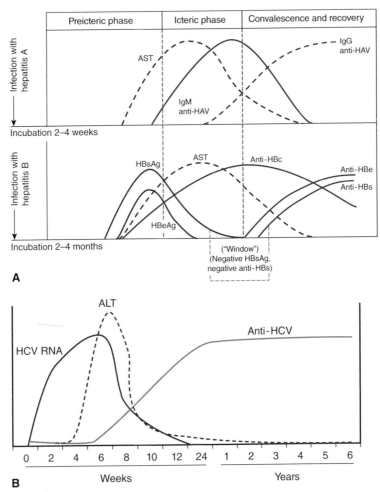

FIGURE 14–11 (**A**) Serum antibody and antigen levels in hepatitis A and hepatitis B. (AST, aspartate aminotransferase, a marker for hepatocellular injury and necrosis; IgM anti-HAV, early antibody response to hepatitis A infection; IgG anti-HAV, late antibody response to hepatitis A infection; HBsAg, hepatitis B surface antigen, a marker of active viral gene expression; HBeAg, hepatitis B early antigen, a marker of infectivity.) Antibodies to the surface or early antigens (anti-HBs or anti-HBe) indicate immunity. (Redrawn, with permission, from Chandrasoma P et al, eds. *Concise Pathology,* 3rd ed. Originally published by Appleton & Lange. Copyright © 1998 by The McGraw-Hill Companies, Inc.) (**B**) Course of acute, resolving HCV infection. (ALT, alanine aminotransferase; HCV RNA, hepatitis C viral load; anti-HCV, HCV antibody.) (Redrawn, with permission, from Hoofnagle JH. Course and outcome of hepatitis C. Hepatology. 2002 Nov;36(5 Suppl 1):S21–9. Copyright © John Wiley and Sons.)

phosphatase is commonly disproportionately elevated relative to AST or ALT. The time course of acute hepatitis is highly variable. In hepatitis A, jaundice is typically seen 4–8 weeks after exposure, whereas in hepatitis B, jaundice usually occurs 8–20 weeks after exposure (see Figure 14–11).

Measuring antigen and antibody titers is a convenient way to assess whether an episode of acute hepatitis is due to viral infection. Moreover, because IgM antibodies are produced early after exposure to antigens (ie, soon after the onset of illness), the presence of IgM antibodies to either HAV or to HBV core antigen (HBcAg) is strong evidence that an episode of acute hepatitis is due to the corresponding viral infection. Several months after the onset of illness, IgM antibody titers wane and are replaced by antibodies of the IgG class, indicating immunity to recurrence of infection by the same virus. The presence of hepatitis B "e" antigen (HBeAg) correlates well with a high degree of infectivity (Table 14–11). However,

more sensitive DNA tests have shown low levels of viral DNA in the blood of many who are HBeAg negative and who are thus still infectious.

Subtle or profound mental status changes are seen in fulminant hepatic necrosis. Encephalopathy is believed to be related in part to a failure to detoxify ammonia, which normally occurs through the urea cycle. Other products such as γ-aminobutyric acid (GABA) may not be metabolized. Although ammonia is a neurotoxin, it remains unclear whether it is the major agent of CNS dysfunction or whether elevated blood levels of GABA (perhaps synergistically with other compounds) may act to alter mental status because of its role as a major inhibitory neurotransmitter. In addition to encephalopathic changes caused by an accumulation of toxins, acute hepatic failure is associated with encephalopathy from cerebral edema caused by increased intracranial pressure, perhaps related to alterations in the blood–brain barrier.

TABLE 14–11   Commonly encountered serologic patterns of hepatitis B infection.

HBsAg	Anti-HBs	Anti-HBc	HBeAg	Anti-HBe	Interpretation
+	–	IgM	+	–	Acute HBV infection, high infectivity[1]
+	–	IgG	+	–	Chronic HBV infection, high infectivity
+	–	IgG	–	+	1. Late acute or chronic HBV infection, low infectivity
					2. HBeAg-negative ("precore-mutant") hepatitis B (chronic or, rarely, acute)
+	+	+	+/–	+/–	1. HBsAg of one subtype and heterotypic anti-HBs (common)
					2. Process of seroconversion from HBsAg to anti-HBs (rare)
–	–	IgM	+/–	+/–	1. Acute HBV infection[1]
					2. Anti-HBc "window"
–	–	IgG	–	+/–	1. Low-level HBV carrier
					2. Remote past HBV infection
–	+	IgG	–	+/–	Recovery from HBV infection
–	+		–	–	1. Immunization with HBsAg (after vaccination)
					2. Remote past HBV infection (?)
					3. False-positive

[1]IgM anti-HBc may reappear during an acute reactivation of chronic hepatitis B.

Reproduced, with permission, from Dienstag JL. Acute viral hepatitis. In: Kasper D et al, eds. *Harrison's Principles of Internal Medicine*, 19th ed. McGraw-Hill, 2015.

Renal dysfunction may complicate fulminant hepatic failure. Affected patients may develop prerenal azotemia when the glomerular filtration rate falls secondary to intravascular volume depletion. A state of intravascular volume depletion can be induced by the combination of decreased oral intake, vomiting, and ascites formation. If uncorrected, this process can lead to acute tubular necrosis and acute kidney injury. Other causes of renal dysfunction in fulminant hepatic failure include toxins (eg, acetaminophen or *Amanita* poisoning) or hepatorenal syndrome. Serum creatinine is a more accurate measure than blood urea nitrogen of renal impairment in fulminant hepatic failure resulting from decreased hepatic urea production. Other complications of fulminant hepatic failure include cardiovascular dysfunction as a result of systemic vasodilation and hypotension, pulmonary edema, coagulopathy, sepsis, and hypoglycemia.

3. **Convalescent phase**—The convalescent phase is characterized by the complete disappearance of constitutional symptoms but persistent abnormalities in liver function tests. Symptoms and signs gradually improve (see Figure 14–11).

Acute hepatitis typically resolves in 3–6 months. Hepatic injury continuing for more than 6 months is arbitrarily defined as chronic hepatitis and suggests, in the absence of continued exposure to a noxious agent, that immune or other mechanisms are at work.

CHECKPOINT

22. Describe the range of clinical presentations of acute hepatitis.
23. Which viruses can cause hepatitis?
24. What are some extrahepatic manifestations of viral hepatitis?
25. What is the basis for the extrahepatic manifestations of viral hepatitis?
26. Describe the spectrum of liver diseases associated with alcohol consumption.
27. What are some ways that ethanol causes liver injury?

CHRONIC HEPATITIS

Chronic hepatitis is a category of disorders characterized by the combination of liver cell necrosis and inflammation of varying severity persisting for more than 6 months. It may be due to viral infection; drugs and toxins; genetic, metabolic, or autoimmune factors; or unknown causes. The severity ranges from an asymptomatic stable illness characterized only by laboratory test abnormalities to a severe, gradually progressive illness culminating in cirrhosis, liver failure, and death. Based on clinical, laboratory, and biopsy findings, chronic hepatitis is best assessed with regard to (1) distribution and severity of

TABLE 14–12   Three simple systems for the histologic grading and staging of chronic hepatitis.

International Association for the Study of the Liver	Batts–Ludwig	Metavir
Grade (activity, inflammation)		
Minimal chronic hepatitis	Grade 1	A1
Mild chronic hepatitis	Grade 2	A1
Moderate chronic hepatitis	Grade 3	A2
Severe chronic hepatitis	Grade 4	A3
Stage (fibrosis)		
Mild: Portal fibrosis	Stage 1	F1
Moderate: Periportal fibrosis	Stage 2	F1
Severe: Bridging fibrosis (few)	Stage 3	F2
Severe: Bridging fibrosis (many)	Stage 3	F3
Cirrhosis	Stage 4	F4

Adapted from Goodman ZD. Grading and staging systems for inflammation and fibrosis in chronic liver diseases. J Hepatol. 2007;47(4):598–607.

inflammation; (2) degree of fibrosis; and (3) etiology, which has important prognostic implications. Table 14–12 presents a simplified scoring system for assessing liver biopsies for chronic hepatitis.

Clinical Presentation

Patients may present with fatigue, malaise, low-grade fever, anorexia, weight loss, mild intermittent jaundice, and mild hepatosplenomegaly. Others are initially asymptomatic and present late in the course of the disease with complications of cirrhosis, including variceal bleeding, coagulopathy, encephalopathy, jaundice, and ascites. In contrast to chronic persistent hepatitis, some patients with chronic active hepatitis, particularly those without serologic evidence of antecedent HBV infection, present with extrahepatic symptoms such as skin rash, diarrhea, arthritis, and various autoimmune disorders (Table 14–13).

Etiology

Either type of chronic hepatitis (persistent or active) can be caused by infection with several hepatitis viruses (eg, hepatitis B, with or without hepatitis D superinfection, and hepatitis C); a variety of drugs and poisons (eg, ethanol, isoniazid, acetaminophen), often in amounts insufficient to cause symptomatic acute hepatitis; genetic and metabolic disorders (eg, α_1-antitrypsin deficiency, Wilson disease); or immune-mediated injury of unknown origin. Table 14–1 summarizes known causes of chronic hepatitis. Less than 5% of otherwise healthy adults with acute hepatitis B remain chronically infected with HBV; the risk is higher in those who are immunocompromised or of young age (ranging from 90% in newborns of HBeAg-positive mothers to

TABLE 14–13   Extrahepatic manifestations of chronic viral hepatitis.

Primarily hepatitis C
Thyroid autoimmune disorders
Diabetes mellitus
Autoimmune thrombocytopenic purpura and hemolytic anemia
Sjögren syndrome and sialadenitis
Arthritis and arthralgias
Essential mixed cryoglobulinemia
Monoclonal gammopathies
B-cell non-Hodgkin lymphoma
Membranoproliferative glomerulonephritis
Porphyria cutanea tarda
Lichen planus
Psoriasis
Leukocytoclastic vasculitis
Primarily hepatitis B
Serum sickness–like syndrome
Polyarteritis nodosa
Immune-complex glomerulonephritis

Data obtained from Sanyal AJ et al, eds. *Zakim and Boyer's Hepatology: A Textbook of Liver Disease*, 7th ed. Elsevier, 2017; and Himoto T et al. Extrahepatic manifestations and autoantibodies in patients with hepatitis C virus infection. Clin Dev Immunol. 2012;2012:871401.

25–30% in infants and children younger than 5 years). Among those chronically infected, about two-thirds develop mild chronic hepatitis and one-third develop severe chronic hepatitis (see later discussion). Those with HDV coinfection progress to chronic hepatitis at higher rates than seen with isolated HBV infection. HDV superinfection is also associated with a high incidence of acute liver failure. Finally, 60–85% of individuals exposed to acute hepatitis C develop chronic hepatitis, and rates are not significantly affected by age, mode of acquisition, or the presence of coinfections.

Pathogenesis

Many cases of chronic hepatitis are thought to represent an immune-mediated attack on the liver occurring as a result of the persistence of certain hepatitis viruses or after prolonged exposure to certain drugs or noxious substances (Table 14–14). In some, no mechanism has been recognized. Evidence that the disorder is immune mediated is that liver biopsies reveal inflammation (lymphocyte infiltration) in characteristic regions of the liver architecture (eg, portal versus lobular). Furthermore,

TABLE 14–14　Drugs implicated in the etiology of chronic hepatitis.

Drug	Use
Acetaminophen	Analgesic
Amiodarone	Antiarrhythmic
Aspirin	Analgesic
Ethanol	Abuse
Isoniazid	Antituberculous therapy
Methyldopa	Antihypertensive
Nitrofurantoin	Antibiotic
Propylthiouracil	Antithyroid therapy
Sulfonamides	Antibiotic

Modified and reproduced, with permission, from Bass NM et al. Drug-induced liver disease. In: Zakim D et al, eds. *Hepatology: A Textbook of Liver Disease*, 2nd ed. Saunders, 1990. Copyright © Elsevier.

a variety of autoimmune disorders occur with high frequency in patients with chronic hepatitis (see Table 14–13).

A. Chronic Viral Hepatitis

Viral hepatitis is the most common cause of chronic liver disease in the United States. In approximately 5% of adult cases of HBV infection and 60–85% of hepatitis C infections, the immune response is inadequate to clear the liver of virus, resulting in persistent infection. The individual becomes a chronic carrier, intermittently producing the virus and hence remaining infectious to others. Biochemically, these patients are often found to have viral DNA integrated into their genomes in a manner that results in the abnormal expression of certain viral proteins with or without the production of intact virus. Viral antigens expressed on the hepatocyte cell surface are associated with class I HLA determinants, thus eliciting lymphocyte cytotoxicity and resulting in hepatitis. The severity of chronic hepatitis depends largely on the activity of viral replication and the response of the host's immune system.

Chronic hepatitis B infection predisposes the patient to the development of hepatocellular carcinoma (HCC). Although in the setting of HBV infection most cases of HCC occur in the presence of cirrhosis, 10–30% of cases occur in the absence of cirrhosis or advanced fibrosis. It remains unclear whether hepatitis B infection is the initiator or simply a promoter of the process of tumorigenesis. In hepatitis C infection, HCC develops exclusively in the setting of cirrhosis.

B. Alcoholic Chronic Hepatitis

Chronic liver disease in response to some poisons or toxins may represent the triggering of an underlying genetic predisposition to immune attack on the liver. In alcoholic hepatitis, however, repeated episodes of acute injury ultimately cause necrosis, fibrosis, and regeneration, leading eventually to cirrhosis (Figure 14–12). As in other forms of liver disease, there

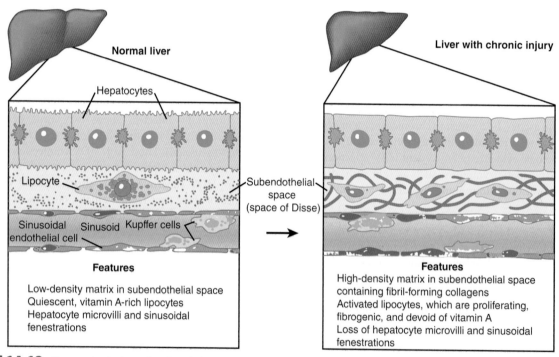

FIGURE 14-12 Changes in the hepatic subendothelial space during fibrosing liver injury. Cellular and matrix alterations in the space of Disse are critical events in the pathogenesis of hepatic fibrosis. The activation of lipocytes, characterized by proliferation and increased fibrogenesis, is associated with the replacement of the normal low-density matrix with a high-density matrix. These alterations are likely to underlie, at least in part, the loss of both endothelial fenestrations (pores) and hepatocytic microvilli typical of chronic liver injury. (Redrawn, with permission, from Bissell DM. Cell-matrix interaction and hepatic fibrosis. Prog Liver Dis 1990;9:143–55. Copyright © Elsevier.)

is considerable variation in the extent of symptoms before cirrhosis develops.

C. Nonalcoholic Fatty Liver Disease

In light of increasing obesity in the United States, there has been a significant increase in the prevalence of nonalcoholic fatty liver disease (NAFLD), a form of chronic liver disease associated with the metabolic syndrome. NAFLD refers to the presence of hepatic steatosis, with or without inflammation and fibrosis, when no other causes of secondary hepatic fat accumulation (eg, heavy alcohol consumption) are present. NAFLD is an umbrella term for a spectrum of liver disease severity, ranging from nonalcoholic fatty liver (NAFL), in which inflammation is minimal, to nonalcoholic steatohepatitis (NASH), in which active inflammation poses a risk for fibrosis and progression to cirrhosis. On biopsy, the inflammation associated with NASH may be histologically indistinguishable from alcoholic steatohepatitis.

NAFLD is prevalent worldwide and is the most common liver disease in industrialized Western countries. In the United States, the estimated prevalence of NAFLD ranges from 10% to 46%, and the prevalence of NASH ranges from 3% to 5%, with variation by age, gender, and ethnicity. NAFLD is strongly associated with metabolic risk factors such as obesity, dyslipidemia, insulin resistance, and type 2 diabetes mellitus, and the rising incidence of NAFLD parallels rising rates of obesity worldwide.

The pathogenesis of NAFLD has not been fully elucidated, but the most widely supported theory implicates insulin resistance as the key mechanism leading to hepatic steatosis and steatohepatitis. Lipid accumulation in hepatocytes results from an increased influx of lipids to the liver or decreased lipid disposal (Figure 14–13).

Lipid accumulation has been shown to lead to toxicity by diverse mechanisms, including increased oxidative stress as a result of the generation of reactive oxygen species by mitochondrial and peroxisomal fatty acid oxidation. In addition, lipotoxicity can result from changes in cell signaling pathways that regulate metabolism and stress responses, promoting a sterile inflammatory response that can potentiate liver cell injury and death. Dying hepatocytes can induce a wound-healing response via DAMPs, cytokines, and hedgehog, which can promote inflammation, fibrogenesis, and hepatocarcinogenesis. Factors that promote lipotoxicity in patients with NAFLD include iron overload, environmental toxins, medications, viral hepatitis, congenital liver disease, alpha-1 antitrypsin deficiency, and Wilson disease.

In general, patients with simple steatosis are at low risk of histologic progression, but patients with NASH can progress to cirrhosis and end-stage liver disease and are at risk for HCC. Long-term studies of patients with NAFL and NASH have revealed that such patients have increased overall mortality and that the most common cause of death in these patients is cardiovascular disease. Moreover, patients with NASH (but not NAFL) have increased rates of liver-related mortality. Management of NAFLD is centered on modifying risk factors and treating metabolic comorbidities. Vitamin E is the only agent that has been shown to improve

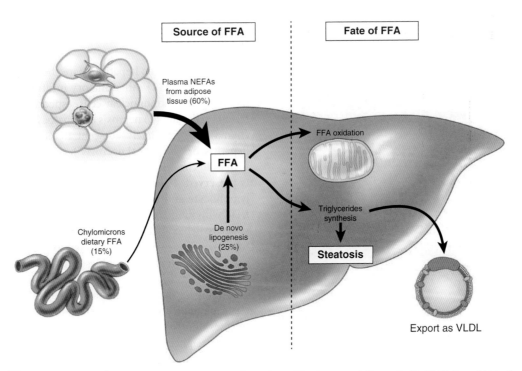

FIGURE 14-13 Pathogenesis of hepatic steatosis. An increased uptake and/or decreased disposal of lipids (fatty acids) in the liver results in an accumulation of fat within hepatocytes. (FFA, free fatty acid; NEFA, non-esterified fatty acid; VLDL, very-low-density lipoprotein.) (Redrawn, with permission, from Machado MV et al. Pathogenesis of nonalcoholic steatohepatitis. Gastroenterology. 2016 Jun;150(8):1769–77. Copyright © Elsevier.)

liver histology in a subgroup of adults who are nondiabetic with biopsy-proven NASH.

D. Other Chronic Hepatitis

Some patients develop chronic hepatitis in the absence of evidence of preceding viral hepatitis or exposure to noxious agents (Figure 14–14). Autoimmune hepatitis is a chronic inflammatory liver disease characterized by a mainly T cell–mediated immune response to as yet unidentified auto-antigen(s). Patients with autoimmune hepatitis demonstrate serologic evidence of disordered immunoregulation, manifested as hyperglobulinemia and circulating autoantibodies, as well as a typical pattern of injury on liver histology characterized by a plasma cell–rich inflammatory infiltrate, interface hepatitis, hepatic rosette formation, and emperipolesis (presence of an intact cell within the cytoplasm of another cell). Nearly 75% of these patients are women, and many have other autoimmune disorders. A genetic predisposition is strongly suggested. Most patients with autoimmune hepatitis show histologic improvement in liver biopsies after treatment with systemic corticosteroids. The clinical response, however, can be variable.

Cholestatic forms of autoimmune liver disease have also been well characterized, including **primary biliary cholangitis** and **primary sclerosing cholangitis**. In primary biliary cholangitis, it is postulated that intralobular bile duct injury is triggered by environmental exposure(s) in a genetically susceptible individual. The persistent activation of innate and adaptive immune responses mediates inflammation and bile duct epithelial damage. The resultant bile duct destruction leads to chronic cholestasis and the intrahepatic accumulation of cytotoxic bile acids. This accumulation causes liver cell injury and a secretion of pro-inflammatory cytokines that induce inflammation and fibrosis in surrounding tissue. The vast majority of individuals with primary biliary cholangitis will have detectable anti-mitochondrial antibody; the diagnosis is also supported by elevated levels of alkaline phosphatase. On liver biopsy, there is histopathological evidence of nonsuppurative cholangitis and destruction of small or medium-sized interlobular bile ducts.

Primary sclerosing cholangitis is characterized by chronic inflammation of the biliary epithelium leading to multifocal intra- and/or extrahepatic biliary strictures and fibrosis; these in turn often lead to biliary cirrhosis and malignancy. The pathogenesis of primary sclerosing cholangitis remains poorly understood, but it is also theorized to occur in genetically susceptible individuals after exposure to an unknown environmental trigger. While immune dysregulation is implicated in its pathogenesis, primary sclerosing cholangitis lacks other classic features of autoimmune disease such as female predominance, pathogenic autoantibodies, and response to immunosuppressive medications. Owing to its definite association with inflammatory bowel disease, a "leaky gut" hypothesis has been postulated, whereby translocation of gastrointestinal flora leads to disruption of biliary epithelial cells and exposes cholangiocytes to bile acid toxicity. Cholangiography showing characteristic bile duct stricturing establishes the diagnosis of primary sclerosing cholangitis.

Pathology

All forms of chronic hepatitis share the common histopathologic features of (1) inflammatory infiltration of hepatic portal areas with mononuclear cells, especially lymphocytes and plasma cells; and (2) necrosis of hepatocytes within the parenchyma or immediately adjacent to portal areas (periportal hepatitis, or "piecemeal necrosis").

In mild chronic hepatitis, the overall architecture of the liver is preserved. Histologically, the liver reveals a characteristic lymphocyte and plasma cell infiltrate confined to the portal triad without disruption of the limiting plate and no evidence of active hepatocyte necrosis. There is little or no fibrosis, and what there is generally is restricted to the portal area; there is no sign of cirrhosis. A "cobblestone" appearance of liver cells is seen, indicating hepatocyte regeneration.

In more severe cases of chronic hepatitis, the portal areas are expanded and densely infiltrated by lymphocytes, histiocytes, and plasma cells. There is necrosis of hepatocytes at the periphery of the lobule, with erosion of the limiting plate surrounding the portal triads (piecemeal necrosis; see Figure 14–14). More severe cases also show evidence of necrosis and fibrosis between portal triads. The normal liver architecture is disrupted by bands of scar tissue and inflammatory

FIGURE 14–14 Chronic hepatitis, showing marked lymphocytic infiltration and fibrosis of the portal areas. The lymphocytes extend into the peripheral part of the lobule through the limiting plate. There is ongoing hepatocyte necrosis in the peripheral part of the lobule (piecemeal necrosis). (Reproduced, with permission, from Chandrasoma P et al, eds. *Concise Pathology*, 3rd ed. Originally published by Appleton & Lange. Copyright © 1998 by The McGraw-Hill Companies, Inc.)

cells that link portal areas to one another and to central areas (bridging necrosis). These connective tissue bridges are evidence of hepatic architecture remodeling, a crucial step in the development of cirrhosis. Fibrosis may extend from the portal areas into the lobules, isolating hepatocytes into clusters and enveloping bile ducts. Hepatocyte regeneration is seen with mitotic figures, multinucleated cells, rosette formation, and regenerative pseudolobules. Progression to cirrhosis is signaled by extensive fibrosis, loss of zonal architecture, and regenerating nodules.

Clinical Manifestations

Some patients with mild chronic hepatitis are entirely asymptomatic and identified only in the course of routine blood testing; others have an insidious onset of nonspecific symptoms such as anorexia, malaise, and fatigue or hepatic symptoms, such as right upper quadrant abdominal discomfort or pain. Fatigue in chronic hepatitis may be related to a change in the hypothalamic–adrenal neuroendocrine axis brought about by altered endogenous opioidergic neurotransmission. Jaundice, if present, is usually mild. There may be mild tender hepatomegaly and occasional splenomegaly. Palmar erythema and spider telangiectases are seen in severe cases. Other extrahepatic manifestations are unusual. By definition, signs of cirrhosis and portal hypertension (eg, ascites, collateral circulation, and encephalopathy) are absent. Laboratory studies show mild to moderate increases in serum aminotransferase, bilirubin, and globulin levels. Serum albumin and the prothrombin time are normal until late in the progression of liver disease.

The clinical manifestations of chronic hepatitis probably reflect the role of a systemic genetically controlled immune disorder in the pathogenesis of severe disease. Acne, hirsutism, and amenorrhea may occur as a reflection of the hormonal effects of chronic liver disease. Laboratory studies in patients with severe chronic hepatitis are invariably abnormal to various degrees. However, these abnormalities do not correlate with clinical severity. Thus, the serum bilirubin, alkaline phosphatase, and globulin levels may be normal and aminotransferase levels only mildly elevated at the same time that a liver biopsy reveals severe chronic hepatitis. However, an elevated prothrombin time usually reflects severe disease.

The natural history and treatment of chronic hepatitis varies depending on its cause. The complications of severe chronic hepatitis are those of progression to cirrhosis: variceal bleeding, encephalopathy, coagulopathy, hypersplenism, and ascites. These are largely due to portosystemic shunting rather than diminished hepatocyte reserve (see later discussion).

CHECKPOINT

28. What are the categories of chronic hepatitis based on histologic findings on liver biopsy?
29. What are the causes of chronic hepatitis?
30. What are the consequences of chronic hepatitis?

CIRRHOSIS

Clinical Presentation

Cirrhosis is an irreversible distortion of normal liver architecture characterized by hepatic injury, fibrosis, and nodular regeneration. The clinical presentations of cirrhosis are a consequence of both progressive hepatocellular dysfunction and portal hypertension (Figure 14–15). As with other presentations of liver disease, not all patients with cirrhosis develop life-threatening complications. Indeed, in nearly 40% of cases of cirrhosis, it is diagnosed at autopsy in patients who did not manifest obvious signs of end-stage liver disease.

Etiology

Table 14–1 lists the causes of cirrhosis. The initial injury can be due to a wide range of processes. A crucial feature is that the liver injury is not acute and self-limited, but rather chronic and progressive. In the United States, alcohol abuse is the most common cause of cirrhosis. In other countries, infectious agents (particularly HBV and HCV) are the most common causes. Other causes include chronic biliary obstruction, drugs, genetic and metabolic disorders, chronic heart failure, and primary (autoimmune) biliary cholangitis.

Pathogenesis

The increased or altered synthesis of collagen and other connective tissue or basement membrane components of the extracellular matrix is implicated in the development of hepatic fibrosis and thus in the pathogenesis of cirrhosis. The role of the extracellular matrix in cellular function is an important area of research, and studies suggest that it is involved in modulating the activities of the cells with which it is in contact. Thus, fibrosis may affect not only the mechanics of blood flow through the liver but also the functions of the cells themselves.

Hepatic fibrosis occurs in three situations: (1) secondary to inflammation and the subsequent activation of immune responses; (2) as part of the process of wound healing; and (3) in response to agents that induce primary fibrogenesis. HBV and *Schistosoma* species are good examples of agents that lead to hepatic fibrosis by stimulating an immune response. Agents such as carbon tetrachloride that attack and kill hepatocytes directly can produce fibrosis as part of wound healing. In both immune responses and wound healing, the fibrosis is triggered indirectly by the effects of cytokines released from invading inflammatory cells. Finally, certain agents such as ethanol and iron may cause primary fibrogenesis by directly increasing collagen gene transcription and thus also increasing the amount of connective tissue secreted by cells.

The actual culprit in all these mechanisms of increased fibrogenesis may be the fat-storing cells (stellate cells) of the hepatic reticuloendothelial system. In response to cytokines, they differentiate from quiescent stellate cells, in which vitamin A is stored, into myofibroblasts, which lose their vitamin

Effects of portal hypertension

- Esophageal varices

  ↓

  Hematemesis

  - Gastropathy

  ↓

- Melena ◄

- Splenomegaly

- Dilated abdominal veins
  (caput medusae)

- Ascites

- Rectal varices
  (hemorrhoids)

Effects of liver cell failure

- Coma

- Fetor hepaticus (breath
  smells like a freshly
  opened corpse)

- Spider nevi

- Gynecomastia

- Jaundice

- Ascites

- Loss of sexual hair

- Testicular atrophy

- Liver "flap" (coarse
  hand tremor)

- Bleeding tendency
  (decreased prothrombin)

- Anemia
  Macrocytic
  Iron deficiency
  (blood loss)

- Ankle edema

FIGURE 14–15 Clinical effects of cirrhosis of the liver. (Redrawn, with permission, from Chandrasoma P et al, eds. *Concise Pathology*, 3rd ed. Originally published by Appleton & Lange. Copyright © 1998 by The McGraw-Hill Companies, Inc.)

A storage capacity and become actively engaged in extracellular matrix production. In addition to the stellate cells, fibrogenic cells also derive from portal fibroblasts, circulating fibrocytes, bone marrow, and epithelial–mesenchymal cell transition. It appears that hepatic fibrosis occurs in two stages (Figure 14–16). The first stage is characterized by a change in extracellular matrix composition from non–cross-linked, non–fibril-forming collagen to collagen that is more dense and subject to cross-link formation. At this stage, liver injury is still reversible. The second stage involves the formation of subendothelial collagen cross-links, the proliferation of myoepithelial cells, and the distortion of hepatic architecture with the appearance of regenerating nodules. Cirrhosis remains a dynamic state in which certain interventions, even at these advanced stages, may yield benefits such as regression of scar tissue and improvements in clinical outcomes.

The manner in which alcohol causes chronic liver disease and cirrhosis is not well understood. However, chronic alcohol abuse is associated with impaired protein synthesis and secretion, mitochondrial injury, lipid peroxidation, formation of acetaldehyde and its interaction with cellular proteins and membrane lipids, cellular hypoxia, and both cell-mediated and antibody-mediated cytotoxicity. The relative importance of each of these factors in producing cell injury is unknown. Genetic, nutritional, and environmental factors (including simultaneous exposure to other hepatotoxins) also influence the development of liver disease in people with chronic alcoholism. Finally, acute liver injury (eg, from exposure to alcohol or other toxins) from which a person with a normal liver would fully recover may be sufficient to produce irreversible decompensation (eg, hepatorenal syndrome) in a patient with underlying hepatic cirrhosis.

Pathology

The liver may be large or small, but it always has a firm and often nodular consistency. Although several noninvasive methods for staging the extent of fibrosis exist, including the use of serum biomarkers and imaging techniques to measure liver stiffness (eg, elastography), these methods are accurate for severe (fibrosis stage F3) and minimal (F1) fibrosis, but not intermediate stages. Liver biopsy remains the only method for definitively diagnosing significant fibrosis (F ≥2) and cirrhosis (F4). Histologically, all forms of cirrhosis are characterized by three findings: (1) marked distortion of hepatic architecture; (2) scarring as a result of increased deposition of fibrous tissue and collagen; and (3) regenerative nodules surrounded by scar tissue. When the nodules are small (<3 mm) and uniform in size, the process is termed **micronodular cirrhosis**. In **macronodular cirrhosis**, the nodules are more than 3 mm and variable in size. Cirrhosis from alcohol abuse is usually micronodular but can be macronodular or both micronodular and macronodular. Scarring may be most severe in central regions, or dense bands of connective tissue may join portal and central areas.

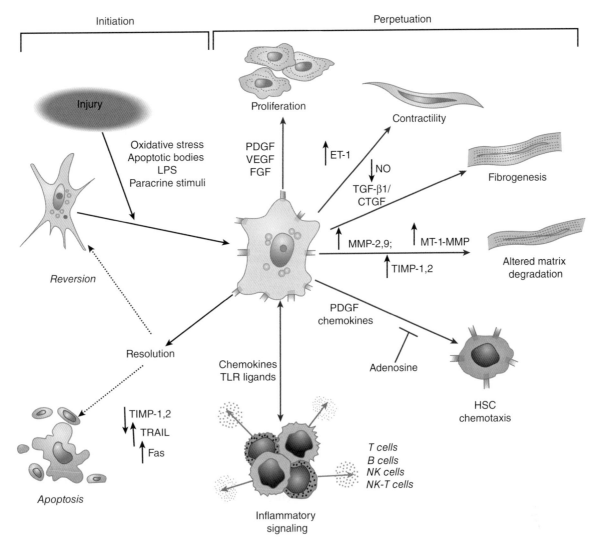

FIGURE 14–16 Pathways of hepatic stellate cell activation. Features of stellate cell activation can be distinguished between those that stimulate initiation and those that contribute to perpetuation. Initiation is provoked by soluble stimuli that include oxidant stress signals (reactive oxygen intermediates), apoptotic bodies, lipopolysaccharide (LPS), and paracrine stimuli from neighboring cell types, including hepatic macrophages (Kupffer cells), sinusoidal endothelium, and hepatocytes. Perpetuation follows, characterized by a number of specific phenotypic changes, including proliferation, contractility, fibrogenesis, altered matrix degradation, chemotaxis, and inflammatory signaling. (CTGF, connective tissue growth factor; ET-1, endothelin-1; FGF, fibroblast growth factor; HSC, hepatic stellate cells; MMP 2, 9, metalloproteinase-2 and -9; MT, membrane type; MT-1-MMP, membrane type 1 metalloproteinase; NK, natural killer; NO, nitric oxide; PDGF, platelet-derived growth factor; TGF-beta 1, transforming growth factor-beta 1; TIMP-1, 2, metallopeptidase inhibitor-1 and -2; TLR, Toll-like receptors; TRAIL, TNF-related apoptosis-inducing ligand; VEGF, vascular endothelial growth factor.) (Adapted, with permission, from Friedman SL. Molecular regulation of hepatic fibrosis, an integrated cellular response to tissue injury. J Biol Chem. 2000 Jan 28:275(4):2247–50. Copyright © American Society for Biochemistry and Molecular Biology.)

More specific histopathologic findings may help establish the cause of cirrhosis. For example, the invasion and destruction of bile ducts by granulomas suggests primary (autoimmune) biliary cirrhosis; extensive iron deposition in hepatocytes and bile ducts suggests hemochromatosis; and alcoholic hyaline and infiltration with polymorphonuclear cells suggest alcoholic cirrhosis.

Clinical Manifestations

The clinical manifestations of progressive hepatocellular dysfunction in cirrhosis are similar to those of acute or chronic hepatitis and include constitutional symptoms and signs: fatigue, loss of vigor, and weight loss; GI symptoms and signs:

nausea, vomiting, jaundice, and tender hepatomegaly; and extrahepatic symptoms and signs: palmar erythema, spider angiomas, muscle wasting, parotid and lacrimal gland enlargement, gynecomastia and testicular atrophy in men, menstrual irregularities in women, and coagulopathy (see Figure 14–15).

Clinical manifestations of portal hypertension include ascites, portosystemic shunting, encephalopathy, splenomegaly, and esophageal and gastric varices with intermittent hemorrhage (see Figure 14–15 and Table 14–15).

A. Portal Hypertension

Portal hypertension is defined by a portal venous pressure gradient greater than 5 mm Hg. Portal hypertension results from

TABLE 14–15   Manifestations of cirrhosis.

Due to portal hypertension with portal-to-systemic shunting
Ascites and increased risk of spontaneous bacterial peritonitis
Increased risk of sepsis
Increased risk of disseminated intravascular coagulation
Splenomegaly with thrombocytopenia
Encephalopathy
Varices
Drug sensitivity
Bile acid deficiency with malabsorption of fat and fat-soluble vitamins
Hyperestrogenemia
Hyperglycemia
Due to loss of hepatocytes
Hypoglycemia
Coagulopathy due to deficient clotting factor synthesis
Peripheral edema due to hypoalbuminemia
Hepatic coma
Other complications
Hepatorenal syndrome
Hepatocellular carcinoma
Hepatopulmonary syndrome

a rise in intrahepatic vascular resistance. The cirrhotic liver loses the physiologic characteristic of a low-pressure circuit for blood flow seen in the normal liver. The increased blood pressure within the sinusoids is transmitted back to the portal vein. Because the portal vein lacks valves, this elevated pressure is transmitted back to other vascular beds, resulting in splenomegaly, portal-to-systemic shunting, and many of the complications of cirrhosis discussed later.

B. Ascites

Ascites refers to the presence of excess fluid within the peritoneal cavity. Patients with ascites develop physical examination findings of increasing abdominal girth, a fluid wave, a ballotable liver, and shifting dullness. Ascites can develop in patients with conditions other than liver disease, including protein-calorie malnutrition (from hypoalbuminemia) and cancer (from lymphatic obstruction). In patients with liver disease, ascites is due to portal hypertension and can be confirmed by the presence of a serum-to-ascites albumin gradient (SAAG) of 1.1 g/dL (11 g/L) or more. Calculating the SAAG involves measuring on the same day the albumin concentration in serum and ascitic fluid (via abdominal paracentesis)

and subtracting the ascitic fluid value from the serum value. Ascites can develop in approximately 50% of patients with compensated cirrhosis over a 10-year follow-up period, and it is associated with significant morbidity and mortality.

It is useful to recognize that liver disease with ascites formation occurs in a wide clinical spectrum. At one end is fully compensated portal hypertension with no ascites present because the volume of ascites generated is less than the approximately 800–1200 mL/d capacity of the peritoneal lymphatic drainage. At the other extreme is the typically fatal hepatorenal syndrome, in which patients with liver disease, usually with massive ascites, succumb to rapidly progressing acute kidney injury. The hepatorenal syndrome seems to be precipitated by intense and inappropriate renal vasoconstriction and is characterized by extreme sodium retention typical of prerenal azotemia, but in the absence of true volume depletion (see Chapter 16). Nonetheless, the presence of clinically apparent ascites in a patient with liver disease is associated with poor long-term survival. Over the years, various mechanisms have been proposed to explain ascites formation. No single hypothesis of pathogenesis easily explains all findings at all points in time during the natural history of portal hypertension. Portal hypertension and inappropriate renal sodium retention are important elements of all theories. The end result of ascites occurs when excess peritoneal fluid exceeds the capacity of lymphatic drainage, leading to increased hydrostatic pressure. The fluid can then be seen to visibly weep from the lymphatics and pool in the abdominal cavity as ascites.

The underfill/vasodilatation hypothesis proposes that the primary event in ascites formation is vascular, with a reduced effective circulating volume leading to the activation of the renin–angiotensin system and subsequent renal sodium retention. The classic underfill hypothesis postulates that elevated hepatic sinusoidal pressure leads to the sequestration of blood in the splanchnic venous bed. This results in underfilling of the central vein with diversion of intravascular volume to the hepatic lymphatics, which, like the central vein, drain the space of Disse. The peripheral arterial vasodilatation or splanchnic vasodilatation hypothesis adds the idea that, with portal-to-systemic shunting, vasodilatory products (eg, nitric oxide) normally cleared by the liver are instead delivered to the systemic circulation, where they cause peripheral arteriolar vasodilation, particularly in the splanchnic arterial bed. The resultant reduced arterial vascular resistance (Figure 14–17) is associated with decreased central filling pressures, decreased renal arterial perfusion, reflex renal arterial vasoconstriction, and increased renal tubular sodium resorption. Sodium retention expands the intravascular volume, which exacerbates portal venous hypertension. The imbalance between hydrostatic versus oncotic pressure in the portal vein results in ascites formation. Although the splanchnic vasodilatation hypothesis accounts for many of the findings in ascites formation, the use of transhepatic intrajugular portal-to-systemic shunting (TIPS) as a means of decompressing the portal vein in patients with ascites provides a counterargument. As a result of the procedure, peripheral arteriolar vasodilation appears to

FIGURE 14–17 Proposed mechanism for ascites formation in cirrhosis according to the splanchnic vasodilation hypothesis. This hypothesis incorporates elements of the underfill and vasodilation theories. (Redrawn, with permission, from Gines P et al. Management of cirrhosis and ascites. N Engl J Med. 2004;350:1646. Copyright © 2004 Massachusetts Medical Society. Reprinted, with permission, from Massachusetts Medical Society.)

increase (perhaps as a result of shunting vasodilators such as nitric oxide that are normally cleared by the liver), yet ascites is generally dramatically improved.

Those who support the overflow hypothesis have proposed that the primary event in the development of ascites is inappropriate renal sodium retention. In this view, ascites is the consequence of fluid overflow from the intravascular volume-expanded portal system into the peritoneal cavity. But what triggers the inappropriate renal sodium retention? One possibility is that there may exist a hepatorenal reflex by which elevated sinusoidal pressure triggers increased sympathetic tone or endothelin-1 secretion. Either of these pathways could cause an inappropriate degree of renal vasoconstriction, a decrease in glomerular filtration rate, and, by tubuloglomerular feedback (see Chapter 16), sodium retention. Note that endothelin-1 is both a renal vasoconstrictor and a stimulant of epinephrine secretion, which in turn stimulates more endothelin-1 secretion. Alternatively, it is possible that an as yet unidentified product from the diseased liver interferes with atrial natriuretic peptide (ANP) action at the kidney or is in some other way responsible for an inappropriate increase in renal sodium retention. Supporters of the overflow hypothesis point to the fact that many cirrhotic patients have sodium handling defects in the absence of ascites and do not have a measurable increase in renin–angiotensin activity. However, studies have shown that the renal sodium retention in these

patients can be reversed by the use of an angiotensin II receptor antagonist.

Most likely, multiple mechanisms contribute to the development of ascites and to its perpetuation, worsening, or improvement in diverse clinical situations. Regardless of the initial events, once fully established, many if not all of the mechanisms described in Figure 14–17 are likely to contribute to ascites formation.

C. Hepatorenal Syndrome

Hepatorenal syndrome refers to a distinct form of kidney injury resulting from renal vasoconstriction that develops in response to the systemic and splanchnic arterial vasodilation in patients with advanced liver disease. The incidence of hepatorenal syndrome in patients who develop decompensated liver disease is 18% within 1 year of diagnosis and up to 40% at 5 years. This disorder generally occurs in patients with cirrhosis and ascites. It is characterized by a progressive rise in serum creatinine (>1.5 mg/dL) with no improvement after 48 hours of withholding diuretics and volume expansion with albumin and in the absence of shock, ingestion of nephrotoxic agents, and underlying parenchymal kidney disease. The urine produced is notable for an extremely low sodium content (<10 mmol/L) and an absence of casts, resembling the findings in prerenal azotemia. Yet, when central venous pressures are measured, the patient does not show intravascular volume depletion, and the disorder does not respond to hydration with normal saline. The renal abnormalities of hepatorenal syndrome appear to be functional because no pathologic changes are identifiable in the kidney. In addition, when a kidney is transplanted from a patient dying of hepatorenal syndrome, it functions well in a recipient without liver disease. While diagnostic criteria for hepatorenal syndrome have been developed (and recently modified), diagnosing and differentiating hepatorenal syndrome from other causes of acute kidney injury in cirrhotic patients can be difficult. Other than hepatorenal syndrome, only acute tubular necrosis and other causes of prerenal azotemia are common in this setting.

Hepatorenal syndrome can be classified into two types, each having different clinical and prognostic characteristics. Type 1 hepatorenal syndrome is rapidly progressive with a doubling of the serum creatinine concentration to a level greater than 2.5 mg/dL in less than 2 weeks. It is associated with multiorgan failure. Patients with type 2 hepatorenal syndrome have less severe and more slowly progressive renal insufficiency, and usually ascites resistant to diuretics. The onset of hepatorenal syndrome can be dramatic or insidious. It can be precipitated by an acute event, such as infection (notably spontaneous bacterial peritonitis) or hypovolemia from GI bleeding or overdiuresis. The prognosis after developing hepatorenal syndrome is dismal (overall survival of 50% at 1 year). Untreated, type 1 patients survive only weeks, type 2 patients, only 4-6 months.

The pathophysiology of hepatorenal syndrome is related to the distinct hemodynamic and circulatory changes that occur in patients with severe hepatic dysfunction. Portal hypertension triggers arterial vasodilation in the splanchnic circulation and a subsequent reduction in systemic vascular resistance, which can no longer be compensated for by an augmented cardiac output. An increased production or activity of vasodilators within the splanchnic circulation, particularly nitric oxide, carbon monoxide, and endogenous cannabinoids, leads to such arterial vasodilation. In advanced cirrhosis, arterial pressure must be maintained through the activation of vasoconstrictor systems, including the renin–angiotensin system and the sympathetic nervous system, as well as by the excess secretion of antidiuretic hormone (arginine vasopressin). These compensatory mechanisms help maintain effective arterial blood volume and relatively normal arterial pressure but lead to intrarenal vasoconstriction and hypoperfusion, which impairs renal function. By the same mechanisms, affected patients may develop further retention of sodium and free water, worsening edema and ascites.

The best approach to the management of hepatorenal syndrome, based on knowledge of its pathogenesis, is the administration of vasoconstrictor drugs. Use of the vasopressin analog, terlipressin, together with albumin, can be considered as initial therapy for hepatorenal syndrome. Terlipressin is effective in approximately 40–50% of patients with type 1

hepatorenal syndrome; data on the use of vasoconstrictors in type 2 hepatorenal syndrome are limited. Renal replacement therapy in the form of hemodialysis or continuous venovenous hemofiltration has been used, particularly in patients awaiting transplantation or in those with acute, potentially reversible hepatorenal syndrome. There is no evidence, however, that renal replacement therapy improves the prognosis of patients with cirrhosis who are not candidates for a liver transplant. Liver transplantation remains the optimal treatment for patients with hepatorenal syndrome.

D. Hypoalbuminemia and Peripheral Edema

The progressive worsening of hepatocellular function in cirrhosis can result in a fall in the concentration of albumin and other serum proteins synthesized by the liver. As the concentration of these plasma proteins decreases, the plasma oncotic pressure is lowered, thereby tilting the balance of hemodynamic forces toward the development of both peripheral edema and ascites.

These hemodynamic changes further contribute to an avid sodium-retaining state despite the total body water and sodium overload seen by urinalysis in the cirrhotic patient. Serum sodium may be low as a result of superimposed water retention caused by antidiuretic hormone release triggered by volume stimuli. There are typically no obvious clinical manifestations until the serum sodium concentration falls below 120 mEq/L, at which point neurologic symptoms can occur. Attempts to raise the serum sodium, including fluid restriction and the administration of vasopressin receptor antagonists (eg, tolvaptan and conivaptan) are generally not recommended owing to adverse effects and lack of clear benefit. Hyponatremia is simply a late manifestation of end-stage liver disease and a strong predictor of mortality in patients with cirrhosis.

A low serum potassium and metabolic alkalosis may be observed as a consequence of elevated aldosterone levels responding to renin release (and angiotensin II release) by the kidneys, which sense afferent intravascular depletion.

E. Spontaneous Bacterial Peritonitis

Spontaneous bacterial peritonitis is defined as infection of ascitic fluid in the absence of an intra-abdominal event (such as a bowel perforation or another surgically treatable source) that would account for the entry of pathogenic organisms into the peritoneal space. This complication carries a high mortality rate and is predictive of poor overall prognosis. The presence of infection is confirmed by an elevated ascitic fluid absolute polymorphonuclear leukocyte count of 250 cells/μL or more and definitively confirmed by a positive ascitic fluid bacterial culture. Symptoms and signs include fever, hypotension, abdominal pain or tenderness, decreased or absent bowel sounds, and an abrupt onset of hepatic encephalopathy in a patient with ascites. Alternatively, patients with spontaneous bacterial peritonitis can have subtle or no symptoms, and hence, a high index of suspicion may be required for timely diagnosis.

Patients with advanced liver disease with large-volume ascites or very low ascitic fluid protein levels, a prior history of spontaneous bacterial peritonitis, and episodes of upper GI bleeding are at increased risk for this complication. Ascitic fluid is an excellent culture medium for a variety of pathogens, including Enterobacteriaceae (chiefly *Escherichia coli*), group D streptococci (enterococci), *Streptococcus pneumoniae*, and viridans streptococci. The greater risk in patients with low ascitic fluid protein levels may be due to a low level of opsonic activity in the fluid.

While the exact pathogenesis of spontaneous bacterial peritonitis is not known, cirrhosis predisposes to the development of GI bacterial overgrowth and increased intestinal permeability. Peritonitis may occur because of bacterial seeding of the ascitic fluid via the blood or lymph or by bacteria traversing the gut wall. Enteric organisms may also enter the portal venous blood via the portosystemic collaterals, bypassing the reticuloendothelial system of the liver.

F. Gastroesophageal Varices and Bleeding

As blood flow through the liver is progressively impeded, hepatic portal venous pressure rises. In response to the elevated portal venous pressure, there is a decrease in blood vessel wall thickness and an enlargement of blood vessels that anastomose with the portal vein, such as those on the surface of the bowel and lower esophagus. These enlarged vessels are termed **gastroesophageal varices**. They eventually develop in approximately 50% of patients with cirrhosis, generally when the portal hypertensive gradient exceeds 12 mm Hg. Physical examination may reveal an enlargement of hemorrhoidal and periumbilical vessels. Gastroesophageal varices are of more significance clinically, however, because of their tendency to rupture. Variceal hemorrhage occurs in 25–40% of patients with cirrhosis and is a leading cause of morbidity and mortality in these individuals. Each episode of active variceal bleeding is associated with a 30% mortality risk, and survivors have a 70% risk of recurrent bleeding within 1 year. GI bleeding from varices and other sources (eg, duodenal ulcer, gastritis) in patients with cirrhosis is often exacerbated by concomitant coagulopathy (see later discussion).

G. Hepatic Encephalopathy

Hepatic encephalopathy presents as a range of reversible neuropsychiatric abnormalities that occur as a consequence of advanced decompensated liver disease or portal-to-systemic shunting. Table 14–16 provides a list of common precipitants. Neuropsychiatric symptoms can be episodic or persistent. Changes in sleep pattern, starting with hypersomnia and progressing to a reversal of the sleep–wake cycle, are often an early sign. Cognitive changes range from mild confusion, apathy, and agitation to marked confusion, obtundation, and even coma. More advanced neurologic features include tremor,

TABLE 14–16   Common precipitants of hepatic encephalopathy.

Increased nitrogen load
Gastrointestinal bleeding
Excess dietary protein
Azotemia
Constipation
Electrolyte imbalance
Hypokalemia
Alkalosis
Hypoxia
Hypovolemia
Drugs
Opioids, tranquilizers, sedatives
Diuretics
Miscellaneous
Infection
Surgery
Superimposed acute liver disease
Progressive liver disease

Reproduced, with permission, from Podolsky DK et al. Cirrhosis of the liver. In: Wilson JD et al, eds. *Harrison's Principles of Internal Medicine*, 12th ed. McGraw-Hill, 1991.

bradykinesia, **asterixis** (flapping motions of outstretched, dorsiflexed hands), hyperactive deep tendon reflexes, and less commonly, transient decerebrate posturing and flaccidity. Cerebral edema, an important accompanying feature in patients with encephalopathy in acute liver disease, is not seen in cirrhotic patients with encephalopathy. Subtle changes of hepatic encephalopathy are present in up to 15% of patients with advanced liver disease and may only be detectable by a number of specialized measures, such as psychometric testing. Such patients have sometimes been referred to as having subclinical or minimal hepatic encephalopathy.

Hepatic encephalopathy is diagnosed by history and clinical features in the appropriate context and after excluding other causes of altered mental status. Common precipitants of encephalopathy are onset of GI bleeding, increased dietary protein intake, and an increased catabolic rate resulting from infection (including spontaneous bacterial peritonitis). Similarly, because of compromised first-pass clearance of ingested drugs, affected patients are exquisitely sensitive to sedatives and other drugs normally metabolized in the liver. Other causes include electrolyte imbalance as a result of diuretics, vomiting, alcohol ingestion or withdrawal, or procedures such as TIPS. TIPS also exacerbates hepatic encephalopathy given the direct bypass of portal venous blood flow into the systemic circulation via the hepatic vein, while bypassing the hepatic parenchyma.

The pathogenesis of hepatic encephalopathy is likely multifactorial and complex. One proposed mechanism is related to toxins in the gut such as ammonia, derived from the metabolic degradation of urea or protein; glutamine, derived from the degradation of ammonia; or mercaptans, derived from the degradation of sulfur-containing compounds; and manganese. Because of anatomic or functional portal–systemic shunts, these toxins bypass the liver's detoxification processes and produce alterations in mental status. Exposure to these toxins can cause astrocyte swelling and structural changes in neurons. In addition, high ammonia levels can result in abnormal cerebral blood flow and glucose metabolism. Increased levels of ammonia, glutamine, and mercaptans can be found in the blood and cerebrospinal fluid. There is also an increase in cerebral manganese deposition in patients with cirrhosis. However, blood ammonia and spinal fluid glutamine levels correlate poorly with the presence and severity of encephalopathy. In addition, the role of manganese in hepatic encephalopathy remains unclear.

Alternatively, there may be impairment in the normal blood–brain barrier, rendering the CNS susceptible to various noxious agents. Increased levels of other substances, including metabolic products such as short-chain fatty acids and endogenous benzodiazepine-like metabolites, have also been found in the blood. Importantly, some patients show improvement in encephalopathy when treated with flumazenil, a benzodiazepine receptor antagonist.

Another proposed mechanism postulates a role for GABA, the principal inhibitory neurotransmitter of the brain. GABA is produced in the gut, and increased levels are found in the blood of patients with liver failure. More recently, cerebral and systematic inflammation has been implicated in the pathogenesis of hepatic encephalopathy. Although the exact mechanisms are unknown, possibilities include cytokine-mediated changes in blood–brain barrier permeability, potential changes in glutamate uptake by astrocytes, and changes in the expression of GABA receptors.

Once the diagnosis is made, it is helpful to grade the severity of hepatic encephalopathy. Stages I through IV are based on degree of behavioral changes, intellectual dysfunction, and alterations in consciousness. Therapy includes the management of potential precipitants and is directed at reducing intestinal ammonia production or increasing the removal of ammonia from the circulation. Nonabsorbable synthetic disaccharides (eg, lactulose) are catabolized by colonic bacteria to short-chain fatty acids, which lower luminal pH. This change in pH favors the formation of ammonium (NH_4^+), which reduces the absorption of ammonia (NH_3) into the circulation. Disaccharides such as lactulose are thus the mainstay of therapy. As discussed above in the section Altered Metabolism of Ammonia, the antibiotic rifaximin

has been used in conjunction with lactulose to treat hepatic encephalopathy.

H. Coagulopathy

Factors contributing to coagulopathy in cirrhosis include loss of hepatic synthesis of clotting factors, some of which have a half-life of just a few hours. Under these circumstances, a minor or self-limited source of bleeding can become massive.

Hepatocytes are also functionally involved in the maintenance of a normal coagulation cascade through the absorption of vitamin K (a fat-soluble vitamin whose absorption depends on bile flow), which is necessary for the activation of some clotting factors (II, VII, IX, X). An ominous sign of the severity of liver disease is the development of a coagulopathy that does not respond to parenteral vitamin K, suggesting deficient clotting factor synthesis rather than impaired vitamin K absorption because of fat malabsorption. Finally, the loss of the liver's capacity to remove activated clotting factors and fibrin degradation products may play a role in the increased susceptibility to **disseminated intravascular coagulation**, a syndrome of coagulation factor consumption that results in uncontrolled simultaneous clotting and bleeding.

I. Splenomegaly and Hypersplenism

Enlargement of the spleen is a consequence of elevated portal venous pressure and the consequent engorgement of the organ. Thrombocytopenia and hemolytic anemia occur because of the sequestering of formed elements of the blood in the spleen, from which they are normally cleared as they age and are damaged.

J. Hepatocellular Carcinoma

The five-year cumulative risk of HCC in patients with cirrhosis ranges from 5% to 30% depending on the patient's sex, ethnicity, cause of liver disease, and stage of cirrhosis. In the United States, the incidence of HCC has been rising over the past few decades, with over 20,000 new cases diagnosed each year, attributable to the increased prevalence of NAFLD, HCV cirrhosis, and chronic HBV infections owing to immigration from high-prevalence regions. Several etiologic factors have been identified in the development of this tumor, although cirrhosis is present in the vast majority (80–90%) of patients who develop HCC.

The risk of developing HCC is increased 100-fold in those with chronic hepatitis B infection, and worldwide, HBV accounts for over 50% of all HCC cases and nearly all childhood cases. While HCC can occur in the absence of cirrhosis, over 70% of HBV-related cases occur in those with advanced fibrosis or cirrhosis. Risk factors for HCC in this population include male sex, older age or longer duration of infection, coinfection (HCV, HDV, HIV), mycotoxin aflatoxin exposure, genotype C, and, in particular, high levels of viral replication, as evidenced by a persistent elevation of HBV viral load.

In patients with chronic hepatitis C, the risk of developing HCC is increased 15- to 20-fold, with risk limited to those with advanced fibrosis and cirrhosis. It has been projected that the incidence of HCV-related HCC cases in the United States will continue to rise over the next several decades. Risk factors for developing HCC include male sex, older age and duration of chronic HCV infection, coinfections (HBV, HIV), heavy alcohol use, obesity, and metabolic factors. Importantly, HCV patients with advanced fibrosis remain at risk for HCC despite cure of infection, and ongoing surveillance for HCC is recommended.

Chronic hepatitis B and C account for 60–70% of all HCC cases in the United States. While any cause of cirrhosis can lead to HCC, alcoholic cirrhosis and nonalcoholic steatohepatitis account for most of the remaining U.S. cases. Obesity and metabolic syndrome are increasingly recognized as risk factors for liver cancer, and patients with NASH who have advanced fibrosis (both stage 3 and 4 fibrosis) have also been shown to be at heightened risk for HCC.

K. Pulmonary Complications

Up to one-third of patients with decompensated cirrhosis have problems associated with oxygenation and may present with shortness of breath. There are three main pulmonary complications of cirrhosis to consider: **hepatopulmonary syndrome**, **portopulmonary syndrome**, and **hepatic hydrothorax**. In addition, mild hypoxemia can be caused by massive ascites, with resulting diaphragmatic elevation and ventilation–perfusion mismatch.

Hepatopulmonary syndrome consists of the triad of advanced liver failure, hypoxemia, and intrapulmonary vascular dilation and shunting. The cause of pulmonary precapillary and capillary vasodilatation is unknown, but substances such as nitric oxide, endothelin, and arachidonic acid are thought to be involved. As a result of ventilation–perfusion mismatch, patients often present with platypnea, dyspnea that worsens in the upright position secondary to preferential perfusion of dilated vessels in the lung bases. Classically, contrast-enhanced echocardiography is used for definitive diagnosis and can reveal opacification of the left heart chambers within three to six cardiac cycles if a right-to-left intrapulmonary shunt is present. Liver transplantation leads to resolution of hepatopulmonary syndrome. However, the development of severe pulmonary hypertension in patients with advanced liver failure may be a contraindication to liver transplantation.

Portopulmonary hypertension refers to the development of pulmonary hypertension in patients with advanced liver disease and advanced portal hypertension. Patients can present with hypoxia, dyspnea on exertion, fatigue, and even signs of right heart failure. Patients have evidence of elevated pulmonary vascular resistance and a transpulmonary gradient in the setting of pulmonary arterial vasoconstriction. Targeted therapy (eg, epoprostenol, vasodilators) and management of right heart failure can delay progression, but prognosis is poor. Liver transplantation is associated with high operative risk when pulmonary hypertension becomes severe.

Individuals with cirrhosis and ascites can develop **hepatic hydrothorax** and present with shortness of breath, cough, or chest discomfort. In this condition, fluid accumulates in the pleural space owing to small defects in the diaphragm, most commonly on the right side. Negative intrathoracic pressure generated during inspiration favors the passage of fluid from the intra-abdominal cavity to the pleural space. Diagnostic thoracentesis should be performed to exclude alternative causes of pleural effusion, particularly infection. Treatment aims to prevent or reduce fluid accumulation with diuretics, a low-sodium diet, and occasionally therapeutic thoracentesis (or paracentesis to decrease pressure from tense ascites) for highly symptomatic patients refractory to or intolerant of conservative measures. TIPS may benefit selected patients (eg, Child–Pugh class A or B with no encephalopathy) who need repeated thoracenteses. If they are otherwise suitable candidates, patients with cirrhosis and persistent hepatic hydrothorax should be referred for liver transplantation.

L. Miscellaneous Manifestations

Other findings on physical examination of patients with cirrhosis include **spider angiomas** (prominent blood vessels with a central arteriole and small vessels radiating from it seen in the skin, particularly on the face and upper trunk), **Dupuytren contractures** (fibrosis of the palmar fascia), testicular atrophy, **gynecomastia** (enlargement of breast tissue in men), palmar erythema, lacrimal and parotid gland enlargement, and diminished axillary and pubic hair (see Figure 14–15). These findings are largely a consequence of estrogen excess resulting from the decreased clearance of endogenous estrogens by the diseased liver combined with the decreased hepatic synthesis of steroid hormone–binding globulin. Both mechanisms result in tissues receiving higher than normal concentrations of estrogens. In addition, the longer half-life of androgens may allow a greater degree of peripheral aromatization (conversion to estrogens by, eg, adipose tissue, hair follicles), further increasing estrogen-like effects in patients with cirrhosis. Xanthomas of the eyelids and extensor surfaces of tendons of the wrists and ankles can occur with chronic cholestasis such as occurs in primary biliary cirrhosis. Finally, profound muscle wasting and cachexia in cirrhosis probably reflect the diminution of the liver's synthesis of carbohydrate, lipid, and amino acids.

CHECKPOINT

31. What are the defining features of cirrhosis?
32. What are the three categories of hepatic fibrosis? Name one agent causing each.
33. What are the two postulated stages of the development of cirrhosis?
34. What are the major clinical manifestations of cirrhosis?
35. For each major clinical manifestation of cirrhosis, suggest a reasonable hypothesis to account for its pathogenesis.

CASE STUDIES

Yeong Kwok, MD

(See Chapter 25, p. 773–74 for answers)

CASE 77

A 28-year-old man, who recently emigrated from the Philippines, was noted to have a positive tuberculin skin test result in the clinic. His chest radiograph showed no active tuberculosis, and he denied any symptoms of this infection, including weight loss, cough, or night sweats. To prevent future disease, daily dosing with isoniazid was recommended for the next 9 months. Two weeks after initiating therapy, the patient reported progressive fatigue, intermittent bouts of nausea, and abdominal pain. He also noticed darkened urine and light-colored stools. His sister noted a gradual yellowing of his eyes and skin. Blood tests showed a marked increase in serum bilirubin and aminotransferases. The isoniazid was discontinued, and his symptoms subsided with his liver enzymes normalizing.

Questions

A. Describe the subtypes of toxic hepatitis.
B. What typical histologic findings are noted during uncomplicated acute hepatitis?
C. What is the pathogenesis of the clinical jaundice seen in this patient?

CASE 78

A 44-year-old man is concerned about abnormal liver tests drawn for his pre-employment physical 6 months ago. His serum aminotransferase levels were two times normal at that time and remain unchanged after repeat testing. On further questioning, he denies regular alcohol use but states that he used to inject heroin. Currently, he reports some fatigue but says he feels well otherwise. His primary care physician orders serologic testing, which reveals HBsAg-positive, anti-HBs-negative, and anti-HBc-positive IgG. Anti-HDV and anti-HCV test results are both negative.

Questions

A. Based on these antigen and antibody test results, what is the patient's diagnosis?
B. What percentage of patients with acute hepatitis B remain chronically infected with HBV? Of those patients, how many develop chronic active disease? What are the significant complications of chronic active infection?
C. What is the significance of hepatitis D superinfection?
D. What evidence exists supporting immune-mediated damage in chronic active hepatitis?

CASE 79

A 63-year-old man with a long history of alcohol use presents to his new primary care physician with a 6-month history of increasing abdominal girth. He has also noted easy bruisability and worsening fatigue. He denies any history of GI bleeding. He continues to drink three or four cocktails a night but says he is trying to cut down. Physical examination reveals a cachectic man who appears older than his stated age. Blood pressure is 108/70 mm Hg. His scleras are anicteric. His neck veins are flat, and chest examination demonstrates gynecomastia and multiple spider angiomas. Abdominal examination is significant for a protuberant abdomen with a detectable fluid wave, shifting dullness, and an enlarged spleen. The liver edge is difficult to appreciate. He has trace pitting pedal edema. Laboratory evaluation shows anemia, mild thrombocytopenia, and an elevated prothrombin time. Abdominal ultrasonogram confirms a shrunken, heterogeneous liver consistent with cirrhosis, significant ascites, and splenomegaly.

Questions

A. Describe possible mechanisms for alcohol-induced cirrhosis.
B. What is the proposed mechanism of portal hypertension, and how does it affect ascites formation?
C. Significant hematologic abnormalities exist in this patient. How might they be explained?

REFERENCES

General

Blasco-Algora S et al. Acute-on-chronic liver failure: pathogenesis, prognostic factors and management. World J Gastroenterol. 2015 Nov 14;21(42):12125–40. [PMID: 26576097]

Gossard AA et al. Cholestatic liver disease. Med Clin North Am. 2014 Jan;98(1):73–85. [PMID: 24266915]

Kim A. Hepatitis C virus. Ann Intern Med. 2016 Sep 6;165(5):ITC33–ITC48. [PMID: 27595226]

Lazaridis KN et al. The cholangiopathies. Mayo Clin Proc. 2015 Jun;90(6):791–800. [PMID: 25957621]

Nakanishi Y et al. Pathophysiology and diseases of the proximal pathways of the biliary system. Arch Pathol Lab Med. 2015 Jul;139(7):858–66. [PMID: 26125426]

Powell LW et al. Haemochromatosis. Lancet. 2016 Aug 13;388(10045):706–16. [PMID: 26975792]

Sanyal AJ et al, eds. *Zakim and Boyer's Hepatology: A Textbook of Liver Disease*, 7th ed. Elsevier, 2017.

Stickel F et al. Pathophysiology and management of alcoholic liver disease: update 2016. Gut Liver. 2017 Mar 15;11(2):173–88. Erratum in: Gut Liver. 2017 May 15;11(3):447. [PMID: 28274107]

Webster DP et al. Hepatitis C. Lancet. 2015 Mar 21;385(9973):1124–35. [PMID: 25687730]

Acute Hepatitis

AASLD/IDSA HCV Guidance Panel. Hepatitis C guidance: AASLD-IDSA recommendations for testing, managing, and treating adults infected with hepatitis C virus. Hepatology. 2015 Sep;62(3):932–54. [PMID: 26111063]

Abdou RM et al. Gut microbiota of nonalcoholic fatty liver disease. Dig Dis Sci. 2016 May;61(5):1268–81. [PMID: 26898658]

Carr RM et al. Nonalcoholic fatty liver disease: pathophysiology and management. Gastroenterol Clin North Am. 2016 Dec;45(4):639–52. [PMID: 27837778]

Dhingra S et al. Liver pathology of hepatitis C, beyond grading and staging of the disease. World J Gastroenterol. 2016 Jan 28;22(4):1357–66. [PMID: 26819505]

Dunn et al. Pathogenesis of alcoholic liver disease. Clin Liver Dis. 2016 Aug;20(3):445–56. [PMID: 27373608]

Farooq MO et al. Pathogenesis and management of alcoholic liver disease. Dig Dis. 2016;34(4):347–55. [PMID: 27170388]

Fisher K et al. Drug-induced liver injury. Arch Pathol Lab Med. 2015 Jul;139(7):876–87. [PMID: 26125428]

Katarey D et al. Drug-induced liver injury. Clin Med (Lond). 2016 Dec;16(Suppl 6):S104–S109. [PMID: 27956449]

Lhomme S et al. Hepatitis E pathogenesis. Viruses. 2016 Aug 5;8(8). pii: E212. [PMID: 27527210]

Liang R et al. Advances in alcoholic liver disease: an update on alcoholic hepatitis. World J Gastroenterol. 2015 Nov 14;21(42):11893–903. [PMID: 26576078]

Mosedale M et al. Drug-induced liver injury: advances in mechanistic understanding that will inform risk management. Clin Pharmacol Ther. 2017 Apr;101(4):469–80. [PMID: 27861792]

Nagy LE et al. Linking pathogenic mechanisms of alcoholic liver disease with clinical phenotypes. Gastroenterology. 2016 Jun;150(8):1756–68. [PMID: 26919968]

Sayed IM et al. Is hepatitis E virus an emerging problem in industrialized countries? Hepatology. 2015 Dec;62(6):1883–92. [PMID: 26175182]

Sureau C et al. The hepatitis delta virus: replication and pathogenesis. J Hepatol. 2016 Apr;64(1 Suppl):S102–16. [PMID: 27084031]

Vescovo T et al. Molecular mechanisms of hepatitis C virus–induced hepatocellular carcinoma. Clin Microbiol Infect. 2016 Oct;22(10):853–61. [PMID: 27476823]

Younossi Z et al. Extrahepatic manifestations of hepatitis C: a meta-analysis of prevalence, quality of life, and economic burden. Gastroenterology. 2016 Jun;150(7):1599–608. [PMID: 26924097]

Zhang YY et al. Rethinking the pathogenesis of hepatitis B virus (HBV) infection. J Med Virol. 2015 Dec;87(12):1989–99. [PMID: 25989114]

Chronic Hepatitis

Aizawa Y et al. Autoimmune hepatitis: current challenges and future prospects. Clin Exp Gastroenterol. 2017 Jan 19;10:9–18. [PMID: 28176894]

Al-Khafaji A et al. Hepatorenal disorders. Chest. 2015 Aug;148(2):550–8. [PMID: 25811649]

Balitzer D et al. Autoimmune hepatitis: review of histologic features included in the simplified criteria proposed by the International Autoimmune Hepatitis Group and proposal for new histologic criteria. Mod Pathol. 2017 May;30(5):773–83. [PMID: 28106105]

Bandiera S et al. Chronic hepatitis C virus infection and pathogenesis of hepatocellular carcinoma. Curr Opin Virol. 2016 Oct;20:99–105. [PMID: 27741441]

Bowles C et al. Primary and secondary sclerosing cholangitis. Chapter 43 in Sanyal AJ et al, eds. *Zakim and Boyer's Hepatology: A Textbook of Liver Disease*, 7th ed. Elsevier, 2017.

Carey EJ et al. Primary biliary cirrhosis. Lancet. 2015 Oct 17;386(10003):1565–75. Erratum in: Lancet. 2015 Oct 17;386(10003):1536. [PMID: 26364546]

Chang KM et al. Chronic hepatitis B: immune pathogenesis and emerging immunotherapeutics. Curr Opin Pharmacol. 2016 Oct;30:93–105. [PMID: 27570126]

Gidwaney NG et al. Pathogenesis and clinical spectrum of primary sclerosing cholangitis. World J Gastroenterol. 2017 Apr 14;23(14):2459–69. [PMID: 28465630]

Lohse AN et al. Autoimmune hepatitis. Chapter 41 in Sanyal AJ et al, eds. *Zakim and Boyer's Hepatology: A Textbook of Liver Disease*, 7th ed. Elsevier, 2017.

Machado MV et al. Pathogenesis of nonalcoholic fatty liver disease. Chapter 25 in Sanyal AJ et al, eds. *Zakim and Boyer's Hepatology: A Textbook of Liver Disease*, 7th ed. Elsevier, 2017.

Machado MV et al. Pathogenesis of nonalcoholic steatohepatitis. Gastroenterology. 2016 Jun;150(8):1769–77. [PMID: 26928243]

Negro F et al. Extrahepatic morbidity and mortality of chronic hepatitis C. Gastroenterology. 2015 Nov;149(6):1345–60. [PMID: 26319013]

Park BJ et al. Chronic liver inflammation: clinical implications beyond alcoholic liver disease. World J Gastroenterol. 2014 Mar 7;20(9):2168–75. [PMID: 24605015]

Patel A et al. Primary biliary cholangitis: disease pathogenesis and implications for established and novel therapeutics. J Clin Exp Hepatol. 2016 Dec;6(4)311–8. [PMID 28003721]

Purohit T et al. Primary biliary cirrhosis: pathophysiology, clinical presentation and therapy. World J Hepatol. 2015 May 8;7(7):926–41. [PMID: 25954476]

Rinella ME. Nonalcoholic fatty liver disease: a systematic review. JAMA. 2015 Jun 9;313(22):2263–73. Erratum in: JAMA. 2015 Oct 13;314(14):1521. [PMID: 26057287]

Sahebjam F et al. Autoimmune hepatitis. Front Med. 2015 Jun;9(2):187–219. [PMID: 25749982]

Sclair SN et al. Primary biliary cirrhosis. Chapter 42 in in Sanyal AJ et al, eds. *Zakim and Boyer's Hepatology: A Textbook of Liver Disease*, 7th ed. Elsevier, 2017.

Sebode M et al. Autoimmune hepatitis: from current knowledge and clinical practice to future research agenda. Liver Int. 2018 Jan;38(1):15–22. [PMID: 28432836]

Valva P et al. Chronic hepatitis C virus infection: serum biomarkers in predicting liver damage. World J Gastroenterol. 2016 Jan 28;22(4):1367–81. [PMID: 26819506]

Cirrhosis

Badillo R et al. Hepatic hydrothorax: clinical features, management, and outcomes in 77 patients and review of the literature. Medicine (Baltimore). 2014 May;93(3):135–42. [PMID: 24797168]

Kalra A et al. Changing prioritization for transplantation: MELD-Na, hepatocellular carcinoma exceptions, and more. Curr Opin Organ Transplant. 2016 Apr;21(2):120–6. [PMID: 26825358]

Peng Y et al. Child-Pugh versus MELD score for the assessment of prognosis in liver cirrhosis: a systematic review and meta-analysis of observational studies. Medicine (Baltimore). 2016 Feb;95(8):e2877. [PMID: 26937922]

Rzouq F et al. New insight into volume overload and hepatorenal syndrome in cirrhosis, "the hepatorenal reflex hypothesis." Am J Med Sci. 2014 Sep;348(3):244–8. [PMID: 24805785]

Tapper EB et al. Preventing and treating acute kidney injury among hospitalized patients with cirrhosis and ascites: a narrative review. Am J Med. 2016 May;129(5):461–7. [PMID: 26724589]

Terrault NA et al. Management of the patient with SVR [sustained virologic response]. J Hepatol. 2016 Oct;65(1 Suppl):S120–9. [PMID: 27641982]

Tsochatzis EA et al. Liver cirrhosis. Lancet. 2014 May 17;383(9930):1749–61. [PMID: 24480518]

Wong F. Renal failure in cirrhosis. Chapter 17 in Sanyal AJ et al, eds. *Zakim and Boyer's Hepatology: A Textbook of Liver Disease*, 7th ed. Elsevier, 2017.

Disorders of the Exocrine Pancreas

Timothy L. Frankel, MD, & Christopher J. Sonnenday, MD, MHS

The pancreas is a gland with both exocrine and endocrine functions. The exocrine pancreas contains **acini**, which secrete pancreatic juice into the duodenum through the pancreatic ducts (Figure 15–1). Pancreatic juice contains a number of enzymes, some of which are initially secreted as zymogens in an inactive form. Once activated, these enzymes help digest food and prepare it for absorption in the intestine. Disorders interfering with normal pancreatic enzyme activity (pancreatic insufficiency) cause fat maldigestion and steatorrhea (fatty stools). Pathology of the exocrine pancreas results from inflammation (acute pancreatitis, chronic pancreatitis), neoplasm (ductal adenocarcinoma, neuroendocrine tumors,

other pancreatic neoplasms), or duct obstruction by stones or abnormally viscid mucus (cystic fibrosis).

The endocrine pancreas is composed of the **islets of Langerhans**. The islets are distributed throughout the pancreas and contain several different hormone-producing cells. The islet cells manufacture hormones such as insulin that are important in nutrient absorption, storage, and metabolism. Dysfunction of the endocrine pancreas may cause diabetes mellitus (see Chapter 18).

Exocrine and endocrine pancreatic dysfunction may occur together in some patients.

NORMAL STRUCTURE & FUNCTION OF THE EXOCRINE PANCREAS

ANATOMY

The pancreas is a solid organ that lies transversely in the retroperitoneum deep within the epigastrium. It is firmly fixed by fibrous attachments anterior to the suprarenal aorta and the first and second lumbar vertebrae. Thus, the pain of acute or chronic pancreatitis is situated deep in the epigastric region and frequently radiates to the back.

The normal pancreas is about 15 cm long and weighs less than 110 g. The organ is covered by a thin capsule of connective tissue that sends septa into it, separating it into lobules. The pancreas can be divided into four parts: the head, including the uncinate process; neck; body; and tail. The head is the thickest part of the gland (2–4 cm) and lies in the "C-loop" or curved space between the first, second, and third portions of the duodenum. The uncinate process is the portion of the head that extends dorsally and to the left, behind the superior mesenteric vessels. The neck connects the head and body and sits immediately ventral to the superior mesenteric vessels.

The body is situated transversely in the retroperitoneal space, bordered superiorly by the splenic artery and dorsally by the splenic vein. The tail of the pancreas is less fixed in the retroperitoneum and extends toward, and often immediately adjacent to, the hilum of the spleen.

Embryologically, the pancreas develops as two separate endodermal buds from the developing foregut. These separate dorsal and ventral elements of the primordial pancreas initially develop opposite each other but, with rotation of the primitive gut, end up fusing together toward the left of the duodenum. The development of the dorsal and ventral buds is regulated by a complex process of intrinsic signals from the endodermal cells themselves, as well as extrinsic signals from surrounding mesoderm. The dorsal bud differentiates into the more cephalad and anterior portion of the pancreatic head, as well as the neck, body, and tail of the pancreas. The dorsal bud contains the accessory pancreatic duct (**duct of Santorini**), which enters the duodenum at the minor papilla. The smaller ventral bud arises adjacent to the bile duct to become the more

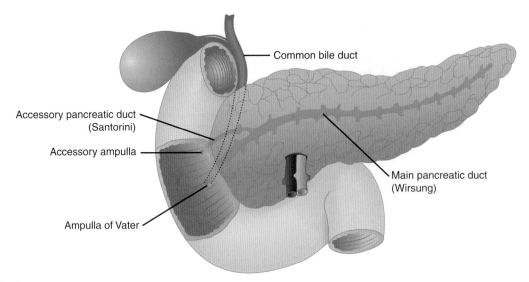

FIGURE 15–1 Anatomy of the pancreas.

caudal portion of the pancreatic head and the uncinate process. The ventral bud contains the major pancreatic duct (**duct of Wirsung**), which enters the duodenum at the **ampulla of Vater** (see Figure 15–1) together with the common bile duct. As cellular and mesenchymal elements differentiate, the dorsal and ventral buds develop a conjoined ductal system, and the whole organ eventually takes its place in the retroperitoneum of the upper abdomen. Primitive neuroendocrine cells arise amid the developing ductal structures and eventually form the interspersed islets of Langerhans.

The major pancreatic duct of Wirsung normally becomes the site of drainage for the majority of the pancreatic parenchyma. This duct is normally about 3–4 mm in diameter. In most individuals, the pancreatic duct enters the duodenum at the duodenal papilla alongside the common bile duct, surrounded by the sphincter of Oddi, which controls the drainage of both ducts. In about one-third of individuals, the duct of Wirsung and the common bile duct join to form a common channel before terminating at the ampulla of Vater (see Figure 15–1).

Pancreas divisum, the most common congenital anomaly of the pancreas, occurs when the embryologic ventral and dorsal components of the pancreas fail to fuse, thus leaving two distinct ductal systems that do not communicate and that separately drain into the duodenum through two different papillae. The smaller system drains through the major papilla, but the dominant dorsal system drains through the minor papilla. This situation can cause a relative obstruction to the flow of pancreatic juice and may be associated with the development of pancreatitis. Pancreas divisum is found in up to 7% of autopsy series.

HISTOLOGY

The exocrine pancreas consists of clusters of enzyme-secreting acini centered around and individually drained by ductules. The islets of Langerhans of the endocrine pancreas

are clusters of a few hundred hormone-secreting cells, each located between the lobules.

Each pancreatic acinus is composed of several acinar cells surrounding a lumen (Figure 15–2). Centroacinar cells are centrally located in the acini, interpositioned between the acinar cells and ductal epithelium. The centroacinar cells are believed to have a primary role in secreting electrolytes and water into the pancreatic ductal system. The acinar cells synthesize and secrete enzymes. On histologic examination, acinar cells are typical exocrine glandular cells. They are pyramidal epithelial cells arranged in rows. Their apexes join to form the lumen of the acinus. **Zymogen granules** containing digestive enzymes or their precursors are found in the acinar cells. These granules are discharged by exocytosis from the apexes of the cells into the lumen. The number of zymogen granules in the cells varies; more are found during fasting and fewer after a meal.

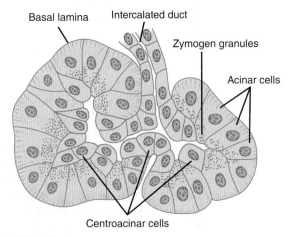

FIGURE 15–2 Schematic drawing of the pancreatic acini. Acinar cells are pyramidal in shape, with zymogen granules at their apexes. (Redrawn, with permission, from Junqueira LC et al, eds. *Basic Histology*, 10th ed. McGraw-Hill, 2003.)

Acini are centered on small branches of the pancreatic duct, which eventually converge to form the continuous lumen of the main pancreatic duct. The mature ducts are lined with a continuous layer of ductal epithelial cells, joined by tight junctions. The ductal epithelium contributes to the secretion of water and electrolytes into pancreatic secretions and forms the important epithelial barrier separating the pancreatic parenchyma from the enzyme-rich ductal secretions. Compromise of this epithelial barrier owing to inflammation or trauma may be associated with significant peripancreatic inflammation and severe clinical sequelae.

PHYSIOLOGY

Composition of Pancreatic Juice

As much as 1500 mL of pancreatic juice is secreted each day by a normal pancreas. Disease states (eg, chronic pancreatitis) may be associated with a marked decrease in exocrine pancreatic secretion. Pancreatic juice contains water, ions, and a variety of proteins. The principal ions in pancreatic juice are HCO_3^-, Cl^-, Na^+, and K^+. Of these, HCO_3^- is particularly important. At maximum flow rates, the concentration of HCO_3^- in pancreatic juice may reach 150 mEq/L (vs. 24 mEq/L in plasma), and the pH of the juice may reach 8.3. The alkaline nature of pancreatic juice plays a major role in neutralizing the gastric acid entering the duodenum with ingested food (chyme) from the stomach. The pH of duodenal contents rises to 6.0–7.0, and by the time the chyme reaches the jejunum, its pH is nearly neutral.

Proteomic analysis suggests that more than 200 proteins exist in pancreatic secretions. Many of these ubiquitous proteins have various roles in cellular growth and signaling, whereas others are engaged in cellular immunology. The remainder of the pancreatic proteins secreted are responsible for the digestive functions of the exocrine pancreas. A primary function of the pancreas is the digestion of proteins, which is mediated by trypsinogen and other secreted proteases. However, the exocrine pancreas also secretes enzymes responsible for metabolism and the absorption of lipids (lipase, colipase) and carbohydrates (amylase, enolase).

Some of the pancreatic enzymes (lipase, amylase, deoxyribonuclease, ribonuclease) are secreted by the acinar cells in their active forms. The remaining enzymes are secreted as inactive proenzymes or **zymogens** (trypsinogen, chymotrypsinogen, proelastase, procarboxypeptidase, and phospholipase A_2) that are activated in the lumen of the proximal intestine. Aberrant activation of zymogens within the acinar cell is hypothesized to lead to acute pancreatitis and pancreatic autodigestion.

When the pancreatic juice enters the duodenum, trypsinogen is converted to the active form trypsin by an enzyme called enteropeptidase, found in the intestinal brush border. Trypsin then converts the remaining proenzymes into active enzymes (eg, chymotrypsinogen into chymotrypsin). Trypsin can also activate its own precursor, trypsinogen, producing the potential for an autocatalytic chain reaction.

When trypsinogen is activated within the pancreas itself, two known protective mechanisms are available. First is the inhibition of activated trypsin by pancreatic secretory trypsin inhibitor (PSTI), also known as serine protease inhibitor, Kazal type 1 (or SPINK1), which can inhibit approximately 20% of trypsin activity. If trypsin activity overwhelms the SPINK1/PSTI inhibitory capacity, trypsin inactivation can then occur through trypsin autolysis.

Regulation of Pancreatic Juice Secretion

Recent advances in our understanding of pancreatic exocrine function reveal hormonal and neural factors as two distinct but interactive elements that regulate secretion. Two hormones in particular appear to have a primary role in the secretion of pancreatic enzymes: **secretin** and **cholecystokinin** (**CCK**). Both hormones are produced by specialized enteroendocrine cells of the duodenal mucosa and act by distinct but synergistic intracellular pathways on the pancreatic acinar cells.

The secretion of secretin is triggered by gastric acid and by the products of protein digestion in the duodenum. Secretin acts chiefly on the pancreatic ductal epithelial, centroacinar, and to a lesser extent acinar cells to produce HCO_3^-, thus raising the pH of pancreatic secretions. The secretion of H_2O also increases in response to secretin, increasing the absolute volume of pancreatic juice. Mechanistic studies have demonstrated that secretin and the related hormone vasoactive intestinal peptide (VIP) act on ductal and acinar cells by activating adenylate cyclase and, subsequently, cAMP-dependent protein kinase A. Proteomic analysis has revealed that secretin does not appear to alter the constituents of pancreatic juice but instead regulates the relative proportions of secreted enzymes.

The secretion of CCK is triggered by the products of protein and fat digestion (peptides, amino acids, fatty acids) when they enter the duodenum. The release of CCK from specific intestinal cells appears to be regulated by a cholecystokinin-releasing peptide in the proximal small intestine that is trypsin sensitive and active in the lumen. CCK controls pancreatic exocrine secretion through two mechanisms: (1) activating neurons located in the dorsal motor nucleus of the vagus motor neurons that control parasympathetic signals; and (2) directly acting on pancreatic acinar cells. CCK release raises intracellular Ca^{2+} concentrations, which lead to the release of pancreatic enzymes from the zymogen granules. The related enteric hormones acetylcholine and gastrin-releasing peptide (GRP) appear to act by similar calcium-dependent pathways. The integrated action of secretin and CCK produces an abundant secretion of enzyme-rich, alkaline pancreatic juice.

When both cAMP and calcium-dependent pathways are stimulated, the effect within the acinar cell is greater than the sum of their individual activities. Thus, CCK and secretin appear to act synergistically in response to a meal to stimulate the production of a large volume of alkaline pancreatic juice rich in digestive enzymes. Recent evidence also implicates a number of other gastrointestinal (GI) hormones and peptides (ghrelin, leptin, melatonin) in the regulation of pancreatic endocrine and exocrine secretion.

Digestive Functions of Pancreatic Juice

The secretion of pancreatic juice aids digestion in several ways. The large amount of bicarbonate in the juice helps to neutralize the acidic chyme from the stomach so that the pancreatic enzymes can function optimally in a neutral pH range.

Each enzyme also has an important digestive function. In digesting carbohydrates, pancreatic **amylase** splits straight-chain glucose polysaccharides (so-called amyloses in starch) into smaller α-limit dextrins: maltose and maltotriose. Brush border enzymes in the small intestine complete the hydrolysis of these smaller sugars into glucose, which is transported across the intestinal epithelium by Na^+-coupled transport. Pancreatic **lipase** contributes to fat metabolism by hydrolyzing triglycerides into fatty acids and a monoglyceride; this activity is most efficient in the presence of bile acids, which serve to emulsify the triglycerides. **Phospholipase A_2** splits a fatty acid off from lecithin to form lysolecithin. **Ribonuclease** and **deoxyribonuclease** attack the nucleic acids. The remaining enzymes help digest proteins. **Trypsin**, **chymotrypsin**, and **elastase** are endopeptidases (ie, they cleave peptide bonds in the middle of polypeptide chains). **Carboxypeptidase** is an exopeptidase (ie, it splits peptide bonds adjacent to the carboxyl terminals of peptide chains). Together, these proteases break down proteins into oligopeptides and free amino acids.

CHECKPOINT

1. What histologic features are associated with the pancreatic secretion of digestive enzymes into the GI tract?
2. What is the volume, composition, and function of pancreatic juice?
3. What are the neural and hormonal controls over exocrine pancreatic function?
4. Why does trypsinogen not self-activate before arriving in the duodenum?

PATHOPHYSIOLOGY OF SELECTED EXOCRINE PANCREATIC DISORDERS

ACUTE PANCREATITIS

Clinical Presentations

Acute pancreatitis is a clinical syndrome resulting from acute inflammation and destructive autodigestion of the pancreas and peripancreatic tissues. Acute pancreatitis is the third most common indication for hospital admission among GI diseases and is associated with significant morbidity and mortality. Data from the National Center for Health Statistics clearly document a near doubling of cases of hospital admissions owing to acute pancreatitis between 1985 and 2005, with a less dramatic but persistent increase over the following decade. Fortunately, the overall survival rate of patients with acute pancreatitis is increasing (less than 1% mortality for all patients with acute pancreatitis admitted to U.S. hospitals), though patients with severe acute pancreatitis continue to face a high mortality rate (20–25%) among patients requiring intensive care unit admission.

Etiology

Acute pancreatitis has many causes, as summarized in Table 15–1. In clinical practice, biliary tract disease and alcohol ingestion account for the majority of cases, with metabolic causes, mechanical etiologies, drug reactions, and traumatic injuries accounting for almost all of the remaining cases. Regardless of etiology, the pathogenesis of pancreatic injury, associated systemic effects, and risk factors for severe acute pancreatitis appear to be similar.

Alcohol use is commonly associated with acute pancreatitis in developed countries. Acute pancreatitis typically occurs after a binge of heavy drinking; chronic heavy alcohol ingestion may lead to chronic pancreatitis and may increase susceptibility to episodes of acute pancreatitis. A number of mechanisms are responsible for alcohol-induced damage to the pancreas. Alcohol or its metabolite, acetaldehyde, can have a direct toxic effect on pancreatic acinar cells, leading to intracellular trypsin activation by the lysosomal enzymes. Additionally, inflammation of the sphincter of Oddi may lead to the retention of hydrolytic enzymes in the pancreatic duct and acini. Alcohol also appears to increase the precipitation of pancreatic secretions to form "protein plugs" in the small ductules. Malnutrition may predispose patients with alcoholism to pancreatic injury. For example, deficiencies of trace elements such as zinc or selenium occur in these patients with alcoholism and are associated with acinar cell injury. Metalloenzymes, such as superoxide dismutase, catalase, and glutathione peroxidase, are important scavengers of free radicals. Interestingly, acute pancreatitis occurs in less than 2–3% of heavy drinkers, suggesting that other cofactors may play a role in the pathogenesis of this disease. Tobacco use has been demonstrated to increase the incidence of acute pancreatitis among heavy drinkers.

In patients who do not drink alcohol, the most common cause of acute pancreatitis is biliary tract disease. In such cases, the hypothesized mechanism is obstruction of the common bile duct and the main pancreatic duct when a gallstone or biliary sludge becomes lodged at the ampulla of Vater. Reflux of bile or pancreatic secretions into the pancreatic duct leads

TABLE 15–1   Causes of acute pancreatitis.

Alcohol ingestion (acute or chronic alcoholism)	**Drugs**
Biliary tract disease	Definite association
Trauma	Immunosuppressives: azathioprine, mercaptopurine
Blunt abdominal trauma	Diuretics: thiazides, furosemide
Postoperative	Antimicrobials: sulfonamides, tetracyclines, pentamidine, didanosine, metronidazole, erythromycin
Post–endoscopic retrograde cannulation of pancreatic duct, injection of pancreatic duct	Steroids: estrogens, oral contraceptives, corticosteroids, ACTH
Post–electric shock	Miscellaneous: valproic acid, metformin, intravenous lipid infusion
Infections	Probable association
Viral: mumps, rubella, coxsackievirus B, echovirus, viral hepatitis A and B, adenovirus, cytomegalovirus, varicella, Epstein–Barr virus, HIV	Immunosuppressives: asparaginase
	Diuretics: ethacrynic acid, chlorthalidone
Bacterial: *Mycoplasma pneumoniae*, *Salmonella typhi*, group A streptococci (scarlet fever), staphylococci, actinomycosis, *Mycobacterium tuberculosis*, *Mycobacterium avium* complex, *Legionella*, *Campylobacter jejuni*, *Leptospira icterohaemorrhagiae*	Miscellaneous: procainamide, cimetidine, ranitidine, sulfasalazine
	Possible association
	Antimicrobials: isoniazid, rifampin, nitrofurantoin
Parasitic: *Ascaris lumbricoides*, hydatid cyst, *Clonorchis sinensis*	Analgesics: acetaminophen, salicylates, sulindac, other NSAIDs
Metabolic	Miscellaneous: methyldopa
Hyperlipidemia, apolipoprotein CII deficiency syndrome, hypertriglyceridemia	**Vascular**
	Vasculitis: systemic lupus erythematosus, polyarteritis nodosa, malignant hypertension, thrombotic thrombocytopenic purpura
Hypercalcemia (eg, hyperparathyroidism)	
Uremia	Shock, hypoperfusion, myocardial or mesenteric infarction
Post–renal transplant	Atheromatous embolism
Pregnancy, eclampsia	**Mechanical**
Hemochromatosis, hemosiderosis	Pancreas divisum with accessory duct obstruction
Malnutrition: kwashiorkor, sprue, post-gastrectomy, Whipple disease	Ampulla of Vater stenosis, tumor, obstruction (regional enteritis, duodenal diverticulum, duodenal surgery, worms, foreign bodies)
Diabetic ketoacidosis	
Hereditary	Choledochocele
Familial pancreatitis	Penetrating duodenal ulcer
Cystic fibrosis	Pancreatic carcinoma
Poisons and toxins	**Idiopathic**
Venom: scorpion (*Tityus trinitatis*)	
Inorganic: zinc, cobalt, mercuric chloride, saccharated iron oxide	
Organic: methanol, organophosphates	

to parenchymal injury. Others have proposed that bacterial toxins or free bile acids travel via lymphatics from the gallbladder to the pancreas, giving rise to inflammation. In either case, acute pancreatitis associated with biliary tract disease is more common in women because gallstones are more common in women.

A significant proportion of "gallstone" pancreatitis is not associated with discrete, measurable gallstones passing through the bile duct and obstructing the ampulla. Instead, biliary sludge, or **microlithiasis**, is believed to play an etiologic role in many cases of pancreatitis previously classified as idiopathic. Endoscopic retrograde cholangiopancreatography

(ERCP) performed in such cases often identifies microlithiasis and viscous particulate bile in the distal common bile duct, which can cause transient biliary obstruction and activate the same mechanistic pathways that lead to pancreatitis as happens with larger gallstones. An alternative mechanism that has been proposed is a recurrent passage of microlithiasis causing papillary stenosis or sphincter of Oddi dysfunction.

Thus, the absence of obvious gallstones on imaging studies does not definitively rule out a biliary cause of acute pancreatitis. Biliary microlithiasis may be suspected when an ultrasound shows low-level echoes that gravitate toward the dependent portion of the gallbladder without the acoustic shadowing typical of gallstones. Microlithiasis is documented when cholesterol monohydrate crystals and calcium bilirubinate granules are found on light microscopy of an endoscopically acquired, centrifuged specimen of bile. In clinical practice, this diagnosis is often made in a patient with an appropriate presentation and with risk factors for biliary microlithiasis including pregnancy, rapid weight loss, critical illness, prolonged fasting, total parenteral nutrition, administration of certain drugs (ceftriaxone, octreotide), and bone marrow or solid organ transplantation.

Acute pancreatitis may result from a variety of infectious agents, including viruses (mumps virus, coxsackievirus, hepatitis A virus, HIV, cytomegalovirus) and bacteria (*Salmonella typhi*, hemolytic streptococci). Patients with HIV infection can develop acute pancreatitis from the HIV infection itself, from related opportunistic infections, or from antiretroviral therapies. In HIV-infected patients, pancreatitis has been associated with intravenous drug abuse, pentamidine therapy, *Pneumocystis jirovecii* and *Mycobacterium avium-intracellulare* infections, and gallstones.

Blunt or penetrating trauma and other injuries may cause acute pancreatitis. Pancreatitis sometimes occurs after surgical procedures near the pancreas (duodenal stump syndrome, pancreatic tail syndrome after splenectomy). Shock and hypothermia may cause decreased perfusion, resulting in cellular degeneration and a release of pancreatic enzymes. Radiation therapy of retroperitoneal malignant neoplasms can sometimes cause acute pancreatitis, likely through injury to the microvasculature and acinar architecture.

Marked hypercalcemia, such as that associated with hyperparathyroidism, sarcoidosis, hypervitaminosis D, or multiple myeloma, causes acute pancreatitis in about 10% of cases. Two mechanisms have been hypothesized. The high plasma calcium concentration may cause calcium to precipitate in the pancreatic duct, leading to ductal obstruction. Alternatively, hypercalcemia may stimulate the activation of trypsinogen in the pancreatic duct.

Pancreatitis is also associated with hyperlipidemia, particularly those types characterized by increased plasma levels of chylomicrons (types I, IV, and V). In these cases, it is postulated that free fatty acids liberated by the action of pancreatic lipase cause gland inflammation and injury. Alcohol abuse or oral contraceptive use increases the risk of acute pancreatitis in patients with hyperlipidemia.

A variety of drugs have been associated with pancreatitis, including corticosteroids, thiazide diuretics, immunosuppressants, and cancer chemotherapeutic agents.

Rarely, acute pancreatitis may be familial, occurring with an autosomal dominant inheritance pattern. **Hereditary pancreatitis** typically presents as recurring acute pancreatitis in childhood, progressing to chronic pancreatitis by young adulthood in more than 50% of cases. Hereditary recurrent acute pancreatitis has been associated with **mutations of the cationic trypsinogen gene** (*protease, serine, 1; PRSS1*) mapped to chromosome 7q35. Two point mutations, R122H and N29I, account for most cases and can be detected by genetic testing. Studies have suggested that the R122H mutation is associated with more severe acute pancreatitis, leading to more frequent attacks and hospital admissions. Other families have mutations in *SPINK1/PSTI*. It appears that mutations in cationic trypsinogen enhance trypsinogen autoactivation by altering calcium-mediated regulatory pathways, and mutations in *SPINK1/PSTI* diminish the inhibition of active trypsinogen. Other mutations eliminate the trypsin autolysis site. Patients demonstrated to have hereditary pancreatitis should be enrolled in a pancreatic cancer surveillance program, and total pancreatectomy should be considered in select cases, as approximately 40% of affected patients develop pancreatic cancer by age 70 years.

In recent years, our understanding of the diagnosis and classification of **autoimmune pancreatitis** has evolved. This chronic disease of fibrosis and lymphoplasmacytic inflammation may cause both acute episodes of pancreatitis as well as chronic injury. Two subtypes have been characterized. **Type I autoimmune pancreatitis** accounts for more than 80% of cases in the United States and is associated with elevated serum levels of IgG4 and with lymphocytic infiltration throughout the pancreatic parenchyma. Many patients with type I autoimmune pancreatitis have extrapancreatic manifestations and are often classified as having IgG4-related disease. Of note, type I autoimmune pancreatitis most commonly presents with distal biliary obstruction and jaundice, mimicking periampullary malignancy. Acute pancreatitis is a less common presentation. **Type II autoimmune pancreatitis** is more common outside the United States and does not appear to be IgG4 mediated. The pathognomonic histopathologic findings in this disease are granulocyte-epithelial lesions with neutrophilic infiltration. Type II autoimmune pancreatitis more often presents with acute pancreatitis compared with type I disease.

In about 15–25% of cases of acute pancreatitis, no etiologic factor can be identified. **Idiopathic acute recurrent pancreatitis** is seen in patients with more than one attack of acute pancreatitis when the underlying cause eludes detection despite a thorough search.

Pathology

The symptoms, signs, laboratory findings, and complications of acute pancreatitis can be explained on the basis of the pathologic damage to the ductules, acini, and islets of the pancreas. However, both the degree of damage and the clinical consequences are quite variable.

When the damage is limited in extent, the pathologic features consist of mild to marked gland swelling, especially in the acini, and mild to marked infiltration with polymorphonuclear neutrophils. However, tissue damage is usually only minimal to moderate, and there is no hemorrhage. In some cases, suppuration may be found along with edema, and this may result in tissue necrosis and abscess formation. In severe cases, massive necrosis and liquefaction of the pancreas occur, predisposing to pancreatic abscess formation. Vascular necrosis and disruption may occur, resulting in peripancreatic hemorrhage. While microvascular hemorrhage involving peripancreatic tissue is common in severe cases of acute pancreatitis, significant bleeding from large-vessel erosion is a rare clinical entity and is more often seen in chronic pancreatitis.

Severe cases of pancreatitis may be associated with the formation of ascites, which is likely a combination of serous fluid excreted by the inflamed peritoneal surface, liquefied peripancreatic fat, blood from peripancreatic tissues, and necrotic pancreatic debris. In rare cases associated with ductal disruption of the pancreas, the ascites may contain frank pancreatic secretions rich in amylase and other pancreatic enzymes. Documentation of amylase-rich peritoneal fluid establishes the diagnosis of so-called pancreatic ascites. In cases of severe acute pancreatitis, the peritoneal surfaces have a characteristic appearance upon surgical exploration or autopsy; fat necrosis, or saponification, may occur in and around the pancreas, omentum, and mesentery, appearing as chalky white foci that may later calcify.

Histologic studies of pancreas tissue obtained from patients with first attacks of acute alcoholic pancreatitis who underwent surgery for complications have found that the acute pancreatitis (pancreatic necrosis, steatonecrosis, infiltration by inflammatory cells) sometimes develops in a gland already affected by chronic pancreatitis (perilobular and intralobular fibrosis, loss of exocrine parenchyma and atrophy of residual lobules, dilated interlobular and intralobular ducts lined with cuboidal or flattened epithelium, and protein plugs within dilated ducts). It has been conjectured that, if acute alcoholic pancreatitis develops in a pancreas already affected by chronic pancreatitis, it is a result of obstruction of the ducts by protein plugs, an early lesion of chronic pancreatitis.

Pathogenesis

The pathogenesis of acute pancreatitis remains only partially understood. The central theory in this disease has long centered on the aberrant activation of trypsinogen and other enzymes within the pancreatic acini, causing autodigestion and a profound systemic inflammatory response. Recent evidence suggests that other events parallel to trypsinogen activation occur, such as the activation of nuclear factor kappa-light-chain-enhancer of activated B cells (NFκB), a protein complex that controls DNA transcription, which can induce acute pancreatitis in experimental models (Figure 15–3). However,

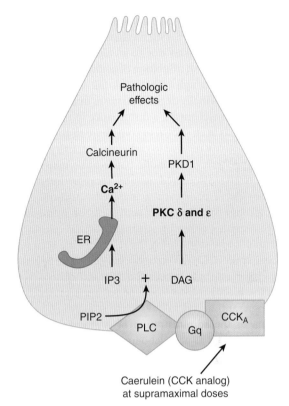

FIGURE 15–3 This schematic shows parallel cell signaling pathways producing the pathologic effects, presumed to be trypsinogen and NFκB activation, leading to pancreatitis. At the bottom, caerulein (a CCK analog) binds to its receptor, cholecystokinin receptor subtype A (CCK$_A$), and leads, via G-protein q subtype (Gq) and phospholipase C (PLC), to the generation of inositol-3 phosphate (IP3) from phosphoinositol 4-phosphate (PIP2) and to the generation of diacylglycerol (DAG). On the left, IP3 opens its endoplasmic reticulum (ER) membrane receptors, receptors implicated in physiologic calcium signaling. The calcium thus released leads caerulein to the pathologic effects inducing pancreatitis. On the right, DAG stimulates the release of two forms of protein kinase C (PKC), which in turn leads to the generation of protein kinase D subtype 1 (PKD1) and the pathologic effects inducing pancreatitis. (Redrawn, with permission, from Sah RP et al. Molecular mechanisms of pancreatic injury. Curr Opin Gastroenterol. 2011 Sept; 27(5):448.)

elegant studies have confirmed that the expression of active trypsin within pancreatic acini is itself sufficient to induce cell death and inflammation in acute pancreatitis. Thus, the in vivo role of alternative mechanisms of pancreatic autodigestion remains unclear.

Trypsinogen activation is associated with a sustained cytosolic influx of calcium (Ca^{2+}) mediated by calcium channels in the plasma membrane as well as by calcium receptors in the endoplasmic reticulum. Calcineurin is a likely downstream target of elevated intracellular Ca^{2+} levels, mediating some of the injury observed in acute pancreatitis via T-cell activation.

Trypsinogen is likely activated within membrane-bound intracellular compartments that exhibit dysregulated autophagy in the setting of acute pancreatitis. While cathepsin B within lysosomes has been shown to activate trypsinogen, this likely occurs only in certain pathologic conditions, such as a low intracellular pH. The mechanism of pH disturbance within acinar cells is likely due to an alteration in cell signaling mechanisms and an inhibition of acinar bicarbonate secretion. Moreover, although cathepsin L (an alternative isoform of cathepsin B) normally degrades trypsin in an important cellular protective mechanism, a disturbance in the intracellular environment has been shown to contribute to an imbalance in cathepsin B activity relative to cathepsin L activity.

The pathogenesis of alcoholic pancreatitis may be unique and may involve disordered agonist–receptor interaction on the membrane of pancreatic acinar cells. According to this theory, alcohol increases the activation of intrapancreatic digestive enzymes, either by sensitizing acinar cells to pathologic stimuli or by stimulating the release of the secretagogue cholecystokinin (CCK) from duodenal cells. The hyperstimulation of pancreatic acinar cells and their muscarinic receptors mimics the mechanism of acute pancreatitis caused by scorpion stings, anti-acetylcholinesterase-containing insecticide poisoning, or the administration of supramaximal doses of secretagogues such as acetylcholine and CCK. CCK receptor activation can initiate different patterns of zymogen activation in pancreatic acinar cells, and the extent of activation is enhanced by a distinct set of short-chain alcohols. Whether ethanol or other alcohols mediate these effects by interfering with acinar cell signaling pathways or by affecting acinar cell membrane fluidity is currently under investigation.

The pathologic changes result from the action of activated trypsin and other pancreatic enzymes on the pancreas and surrounding tissues. Activated trypsin in turn activates the proenzymes of chymotrypsin, elastase, and phospholipase A_2, and those enzymes cause damage in several ways (Figure 15–4). For example, chymotrypsin activation leads to edema and vascular damage. Similarly, elastase, once activated from proelastase, digests the elastin in blood vessel walls and causes vascular injury and hemorrhage; damage to peripancreatic blood vessels can lead to hemorrhagic pancreatitis.

Phospholipase A_2 splits a fatty acid off lecithin, forming lysolecithin, which is cytotoxic to erythrocytes and damages cell membranes. The formation of lysolecithin from the lecithin in bile may contribute to the disruption of the pancreas and the necrosis of surrounding fat. Phospholipase A_2 also liberates arachidonic acid, which is then converted to prostaglandins, leukotrienes, and other mediators of inflammation, contributing to coagulation necrosis. Pancreatic lipase, released as a direct result of pancreatic acinar cell damage, acts enzymatically on surrounding adipose tissue, causing the characteristic peripancreatic fat necrosis seen in severe acute pancreatitis (see Figure 15–4).

Furthermore, trypsin and chymotrypsin activate kinins, complement, coagulation factors, and plasmin, leading to edema, inflammation, thrombosis, and hemorrhage within the gland. For example, trypsin activation of the kallikrein–kinin system leads to the release of bradykinin and kallidin, causing vasodilation, increased vascular permeability, edema, and inflammation (see Figure 15–4), which all contribute to the systemic inflammatory response syndrome characteristic of acute pancreatitis. Circulating phospholipases interfere with the normal function of pulmonary surfactant, contributing to the development of an adult respiratory distress syndrome in some patients with acute pancreatitis. Elevated serum lipase levels are sometimes associated with fat necrosis outside the abdomen.

Experimental models of acute pancreatitis suggest that NFκB activation occurs in parallel with trypsinogen activation. A pathologic Ca^{2+} influx appears to play a role in NFκB activation and may be a common activator of both parallel pathways of pancreatic injury. Moreover, as a downstream effector of CCK action, protein kinase C isoforms appear to play a role in NFκB activation, consistent with the parallel activation of the zymogen and NFκB pathways.

Finally, during acute pancreatitis, both the CC and CXC families of cytokines are implicated in the pathogenesis of the local and systemic inflammatory response. Cytokines

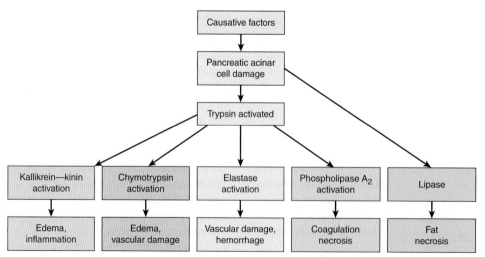

FIGURE 15–4 Hypothesized pathogenesis of acute pancreatitis. (Redrawn, with permission, from Marshall JB. acute pancreatitis: A review with an emphasis on new developments. Arch Intern Med. 1993;153:1188. Copyright © 1993 American Medical Association. All rights reserved.)

and other inflammatory mediators, such as tumor necrosis factor (TNF), interleukins (especially IL-1, IL-6, and IL-8), platelet-activating factor (PAF), and endotoxin, are released rapidly and predictably from inflammatory cells. This release appears to be in response to the presence of active digestive enzymes, independent of the underlying cause. The production of cytokines during clinical pancreatitis begins shortly after pain onset and peaks 36–48 hours later. These agents are now thought to be principal mediators in the transformation of acute pancreatitis from a local inflammatory process to a systemic illness (Figure 15–5). The degree of TNF-induced inflammation correlates with the severity of the pancreatitis. Cytokines rapidly enter the systemic circulation from the peritoneal cavity via the thoracic duct. In the systemic circulation, the cytokines affect many body systems and can produce the systemic inflammatory response syndrome (SIRS) and the multiorgan dysfunction syndrome typical of severe acute pancreatitis. Systemic complications of acute pancreatitis, such as respiratory failure, shock, and even multisystem organ failure, are accompanied by significant increases in monocyte secretion of TNF, IL-1, IL-6, and IL-8, as well as an upregulation in the number of receptors for these cytokines on target cells. This finding suggests that TNF, IL-1, IL-6, and IL-8 play a central role in the pathophysiology of these manifestations.

Studies also suggest that substance P acting via neurokinin-1 (NK-1) receptors, PAF, and chemokines interacting with CCR1 receptors play important pro-inflammatory roles in determining the severity of acute pancreatitis. In particular, substance P and NK-1 are involved in mediating acute lung injury. Substance P, a neuropeptide released from sensory afferent nerve endings, binds to the NK-1 receptor on the surface of effector cells and increases the permeability of vascular endothelium. The amount of substance P in the pancreas increases during episodes of acute pancreatitis, and acinar cell expression of NK-1 receptors is markedly upregulated. Substance P appears to be a powerful pro-inflammatory mediator of both pancreatitis and associated lung injury. PAF also appears to play an important role in the development of pancreatitis and associated lung injury. Chemokines are chemoattractant cytokines involved in activating and trafficking various inflammatory cells. Chemokines acting via the chemokine receptor CCR1 appear to have a role in determining the severity of pancreatitis-associated lung injury but have no effect on the severity of the pancreatitis itself. On the other hand, complement factor 5a (C5a) appears to act as an anti-inflammatory agent during the development of pancreatitis.

Various factors play active roles as pro-inflammatory or anti-inflammatory agents in acute pancreatitis. Drugs or other interventions to counteract pro-inflammatory agents (eg, TNF, IL-1, IL-6, IL-8, PAF) or to stimulate those that are anti-inflammatory (eg, IL-10) may eventually prove useful in treating patients with clinical pancreatitis to prevent severe injury to the pancreas and to prevent associated systemic manifestations, such as lung injury.

Clinical Manifestations

Acute pancreatitis may present in a highly variable manner, with the severity of inflammation and associated morbidity differing markedly among patients. Approximately 85% of patients experience a mild, self-limited illness of 2–3 days with no significant sequelae, but the remainder may develop severe acute pancreatitis, a life-threatening illness defined by the presence of associated organ system failure (typically affecting the pulmonary, cardiovascular, and/or renal systems). Acute pancreatitis may recur, depending primarily on its cause. With repeated attacks, the gland may eventually become permanently damaged, resulting in chronic pancreatitis or, sometimes, pancreatic insufficiency (see below). The distinction between acute pancreatitis and an acute exacerbation of chronic pancreatitis is determined by the clinical history and the characteristic findings of chronic pancreatitis on imaging. Acute and chronic pancreatitis have notably different management paradigms, so this distinction is important.

Recent consensus criteria require two of the following three criteria for the diagnosis of acute pancreatitis: abdominal pain, elevation of serum amylase or lipase (>3 times the upper limit of normal), and characteristic findings on computed tomography (CT) (or magnetic resonance imaging [MRI] or ultrasound). In practice, the first two elements are often present and sufficient to make to the clinical diagnosis. Nonetheless, cross-sectional imaging (eg, contrast-enhanced CT) may be

FIGURE 15–5 The inflammatory mediators of acute pancreatitis include interleukin-1B (IL-1) and tumor necrosis factor (TNF). As depicted, these two cytokines can induce other inflammatory mediators, such as IL-2, IL-6, IL-8, and IL-10; nitric oxide (NO); platelet activating factor (PAF); and interferon (INF)-α and INF-γ, while at the same time producing a direct noxious effect on the pancreas itself. Each of the mediators shown plays a role in the development of the systemic manifestations of acute pancreatitis. (ARDS, acute respiratory distress syndrome; ATN, acute tubular necrosis.) (Redrawn, with permission, from Norman J. The role of cytokines in the pathogenesis of acute pancreatitis. Am J Surg. 1998;175:76. Copyright © Elsevier.)

FIGURE 15–6 Acute pancreatitis on CT. Findings include enlargement and edema of the pancreas plus peripancreatic inflammatory change and fluid collections (arrow). (Used, with permission, from Henry I. Goldberg.)

useful in severe acute pancreatitis to assess the extent of associated pancreatic necrosis and other associated complications of the disease (Figure 15–6).

A. Signs and Symptoms at Presentation

Abdominal pain is nearly universal and a hallmark presentation of acute pancreatitis. In rare cases, patients may present with occult pancreatic inflammation evident by hyperamylasemia; for example, following pancreatic trauma, medication administration, or other known precipitants. However, such presentations are unlikely to be associated with clinically significant pancreatitis.

The pain of acute pancreatitis is characteristic, often described as an intense, deep, searing pain that radiates to the back. Frank peritoneal inflammation may lead to diagnostic confusion with other, more immediate surgical emergencies such as a perforated peptic ulcer, appendicitis, or diverticulitis.

The pain of acute pancreatitis is thought to derive in part from stretching of the pancreatic capsule by distended ductules and parenchymal edema, inflammatory exudate, digested proteins and lipids, and hemorrhage. In addition, these materials may seep out of the parenchyma into the retroperitoneum and lesser sac, where they irritate retroperitoneal and peritoneal sensory nerve endings and produce intense back and flank pain. The clinical findings of generalized peritonitis may follow.

Stretching of the pancreatic capsule may also produce **nausea and vomiting**. Increasing abdominal pain, peritoneal irritation, and electrolyte imbalance (especially hypokalemia) may cause a paralytic **ileus** with marked abdominal distention. If gastric motility is inhibited and the gastroesophageal sphincter is relaxed, there may be emesis. Both the small and large bowel often dilate during an acute attack. Sometimes only a localized segment of bowel dilates. For example, there may be localized dilation of a segment of jejunum overlying the pancreas. In such cases, a plain x-ray film of the abdomen shows thickening of the valvulae conniventes and air–fluid levels ("sentinel loop"). In other cases, there may be segmental

dilation of a portion of the overlying transverse colon. The x-ray film shows a sharply demarcated area of localized colonic dilation and edema ("colon cutoff sign").

Almost two-thirds of patients with acute pancreatitis develop **fever**. The pathophysiologic mechanism responsible for fever involves the extensive tissue injury, inflammation, and necrosis and release of endogenous pyrogens, principally IL-1, from polymorphonuclear leukocytes into the circulation. In most cases of acute pancreatitis, fever does not indicate a bacterial infection. However, persistent fever beyond the fourth or fifth day of illness—or spiking temperatures to 40°C or more—may signify the development of infectious complications such as infected peripancreatic fluid collections, infected pancreatic necrosis, or ascending cholangitis.

The cardinal laboratory finding in acute pancreatitis is an elevation of the **serum amylase**, often up to 10- to 20-fold. The serum amylase elevation occurs almost immediately (within hours), but it usually returns to normal within 48–72 hours even if symptoms continue. The sensitivity of the serum amylase in acute pancreatitis is estimated to be 70–95%, meaning that 5–30% of patients with acute pancreatitis have normal or minimally elevated serum amylase values. The specificity of the test is considerably lower. Patients with marked (more than 3-fold) elevations of serum amylase usually have acute pancreatitis. Patients with lesser elevations of serum amylase often have one of a variety of other conditions.

The serum amylase concentration reflects the steady state between the rates of amylase entry into and removal from the blood. Hyperamylasemia can result from either an increased rate of entry or a decreased rate of metabolic clearance of amylase in the circulation. The pancreas and salivary glands have much higher concentrations of amylase than any other organ and probably contribute almost all of the serum amylase activity in healthy persons. Amylase of pancreatic origin can now be distinguished from that of salivary origin by a variety of techniques. Pancreatic hyperamylasemia results from injuries to the pancreas, ranging from minor (cannulation of the pancreatic duct) to severe (pancreatitis). In addition, injuries to the bowel wall (infarction or perforation) cause pancreatic hyperamylasemia as a result of enhanced amylase absorption from the intestinal lumen. Salivary hyperamylasemia is observed in salivary gland diseases such as mumps parotitis, but also (inexplicably) in a host of unrelated conditions such as chronic alcoholism, postoperative states (particularly after coronary artery bypass graft surgery), lactic acidosis, anorexia nervosa or bulimia nervosa, and certain malignancies. Hyperamylasemia can also result from the decreased metabolic clearance of amylase caused by renal failure or macroamylasemia, a condition in which abnormally high-molecular-weight complexes of amylase are bound to abnormal immunoglobulins in the serum.

Determining the **serum lipase** level is often helpful diagnostically. In acute pancreatitis, the serum lipase level is elevated, usually about 72 hours after the onset of symptoms. The serum lipase measurement may be a better diagnostic test than serum amylase because it is just as easy to perform, may be more sensitive (85% vs. 79% sensitivity), is more specific for acute pancreatitis, and decreases to normal more slowly.

B. Early Complications of Acute Pancreatitis

Shock may occur in severe acute pancreatitis as a result of several interrelated factors. Hypovolemia results from a massive exudation of plasma and hemorrhage into the retroperitoneal space and from fluid accumulation in the gut as a result of ileus. Hypotension and shock may also result from the release of kinins into the general circulation. For example, activation during acute inflammation of the proteolytic enzyme kallikrein results in peripheral vasodilation via liberation of the vasoactive peptides, bradykinin and kallidin. This vasodilation causes the pulse rate to rise and the blood pressure to fall. Cytokines like PAF, a very potent vasodilator and leukocyte activator, have been implicated in the development of shock and other manifestations of SIRS. The contracted intravascular volume combined with hypotension may lead to myocardial and cerebral ischemia, respiratory failure, metabolic acidosis, and decreased urinary output or renal failure as a result of acute tubular necrosis.

Tissue factor release and expression during proteolysis may activate the plasma coagulation cascade and may lead to **disseminated intravascular coagulation (DIC)**. In other cases, blood hypercoagulability is thought to be due to elevated concentrations of several coagulation factors, including factor VIII, fibrinogen, and perhaps factor V. Clinically affected patients may present with hemorrhagic discoloration (purpura) in the subcutaneous tissues around the umbilicus (Cullen sign) or in the flanks (Grey Turner sign). The splenic and portal veins are in close proximity to the pancreas and thus can become involved in the inflammatory process. Splenic vein thrombosis occurs in approximately 11% and portal vein thrombosis in approximately 2% of patients. Most thrombi are asymptomatic, but they may be associated with the development of venous hypertension and the formation of varices over time.

Pulmonary complications are a dreaded manifestation of severe acute pancreatitis and occur in 15–50% of patients. The severity of pulmonary complications can vary from mild hypoxia to respiratory failure (acute respiratory distress syndrome [ARDS]). It is estimated that 50% of early deaths in patients with severe acute pancreatitis are associated with respiratory failure owing to profound acute lung injury. The pathophysiology of this acute lung injury appears to involve an increase in the permeability of the alveolar–capillary membrane. The endothelial cell destruction in the alveolar capillaries may be mediated by circulating activated pancreatic enzymes including elastase and phospholipase A_2. Pulmonary surfactant, another important alveolar barrier, appears to be destroyed by phospholipase A_2. Additional pulmonary injury appears to be mediated by inflammatory leukocytes sequestered in the alveoli and interstitial tissues, with the subsequent release of pro-inflammatory cytokines and chemokines that lead to further tissue destruction. Elevated serum levels of

IL-6 have been associated with the severity of lung injury in acute pancreatitis, an effect mediated by NFκB activation in pancreatic acinar cells. IL-6 and other inflammatory signaling pathways may prove to be appropriate therapeutic targets in severe acute pancreatitis, although to date no therapeutic agents have been found effective in clinical trials.

Acute pancreatitis may be accompanied by a small (usually left-sided) **pleural effusion**. The effusion may be reactive and hence secondary to a direct effect of the inflamed, swollen pancreas on the pleura abutting the diaphragm (typically transudative). Alternatively, in cases of severe acute pancreatitis, an effusion can be due to the tracking of exudative fluid from the pancreatic bed retroperitoneally into the pleural cavity through defects in the diaphragm. Characteristically, the pleural fluid in this latter circumstance is an exudate with high levels of protein, lactate dehydrogenase, and amylase. The effusion may contribute to segmental atelectasis of the lower lobes, leading to ventilation–perfusion mismatch and hypoxia.

Given the protean presentations of acute pancreatitis, there has been confusion regarding the classification of acute pancreatitis and its associated complications. Recent consensus guidelines have provided accurate criteria to aid in its diagnosis, treatment, and prognosis. The 2012 revision of the Atlanta classification represents the most recent standardized definitions for the characterization of acute pancreatitis.

Acute pancreatitis is recognized to exist in two primary forms: **interstitial edematous pancreatitis** and **necrotizing pancreatitis**.

Interstitial edematous acute pancreatitis is characterized by an enlargement of the pancreatic parenchyma with associated peripancreatic fluid but with uniform enhancement of the pancreatic parenchyma on contrast-enhanced CT. This form of the disease typically is clinically less severe, with symptoms routinely resolving within a week of presentation.

Necrotizing pancreatitis (necrosis of the pancreatic and peripancreatic tissues) occurs in approximately 5–10% of patients. While the degree of pancreatic necrosis is often detected by the lack of uniform parenchymal enhancement of contrast-enhanced CT, this process typically evolves over the first 1–2 weeks of illness, thereby rendering early imaging unreliable in predicting disease severity. The natural history of patients with necrotizing pancreatitis varies depending on whether pancreatic/peripancreatic necrosis remains solid or liquefies, becomes infected, persists, or resolves.

Infected pancreatic necrosis is a late complication of necrotizing pancreatitis. Rarely occurring in the first week of illness, procedures to diagnose this complication should be reserved for later in the patient's clinical course. Infected pancreatic necrosis should be suspected when there is progressive clinical collapse with shock and end organ failure or failure to improve following initial stabilization. Infected pancreatic necrosis is suggested by the presence of pancreatic or peripancreatic necrosis with extraluminal gas on contrast-enhanced CT. However, it is important to document infected pancreatic necrosis by image-guided fine-needle aspiration (percutaneous or endoscopic) and subsequent positive aspirate cultures because most pancreatic necrosis is in fact sterile. Infected pancreatic necrosis is a very serious complication of severe acute pancreatitis with a mortality rate of 25–50%. Consequently, it requires early pancreatic debridement.

Early complications of acute pancreatitis include both systemic and local problems. Systemic complications include the presence of organ failure, which defines severe acute pancreatitis. Organ failure may be transient (resolving within 48 hours) or persistent (affecting prognosis). Early local complications of acute pancreatitis are defined by their presence within the first 4 weeks of disease onset. **Acute peripancreatic fluid collections** develop in the early phase of acute pancreatitis and may occur in the absence of pancreatic necrosis. On contrast-enhanced CT, these collections often have a poorly defined wall or boundary. These fluid collections are sterile and typically resolve without intervention. **Acute necrotic collections** occur in necrotizing pancreatitis and appear on contrast-enhanced CT as heterogeneous collections with variable amounts of fluid and solid debris. Sequential imaging studies may be necessary to define the evolution of these lesions. They may variably communicate with the pancreatic duct when necrosis is associated with ductal disruption, and they may become secondarily infected.

C. Late Complications of Acute Pancreatitis

Late complications of acute pancreatitis may similarly be divided into systemic and local effects. Systemic complications include persistent organ failure and the need for prolonged intensive care, factors that portend a poor prognosis. Local complications are defined by their presence beyond 4 weeks from the onset of illness and are typically characterized by serial imaging that documents their evolution.

Pancreatic pseudocysts are non-epithelium-lined cavities that contain plasma, blood, pus, and pancreatic juice. They are the product of inflammatory fibrous or granulation tissue walling off a peripancreatic fluid collection. By definition, pseudocysts are distinguished from acute peripancreatic fluid collections by their persistence more than 4 weeks following an episode of acute pancreatitis. Pseudocysts generally occur after recovery from the acute attack and are the result of both parenchymal destruction and ductal obstruction or disruption. Some acini continue to secrete pancreatic juice, but because the juice cannot drain normally, it collects in an area of necrotic tissue, forming the ill-defined pseudocyst (Figure 15–7). As more juice is secreted, the cyst may grow larger and may compress nearby structures, such as the portal vein (producing portal hypertension), common bile duct (producing jaundice or cholangitis), or gut (producing gastric outlet or bowel obstruction). Pancreatic pseudocysts are distinguished by their lack of solid debris, appearing as homogenous, fluid-filled cavities on imaging studies.

Most pancreatic pseudocysts resolve spontaneously, and no specific intervention is required when asymptomatic. Indications for surgical, endoscopic, or percutaneous intervention include persistent symptoms or associated complications (bowel or bile duct obstruction, hemorrhage, secondary infection). Treatment options for pseudocysts include external drainage either by surgical or percutaneous techniques or internal drainage to the GI tract by surgical or endoscopic means. An infected pancreatic pseudocyst is typically designated a **pancreatic abscess**. As such, it is typically confined to a solitary cyst and occurs late in the course of disease. A pancreatic abscess can often be treated successfully. Percutaneous drainage is the mainstay of therapy, with surgical or endoscopic drainage reserved for refractory cases.

FIGURE 15–7 Pancreatic pseudocyst on CT. (Reproduced, with permission, from Way LW, ed. *Current Surgical Diagnosis & Treatment*, 10th ed. Originally published by Appleton & Lange. Copyright © 1994 by The McGraw-Hill Companies, Inc.)

Walled-off pancreatic necrosis is a mature, encapsulated collection of debris with a well-defined inflammatory rind that occurs beyond 4 weeks from the onset of necrotizing pancreatitis. Sometimes, walled-off necrosis may be difficult to distinguish from a pancreatic pseudocyst, and contrast-enhanced CT may underestimate the amount of solid debris present in the walled-off necrosis. MRI and/or endoscopic ultrasound (EUS) may more reliably distinguish between these two entities and help define treatment strategies. In patients with persistent symptoms, with failure to improve clinically or with secondary infection, intervention for walled-off necrosis may be necessary. Surgical necrosectomy, which may be done by open or minimally invasive techniques, or endoscopic transgastric necrosectomy may be considered.

Pancreatic ascites occurs when a direct connection develops between the pancreatic duct and the peritoneal cavity. Given its origin, it is unsurprising that the ascitic fluid resembles pancreatic juice, characteristically an exudate with high protein and extremely high amylase levels. Left untreated, massive pancreatic ascites may lead to pleural effusions, subcutaneous fat necrosis, or abdominal compartment syndrome. Treatment typically involves draining the ascites and controlling the pancreatic ductal disruption, either by endoscopic pancreatic duct stent placement or by surgical therapy.

Pancreatic fistulas, caused by disruption of the pancreatic duct, should be suspected in patients who develop pancreatic ascites or pleural effusions. Fistulas can be internal, connecting to pleural or pericardial spaces, the colon, the small intestine, or the biliary tract, or external, draining through the skin.

Course & Prognosis

Most patients with acute pancreatitis recover completely with supportive medical management. The pancreas then regenerates and returns to normal except for some mild residual scarring. Diabetes mellitus almost never occurs after a single attack of pancreatitis, but either endocrine or exocrine insufficiency may occur following an episode of severe acute pancreatitis or repeated episodes of acute pancreatitis.

The initial course of alcoholic pancreatitis is characterized by recurrent acute exacerbations and the later course by progressive pancreatic insufficiency. However, among individuals with recurrent acute alcoholic pancreatitis, two groups can be distinguished in terms of prognosis. About 75% of cases progress to advanced chronic pancreatitis, typically with pancreatic calcification and pancreatic insufficiency. The remainder do not progress and do not develop pancreatic duct dilation. The factors responsible for progression have not yet been elucidated.

The severity of acute pancreatitis can be estimated by various methods: clinical assessment, biochemical tests, peritoneal lavage, CT, and prognostic criteria (Table 15–2).

Studies have shown that important predictors of mortality are (1) failure of more than one organ system in the early phase of acute pancreatitis; and (2) pancreatic necrosis associated with the later development of multiple-organ failure. Organ failure may be defined by the modified Marshall scoring system, which includes an assessment of respiratory failure (measured by the PaO_2/FiO_2 ratio and the need for supplemental oxygen), cardiovascular collapse (defined by systolic blood pressure, the need for fluid resuscitation, and blood pH on arterial blood gases), and renal failure (defined by serum creatinine). Multiple-organ failure is defined as a syndrome of progressive but potentially reversible organ failure, involving two or more systems remote from the original insult. Persistent organ failure beyond 48 hours of presentation may be associated with a mortality as high as 36–50%.

Improvements in recent years in the survival of severe acute pancreatitis reflect improvements in critical care medicine, as well as the evolution of evidence-based management approaches to pancreatitis patients. Pharmacologic therapies (eg, anti-inflammatory agents, immune mediators) for severe acute pancreatitis have to date proven largely ineffective in changing clinical outcomes. Prophylactic antibiotic therapy is ineffective but indicated when sources of infection are documented or highly suspected (eg, infected pancreatic necrosis). Early enteral nutrition has proven to be a key intervention in severe acute pancreatitis, with the expedited (first 72 hours after presentation) placement of a nasojejunal tube and the initiation of enteral liquid artificial nutrition as a key early management principle. Parenteral nutrition use should be minimized and restricted to patients unable to achieve adequate enteral nutrition. Endobiliary interventions (endoscopic retrograde cholangiopancreatography [ERCP]) are indicated only in patients with acute pancreatitis and evidence of ascending cholangitis or persistent biliary obstruction. Finally, surgical interventions for complications of severe acute pancreatitis should rarely be performed. Asymptomatic acute peripancreatic fluid collections, acute pancreatic necrosis, and walled-off pancreatic necrosis do not require intervention and should be aspirated for sampling and culture only when concern for infection exists. In symptomatic or infected pancreatic pseudocysts or walled-off pancreatic necrosis, surgical or endoscopic interventions should be delayed in stable patients until at least 4 weeks after presentation to allow development of a mature wall around the focal collection.

CHECKPOINT

5. What are the presenting symptoms and signs of acute pancreatitis?
6. What are the most common causes of acute pancreatitis?
7. Which drugs are commonly associated with pancreatitis?
8. What is the pathophysiologic mechanism by which hemorrhagic pancreatitis occurs?
9. What are the complications of severe pancreatitis?
10. What are the pathophysiologic mechanisms by which each of the complications of severe pancreatitis occurs?

TABLE 15–2   Adverse prognostic signs in acute pancreatitis.

I. Ranson criteria of severity of acute pancreatitis[1]	
Criteria present at diagnosis or admission	Criteria developing during first 48 hours[2]
Age >55 years	Hemoglobin falls below 10 g/dL
White blood cell count >16,000/µL	Blood urea nitrogen rises by >5 mg/dL
Blood glucose >200 mg/dL	Serum calcium <8 mg/dL
Serum LDH >350 IU/L	Arterial Po$_2$ <60 mm Hg
Serum AST >250 IU/L	Base deficit >4 mEq/L
	Estimated fluid sequestration >6 L

1 point for each factor listed

Score >3 indicates severe acute pancreatitis

Mortality rates correlate with number of criteria present

Number of points	Mortality rate
0–2	1%
3–4	16%
5–6	40%
7–8	100%

II. Poor prognostic indicators in severe acute pancreatitis (revised Atlanta Classification)[3]	
A. Early phase: Signs of systemic inflammatory response syndrome (SIRS)	B. Grades of severity
1. Heart rate >90 beats/min	1. Mild acute pancreatitis
2. Core temperature <36°C or >38°C	a. No organ failure
3. White blood count <4000 or >12,000/mm^3	b. No local or systemic complications
4. Respirations >20/min or PCO$_2$ <32 mm Hg	2. Moderately severe acute pancreatitis
	a. Organ failure that resolves within 48 hours and/or
	b. Local or systemic complications without persistent organ failure
	3. Severe acute pancreatitis
	a. Persistent organ failure >48 hours, single
	b. Persistent organ failure >48 hours, multiple

[1]Modified, with permission, from Oropello JM et al, eds. *Critical Care*. McGraw-Hill, 2017. [Table 35–1]

[2]Requires 48 h to calculate entire score.

[3]Modified, with permission, from BMJ Publishing Group Ltd. From Banks PA et al; Acute Pancreatitis Classification Working Group. Classification of acute pancreatitis—2012: revision of the Atlanta classification and definitions by international consensus. Gut. 2013 Jan;62(1):102–11.

CHRONIC PANCREATITIS

Clinical Presentations

Chronic pancreatitis is a relapsing disorder causing severe abdominal pain, exocrine and endocrine pancreatic insufficiency, severe duct abnormalities, and pancreatic calcifications. The prevalence of the disorder is about 30 cases per 100,000 individuals, and the yearly incidence ranges from 3.5 to 10 cases per 100,000. In chronic pancreatitis, the parenchyma is chronically inflamed, leading to the progressive destruction of the acini, stenosis and dilation of the ductules, and fibrosis of the gland. Eventually, the gland's exocrine function becomes impaired (see Pancreatic Insufficiency later), and, in severe cases, a loss of endocrine function as well (Chapter 18).

Etiology

It was once believed that chronic pancreatitis resulted simply from recurrent attacks of acute pancreatitis. However, there is some evidence that acute and chronic pancreatitis are distinct pathogenetic entities. Patients developing acute pancreatitis are a mean 13 years older than those with the onset of chronic calcified pancreatitis. Furthermore, the two diseases

TABLE 15–3   Causes of chronic pancreatitis.

Alcohol abuse
Duct obstruction (eg, gallstones)
Pancreas divisum[1]
Tropical (malnutrition, toxin)
Hypercalcemia (eg, hyperparathyroidism)
Hyperlipidemia
Drugs
Trauma
Autoimmune
Hereditary
Cystic fibrosis (mucoviscidosis)
Idiopathic

[1]An anatomic variant that occurs when normal fusion between the dorsal and ventral pancreatic ducts fails.

have been linked to different causes. Finally, in acute pancreatitis, the pancreas is normal before the attack and the pathologic changes are completely reversible if the patient survives, whereas in chronic pancreatitis the gland is abnormal before the attack and the pathologic changes are not reversible.

The major cause of chronic pancreatitis is chronic alcoholism, which accounts for about 70–80% of cases. The remainder are due to the diverse causes listed in Table 15–3. In 1788, Cawley first reported the association of alcoholism with chronic pancreatitis. He described a "free living young man" with diabetes and emaciation. At autopsy, his pancreas was "full of stones." Patients with chronic pancreatitis resulting from alcohol abuse usually have a long history (6–12 years) of heavy alcohol consumption (150–175 g/d) before disease onset. In individuals with alcoholism, deficiencies of zinc and selenium may inhibit the quenching of oxygen free radicals.

Recent epidemiologic evidence identifies cigarette smoking as a strong independent risk factor for the development of chronic pancreatitis. Moreover, tobacco exposure appears to have a dose-dependent relationship with its incidence. The number of cigarettes smoked daily and the duration of tobacco smoke exposure both appear to be important risk factors. Last, the combination of significant alcohol and cigarette use appears to be synergistic in augmenting the risk of chronic pancreatitis.

Long-term obstruction of the pancreatic duct can also cause chronic pancreatitis. The obstruction can be caused by a neoplasm, papillary stenosis, cystic lesions (cystic tumors or pseudocysts), scarring or stricture, or trauma. Pancreas divisum can cause chronic pancreatitis as a result of obstruction at the lesser papilla. Tropical chronic pancreatitis is a juvenile form of chronic calcific nonalcoholic pancreatitis, thought to be caused by protein or micronutrient deficiencies, which may

cause impaired free radical clearance, or by ingesting a toxic substance, such as cyanogens in cassava root. Chronic hypercalcemia may cause pancreatitis, as seen in 10–15% of patients with hyperparathyroidism. The intraductal precipitation of calcium and stimulation of pancreatic enzyme secretion are thought to be important in pathogenesis. In some cases of chronic pancreatitis with features of Sjögren syndrome, an autoimmune mechanism may be involved. Chronic hereditary pancreatitis, characterized by recurrent episodes of abdominal pain beginning in childhood, accounts for about 1% of cases. It is transmitted as an autosomal dominant genetic disorder with incomplete (~80%) penetrance. Hereditary chronic pancreatitis has also been associated with mutations in the cationic trypsinogen gene *PRSS1* or in the *SPINK1/PSTI* gene (discussed previously). Some cases are due to cystic fibrosis (mucoviscidosis; see later discussion). In some cases, no cause can be identified, and the disease is termed idiopathic chronic pancreatitis.

Pathology

Pathologically, chronic pancreatitis is characterized by scarring and shrinkage of the pancreas resulting from acinus fibrosis and atrophy, and by ductule stenosis and dilation. Grossly, the process usually involves the whole gland, but in about one-third of cases it is localized, most often involving the head and body of the gland. The ductules and ducts are often filled with inspissated secretions or calculi. Between 36% and 87% of patients with chronic pancreatitis have ductal stones. The gland may be rock hard as a result of diffuse sclerosis and calcification, and biopsy may be required to differentiate chronic pancreatitis from pancreatic carcinoma. Microscopically, acinus loss, ductile dilation, marked fibrosis, and a lymphocytic infiltrate are seen. The islets of Langerhans are usually well preserved.

In the early stage of chronic pancreatitis, pseudocysts are present in approximately half (52%) of patients. A focally accentuated, perilobular fibrosis and a lesser degree of intralobular fibrosis are typically observed. Although intralobular fibrosis and peri-lobular fibrosis of the pancreas are hallmarks of alcoholic pancreatitis, they are also common among patients with alcohol dependence and abuse who have no history of pancreatitis. Marked fibrosis, ductal distortions, and the presence of intraductal calculi are the main features of advanced chronic pancreatitis. Pseudocysts occur less frequently (36%). CD4 and CD8 T lymphocytes are the predominant T-cell subsets in the inflammatory infiltrates in chronic pancreatitis.

In clinical practice, an important distinction must be made between patients with chronic pancreatitis who have "large-duct" versus "small-duct" disease. The presence of a dilated main pancreatic duct, secondary to obstruction resulting from intraductal calculi and/or ductal strictures, is identified as large-duct disease and is thought to produce symptoms of abdominal pain secondary to ductal hypertension. Such patients may be candidates for surgical decompression procedures, as described below. Patients with small-duct disease tend to have small atrophic glands, often riddled with calcifications but without focal ductal abnormalities or dilatation. The pain syndrome in patients with small-duct disease is attributed to local enzymatic activity and the destruction of the perineural sheath, exposing axons to cytokines released by inflammatory cells and ultimately causing perineural fibrosis.

Pathogenesis

Table 15–4 presents a classification of pancreatitis based on pathogenesis, emphasizing the fundamental differences between acute and chronic pancreatitis. Table 15–5 lists proposed pathogenetic mechanisms for chronic pancreatitis, emphasizing the differences between large-duct and small-duct pathologies and their associated causes.

As with acute pancreatitis, an increasing understanding of the genetic profiles of patients with chronic pancreatitis and more sophisticated knowledge of cell-signaling pathways have led to the appreciation of chronic pancreatitis as a complex genetic disorder. While a minority of patients have mendelian disorders with single mutations that lead to pancreatitis (eg, hereditary pancreatitis, cystic fibrosis), the majority of patients likely have genetic susceptibilities that interact with environmental exposures to produce the clinical syndrome. At least five genes conveying susceptibility to pancreatitis have been identified, including variants in the cationic trypsinogen gene (*PRSS1*), the cystic fibrosis transmembrane conductance regular gene (*CFTR*), the pancreatic secretory trypsin inhibitor gene (*SPINK1*), the chymotrypsinogen C gene (*CTRC*), and the calcium-sensing receptor gene (*CASR*). Evidence suggests

TABLE 15–5   Proposed pathogenetic mechanisms of chronic pancreatitis.

"Large-duct" mechanisms
Biliary–pancreatic reflux
Sphincter of Oddi obstruction or hypersecretion
Increased ductal permeability
"Small-duct" mechanisms
Increased viscosity or protein hypersecretion
Increased lactoferrin
Decreased lithostathine (pancreatic stone protein)
Acinar cell mechanisms
Toxic metabolites
Unopposed free radical injury
Leukocyte hyperstimulation
Lysosomal hyperactivity
Cholinergic hyperactivity
Abnormal protein trafficking
Stellate cell-induced fibrosis
Necrosis–fibrosis sequence

Data from Pitchumoni CS. Pathogenesis of alcohol-induced chronic pancreatitis: facts, perceptions, and misperceptions. Surg Clin North Am. 2001;81:379.

TABLE 15–4   Pathogenetic classification of pancreatitis.

Pathogenetic Class	Subclassification	Pathologic Features
Acute pancreatitis	Mild pancreatitis	Fat necrosis
	Severe (necrotizing) pancreatitis	Coagulation necrosis
		Hemorrhagic necrosis
Chronic pancreatitis	Lithogenic pancreatitis	Protein plugs
	Obstructive pancreatitis	Calculi
	Inflammatory pancreatitis	Obstruction of main pancreatic duct
	Pancreatic fibrosis	Mononuclear cell infiltration
		Acinar cell necrosis
		Diffuse perilobular fibrosis

Modified, with permission, from BMJ Publishing Group Ltd. From Sidhu SS et al. The pathogenesis of chronic pancreatitis. Postgrad Med J. 1995;71:67.

that these genes interact with each other as well as with environmental (eg, alcohol, tobacco) exposures in heterogeneous ways. The clinical observations that alcohol-related chronic pancreatitis does not always correlate with degree or duration of alcohol exposure and that other end-organ damage due to alcohol abuse (eg, cirrhosis) does not always correlate with the appearance of chronic pancreatitis suggest that genetic cofactors may play an important role in the disease.

Mutations of the *CFTR* gene located on chromosome 7q32 are arguably the most well understood of the genetic susceptibilities to pancreatitis. In cystic fibrosis patients with chronic pancreatitis, a mutation of the *CFTR* gene causes the inadequate function of CFTR, the chloride channel located on the luminal surface of the pancreatic duct cell that is highly involved in bicarbonate secretion. Major mutations in both alleles lead to loss of *CFTR* function and the inability to hydrate mucus, resulting in inspissated secretions and ductal obstruction. Because pancreatic function may be maintained with CFTR function as little as 1% of normal, only severe *CFTR* mutations yielding little or no functional protein produce chronic pancreatitis and pancreatic insufficiency.

Chronic pancreatitis appears to occur in the context of one of several pathogenic pathways. In patients with large-duct obstruction, the ductal lesion likely predates the development of pancreatic parenchymal abnormalities. The pathogenesis probably involves elevated pressures in the pancreatic duct, resulting in ischemia, necrosis, and inflammation of the acinar cells. However, the ductal epithelium is preserved. Calcified protein plugs and stones are less often present, although some patients with lithogenic pancreatitis may develop secondary ductal obstruction and large-duct disease over time. Many patients with idiopathic chronic pancreatitis also have ductal hypertension.

For chronic lithogenic pancreatitis, several different pathogenetic mechanisms have been postulated. One theory postulates **acinar protein (trypsinogen) hypersecretion** as an initial event (Figure 15–8A). Ultrastructural studies of exocrine pancreatic tissue from patients with chronic pancreatitis show signs of protein hypersecretion, including a larger diameter of cells, nuclei, and nucleoli; increased length of the endoplasmic reticulum; increased numbers of condensing vacuoles; and decreased numbers of zymogen granules. The hypersecretion of protein occurs without increased fluid or bicarbonate secretion by ductal cells. At the same time, there is an increase in the ratio of lysosomal hydrolases (cathepsin B) to digestive hydrolases (trypsinogen), resulting in trypsinogen activation. The precipitation of intraductal protein into plugs is then

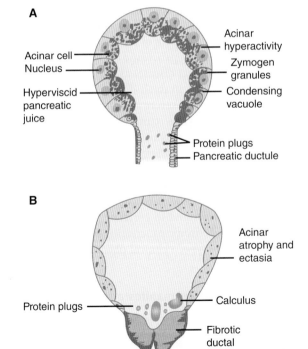

FIGURE 15–8 Proposed pathogenetic model of chronic pancreatitis emphasizing acinar protein hypersecretion. **A:** Early chronic pancreatitis is characterized by acinar cell hyperactivity and the secretion of a hyperviscid pancreatic juice with an imbalance of pancreatic stone promoters and inhibitors, resulting in protein plug formation. **B:** Advanced chronic pancreatitis is characterized by acinar cell atrophy, ductal strictures and ectasia, and intraductal stones. (Redrawn, with permission, from BMJ Publishing Group Ltd. From Sidhu SS et al. The pathogenesis of chronic pancreatitis. Postgrad Med J. 1995;71:67.)

thought to occur in the following fashion: **Lithostathines** (formerly called **pancreatic stone proteins [PSPs]**) are peptides secreted into pancreatic juice that normally inhibit the formation of protein plugs and the aggregation of calcium carbonate crystals to form stones. Acinar cell secretion of lithostathine is impaired by alcohol. Furthermore, when hydrolyzed by trypsin and cathepsin B, lithostathine H2/PSP-S1 is created. This insoluble peptide polymerizes into fibrils that form the matrix of protein plugs. At the same time, there is a hypersecretion of calcium into the pancreatic juice. The calcium hypersecretion is first triggered by neural (cholinergic, vagally mediated) or hormonal stimuli. Later, as the basal lamina of the pancreatic duct is eroded by contact with the protein plugs, there is a transudation of serum protein and calcium into the pancreatic juice. The formation of a protein plugs in pancreatic juice that is thick, viscid, protein rich, and supersaturated with calcium carbonate leads to the formation of **calculi** (stones) (Figure 15–8B). Lithostathine deficiency is unexplained but may be hereditary or acquired. Chronic alcoholism and malnutrition are acquired causes of lithostathine deficiency. Decreased levels of other nucleation-inhibitory factors, such as local trypsin inhibitor and citrate, in pancreatic juice further enhance the formation of pancreatic plugs and stones. Lactoferrin, an iron-containing macromolecular protein, is elevated in the pancreatic secretions of alcoholic patients with pancreatitis. Lactoferrin can produce an aggregation of large acidophilic proteins, such as albumin, and thus may be partly responsible for the formation of protein plugs. Similarly, GP2, a glycosylphosphatidylinositol-anchored protein, might have a role in protein plug formation. GP2 is released from the apical surface of acinar cells into the pancreatic ducts in relatively high concentrations. GP2 aggregates at a pH <7.0, and pancreatic juice from patients with chronic pancreatitis usually has a pH <7.0. Eventually, the stones provoke the formation of fibrotic ductal strictures and ductal ectasia, acinar cell atrophy, and parenchymal atrophy distal to obstructed ducts in the advanced stages of chronic pancreatitis.

Another theory postulates a necrosis–fibrosis sequence, in which focal necrosis during recurrent attacks of acute pancreatitis induces scarring and fibrosis, leading to chronic lithogenic pancreatitis (Figure 15–9A). In this scenario, vascular damage in acute pancreatitis causes cellular anoxia, necrosis, chronic inflammation, and subsequent fibrosis. In particular, periacinar and periductal fat necrosis induce periductal fibrosis, which partially obstructs the interlobular ducts. Stasis within the ductules then leads to protein plug and stone formation in the pancreatic juice (Figure 15–9B). Subsequently, total ductal obstruction by calculi induces acinar cell necrosis, inflammation, and fibrosis (Figure 15–9C). Transforming growth factor-β (TGF-β) appears to be a mediator of collagen synthesis after pancreatic injury.

Pathophysiology

Maldigestion in chronic pancreatitis results from several factors. Long-standing inflammation and fibrosis of the

A

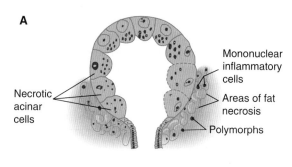

Necrotic acinar cells

Mononuclear inflammatory cells

Areas of fat necrosis

Polymorphs

B

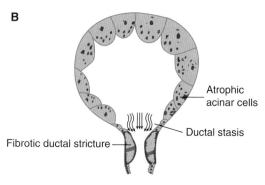

Atrophic acinar cells

Ductal stasis

Fibrotic ductal stricture

C

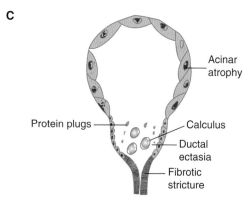

Acinar atrophy

Protein plugs

Calculus

Ductal ectasia

Fibrotic stricture

FIGURE 15–9 Proposed pathogenetic model of chronic pancreatitis emphasizing the sequence of acute pancreatitis followed by chronic pancreatitis. **A:** Acute pancreatitis is characterized by acinar cell and fat necrosis and inflammatory cell infiltration. **B:** Later, healing and fibrosis occur. **C:** Finally, changes characteristic of chronic pancreatitis appear, including acinar cell atrophy, protein plugs and calculus formation, and ductal strictures and ectasia. (Redrawn, with permission, from BMJ Publishing Group Ltd. From Sidhu SS et al. The pathogenesis of chronic pancreatitis. Postgrad Med J. 1995;71:67.)

pancreas can destroy exocrine tissue, leading to inadequate delivery of digestive enzymes to the duodenum in the prandial and postprandial periods. This maldigestion is worsened by an inadequate delivery of bicarbonate to the duodenum, with consequent gastric acid inactivation of enzymes and bile acids. Gastric dysmotility and mechanical obstruction from fibrosis in the pancreatic head may also contribute. Chronic pancreatitis may thus result in the profound steatorrhea of pancreatic insufficiency. There is a direct correlation between severity of histologic findings and exocrine pancreatic dysfunction as estimated by the CCK-secretin test (see later discussion).

Studies of patients with chronic pancreatitis have found no abnormalities in basal plasma CCK and pancreatic polypeptide (PP) levels, but impaired interdigestive cycling and postprandial CCK and PP release have been noted. Chronic pancreatitis does not seem to have any effect on intestinal motility.

In chronic pancreatitis, fecal bile acid excretion has been found to be three times that of healthy individuals. Bile acid malabsorption is related to an impairment of pancreatic bicarbonate secretion; it is generally not observed until bicarbonate output is markedly reduced (<0.05 mEq/kg/h). Such bile acid malabsorption may cause the hypocholesterolemia seen in patients with chronic pancreatitis.

The impairment of exocrine function in chronic pancreatitis may also lead to increased CCK-mediated stimulation of the pancreas.

Hepatic insulin resistance has been demonstrated in patients with chronic pancreatitis, perhaps related to a decrease in high-affinity insulin receptors on the hepatocyte cell membrane. In rats, insulin binding improves after administering pancreatic polypeptide.

Clinical Manifestations

Table 15–6 lists the clinical manifestations of chronic pancreatitis. The major symptom of chronic pancreatitis is severe abdominal pain that can be either constant or intermittent. The abdominal pain often radiates to the midback or scapula and increases after eating. The pain of chronic pancreatitis is multifactorial, likely reflecting pancreatic ductal hypertension (eg, in patients with large-duct disease) as well as chronic inflammatory neural injury (eg, in small-duct disease). Patients may have recurrent attacks of severe abdominal pain, vomiting, and elevated serum amylase (chronic relapsing pancreatitis). Continued alcohol intake may increase the frequency of painful episodes, at least when there is still relatively preserved pancreatic function; in severe pancreatic insufficiency, alcohol intake appears to have less influence on the development of abdominal pain. Pancreatic parenchymal pressure measurements have not been found to correlate with pain. Of note, patients with painful chronic pancreatitis can over time evolve to a "painless" phenotype, a clinical phenomenon thought to

TABLE 15–6 Clinical manifestations of chronic pancreatitis.

Abdominal pain
Nausea
Vomiting
Weight loss
Malabsorption
Hyperglycemia, diabetes mellitus
Jaundice

be secondary to ongoing neural injury resulting in the abla-tion of pain pathways. Furthermore, a proportion of patients who undergo total pancreatectomy for refractory pain owing to chronic pancreatitis will have residual pain, suggesting that neural remodeling and central signaling changes account for some of the pain experienced by chronic pancreatitis patients. From 10% to 20% of patients have "painless pancreatitis," pre-senting with diabetes, jaundice, maldigestion, malabsorption, or steatorrhea. Anorexia and weight loss occur frequently, related to both poor nutrition and malabsorption from pan-creatic insufficiency.

The diagnosis of chronic pancreatitis is based mainly on symptoms and signs. Serum amylase and lipase levels are elevated in only a minority of cases. In the remaining cases, amylase and lipase levels are normal or low, probably because there is little residual functional pancreatic tissue and true acute inflammation is rare. The pancreatic parenchymal and main duct calcifications seen on CT or plain-film x-rays are pathognomonic of chronic pancreatitis. The calcifications are actually the intraductal pancreatic calculi composed of cal-cium carbonate and lithostathines. Pseudocyst formation may also be evident on CT imaging.

EUS has become the test of choice for evaluating patients with early or mild chronic pancreatitis. Studies correlating histologic findings with EUS scoring of chronic pancreatitis changes have confirmed the excellent sensitivity (85–91%) and specificity (70–86%) of EUS. The value of EUS is most appar-ent in patients without calcific disease, because those patients can have a definitive diagnosis made on CT and because they often have more severe or long-standing symptoms. A consen-sus conference established the Rosemont criteria as a scoring system composed of major and minor parenchymal and duc-tal features that has provided standardized criteria for diag-nosing chronic pancreatitis.

About 5% of patients develop severe sclerosing pancreati-tis involving the head of the pancreas, leading to obstruction of the common bile and pancreatic ducts. Obstruction of the common bile duct in the setting of chronic pancreatitis typi-cally appears as a smooth, tapering stricture, rather than an abrupt cutoff, as is seen in bile duct obstruction owing to pan-creatic cancer. Obstruction may also be caused by a pseudocyst in the head of the pancreas. Common bile duct obstruction results in profound and persistent jaundice, resembling that produced by pancreatic carcinoma. The serum bilirubin and alkaline phosphatase are elevated.

Magnetic resonance cholangiopancreatography (MRCP) is the most appropriate initial test to assess the severity and extent of ductal changes, particularly in the setting of associ-ated or suspected distal biliary obstruction. Imaging findings can include dilated ducts, frequently with adjacent areas of stricture, yielding a "chain of lakes" or "string of pearls" appear-ance, or ducts of normal caliber, with adjacent small ducts lacking side branches, yielding a "tree in winter" appearance. MRCP can be suggestive of focal-dominant strictures, and/or associated calculi, that may be targets for intervention. ERCP offers direct visualization of ductal abnormalities in chronic

pancreatitis and is most appropriately used when specific focal abnormalities appear to correlate with clinical symptoms (eg, biliary obstruction, pancreatic ductal disruption).

Failure to secrete pancreatic juice results in the malabsorp-tion of fat (steatorrhea) and fat-soluble vitamins, leading to weight loss. Impairment of exocrine function is manifested by pancreatic insufficiency (see later discussion). Studies screening patients with chronic pancreatitis have found that the majority develop exocrine dysfunction over time. One study documented that 63% developed exocrine dysfunction within 5 years and 94% after 10 years. Diabetes mellitus is a late complication of chronic pancreatitis and is not apparent until 80–90% of the gland is severely damaged.

The treatment of chronic pancreatitis is mainly symptom-atic and directed toward relieving pain and treating exocrine and endocrine insufficiency (see below). Pain in these patients is often a serious clinical problem, leading to a significant compromise of quality of life and potential opioid tolerance and even addiction. If a precipitating factor such as an ana-tomic abnormality or metabolic condition is present, it may be treated with surgical or medical intervention. Methods of pain relief include abstinence from alcohol and the use of conventional analgesics. If pain is not relieved, opioids may be necessary. Invasive procedures, such as celiac plexus block, endoscopic procedures, and surgical drainage or resection may be indicated in select patients with debilitating symptoms.

The major complications of chronic pancreatitis are pseu-docyst formation and mechanical obstruction of the common bile duct and duodenum. Less common complications include pancreatic fistulas with pancreatic ascites, pleural effusion, or sometimes pericardial effusion; splenic vein thrombosis and the development of gastric varices; and the formation of a pseudoaneurysm, with hemorrhage or pain resulting from expansion and pressure on adjacent structures. Fistulas result from disruption of the pancreatic duct. Splenic vein throm-bosis occurs because the splenic vein, which courses along the posterior surface of the pancreas, may become involved in peripancreatic inflammation. Pseudoaneurysms may affect any of the arteries in proximity to the pancreas, most com-monly the splenic, hepatic, gastroduodenal, and pancreatico-duodenal arteries.

In patients monitored for more than 10 years, the mortal-ity rate is 22%; pancreatitis-induced complications account for 13% of the deaths. Older age at diagnosis, cigarette smoking, and alcohol intake are major predictors of mortality among individuals with chronic pancreatitis. Chronic pancreatitis of any cause has been associated with a 25-year cumulative risk of approximately 4% for the development of pancreatic cancer.

PANCREATIC INSUFFICIENCY

Clinical Presentations

Pancreatic exocrine insufficiency is a syndrome of maldiges-tion resulting from disorders interfering with effective pan-creatic enzyme activity. Because pancreatic lipase is essential

TABLE 15–7   Causes of pancreatic insufficiency.

Primary

A. Acquired decreased enzyme secretion

    Chronic pancreatitis (alcohol abuse, trauma, hereditary, idiopathic)

    Pancreatic, ampullary, and duodenal neoplasms

    Pancreatic resection

    Severe protein-calorie malnutrition, hypoalbuminemia

B. Congenital decreased enzyme secretion

    Cystic fibrosis

    Hemochromatosis

    Shwachman–Diamond syndrome (pancreatic insufficiency with anemia, neutropenia, and bony abnormalities)

    Enzyme deficiencies (trypsinogen, enterokinase, amylase, lipase, protease, and α_1-antiprotease deficiency)

Secondary

A. Intraluminal enzyme destruction: gastrinoma (Zollinger–Ellison syndrome)

B. Decreased pancreatic stimulation: small intestinal mucosal disease (nontropical sprue)

C. Mistiming of enzyme secretion: gastric surgery

    1. Subtotal gastrectomy with Billroth I anastomosis

    2. Subtotal gastrectomy with Billroth II anastomosis

    3. Truncal vagotomy and pyloroplasty

for fat digestion, its absence leads to steatorrhea (the occurrence of greasy, bulky, light-colored stools). On the other hand, although pancreatic amylase and trypsin are important for carbohydrate and protein digestion, other enzymes in gastric and intestinal juice can usually compensate for their loss. Thus, patients with pancreatic insufficiency seldom present with maldigestion of carbohydrate and protein (nitrogen loss).

Etiology

Pancreatic insufficiency usually results from chronic pancreatitis in adults or cystic fibrosis (mucoviscidosis) in children (Table 15–7). In some cases, it is a consequence of pancreatic resection or carcinoma of the pancreas. Pancreatic insufficiency occurs after bone marrow transplantation and appears to be related to prior acute or chronic graft-versus-host disease. Each of these conditions markedly reduces the amount of pancreatic enzymes secreted, often to less than 5% of normal.

Pancreatic exocrine insufficiency is also a common occurrence in patients recovering from severe acute pancreatitis, and its severity correlates with the extent of pancreatic necrosis. Its severity also correlates with the severity of concomitant endocrine insufficiency, manifested by the new onset of diabetes mellitus.

Less commonly, pancreatic insufficiency results from disease states that cause the hypersecretion of gastric acid. For example, excessive gastrin secretion from a gastrinoma (an islet cell neoplasm composed of G cells) leads to the continuous

hypersecretion of gastric acid and a very low gastric juice pH. In affected patients, the excess gastric acid overwhelms the normal pancreatic bicarbonate production and results in an abnormally acidic pH in the duodenum. This acidic pH, in turn, causes a decrease in the activity of other types of pancreatic enzymes.

Pathology & Pathogenesis

Normally, the activities of the various pancreatic enzymes decrease during their passage from the duodenum to the terminal ileum. However, the degradation rates of individual enzymes vary; lipase activity is lost rapidly, and protease and amylase activities are lost slowly. Lipase activity is usually destroyed by proteolysis, mainly by the action of residual chymotrypsin. This mechanism persists in patients with pancreatic insufficiency, helping to explain why fat malabsorption develops earlier than protein or starch malabsorption.

Patients with destruction of the exocrine pancreas develop impaired digestion and fat absorption. Clinically, fat malabsorption is manifested as steatorrhea. Although the steatorrhea is caused mostly by the deficiency of pancreatic lipase, the absence of pancreatic bicarbonate secretion also contributes to its occurrence. Without bicarbonate, acidic chyme from the stomach inhibits the activity of pancreatic lipase and causes a precipitation of bile salts. Bile salt deficiency in turn causes failure of micelle formation and interference with fat absorption.

Pathophysiology

Causes of maldigestion from exocrine pancreatic insufficiency include chronic pancreatitis, cystic fibrosis, pancreatic cancer, partial or total gastrectomy, and pancreatic resection. Each of these causes is associated with specific related changes in GI physiology, including changes in intraluminal pH, bile acid metabolism, gastric emptying, and intestinal motility.

For example, during the course of chronic pancreatitis, there is a close relationship among gastric acidity, exocrine pancreatic insufficiency, and impaired digestion. Postprandial gastric acidification has been found to be significantly greater among patients with severe pancreatic insufficiency than among those with mild or no insufficiency. The inhibition of gastric acid secretion by H_2 blockers such as cimetidine or proton pump inhibitors such as omeprazole improves the response to pancreatic enzyme replacement and decreases fecal fat excretion. However, it does not lead to the complete elimination of steatorrhea.

On the other hand, stomach loss can cause considerable change in the function of the exocrine pancreas. After total gastrectomy, patients frequently develop severe primary exocrine pancreatic insufficiency with maldigestion and weight loss. Postoperatively, pancreatic juice volume, bicarbonate output, and enzyme (amylase, trypsin, chymotrypsin) secretion are reduced significantly compared with preoperative levels. These reductions probably result from changes in GI hormone secretion, altering the regulation of pancreatic function. For

TABLE 15–8   Clinical manifestations of pancreatic insufficiency.

Symptoms and Signs
Weight loss, muscle wasting, loss of subcutaneous fat
Steatorrhea (stool fat >6 g/d)
Flatulence, abdominal distension, cramps
Hypoproteinemia, peripheral edema, ascites
Weakness, fatigue
Orthostatic hypotension
Anemia due to malabsorption of vitamin B_{12} or iron
Ecchymoses due to vitamin K deficiency
Osteoporosis or osteomalacia; hypocalcemia or secondary hypoparathyroidism (with Chvostek sign and/or Trousseau sign), caused by vitamin D deficiency
Pellagra, alopecia, or seborrheic dermatitis

example, after gastrectomy, most patients exhibit decreased baseline and postprandial gastrin and pancreatic polypeptide secretion and increased postprandial CCK secretion.

Clinical Manifestations

The symptoms and signs exhibited by patients with pancreatic insufficiency (Table 15–8) vary to some extent with the underlying disease.

A. Steatorrhea

Patients with steatorrhea usually describe their stools as voluminous or bulky, foul-smelling, greasy, frothy, pale yellow, and floating. However, significant steatorrhea may occur without any of these characteristics. A 24-hour quantitative fecal fat test showing an excretion of more than 6 g is necessary for the definitive diagnosis of steatorrhea. Steatorrhea responds, often dramatically, to treatment with oral pancreatic enzymes, ingested with each meal and with snacks. In severe cases of fat malabsorption, deficiencies of the fat-soluble vitamins (vitamins A, D, E, K) may occur and require parenteral supplementation.

B. Diarrhea

In patients with fat malabsorption, diarrhea may result from the cathartic action of hydroxylated fatty acids. These fatty acids inhibit the absorption of sodium and water by the colon. Less commonly, watery diarrhea, abdominal cramping, and bloating are due to carbohydrate malabsorption. Indeed, because salivary amylase production remains undisturbed and because pancreatic amylase production must be markedly reduced before intraluminal starch digestion is slowed,

symptomatic carbohydrate malabsorption is uncommon in pancreatic insufficiency.

C. Hypocalcemia

Hypocalcemia, hypophosphatemia, tetany, osteomalacia, osteopenia (low bone mineral density), and osteoporosis can occur both from deficiency of the fat-soluble vitamin D and from the binding of dietary calcium to unabsorbed fatty acids, forming insoluble calcium–fat complexes (soaps) in the gut.

D. Nephrolithiasis

The formation of insoluble calcium soaps in the gut also prevents the normal binding of dietary oxalate to calcium. Dietary oxalate remains in solution and is absorbed from the colon, causing hyperoxaluria and predisposing to nephrolithiasis.

E. Vitamin B_{12} Deficiency

About 40% of patients with pancreatic insufficiency demonstrate malabsorption of vitamin B_{12} (cobalamin), although clinical manifestations of vitamin B_{12} deficiency (anemia, subacute combined degeneration of the spinal cord, dementia) are rare. The malabsorption of vitamin B_{12} appears to result from reduced degradation by pancreatic proteases of the normal complexes of vitamin B_{12} and its binding protein (R protein), resulting in less free vitamin B_{12} to bind to intrinsic factor in the small intestine.

F. Weight Loss

Long-standing malabsorption leads to protein catabolism and consequent weight loss, muscle wasting, fatigue, and edema. At times, weight loss occurs in patients with chronic pancreatitis because eating exacerbates their abdominal pain or because opioids used to control pain cause anorexia. In patients who develop diabetes mellitus, weight loss may be due to glycosuria.

Laboratory Tests & Evaluation

Because there is a direct correlation between duodenal (and therefore fecal) output of elastase 1 and duodenal output of lipase, amylase, trypsin, and bicarbonate, the measurement of fecal elastase concentrations has been used as a screening test for exocrine pancreatic insufficiency. The test appears most helpful in diagnosising severe pancreatic exocrine insufficiency, but may be insufficiently sensitive in mild or moderate cases. In addition, patients with other diarrheal illnesses (eg, irritable bowel syndrome) can produce spurious results. Other noninvasive tests may be considered (bentiromide test, pancreolauryl test, cholesteryl-[^{14}C]octanoate breath test), but these tests are not widely available. The ^{13}C breath test with mixed-chain triglycerides is an alternative study that is more readily available and has been shown to be helpful in following the response to pancreatic enzyme administration. In clinical practice, steatorrhea and associated weight loss are the most common and striking signs of exocrine pancreatic insufficiency. Therefore, providers must document and treat steatorrhea prior to proceeding with more specialized diagnostic testing.

CARCINOMA OF THE PANCREAS

Epidemiology & Etiology

Pancreatic carcinoma has become the third leading cause of cancer-related death in the United States, with a 2017 estimated incidence rate of 53,760 new cases and death rate of 43,090 individuals. Delay in diagnosis, relative resistance to chemotherapy and radiation, and intrinsic biological aggressiveness manifested by early metastatic disease all contribute to the abysmal prognosis associated with pancreatic adenocarcinoma. Pancreatic cancer typically occurs after age 50 years and increases in incidence with age, with most patients diagnosed between 60 and 80 years of age. It is somewhat more frequent in men than in women, and its incidence in both sexes is continuing to rise. Autopsy series document that pancreatic cancer has been identified in up to 2% of individuals undergoing a postmortem examination. Despite expanded awareness and advances in our understanding of the disease, diagnostic

procedures, and surgical and medical therapies, the overall 5-year survival for pancreatic adenocarcinoma remains approximately 9%.

Many risk factors for pancreatic adenocarcinoma have been identified. Cigarette smoking has the strongest overall association and is thought to account for one-quarter of cases diagnosed. The association between cigarette smoking and pancreatic cancer is thought to be related to the N-nitroso compounds present in cigarette smoke. Exposure to these agents leads to pancreatic ductal hyperplasia, a possible precursor to adenocarcinoma.

Other factors associated with an increased risk of pancreatic adenocarcinoma include a high dietary intake of saturated fat, exposure to nonchlorinated solvents, and the pesticide dichlorodiphenyl trichloroethane (DDT), although the overall contribution of these factors is likely small. The role of other dietary factors (coffee, high fat intake, alcohol use) is much debated, though diets containing fresh fruits and vegetables are thought to be protective. Diabetes mellitus has also recently been identified as a risk factor for the disease, though the exact pathophysiology is unknown. Chronic pancreatitis increases the risk of developing pancreatic adenocarcinoma by 10- to 20-fold. There is also an increased incidence of pancreatic cancer among patients with hereditary pancreatitis, particularly among those who develop pancreatic calcifications. Both highlight the important role of inflammation in pancreatic tumorigenesis. Rarely, pancreatic carcinoma is inherited in an autosomal dominant fashion in association with diabetes mellitus and exocrine pancreatic insufficiency. A genetic predisposition has also been identified in a number of familial cancer syndromes, including the syndromes listed in Table 15–9.

TABLE 15–9   Genetic syndromes associated with pancreatic cancer.

Syndrome	Mode of Inheritance	Gene	Chromosomal Locus	Risk Ratio
Hereditary pancreatitis	AD	PRSS1 (cationic trypsinogen), SPINK1	7q35	50–80
Hereditary nonpolyposis colorectal cancer (Lynch Syndrome)	AD	MSH2	2p	9
		MLH1	2p	
		PMS2	7p	
		PMS1	2q	
Familial breast and ovarian cancer	AD	BRCA2	13q	3.5–10
Familial atypical multiple-mole melanoma	AD	CDKN2A (P16)	9p	9–47
Ataxia-telangiectasia	AR	ATM	11q22–23	Unknown
Familial pancreatic cancer	AD	PALB2	16p	6
Peutz–Jeghers syndrome	AD	STK11 (LKB1)	19p	132
Cystic fibrosis	AD	CFTR	7	

AD, autosomal dominant; AR, autosomal recessive.

Modified from Kamisawa T et al. Pancreatic cancer. Lancet 2016;388(10039):73–85.

A number of genes linked with the familial syndromic and sporadic pancreatic cancer have been described. However, the penetrance of the disease in gene carriers is highly variable, and individual gene mutations have been variably linked to pancreatic oncogenesis. Importantly, the vast majority of pancreatic adenocarcinoma patients develop the disease without any recognized genetic mutation or putative or established risk factor.

Pathology

Carcinomas occur more often in the head (70%) and body (20%) than in the tail (10%) of the pancreas. Grossly, pancreatic cancer presents as a profoundly desmoplastic, infiltrative tumor that obstructs the pancreatic duct and thus often causes fibrosis and atrophy of the distal gland. Carcinomas of the head of the pancreas tend to obstruct the common bile duct early in their course, with resulting jaundice, and can extend into the uncinate process to involve the superior mesenteric artery and vein, thus compromising surgical resectability. Lesions tend to display vascular and neural tropism and can often be seen spreading along arteries and splanchnic nerves. Tumors of the body and tail tend to present later in their course, as they cause few symptoms until they become quite large.

Microscopically, 90% of pancreatic cancers are adenocarcinomas; the remainder are adenosquamous, anaplastic, or acinar cell carcinomas. Recently, whole genome sequencing has allowed for more accurate tumor classification and has identified unique subtypes based on genetic signature. Pancreatic cancer tends to spread into surrounding tissues, invading neighboring organs along the perineural fascia, causing severe pain, and via the lymphatics and bloodstream, causing metastases in regional lymph nodes, the liver, and other more distant sites (Figure 15–10).

Pancreatic adenocarcinomas consist of multiple cell types that each contribute to the clinical behavior of the disease. While mature cells in various stages of differentiation constitute the majority of the cellular elements, a small proportion of cancer stem cells account for the resistance to chemotherapy and radiation often characteristic of pancreatic cancer. A rich immune infiltrate of regulatory lymphocytes and immature myeloid cells is also present and creates an immunosuppressive barrier, limiting immune-mediated tumor destruction. Finally, pancreatic adenocarcinomas often have dense desmoplastic stromal elements that account for the tumor's infiltrative and fibrotic nature.

Pathogenesis

As with other epithelial malignancies, pancreatic adenocarcinoma appears to develop through a series of progressive genetic mutations within the pancreatic ductal epithelium (Figure 15–11). These sequential genetic and epigenetic events correlate with the evolution from premalignant ductal lesions

Hematogenous
• Liver
• Lungs
• Other

Lymph nodes
• Peripancreatic
• Para-aortic
• Extra-abdominal

Metastasis
• Early in adenocarcinoma
• Late in islet-cell carcinoma

Direct invasion
• Determines resectability
• Superior mesenteric vessels
• Portal vein
• Retroperitoneum, peritoneum
• Adjacent organs

Adenocarcinoma, head of pancreas
• 70% of pancreatic carcinomas
• Obstructs common bile duct
• Obstructive jaundice
• Tumor small at presentation

Adenocarcinoma, body and tail of pancreas
• Body: 20%; tail: 10% of pancreatic carcinomas
• Presents late
• Tumors large at presentation

FIGURE 15–10 Pancreatic cancer: location and pattern of spread. (Redrawn, with permission, from Chandrasoma P et al, eds. *Concise Pathology*, 3rd ed. Originally published by Appleton & Lange. Copyright © 1998 by The McGraw-Hill Companies, Inc.)

FIGURE 15–11 Model for the histological and genetic progression from normal cells (far left) through pancreatic intraepithelial neoplasia (PanIN) lesions (center), to invasive pancreatic cancer (far right). (Redrawn, with permission, from Maitra A et al. Pancreatic cancer. Annu Rev Pathol: Mechanisms Dis. 2008;3:157–88. Copyright © by Annual Reviews. www.annualreviews.org.)

to invasive carcinoma. Pancreatic intraepithelial neoplasia (PanIN) is the most well-characterized precursor to pancreatic adenocarcinoma. The evolution from minimal dysplasia (PanIN 1a and b) to severe dysplasia (PanIN 2 and 3) to adenocarcinoma appears to track with the stepwise accumulation of genetic mutations, including the activation of the K-ras2 oncogene, inactivation of the tumor suppressor gene *CDKN2a/INK4a*, and finally, inactivation of the tumor suppressor genes *TP53* and *DPC4/SMaD4*. Other precursor lesions of pancreatic adenocarcinoma likely exist in the form of mucin-producing pancreatic cystic neoplasms such as intraductal papillary mucinous neoplasms and mucinous cystic neoplasms.

Invasive pancreatic adenocarcinomas usually have one or more characteristic genetic mutations. Activating point mutations in the proto-oncogene K-ras at codon 12 have been identified in more than 90% of pancreatic cancers. Mutation in the *TP53* tumor suppressor gene has been detected in 50–75% of adenocarcinomas of the pancreas. The concurrent loss of *TP53* and K-ras function may contribute to the clinical aggressiveness of the cancer. In addition, in approximately 90% of cases, the *P16* tumor suppressor gene, located on chromosome 9p, is inactivated. DPC4 deletion is present in up to 50% of pancreatic adenocarcinomas and has been associated with increased metastatic potential.

Despite these prevalent mutations, comprehensive genomic analysis of human pancreatic cancer specimens has revealed tremendous genetic heterogeneity. Point mutations occur in numerous cellular pathways associated with neoplastic behavior, but few tumors share the same mutations or have defects in all pathways. Unfortunately, few targets susceptible to currently available drugs have been identified. Analyses of pancreatic cancer metastases have also revealed that the cellular clones that give rise to metastatic lesions may be distinct from the genetic fingerprint of the primary tumor. Although these characteristics complicate pancreatic cancer treatment, recent studies have attempted to identify tumor subtypes that differ in their response to various chemotherapy regimens, potentially facilitating a future customized treatment regimen for individual tumor genotypes.

Mutations in DNA mismatch repair genes can also give rise to pancreatic cancer, though multiple mutations must occur

for pancreatic cancer to develop. Familial pancreatic cancer syndromes arise from germline mutations such as *STK11* in Peutz–Jeghers syndrome. The mismatch repair gene *BRCA2* is inactivated in approximately 7–10% of pancreatic cancers. This creates a therapeutic opportunity, as cancers with deficient *BRCA2* rely on alternative DNA damage repair machinery for cell survival. Inhibition of Poly (ADP-ribose) polymerase (PARP), a protein involved in single-strand DNA break repair, has shown efficacy in *BRCA2*-mutated pancreatic cancers. Table 15–9 summarizes familial syndromes and genetic alterations associated with pancreatic cancer. A 2012 consensus conference defined a group of high-risk individuals deemed appropriate for pancreatic cancer screening: first-degree relatives of patients with pancreatic cancer from a familial kindred (at least two affected first-degree relatives); patients with Peutz–Jeghers syndrome; and *p16*, *BRCA2*, and hereditary nonpolyposis colorectal cancer (*HNPCC*) mutation carriers with one or more affected first-degree relative(s).

The tumor microenvironment (internal and surrounding stromal elements of pancreatic adenocarcinoma) is increasingly recognized both as central to the pathogenesis of the disease and as a potential target for therapy. Pancreatic stellate cells (myofibroblasts) responsible for stromal growth and turnover express growth factors and other peptides that may be associated with tumor behavior and prognosis.

In chronic pancreatitis, a common pathway for the development of pancreatic cancer may be through the chronic inflammatory process, including a pronounced stromal reaction. Mediators of chronic inflammation in the stroma likely support a transformation to malignancy, although the exact mechanisms remain unknown. Cytokines produced by the activated stroma appear to promote the aggressive behavior of pancreatic cancer cells.

Pancreatic cancer has a unique immune cell infiltrate that locally suppresses the immune system, contributing to tumor growth. As PanIN progresses to invasive cancer, there is an influx of myeloid-derived suppressor cells, regulatory T lymphocytes, and tumor-associated macrophages. These all serve to inhibit the destructive capability of cytotoxic T lymphocytes and represent a major barrier to immunotherapy for pancreatic cancer.

Clinical Manifestations

The clinical manifestations (Table 15–10) of pancreatic cancer vary with location and histologic tumor type.

Patients with carcinoma of the head of the pancreas usually present with painless, progressive jaundice resulting from common bile duct obstruction (see Figure 15–10). In addition to jaundice, distal obstruction caused by carcinoma can result in a dilated gallbladder, palpable in the right upper quadrant (**Courvoisier law**). Patients with carcinoma of the body or tail of the pancreas typically present with epigastric abdominal pain, profound weight loss, abdominal mass, and early satiety. Because of the vague nature of these symptoms, patients tend to present at later stages, often with distant metastases, particularly in the liver. Splenic vein thrombosis may occur as a complication of cancers in the body or tail of the gland, leading to splenomegaly and the development of intra-abdominal varices.

About 70% of patients with pancreatic cancer have impaired glucose tolerance or frank diabetes mellitus. While this may result from proximal ductal obstruction and atrophy of the distal gland, some patients appear to experience a resolution of impaired glucose tolerance or diabetes with surgical resection, suggesting that pancreatic cancers elaborate a yet unidentified diabetogenic substance. The relationship between pancreatic cancer and diabetes remains the subject of intense investigation.

A variety of tumor markers, such as carcinoembryonic antigen (CEA), CA 19-9, α-fetoprotein, pancreatic oncofetal antigen, and galactosyl transferase II, can be found in the serum of patients with pancreatic cancer. However, none of these tumor markers have sufficient specificity or predictive value to be useful in screening for the disease. CA 19-9 may be useful in predicting recurrence in patients following surgical resection or to follow disease burden in patients being treated with systemic chemotherapy.

In evaluating patients suspected of having pancreatic cancer, the initial diagnostic test of choice is a contrast-enhanced, thin-cut, helical CT scan. In addition to aiding in diagnosis, helical CT is useful for delineating the regional vascular anatomy, looking for major vascular invasion by tumor (a sign of unresectability), and determining the presence of metastatic disease. Tumors most often appear as hypodense, ill-defined structures with pancreatic duct dilation proximal to the mass. In cancers of the head of the pancreas, dilation of the main pancreatic duct often coincides with dilation of the common bile duct, creating a "double duct" sign. For patients with an inconclusive CT scan, or in cases where tissue is needed, EUS with fine-needle aspiration may aid in diagnosis. This is often important in cancers arising in the setting of chronic pancreatitis, since the clinical presentation may be indistinguishable and since inflammatory changes often obscure imaging. Endoscopic retrograde cholangiography (ERC) with endobiliary stent placement is typically used to palliate obstructive jaundice when present. In patients with pancreatic head lesions, brushing the biliary or pancreatic duct during ERCP may confirm the diagnosis of pancreatic adenocarcinoma.

Treatment with curative intent for pancreatic adenocarcinoma involves a multidisciplinary approach of surgical resection, systemic chemotherapy, and radiation therapy. Unfortunately, only 15–20% of patients are eligible for treatment with curative intent; all other patients with unresectable locally advanced pancreatic cancer and/or metastatic disease are candidates for palliative chemotherapy with the goal of improving survival. Advances in surgical strategies, such as vascular resection and reconstruction, resection in elderly

TABLE 15–10   Clinical manifestations of pancreatic carcinoma.

Symptoms and signs
Abdominal pain
Anorexia
Weight loss
Jaundice[1]
Diarrhea (irritable bowel symptoms)
Weakness
Palpable gallbladder
Constipation
Hematemesis or melena
Vomiting
Abdominal mass
Migratory thrombophlebitis
New onset mood changes
Abnormal laboratory tests
↑ Serum alkaline phosphatase
↑ Serum 5′-nucleotidase
↑ Serum LDH
↑ Serum AST
↑ Serum bilirubin
↑ Serum amylase
↑ Serum α-fetoprotein
↑ Serum carcinoembryonic antigen (CEA)
↑ Serum CA 19-9
↓ Serum albumin
New onset diabetes mellitus after age 50 years

[1]With carcinoma of the head of the pancreas.

Modified, with permission, from Greenberger NJ et al. *Current Diagnosis & Treatment: Gastroenterology, Hepatology, & Endoscopy*, 3rd ed. McGraw-Hill, 2016.

patients, minimally invasive pancreatectomy, and neoadjuvant chemoradiation regimens, have all attempted to expand the population of patients eligible for surgical resection. However, the invasive growth behavior of pancreatic cancer into perineural and retroperitoneal tissues often makes achieving a negative microscopic margin challenging, and operations that leave even microscopic disease behind afford no real chance for long-term survival.

Techniques in surgical resection vary by tumor location. Tumors arising from the head of the pancreas are treated with pancreaticoduodenectomy (**Whipple procedure**), in which the tumor-containing pancreatic head, duodenum, distal common bile duct, and surrounding lymph nodes are removed. Gastrointestinal continuity is re-established by connecting a portion of intestine to the bile duct, remaining pancreatic body/tail, and the stomach or duodenum. Lesions in the body and tail are treated with a distal pancreatectomy, often with the concomitant removal of the spleen.

Of patients eligible for surgical resection, the overall 5-year survival rate is approximately 20%, while select patients with small tumors, negative lymph nodes, and a negative microscopic margin have a slightly better prognosis. Patients with unresectable locally advanced disease may survive 12–24 months with modern multimodality palliative regimens. Patients with metastatic disease at presentation have a median survival of 6 months or less. These ominous outcomes indicate the need for improved treatment strategies. Given the significant expansion in our understanding of the genetic characteristics and cellular compartments of pancreatic adenocarcinoma, there is now more optimism that targeted agents, immunotherapy, and personalized treatment strategies will ultimately lead to improved survival for patients stricken with this aggressive disease.

CHECKPOINT

13. What are the risk factors for pancreatic cancer?
14. What are common symptoms and signs of pancreatic cancer?
15. How can you make the diagnosis of pancreatic cancer in a patient with suggestive symptoms and signs?

CASE STUDIES

Yeong Kwok, MD

(See Chapter 25, p. 774–75 for answers)

CASE 80

An admitting physician is called to the emergency department to evaluate a 58-year-old woman presenting with a 2-day history of fever, anorexia, nausea, and abdominal pain. Suspecting pancreatitis, the physician enquires about a history of similar symptoms. The patient was seen 2 months ago in the emergency department for an episode of unrelenting, achy right upper quadrant abdominal pain, at which time ultrasound imaging demonstrated multiple gallstones without evidence of cystic duct obstruction or gallbladder wall edema. At this time, serum amylase and lipase levels are both grossly elevated. On day 3 of the patient's hospital course, the physician is called urgently to evaluate her for hypotension, increased shortness of breath, and ensuing respiratory failure. She requires endotracheal intubation and mechanical ventilation. A chest radiograph and severe hypoxia support the diagnosis of acute respiratory distress syndrome.

Questions

A. By what mechanism can biliary stones cause pancreatitis?
B. At the time of admission, what additional historic features and laboratory studies should be obtained to further clarify the etiology of the patient's pancreatitis?
C. Describe how acute pancreatitis may be complicated by acute respiratory distress syndrome.

CASE 81

A 52-year-old man with a 20-year history of alcohol abuse presents to his primary care provider complaining of recurrent episodes of epigastric and left upper quadrant abdominal pain. Over the past month, the pain has become almost continuous, and he has requested morphine for better pain control. He has a history of alcohol-related acute pancreatitis. Examination reveals a 10-pound weight loss over the past 6 months. He has some mild muscle guarding over the epigastrium with tenderness to palpation. Bowel sounds are somewhat decreased. Serum amylase and lipase are mildly elevated. A plain film of the abdomen demonstrates pancreatic calcifications.

Questions

A. How often do heavy drinkers develop chronic pancreatitis?
B. What are the proposed mechanisms of alcohol-induced chronic pancreatitis?
C. Why may a proton pump inhibitor be helpful for this patient?

CASE 82

A 15-year-old boy with a history of cystic fibrosis comes to see you because of worsening diarrhea and weight loss. His lung disease has been relatively well controlled, but recently he has lost 5 kg unintentionally. His stools have also become loose and are very bulky, greasy, and foul smelling, especially after fatty meals. On examination, he is thin but otherwise normal appearing with a weight of 45 kg and height of 160 cm. Lung examination is notable for scattered rhonchi and crackles, but the rest of the examination, including the abdominal exam, is normal. Stool collection verifies the presence of steatorrhea. He is started on pancreatic enzymes with resolution of his gastrointestinal symptoms.

Questions

A. Why is fat malabsorption such a prominent finding in pancreatic insufficiency?
B. What are other consequences of pancreatic insufficiency?

CASE 83

During a family reunion, a 62-year-old widower describes to his son a 1-month history of lethargy. He attributed it to the stress of a recent move from a large three-bedroom house into an apartment. His granddaughter comments that his eyes appear "yellow" and that he has lost a significant amount of weight since their last visit with him. Corroborating the finding of painless jaundice, his internist orders a contrast-enhanced spiral CT, revealing a 3 cm mass in the head of the pancreas.

Questions

A. On physical examination, the patient has a palpable and mildly tender gallbladder. What is the significance of this finding?
B. What hematologic abnormalities may be associated with pancreatic cancer?
C. What are some important clinical prognostic factors?

REFERENCES

Anatomy

Pan FC et al. Pancreas organogenesis: from bud to plexus to gland. Dev Dyn. 2011 Mar;240(3):530–65. [PMID: 21337462]

Physiology

Chandra R et al. Recent advances in pancreatic endocrine and exocrine secretion. Curr Opin Gastroenterol. 2011 Sep;27(5):439–43. [PMID: 21778879]

Doyle CJ et al. The proteome of normal pancreatic juice. Pancreas. 2012 Mar;41(2):186–94. [PMID: 22129531]

Acute Pancreatitis

Bendersky VA et al. Necrotizing pancreatitis: challenges and solutions. Clin Exp Gastroenterol. 2016 Oct 31;9:345–50. [PMID: 27826206]

Fisic E et al. The role of IL-6, 8, and 10, sTNFr, CRP, and pancreatic elastase in the prediction of systemic complications in patients with acute pancreatitis. Gastroenterol Res Pract. 2013;2013:282645. [PMID: 23476635]

Hegyi P et al. The role of pancreatic ducts in the pathogenesis of acute pancreatitis. Pancreatology. 2015 Jul;15(4 Suppl):S13–7. [PMID: 25921231]

Italian Association for the Study of the Pancreas (AISP), Pezzilli R et al. Consensus guidelines on severe acute pancreatitis. Dig Liver Dis. 2015 Jul;47(7):532–43. [PMID: 25921277]

Lankisch PG et al. Acute pancreatitis. Lancet. 2015 Jul 4;386(9988):85–96. [PMID: 25616312]

Madhani K et al. Autoimmune pancreatitis: an update on diagnosis and management. Gastroenterol Clin North Am. 2016 Mar;45(1):29–43. [PMID: 26895679]

Peery AF et al. Burden of gastrointestinal, liver, and pancreatic diseases in the United States. Gastroenterology. 2015;149(7):1731–41. [PMID: 26327134]

Singh P et al. Pathophysiological mechanisms in acute pancreatitis: current understanding. Indian J Gastroenterol. 2016 May;35(3):153–66. [PMID: 27206712]

Tenner S et al. American College of Gastroenterology guideline: management of acute pancreatitis. Am J Gastroenterol. 2013 Sep;108(9):1400–15. [PMID: 23896955]

Testoni PA. Acute recurrent pancreatitis: etiopathogenesis, diagnosis and treatment. World J Gastroenterol. 2014 Dec 7;20(45):16891–901. [PMID: 25493002]

Windsor JA et al. Classifying the severity of acute pancreatitis: towards a way forward. Pancreatology. 2015 Mar-Apr;15(2):101–4. [PMID: 25683639]

Yang CJ et al. Predictors of severe and critical acute pancreatitis: a systematic review. Dig Liver Dis. 2014 May;46(5):446–51. [PMID: 24646880]

Chronic Pancreatitis

Aghdassi AA et al. Genetic susceptibility factors for alcohol-induced chronic pancreatitis. Pancreatology. 2015 Jul;15(4 Suppl):S23–31. [PMID: 26149858]

Ketwaroo GA et al. Approach to patients with suspected chronic pancreatitis: a comprehensive review. Pancreas. 2015 Mar;44(2):173–80. [PMID: 25675419]

Majumder S et al. Chronic pancreatitis. 2016 May 7;387(10031):1957–66. [PMID: 26948434]

Whitcomb DC. Genetics of alcoholic and nonalcoholic pancreatitis. Curr Opin Gastroenterol. 2012 Sep;28(5):501–6. [PMID: 22885947]

Pancreatic Insufficiency

Domínguez-Muñoz JE et al. Potential for screening for pancreatic exocrine insufficiency using the fecal elastase-1 test. Dig Dis Sci. 2017 May;62(5):1119–30. [PMID: 28315028]

Lohr JM et al. Synopsis of recent guidelines on pancreatic exocrine insufficiency. United European Gastroenterol J. 2013 Apr;1(2):79–83. [PMID: 24917944]

Phillips ME. Pancreatic exocrine insufficiency following pancreatic resection. Pancreatology. 2015 Sep-Oct;15(5):449–55. [PMID: 26145836]

Ramsey ML et al. Complications of chronic pancreatitis. Dig Dis Sci. 2017 Jul;62(7):1745–50. [PMID: 28281169]

Struyvenberg MR et al. Practical guide to exocrine pancreatic insufficiency - breaking the myths. BMC Med. 2017 Feb 10;15(1):29. [PMID: 28183317]

Tseng DS et al. Pancreatic exocrine insufficiency in patients with pancreatic or periampullary cancer: a systematic review. Pancreas. 2016 Mar;45(3):325–30. [PMID: 26495777]

Pancreatic Cancer

Fogel EL et al. A multidisciplinary approach to pancreas cancer in 2016: a review. Am J Gastroenterol. 2017 Apr;112(4):537–54. [PMID: 28139655]

Kamisawa T et al. Pancreatic cancer. Lancet. 2016 Jul 2;388(10039):73–85. [PMID: 26830752]

Klein AP. Identifying people at a high risk of developing pancreatic cancer. Nat Rev Cancer. 2013 Jan;13(1):66–74. [PMID: 23222481]

Noone AM et al. SEER cancer statistics review, 1975–2015, National Cancer Institute. Bethesda, MD. https://seer.cancer.gov/csr/1975_2015/, based on November 2017 SEER data submission, posted to the SEER web site, April 2018.

Pinho DF et al. PET-computed tomography and precision medicine in pancreatic adenocarcinoma and pancreatic neuroendocrine tumors. PET Clin. 2017 Oct;12(4):407–21. [PMID: 28867112]

Whitcomb DC et al. Genetics and genetic testing in pancreatic cancer. Gastroenterology. 2015 Oct;149(5):1252–64. [PMID: 26255042]

Wörmann SM et al. The immune network in pancreatic cancer development and progression. Oncogene. 2014 Jun 5;33(23):2956–67. [PMID: 23851493]

Renal Disease

Rachel L. Perlman, MD,
& Michael Heung, MD, MS

Kidney disease contributes significantly to the global burden of disease, both in developing and developed countries. The Centers for Disease Control and Prevention estimate that in the United States, more than 10% of people 20 years of age and older (more than 20 million individuals) have chronic kidney disease. In addition, many more people suffer from acute kidney injury and other forms of kidney disease annually. Thus, clinicians of all specialties will encounter patients with renal disorders, and it behooves us to be aware of the various risk factors and causes of kidney disease. This is particularly important because with early detection and appropriate management, most forms of kidney disease can be treated to prevent or at least slow the rate of progression to kidney failure or other complications.

The kidneys serve a crucial role in filtering blood, and a wide range of diseases of other organ systems and systemic diseases may be manifested in the kidney. For example, renal disease is a prominent presentation of long-standing diabetes mellitus and hypertension and of autoimmune disorders such as systemic lupus erythematosus.

A particular challenge is that patients are typically asymptomatic until relatively advanced kidney failure is present. There are no pain receptors within the substance of the kidney, so pain is not a prominent presenting complaint, except in those renal diseases in which there is involvement of the ureter (eg, nephrolithiasis) or the renal capsule (eg, renal cell carcinoma). In early stages of kidney disease, patients may have only abnormalities of urine volume or composition (eg, presence of red blood cells and/or protein). Later, they may manifest systemic symptoms and signs of lost renal function (eg, edema, fluid overload, electrolyte abnormalities, anemia). Depending on the nature of the renal disease, they may progress to display a wide range of chronic complications resulting from inadequate renal function.

The kidneys play multiple roles in the body, including blood filtration, metabolism and excretion of endogenous and exogenous compounds, and endocrine functions. Perhaps most significantly, the kidneys are the primary regulators of fluid, acid–base, and electrolyte balances in the body, and this remarkable pair of organs maintains homeostasis across a broad array of dietary and environmental changes. An understanding of each of these roles is required to illuminate the pathophysiologic basis behind the many manifestations of kidney disease.

CHECKPOINT

1. What are some important causes of renal disease?
2. What are some consequences of renal failure?

NORMAL STRUCTURE & FUNCTION OF THE KIDNEY

ANATOMY, HISTOLOGY & CELL BIOLOGY

A remarkable attribute of the kidneys is their ability to maintain homeostasis while functioning under a broad range of environmental water and salt availabilities. For example, the kidneys have the capacity to excrete free water in freshwater fish, widely varying amounts of water and solute in humans, and an extremely concentrated urine in the kangaroo rat, which can live its entire life without access to water. The kidneys are a pair of encapsulated organs located in the retroperitoneal area (Figure 16–1). A renal artery enters and a renal vein exits from each kidney at the hilum. Approximately 20% of cardiac output goes to the kidneys. Blood is filtered in the

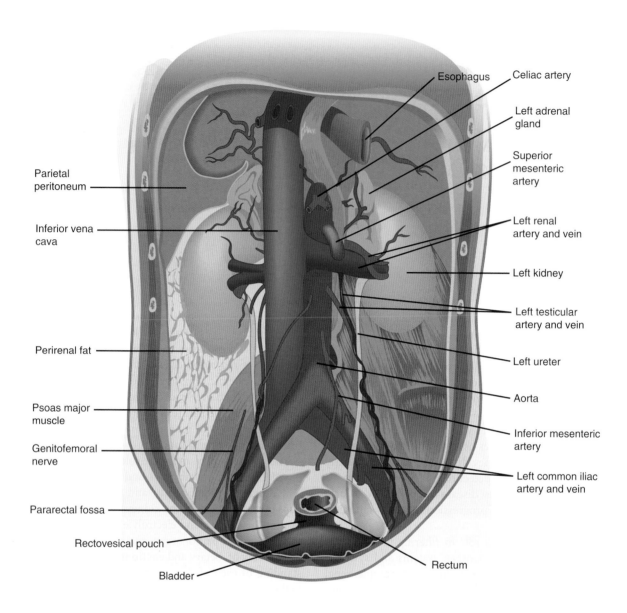

FIGURE 16–1 Vessels and organs of the retroperitoneum. (Redrawn, with permission, from Lindner HH. *Clinical Anatomy*. Originally published by Appleton & Lange. Copyright © 1989 by The McGraw-Hill Companies, Inc.)

kidneys, removing wastes—in particular urea and nitrogen-containing compounds—and regulating extracellular electrolytes and intravascular volume. Because renal blood flow is from the cortex to the medulla, and because the medulla has a relatively low rate of blood flow for a high rate of metabolic activity, the normal oxygen tension in the medulla is lower than in other parts of the kidney. This makes the medulla particularly susceptible to ischemic injury.

The **nephron** is the basic structural and functional unit of the kidney. Each nephron consists of a tuft of capillaries termed the **glomerulus**, the site at which blood is filtered, and a **renal tubule** from which water and salts in the filtrate are reclaimed (Figure 16–2). Each human kidney has approximately 1 million nephrons.

A glomerulus consists of an **afferent** and an **efferent arteriole** and an intervening tuft of capillaries lined with endothelial cells and covered with epithelial cells that form a continuous layer with those of the **Bowman capsule** and the renal tubule. The space between capillaries in the glomerulus is called the **mesangium**. Material comprising a basement membrane is located between the capillary's endothelial cells and the glomerular epithelial cells (on the other side of the basement membrane) (Figure 16–2C).

A closer examination of glomerular histology and cell biology reveals unique features not found in most peripheral capillaries (see Figure 16–2). First, the glomerular capillary endothelium is fenestrated (see Figure 16–2C). However, because the endothelial cells have a coat of negatively charged glycoproteins and glycosaminoglycans, they normally exclude plasma proteins

FIGURE 16–2 Structures of the kidney. **A:** Landmarks of the normal kidney. **B:** Glomerulus and glomerular capillary. **C:** Detailed structure of the glomerulus and the glomerular filtration membrane composed of endothelial cell, basement membrane, and podocyte. Note that, for clarity, the distal tubule is separated from the glomerulus in **A;** however, its true anatomic relationship, which is essential for physiologic function, is illustrated in **B.** (Redrawn, with permission, from Chandrasoma P et al, eds. *Concise Pathology*, 3rd ed. Originally published by Appleton & Lange. Copyright © 1998 by The McGraw-Hill Companies, Inc.)

such as albumin. On the other side of the glomerular basement membrane are the epithelial cells. Termed **podocytes** because of their numerous extensions, or foot processes, these cells are connected to one another by modified desmosomes.

The mesangium is an extension of the glomerular basement membrane but is less dense and consists of two distinct cell types: intrinsic glomerular cells and tissue macrophages. Both cell types contribute to the development of immune-mediated

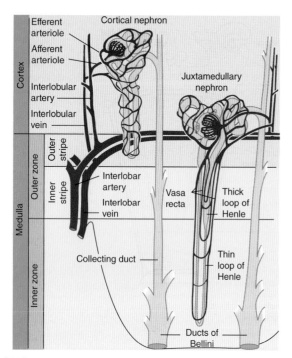

FIGURE 16–3 The vascular supply of the cortical and juxtamedullary nephrons. (Redrawn, with permission, from Pitts RF. *Physiology of the Kidney and Body Fluids*, 3rd ed. Year Book, 1963. Copyright © Elsevier.)

glomerular disease by their production of, and response to, cytokines such as transforming growth factor-β (TGF-β).

Understanding the complex organization of the glomerulus is crucial for understanding normal renal function and also the characteristics of different glomerular diseases. Thus, in some conditions, immune complexes may accumulate under the epithelial cells, whereas in others, they may accumulate under the endothelial cells. Likewise, because immune cells are unable to cross the glomerular basement membrane, immune complex deposition under the epithelial cells is generally not accompanied by a cellular inflammatory reaction (see later discussion).

The renal tubule itself has a number of different structural regions: the **proximal convoluted tubule**, from which most of the electrolytes and water are reclaimed; the **loop of Henle**; and a **distal convoluted tubule** and **collecting duct** (Figure 16–3), where urine is concentrated and additional electrolyte and water changes are made in response to hormonal control.

PHYSIOLOGY

Glomerular Filtration & Tubular Resorption

Approximately 100–120 mL/min of glomerular filtrate is generated in a normal adult with two fully functional kidneys. The approximate mass cutoff of substances for filtration is 70 kDa. However, substances smaller than this are often retained, either because of electric charge effects or because they are tightly bound to other proteins, giving them a larger effective size.

After filtration at the glomerulus, there is extensive reabsorption of filtered substances along the renal tubular network. The degree of reabsorption varies by substance and anatomic location in the tubules, thus allowing for differential regulation of constituent components. Most (60–70%) of the filtered Na⁺—and, under normal conditions, almost all the K⁺ and glucose—is actively resorbed from the tubular fluid via co-transporter mechanisms in the proximal tubule. Water is resorbed passively and along osmotic gradients established by the reabsorption of Na⁺. In addition to absorption, a number of substances are secreted into the tubular fluid through the action of transporters along the renal tubule. Examples of substances secreted include organic anions and cations such as creatinine, histamine, and many drugs and toxins.

Normally, about 30 mL/min of isotonic filtrate is delivered to the loop of Henle, where a countercurrent multiplier mechanism achieves concentration of the urine. The loop of Henle passes down into the medulla of the kidney, where secretion of Na⁺ from the cells in the thick ascending limb establishes a hypertonic concentration gradient to reabsorb water from the tubular fluid across the cells of the descending limb.

Under normal circumstances, no more than 5–10 mL/min of glomerular filtrate is delivered to the collecting ducts. Water absorption in the collecting ducts occurs directly through water channels controlled by **vasopressin** (also known as **antidiuretic hormone [ADH]**). Under the control of aldosterone, Na⁺ resorption from tubular fluid and K⁺ and H⁺ transport into tubular fluid occur in different types of cells in the renal collecting ducts. Even though it deals with less than one-tenth of the total glomerular filtrate, the collecting duct is the site of urine volume regulation and the site at which water, Na⁺, acid–base, and K⁺ balance is achieved. The crucial role of the collecting duct in regulating kidney function depends on two features. First, the collecting duct is under hormonal control, in contrast to the proximal tubule, whose actions are generally a simple function of volume and the composition of tubular fluid and constitutively active transporters. Second, the collecting duct is the last region of the renal tubule traversed before the remaining 1–2 mL/min of the original glomerular filtrate exits into the ureters as urine.

Renal Regulation of Blood Pressure & Blood Volume

The kidney plays an important role in blood pressure regulation through their effect on Na⁺ and water balance, which are major determinants of blood pressure. First, the Na⁺ concentration in the proximal tubular fluid is sensed at the macula densa (see Figure 16–2), part of the **juxtaglomerular apparatus**. The juxtaglomerular apparatus also assesses the perfusion pressure of the blood, an important indicator of intravascular volume status under normal circumstances. Through the action of these two sensors, either low Na⁺ or low perfusion pressure acts as a stimulus for renin release. **Renin**, a protease made in the juxtaglomerular cells, cleaves angiotensinogen in the blood to generate **angiotensin I**, which is then cleaved to **angiotensin II** by **angiotensin-converting enzyme** (ACE). Angiotensin II raises blood pressure by directly triggering vasoconstriction and by stimulating aldosterone production and secretion in the adrenal cortex, resulting in Na$^+$ and water retention by the collecting duct (see Chapter 21). All these effects expand the extracellular fluid (ECF) and thus renal perfusion pressure, completing a homeostatic negative feedback loop that alleviates the initial stimulus for renin release. However, these mechanisms can also be maladaptive and contribute to the pathophysiology of various disease states.

Notably, the trigger activating the renin–angiotensin-aldosterone system is the physiologic signal of **low effective circulating volume**, which may not be synonymous with low total body volume. Edematous states (eg, heart failure, nephrotic syndrome, cirrhosis) develop owing to a pathophysiologic factor favoring fluid movement out of the intravascular space and into the interstitium or third spaces (eg, peritoneal cavity, pleural space). In the case of heart failure, this factor is an elevated hydrostatic component related to cardiac congestion. In nephrotic syndrome, it is a fall in oncotic pressure owing to a loss of protein in the urine. In cirrhosis, there can be a combination of lower oncotic pressures from decreased protein production and increased hydrostatic pressure from hepatic congestion, leading to third-spacing of fluid. In all these conditions, the resultant decreased effective circulating volume signals the kidneys to progressively retain Na$^+$ and water until a new equilibrium is established between the vascular space and interstitial space.

Another trigger activating the renin–angiotensin-aldosterone system is renovascular disease, an important cause of secondary hypertension. In renovascular disease, a fixed vascular abnormality in the renal arterial circulation (most commonly atherosclerosis) results in impaired blood flow, generating the signal for low effective circulating volume despite a normal circulating volume. The resultant activation of the renin–angiotensin-aldosterone system leads to hypertension because of the direct vascular effects of angiotensin and because of the increased circulating volume resulting from an aldosterone-mediated increase in Na$^+$ reabsorption.

Intravascular volume depletion also triggers vasopressin release. Receptors in the carotid body and elsewhere sense a fall in blood pressure and activate autonomic neural pathways, including fibers that go to the hypothalamus, where vasopressin release is controlled. Vasopressin is released and travels via the bloodstream throughout the body. At the collecting duct, vasopressin facilitates insertion of water channels into the cell membranes, allowing for the passive reabsorption of free water based on the medullary interstitial osmotic gradient. Chapter 19 provides further discussions of water balance and the role of vasopressin.

Renal Regulation of Acid–Base Balance

Along with the pulmonary system, the kidneys play a primary role in acid–base homeostasis. In normal conditions, the arterial blood pH is maintained within the range of 7.35–7.45 through a buffering system in which bicarbonate plays a key role:

$$H^+ + HCO_3^- \leftrightarrow H_2CO_3 \leftrightarrow H_2O + CO_2$$

For example, a drop in pH (increase in H$^+$ concentration) leads to an increase in CO$_2$, which can be exhaled from the lungs. This immediate buffering effect depletes the body's stores of bicarbonate. The kidneys subsequently excrete additional H$^+$ and thus serve to replete bicarbonate stores. In this system, the pulmonary response to an acid–base imbalance is rapid (seconds to minutes), whereas the kidney's response is delayed (hours to days). However, the lungs can excrete only volatile acids, and the removal of nonvolatile ("fixed") acids relies on the kidneys.

During the ingestion of a normal daily diet, humans generate an obligate acid load through protein metabolism. To maintain homeostasis, this acid load is excreted by the kidneys. The primary site of acid excretion is the distal collecting duct, where H$^+$ is secreted into the tubular lumen, where it combines primarily with ammonia (NH$_3$) to form ammonium (NH$_4^+$), which is subsequently excreted in the urine.

In addition to acid excretion, the kidneys regulate acid–base balance through the reabsorption and regeneration of bicarbonate, primarily in the proximal tubule. Insight into the functional roles of the proximal and distal renal tubules in maintaining acid–base balance can be seen in the clinical features of the various forms of renal tubular acidosis (Table 16–1).

Metabolic acidosis is a common and potentially severe condition that warrants careful evaluation in the clinical setting. Several mechanisms can lead to the development of metabolic acidosis. First, the excess production of endogenous acids can exceed the ability of the kidneys to excrete H$^+$. This can occur in advanced kidney failure, as the kidneys' ability to generate ammonium is diminished. Conversely, metabolic acidosis can develop from the excess production of endogenous acids even in the face of intact renal function (eg, in lactic acidosis from tissue ischemia or in diabetic ketoacidosis). Second, metabolic acidosis can result from the ingestion of exogenous acids (eg, in intoxication with methanol or ethylene glycol, which are metabolized to formic acid and oxalic acid, respectively). Third, metabolic acidosis can develop through the loss of bicarbonate, which can occur from a failure to reabsorb bicarbonate in the kidney (ie, proximal renal tubular acidosis) or from the gastrointestinal (GI) loss of bicarbonate-rich fluids (eg, severe diarrhea, pancreatic fistula). Fourth, the administration of large amounts of bicarbonate-depleted solution (such as 0.9% normal saline) to patients can lead to a dilutional acidosis.

Renal Regulation of Potassium Balance

Potassium balance is primarily regulated in the distal collecting duct, where it is secreted into the lumen in response to aldosterone-mediated Na$^+$ reabsorption. Therefore, aldosterone is the primary hormonal regulator of K$^+$. Indeed, in addition to the angiotensin-mediated stimulus discussed above,

TABLE 16–1   **Characteristics of renal tubular acidosis.**

	Type 1 (Distal)	Type 2 (Proximal)	Type 4
Basic defect	Decreased distal acidification	Diminished proximal HCO_3^- reabsorption	Aldosterone deficiency or resistance
Etiology	Autoimmune disease, genetic, medication	Light chain excretion, genetic, medication, idiopathic	Diabetes mellitus, medication, adrenal insufficiency, genetic
Urine pH	>5.3	Variable: >5.3 if above reabsorptive threshold; <5.3 if below	Usually <5.3
Plasma [HCO_3^-], untreated	Often extremely low, ~10 mEq/L	Usually 14–20 mEq/L	Usually >15 mEq/L
Fractional excretion of HCO_3^- at normal plasma [HCO_3^-]	<3% in adults; may reach 5–10% in young children	>15–20%	<3%
Plasma [K^+]	Usually reduced, although a hyperkalemic form exists	Usually reduced	Elevated
Dose of HCO_3^- to normalize plasma [HCO_3^-], mEq/kg per day	1–2 in adults; 4–14 in children	10–15	1–3; may require no alkali if hyperkalemia corrected
Nonelectrolyte complications	Nephrocalcinosis, nephrolithiasis, osteopenia	Rickets or osteomalacia	None

hyperkalemia is a signal for aldosterone release, whereas hypokalemia provides negative feedback for such release (see Chapter 21). The kidneys' ability to regulate K^+ balance is such that K^+ excretion can be upregulated to exceed even the amount filtered in the glomerulus.

Hypokalemia can develop from three main mechanisms: shifting of K^+ from the extracellular to intracellular compartments (eg, alkalosis, use of β-agonist therapy), extrarenal losses (eg, diarrhea), or renal losses. In general, increased delivery of Na^+ to the distal tubules/collecting duct will result in increased K^+ secretion, with the most common causes of renal K^+ wasting being diuretic use and osmotic kaliuresis. Hyperaldosteronism, either primary aldosteronism from an adrenal tumor (ie, Conn syndrome) or secondary (eg, hyperreninemic) hyperaldosteronism, frequently presents with hypokalemia owing to unchecked Na^+ reabsorption with the resultant secretion of both K^+ and H^+. Therefore, the clinical presentation of hypokalemia with hypertension and metabolic alkalosis should prompt an evaluation for a state of aldosterone excess. Chapter 21 provides a further discussion of the role of the renin–angiotensin–aldosterone system in regulating potassium and intravascular volume.

Hyperkalemia can occur from extracellular potassium shifting (eg, acidosis), cellular potassium release (eg, hemolysis), increased potassium ingestion, or decreased renal potassium excretion (eg, renal insufficiency or kidney failure). Numerous drugs can also interfere with renal K^+ excretion.

Renal Regulation of Ca^{2+} Metabolism

The kidney plays a number of important roles in Ca^{2+} and phosphate homeostasis. First, the kidney is the site of 1α-hydroxylation or 24-hydroxylation of 25-hydroxycholecalciferol, the hepatic metabolite of vitamin D_3. This produces calcitriol (1,25-dihydroxy vitamin D), the biologically active form of vitamin D that increases Ca^{2+} absorption from the gut. Second, the kidney is a site of action for **parathyroid hormone** (**PTH**), resulting in Ca^{2+} retention and phosphate wasting in the urine. Chapter 17 provides a further discussion of the role of the kidney in Ca^{2+} and phosphate homeostasis.

Renal Regulation of Erythropoiesis

The kidney is the main site of production of the hormone **erythropoietin**, which stimulates the bone marrow production and maturation of red blood cells. The signal for erythropoietin production is thought to be the level of blood oxygenation, which is monitored in the kidney. With progressive renal insufficiency, the capacity to produce erythropoietin becomes impaired and anemia can develop. Anemia typically begins to occur when the glomerular filtration rate (GFR) has fallen to 30–45 mL/min or less, and it is nearly universally observed in patients with end-stage renal disease. Although common, anemia of chronic kidney disease is a diagnosis of exclusion. Iron deficiency and other underlying abnormalities should be investigated and corrected if possible. The primary management of severe anemia of chronic kidney disease is hormone replacement therapy with a recombinant analog of erythropoietin. Chapter 6 provides additional discussion of the role of erythropoietin in the regulation of red blood cell mass.

Regulation of Renal Function

There are a variety of physical, hormonal, and neural mechanisms by which the functions of the kidney are controlled.

Vasopressin, together with the physics of the countercurrent multiplier in the loop of Henle and the hypertonic medullary interstitium, makes it possible to concentrate the urine under normal circumstances. This confers on the healthy kidney the ability to maintain fluid homeostasis under widely diverse conditions (by generating either a concentrated or dilute urine, depending on whether the body needs to conserve or excrete salt and water).

Tubuloglomerular feedback refers to the ability of the kidney to regulate the GFR in response to the solute concentration in the distal renal tubule. When an excessive concentration of Na^+ in the tubular fluid is sensed by the **macula densa**, afferent arteriolar vasoconstriction is triggered. This diminishes the GFR so that the renal tubule has a smaller solute load per unit time, allowing Na^+ to be more efficiently reclaimed from tubular fluid. A variety of vasoactive substances, including adenosine, prostaglandins, nitric oxide, and peptides such as endothelin and bradykinin, contribute to the humoral control of tubuloglomerular feedback.

Another important challenge for the kidney is regulating renal cortical versus medullary blood flow. Renal cortical blood flow needs to be sufficient to maintain a GFR high enough to clear renally excreted wastes efficiently without exceeding the capacity of the renal tubules for solute reabsorption. Likewise, medullary blood flow must be closely regulated. Excessive medullary blood flow can disrupt the osmolar gradient achieved by the countercurrent exchange mechanism. Insufficient medullary blood flow can result in anoxic injury to the renal tubule. From the perspective of individual nephrons, redistribution of blood flow from the cortex to the medulla involves preferentially supplying blood (and therefore oxygen) to those nephrons with long loops of Henle that dip down into the inner medulla.

Adaptations of the kidney to injury can also be thought of as a form of regulation. Thus, nephron loss results in compensatory **glomerular hyperfiltration** (increased GFR per nephron) and renal hypertrophy. Although hyperfiltration may be adaptive in the short term, allowing maintenance of the total renal GFR, it has been implicated as a common inciting event in further nephron destruction from a variety of causes.

There are other clinically important adaptations to injury. Poor renal perfusion from any cause results in responses that improve perfusion through afferent arteriolar vasodilation and efferent arteriolar vasoconstriction in response to hormonal and neural cues. These regulatory effects are reinforced by inputs sensing Na^+ balance. Altering the Na^+ balance is another way to influence blood pressure and hence renal perfusion pressure. Sympathetic innervation by the renal nerves influences renin release. Renal prostaglandins play an important role in vasodilation, especially in patients with chronically poor renal perfusion.

CHECKPOINT

3. What are the parts of the nephron, and what role does each play in renal function?
4. How is renal function regulated?
5. What are the nonexcretory functions of the kidney?
6. What are the relationships, if any, between each nonexcretory function named previously and the kidney's role in fluid, electrolyte, and blood pressure regulation?

OVERVIEW OF RENAL DISEASE

ALTERATIONS OF KIDNEY STRUCTURE & FUNCTION IN DISEASE

Renal disease can be categorized either by the site of the lesion (eg, glomerulopathy vs. tubulointerstitial disease) or by the nature of the factors leading to kidney disease (eg, immunologic, metabolic, infiltrative, infectious, hemodynamic, toxic).

Glomerular disease can be further categorized according to clinical presentation. Thus, some disorders present with profound proteinuria but no evidence of a cellular inflammatory reaction (nephrotic disorders), whereas others have variable degrees of proteinuria associated with red and white blood cells in the urine (nephritic disorders).

Nephrotic disorders typically show immune complex deposition at or under the epithelial cells, often with morphologic changes in the foot processes (Figure 16–4). This probably reflects damage to the selective nature of the glomerular filter (eg, by immune complex formation) or the deposition of preformed complexes, in some cases with complement activation but without concomitant activation of a cellular immune response. Although the lack of a cellular immune response may limit the damage done, it also slows the resolution of the disorder, with proteinuria taking months or years to resolve even when the underlying disease has been brought under control.

Nephritic disorders show immune complex deposits either in a subendothelial location or in the glomerular basement membrane or mesangium (see Figure 16–4). The cellular immune system has ready access to all these locations, and the resulting inflammatory reaction can be a "double-edged sword." Thus, when the underlying process can be controlled, phagocytosis of the subendothelial deposits speeds recovery. On the other hand, an uncontrolled or prolonged inflammatory response can result in a greater degree of destruction of the glomerular architecture, in part because of the local production and action of cytokines.

FIGURE 16–4 The anatomy of a normal glomerular capillary is shown on the left. Note the fenestrated endothelium (EN), glomerular basement membrane (GBM), and the epithelium with its foot processes (EP). The mesangium is composed of mesangial cells (MC) surrounded by extracellular matrix (MM) in direct contact with the endothelium. Ultrafiltration occurs across the glomerular wall and through channels in the mesangial matrix into the urinary space (US). The typical localization of immune deposits and other pathologic changes is depicted on the right. (1) Uniform subepithelial deposits as in membranous nephropathy. (2) Large, irregular subepithelial deposits or "humps" seen in acute postinfectious glomerulonephritis. (3) Subendothelial deposits as in diffuse proliferative lupus glomerulonephritis. (4) Mesangial deposits characteristic of immunoglobulin A nephropathy. (5) Antibody binding to the glomerular basement membrane (as in Goodpasture syndrome) does not produce visible deposits, but a smooth linear pattern is seen on immunofluorescence. (6) Effacement of the epithelial foot processes is common in all forms of glomerular injury with proteinuria.

Specific regions of the kidney are particularly susceptible to certain kinds of injury: (1) Hemodynamic factors regulating blood flow have profound effects on the kidney, both because the GFR, a primary determinant of renal function, depends on renal blood flow and because the kidney is susceptible to hypoxic injury; (2) the renal medulla is a low-oxygen-tension environment, which makes it very susceptible to ischemic injury; and (3) the glomerulus is the initial filter of blood entering the kidney and thus is a prominent site of injury related to immune complex deposition and complement fixation.

One useful organizing scheme that combines a consideration of both the site and cause of renal disease in approaching patients with new renal failure is to first categorize the cause of the patient's renal failure as prerenal, intrarenal, or postrenal and then to subdivide each of these categories according to specific causes and anatomic locations (Table 16–2).

MANIFESTATIONS OF ALTERED KIDNEY FUNCTION

Decreased kidney function leads to an accumulation of urea and an inability to maintain electrolyte, water, and acid–base balance. The failure to adequately excrete urea, manifested as a progressive elevation of blood urea nitrogen (BUN), serum creatinine, and other poorly defined toxins, results in uremia (see Chronic Kidney Disease, below). Uremia is a syndrome characterized by a constellation of symptoms, physical examination findings, and laboratory abnormalities (Table 16–3), presumably caused by a buildup of one or more uncharacterized toxins. In the absence of adequate renal clearance, ingesting excess amounts of Na^+, K^+, water, or acids results in electrolyte, volume, and acid–base abnormalities that can be life threatening. Furthermore, excess Na^+ ingestion in a patient with renal insufficiency results in intravascular volume expansion, which in turn can lead to hypertension and heart failure.

CHECKPOINT

7. What characteristics of various parts of the nephron make it particularly susceptible to certain types of injury?

8. What is uremia, and what are its most prominent symptoms and signs?

TABLE 16–2   Kidney diseases by site of injury.

Prerenal disease		Tubular
True volume depletion		Acute
Gastrointestinal, renal, or cutaneous fluid losses		Acute tubular necrosis
Hemorrhage		Multiple myeloma
Decreased effective circulating volume		Uric acid nephropathy
Heart failure (including cardiorenal syndrome)		Chronic
Cirrhosis (including hepatorenal syndrome)		Polycystic kidney disease
Nephrotic syndrome (especially with diuretic therapy for edema)		Medullary sponge kidney
Hypotension		Interstitial
Nonsteroidal anti-inflammatory drugs		Acute
Bilateral renal artery stenosis (especially in the presence of an angiotensin-converting enzyme inhibitor)		Interstitial nephritis (often drug-induced)
		Pyelonephritis
Intrarenal disease		Chronic
Vascular		Chronic interstitial nephritis (due to malignancy, infection, rheumatic disease)
Acute		Pyelonephritis
Vasculitis		Analgesic nephropathy (papillary necrosis and interstitial nephritis)
Malignant hypertension		**Postrenal disease**
Scleroderma		Acute or chronic
Thromboembolic disease		Obstructive uropathy (intrinsic or extrinsic compression of ureter, bladder, or urethra, typically due to nephrolithiasis, malignancy, retroperitoneal fibrosis, prostatic hypertrophy)
Chronic		
Hypertensive nephrosclerosis		Mechanical (medications, neurogenic bladder)
Glomerular		Acute
Glomerulonephritis		Renal vein thrombosis
Nephrotic syndrome		

PATHOPHYSIOLOGY OF SELECTED RENAL DISEASES

ACUTE KIDNEY INJURY

Clinical Presentation

Acute kidney injury is a syndrome characterized by a rapid deterioration of renal function (typically within days to a week), resulting in the accumulation of nitrogenous wastes in the blood that would normally be excreted in the urine. The patient presents with a rapidly rising BUN (ie, azotemia) and serum creatinine. Depending on the cause and when the patient comes to medical attention, there may be other presenting features as well (Table 16–4). Thus, diminished urine volume (oliguria) is commonly but not always seen. Urine volume may be normal early or indeed at any time in milder forms of acute kidney injury. Patients presenting relatively late may display any of the clinical manifestations described later.

The most widely accepted definition of acute kidney injury is a rise in serum creatinine of 0.3 mg/dL or more within a 48-hour period or a fall in urine output to less than 0.5 mL/kg/h for at least 6 hours. However, in patients who develop acute kidney injury outside the hospital setting, the time course of serum creatinine rise may be difficult to ascertain, and an empiric diagnosis may be required.

TABLE 16-3   Clinical abnormalities in uremia.[1]

Fluid and electrolyte	
Volume expansion (I)	Coma (I)
Hyponatremia (I)	Muscle cramps (P or D)
Hyperkalemia (I)	Dialysis disequilibrium syndrome (D)
Hyperphosphatemia (I)	Myopathy (P or D)
Secondary hyperparathyroidism (I or P)	**Cardiovascular/pulmonary**
Adynamic bone (D)	Arterial hypertension (I or P)
Vitamin D–deficient osteomalacia (I)	Heart failure or pulmonary edema (I)
Carbohydrate resistance (I)	Pericarditis (I)
Hyperuricemia (I or P)	Hypertrophic or dilated cardiomyopathy (I, P, or D)
Hypertriglyceridemia (P)	Uremic lung (I)
Increased Lp(a) level (P)	Accelerated atherosclerosis (P or D)
Decreased high-density lipoprotein level (P)	Hypotension and arrhythmias (D)
Protein-calorie malnutrition (I or P)	Vascular calcification (P or D)
Impaired growth and development (P)	**Skin**
Infertility and sexual dysfunction (P)	Pallor (I)
Amenorrhea (P)	Hyperpigmentation (I, P, or D)
β_2-microglobulin amyloidosis (P or D)	Pruritus (P)
Neuromuscular	Ecchymoses (I or P)
Fatigue (I)	Uremic frost (I)
Sleep disorders (P)	**Gastrointestinal**
Headache (P)	Anorexia (I)
Impaired mentation (I)	Nausea and vomiting (I)
Lethargy (I)	Gastrointestinal bleeding (I, P, or D)
Asterixis (I)	Idiopathic ascites (D)
Muscular irritability (I)	Peritonitis (D)
Peripheral neuropathy (I or P)	**Hematologic**
Restless legs syndrome (I or P)	Anemia (I)
Myoclonus (I)	Bleeding diathesis (I or D)
Seizures (I or P)	Increased susceptibility to infection (I or P)

[1]Virtually all the abnormalities contained in this table are completely reversed in time by successful renal transplantation. The response of these abnormalities to hemodialysis or peritoneal dialysis therapy is more variable. I denotes an abnormality that usually improves with an optimal program of dialysis and related therapy. P denotes an abnormality that tends to persist or even progress, despite an optimal program. D denotes an abnormality that develops only after the initiation of dialysis therapy.

Reproduced, with permission, from Bargman JM et al. Chronic kidney disease. In: Longo D et al, eds. *Harrison's Principles of Internal Medicine*, 18th ed. McGraw-Hill, 2012.

TABLE 16–4   **Initial clinical and laboratory data base for defining major syndromes in nephrology.**

Syndrome	Important Clues to Diagnosis	Common Findings Not of Diagnostic Value
Acute or rapidly progressive renal failure	Anuria	Hypertension
	Oliguria	Hematuria, proteinuria, pyuria, casts
	Documented recent decline in GFR	Edema
Acute nephritis	Hematuria, red cell casts	Proteinuria, pyuria
	Azotemia, oliguria	Circulatory congestion
	Edema, hypertension	
Chronic renal failure	Azotemia for >3 months	Hematuria, proteinuria, casts
	Prolonged symptoms or signs of uremia	Oliguria, polyuria, nocturia
	Symptoms or signs of renal osteodystrophy	Edema, hypertension
	Kidneys reduced in size bilaterally	Electrolyte disorders
	Broad casts in urinary sediment	
Nephrotic syndrome	Proteinuria >3.5 g/1.73 m² per 24 h	Casts
	Hypoalbuminemia	Edema
	Hyperlipidemia	
	Lipiduria	
Asymptomatic urinary abnormalities	Hematuria	
	Proteinuria (below nephrotic range)	
	Sterile pyuria, casts	
Urinary tract infection	Bacteriuria >10⁵ colonies/mL	Hematuria
	Other infectious agent documented in urine	Mild azotemia
	Pyuria, leukocyte casts	Mild proteinuria
	Frequency, urgency	Fever
	Bladder tenderness, flank tenderness	
Renal tubular defects	Electrolyte disorders	Hematuria
	Polyuria, nocturia	Mild azotemia
	Symptoms or signs of renal osteodystrophy	Mild proteinuria
	Large kidneys	Fever
	Renal transport defects	
Hypertension	Systolic/diastolic hypertension	Proteinuria
		Casts
		Azotemia
Nephrolithiasis	History of stone passage or removal	Hematuria
	Stone seen by x-ray	Pyuria
	Renal colic	Frequency, urgency
Urinary tract obstruction	Azotemia, oliguria, anuria	Hematuria
	Polyuria, nocturia, urinary retention	Pyuria
	Slowing of urinary stream	Enuresis, dysuria
	Large prostate, large kidneys	
	Flank tenderness, full bladder after voiding	

Reproduced, with permission, from Lin J et al. Azotemia and urinary abnormalities. In: Longo D et al, eds. *Harrison's Principles of Internal Medicine*, 18th ed. McGraw-Hill, 2012.

Etiology

Table 16–5 presents the major causes of acute kidney injury.

A. Prerenal Causes

As demonstrated by the Starling equation, filtration across a glomerulus is determined by the hydrostatic and oncotic pressures in both the glomerular capillary and its surrounding tubular lumen as described by the following relationship:

$$\text{Filtration} = K_f [P_c - P_t] - \sigma[\pi_c - \pi_t]$$

K_f and σ are constants determined by the permeability of a given glomerulus and the effective contribution of osmotic pressure, respectively; P_c = intracapillary hydrostatic pressure; π_c = intracapillary oncotic pressure; P_t = intratubular

TABLE 16–5   **Major causes of acute kidney injury.**

Disorder	Examples
Hypovolemia	Volume loss via the skin, gastrointestinal tract, or kidney; hemorrhage; sequestration of extracellular fluid (burns, pancreatitis, peritonitis)
Cardiovascular failure	Impaired cardiac output (infarction, tamponade); vascular pooling (anaphylaxis, sepsis, drugs)
Extrarenal obstruction	Urethral occlusion: vesical, pelvic, prostatic, or retroperitoneal neoplasms; surgical accident; medication; calculi; pus, blood clots
Intrarenal obstruction	Crystals (uric acid, oxalic acid, sulfonamides, methotrexate)
Bladder rupture	Trauma
Vascular diseases	Vasculitis; malignant hypertension; thrombotic thrombocytopenia purpura; scleroderma; arterial or venous occlusion
Glomerulonephritis	Immune complex disease; anti-GBM disease; ANCA or pauci-immune disease
Interstitial nephritis	Drugs; hypercalcemia; infections; idiopathic
Pigment-induced	Hemolysis (transfusion reaction, malaria); rhabdomyolysis (trauma, muscle disease, coma, heat stroke, severe exercise, potassium or phosphate depletion)
Poison-induced	Antibiotics; contrast material; anesthetic agents; heavy metals; organic solvents
Pregnancy-related	Septic abortion; uterine hemorrhage; eclampsia

ANCA, anti-neutrophil cytoplasmic antibody; GBM, glomerular basement membrane.

Modified, with permission, from Andersen RJ et al. Acute renal failure. In: Wilson JD et al, eds. *Harrison's Principles of Internal Medicine*, 12th ed. McGraw-Hill, 1991.

hydrostatic pressure; and π_t = intratubular oncotic pressure. Perturbations in any of the above factors may alter renal filtration. Of particular importance is the intracapillary hydrostatic pressure, which is determined by relative blood flow into and out of the glomerular capillary. A normal kidney has the unique ability to autoregulate blood flow both in and out of the glomerular capillary through alterations in the resistance of the afferent and efferent arterioles across a wide range of systemic blood pressures. (Most capillary beds possess only the ability to regulate blood flow in to the bed.) Lower relative flows into the glomerulus with decreased renal blood flow or afferent artery constriction may lower intracapillary hydrostatic pressure and diminish filtration. Likewise, higher relative flows out of the glomerulus with efferent artery dilation may also lower intracapillary hydrostatic pressure.

Despite the ability of the kidney to autoregulate and maintain the GFR, more advanced volume depletion can result in the development of azotemia. This can result from excessive volume losses (renal, GI, or cutaneous in origin), low fluid intake, or low effective circulating volume. An example of the latter is decompensated heart failure with poor cardiac output and diminished renal perfusion (termed cardiorenal syndrome).

Drugs are another important cause of prerenal acute kidney injury. Some patients who are dependent on prostaglandin-mediated vasodilation to maintain renal perfusion can develop renal failure from ingesting nonsteroidal anti-inflammatory drugs (NSAIDs). Similarly, patients with renal hypoperfusion (eg, renovascular disease) who are dependent on angiotensin II–mediated vasoconstriction of the efferent renal arterioles to maintain renal perfusion pressure may develop acute kidney injury on ingesting ACE inhibitors.

B. Intrarenal Causes

The intrarenal causes of acute kidney injury can be further divided into specific **inflammatory diseases** (eg, vasculitis, glomerulonephritis [GN], drug-induced injury) and **acute tubular necrosis** resulting from many causes (including ischemia and endogenous or exogenous toxic injury).

Notable among intrarenal causes are the toxic effects of aminoglycoside antibiotics and rhabdomyolysis, in which myoglobin, released into the bloodstream after a crush injury to muscle, precipitates in the renal tubules. Drug toxicity may be mitigated by closely monitoring renal function during antibiotic therapy, especially in elderly patients and those with some degree of underlying renal compromise. Rhabdomyolysis may be detected by obtaining a serum creatine kinase level in patients admitted to the hospital with trauma or altered mental status and may be mitigated by maintaining a vigorous alkaline diuresis to prevent myoglobin precipitation in the tubules.

Sepsis is one of the most common causes of acute kidney injury, and the injury results from a combination of prerenal and intrarenal factors. The prerenal factor is renal hypoperfusion owing to the hypotensive, low systemic vascular resistance of the septic state. The intrarenal component may be a consequence of the cytokine dysregulation that characterizes sepsis syndrome (see Chapter 4), including elevated blood levels of tumor necrosis factor, interleukin-1, and interleukin-6, which contribute to intrarenal inflammation, sclerosis, and obstruction. Patients with sepsis are often also exposed to nephrotoxic drugs such as aminoglycoside antibiotics or iodinated intravenous contrast for computed tomography imaging.

C. Postrenal Causes

The postrenal causes of acute kidney injury are those resulting in urinary tract obstruction, which may occur at any level of the urinary tract. Obstruction can be either intrinsic (eg, nephrolithiasis causing ureteral obstruction) or extrinsic (eg, retroperitoneal mass compressing a ureter). For obstruction occurring above the level of the bladder, bilateral obstruction is typically required to cause acute kidney injury unless the patient has only one functioning kidney.

Pathology & Pathogenesis

Regardless of their origin, all forms of acute kidney injury, if untreated, result in acute tubular necrosis, with sloughing of the epithelial cells that make up the renal tubule.

The precise molecular mechanisms responsible for the development of acute tubular necrosis remain unknown. Theories favoring either a tubular or vascular basis have been proposed (Figure 16–5). According to the tubular theory, cellular debris occludes the tubular lumen, forming a cast that increases intratubular pressure sufficiently to offset perfusion pressure and decrease or abolish net filtration pressure. The vascular theory proposes that decreased renal perfusion pressure from the combination of afferent arteriolar vasoconstriction and efferent arteriolar vasodilation reduces glomerular perfusion pressure and, therefore, glomerular filtration. It may be that both mechanisms act to produce acute kidney injury, varying in relative importance in different individuals depending on the

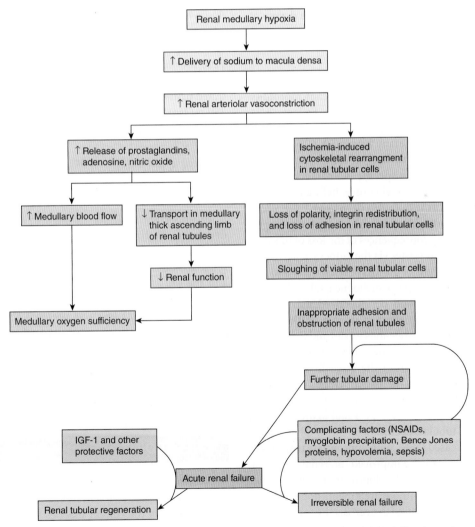

FIGURE 16–5 Pathophysiology of ischemia-induced acute kidney injury. Mild or uncomplicated medullary hypoxia results in tubuloglomerular reflex adjustments that restore medullary oxygen sufficiency at the price of diminished renal function. However, in the event of extreme renal medullary hypoxia or when associated with complicating factors such as those indicated in the figure, full-blown acute kidney injury develops. Whether acute kidney injury is reversible or irreversible depends on a balance of reparative and complicating factors. (IGF-1, insulin-like growth factor 1; NSAID, nonsteroidal anti-inflammatory drug.)

cause and time of presentation. Studies suggest that one consequence of hypoxia is the disordered adhesion of renal tubular epithelial cells, resulting both in their exfoliation and subsequent adhesion to other cells of the tubule, thereby contributing to tubular obstruction (see Figure 16–5). Another consequence may be a dysregulation of elements that secure tubular cells together, resulting in a leak of filtrate out of the tubular lumen and an abnormal sorting of cellular transmembrane channels required for the normal function of the nephron. Renal damage, whether caused by tubular occlusion or vascular hypoperfusion, is potentiated by the hypoxic state of the renal medulla, which increases the risk of ischemia. Research has implicated cytokines and endogenous peptides, such as endothelins, and the regulation of their production as possible explanations for why, subjected to the same toxic insult, some patients develop acute kidney injury and others do not, and why some with acute kidney injury recover and others do not. It appears that these products, together with the activation of complement and neutrophils, increases vasoconstriction in the already ischemic renal medulla and, in that way, exacerbate the degree of hypoxic injury occurring in acute kidney injury.

Clinical Manifestations

Acute kidney injury can contribute to significant morbidity and is an independent predictor of mortality. Patients hospitalized in an intensive care setting who develop acute kidney injury requiring dialysis therapy have a 50–60% hospital mortality rate. Thus, in recent years, significant research effort has been focused on identifying specific biomarkers of acute kidney injury earlier in the hospital course, before the serum creatinine is elevated or urine output is decreased.

The initial symptoms of kidney injury are typically fatigue and malaise, probably early consequences of the loss of the ability to excrete water, salt, and wastes via the kidneys. Later, more profound symptoms and signs of the loss of renal water and salt excretory capacity develop: dyspnea, orthopnea, rales, a prominent third heart sound (S_3), and peripheral edema. Altered mental status reflects the toxic effect of uremia on the brain, with elevated blood levels of nitrogenous wastes and fixed acids.

The clinical manifestations of acute kidney injury depend not only on the cause but also on the stage in the natural history of the disease at which the patient comes to medical attention. Patients with renal hypoperfusion (prerenal causes of acute kidney injury) first develop **prerenal azotemia** (elevated BUN without tubular necrosis), a direct physiologic consequence of a decreased GFR. With appropriate treatment, renal perfusion can typically be improved, prerenal azotemia can be readily reversed, and the development of acute tubular necrosis can be prevented. Without treatment, prerenal azotemia may progress to acute tubular necrosis. Recovery from acute tubular necrosis, if it occurs, will then follow a more protracted course, potentially requiring supportive dialysis before adequate renal function is regained.

A variety of clinical tests can help determine whether a patient with signs of acute kidney injury is in the early phase of prerenal azotemia or has progressed to full-blown acute tubular necrosis. However, the overlap in clinical presentation along the continuum between prerenal azotemia and acute tubular necrosis is such that the results of any one of these tests must be interpreted in the context of other findings and the clinical history.

Perhaps the earliest manifestation of prerenal azotemia is an elevated ratio of BUN to serum creatinine. Normally 10–15:1, this ratio may rise to 20–30:1 in prerenal azotemia, with a normal or near-normal serum creatinine. If the patient proceeds to acute tubular necrosis, this ratio may return to normal but with a progressively elevated serum creatinine.

Urinalysis is a simple and inexpensive test that serves as an important tool in the initial evaluation of the patient with acute kidney injury. The presence of hematuria and proteinuria should prompt an evaluation for GN. There are no typical abnormal findings in simple prerenal azotemia, whereas granular casts, tubular epithelial cells, and epithelial cell casts suggest acute tubular necrosis. Casts are formed when debris in the renal tubules (protein, red cells, epithelial cells) takes on the cylindrical, smooth-bordered shape of the tubule. Likewise, because hypovolemia is a stimulus to vasopressin release (see Chapter 19), the urine is maximally concentrated (up to 1200 mOsm/L) in prerenal azotemia. However, with progression to acute tubular necrosis, the ability to generate a concentrated urine is largely lost. Thus, a urine osmolality of less than 350 mOsm/L is a typical finding in acute tubular necrosis.

Finally, the fractional excretion of Na^+

$$FE_{Na^+}[\%] = \frac{Urine_{Na^+}/Plasma_{Na^+}}{Urine_{Cr}/Plasma_{Cr}} \times 100$$

is an important indicator in oliguric acute kidney injury to determine whether a patient has progressed from simple prerenal azotemia to frank acute tubular necrosis. In simple prerenal azotemia, more than 99% of filtered Na^+ is reabsorbed, and the FE_{Na^+} will be less than 1% (except when the patient is on a diuretic). This value allows accurate identification of Na^+ retention states (such as prerenal azotemia) even when there is water retention as a result of vasopressin release. With the progression of prerenal azotemia to acute kidney injury with acute tubular necrosis, this ability of the kidney to avidly retain sodium is generally lost. However, there are some conditions in which the FE_{Na^+} is less than 1% in patients with acute tubular necrosis (Table 16–6).

CHECKPOINT

9. What are the features that distinguish prerenal, intrarenal, and postrenal causes of renal failure?

10. What are the current theories for the development of acute tubular necrosis?

11. What clues are helpful in determining whether newly diagnosed renal failure is acute or chronic?

12. What is the natural history of acute kidney injury?

TABLE 16–6   Causes of acute kidney injury in which FE$_{Na+}$ may be below 1%.

Prerenal disease
Acute tubular necrosis
10% of nonoliguric cases
Superimposed upon chronic prerenal state
Cirrhosis
Heart failure
Severe burns
Myoglobinuria or hemoglobinuria
Radiocontrast media
Sepsis
Acute glomerulonephritis or vasculitis
Acute obstructive uropathy
Acute interstitial nephritis

Reproduced, with permission, from Rose BD. Acute renal failure—prerenal disease vs acute tubular necrosis. In: *Pathophysiology of Renal Disease*, 2nd ed. McGraw-Hill, 1987.

CHRONIC KIDNEY DISEASE

Clinical Presentation

Patients with chronic kidney disease (CKD) and uremia show a constellation of symptoms, signs, and laboratory abnormalities in addition to those observed in acute kidney injury. This reflects the long-standing and progressive nature of their renal disease and its systemic effects. A clinical pearl is to always assume that renal failure is acute—this gives clinicians the opportunity to identify and treat acute kidney injury in a timely fashion while it still has the potential to respond to treatment. However, osteodystrophy, neuropathy, bilateral small kidneys on imaging, and anemia are typical initial findings that suggest a chronic course for a patient newly diagnosed with renal failure on the basis of elevated BUN and serum creatinine.

Etiology

In developed nations, the most common cause of CKD is diabetes mellitus (see Chapter 18), followed by hypertension; GN is a distant third cause (Table 16–7). Polycystic kidney disease, obstruction, and infection are significant but less common causes of CKD. In addition, episodes of acute kidney injury are associated with an increased risk for later development of CKD and end-stage renal disease.

Pathology & Pathogenesis

A. Development of Chronic Kidney Disease

The pathogenesis of acute renal disease is very different from that of CKD. Whereas acute injury to the kidney leads to

TABLE 16–7   Prevalence by etiology for U.S. Medicare–treated end-stage renal disease for 2014.

	Prevalence, n = 678,383	
	Count	Percentage
Diabetes mellitus	256,828	37.9
Hypertension	171,155	25.2
Glomerulonephritis	108,624	16.0
Cystic disease	31,846	4.7

Data from United States Renal Data System, 2016 USRDS annual data report: epidemiology of kidney disease in the United States. National Institutes of Health, National Institute of Diabetes and Digestive and Kidney Diseases, Bethesda, MD, 2016. https://www.usrds.org/default.aspx.

death and sloughing of tubular epithelial cells, often followed by their regeneration with the re-establishment of normal architecture, chronic injury results in the irreversible loss of nephrons. As a result, a greater functional burden is borne by fewer nephrons, leading to an increase in glomerular filtration pressure and hyperfiltration. For reasons not well understood, this compensatory hyperfiltration, which can be thought of as a form of "hypertension" at the level of the individual nephron, predisposes to fibrosis and scarring (**glomerular sclerosis**). As a result, the rate of nephron destruction and loss increases, thus speeding the progression to **uremia**, the complex of symptoms and signs that occurs when residual renal function is inadequate (see Table 16–3).

The kidneys have a tremendous functional reserve—up to 50% of nephrons can be lost without any short-term evidence of functional impairment. This is why individuals with two healthy kidneys are able to donate one for transplantation. When the GFR is further reduced, leaving only about 20% of initial renal capacity, some degree of azotemia (elevated blood levels of products normally excreted by the kidneys) is observed. Nevertheless, patients may be largely asymptomatic because a new steady state is achieved in which the blood levels of these products are not high enough to cause overt toxicity. However, even at this apparently stable level of renal function, hyperfiltration-accelerated evolution to end-stage chronic kidney disease is in progress. Furthermore, because patients with this level of GFR have little functional reserve, they can easily become uremic with any added stress (eg, infection, obstruction, dehydration, use of nephrotoxic drugs) or with any catabolic state associated with an increased turnover of nitrogen-containing products. Thus, patients with CKD are at significant risk for superimposed acute kidney injury.

B. Pathogenesis of Uremia

The pathogenesis of uremia derives in part from a combination of the toxic effects of (1) retained products normally excreted by the kidneys (eg, nitrogen-containing products of protein metabolism); (2) normal products such as hormones now present in increased amounts; and (3) the loss of normal products of the kidney (eg, loss of erythropoietin).

Excretory failure also leads to fluid shifts, with increased intracellular Na^+ and water and decreased intracellular K^+. These alterations may contribute to subtle alterations in the function of a host of enzymes, transport systems, and so on. Regardless of the etiology, CKD tends to have an impact on many other organ systems and thus is truly a systemic disease.

Clinical Manifestations

A. Na⁺ Balance and Volume Status

Patients with CKD typically have some degree of excess Na^+ and water, reflecting loss of the renal route of salt and water excretion. A moderate degree of Na^+ and water retention may occur without objective signs of extracellular fluid excess. However, continued excessive Na^+ ingestion (as found in a typical Western diet) leads to further fluid retention and contributes to heart failure, hypertension, peripheral edema, and weight gain. On the other hand, excessive water ingestion contributes to hyponatremia. A common recommendation for the patient with chronic kidney disease is to limit sodium to 2 g/d or less and to restrict fluid intake so that it equals urine output plus 500 mL (to compensate for insensible losses). Further adjustments in volume status can be made either through the use of diuretics (in a patient who still makes urine) or at dialysis.

Because these patients also have impaired renal salt and water conservation mechanisms, they are more sensitive than normal to sudden extrarenal Na^+ and water losses (eg, via vomiting, diarrhea, or increased cutaneous losses such as with fever). Under these circumstances, they more easily develop ECF depletion, a further deterioration of renal function (which may not be reversible), and even vascular collapse and shock. Dry mucous membranes, tachycardia, hypotension, and dizziness all suggest volume depletion.

B. K⁺ Balance

Hyperkalemia is a potentially life-threatening complication of CKD, especially with advanced renal impairment (eg, GFR <15 mL/min). Early in CKD, as the GFR falls, aldosterone-mediated K^+ transport in the distal tubule increases in a compensatory fashion to maintain normal potassium levels. However, treatment with K^+-sparing diuretics, ACE inhibitors, or β-blockers—drugs that may impair aldosterone-mediated K^+ transport—can precipitate dangerous hyperkalemia in a patient with CKD.

Patients with diabetes mellitus may develop a syndrome of **hyporeninemic hypoaldosteronism (type 4 RTA)**. Decreased renin production by the kidney leads to decreased levels of angiotensin II and thus impairs aldosterone secretion. As a result, affected patients are unable to compensate for the falling GFR by enhancing their aldosterone-mediated K^+ transport and, therefore, have relative difficulty excreting K^+. This

difficulty is usually manifested as hyperkalemia long before the GFR has fallen below 15 mL/min.

Patients with CKD are also at greater risk of hyperkalemia in the face of sudden loads of K^+ from either endogenous sources (eg, hemolysis, infection, trauma) or exogenous sources (eg, K^+-rich foods, blood transfusions, K^+-containing medications).

C. Metabolic Acidosis

The diminished capacity to excrete acid and generate base in CKD results in metabolic acidosis. In most cases when the GFR is above 20 mL/min, only moderate acidosis develops before a new steady state of buffer production and consumption is re-established. The fall in blood pH in these individuals can usually be corrected with 20–30 mmol (2–3 g) of sodium bicarbonate by mouth daily. However, these patients are highly susceptible to acidosis in the event of either a sudden acid load (eg, ketoacidosis, lactic acidosis, toxic ingestions) or bicarbonate loss (eg, diarrhea).

D. Mineral and Bone

Several disorders of phosphate, Ca^{2+}, and bone metabolism are observed in CKD as a result of a complex series of events (Figure 16–6). The key factors in the pathogenesis of these disorders include (1) diminished absorption of Ca^{2+} from the gut; (2) overproduction of PTH; (3) disordered vitamin D metabolism; (4) retention of phosphorus; and (5) chronic metabolic acidosis. All these factors contribute to enhanced bone resorption. Hyperphosphatemia contributes to the development of hypocalcemia and thus serves as an additional trigger for secondary hyperparathyroidism, elevating blood PTH levels. The elevated blood PTH further depletes bone Ca^{2+} and contributes to osteomalacia of CKD (see later discussion).

E. Cardiovascular and Pulmonary Abnormalities

Heart failure and pulmonary edema can develop in the context of volume and salt overload. Hypertension is a common finding in CKD and is often due to fluid and Na^+ overload. However, hyperreninemia, in which decreased renal perfusion triggers the failing kidney to overproduce renin, can also elevate systemic blood pressure.

Pericarditis can develop from irritation and inflammation of the pericardium by uremic toxins. In developed countries, this complication has become less common because of the availability of dialysis.

An increased incidence of cardiovascular disease is observed in patients with CKD and remains the leading cause of mortality in this population. Cardiovascular risk factors in CKD patients include hypertension, hyperlipidemia, glucose intolerance, chronic elevated cardiac output, and valvular and myocardial calcification, as well as other, less well-characterized factors of the uremic milieu. As a result, an increased burden of myocardial infarction, stroke, and peripheral vascular disease is observed in CKD.

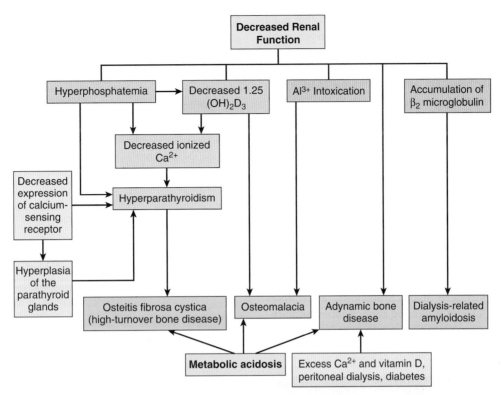

FIGURE 16–6 Pathogenesis of bone diseases in chronic kidney disease. (Redrawn, with permission, from Brenner BM et al. Chronic renal failure. In: Kasper DL et al, eds. *Harrison's Principles of Internal Medicine*, 16th ed. McGraw-Hill, 2005.)

F. Hematologic Abnormalities

Patients with CKD have marked abnormalities in red blood cell count, white blood cell function, and clotting parameters. The normochromic and normocytic anemia is due chiefly to the decreased production of erythropoietin, resulting in decreased erythropoiesis. Additional causes of anemia may include the bone marrow suppressive effects of uremic toxins, bone marrow fibrosis owing to elevated blood PTH, the toxic effects of aluminum (historically, these effects occurred from aluminum-based phosphate-binding antacids and from contaminated dialysis solutions), and dialysis-associated hemolysis and blood loss.

Patients with CKD display abnormal hemostasis manifested as increased bruising, decreased clotting, and an increased incidence of spontaneous GI and cerebrovascular hemorrhage (including both hemorrhagic stroke and subdural hematoma). Laboratory abnormalities include prolonged bleeding time, decreased platelet factor III, abnormal platelet aggregation and adhesiveness, and impaired prothrombin consumption, none of which is completely reversible, even in well-dialyzed patients.

Uremia is associated with an increased susceptibility to infections, likely owing to leukocyte suppression by uremic toxins. Chemotaxis, the acute inflammatory response, and delayed hypersensitivity are all suppressed. Acidosis, hyperglycemia, malnutrition, and hyperosmolality are also believed to contribute to immunosuppression in CKD. The invasiveness of dialysis and the use of immunosuppressive drugs in renal transplant patients further contribute to an increased incidence of infections.

G. Neuromuscular Abnormalities

Neurologic symptoms and signs of uremia range from mild sleep disorders and impaired mental concentration, loss of memory, errors in judgment, and neuromuscular irritability (manifested as hiccups, cramps, fasciculations, and twitching) to asterixis, myoclonus, stupor, seizures, and coma in end-stage uremia. Asterixis is involuntary hand flapping when the arms are extended and the wrists are held back to "stop traffic." It is due to altered nerve conduction in metabolic encephalopathy from a wide variety of causes, including renal failure.

Peripheral neuropathy, typified by restless legs syndrome (a poorly localized sense of discomfort and involuntary movements of the lower extremities), is a common finding in CKD.

H. GI Abnormalities

Nonspecific GI findings in uremic patients include anorexia, hiccups, nausea, and vomiting. Although their precise pathogenesis is unclear, many of these symptoms improve with dialysis.

I. Endocrine and Metabolic Abnormalities

Many women with uremia have low estrogen levels, which perhaps explains the high incidence of amenorrhea and decreased fertility and the observation that such individuals are rarely able to carry a pregnancy to term. Regular menses—but not a higher rate of successful pregnancies—-typically return with frequent dialysis.

Similarly, low testosterone levels, impotence, oligospermia, and germinal cell dysplasia are common findings in men with chronic kidney disease.

In CKD, the kidney's role in insulin degradation decreases, increasing the half-life of insulin. This often has a stabilizing effect on diabetic patients whose blood glucose was previously difficult to control and can lead to a decreased need for insulin and other hypoglycemic medications.

J. Dermatologic Abnormalities

Skin changes are common and arise from many of the effects of CKD already discussed. Patients with CKD may display pallor because of anemia, skin color changes related to accumulated pigmented metabolites, or a gray discoloration resulting from transfusion-mediated hemochromatosis, ecchymoses and hematomas as a result of clotting abnormalities, and pruritus and excoriations as a result of Ca^{2+} deposits from secondary hyperparathyroidism.

CHECKPOINT

13. What is the mechanism by which altered sodium, potassium, and volume status develop in chronic kidney disease?

14. What are the most common causes of chronic kidney disease?

GLOMERULONEPHRITIS & NEPHROTIC SYNDROME

Clinical Presentation & Etiology

Glomerular disorders can originate in the kidney or be manifestations of systemic diseases in which the kidney is prominently involved. Glomerulonephritis (GN) is currently characterized by both clinical and microscopic features. Renal biopsy is often the only way to correctly diagnose the cause of GN and hence determine the appropriate treatment.

Disorders resulting in glomerular disease typically fall into one of several categories of clinical presentation. However, there can be overlap among these categories:

1. **Acute GN**, characterized by the abrupt onset of hematuria and proteinuria with a reduced GFR and renal salt and water retention. Acute GN often occurs in the setting of infectious diseases, classically pharyngeal or cutaneous infections with certain "nephritogenic" strains of group A β-hemolytic streptococci. However, other pathogens have also been implicated (Table 16–8). **Rapidly progressive glomerulonephritis (RPGN)** is a subset of acute GN characterized by a progressive and

---

TABLE 16–8   Causes of acute glomerulonephritis.

Poststreptococcal glomerulonephritis
Infective endocarditis (IE)
Systemic lupus erythematosus (SLE) nephritis
Class I minimal mesangial
Class II mesangial proliferative
Class III focal nephritis
Class IV diffuse nephritis
Class V membranous nephritis
Class VI sclerotic nephritis
Rheumatoid arthritis (with vasculitis)
Relapsing polychondritis
IgA nephropathy
ANCA small-vessel vasculitis
Granulomatosis with polyangiitis
Microscopic polyangiitis
Eosinophilic granulomatosis with polyangiitis
Henoch–Schönlein purpura
Cryoglobulinemia
Membranoproliferative glomerulonephritis
Type I: idiopathic, IE, SLE, hepatitis C ± cryoglobulinemia, mixed cryoglobulinemia, hepatitis B, cancer (lung, breast, ovary [germinal])
Type II: idiopathic, C3 nephritic factor–associated, partial lipodystrophy
Type III: idiopathic, complement receptor deficiency
Mesangioproliferative glomerulonephritis
Drugs (penicillamine, hydralazine, allopurinol, rifampin)

ANCA, anti-neutrophil cytoplasmic antibody.

Modified, with permission, from Lewis JB et al. Glomerular diseases. In: Longo D et al, eds. *Harrison's Principles of Internal Medicine*, 18th ed. McGraw-Hill, 2012.

---

dramatic decline (weeks to months) in renal function, often leading to complete renal failure and oliguria if left untreated. RPGN is also often called "crescentic GN," as the characteristic finding on biopsy is cellular "crescents" in the Bowman space. Cellular crescents, visible on light microscopy, form in response to severe damage to the glomerular capillaries. This appears to be a nonspecific final pathway in a variety of glomerular diseases, and recovery without specific treatment is rare.

2. **Chronic glomerulonephritis** is characterized by persistent urinary abnormalities and a slowly progressive

(years) decline in renal function. Chronic GN does not typically resolve. Progressive renal deterioration in patients with chronic GN proceeds inexorably, resulting in end-stage renal disease up to 20 years after the initial discovery of an abnormal urinary sediment.

3. **Nephrotic syndrome** manifests as marked proteinuria, particularly albuminuria (24-hour urine protein excretion >3.5 g), hypoalbuminemia, hyperlipidemia, and edema. Nephrotic syndrome may be either isolated (eg, minimal-change disease) or part of some other glomerular syndrome (eg, with hematuria and casts). The underlying causes of the nephrotic syndromes are very often unclear, and these syndromes are distinguished instead by their histologic features (discussed below). Each type of nephrotic syndrome may be primary (ie, idiopathic), or it may be secondary to a specific cause (eg, medication induced) or systemic syndrome (eg, systemic lupus erythematosus, malignancy). Some cases of nephrotic syndrome are variants of acute GN, RPGN, or chronic GN in which massive proteinuria is a presenting feature. Other cases of nephrotic syndrome fall into the category of **minimal-change disease**, in which many of the pathologic consequences result from proteinuria.

4. **Asymptomatic urinary abnormalities** include hematuria and proteinuria (usually in amounts significantly below that seen in nephrotic syndrome) but with no functional abnormalities associated with reduced GFR, edema, or hypertension. Many patients with these findings will slowly develop progressive renal dysfunction over decades. The most common causes of asymptomatic urinary abnormalities are **immunoglobulin A (IgA) nephropathy**, an immune complex disease characterized by diffuse mesangial IgA deposition, and **thin basement membrane nephropathy**, a familial disorder characterized by a defect in collagen synthesis. Table 16–9 lists other causes.

Pathology & Pathogenesis

The different forms of GN and nephrotic syndrome probably represent differences in the nature, extent, and specific cause of immune-mediated renal damage. Genetic predisposition and poorly understood environmental triggers are likely involved and lead to the activation of an immune response. Leukocyte activation, complement deposition, and cytokines—in particular transforming growth factor-1 (TGF-1) and platelet-derived growth factor (PDGF)—synthesized by mesangial cells, incite an inflammatory reaction and subsequent glomerular injury in many forms of glomerular disease. Histologic patterns can be nonspecific; however, classic associations between the natural history and defining immunofluorescence and electron microscopic observations have been made (see Figure 16–4; Table 16–10). However, because it is not yet known exactly how the various forms of immune-mediated renal damage occur, each category is described separately with its associated findings.

TABLE 16–9 Glomerular causes of asymptomatic urinary abnormalities.

Hematuria with or without proteinuria
Primary glomerular diseases
IgA nephropathy[1]
Mesangiocapillary glomerulonephritis
Other primary glomerular hematurias accompanied by "pure" mesangial proliferation, focal and segmental proliferative glomerulonephritis, or other lesions
"Thin basement membrane" disease (? "forme fruste" of Alport syndrome)
Associated with multisystem or heredofamilial diseases
Alport syndrome and other "benign" familial hematurias
Fabry disease
Sickle cell disease
Associated with infections
Resolving poststreptococcal glomerulonephritis[1]
Other postinfectious glomerulonephritides[1]
Isolated non-nephrotic proteinuria
Primary glomerular diseases
"Orthostatic" proteinuria[1]
Focal and segmental glomerulosclerosis[1]
Membranous glomerulonephritis[1]
Associated with multisystem or heredofamilial diseases
Diabetes mellitus[1]
Amyloidosis[1]
Nail-patella syndrome

[1]Most common causes.

Reproduced, with permission, from Glassock RJ et al. The major glomerulopathies. In: Wilson JD et al, eds. *Harrison's Principles of Internal Medicine*, 12th ed. McGraw-Hill, 1991.

A. Acute and Rapidly Progressive Glomerulonephritis

There are several ways to classify acute GN. Light microscopy is essential for establishing areas of injury. Circulating autoantibodies and measures of complement deposition combined with immunofluorescence studies and electron microscopy allow GN to be categorized into subgroups correlating with other features of the disease. Three patterns emerge:

1. **Antiglomerular basement membrane (anti-GBM) antibody disease** (eg, Goodpasture syndrome): This disease results from the development of circulating antibodies to an antigen intrinsic to the glomerular

TABLE 16–10   Location of electron-dense deposits in glomerular disease.

Subepithelial
Amorphous (epimembranous) deposits
Membranous nephropathy
Systemic lupus erythematosus
Humps
Acute postinfectious glomerulonephritis (eg, poststreptococcal glomerulonephritis, bacterial endocarditis)
Intramembranous
Membranous nephropathy
Membranoproliferative glomerulonephritis type II
Subendothelial
Systemic lupus erythematosus
Membranoproliferative glomerulonephritis type I
Less commonly, bacterial endocarditis, IgA nephropathy, Henoch–Schönlein purpura, mixed cryoglobulinemia
Mesangial
Focal glomerulonephritis
IgA nephropathy
Henoch–Schönlein purpura
Systemic lupus erythematosus
Mild or resolving acute postinfectious glomerulonephritis
Subepithelial and subendothelial
Systemic lupus erythematosus
Membranoproliferative glomerulonephritis, type III
Postinfectious glomerulonephritis

Reproduced, with permission, from Rose BD. Pathogenesis, clinical manifestations and diagnosis of glomerular disease. In: *Pathophysiology of Renal Disease*, 2nd ed. McGraw-Hill, 1987.

basement membrane. The binding of these pathologic anti-GBM antibodies to the glomerular basement membrane causes a cascade of inflammation. Light microscopy shows crescentic GN, and a characteristic linear immunoglobulin deposition in the glomerular capillaries is seen on immunofluorescence.

2. **Immune complex glomerulonephritis**: Immune complex deposition can be seen in a variety of diseases. On renal biopsy, granular immunoglobulin deposits are suggestive of immune complexes from the underlying systemic disease. A classic example is postinfectious GN in which there is cross-reactivity between an antigen of the infecting organism and a host antigen, resulting in the deposition of immune complexes and complement in the glomerular capillaries and the mesangium. Resolution of glomerular disease typically occurs weeks after treatment of the original infection. Other examples are IgA nephropathy, lupus nephritis, and membranoproliferative GN.

3. **Anti-neutrophil cytoplasmic antibody (ANCA) disease** or **pauci-immune GN**: Characterized by a necrotizing GN but few or no immune deposits (hence, pauci-immune) seen on immunofluorescence or electron microscopy, this pattern is typical of granulomatosis with angiitis, microscopic polyangiitis, or eosinophilic granulomatosis with polyangiitis. ANCA-negative pauci-immune necrotizing GN occurs less frequently but is also a well-described clinical entity.

B. Chronic Glomerulonephritis

Some patients with acute GN develop CKD slowly over a period of 5–20 years. Cellular proliferation, in either the mesangium or the capillary, is a pathologic structural hallmark in some of these cases, whereas others are notable for the obliteration of glomeruli (**sclerosing chronic GN**, which includes both focal and diffuse subsets), and yet others display irregular subepithelial proteinaceous deposits with uniform involvement of individual glomeruli (**membranous GN**).

C. Nephrotic Syndrome

In patients with nephrotic syndrome, the podocyte is the usual target of injury. On light microscopy, the glomerulus may appear intact or only subtly altered, without a cellular infiltrate as a manifestation of inflammation. Immunofluorescence with antibodies to IgG often demonstrates the deposition of antigen–antibody complexes in the glomerular basement membrane. In the subset of patients with minimal-change disease, in which proteinuria is the sole urinary sediment abnormality and in which (often) no changes can be seen by light microscopy, electron microscopy reveals the obliteration of epithelial foot processes and slit diaphragm disruption (Table 16–11).

Clinical Manifestations

In glomerulonephritic diseases, damage to the glomerular capillary wall results in the leakage of red blood cells and proteins, which are normally too large to cross the glomerular capillary, into the renal tubular lumen, giving rise to hematuria and proteinuria. The GFR falls either because glomerular capillaries are infiltrated with inflammatory cells or because contractile cells (eg, mesangial cells) respond to vasoactive substances by restricting blood flow to many glomerular capillaries. The decreased GFR leads to fluid and salt retention that clinically manifests as edema and hypertension.

A fall in serum complement is observed as a result of immune complex and complement deposition in the glomerulus, as can be seen with lupus nephritis, membranoproliferative GN, and postinfectious GN.

TABLE 16–11 Clinical and histologic features of idiopathic nephrotic syndrome.

Glomerular Disease	Distinguishing Clinical and Laboratory Findings	Characteristic Morphologic Features
Minimal-change disease	Commonest cause in children (75%); steroid or cyclophosphamide sensitive (80% of cases); nonprogressive; normal renal function; scant hematuria	**LM:** Normal **IF:** Negative to trace IgM **EM:** Podocyte effacement; no immune deposits
Focal and segmental glomerulosclerosis	Early-onset hypertension; microscopic hematuria; progressive renal failure (75% of cases)	**LM:** Early, segmental sclerosis in some glomeruli with tubular atrophy; late, sclerosis of most glomeruli **IF:** Focal and segmental IgM, C3 **EM:** Foot process fusion, sclerosis, hyalin
Membranous nephropathy	Commonest cause in adults (40–50%); peak incidence in fourth and sixth decades; male-to-female ratio, 2–3:1; microscopic hematuria (55%); early hypertension (30%); spontaneous remission (20%); progressive renal failure (30–40%)	**LM:** Early, normal; late, GBM thickening **IF:** Granular IgG and C3 **EM:** Subepithelial deposits and GBM expansion
Membranoproliferative glomerulonephritis	Peak incidence in second and third decades; mixed nephrotic–nephritic features; slowly progressive in most, rapid in some; hypocomplementemia	**LM:** Hypercellular glomeruli with duplicated GBM ("tram tracks") **IF:** Type I, diffuse C3, variable IgG and IgM; type II, C3 capillary wall and mesangial nodules **EM:** Type I, subendothelial immune deposits; type II, dense GBM

EM, electron microscopy; GBM, glomerular basement membrane; IF, immunofluorescence; LM, light microscopy.

Data from Glassock RJ et al. The major glomerulopathies. In: Isselbacher KJ et al, eds. *Harrison's Principles of Internal Medicine*, 13th ed. McGraw-Hill, 1994; and data from Hall PM. Nephrology and hypertension. In: *Medical Knowledge Self-Assessment Program 13*. American College of Physicians, 2003.

An elevated titer of antibody to streptococcal antigens is observed in cases associated with group A β-hemolytic streptococcal infections. Another characteristic of the clinical course in poststreptococcal acute GN is a lag between clinical signs of infection and the development of clinical signs of nephritis.

Patients with nephrotic syndrome have hypoalbuminemia and profoundly decreased plasma oncotic pressures because of the loss of serum proteins in the urine. This leads to intravascular volume depletion and the activation of the renin–angiotensin–aldosterone system and the sympathetic nervous system. Vasopressin secretion is also increased. Such patients also have altered renal responses to atrial natriuretic peptide. Despite signs of volume overload such as edema or anasarca, patients may develop signs of intravascular volume depletion, including syncope, shock, and acute kidney injury. Hyperlipidemia associated with nephrotic syndrome appears to be a result of decreased plasma oncotic pressure, which stimulates hepatic very-low-density lipoprotein synthesis and secretion.

Hypercoagulability is a clinically significant manifestation of nephrotic syndrome and is caused by renal losses of proteins C and S and antithrombin, as well as elevated serum fibrinogen and lipid levels.

The loss of other plasma proteins besides albumin in nephrotic syndrome may present as any of the following: (1) a defect in bacterial opsonization and thus increased susceptibility to infections (eg, as a result of loss of IgG); (2) a vitamin D deficiency state and secondary hyperparathyroidism (eg, resulting from loss of vitamin D–binding proteins); and (3) altered thyroid function tests without any true thyroid abnormality (resulting from reduced levels of thyroxine-binding globulin).

CHECKPOINT

15. What are the categories of glomerulonephritis, and what are their common and distinctive features?

16. What are the pathophysiologic consequences of nephrotic syndrome?

RENAL STONES

Clinical Presentation

Patients with renal stones present with flank pain that may radiate to the groin region and hematuria that may be macroscopic or microscopic. Depending on the level of the stone and the patient's underlying anatomy (eg, if there is only a single functioning kidney or significant pre-existing renal disease), the presentation may be complicated by obstruction (Table 16–12), with decreased or absent urine production.

TABLE 16–12   Common mechanical causes of urinary tract obstruction.

Ureter	Bladder outlet
Ureteropelvic junction narrowing or obstruction	Bladder neck obstruction
Ureterovesical junction narrowing or obstruction	Ureterocele
Ureterocele	Benign prostatic hypertrophy
Retrocaval ureter	Cancer of prostate
Calculi	Cancer of bladder
Inflammation	Calculi
Trauma	Diabetic neuropathy
Sloughed papillae	Spinal cord disease
Tumor	Carcinoma of cervix, colon
Blood clots	Trauma
Uric acid crystals	**Urethra**
Pregnant uterus	Posterior urethral valves
Retroperitoneal fibrosis	Anterior urethral valves
Aortic aneurysm	Stricture
Uterine leiomyomas	Meatal stenosis
Carcinoma of uterus, prostate, bladder, colon, rectum	Phimosis
Retroperitoneal lymphoma	Tumor
Accidental surgical ligation	Calculi
	Trauma

Reproduced, with permission, from Seifter JL. Urinary tract obstruction. In: Longo D et al, eds. *Harrison's Principles of Internal Medicine*, 18th ed. McGraw-Hill, 2012.

Etiology

Although a variety of disorders may result in the development of renal stones (Table 16–13), at least 75% of renal stones contain calcium. Most cases of calcium stones are due to idiopathic hypercalciuria, with hyperuricosuria and hyperparathyroidism as other major causes. Uric acid stones are typically caused by hyperuricosuria, especially in patients with a history of gout or excessive purine intake (eg, a diet high in organ meat). Defective amino acid transport, as occurs in cystinuria, can result in stone formation. Finally, struvite stones, made of magnesium, ammonium, and phosphate salts, are a result of chronic or recurrent urinary tract infection by urease-producing organisms (typically *Proteus*).

Pathology & Pathogenesis

Renal stones result from alterations in the solubility of various substances in urine, which lead to the nucleation and precipitation of salts. A number of factors can tip the balance in favor of stone formation.

Dehydration favors stone formation, and a high fluid intake to maintain a daily urine volume of 2 L or more appears to be protective. The precise mechanism of this protection is unknown. Hypotheses include the dilution of unknown substances that predispose to stone formation and decreased transit time of Ca^{2+} through the nephron, minimizing the likelihood of precipitation.

A high-protein diet predisposes to stone formation in susceptible individuals. A dietary protein load causes transient metabolic acidosis and an increased GFR. Although serum Ca^{2+} is not detectably elevated, there is probably a transient increase in calcium resorption from bone, an increase in glomerular calcium filtration, and an inhibition of distal tubular calcium resorption. This effect appears to be greater in known stone formers than in healthy controls.

A high-Na^+ diet predisposes to Ca^{2+} excretion and calcium oxalate stone formation, whereas a low dietary Na^+ intake has the opposite effect. Furthermore, urinary Na^+ excretion increases the saturation of monosodium urate, which can act as a nidus for Ca^{2+} crystallization.

Despite the fact that most stones are calcium oxalate stones, oxalate concentration in the diet is generally too low to support a recommendation to avoid oxalate to prevent stone formation. Similarly, calcium restriction, formerly a major dietary recommendation to calcium stone formers, is beneficial only to the small subset of patients whose hypercalciuria is diet dependent. In others, decreased dietary calcium may actually increase oxalate absorption in the GI tract and thus predispose to stone formation. Therefore, calcium restriction is not recommended for stone prevention.

A number of factors are protective against stone formation. In order of decreasing importance, fluids, citrate, magnesium, and dietary fiber appear to have a protective effect. Citrate decreases the likelihood of stone formation by chelating calcium in solution and forming highly soluble complexes compared with calcium oxalate and calcium phosphate. Although pharmacologic supplementation of the diet with potassium citrate has been shown to increase urinary citrate and pH and to decrease the incidence of recurrent stone formation, the benefits of a naturally high-citrate diet are less clear. However, some studies suggest that vegetarians have a lower incidence of stone formation. Presumably, they avoid the stone-forming effect of high protein and Na^+ in the diet and benefit from the protective effects of fiber and other factors.

Stone formation per se within the renal pelvis is painless until a fragment breaks off and travels down the ureter, precipitating ureteral colic. Hematuria and renal damage can occur in the absence of pain.

Clinical Manifestations

The pain associated with renal stones results from distention of the ureter, renal pelvis, or renal capsule. The severity of pain is related to the degree of distention that occurs and thus is extremely severe in acute obstruction. Anuria and azotemia are suggestive of bilateral obstruction or the unilateral

TABLE 16–13   Major causes of renal stones.

Stone Type and Causes	All Stones (%)	Occurrence of Specific Causes[1]	M:F Ratio	Etiology	Diagnosis	Treatment
Calcium stones	75–85%		2:1 to 3:1			
Idiopathic hypercalciuria		50–55%	2:1	Possible hereditary	Normocalcemia, unexplained hypercalciuria[2]	Thiazide diuretic agents; low-sodium, low-protein diet
Hyperuricosuria		20%	4:1	Diet	Urine uric acid >750 mg/24 h (women); >800 mg/24 h (men)	Allopurinol or febuxostat, or low-purine diet
Primary hyperparathyroidism		3–5%	3:10	Neoplasia	Hypercalcemia with nonsuppressed parathyroid hormone level	Surgery
Distal renal tubular acidosis		Rare	1:1	Hereditary or acquired	Hyperchloremic acidosis, minimum urine pH >5.5	Alkali replacement
Dietary hyperoxaluria		10–30%	1:1	High-oxalate or low-calcium diet	Urine oxalate >40 mg/24 h	Low-oxalate, normal-calcium diet
Intestinal hyperoxaluria		≈1–2%	1:1	Bowel surgery	Urine oxalate >75 mg/24 h	Low-oxalate diet and oral calcium
Primary hyperoxaluria		Rare	1:1	Hereditary	Urine oxalate and glycolic or L-glyceric acid increased	Fluids, pyridoxine, citrate, and neural phosphate
Hypocitraturia		20–40%	1:1 to 2:1	Diet, possible hereditary	Urine citrate <320 mg/24 h	Alkali supplements
Idiopathic stone disease		20%	2:1	Unknown	None of the above	Oral phosphate, fluids
Uric acid stones	5–10%					
Metabolic syndrome		~30	1:1	Diet	Glucose intolerance, obesity, hypertriglyceridemia	Alkali and allopurinol or febuxostat if daily urine uric acid >1000 mg
Gout		≈ 50%	3:1 to 4:1	Hereditary	Clinical diagnosis	Alkali and allopurinol or febuxostat
Idiopathic		≈ 50%	1:1	Possible hereditary	Uric acid stones, no gout	Allopurinol or febuxostat if daily urine uric acid >1000 mg
Dehydration			1:1	Intestinal, habit	History, intestinal fluid loss	Alkali, fluids, reversal of cause
Lesch–Nyhan syndrome		Rare	Males only	Hereditary	Reduced hypoxanthine-guanine phosphoribosyl transferase level	Allopurinol or febuxostat
Cystine stones	1%		1:1	Hereditary	Stone type; elevated cystine excretion	Massive fluids, alkali, D-penicillamine if needed
Struvite stones	5%		1:3	Infection	Stone type	Antimicrobial agents and judicious surgery

[1]Values are percentages of patients who form a particular type of stone and who display each specific cause of stones.

[2]Urine calcium >300 mg/24 h (men), >250 mg/24 h (women), or >4 mg/kg/24 h (either sex). Hyperthyroidism, Cushing syndrome, sarcoidosis, malignant tumors, immobilization, vitamin D intoxication, rapidly progressive bone disease, and Paget disease all cause hypercalciuria and must be excluded in the diagnosis of idiopathic hypercalciuria.

Modified, with permission, from Asplin JR et al. Nephrolithiasis. In: Longo D et al, eds. *Harrison's Principles of Internal Medicine*, 18th ed. McGraw-Hill, 2012.

obstruction of a single functioning kidney. The pain, hematuria, and even ureteral obstruction caused by a renal stone are typically self-limited. For smaller stones, passage usually requires only fluids, bed rest, and analgesia. The major complications are (1) hydronephrosis and potentially permanent renal damage as a result of complete ureter obstruction, with its resulting urine backup and pressure buildup; (2) infection or abscess formation behind a partially or completely obstructing stone; (3) renal damage subsequent to repeated

kidney stones; and (4) hypertension resulting from increased renin production by the obstructed kidney.

CHECKPOINT

17. How do patients with renal stones present?
18. Why do renal stones form?
19. What are the common categories of renal stones (by composition)?

CASE STUDIES

Yeong Kwok, MD

(See Chapter 25, p. 775–76 for answers)

CASE 84

A healthy 26-year-old woman sustained a significant crush injury to her right upper extremity while on the job at a local construction site. She was brought to the emergency department and subsequently underwent pinning and reconstructive surgery and received perioperative broad-spectrum antibiotics. Her blood pressure remained normal throughout her hospital course. On the second hospital day, a medical consultant noted a marked increase in her creatinine, from 0.8 to 1.9 mg/dL. Her urine output dropped to 20 mL/h. Serum creatine kinase was ordered and reported as 3400 units/L.

Questions

A. What are the primary causes of this patient's acute kidney injury? How should her kidney injury be categorized (as prerenal, intrarenal, or postrenal)?
B. Which two types are most likely in this patient? How might they be distinguished clinically?
C. How should the patient be treated?

CASE 85

A 58-year-old obese woman with hypertension, type 2 diabetes, and chronic kidney disease is admitted to hospital after a right femoral neck fracture sustained in a fall. Recently, she had been complaining of fatigue and was started on epoetin alfa subcutaneous injections. Her other medications include an angiotensin-converting enzyme inhibitor, a β-blocker, a diuretic, calcium supplementation, and insulin. On review of systems, she reports mild tingling in her lower extremities. On examination, her blood pressure is 148/60 mm Hg. She is oriented and able to answer questions appropriately. There is no evidence of jugular venous distention or pericardial friction rub. Her lungs are clear, and her right lower extremity is in Buck traction in preparation for surgery. Asterixis is absent.

Questions

A. Describe the pathogenesis of bone disease in chronic kidney disease. How could this explain the patient's increased likelihood of sustaining a fracture after a fall?
B. Why was erythropoietin therapy initiated?
C. What is the significance of a pericardial friction rub in the setting of chronic kidney disease?

CASE 86

A 28-year-old nursery school teacher developed a marked change in the color of her urine ("cola-colored") 1 week after she contracted impetigo from one of her students. She also complained of a new onset of global headaches and fluid retention in her legs. Examination revealed a blood pressure of 158/92 mm Hg, resolving honey-crusted pustules over her right face and neck, 1+ pitting edema of her ankles, and no cardiac murmur. Urinalysis revealed 2+ protein and numerous red cells and red cell casts. Her serum creatinine was elevated at 1.9 mg/dL. Serum complement levels (CH50, C3, and C4) were low. She was diagnosed with poststreptococcal glomerulonephritis.

Questions

A. What is the relationship between the patient's skin infection and the subsequent development of glomerulonephritis?
B. Describe the pathogenesis of this disorder.
C. What is the natural history of this form of immune complex vasculitis?

CASE 87

A 40-year-old man with Hodgkin lymphoma is admitted to the hospital because of anasarca. He has no known history of renal, liver, or cardiac disease. His serum creatinine level is slightly elevated at 1.4 mg/dL. His serum albumin level is 2.8 g/dL. Liver function test results are normal. Urinalysis demonstrates no red or white blood cell casts, but 3+ protein is noted and a 24-hour urine collection shows a protein excretion of 4 g/24 h. He is diagnosed with nephrotic syndrome, and renal biopsy suggests minimal-change disease. Steroids and diuretics are instituted, with gradual improvement of edema. The hospital course is complicated by deep venous thrombosis of the left calf and thigh that requires anticoagulation.

Questions

A. This patient suffers from generalized body edema (anasarca). By what mechanism does the edema form?
B. What are the characteristic morphologic features seen in minimal-change disease? How does this differ from other forms of glomerulonephritis?
C. How does nephrotic syndrome predispose this patient to thromboembolic disease?

CASE 88

A 48-year-old white man presents to the emergency department with unremitting right flank pain. He denies dysuria and fever. He reports significant nausea without vomiting. He has never experienced anything like this before. On examination, he is afebrile, and his blood pressure is 160/80 mm Hg with a pulse rate of 110/min. He is writhing on the gurney, unable to find a comfortable position. His right flank is mildly tender to palpation, and abdominal examination is benign. Urinalysis is significant for 1+ blood, and microscopy reveals 10–20 red blood cells per high-power field. Nephrolithiasis is suspected, and the patient is intravenously hydrated and given pain medication with temporary relief.

Questions

A. What is the most likely cause of this patient's renal stone disease?
B. Describe your discharge instructions to the patient, reflecting on the pathogenesis of stone disease.
C. Why is this disorder painful?

REFERENCES

General

Farooq U et al. 2014 Guideline for the management of high blood pressure (Eighth Joint National Committee): take-home messages. Med Clin North Am. 2015 Jul;99(4):733–8. [PMID: 26042879]

Kuroda N et al. IgG4-related renal disease: clinical and pathological characteristics. Int J Clin Exp Pathol. 2014 Aug 15;7(9):6379–85. [PMID: 25337295]

Levey AS et al. Glomerular filtration rate and albuminuria for detection and staging of acute and chronic kidney disease in adults: a systematic review. JAMA. 2015 Feb 24;313(8):837–46. [PMID: 25710660]

United States Renal Data System. 2017 USRDS annual data report: epidemiology of kidney disease in the United States. Volume 1: Chronic-kidney-disease in the United States, and Volume 2: End-stage renal disease in the United States. National Institutes of Health, National Institute of Diabetes and Digestive and Kidney Diseases, Bethesda, MD, 2017. https://www.usrds.org/adr.aspx.

Zager RA. Progression from acute kidney injury to chronic kidney disease: clinical and experimental insights and queries. Nephron Clin Pract. 2014;127(1–4):46–50. [PMID: 25343820]

Acute Kidney Injury

Al-Khafaji A et al. Hepatorenal disorders. Chest. 2015 Aug;148(2):550–8. [PMID: 25811649]

Hadjiphilippou S et al. Cardiorenal syndrome: review of our current understanding. J R Soc Med. 2016 Jan;109(1):12–7. [PMID: 26609123]

Hobson C et al. Acute kidney injury in the surgical patient. Crit Care Clin. 2015 Oct;31(4):705–23. [PMID: 26410139]

Kanagasundaram NS. Pathophysiology of ischaemic acute kidney injury. Ann Clin Biochem. 2015 Mar;52(Pt 2):193–205. [PMID: 25293591]

Karvellas CJ et al. Acute kidney injury in cirrhosis. Crit Care Clin. 2015 Oct;31(4):737–50. [PMID: 26410141]

Kellum JA. Diagnostic criteria for acute kidney injury: present and future. Crit Care Clin. 2015 Oct;31(4):621–32. [PMID: 26410133]

Marenzi G et al. Acute kidney injury in patients with acute coronary syndromes. Heart. 2015 Nov;101(22):1778–85. [PMID: 26243789]

Shum HP et al. Recent knowledge on the pathophysiology of septic acute kidney injury: a narrative review. J Crit Care. 2016 Feb;31(1):82–9. [PMID: 26475099]

Umbro I et al. Recent advances in pathophysiology and biomarkers of sepsis-induced acute kidney injury. J Infect. 2016 Feb;72(2):131–42. [PMID: 26702738]

Zuk A et al. Acute kidney injury. Annu Rev Med. 2016;67:293–307. [PMID: 26768243]

Chronic Kidney Disease

Kiefer MM et al. Primary care of the patient with chronic kidney disease. Med Clin North Am. 2015 Sep;99(5):935–52. [PMID: 26320040]

Noone D et al. Chronic kidney disease: a new look at pathogenetic mechanisms and treatment options. Pediatr Nephrol. 2014 May;29(5):779–92. [PMID: 23471475]

Re RN. A reassessment of the pathophysiology of progressive cardiorenal disorders. Med Clin North Am. 2017 Jan;101(1):103–15. [PMID: 27884222]

Sternlicht H et al. The kidney in hypertension. Med Clin North Am. 2017 Jan;101(1):207–17. [PMID: 27884230]

Vassalotti JA et al; National Kidney Foundation Kidney Disease Outcomes Quality Initiative. Practical approach to detection and management of chronic kidney disease for the primary care clinician. Am J Med. 2016 Feb;129(2):153–62. [PMID: 26391748]

Glomerulonephritis

Floege J et al. Primary glomerulonephritides. Lancet. 2016 May 14;387(10032):2036–48. [PMID: 26921911]

Fogo AB. Causes and pathogenesis of focal segmental glomerulosclerosis. Nat Rev Nephrol. 2015 Feb;11(2):76–87. [PMID: 25447132]

François H et al. Renal involvement in primary Sjögren syndrome. Nat Rev Nephrol. 2016 Feb;12(2):82–93. [PMID: 26568188]

Gupta A et al. Glomerular diseases associated with hepatitis B and C. Adv Chronic Kidney Dis. 2015 Sep;22(5):343–51. [PMID: 26311595]

Lorenz G et al. Lupus nephritis: update on mechanisms of systemic autoimmunity and kidney immunopathology. Curr Opin Nephrol Hypertens. 2014 May;23(3):211–7. [PMID: 24662982]

Markowitz GS et al. Drug-induced glomerular disease: direct cellular injury. Clin J Am Soc Nephrol. 2015 Jul 7;10(7):1291–9. [PMID: 25862776]

Pillai U et al. Immunoglobulin A nephropathy: a review of current literature on emerging pathophysiology. Am J Med Sci. 2014 Mar;347(3):249–53. [PMID: 23719511]

Syed R et al. Pauci-immune crescentic glomerulonephritis: an ANCA-associated vasculitis. Biomed Res Int. 2015;2015:402826. [PMID: 26688808]

Kidney Stones

Arcidiacono T et al. Idiopathic calcium nephrolithiasis: a review of pathogenic mechanisms in the light of genetic studies. Am J Nephrol. 2014;40(6):499–506. [PMID: 25504362]

Arrabal-Polo MA et al. Calcium nephrolithiasis and bone demineralization: pathophysiology, diagnosis, and medical management. Curr Opin Urol. 2014 Nov;24(6):633–8. [PMID: 25188231]

Flannigan R et al. Renal struvite stones—pathogenesis, microbiology, and management strategies. Nat Rev Urol. 2014 Jun;11(6):333–41. Erratum in: Nat Rev Urol. 2014 Jun;11(6):page after 341. [PMID: 24818849]

Mohebbi N et al. Tubular and genetic disorders associated with kidney stones. Urolithiasis. 2017 Feb;45(1):127–37. [PMID: 27896392]

Sakhaee K. Epidemiology and clinical pathophysiology of uric acid kidney stones. J Nephrol. 2014 Jun;27(3):241–5. [PMID: 24497296]

Vestergaard P. Primary hyperparathyroidism and nephrolithiasis. Ann Endocrinol (Paris). 2015 May;76(2):116–9. [PMID: 25911000]

Disorders of the Parathyroids & Calcium and Phosphorus Metabolism

Dolores M. Shoback, MD

This chapter presents a general overview of the key hormones involved regulating calcium, phosphate, and bone mineral metabolism. These include **parathyroid hormone**, **vitamin D**—principally the 1,25-(OH)$_2$ vitamin D metabolite (1,25-dihydroxycholecalciferol)—**calcitonin**, and **fibroblast growth factor (FGF)-23**. The cycle of bone remodeling is described as a basis for understanding the normal maintenance of skeletal integrity in adults and of mineral homeostasis. The symptoms and signs caused by an excess or deficiency of the calciotropic hormones are presented, along with the natural histories of **primary hyperparathyroidism, familial hypocalciuric hypercalcemia, hypercalcemia of malignancy,** different forms of **hypoparathyroidism,** and **medullary carcinoma of the thyroid.** Two of the most commonly encountered causes of low bone mass—**osteoporosis** and **osteomalacia**—are reviewed, and the pathogenesis of these conditions is discussed.

NORMAL REGULATION OF CALCIUM & PHOSPHORUS METABOLISM

PARATHYROID GLANDS

Anatomy

Normal parathyroid glands each weigh 30–40 mg and are gray-tan to yellow-gray. Each person typically has four glands, so that the average total parathyroid tissue mass in the adult is 120–160 mg.

The superior pair of parathyroid glands arise from the fourth branchial pouches in the embryo. These glands are located near the point of intersection of the middle thyroid artery and the recurrent laryngeal nerve. The superior parathyroid glands may be attached to the thyroid capsule posteriorly or, rarely, embedded in the thyroid gland itself. Alternative locations include the tracheoesophageal groove and the retroesophageal space. The blood supply to the superior parathyroid glands is from the inferior thyroid artery or, less commonly, the superior thyroid artery.

The inferior parathyroid glands develop from the third branchial pouch, as does the thymus gland. These glands typically lie at or near the lower pole of the thyroid gland, lateral to the trachea. The inferior glands receive their blood supply from the inferior thyroid arteries. The location of the inferior parathyroid glands is variable. When there are ectopic glands, they are typically found in association with thymic remnants. A common site for ectopic glands is the anterior mediastinum. Less common ectopic locations are the carotid sheath, pericardium, and pharyngeal submucosa. About 10% of people have additional (supernumerary) parathyroid glands. This becomes a critically important issue when such ectopic glands develop hyperparathyroidism and need to be localized and removed.

Histology

The parathyroid gland is composed of three different cell types: chief cells, clear cells, and oxyphil cells. **Chief cells** are small in diameter (4–8 μm) with central nuclei and are thought to be the main source of **parathyroid hormone (PTH)**. In their active state, they have prominent endoplasmic reticula and dense Golgi regions where PTH is synthesized and packaged for secretion. **Clear cells** are probably chief cells with an increased glycogen content. **Oxyphil cells** appear in the parathyroid glands after puberty. They are larger than chief cells (6–10 μm), and their number increases with age. Whether these cells secrete PTH and whether they are derived from chief cells remains unclear.

The normal adult parathyroid gland contains fat. The relative contribution of fat to the glandular mass increases with age and may reach 60–70% of gland volume in the elderly. If hyperplasia or an adenoma develops, the glandular fat content decreases dramatically. Hypercellularity of the parathyroid gland is typically the pathologic feature distinguishing the abnormal from the normal gland(s).

Physiology

Approximately 99% of total body calcium is found in the skeleton and teeth; the remainder is in the extracellular fluids. Calcium in these fluids exists in three forms: ionized, protein bound, and complexed. About 47% of total blood calcium is protein bound, predominantly to albumin but also to globulins. A similar fraction is ionized. The remainder is complexed to organic ions such as citrate, phosphate, and bicarbonate. Serum ionized calcium controls vital cellular functions such as hormone secretion and action, muscle contraction, neuromuscular transmission, and blood clotting. The binding of calcium to albumin is pH dependent, increasing with alkalosis and decreasing with acidosis. Thus, if the ionized calcium is low, acidosis tends to protect against symptomatic hypocalcemia. Conversely, alkalosis predisposes to symptomatic hypocalcemia.

Circulating levels of PTH can change within seconds after an alteration in serum calcium. PTH secretory rates are controlled by the serum ionized calcium concentration as reflected in an inverse sigmoidal relationship (Figure 17–1). Low ionized calcium concentrations maximally stimulate secretion, whereas increases in calcium suppress the transcription of the *prepro-PTH* gene and the subsequent production of PTH. PTH secretion is exquisitely sensitive to very small changes in serum calcium concentration, which has substantial effects on the rate of hormone synthesis and release.

The extracellular calcium-sensing receptor (CaSR) is expressed by parathyroid and many other types of cells. Its job is to detect changes in the extracellular calcium concentration. This receptor is activated by increases in calcium concentration and couples to intracellular pathways, which inhibits hormone secretion (Figure 17–2) and parathyroid cell proliferation. CaSRs are also expressed in the kidney, thyroid C cells, brain, and many other tissues. CaSRs also sense hypocalcemia and stimulate PTH secretion in response. Chronic hypocalcemia stimulates parathyroid cell proliferation, which eventually results in glandular hyperplasia. Thus, the CaSR controls secretion and proliferation in appropriate directions to respond to physiologic needs.

PTH is produced in the parathyroid glands as a 115-amino-acid precursor molecule (preproPTH) that is successively cleaved within the cell to form the mature 84-amino-acid peptide PTH(1–84) (Figure 17–3). This form of the hormone is

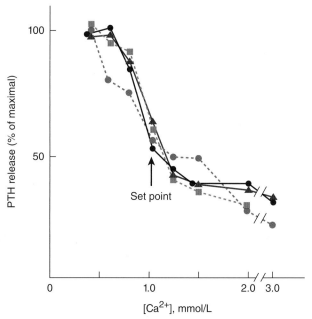

FIGURE 17–1 Inverse sigmoidal relationship between parathyroid hormone (PTH) release and extracellular calcium concentration in human studies (upper panel) and in vitro in human parathyroid cells (bottom panel). The studies shown in the upper panel were performed by infusing calcium and the calcium chelator EDTA into normal subjects. Serum intact PTH was measured by a two-site immunoradiometric assay. In the lower panel, PTH was measured in the medium surrounding parathyroid cells in vitro by an assay for intact PTH. The midpoint between the maximal and minimal secretory rates is defined as the set point for secretion. (Redrawn, with permission, from Brown E. Extracellular Ca²⁺ sensing, regulation of parathyroid cell function, and role of Ca²⁺ and other ions as extracellular [first] messengers. Physiol Rev. 1991;71:371.)

packaged into secretory granules and released into the circulation. PTH(1–84) is the biologically active form of PTH at target cells and has a very short half-life in vivo of approximately 10 minutes. PTH(1–84) is metabolized in the liver and other tissues to midregion and carboxyl terminal forms that are probably biologically inactive. These circulating fragments accumulate to very high levels in patients with renal failure, because the kidney is an important site for clearing PTH from

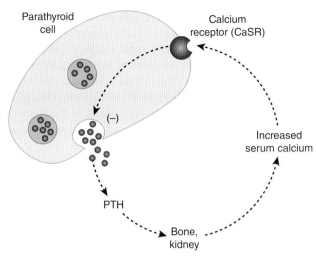

FIGURE 17–2 Sequence of events by which the calcium ion concentration is sensed by the parathyroid calcium-sensing receptor (CaSR). Activation of this receptor is eventually linked through intracellular signal transduction pathways to the inhibition of PTH secretion and parathyroid cell proliferation. (Redrawn, with modifications, from Taylor R. A new receptor for calcium ions. J NIH Res. 1994;6:25.)

FIGURE 17–3 Biosynthetic events in the production of parathyroid hormone (PTH) within the parathyroid cell. The *PreproPTH* gene is transcribed to its mRNA, which is translated on the ribosomes to preproPTH (amino acids −29 to +84). The presequence is removed within the endoplasmic reticulum, yielding proPTH (−6 to +84). An additional six-amino-acid fragment is removed in the Golgi. Mature PTH(1–84) released from the Golgi is packaged in secretory granules and released into the circulation in the presence of hypocalcemia. The calcium-sensing receptor (CaSR or CaR) is proposed to sense changes in extracellular calcium levels that affect both the release of PTH and the transcription of *preproPTH*. High extracellular calcium concentrations also promote the intracellular degradation of PTH. (Redrawn, with permission, from Habener JF et al. Biosynthesis of parathyroid hormone. Recent Prog Horm Res. 1977;33:249. Copyright © Elsevier.)

FIGURE 17–4 Schematic representation of the principle of the two-site assay for parathyroid hormone (PTH), in this case full-length, biointact PTH(1–84). The label may be a luminescent probe or ^{125}I in the immunochemiluminometric or immunoradiometric assay, respectively. Two different region-specific antibodies are used (Ab$_1$ and Ab$_2$). The epitope for Ab$_1$ is at the extreme N-terminus ensuring that only the hormone species containing both N- and C-terminal/midregion immunodeterminants are counted in the assay.

the body. Intact PTH assays in routine use measure PTH(1–84) using immunoradiometric or immunochemiluminometric methods that employ two antibodies: one directed against an amino terminal epitope, which is labeled, and the other directed against a carboxyl terminal epitope of PTH(1–84), which is immobilized (Figure 17–4). It is now clear that these "intact" PTH assays also detect amino-terminally truncated fragments of hormone such as PTH(7–84), which can accumulate, particularly in the serum of uremic patients. It is estimated that 30–50% of circulating "intact PTH" in uremic sera may represent these amino terminal fragments. This finding led to the development of "whole PTH" assays that detect only PTH(1–84). The amino terminal antibody in these assays specifically recognizes the first six amino acids of PTH(1–84). Such assays, however, have not replaced the original intact assays for routine clinical use.

Mechanism of Parathyroid Hormone Action

There are two types of PTH receptor. The type 1 receptor recognizes PTH and parathyroid hormone–related peptide (PTHrP) and is also called the PTH-1 receptor. The type 2 receptor is specific for PTH. PTH and PTHrP (described later)

FIGURE 17–5 Signal transduction pathways activated by parathyroid hormone (PTH) binding to the PTH-1 receptor (PTH-R) in a target cell. PTH interacting with its receptor enhances guanosine triphosphate binding to the stimulatory G protein of adenylyl cyclase G_s, which activates the enzyme. Cyclic adenosine monophosphate (cAMP) is formed. The PTH-receptor interaction also increases the G protein–dependent activation of phospholipase C (PLC). This activation catalyzes the breakdown of the membrane phospholipid phosphatidylinositol 4,5-bisphosphate (PIP_2). This breakdown produces the second messengers inositol trisphosphate (1,4,5-InsP$_3$) and diacylglycerol. 1,4,5-InsP$_3$ mobilizes intracellular calcium, and diacylglycerol activates protein kinase C.

bind to the type 1 receptor through residues in their amino terminal domains. PTH activates adenylyl cyclase and produces the second messenger cAMP (Figure 17–5). The type 1 receptor also couples to produce stimulation of phospholipase C activity, leading to the generation of inositol trisphosphate and diacylglycerol (see Figure 17–5). Activation of this signal transduction pathway induces intracellular calcium mobilization and protein kinase C activation in PTH- and PTHrP-responsive cells. The type 2 PTH receptor is expressed in nonclassic PTH target tissues (ie, brain, pancreas, testis, placenta). This receptor is not thought to be involved in mineral balance, and its natural ligand may be a hypothalamic peptide called tubuloinfundibular peptide.

Effects of Parathyroid Hormone

The serum ionized calcium and phosphate concentrations reflect the net transfer of these ions from bone, the gastrointestinal (GI) tract, and glomerular filtrate. PTH and 1,25-(OH)$_2$D play key roles in regulating the calcium and phosphate balance (Figure 17–6). When the serum calcium concentration falls, PTH is rapidly released and acts quickly to promote calcium reabsorption in the distal tubule and the medullary thick ascending limb of the Henle loop. PTH also stimulates the release of calcium from bone. These actions serve to restore serum calcium levels to normal.

The renal action of PTH is rapid, occurring within minutes after an increase in the hormone. The overall effect of PTH on the kidney, however, depends on several factors. When

hypocalcemia is present and PTH is elevated, urinary calcium excretion is low. This reflects the full expression of the primary renal effect of PTH to enhance renal calcium reabsorption. When PTH levels are high in primary hyperparathyroidism, hypercalcemia results from the increased mobilization of calcium from bone and enhanced intestinal calcium absorption. These events increase the delivery of calcium to the glomerular filtrate. Because more calcium is filtered, more is excreted in the urine, despite the high PTH levels. If the filtered load of calcium is normal or low in a patient with primary hyperparathyroidism—because of a low dietary calcium intake or demineralized bone—urinary calcium excretion may be normal or even low. Thus, there may be considerable variability in calcium excretion among patients with hyperparathyroidism.

If kidney function is normal, chronic elevation in serum PTH increases renal 1,25-(OH)$_2$D production. This steroid hormone stimulates both calcium and phosphate absorption across the small intestine (see Figure 17–6). The effect requires at least 24 hours to develop fully and begin to restore normal calcium levels. Achievement of eucalcemia then leads to a downward readjustment in the PTH secretory rate. Any increase in 1,25-(OH)$_2$D serves to inhibit further PTH synthesis by binding to vitamin D receptors in the parathyroid.

The major effect of PTH on phosphate handling is to promote its excretion by inhibiting sodium-dependent phosphate transport in the proximal tubule. Serum phosphate levels are thought to affect PTH secretion rates directly, with hyperphosphatemia serving to stimulate PTH secretion by an uncertain mechanism, possibly through the CaSR. Hypophosphatemia enhances the conversion of 25-(OH)D to 1,25-(OH)$_2$D in the kidney, which through its intestinal and renal effects promotes phosphate retention. Hyperphosphatemia also inhibits 1,25-(OH)$_2$D production (see below) and lowers serum calcium by complexing with it in the circulation.

PTH also increases the urinary excretion of bicarbonate through its action on the proximal tubule. This can produce proximal renal tubular acidosis. These physiologic responses to PTH are the basis for the hypophosphatemia and hyperchloremic acidosis commonly observed in patients with hyperparathyroidism. Dehydration is also common in moderate to severe hypercalcemia of any origin. This is due to the effect of hypercalcemia on vasopressin action in the medullary thick ascending limb of the kidney. High calcium levels, presumably by interacting with renal CaSRs, blunt the ability of endogenous vasopressin to stimulate water reabsorption. Thus, hypercalcemia induces vasopressin-resistant nephrogenic diabetes insipidus.

In conjunction with 1,25-(OH)$_2$D, PTH increases bone resorption to restore normocalcemia (see below). PTH enhances osteoclastic activity by stimulating the receptor activator of nuclear factor kappa B ligand (RANK-L), which is expressed by cells of the osteoblastic lineage (including stromal cells and osteoblasts). RANK-L interacts with its receptor, RANK, on cells of the osteoclast lineage to stimulate their differentiation and functional responses, particularly bone resorption (Figure 17–7). Once resorption ceases, bone

FIGURE 17–6 Main actions of parathyroid hormone (PTH) and 1,25-(OH)$_2$D in the maintenance of calcium and phosphate homeostasis. (Redrawn, with permission, from Chandrasoma P et al, eds. *Concise Pathology*, 3rd ed. Originally published by Appleton & Lange. Copyright © 1998 by The McGraw-Hill Companies, Inc.)

formation ensues, because the processes of resorption and formation are coupled. In primary and secondary hyperparathyroidism, when PTH production rates are excessive, net bone loss may occur over time, perhaps because even though the processes of formation and resorption are coupled, they may not occur with 100% efficiency.

PARATHYROID HORMONE–RELATED PEPTIDE

PTHrP is a 141-amino-acid peptide that is homologous with PTH at its amino terminal region (Figure 17–8) and binds to

FIGURE 17-7   Cell–cell interactions and molecules essential for the differentiation and activation of osteoclasts. A cell surface molecule known as **RANK-L** on osteoblastic bone marrow stromal cells can interact with osteoclastic precursor cells in the bone marrow (derived from cells of the monocytic lineage) through their cell surface molecules designated **RANK**. This interaction, in the presence of sufficient macrophage colony-stimulating factor (M-CSF), promotes the differentiation and fusion of these cells eventually to form mature osteoclasts and enables the activation of otherwise quiescent osteoclasts to resorb bone. These pathways are interfered with by the elaboration of a secreted decoy receptor molecule for RANK-L known as **osteoprotegerin** (**OPG**), which blocks the activation and differentiation of osteoclasts. (Oc, osteoclast.) (Redrawn, with permission, from Goltzman D. Osteolysis and cancer. J Clin Invest. 2001;107:1219.)

the type 1 PTH receptor. Consequently, PTHrP has effects on bone and kidney similar to those of PTH; it increases bone resorption, increases phosphate excretion, and decreases renal calcium excretion. PTHrP is secreted by tumor cells and was originally identified as the cause of hypercalcemia of malignancy, a syndrome that can mimic primary hyperparathyroidism (see later discussion).

Unlike PTH, which is exclusively produced by parathyroid cells, PTHrP is produced in many normal tissues. It functions mainly as a tissue growth and differentiation factor at the local level and a regulator of smooth muscle tone. In the normal development of cartilage and bone, PTHrP stimulates the proliferation of chondrocytes and inhibits the mineralization of cartilage. Embryos without PTHrP are nonviable, with multiple abnormalities of bone and cartilage. PTHrP also appears to regulate the normal development of skin, hair follicles, teeth, and the breast. PTHrP plays an important role in determining the calcium content of the milk from lactating animals.

Despite PTHrP binding to the same PTH-1 receptor (see above) to achieve most of its physiologic effects, new studies indicate that the consequences of PTH and PTHrP interacting with the receptor are surprisingly different. Each peptide has different effects on the conformational state and the extent of

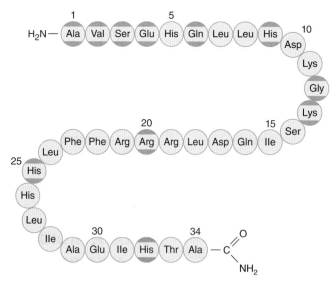

FIGURE 17-8   The amino acid sequence of the 34 amino acid residue at the N-terminal parathyroid hormone (PTH)–related peptide. Amino acids that are identical to those in PTH are shown with dark yellow borders. (Redrawn, with permission, from Felig P et al, eds. *Endocrinology and Metabolism*, 3rd ed. McGraw-Hill, 1995.)

activation of the receptor, particularly in terms of the intensity and duration of the downstream cyclic AMP signaling response.

CHECKPOINT

1. Describe the types of cells in the parathyroid gland.

2. How do serum albumin concentration and blood pH influence the distribution of calcium into ionized and protein-bound fractions?

3. What advances have occurred in two-site immunoassays for PTH that affect uremic patients?

4. What are the actions of PTH and 1,25-(OH)$_2$D on bone, kidney, and the GI tract?

5. What is PTHrP? How is its action similar to and different from that of PTH?

BONE

Most bones contain two types of tissue. On the outside is **cortical** or **compact** bone, which makes up 80% of the skeletal mass and plays a significant role in giving bone its strength. Inside is **trabecular** or **cancellous** bone, which makes up 20% of skeletal mass. Trabecular bone consists of interconnected plates, the trabeculae, which are covered by bone cells and are sites of active remodeling. The spaces in this irregular honeycomb are filled with bone marrow: either red marrow, in which hematopoiesis is active, or white marrow, which is mainly fat. Because of its high surface-to-volume ratio and abundant cellular activity, trabecular bone is remodeled more rapidly than cortical bone. Because of the low ratio of surface to volume, cortical bone is remodeled slowly.

To understand the remodeling process, it is important to know something about bone cells. **Osteocytes**, the most abundant cells in bone (~95% of all cells), are in the osteoblast lineage and reside deep in the matrix. Among the functions of osteocytes are mechanoreception and the transduction of loading signals that induce changes in bone remodeling. **Osteoclasts**, multinucleated giant cells specialized for bone resorption, are terminally differentiated cells that arise continuously from hematopoietic precursors in the macrophage/monocyte lineage. The formation of osteoclasts requires the hematopoietic growth factor macrophage colony-stimulating factor (M-CSF) and a signal from marrow stromal cells. The critical signal, RANK-L, either resides on the surface of bone marrow stromal cells and osteoblastic cells or is secreted in the extracellular environment. This molecule, required for osteoclast differentiation and activation, binds to its receptor, **RANK**, on osteoclast precursors and signals to the cell interior. A variety of cells, including those from the marrow, produce a soluble, secreted decoy receptor, **osteoprotegerin (OPG)**, that binds RANK-L, thereby preventing its interaction with RANK and halting osteoclast differentiation and activation (see Figure 17–7). As osteoclasts mature, they acquire the

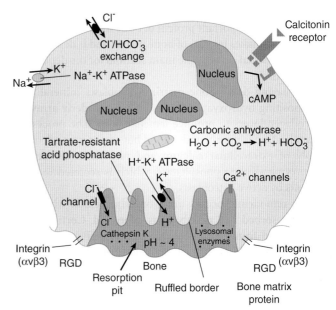

FIGURE 17–9 Schematic view of an active osteoclast. Calcitonin receptors, the ruffled border, enzymes, and channels involved in secreting acid onto the bone surface are shown. Integrins (alpha V, beta 3) are transmembrane-spanning receptors on osteoclasts, which bind to determinants (RGD) in bone matrix proteins such as fibronectins. The integrins are responsible for the tight attachment of osteoclasts to the bone surface. Cathepsin K and other lysosomal enzymes are secreted into the resorption pit to dissolve the matrix. (Modified from Gardner DG et al, eds. *Greenspan's Basic & Clinical Endocrinology*, 10th ed. McGraw-Hill, 2017. Redrawn, with permission, from Felig P et al, eds. In: *Endocrinology and Metabolism*, 3rd ed. Copyright © 1995 by The McGraw-Hill Companies, Inc.)

capacity to produce osteoclast-specific enzymes and fuse to become a mature multinucleated cell. The maturation process is accelerated by bone-resorbing hormones, such as PTH and 1,25-(OH)$_2$D, presumably through their effects on the RANK-L/OPG system.

To resorb bone, the mature osteoclast alights on bone surface and seals off an area by forming an adhesive ring in which cellular integrins bind to receptor proteins in the bone matrix (Figure 17–9). Above an isolated area of bone surface, the osteoclast develops an elaborately invaginated plasma membrane structure called the **ruffled border**. The ruffled border is a distinctive organelle, but it acts essentially as a huge lysosome, dissolving bone mineral by secreting acid onto the isolated bone surface, and simultaneously breaking down the bone matrix by secreting collagenase and proteases. The resulting collagen peptides have cross-links that can be assayed in urine as a measure of bone resorption rates. The main way that bone resorption can be controlled is by regulating the formation of mature osteoclasts and by regulating their activity. The **osteoblast**, or bone-forming cell, arises from a mesenchymal stem cell induced to differentiate in the bone marrow microenvironment. When actively forming bone, the osteoblast is a tall, plump cell with an abundant Golgi apparatus. On active bone-forming surfaces, osteoblasts are found side by side, laying down bone matrix by secreting proteins and proteoglycans. The most important protein of bone matrix is type I collagen, which makes up 90% of bone matrix and is deposited in regular layers that serve as the main scaffold for the deposition of minerals.

After laying down bone matrix, osteoblasts mineralize it by depositing hydroxyapatite crystals in an orderly array on the collagen layers to produce lamellar bone. The process of mineralization is poorly understood but requires an adequate supply of extracellular calcium and phosphate, as well as the enzyme alkaline phosphatase, which is secreted in large amounts by active osteoblasts.

Bone remodeling occurs in an orderly cycle in which old bone is resorbed and new bone is deposited. Cortical bone is remodeled from within by cutting cones (Figure 17–10), groups of osteoclasts that cut tunnels through the compact bone. They are followed by trailing osteoblasts, lining the tunnels and laying down a cylinder of new bone on their walls, so that the tunnels are progressively narrowed until all that remains are the tiny haversian canals, by which the cells that are left behind as resident osteocytes are fed.

In trabecular bone, the remodeling process occurs on the surface (Figure 17–11). Osteoclasts first excavate a pit, which is then filled in with new bone by osteoblasts. In a normal adult,

1. Osteoclast recruitment and activation

2. Resorption and osteoblast recruitment

3. Osteoblastic bone formation

4. Completed remodeling cycle

FIGURE 17–11 Sequential steps in trabecular bone remodeling. (Redrawn, with permission, from Felig P et al, eds. *Endocrinology and Metabolism*, 3rd ed. McGraw-Hill, 1995.)

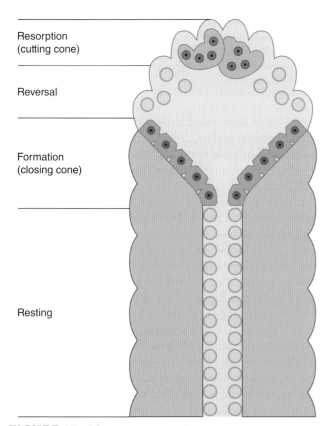

FIGURE 17–10 A cutting cone remodeling cortical bone. (Modified from Gardner DG et al, eds. *Greenspan's Basic & Clinical Endocrinology*, 10th ed. McGraw-Hill, 2017. Redrawn, with permission, from Felig P et al, eds. In: *Endocrinology and Metabolism*, 3rd ed. Copyright © 1995 by The McGraw-Hill Companies, Inc.)

this cycle takes approximately 200 days. At each remodeling site, bone resorption and new bone formation are ordinarily tightly coupled, so that in a state of zero net bone balance, the amount of new bone formed is precisely equivalent to the amount of old bone resorbed. This degree of balance is brief, however. From approximately 20 to 30 years of age, bone mass is consolidated following gains in growth and mineral deposition achieved during adolescence. Beginning at age 30–35 years, adult females begin to lose bone slowly.

How osteoclasts and osteoblasts communicate to achieve the coupling that ensures perfect (or near-perfect) bone balance is not fully known. It appears that the important signals are local, not systemic. Although they have not been identified with certainty, one candidate is RANK-L (described above). RANK-L on the cell surface or as a soluble molecule binds to osteoclast precursors and supports their development and differentiation. RANK-L also binds to RANK on mature osteoclasts and mediates the resorptive process. Bone remodeling does not absolutely require systemic hormones, except to ensure an adequate supply of calcium and phosphate. However, systemic hormones use the bone as a source of minerals to regulate extracellular calcium homeostasis. Osteoblasts have receptors for PTH and 1,25-$(OH)_2$D, but osteoclasts do not. Isolated osteoclasts do not respond to PTH or vitamin D, except in the presence of osteoblasts.

This coupling mechanism ensures that when bone resorption is activated by PTH (eg, to provide calcium to correct hypocalcemia), bone formation will also increase, tending to replenish lost bone.

CHECKPOINT

6. Describe the two types of bone tissue.
7. How is bone resorption by osteoclasts controlled?
8. What is the role of osteoblasts in bone formation? How are the actions of osteoblasts and osteoclasts coupled?

VITAMIN D

Vitamin D is actually a prohormone produced in the dermis in response to ultraviolet B (UVB) exposure and metabolized to its active forms in the liver first, then in the kidney. The amount of sunlight exposure necessary to produce sufficient vitamin D is difficult to estimate because of individual differences in skin pigmentation, latitude, and time of day. Dietary sources are relatively modest in vitamin D content.

Physiology

7-Dehydrocholesterol, stored in the epidermis, is converted to vitamin D_3 (cholecalciferol) by ultraviolet light (wavelengths of 280–310 nm) (Figure 17–12). This step involves breaking the B ring of the cholesterol structure to produce a secosteroid; hormones with an intact cholesterol nucleus (eg, estrogen) are called steroids. A similar process occurs in plants with one small structural difference, resulting in vitamin D_2 rather than vitamin D_3. Vitamin D_2 is activated similarly to D_3 in humans but does appear to have a decreased binding affinity for vitamin D–binding protein (DBP), resulting in enhanced clearance. This is particularly evident when large intermittent doses (ie, once weekly) rather than single daily doses are used medically in the treatment of vitamin D deficiency.

Although the cutaneous synthesis of vitamin D can be sufficient to prevent rickets (the overt skeletal manifestation of vitamin D deficiency), it is not clear that sunlight exposure can be obtained in sufficient quantities to optimize vitamin D stores without untoward skin consequences. Further, at most latitudes in the United States, there is insufficient UVB radiation in the sunlight during the winter months to induce the cutaneous production of vitamin D. In 2011, the Institute of Medicine revised the recommended intakes of vitamin D, recommending consumption of 400 IU/d up to 1 year of age, 600 IU/d for individuals 1–70 years of age, and 800 IU/d for individuals older than 70 years. In the United States, milk is supplemented with 400 IU of vitamin D per quart. Dietary supplements of vitamin D consist of vitamin D_2 (ergocalciferol) and vitamin D_3 (cholecalciferol).

FIGURE 17–12 The formation and activation of vitamin D. (Redrawn, with permission, from Felig P et al, eds. *Endocrinology and Metabolism*, 3rd ed. McGraw-Hill, 1995.)

While there is minimal regulation of vitamin D production in the skin, enhanced sun exposure does not result in vitamin D toxicity, as vitamin D is photo-converted to inactive metabolites when skin levels of vitamin D rise. Vitamin D formed in the skin is a lipophilic substance that is transported to the liver bound to albumin and a specific DBP. Ingested vitamin D is transported to the liver via chylomicrons. In the liver, vitamin D is hydroxylated to produce 25-hydroxyvitamin D (25-[OH]D) (see Figure 17–12). This process is not closely regulated. 25-(OH)D is transported by DBP in the serum to target tissues and is stored in the liver and adipose tissues. The clinical test for vitamin D deficiency is a measurement of the serum level of 25-(OH)D.

The final metabolic processing step in the synthesis of the circulating active hormone, 1,25-(OH)$_2$D, takes place principally in the kidney, although many tissues can locally activate vitamin D for paracrine and autocrine functions. The conversion of 25-(OH)D to 1,25-(OH)$_2$D by the 25-(OH)D 1-hydroxylase in the renal cortex is tightly regulated. The synthesis of 1,25-(OH)$_2$D is increased by PTH, thus linking the formation of 1,25-(OH)$_2$D closely to PTH in the integrated control of calcium homeostasis. The production of 1,25-(OH)$_2$D is also stimulated by hypophosphatemia and hypocalcemia. On the other hand, the production of 1,25-(OH)$_2$D is reduced by increased serum calcium, phosphate and fibroblast growth factor (FGF)-23 and by decreased serum PTH. As an additional control, 1,25-(OH)$_2$D induces the enzyme 24-hydroxylase, which catabolizes 25-(OH)D and 1,25-(OH)$_2$D, thus reducing their levels. The coordinated control by PTH, blood mineral levels, and vitamin D supply is very efficient. Serum levels of 1,25-(OH)$_2$D vary only slightly over an enormous range of vitamin D production rates but respond precisely to changes in the serum levels of calcium and phosphate within the normal range.

Vitamin D Action

The vitamin D receptor is a member of the steroid receptor superfamily of DNA-binding nuclear receptors. Upon ligand binding, the receptor attaches to enhancer sites in target genes and directly regulates their transcription. Thus, many of the effects of vitamin D involve new RNA and protein synthesis. Although many vitamin D metabolites are recognized by the receptor, 1,25-(OH)$_2$D has an affinity approximately 1000-fold greater than that of 25-(OH)D. 25-(OH)D is present in the circulation at nanogram quantities, whereas 1,25-(OH)$_2$D circulates in picogram quantities; thus, other vitamin D metabolites besides 1,25-(OH)$_2$D may interact with the vitamin D receptor to produce clinical effects.

The primary target organs for 1,25-(OH)$_2$D are intestine and bone. The most essential action of 1,25-(OH)$_2$D is to stimulate the active intestinal transport of calcium in the duodenum. Calcium also can be absorbed passively through a paracellular route throughout the small intestine. However, particularly at low calcium intakes, the majority of gastrointestinal calcium absorption is mediated by the active vitamin D–mediated process. 1,25-(OH)$_2$D also induces the active transport of phosphate, but passive absorption dominates this process, and the net effect of 1,25-(OH)$_2$D is small.

In bone, 1,25-(OH)$_2$D regulates a number of osteoblastic functions. Vitamin D deficiency leads to rickets, a defect in mineralization. However, the defect in mineralization results mainly from a decrease in the delivery of calcium and phosphate to sites of mineralization. 1,25-(OH)$_2$D also stimulates osteoclasts to resorb bone, releasing calcium to maintain the extracellular calcium concentration. This resorption likely results from activation of the RANK-L/RANK signaling pathway by 1,25-(OH)$_2$D.

To demonstrate the interplay among calcium, phosphorus, PTH, and vitamin D, consider a person who switches from a high normal to a low intake of calcium and phosphate: from 1200 to 300 mg/d of calcium (the equivalent of leaving three glasses of milk out of the diet). The net absorption of calcium falls sharply, causing a transient decrease in the serum calcium level. This activates a homeostatic response led by an increase in PTH. The increased PTH level stimulates the release of calcium from bone and the retention of calcium by the kidney. In addition, the increase in PTH, the fall in calcium, and the concomitant fall in the serum phosphate level (because of both decreased intake and PTH-induced phosphaturia) activate renal 1,25-(OH)$_2$D synthesis. 1,25-(OH)$_2$D increases the fraction of calcium absorbed from the intestine, further increases calcium release from bone, and restores the serum calcium to normal. 1,25-(OH)$_2$D also promotes the intestinal absorption of phosphorus, although phosphorus absorption is much less regulated than calcium absorption. While these mechanisms can compensate for a low dietary calcium intake and maintain normal serum calcium and phosphorus levels, this is at the expense of mobilizing stored calcium from bone and maintaining an elevated PTH level. Over the long term, these compensatory mechanisms will result in depletion of skeletal calcium, increased bone resorption, and compromised skeletal integrity.

FIBROBLAST GROWTH FACTOR–23 (FGF-23)

FGF-23 Biochemistry

FGF-23 is a member of the large family of FGFs, typically local factors important in the control of cell proliferation and differentiation. FGF-23, in contrast to other FGF family members, plays a central role in regulating systemic phosphate homeostasis, vitamin D metabolism, and bone mineralization. Studies of kindreds with rare genetic disorders, as well as transgenic and knockout mouse models that target essential molecules in FGF-23 signaling cascades, have demonstrated

FIGURE 17–13 Phosphate homeostasis is maintained by the coordinated actions of FGF-23 and 1,25(OH)$_2$D. Low serum phosphate (PO$_4^{3-}$) levels suppress FGF-23 production, which increases 1,25(OH)$_2$D production and the expression of renal and intestinal phosphate transporters (NaPi 2a, 2c). As a result, intestinal and renal phosphate reabsorption rises to restore serum phosphate back to normal. When serum phosphate levels increase, FGF-23 levels rise, thereby suppressing these same biochemical pathways and restoring the serum phosphate balance.

the importance of FGF-23 in phosphate metabolism and skeletal mineralization.

Physiology of FGF-23

FGF-23 is produced by many tissues in the body, but its primary source is bone and, in particular, osteocytes. A critical regulator of FGF-23 production is the serum phosphate level (Figure 17–13). Under normal physiologic conditions, when phosphate levels rise (eg, high-phosphate diet, renal failure), FGF-23 levels increase. When serum phosphate levels fall (eg, phosphate depletion, low-phosphate diet), serum FGF-23 levels decrease. In states of phosphate excess, FGF-23 reduces the expression of the sodium phosphate co-transporters (NaPi 2a and 2c) in the kidney and intestine. This leads to the rapid excretion of phosphate by the kidney and reduced intestinal phosphate absorption, which in turn restore the serum phosphate level to normal. To further control the amount of phosphate being delivered to the circulation, FGF-23 also inhibits the renal production of 1,25-(OH)$_2$D (see Figure 17–13), further decreasing intestinal phosphorus absorption. These direct actions of FGF-23 are mediated by FGF receptors and their co-receptor transmembrane protein klotho. This co-receptor complex becomes a high-affinity receptor for FGF-23 in its target tissues.

Role of FGF-23 in Disease

The study of several rare disorders has defined the key actions of FGF-23 in phosphate and vitamin D metabolism. Disorders of FGF-23 excess include **X-linked hypophosphatemic rickets**, **autosomal dominant hypophosphatemic rickets**, and **tumor-induced osteomalacia** (Table 17–12; see also the **Osteomalacia** section, below). Hypophosphatemia and osteomalacia, resulting from phosphate wasting with a low or inappropriately normal serum 1,25-(OH)$_2$D level, are the hallmarks of these disorders. In contrast, the loss of FGF-23 function, owing to rare genetic disorders, is associated with syndromes of ectopic calcification, abnormal mineralization, and hyperphosphatemia. FGF-23 levels rise progressively as chronic kidney disease (CKD) worsens. Temporally, it appears that FGF-23 levels rise earlier in CKD than do PTH levels and that FGF-23 may be important in the suppression of 1,25-(OH)$_2$D in CKD.

CHECKPOINT

9. How is vitamin D produced from 7-dehydrocholesterol?
10. Where is vitamin D stored?
11. Where does the final step in the activation of vitamin D take place, and how is it regulated?
12. What are the actions of vitamin D?

PARAFOLLICULAR CELLS (C CELLS)

Anatomy & Histology

The C cells of the thyroid gland secrete the peptide hormone calcitonin. They constitute 0.1% or less of thyroid cell mass

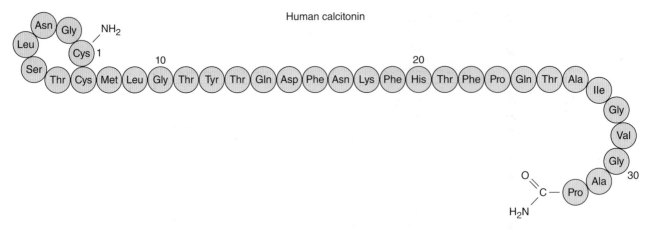

FIGURE 17–14 The amino acid sequence of human calcitonin, demonstrating its biochemical features, including an amino terminal disulfide bridge and carboxyl terminal prolineamide.

and are distributed in the central parts of the lateral lobes of the thyroid, especially between the upper and middle thirds of the lobes. C cells are neuroendocrine cells derived from the ultimobranchial body, a structure that fuses with the thyroid.

C cells are small, spindle-shaped or polygonal cells distributed throughout the thyroid. They contain abundant granules, mitochondria, and Golgi. They may be present as single cells or arranged in nests, cords, and sheets within the thyroid parenchyma. They are often found within thyroid follicles, are larger than follicular cells, and stain positively for calcitonin.

Physiology

Calcitonin is a 32-amino-acid peptide hormone with a seven-member amino terminal disulfide ring and carboxyl terminal prolineamide (Figure 17–14). Differential processing of the calcitonin gene can lead to the production of either calcitonin in C cells or calcitonin gene-related peptide in neurons. Although both calcitonin and calcitonin gene-related peptide have demonstrated clinical effects in pharmacologic doses, the function of the peptides at normal physiologic levels is unknown. C-cell tumors may release both peptides.

Hypercalcemia stimulates the release of calcitonin through the activation of CaSRs in C cells. Substantial changes in serum calcium are normally required to modulate the release of calcitonin. It is not known whether small physiologic changes in serum calcium, which rapidly modulate PTH secretion, elicit significant changes in calcitonin levels. The GI hormones cholecystokinin and gastrin are also secretagogues for calcitonin. Calcitonin secretion in vivo is assessed by measuring serum levels with a two-site radioimmunoassay.

Actions of Calcitonin

Calcitonin interacts with receptors in kidney and bone. This interaction stimulates adenylyl cyclase activity and the generation of cAMP (as shown in Figure 17–5 for PTH). In the kidney, receptors for calcitonin are localized in the cortical ascending limb of the Henle loop, whereas in bone, calcitonin receptors are found on osteoclasts.

The main function of calcitonin is to lower serum calcium, and this hormone is rapidly released in response to hypercalcemia. Calcitonin inhibits osteoclastic bone resorption and rapidly blocks the release of calcium and phosphate from bone. The latter effect is apparent within minutes after the administration of calcitonin. These effects ultimately lead to a fall in serum calcium and phosphate.

Calcitonin acts directly on osteoclasts and blocks the resorption of bone induced by hormones like PTH and vitamin D. The potency of calcitonin depends on the underlying rate of bone resorption. Calcitonin also has a modest effect on the kidney to produce mild phosphaturia. With continued administration of calcitonin, an "escape" from its effects on serum calcium occurs.

The overall importance of calcitonin in the maintenance of calcium homeostasis is unclear. Serum calcium concentrations are normal in patients after thyroidectomy, which removes all functioning C cells. Similarly, calcitonin typically rises to very high levels in patients with medullary carcinoma of the thyroid with no apparent effect on serum calcium levels.

CHECKPOINT

13. What are the actions of calcitonin?
14. What is the effect of thyroidectomy on serum calcium?

PATHOPHYSIOLOGY OF SELECTED DISORDERS OF CALCIUM METABOLISM

PRIMARY & SECONDARY HYPERPARATHYROIDISM

Etiology

Primary hyperparathyroidism is due to the excessive production and release of PTH by the parathyroid glands. The prevalence of hyperparathyroidism is approximately 1:1000 in the United States, and the incidence of the disease increases with age. The patient group most frequently affected is postmenopausal women.

Primary hyperparathyroidism may be caused by any of the following: adenoma, hyperplasia, or carcinoma (Table 17–1). **Chief cell adenomas** are the most common cause, accounting for almost 85% of all cases. The vast majority of parathyroid adenomas occur sporadically and are solitary.

Parathyroid hyperplasia refers to an enlargement or abnormality of all four glands. In atypical forms of hyperplasia, only one gland may be enlarged, but the other three glands typically show at least slight microscopic abnormalities, such as increased cellularity and reduced fat content. Distinguishing between hyperplasia and multiple adenomas is challenging and usually requires the examination of all four glands. Key characteristics for judging whether a gland is normal or not are its size, weight, and histologic features.

Parathyroid hyperplasia may be part of the autosomal dominant **multiple endocrine neoplasia (MEN)** syndromes (Table 17–2). In patients with MEN-1, caused by mutations in the *MEN1* gene, which encodes the protein **menin**, there is a high penetrance of hyperparathyroidism, affecting as many as 95% of patients. When their glands are examined microscopically, there are usually abnormalities in all four glands. Recurrent hyperparathyroidism, even after initially successful surgery, is common in these patients. Hyperparathyroidism also occurs in MEN-2A, although at a much lower frequency (about 20%). Familial hyperparathyroidism, without other features of MEN syndromes, characteristically involves all four glands, but there is often asynchrony in the presentation of the hyperparathyroidism. Kindreds with isolated hyperparathyroidism and mutations in *menin* are considered to be allelic variants of MEN-1. The hyperparathyroidism–jaw tumor syndrome and familial isolated hyperparathyroidism are other causes of autosomal dominant hyperparathyroidism. The former often includes ossifying fibromas of the jaw and renal tumors and is caused by inactivating germline mutations in the *HRPT2* gene that encodes the protein **parafibromin**.

Parathyroid carcinoma is a rare malignancy, but the diagnosis should be considered in a patient with severe hypercalcemia and a palpable cervical mass. At surgery, cancers are firmer than adenomas and more likely to be attached to adjacent structures. It is sometimes difficult to distinguish parathyroid carcinomas from adenomas on histopathologic grounds. Vascular or capsular invasion by tumor cells is a

TABLE 17–2   Clinical features of multiple endocrine neoplasia (MEN) syndromes.

MEN-1
Benign parathyroid tumors (very common)
Pancreatic tumors (benign or malignant)
Gastrinoma
Insulinoma
Glucagonoma, VIPoma (both rare)
Pituitary tumors
Growth hormone–secreting
Prolactin-secreting
ACTH-secreting
Other tumors: lipomas, carcinoids, adrenal and thyroid adenomas

MEN-2A
Medullary carcinoma of the thyroid
Pheochromocytoma (benign or malignant)
Hyperparathyroidism (uncommon)

MEN-2B
Medullary carcinoma of the thyroid
Pheochromocytoma
Mucosal neuromas, ganglioneuromas
Marfanoid habitus

ACTH, adrenocorticotropic hormone; VIP, vasoactive intestinal polypeptide.

TABLE 17–1   Causes of primary hyperparathyroidism.

Solitary adenomas	80–85%
Hyperplasia	10%
Multiple adenomas	≈2%
Carcinoma	≈2–5%

good indicator of malignancy, but these features are not always present. In many cases, local recurrences or distant metastases to liver, lung, or bone are the clinical findings that support this diagnosis. Approximately 20% of patients with hyperparathyroidism–jaw tumor syndrome and germline mutations in the *HRPT2* gene (described above) develop parathyroid cancer. Furthermore, mutations in *HRPT2* have also been found in familial isolated hyperparathyroidism and in sporadic parathyroid cancers. The normal cellular function of parafibromin is unknown.

Secondary hyperparathyroidism implies diffuse glandular hyperplasia resulting from a defect outside the parathyroids. Secondary hyperparathyroidism in patients with normal kidney function may be observed in patients with severe calcium and vitamin D deficiency states (see below). In patients with CKD, many causative factors contribute to the often dramatic enlargement of the parathyroid glands. These include decreased 1,25-$(OH)_2$D production, reduced intestinal calcium absorption, skeletal resistance to PTH, renal phosphate retention, and chronically high FGF-23 levels.

Pathogenesis

PTH secretion in primary hyperparathyroidism is excessive, given the level of serum calcium. At the cellular level, there is both increased cell mass and a secretory defect. The latter is characterized by reduced sensitivity of PTH secretion to suppression by the elevated serum calcium concentration. This qualitative regulatory defect is more common than truly autonomous secretion. Thus, the parathyroid glands of patients with primary hyperparathyroidism are typically enlarged and, in vitro, demonstrate a "shift to the right" in their calcium set-point for secretion (Figure 17–15). How these two defects interact in the pathogenesis of the disease remains to be fully elucidated.

The genetic defects responsible for primary hyperparathyroidism have received considerable attention. Genes that regulate the cell cycle are thought to be important in the pathogenesis of a significant subset of parathyroid tumors. The *PRAD1* gene (parathyroid rearrangement adenoma), whose product is a D1 cyclin, has been implicated in parathyroid tumor development and also in the pathogenesis of several malignant tumors (B-cell lymphomas, breast and lung cancers, and squamous cell cancers of the head and neck). Cyclins are cell cycle regulatory proteins. The *PRAD1* gene is located on the long arm of chromosome 11, as is the gene encoding PTH. Analysis of parathyroid tumor DNA suggests that a chromosome inversion event occurs, which leads to the juxtaposition of the 5′-regulatory domain of the *PTH* gene upstream of the *PRAD1* gene (Figure 17–16). Because regulatory sequences in the *PTH* gene are responsible for its cell-specific transcription, this inversion was initially postulated to lead to a parathyroid cell-specific overproduction of the *PRAD1* gene product. Excessive cyclin D1 would enhance the proliferative potential of the cells bearing this inversion and, given sufficient time, could induce PTH excess. A transgenic

FIGURE 17–15 PTH secretion in vitro from human parathyroid cells from patients with parathyroid adenomas and hyperplasia. The set point for secretion is the calcium concentration at which PTH release is suppressed by 50%. This is shifted to the right in the majority of parathyroid adenomas compared to normal tissues, in which the set point is approximately 1.0 mmol/L ionized calcium. (Redrawn, with permission, from Brown EM et al. Dispersed cells prepared from human parathyroid glands: distinct calcium sensitivity of adenomas vs primary hyperplasia. J Clin Endocrinol Metab. 1978;46:267. By permission of Oxford University Press on behalf of the Endocrine Society.)

mouse model in which cyclin D1 is overexpressed in parathyroid tissue under the control of the *PTH* gene promoter provides proof for this pathogenetic mechanism of primary hyperparathyroidism.

The gene responsible for MEN-1, which produces the protein product menin, was identified in 1997. It is thought to function as a tumor suppressor gene. In keeping with the "two-hit" hypothesis of oncogenesis, patients with MEN-1 inherit an abnormal or inactivated *MEN1* allele from one parent. This germline defect is present in all cells. During postnatal life, the other *MEN1* allele in a parathyroid cell, for example, undergoes spontaneous mutation or deletion. If this second mutation confers a growth advantage on the descendant cells, there is clonal outgrowth of cells bearing the second mutation, and eventually a tumor results. In approximately 25% of nonfamilial benign parathyroid adenomas, there is allelic loss of DNA from chromosome 11, where the *MEN1* gene is located.

Menin localizes to the nucleus, where it binds to the transcription factor JunD in vitro and suppresses transcription. The role of menin in normal physiology and the mechanisms by which it promotes tumor formation in the pituitary, pancreas, and parathyroid glands are unknown. Mice with targeted deletion of both genes encoding the murine menin homologues (or *Men1*) die in utero. Mice that are heterozygous for *Men1* deletion survive but develop tumors in their pancreatic islets and adrenal cortices and in their parathyroid, thyroid, and pituitary glands as they age, serving as a model for MEN-1 syndrome.

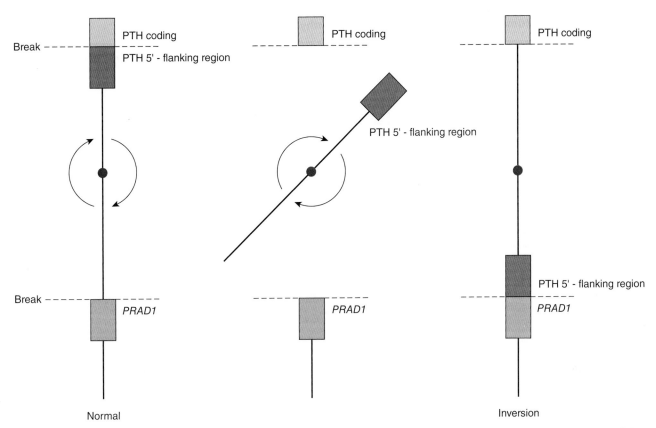

FIGURE 17–16 Proposed genetic rearrangement of chromosome 11 in a subset of sporadic parathyroid adenomas. An inversion of the DNA sequence near the centromere of chromosome 11 places the 5′-regulatory region of the *PTH* gene (also on chromosome 11) adjacent to the *PRAD1* gene, whose product is involved in cell cycle control. This places the *PRAD1* gene under the control of *PTH* regulatory sequences, which would be predicted to be highly active in parathyroid cells. (Redrawn, with permission, from Arnold A. Molecular genetics of parathyroid gland neoplasia. J Clin Endocrinol Metab. 1993;77:1109. By permission of Oxford University Press on behalf of the Endocrine Society.)

Genetic testing is available to detect mutations in the *MEN1* gene so that appropriate case management and genetic counseling can be done.

Hyperparathyroidism in MEN-2A is caused by mutations in *RET*. The RET protein, a receptor tyrosine kinase, plays an important role in the pathogenesis of the other endocrine tumors in these syndromes, as well as in familial medullary carcinoma of the thyroid (see below). How mutant RET protein alters parathyroid cell growth or PTH secretion has not been elucidated.

Clinical Manifestations

Hyperparathyroidism may present in a variety of ways. Patients with this disease may be asymptomatic, their diagnosis being made by screening laboratory tests. Other patients may have skeletal complications or nephrolithiasis. Because calcium affects the functioning of nearly every organ system, the symptoms and signs of hypercalcemia are protean (Table 17–3). Depending on the nature of the complaints, the patient with primary hyperparathyroidism may be suspected of having a psychiatric disorder, a malignancy, or, less

commonly, a granulomatous disease such as tuberculosis or sarcoidosis.

Primary hyperparathyroidism is a chronic disorder in which longstanding PTH excess and hypercalcemia may produce increasing symptomatology, especially symptoms from renal stones or low bone mass. Recurrent stones containing calcium phosphate or calcium oxalate occur in 10–15% of patients with primary hyperparathyroidism. Nephrolithiasis may be complicated by urinary outflow tract obstruction, infection, and progressive renal insufficiency. Patients with significant PTH excess may experience increased bone turnover and progressive loss of bone mass, especially in postmenopausal women. This is reflected in subperiosteal resorption, osteoporosis (particularly of cortical bone), and even pathologic fractures.

A sizable proportion of patients with primary hyperparathyroidism (50–80%), however, are asymptomatic. These patients may experience no clinical deterioration if their hyperparathyroidism is monitored rather than treated surgically. Because it is difficult to identify these patients with certainty when the diagnosis of hyperparathyroidism is made, regular follow-up is mandatory. Recent studies indicate that

TABLE 17–3   Symptoms and signs of primary hyperparathyroidism.

Systemic	Ocular	Skeletal and rheumatologic
Weakness	Band keratopathy	Osteopenia
Easy fatigue	**Cardiac**	Pathologic fractures[1]
Weight loss[1]	Shortened QT interval	Brown tumors of bone[1]
Anemia[1]	Hypertension	Bone pain[1]
Anorexia	**Renal**	Gout
Pruritus[1]	Stones	Pseudogout
Ectopic calcifications	Polyuria, polydipsia	Chondrocalcinosis
Neuropsychiatric and neuromuscular	Metabolic acidosis	Osteitis fibrosa cystica[1]
Depression	Concentrating defects	**Gastrointestinal**
Poor concentration	Nephrocalcinosis	Peptic ulcer disease
Memory deficits		Pancreatitis
Peripheral sensory neuropathy		Constipation
Motor neuropathy		Nausea
Proximal and generalized muscle weakness		Vomiting

[1]If moderate or severe hyperparathyroidism is present.

bone mass may deteriorate significantly, especially at cortical sites (ie, hip, forearm) after conservative follow-up beyond 8–10 years. These observations have reopened the issue of the advisability of long-term medical observation in this condition. By comparison, patients with mild disease who undergo definitive parathyroid surgery will experience improvements in bone mass over time. These data raise the question of how a mild primary hyperparathyroidism presumed to be innocuous may be deleterious to the skeleton.

The radiologic features of primary hyperparathyroidism are caused by the chronic effects of excess PTH on bone. These include subperiosteal resorption (evident most strikingly in the clavicles and distal phalanges), generalized low bone mass, and the classic, but now rare, brown tumors. Uncommonly, osteosclerosis may result from excessive PTH action on bone. Abdominal films or computed tomography may show nephrocalcinosis or nephrolithiasis.

The complete differential diagnosis of hypercalcemia should be considered in all patients with this abnormality (Table 17–4). Primary hyperparathyroidism accounts for most cases of hypercalcemia in the outpatient setting (>90%). The diagnosis of primary hyperparathyroidism is confirmed by at least two simultaneous measurements of calcium and intact PTH. An elevated or inappropriately normal PTH in the setting of hypercalcemia is the key feature in making the diagnosis of primary hyperparathyroidism—the most common cause of PTH-dependent hypercalcemia (Table 17–5).

Patients with secondary hyperparathyroidism may have normal or subnormal calcium levels (see below). If renal function is normal, serum phosphate is also often reduced, owing to the phosphaturic effects of the high PTH levels. Although serum PTH is elevated, the demineralized state of the bone and the chronic vitamin D deficiency combine to produce a low filtered load of calcium. Hence, urinary calcium excretion is often quite low. The 25-(OH)D level is also low or undetectable in vitamin D deficiency resulting from a variety of causes.

FAMILIAL HYPOCALCIURIC HYPERCALCEMIA

Etiology

In patients with asymptomatic hypercalcemia, the diagnosis of **familial hypocalciuric hypercalcemia** types 1 to 3 should be considered. Individuals with familial hypocalciuric hypercalcemia typically have elevated serum calcium and magnesium, normal or mildly elevated PTH levels, and hypocalciuria (see Table 17–5). Familial hypocalcuric hypercalcemia type 1 and 2 are due to mutations in genes encoding proteins involved in extracellular calcium sensing. Familial hypocalciuric hypercalcemia type 1 is due to point mutations in the *CASR*, whereas familial hypocalciuric hypercalcemia type 2 is caused by mutations in the G-protein alpha subunit *GNAS11*. G alpha 11 couples the CaSR to downstream phospholipase C signaling. Familial hypocalciuric hypercalcemia type 3 is due to mutations in a subunit of an adapter protein, AP2S1. All three disorders are inherited in an autosomal dominant

TABLE 17–4 Differential diagnosis of hypercalcemia.

Primary hyperparathyroidism
Adenoma
Carcinoma
Hyperplasia
Familial hypocalciuric hypercalcemia
Inherited: *CASR*, *GNA11*, and *AP2S1* mutations
Acquired: autoantibodies blocking CaSR sensing of calcium or signal transduction
Malignancy-associated hypercalcemia
Solid tumors (majority with excess PTHrP production)
Local osteolytic metastases
Plasma cell myeloma
Adult T-cell leukemia and lymphoma
Other lymphomas
Thyrotoxicosis
Drugs
Thiazides
Lithium
Vitamin D or A intoxication
Elevated $1,25(OH)_2D$
Granulomatous diseases
Sarcoidosis
Tuberculosis
Histoplasmosis (and other fungal diseases)
Mutations in *CYP2A41* reducing catabolism of $1,25(OH)_2D$
Milk–alkali syndrome

AP2S1, adapter protein 2 subunit 1; CaSR, calcium-sensing receptor; *GNA11*, alpha subunit of G 11; PTHrP, parathyroid hormone–related peptide.

fashion. In families with familial hypocalciuric hypercalcemia type 1, which is typically heterozygous and benign, there are rare occurrences of **neonatal severe primary hyperparathyroidism**. Infants with this form of hyperparathyroidism, usually the result of consanguinity, generally have inherited two copies of mutant CaSR genes.

Pathogenesis

The CaSR is a member of the G protein–coupled receptor superfamily and is highly expressed in the parathyroid gland and kidney. In the parathyroid, the molecule functions to detect changes in the ambient serum calcium concentration and then adjust the rate of PTH secretion accordingly. In the kidney, the CaSR sets the level of urinary calcium excretion, based on its perception of the serum calcium concentration.

In familial hypocalciuric hypercalcemia and neonatal severe hyperparathyroidism, the ability to detect serum calcium is faulty in both the kidney and parathyroid. Familial hypocalciuric hypercalcemia is due to a partial reduction—and neonatal hyperparathyroidism to a marked reduction—in the ability to sense extracellular calcium. Parathyroid chief cells missense the serum calcium as "low," and PTH secretion occurs when it should be suppressed (see Figure 17–2). This produces inappropriately normal or slightly high PTH levels. In the kidney, serum calcium concentrations are also detected (inappropriately) as low, and calcium is retained. This produces the hypocalciuria typical of this condition. Depending on the mutant gene dosage, the clinical symptoms tend to be mild in familial hypocalciuric hypercalcemia and profound and life-threatening in neonatal severe hyperparathyroidism.

Clinical Manifestations

Patients with familial hypocalciuric hypercalcemia typically have lifelong asymptomatic elevations in serum calcium. However, they generally do not suffer the consequences of end-organ dysfunction characteristic of long-standing hyperparathyroidism and hypercalcemia. They do not have nephrolithiasis, low bone mass, or renal dysfunction, which can occur in patients with primary hyperparathyroidism. Individuals with familial hypocalciuric hypercalcemia do not benefit from parathyroidectomy. Surgery is not recommended because the condition is generally benign and the hypercalcemia does not remit even with total parathyroidectomy.

In contrast, infants with neonatal severe hyperparathyroidism have marked hypercalcemia, dramatic elevations in serum PTH, bone demineralization at birth, hypotonia, and failure to thrive. These infants usually require total parathyroidectomy in the newborn period to survive.

In the asymptomatic hypercalcemic patient, a careful family history should be obtained in an effort to document hypercalcemia or the occurrence of failed parathyroidectomies in other family members. Simultaneous serum and urinary calcium and creatinine levels should be measured to rule out familial hypocalciuric hypercalcemia. In this condition, urinary calcium levels are typically low and almost always less than 100 mg/24 h (see Table 17–5). The calcium–creatinine clearance ratio derived from 24-hour urine collections is often below 0.01 but can be as high as 0.02. The ratio is calculated as urine calcium (mg/dL) × serum creatinine (mg/dL)/serum calcium (mg/dL) × urine creatinine (mg/dL). Genetic testing for *CASR* mutations is commercially available in several reference laboratories and is the best approach to achieving a definitive diagnosis of familial hypocalciuric hypercalcemia type 1.

TABLE 17–5 **Laboratory findings in hypercalcemia from various causes.**

	Serum Ca^{2+}	Serum PO_4^{3-}	Intact PTH	PTHrP	Serum 1,25-$(OH)_2D$	Urine Ca^{2+}
Primary hyperparathyroidism	↑	↓, N	↑, N	N, Und	N, ↑	N, ↑[1]
Malignancy-associated hypercalcemia	↑	↓, N	Und	↑[2]	N, ↓	↑
Familial hypocalciuric hypercalcemia	↑	N	N, ↑[3]	Und	N	↓
Vitamin D–dependent hypercalcemia	↑	N, ↑	↓	Und	N, ↑[4]	↑

N, normal; Und, undetectable; PTH, parathyroid hormone; PTHrP, PTH-related peptide.

[1]Can also be low depending on dietary calcium and the filtered load of calcium.

[2]In the 70–80% of patients with cancer and a humoral basis for hypercalcemia.

[3]Mild increases in PTH have been reported in up to 25% of patients.

[4]1,25-$(OH)_2D$ may not be frankly elevated in patients with vitamin D_2 or D_3 intoxication.

HYPERCALCEMIA OF MALIGNANCY

Etiology

Hypercalcemia occurs in approximately 10% of all malignancies. It is commonly seen in solid tumors, particularly squamous cell carcinomas (eg, lung, esophagus), renal carcinoma, and breast carcinoma. Hypercalcemia occurs in more than one-third of patients with plasma cell myeloma but is unusual in lymphomas and leukemias.

Pathogenesis

Solid tumors usually produce hypercalcemia by secreting PTHrP, whose properties have been described previously. This is humoral hypercalcemia, which mimics primary hyperparathyroidism and results from a diffuse increase in bone resorption induced by high circulating levels of PTHrP. The syndrome is exacerbated by the ability of PTHrP to reduce the renal excretion of calcium and the ability of hypercalcemia (acting via renal CaSRs) to blunt renal concentrating ability, which results in progressive dehydration.

Plasma cell myeloma can present with hypercalcemia that in many cases is mediated by a different mechanism; myeloma cells induce local bone resorption or osteolysis in the bone marrow by releasing proresorptive cytokines with bone-resorbing activity, such as interleukin-1 and tumor necrosis factor. Along with the hypercalcemia of progressive renal insufficiency that occurs frequently in the disease, myeloma cells can also produce PTHrP, indicating that multiple mechanisms can contribute to the hypercalcemia in plasma cell myeloma. Rarely, lymphomas produce hypercalcemia by secreting 1,25-$(OH)_2D$. Finally, patients with a variety of solid malignancies develop hypercalcemia because of bone metastases and the resultant bone resorption. This occurs in a minority of cases and is called local osteolytic hypercalcemia, owing to local metastases being central to the pathogenesis, rather than circulating PTHrP being responsible.

Clinical Manifestations

Unlike patients with primary hyperparathyroidism, who often are minimally symptomatic, patients with hypercalcemia of malignancy are typically very ill. Hypercalcemia typically occurs in advanced malignancy—the average survival of hypercalcemic patients is usually several weeks to months—and the tumor is almost invariably obvious on examination of the patient. In addition, hypercalcemia is often severe and symptomatic, with nausea, vomiting, dehydration, confusion, or coma. Biochemically, malignancy-associated hypercalcemia is characterized by a decreased serum phosphate level and a suppressed level of intact PTH (see Table 17–5). With most solid tumors, the serum level of PTHrP is increased. These findings, together with the differences in clinical presentation, usually make the differentiation of this syndrome from primary hyperparathyroidism easy.

HYPOPARATHYROIDISM & PSEUDOHYPOPARATHYROIDISM

Etiology

The total serum calcium includes the ionized, protein-bound, and complexed forms of calcium. It should be recognized, however, that symptoms of hypocalcemia occur only if the ionized fraction of calcium is reduced. Furthermore, only patients with low ionized calcium levels should be evaluated for the possibility of a hypocalcemic disorder.

A common cause of low total serum calcium is hypoalbuminemia. A low serum albumin lowers only the protein-bound, and not the ionized, calcium. Thus, such patients need not be evaluated for mineral disorders. To determine whether a hypoalbuminemic patient has low ionized calcium, this parameter can be measured directly. If this laboratory test is not readily available, a reasonable alternative is to correct the serum total calcium for the low serum albumin. This is done by adjusting the serum total calcium upward by 0.8 mg/dL for each 1 g/dL reduction in serum albumin. This simple correction usually brings the adjusted total serum calcium into the normal range.

The differential diagnosis of low ionized calcium is lengthy (Table 17–6). Hypocalcemia can result from reduced PTH secretion caused by **hypoparathyroidism** or hypomagnesemia. It can also be due to decreased end-organ responsiveness to PTH despite adequate or even excessive levels of the hormone; this is termed **pseudohypoparathyroidism**.

All forms of hypoparathyroidism are uncommon (Table 17–7). Most cases are the result of inadvertent trauma to, the removal of, or the devascularization of the parathyroid glands during thyroid or parathyroid surgery. The incidence of postoperative hypoparathyroidism (range: 0.2–30%) depends on the extent of the antecedent surgery and the surgeon's skill in identifying and leaving undisturbed normal parathyroid tissue and preserving its blood supply. Postoperative hypocalcemia may be transient (75%) or permanent (25%). Some patients may also be left with a diminished parathyroid reserve.

A variety of causes other than postsurgical complications may produce absolute or relative PTH deficiency (see Table 17–7). These include autoimmune destruction of the glands, magnesium depletion, and autosomal dominant or recessive or X-linked hypoparathyroidism. Hypoparathyroidism resulting from activating *CASR* mutations is called autosomal dominant hypocalcemia type 1, wherease activating *GNA11* mutations produce autosomal dominant hypocalcemia type 2. Stimulating autoantibodies directed against the CaSR can suppress PTH secretion (see below), and hypoparathyroidism can also result from iron overload or Wilson disease. Abnormal gland development resulting in varying degrees of severity of hypoparathyroidism is seen in **DiGeorge syndrome**. This syndrome can present in infancy, childhood, or even adulthood and may be accompanied by defective cell-mediated immunity and other congenital anomalies (see Table 17–7). Mutations in the gene for transcription factor

TABLE 17–6   Differential diagnosis of hypocalcemia.

Failure to secrete parathyroid hormone (PTH)
Hypoparathyroidism (see Table 17–7)
Resistance to PTH action
Pseudohypoparathyroidism (types 1a, 1b, 2)
Sepsis-associated hypocalcemia
Failure to secrete PTH and resistance to PTH action
Chronic magnesium depletion as a result of
Diarrhea, malabsorption
Alcoholism
Drugs: aminoglycoside antibiotics, loop diuretics, cisplatin, amphotericin B
Parenteral nutrition
Primary renal magnesium wasting
Reduction in 1,25-(OH)$_2$D production
Renal failure
Vitamin D deficiency
Nutritional deficiency
Pancreatic insufficiency
Liver disease
Cholestasis
Small intestinal disorders or surgery causing malabsorption
Renal failure
Vitamin D–dependent rickets type 1: defective 1α-hydroxylase activity (very rare)
Tumor-induced osteomalacia
Resistance to 1, 25-(OH)$_2$D action
Vitamin D–dependent rickets type 2: defect in vitamin D receptor (rare)
Acute challenges to the homeostatic mechanisms
Pancreatitis (formation of calcium salts in retroperitoneal fat)
Drug-induced (eg, EDTA, citrate, bisphosphonates, denosumab, phosphate, foscarnet)
Liver transplantation (citrate is not metabolized, resulting in the formation of calcium citrate complexes and a lowered ionized calcium)
Rhabdomyolysis
Hungry bone syndrome (increased deposition into demineralized bone)
Osteoblastic metastases (eg, breast and prostate cancer)
Tumor lysis syndrome (acute phosphate load released from tumor cells as a result of cytolytic therapy)

EDTA, ethylenediamine tetraacetic acid.

TABLE 17–7   Causes of hypoparathyroidism.

Complication of thyroid, parathyroid, or laryngeal surgery
Autoimmune destruction
Autoimmune polyendocrine failure syndrome type 1 (APS-1)
Secondary to magnesium depletion or hypermagnesemia
Post-^{131}I therapy for Graves disease or thyroid cancer
Secondary to the accumulation of iron (thalassemia, hemochromatosis) or copper (Wilson disease)
Genetic forms of hypoparathyroidism
DiGeorge or 22q deletion syndrome
Autosomal recessive or autosomal dominant mutations in *pre-proPTH*
X-linked hypoparathyroidism
Mutations in transcription factors involved in parathyroid development (eg, *GCMB*, *GATA3*)
Mitochondrial DNA mutations
Activating mutations of the *CASR* or *GNA11* genes causing autosomal dominant hypocalcemia type 1 and 2
Acquired autoimmune syndrome caused by autoantibodies activating the calcium-sensing receptor (CaSR)
Tumor invasion (very rare)

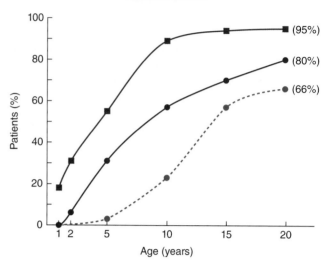

- ■ Mucocutaneous candidiasis
- ● Hypoparathyroidism
- ● Addison's disease

FIGURE 17–17 Cumulative incidence of three common manifestations of autoimmune polyglandular failure type 1 (APS-1) compared with age at onset in a cohort of 68 patients. The figures in parentheses reflect incidences at age 20. (Data plotted from Ahonen P et al. Clinical variation of autoimmune polyendocrinopathy-candidiasis-ectodermal dystrophy [APECED] in a series of 68 patients. N Engl J Med. 1990;322:1829.)

GCMB (glial cell missing-B), which is essential to the development of the parathyroid glands, are linked to familial isolated hypoparathyroidism. Mutations in the transcription factor *GATA3* cause abnormal otic vesicle, renal, and parathyroid gland development resulting in deafness, renal anomalies, and hypoparathyroidism.

There are two syndromes of **autoimmune polyendocrine failure syndrome (APS)**. Patients with APS-1 commonly have mucocutaneous candidiasis, Addison disease (adrenal insufficiency), and hypoparathyroidism and, less commonly, ovarian failure and thyroid dysfunction. Various components of APS-1 present by the teens or early 20s (Figure 17–17).

APS-1 is typically an autosomal recessive disorder resulting from mutations in the autoimmune regulator (*AIRE*) gene. *AIRE* is expressed normally in a subpopulation of epithelial cells in the thymus thought to be involved in the negative selection of autoreactive T cells during clonal selection. These T-cell clones are involved in self-recognition, and the failure to delete these T-cell clones is thought to underlie the autoimmune destruction of the endocrine cells affected in APS-1. Excellent clinical markers of APS-1 are autoantibodies to type 1 interferons (alpha and omega), which can be present even before disease manifestations are clinically evident.

APS-2, or **Schmidt syndrome**, is characterized by hypothyroidism and adrenal insufficiency and does not involve the parathyroid glands (see Chapter 21).

Pathogenesis

The pathogenesis of hypoparathyroidism is straightforward. The mineral disturbance occurs because the amount of PTH released is inadequate to maintain normal serum calcium concentrations, mainly due to the loss of the renal calcium-conserving effects of PTH and the inability to generate 1,25-$(OH)_2$D sustainably. Hypocalcemia results, and hyperphosphatemia is also observed because the proximal tubular effect of PTH to promote phosphate excretion is lost. Because PTH is required to stimulate the renal production of 1,25-$(OH)_2$D, levels of 1,25-$(OH)_2$D are low in patients with hypoparathyroidism. Hyperphosphatemia further suppresses 1,25-$(OH)_2$D synthesis. Low 1,25-$(OH)_2$D levels lead to reduced intestinal calcium absorption. In the absence of adequate 1,25-$(OH)_2$D and PTH, the mobilization of calcium from bone is abnormal. Because PTH is deficient, urinary calcium excretion is often high, despite the hypocalcemia.

Magnesium depletion is a common cause of hypocalcemia. The pathogenesis of hypocalcemia in this clinical setting relates to a functional and reversible state of hypoparathyroidism. There is also decreased renal and skeletal responsiveness to PTH. Magnesium depletion may occur from a variety of causes, including chronic alcoholism, diarrhea, and drugs such as loop diuretics, aminoglycoside antibiotics, amphotericin B, and cisplatin (see Table 17–6). Magnesium is required to maintain normal PTH secretory responses. Once body magnesium stores are replete, PTH levels rise appropriately in response to the hypocalcemia, and the mineral imbalance is corrected.

In **pseudohypoparathyroidism**, PTH levels are usually elevated, but the ability of target tissues (particularly kidney) to respond to the hormone is subnormal. In pseudohypoparathyroidism type 1, the ability of PTH to generate an increase in the second messenger cAMP is reduced. In patients with type 1a, this is due to a deficiency in the levels of the α subunit of the stimulatory G protein ($G_{s-\alpha}$), which couples the PTH receptor to the adenylyl cyclase enzyme. Type 1b is characterized by altered transcription of the $G_{s-\alpha}$ gene (*GNAS*) owing to abnormal DNA methylation at this locus. In patients with pseudohypoparathyroidism type 2, urinary cAMP is normal, but the phosphaturic response to infused PTH is reduced. The pathogenesis of this even rarer form of PTH resistance remains obscure.

Patients with activating mutations of *CASR* typically present with autosomal dominant hypocalcemia and hypercalciuria. Both defects are due to overly sensitive CaSRs, which turn off PTH secretion and renal calcium reabsorption at subnormal serum calcium levels. These individuals rarely experience symptoms of their often mild hypocalcemia, but if given vitamin D, they are prone to developing marked hypercalciuria, nephrocalcinosis, and even renal failure.

Clinical Manifestations

The symptoms and signs of hypocalcemia are similar, regardless of the underlying cause (Table 17–8). Patients may be asymptomatic or may have latent or overt tetany. **Tetany** is defined as spontaneous tonic muscular contractions. Painful carpal spasms and laryngeal stridor are striking manifestations of tetany. Latent tetany may be demonstrated by testing for the Chvostek and Trousseau signs. The **Chvostek sign** is elicited by tapping on the facial nerve anterior to the ear. Twitching of the ipsilateral facial muscles indicates a positive test. A positive **Trousseau sign** is demonstrated by inflating the sphygmomanometer with the cuff around the arm above the systolic blood pressure for 3 min. In hypocalcemic individuals, this causes painful carpal muscle contractions and spasms (Figure 17–18). If hypocalcemia is severe and unrecognized, airway compromise, altered mental status, generalized seizures, and even death may occur.

Chronic hypocalcemia is associated with intracranial calcifications, especially in the basal ganglia, that are detected by CT scanning, MRI, or skull radiographs. Chronic hypocalcemia is also associated with the premature formation of cataracts.

In addition to the symptoms and signs of hypocalcemia, patients with pseudohypoparathyroidism type 1a may have a constellation of features collectively known as **Albright hereditary osteodystrophy**. These include short stature, obesity, mental retardation, round facies, shortened fourth and fifth metacarpal and metatarsal bones, and subcutaneous ossifications. In considering the differential diagnosis of hypocalcemia, one must be guided by the clinical setting. A positive family history is very important in supporting a diagnosis of pseudohypoparathyroidism and other hereditary forms of hypoparathyroidism (see Table 17–7). The patient with hypocalcemia, hyperphosphatemia, and a normal serum creatinine

TABLE 17–8   Symptoms and signs of hypocalcemia.

Systemic	Confusion
	Weakness
	Behavioral changes
Neuromuscular	Paresthesias
	Psychosis
	Seizures
	Carpopedal spasms
	Chvostek and Trousseau signs
	Depression
	Muscle cramping
	Parkinsonism
	Irritability
	Basal ganglia calcifications
Cardiac	Prolonged QT interval on electrocardiogram
	ST-T wave changes on electrocardiogram
	Heart failure
Ocular	Cataracts
	Papilledema
Dental	Enamel hypoplasia of teeth
	Defective root formation
	Failure of adult teeth to erupt
Respiratory	Laryngospasm
	Bronchospasm
	Stridor

most likely has hypoparathyroidism. A history of neck surgery should be sought. There may be a long latent period before symptomatic hypocalcemia presents in postsurgical hypoparathyroidism. The physical examination can be helpful if it identifies signs of hypocalcemia, stigmata of Albright hereditary osteodystrophy, or other features of APS-1 (ie, vitiligo,

FIGURE 17–18 Position of fingers in carpal spasm resulting from hypocalcemic tetany. (Redrawn, with permission, from Ganong WF: *Review of Medical Physiology*, 16th ed. Appleton & Lange. Copyright © 1993 by The McGraw-Hill Companies, Inc.)

TABLE 17–9   Laboratory findings in hypocalcemia.

	Serum Ca^{2+}	Serum PO_4^{3-}	Intact PTH	25-$(OH)D_3$	Urinary cAMP Response to PTH Infusion
Hypoparathyroidism	↓	↑, N	↓, N[1]	N	N
Pseudohypoparathyroidism	↓	↑, N	↑	N	↓[2]
Magnesium depletion	↓	N	↓, N[1]	N	N
Vitamin D deficiency	↓	N, ↓	↑	↓	N

cAMP, cyclic adenosine monophosphate; N, normal; PTH, parathyroid hormone.

[1]May be normal but inappropriate to level of serum calcium.

[2]Urinary cAMP responses to PTH infusion are subnormal in pseudohypoparathyroidism type 1a and 1b.

mucocutaneous candidiasis, adrenal insufficiency). Patients with pseudohypoparathyroidism type 1a often have other endocrine abnormalities, such as primary hypothyroidism or gonadal failure.

In the differential diagnosis of hypocalcemia, laboratory findings are extremely useful (Table 17–9). Serum phosphate is often (but not invariably) elevated in hypoparathyroidism and pseudohypoparathyroidism. In magnesium depletion, serum phosphate is usually normal. In secondary hyperparathyroidism not due to renal failure, serum phosphate is typically low. Serum PTH levels are crucial in determining the cause of hypocalcemia. PTH is classically elevated in untreated pseudohypoparathyroidism but not in hypoparathyroidism or magnesium depletion. Intact PTH may be undetectable, low, or normal in patients with hypoparathyroidism depending on the parathyroid functional reserve. In patients with secondary hyperparathyroidism resulting from defects in the production or bioavailability of vitamin D, the clinical setting often suggests a problem with vitamin D (eg, regional enteritis, bowel resection, liver disease). The presence of low 25-(OH)D and increased PTH levels confirms this diagnosis.

Measuring serum magnesium is the first step in ruling out magnesium depletion as the cause of hypocalcemia and should be part of the initial evaluation. If urinary magnesium is inappropriately high relative to the serum magnesium, renal magnesium wasting by definition is present. PTH levels in this setting are typically low or normal. Normal PTH levels, however, are inappropriate in the presence of hypocalcemia.

Patients with autoimmune hypoparathyroidism due to *AIRE* mutations can be suspected clinically when the patient has at least two of the three features of the syndrome. Recent work indicates that autoantibodies to interferon-α or interferon-ω are present in more than 95% of patients with APS-1 and are an excellent screening test for the disorder along with *AIRE* gene sequencing.

The diagnosis of pseudohypoparathyroidism can be confirmed by infusing synthetic human PTH(1–34) and measuring urinary cAMP and phosphate responses. This maneuver is designed to prove end-organ resistance to PTH and to determine whether the diagnosis is pseudohypoparathyroidism type 1 or type 2.

Hypoparathyroidism may vary in its severity and, therefore, in the need for therapy. In some patients with decreased PTH reserve, only situations of increased stress on the glands, such as pregnancy or lactation, induce hypocalcemia. In other patients, PTH deficiency is a chronic symptomatic disorder necessitating lifelong therapy with calcium supplements and vitamin D analogues. All patients so treated should have periodic monitoring of serum calcium, urinary calcium, and renal function. Patients with autoimmune hypoparathyroidism should also be examined regularly for the development of adrenal insufficiency and malabsorption, chronic hepatitis, keratitis, pernicious anemia, alopecia, vitiligo, and other endocrine and nonendocrine complications of APS-1.

CHECKPOINT

22. What are the causes of hypoparathyroidism?
23. What are the mechanisms responsible for pseudohypoparathyroidism?
24. What are the symptoms and signs of hypocalcemia?
25. How can laboratory studies be used to distinguish the various causes of hypocalcemia?

MEDULLARY CARCINOMA OF THE THYROID

Etiology

Medullary carcinoma of the thyroid gland, a C-cell neoplasm, accounts for only 5–10% of all thyroid malignancies. Approximately 80% are sporadic and 20% are familial, occurring in autosomal dominant MEN-2A and MEN-2B and in non-MEN syndromes. In sporadic cases, the tumor is usually unilateral. In hereditary forms, however, tumors are often bilateral and multifocal. Germline activating mutations in the *RET* proto-oncogene on chromosome 10 are known to play a causal role in three forms of medullary carcinoma. These include cases of familial isolated medullary thyroid cancer, MEN-2A, and MEN-2B. More than half of sporadically occurring medullary thyroid carcinomas have a somatic mutation identical to that causing the familial syndromes; however, because the mutation is present only in the tumor and not in the genomic DNA, these cases are not heritable.

Pathogenesis

The growth pattern of medullary carcinoma is slow but progressive, and local invasion of adjacent structures is common. The tumor spreads hematogenously, with metastases typically to lymph nodes, bone, and lung. The clinical progression of this cancer is variable. Although there may be early metastases to cervical and mediastinal lymph nodes in as many as 70% of patients, the tumor still usually behaves in an indolent fashion. In a minority of cases, a more aggressive pattern of tumor growth has been noted. Early detection in high-risk individuals, such as those with a family history of medullary carcinoma or MEN-2A or MEN-2B, is crucial to prevent advanced disease and distant metastases. Overall survival is estimated to be 80% at 5 years and 60% at 10 years. Some studies suggest that individuals younger than 40 years at the time of diagnosis may have higher survival rates than older individuals. The *RET* proto-oncogene mutation on codon 918, seen in nearly 95% of MEN-2B cases, portends a worse prognosis.

Patients with MEN-2 develop medullary carcinoma at frequencies approaching 100%. In MEN-2A and MEN-B, the thyroid lesions are malignant. C-cell hyperplasia typically precedes the development of cancer, allowing for premalignancy detection and the consideration of prophylactic thyroidectomy. The pheochromocytomas associated with either MEN-2A or MEN-2B are infrequently malignant. Hyperparathyroidism in MEN-2A, which is uncommon, is usually due to diffuse hyperplasia rather than malignancy of the parathyroids. Chronic hypercalcitoninemia as a result of the tumor may contribute to the pathogenesis of parathyroid hyperplasia. Parathyroid hyperplasia is rarely seen in patients with either MEN-2B or sporadic medullary carcinoma.

Clinical Manifestations

Sporadic medullary carcinoma occurs with about equal frequency in males and females and typically occurs in patients older than 50 years. In MEN-2A or MEN-2B, the tumor occurs at a much younger age, often in childhood. In fact, medullary carcinoma in a patient younger than 40 years suggests familial medullary carcinoma or MEN-2A or MEN-2B. Medullary carcinoma may present as a single nodule or as multiple thyroid nodules. Patients with sporadic medullary carcinoma often have palpable cervical lymphadenopathy.

Because C cells are neuroendocrine cells, these tumors have the capacity to release calcitonin and other hormones such as prostaglandins, serotonin, adrenocorticotropin, somatostatin, and calcitonin gene-related peptide. Serotonin, calcitonin, or the prostaglandins have been implicated in the pathogenesis of the secretory diarrhea observed in approximately 25% of patients with medullary carcinoma. Diarrhea usually indicates

a large tumor burden or metastatic disease. Patients may also have flushing, which has been ascribed to the tumor producing substance P or calcitonin gene-related peptide, both of which are vasodilators.

In a patient suspected of having medullary carcinoma, the nodules are solid on ultrasonography. Fine-needle aspiration biopsy shows the characteristic C-cell lesion with positive immunostaining for calcitonin. Fine-needle aspiration may be nondiagnostic in more than half of individuals with medullary thyroid carcinoma. Staining for calcitonin may improve diagnostic sensitivity; however, the diagnosis of medullary thyroid carcinoma may not be evident until an examination of frozen-section specimen slides during surgery or, later, of final pathological slides from the resected thyroid. The tumor has the propensity to contain large calcifications, which can be seen on x-ray films of the neck. Bone metastases may be lytic or sclerotic in their appearance, and pulmonary metastases may be surrounded by fibrotic reactions.

The most important laboratory test in determining the presence and extent of medullary carcinoma is the serum calcitonin level. Circulating calcitonin levels are typically elevated in most patients, and serum levels correlate with tumor burden. In C-cell hyperplasia, basal calcitonin may or may not be elevated. However, these patients usually demonstrate abnormal provocative testing. Intravenous calcium gluconate (2 mg/kg of elemental calcium) is injected over 1 minute, followed by pentagastrin (0.5 μg/kg) over 5 seconds. Provocative testing is based on the ability of calcium and the synthetic gastrin analogue pentagastrin to hyperstimulate calcitonin release in patients with increased C-cell mass resulting from either hyperplasia or carcinoma. Provocative testing to detect C-cell hyperplasia (and hence serum calcitonin elevation) in relatives of patients with medullary thyroid carcinoma has largely been replaced by genetic testing for germline mutations known to cause MEN or familial medullary thyroid carcinoma syndromes.

Serial calcitonin levels are useful for monitoring therapeutic responses in patients with medullary carcinoma or for diagnosing a recurrence, along with clinical examination and imaging procedures. Calcitonin levels usually reflect the extent of disease. If the tumor becomes less differentiated, calcitonin levels may no longer reflect tumor burden. Another useful tumor marker for medullary carcinoma is the serum carcinoembryonic antigen (CEA). This antigen is frequently elevated in patients with medullary carcinoma and is present at all stages of the disease. Rapid increases in CEA predict a worse clinical course.

Surgery is the mainstay of therapy for patients with medullary thyroid carcinoma. Total thyroidectomy is advocated because the tumors are often multicentric. Patients should be monitored indefinitely for recurrences because these tumors may be very indolent. All patients with medullary carcinoma of the thyroid, whether familial or sporadic, should be tested for *RET* oncogene mutations. More than 95% of patients with MEN-2 have been found to harbor *RET* mutations. Sporadic cases of medullary carcinoma of the thyroid should also be tested to detect the occurrence of a new mutation for which other family members can then be screened. Properly performed DNA testing is essentially unambiguous in predicting gene carrier status and can be used prospectively to recommend prophylactic thyroidectomy in young patients and children with MEN-2 before the development of C-cell hyperplasia or frank carcinoma.

Patients with either MEN-2A or MEN-2B, even in the absence of symptoms, should undergo screening tests for the possibility of pheochromocytoma, whereas only patients with MEN-2A need to be screened for hyperparathyroidism before thyroid surgery. These tests include the determination of serum calcium and PTH together with plasma fractionated metanephrines and additional biochemical testing or imaging as needed. Pheochromocytomas may be clinically silent at the time medullary carcinoma is diagnosed, and they should be removed before thyroidectomy to prevent potentially serious surgical complications from uncontrolled catecholamine secretion. If hyperparathyroidism is present, it should be treated surgically at the time of thyroidectomy to avoid a second neck operation (see Chapter 12).

FIGURE 17–19 Bone mass in women as a function of age, demonstrating the potential effect of suboptimal nutrition and physical activity during the critical time of bone accrual in childhood and adolescence. (Redrawn, with permission, from Heaney RP et al. Peak bone mass. Osteo Int. 2000;11:985.)

CHECKPOINT

26. How can you make the diagnosis of medullary carcinoma of the thyroid?
27. What is the treatment for medullary carcinoma?
28. Which patients are at high risk for medullary carcinoma?

OSTEOPOROSIS

Etiology

Osteoporosis is defined as a state of low bone mass with microarchitectural deterioration of bone structure leading to compromised bone strength with an attendant propensity to fragility fracture. The bone is normal in composition but reduced in amount. Bone mass accrues rapidly throughout childhood and very rapidly in adolescence; half of adult bone mineral density is achieved during the teenage years (Figure 17–19). Peak bone mass is reached late in the third decade of life. Bone mass then remains relatively stable through the adult years, followed by a rapid loss of bone in women at the time of menopause. In the later stages of life, both men and women continue to lose bone, although at a slower rate than that seen at the time of menopause.

Achieving maximum peak bone mass depends on optimal nutrition, physical activity, general health, and hormonal exposure throughout childhood and adolescence. Inadequacies in nutrition, weight-bearing exercise, and gonadal steroid exposure all have a negative impact on the acquisition of peak bone mass. After bone growth is completed, bone mass is determined by the level of peak bone mass attained and the subsequent rate of loss. Genetics are very important in determining bone mass. Black individuals have greater peak bone mass than white individuals and those of Asian descent and are relatively protected from osteoporosis. It now appears that, within the Caucasian population, about half the variance in bone mass is genetically determined. However, a number of hormonal and environmental factors can reduce the genetically determined peak bone mass or hasten the loss of bone mineral and thus represent important risk factors for osteoporosis (see Figure 17–19).

The most important etiologic factor in osteoporosis is gonadal steroid deficiency. The estrogen deficiency that occurs after menopause accelerates the loss of bone mass; postmenopausal women consistently have lower bone mass than men and a higher incidence of osteoporotic fractures. With respect to bone remodeling in men, testosterone serves some of the same functions as estrogen in women, but estradiol generated from the peripheral aromatization of testosterone is the critical gonadal steroid mediating the development and preservation of male bone mass. Hypogonadal men experience accelerated bone loss. Men on androgen deprivation therapy for prostate cancer are at increased risk for bone loss and fracture. Other important risk factors for bone loss are the use of corticosteroids and the endogenous cortisol excess seen in Cushing syndrome. Glucocorticoid-induced osteoporosis is one of the most devastating complications of chronic therapy with these agents. Certain other medications, including excessive thyroid hormone, replacement, anticonvulsants, and chronic heparin therapy; immobilization; alcohol abuse; and smoking are also risk factors for osteoporosis. Diet is important as well. As discussed below, an adequate intake of calcium and vitamin D is necessary to optimally build peak bone mass and to minimize the rate of loss. Many additional disorders affecting the gastrointestinal, hematologic, and connective tissue systems can also contribute to the development of osteoporosis (Table 17–10).

Pathogenesis

Because bone remodeling involves the coupled resorption of bone by osteoclasts and the deposition of new bone by

TABLE 17–10   Secondary causes of osteoporosis.

Connective tissue diseases
Osteogenesis imperfecta
Homocystinuria
Ehlers–Danlos syndrome
Marfan syndrome
Drug-induced
Corticosteroids
Alcohol
Excessive thyroid hormone replacement
Chronic heparin
Anticonvulsants
Hematologic
Plasma cell myeloma
Systemic mastocytosis
Immobilization
Endocrine
Hypogonadism
Hypercortisolism
Hyperthyroidism
Hyperparathyroidism
Types 1 and 2 diabetes mellitus
Gastrointestinal disorders
Subtotal gastrectomy
Post–bariatric surgery
Malabsorption syndromes
Obstructive jaundice
Biliary cirrhosis
Rheumatologic disorders
Rheumatoid arthritis
Ankylosing spondylitis
Idiopathic (young adults)

osteoblasts, bone loss can result from increased bone resorption, decreased bone formation, or a combination of both processes. Younger individuals with low bone mass typically have experienced low bone formation and insufficient bone accrual, whereas postmenopausal osteoporosis is the consequence of accelerated bone resorption. The urinary excretion of calcium and breakdown products of type 1 collagen (eg, N and C telopeptides) increases, as do the number of osteoclasts and resorption surfaces. The rate of bone formation is also enhanced, with increases in serum alkaline phosphatase and serum N-terminal propeptide of type 1 collagen, both reflecting increased osteoblastic activity. Bone formation, while increased, does not keep pace with bone resorption, and there is a net loss of bone mass at the time of menopause. This high-turnover state is the direct result of estrogen deficiency and can be reversed by estrogen replacement therapy or the use of a potent antiresorptive drug such as a bisphosphonate.

The accelerated phase of estrogen-deficient bone loss begins immediately at the time of menopause (natural or surgical). It is most evident in trabecular bone, the compartment remodeled most rapidly. As much as 5–10% of spinal trabecular bone mineral is lost yearly in early postmenopausal women; osteoporotic fractures in such early postmenopausal women are often in the spine, a site of primarily trabecular bone. After 5–15 years, the rate of bone loss slows, so that after age 65, the annual rate of bone loss is similar in both sexes.

The cellular basis for the activation of bone resorption in the estrogen-deficient state is not fully understood. Clearly, it involves an increased release of cytokines such as (eg, interleukin-6) from cells in the bone microenvironment in estrogen deficiency. These cytokines increase the expression of RANK-L and decrease the expression of OPG on stromal cells and osteoblasts. These critical changes together promote an imbalance in bone remodeling that favors increased osteoclastogenesis and bone resorption.

The pathogenesis of age-related bone loss is less certain. Bone mass is relatively stable in the fourth and fifth decades of life; the bone mass accelerates for 5–10 years in women at the time of menopause, and subsequently continues throughout life at a slower rate that is similar in men and women.

One important factor in the pathogenesis of age-related bone loss is a relative deficiency of calcium and $1,25\text{-}(OH)_2D$. The capacity of the intestine to absorb calcium diminishes with age. Because renal losses of calcium are obligatory, a decreased efficiency of calcium absorption means that dietary calcium intake must be increased to prevent a negative calcium balance. It is estimated that about 1200 mg/d of elemental calcium is required to maintain calcium balance in people over age 65 (Table 17–11). American women in this age group typically ingest far less calcium (500–600 mg/d); calcium intake in men is somewhat higher. In addition, older individuals may be deficient in vitamin D, further impairing their ability to absorb calcium. $25\text{-}(OH)D$ shows seasonal variability, with lower levels and mild secondary hyperparathyroidism evident by the end of winter.

The PTH level increases with age owing to changes in multiple organ systems with aging. There is a decrease in the mass of functioning renal tissue with age that could lead to the decreased renal synthesis of $1,25\text{-}(OH)_2D$, which would directly release PTH secretion from its normal inhibition by $1,25\text{-}(OH)_2D$. The reduced $1,25\text{-}(OH)_2D$ level decreases calcium absorption, exacerbating an intrinsic inability of the aging intestine to absorb calcium normally. Secondary hyperparathyroidism results from the dual effects of $1,25\text{-}(OH)_2D$

TABLE 17–11   **Recommended calcium and vitamin D intakes.**

Age	Calcium (mg/d)	Vitamin D (IU/d)
0–6 months	200	400
6–12 months	260	400
1–3 years	700	600
4–8 years	1000	600
9–13 years	1300	600
14–18 years	1300	600
19–30 years	1000	600
31–50 years	1000	600
51–70 years (women)	1200	600
51–70 years (men)	1000	600
70+ years	1200	800

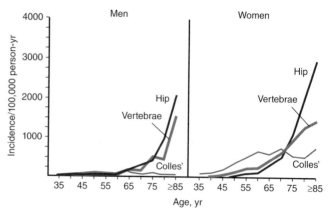

FIGURE 17–20 Age-specific incidences of wrist, hip, and vertebral fractures in men and women, derived from Rochester, Minnesota, data. (Redrawn, with permission, from Cooper C et al. Epidemiology of osteoporosis. Trends Endocrinol Metab. 1992;3:224. Copyright © Elsevier.)

deficiency on the parathyroid gland and the intestine. In addition, the responsiveness of the parathyroid gland to inhibition by calcium is reduced with aging. The secondary hyperparathyroidism of aging may thus result from the combined effects of age on the kidney, intestine, and parathyroid glands.

Dietary supplementation with adequate vitamin D modestly reduces the rate of age-related bone loss and protects against fracture. This suggests that reduced calcium absorption and secondary hyperparathyroidism play significant roles in the pathogenesis of osteoporosis in the elderly. However, calcium and vitamin D supplements alone do not completely ameliorate fracture risk.

In secondary osteoporosis associated with glucocorticoid administration or alcoholism, there is a marked reduction in bone formation rates. It is likely that glucocorticoids dramatically increase fracture risk because of the rapid loss of bone that results from frankly depressed bone formation in the face of normal or even increased bone resorption. Additionally, glucocorticoids decrease intestinal calcium absorption and increase urine calcium losses.

The secondary osteoporosis associated with immobilization is another example of a resorptive state with marked uncoupling of bone resorption and bone formation; it is characterized by hypercalciuria and PTH suppression. When individuals with a high pre-existing state of bone remodeling (eg, adolescents, patients with hyperthyroidism or Paget disease) are immobilized, bone resorption may be accelerated enough to produce hypercalcemia.

Clinical Manifestations

Osteoporosis is asymptomatic until it produces fractures with their attendant disability. Typical osteoporotic fractures occur in the spine, hip, and wrist (Colles fracture). In women, wrist fractures increase in incidence at menopause and then stay relatively stable at this increased rate with age. The incidence of hip and vertebral fractures increases rapidly with aging in both men and women (Figure 17–20). The vertebral bodies may be crushed, resulting in a loss of height, or may be wedged anteriorly, resulting in height loss and kyphosis. The dorsal kyphosis of elderly women ("dowager's hump") results from the anterior wedging of multiple thoracic vertebrae. Spinal fractures may be acute and painful or may occur gradually and manifest only as kyphosis or loss of height.

The complication of osteoporosis with the highest rate of morbidity and mortality is hip fracture. Hip fractures typically occur in the elderly, with a sharply rising incidence in both sexes after age 80 years. This is due to a variety of factors, including the tendency for a slower rate of bone loss in the cortical bone that makes up the hip compared with the predominantly trabecular bone of the spine, as well as the diminished motor and visual function that comes with aging that results in more frequent falls. The personal and societal costs of hip fracture are enormous. One-third of American women who survive past age 80 years will suffer a hip fracture. The 6-month mortality rate is approximately 20%, much of it resulting from the complications of immobilizing frail persons in bed. Complications include pulmonary embolus and pneumonia. About half of elderly people with a hip fracture will never walk freely again.

The diagnosis of osteoporosis is sometimes made radiologically, but, in general, x-rays are imprecise diagnostic tools for this disease. A chest x-ray will miss 30–50% of cases of spinal osteoporosis and, if over-penetrated, may lead to the diagnosis of osteoporosis in someone with normal bone mass. The best way to diagnose osteoporosis is by measuring bone mineral density by dual-energy x-ray absorptiometry (DXA). The technique is precise, rapid, and inexpensive. The relationship between bone mineral density and fracture risk is a continuous one (ie, the lower the bone mineral density, the higher the fracture risk). Osteoporosis has been defined by the World Health Organization (WHO) as a bone mineral density value 2.5 standard deviations or more below the young adult normal value (ie, a T score of −2.5 or less). This cutoff was selected based on the observation that 16% of postmenopausal Caucasian women at age 50 years will have femoral neck bone density values below −2.5, and this population has a 16% lifetime risk of hip fracture. However, it should be remembered that there is no threshold at this value and that bone mineral density measurements need to be interpreted in light of other risk factors for fracture such as age and propensity for falls. An absolute 10-year fracture risk calculation algorithm (termed FRAX) was developed by the WHO and is widely used. The algorithm incorporates femoral neck bone mineral density values and several clinical risk factors to determine two separate 10-year probabilities: one for a major osteoporotic fracture (hip, clinical spine, forearm, and proximal humerus) and the second for a hip fracture. The URL https://www.sheffield.ac.uk/FRAX/ provides access to the WHO absolute fracture risk calculator. This tool is useful for determining the need for treatment in addition to the bone density values.

It is additionally important to realize that not all the risk for fracture is captured by measurements of bone mineral density, because bone strength is also a function of bone quality. Bone quality, determined by the microarchitecture of a bone, its mechanical strength, its material properties, and its ability to withstand stress, may be substantially different in two individuals with the same bone mineral density. Techniques to assess bone quality noninvasively are being actively investigated.

Elderly persons with osteoporosis are unlikely to sustain a hip fracture unless they fall. Risk factors for falling include muscle weakness, impaired vision, impaired balance, sedative use, and environmental factors. Therefore, strategies to prevent falls are an important part of the approach to the osteoporotic patient.

Individuals at risk for osteoporosis benefit from a total calcium intake of about 1200 mg/d. This can be accomplished with dairy products or other calcium-rich foods, with calcium-fortified foods, or with a calcium supplement such as calcium carbonate or calcium citrate. Vitamin D should also be provided in age-appropriate doses (600–800 IU/d). The serum level of 25-(OH)D that represents sufficiency remains controversial, with the Health and Medicine Division of the National Academies of Sciences, Engineering, and Medicine (formerly the Institute of Medicine) recommending a level of 20 ng/mL and many metabolic bone disease experts recommending a level of more than 32 ng/mL. Table 17–11 provides the current recommended intake for calcium and vitamin D. Calcium supplementation in younger individuals may increase peak bone mass and decrease premenopausal bone loss, but its optimal role in this age group has not been determined. Estrogen replacement reduces bone loss, relieves hot flushes after menopause, and reduces fracture risk. It requires the concomitant use of progestins in women who have not had a hysterectomy to prevent endometrial carcinoma; however, it also increases the risk of breast cancer,

stroke, myocardial infarction, and venous thromboembolism. The side effect profile of estrogen has limited its use to short-term therapy at the time of menopause, typically in women suffering from hot flushes. Other antiresorptive agents available for the treatment of osteoporosis include alendronate, risedronate, ibandronate, zoledronic acid, calcitonin, raloxifene, and denosumab. The first four agents are bisphosphonates that directly inhibit osteoclastic bone resorption. Given therapeutically, calcitonin decreases bone resorption and may protect against bone loss and vertebral fractures. Raloxifene, a selective estrogen response modulator, inhibits bone resorption as estrogen does. Raloxifene does not induce endometrial changes, and it has estrogen antagonist actions in breast cells that may decrease the incidence of breast carcinoma in postmenopausal women. Denosumab is a monoclonal antibody to RANK ligand and inhibits osteoclast development and activation. Two other agents that stimulate bone formation are parathyroid hormone (PTH1-34; teriparatide) and a PTHrP analog called abaloparatide. In contrast to the bone resorption caused by continuous PTH elevations such as that occuring in hyperparathyroidism or the hypercalcemia of malignancy, daily injections of PTH or PTHrP stimulate bone formation and, to a lesser extent, bone resorption, resulting in net gains in bone density and decreased fracture risk.

CHECKPOINT

29. What is the relative importance of hereditary versus environmental or hormonal factors in contributing to osteoporosis?

30. What are the risk factors for osteoporosis?

31. What are the symptoms and signs of osteoporosis?

32. What are the risk factors for fracture in a patient with osteoporosis?

33. What treatments can prevent bone loss?

OSTEOMALACIA

Etiology

Osteomalacia is defined as a defect in the mineralization of bone. When it occurs in growing individuals, it also affects the mineralization of cartilage in the growth plate, a disorder called **rickets**. Osteomalacia can result from a deficiency of vitamin D, a deficiency of phosphate, an inherited deficiency in alkaline phosphatase (hypophosphatasia), or agents that have adverse effects on bone (Table 17–12). Surprisingly, dietary calcium deficiency rarely produces osteomalacia, although such cases have been reported.

Vitamin D deficiency is becoming more common in the United States because of decreased sunlight exposure, the increased use of sunscreen, and limited dietary sources of vitamin D. Individuals of dark-skinned ethnicities are particularly vulnerable because they experienc less cutaneous synthesis of

TABLE 17–12   Causes of osteomalacia.

Vitamin D deficiency
Nutritional
Malabsorption
Hereditary vitamin D–dependent rickets
Renal 1α-hydroxylase deficiency
Hereditary vitamin D–resistant rickets (absent or defective vitamin D receptor)
Phosphate deficiency
Renal phosphate wasting
X-linked hypophosphatemia
Autosomal dominant hypophosphatemic rickets
Autosomal recessive hypophosphatemic rickets
Hereditary hypophosphatemic rickets with hypercalciuria
Fanconi syndrome
Renal tubular acidosis (type II)
Tumor-induced osteomalacia (acquired, associated with mesenchymal tumors and prostate cancer)
Phosphate-binding antacids
Deficient alkaline phosphatase: hereditary hypophosphatasia
Drug toxicity
Fluoride
Aluminum (chronic kidney disease)
Etidronate disodium
Tenofovir, adefovir, cidofovir
Chronic kidney disease

vitamin D in response to sunlight. Fortified milk is the main food source of vitamin D, but at 100 IU/cup of milk, it can be difficult to achieve the daily recommended intake of 600–800 IU of vitamin D for adults. Some cereals and other foods have been also been fortified with vitamin D. In addition to insufficient intake, vitamin D deficiency can be the result of malabsorption of this fat-soluble vitamin. Severe rickets also occurs as part of two rare heritable disorders of vitamin D production or action: renal 1α-hydroxylase deficiency, in which vitamin D is not converted to $1,25\text{-}(OH)_2D$, and hereditary 1,25-dihydroxyvitamin D-resistant rickets (also known as vitamin D dependent rickets type 2), a disorder characterized by mutant vitamin D receptors with reduced activity.

Phosphate deficiency with osteomalacia is usually caused by inherited or acquired renal phosphate wasting. Three hereditary forms of renal phosphate wasting include X-linked, autosomal dominant, or autosomal recessive hypophosphatemic

rickets. Osteomalacia and hypophosphatemia can also result from tumors that are typically mesenchymal in origin and often located in the head-and-neck region. Many of these tumors overproduce FGF-23 (see above) and induce renal phosphate wasting and low $1,25\text{-}(OH)_2D$ levels, eventually leading to osteomalacia. The *FGF23* gene is mutated in kindreds with autosomal dominant hypophosphatemic rickets. Families with X-linked hypophosphatemic rickets have mutations in the *PHEX* gene, which encodes an endopeptidase called PHEX. This endopeptidase is involved in the production and degradation of FGF-23. In X-linked hypophosphatemic rickets, FGF-23 levels are elevated and appear to be responsible for the hypophosphatemic phenotype, although the exact role of PHEX in FGF-23 metabolism remains to be elucidated.

Pathogenesis

Vitamin D deficiency produces osteomalacia in stages. In the early stage, reduced calcium absorption produces secondary hyperparathyroidism, preventing hypocalcemia at the cost of increased renal phosphate excretion and hypophosphatemia. In later stages, hypocalcemia ensues, and hypophosphatemia progresses because of the combined effects of reduced absorption and the phosphaturic action of PTH. The poor delivery of minerals to bone (possibly coupled with the absence of direct effects of vitamin D on bone) impairs the mineralization of bone matrix. Since osteoblasts continue to synthesize bone matrix, unmineralized matrix, or osteoid, accumulates at bone-forming surfaces.

Clinical Manifestations

Patients with osteomalacia experience bone pain, muscle weakness, and a waddling gait. Radiologically, they may have reduced bone mass, detectable by both x-ray and bone densitometry. The hallmark of the disorder, however, is the pseudofracture: local bone resorption that has the appearance of a nondisplaced fracture, classically in the pubic rami, clavicles, or scapulas. In children with rickets, the leg bones are bowed (osteomalacia means "softening of bones"), the costochondral junctions are enlarged ("rachitic rosary"), and the growth plates are widened and irregular, reflecting the increase in unmineralized cartilage that bends under the child's weight, resulting in the bowing. Biochemically, the hallmarks of vitamin D–deficient osteomalacia are hypophosphatemia, hyperparathyroidism, variable hypocalcemia, and marked reductions in urinary calcium to less than 50 mg/d. The 25-(OH)D level is reduced, indicative of decreased body stores of vitamin D. In vitamin D deficiency and other forms of osteomalacia, the alkaline phosphatase level is often increased.

Although the disorder can be suspected strongly on clinical grounds and the biochemical changes summarized previously are confirmatory, a firm diagnosis of osteomalacia requires either the radiologic appearance of rickets or pseudofractures or a characteristic bone biopsy. If bone is biopsied for quantitative histomorphometry, thickened osteoid seams and a reduction in the mineralization rate are found. Treatment with vitamin D or aggressive phosphate replacement in patients with renal phosphate wasting will reverse osteomalacia and heal rickets. In renal disease, and in the FGF-23–mediated disorders, calcitriol also must be provided to mineralize bone because in these disorders, endogenous synthesis is either absent (renal disease) or suppressed (FGF-23 disorders).

CHECKPOINT

34. What are the causes of osteomalacia?
35. What are the two stages in which vitamin D deficiency produces osteomalacia?
36. What are the symptoms and signs of osteomalacia?

CASE STUDIES

Yeong Kwok, MD

(See Chapter 25, p. 776–79 for answers)

CASE 89

A 56-year-old woman presents to her primary care physician complaining of progressive fatigue, weakness, and diffuse bony pain. She says that her symptoms have been getting worse over the past 2 months. Her medical history is notable for well-controlled hypertension and recurrent renal stones. The physical examination is unremarkable. The serum calcium level is elevated.

Questions

A. What are some common causes of hypercalcemia? Which do you suspect in this patient, and why?
B. What is the pathogenesis of primary hyperparathyroidism? What genes have been implicated?
C. How would you make the diagnosis of primary hyperparathyroidism?

CASE 90

A 40-year-old woman comes to clinic to discuss some unexpected laboratory test abnormalities. She underwent these tests as part of a life insurance examination and was noted to have a mildly elevated serum calcium level. She has been healthy with no medical problems. She feels well and denies fatigue and pain. She does not take any medications or dietary supplements. There is no significant family history. Her physical examination is unremarkable. Repeated laboratory testing confirms a mildly elevated serum calcium level but also shows a normal serum phosphorus level and intact parathyroid hormone (PTH) and 1,25-OH$_2$D levels. A 24-hour urinary calcium test returns low, at 60 mg/24 h.

Questions

A. What is the likely diagnosis in this patient?
B. What is the underlying pathophysiology of this disorder, and how does this lead to the elevated serum calcium?

CASE 91

A 69-year-old man presents to his primary care physician complaining of fatigue, nausea, weakness, and diffuse bony pain. He states his symptoms have been getting progressively worse over the past 2 months. In addition, he has noted a 15-pound weight loss over approximately the same time span. His wife, who has accompanied him, also notes that he seems increasingly confused. His medical history is notable for well-controlled hypertension and chronic obstructive pulmonary disease. He has a 100-pack-year smoking history. On physical examination, he appears chronically ill and thin. Vital signs are notable for a blood pressure of 120/85 mm Hg, a heart rate of 98 bpm, and a respiratory rate of 16/min. The lungs have an increased expiratory phase, with a mild expiratory wheeze. He has decreased breath sounds at the left base. The remainder of his examination is unremarkable. The serum calcium level is markedly elevated. Hypercalcemia of malignancy is suspected.

Questions

A. What tumors commonly cause hypercalcemia? Which is likely in this patient?
B. What would you expect his serum PTH level to be? What about his serum PTHrP? Why?
C. How does PTHrP secretion cause hypercalcemia?

CASE 92

A 32-year-old woman presents to the emergency department with complaints of involuntary hand spasms. She states that as she was folding laundry, she experienced a sudden severe spasm in her right hand such that her fingers flexed. The spasm was quite painful and lasted several minutes, resolving spontaneously. She is 6 months pregnant. Her medical history is otherwise notable for thyroid tumor status post-thyroidectomy 3 years ago. She is taking synthetic thyroid hormone and a prenatal multivitamin. Her family history is unremarkable. On physical examination, she has positive Chvostek and Trousseau signs. The examination is otherwise unremarkable. Her serum calcium level is low. Hypoparathyroidism as a complication of thyroid surgery is suspected.

Questions

A. What is the mechanism by which thyroid surgery can result in hypocalcemia? Why may the patient only now be symptomatic?
B. What are the Chvostek and Trousseau signs? What does each represent?
C. What would you expect this patient's serum phosphate and PTH levels to be? Why?

CASE 93

A 23-year-old woman presents to her primary care physician complaining of diarrhea. The diarrhea is described as profuse and watery and has been getting progressively worse over the last 2 months. She has had no bloody or black bowel movements. The condition is not made worse by food and is not associated with fever, chills, sweats, nausea, or vomiting. On review of systems, she notes a 5-pound weight loss in the last 3 months. She also notes occasional flushing. She denies any significant family history. On physical examination, she is a thin white woman in no acute distress. She is afebrile, with a blood pressure of 100/60 mm Hg, heart rate of 100 bpm, and respiratory rate of 14/min. The head examination is unremarkable. The neck examination reveals bilateral hard nodules of the thyroid: a 2 cm nodule on the right upper pole and a 1.5 cm nodule on the left upper pole. She has a firm 1 cm lymph node in the right anterior cervical chain. The lungs are clear. On cardiac examination, she is mildly tachycardiac, with a regular rhythm and no extra sounds. The abdomen has hyperactive bowel sounds and is soft, nontender, nondistended, and without masses. The skin examination discloses no rashes. Medullary carcinoma of the thyroid is suspected.

Questions

A. What is the cause of this patient's diarrhea and flushing?
B. How would you make a diagnosis of medullary carcinoma of the thyroid?
C. What other tests would you like to order? Why?

CASE 94

A 72-year-old woman presents to the emergency department after falling in her home. She had slipped on spilled water in her kitchen. She was unable to get up after her fall and was found by her son, stopping by after work. She complains of severe right hip pain. On examination, she has bruising over her right hip. Range of motion in her right hip is markedly decreased, with pain on both internal and external rotation. X-ray film reveals a hip fracture and probable low bone mass. The situation raises concern for osteoporosis.

Questions

A. What are some important causes of osteoporosis?
B. What are the likely causes of osteoporosis in this patient? What is the underlying pathogenesis of each?
C. What are the risk factors for fracture in patients with osteoporosis?
D. What are common complications of hip fractures?
E. What treatments are available to prevent bone loss?

CASE 95

A 93-year-old woman is brought to the emergency department by ambulance for "failure to thrive." She has been bed-bound, living in a basement apartment without any real sunlight exposure. Today the woman's daughter was attempting to roll her to clean her, and the patient fell from the bed to the floor. She had been a strict vegetarian, avoiding all dairy products. And for many months, the patient has been eating only broth because of difficulty chewing and swallowing. On examination, she is pale, with central obesity, wasting of her extremities, and flexion contractures of her right upper and lower extremities. On head-and-neck examination, she has temporal wasting, right facial droop, pale conjunctivas, and dry mucous membranes. The lungs are clear to auscultation. The cardiac examination is notable for an S4 gallop. The patient moans when her extremities are palpated. Laboratory reports show hypocalcemia, hypophosphatemia, and elevated alkaline phosphatase. X-ray films of her pelvis reveal low bone mass and pseudofracture of the pubic rami. Osteomalacia is suspected.

Questions

A. What are the causes of osteomalacia? Which do you suspect in this patient? Why?
B. What is the pathogenesis of osteomalacia in this patient?
C. What would you expect to see on a bone biopsy for quantitative histomorphometry?

REFERENCES

General Bone and Mineral Metabolism, Calciotropic Hormones & Vitamin D

Abrams SA et al. Vitamin D: effects on childhood health and disease. Nat Rev Endocrinol. 2013 Mar;9(3):162–70. [PMID: 23381033]

Carmeliet G et al. Vitamin D signaling in calcium and bone homeostasis: a delicate balance. Best Pract Res Clin Endocrinol Metab. 2015 Aug;29(4):621–31. [PMID: 26303088]

Cauley JA. Estrogen and bone health in men and women. Steroids. 2015 Jul;99(Pt A):11–5. [PMID: 25555470]

Chapurlat RD et al. Novel biological markers of bone: from bone metabolism to bone physiology. Rheumatology (Oxford). 2016 Oct;55(10):1714–25. [PMID: 26790456]

Cheloha RW et al. PTH receptor-1 signalling – mechanistic insights and therapeutic prospects. Nat Rev Endocrinol. 2015 Dec;11(12):712–24. [PMID: 26303600]

Christakos S et al. Vitamin D: metabolism, molecular mechanism of action, and pleiotropic effects. Physiol Rev. 2016 Jan;96(1):365–408. [PMID: 26681795]

Khundmiri SJ et al. PTH and vitamin D. Compr Physiol. 2016 Mar 15;6(2):561–601. [PMID: 27065162]

Martin TJ. Parathyroid hormone-related protein, its regulation of cartilage and bone development, and role in treating bone diseases. Physiol Rev. 2016 Jul;96(3):831–71. [PMID: 27142453]

Miller WL. Genetic disorders of vitamin D biosynthesis and degradation. J Steroid Biochem Mol Biol. 2017 Jan;165(Pt A):101–8. [PMID: 27060335]

Rizzoli R. Nutritional aspects of bone health. Best Pract Res Clin Endocrinol Metab. 2014 Dec;28(6):795–808. [PMID: 25432353]

Siddiqui JA et al. Physiological bone remodeling: systemic regulation and growth factor involvement. Physiology (Bethesda). 2016 May;31(3):233–45. [PMID: 27053737]

Hyperparathyroidism

Bilezikian JP et al. Guidelines for the management of asymptomatic primary hyperparathyroidism: summary statement from the Fourth International Workshop. J Clin Endocrinol Metab. 2014 Oct;99(10):3561–9. [PMID: 25162665]

Bilezikian JP et al. Primary hyperparathyroidism. Nat Rev Dis Primers. 2016;2:1–16. [PMID: 27194212]

Duan K et al. Clinicopathological correlates of hyperparathyroidism. J Clin Pathol. 2015;68:771–87. [PMID: 26163537]

Eastell R et al. Diagnosis of asymptomatic primary hyperparathyroidism: proceedings of the Fourth International Workshop. J Clin Endocrinol Metab. 2014 Oct;99(10):3570–9. [PMID: 25162666]

Li Y et al. Endocrine neoplasms in familial syndromes of hyperparathyroidism. Endocrine-Related Cancer. 2016;23:R229–47. [PMID: 27207564]

Marcocci C et al. Medical management of primary hyperparathyroidism: proceedings of the Fourth International Workshop on the management of asymptomatic primary hyperparathyroidism. J Clin Endocrinol Metab. 2014 Oct;99(10):3607–18. [PMID: 25162668]

Silverberg SJ et al. Current issues in the presentation of asymptomatic primary hyperparathyroidism: proceedings of the Fourth International Workshop. J Clin Endocrinol Metab. 2014 Oct;99(10):3580–94. [PMID: 25162667]

Simonds WF. Genetics of hyperparathyroidism, including parathyroid cancer. Endocrinol Metab Clin North Am. 2017 Jun;46(2):405–18. [PMID: 28476229]

Udelsman R et al. The surgical management of asymptomatic primary hyperparathyroidism: proceedings of the Fourth International Workshop. J Clin Endocrinol Metab. 2014;99(10):3595–606. [PMID: 25162669]

Verdelli C et al. Mechanisms in endocrinology: kidney involvement in patients with primary hyperparathyroidism: an update on clinical and molecular aspects. Eur J Endocrinol. 2017 Jan;176(1):R39–52. [PMID: 27601015]

Vestergaard P. Primary hyperparathyroidism and nephrolithiasis. Ann Endocrinol (Paris). 2015 May;76(2):116–9. [PMID: 25911000]

Familial Hypocalciuric Hypercalcemia

Hannan FM et al. Adapter protein-2 sigma subunit mutations causing familial hypocalciuric hypercalcaemia type 3 (FHH3) demonstrate genotype-phenotype correlations, codon bias and dominant negative effects. Hum Mol Genet. 2015 Sept 15;24(18):5079–92. [PMID: 26082470]

Hendy GN et al. Calcium-sensing receptor, proinflammatory cytokines and calcium homeostasis. Semin Cell Dev Biol. 2016 Jan;49:37–43. [PMID: 26612442]

Mayr B et al. Genetics In Endocrinology: Gain and loss of function mutations of the calcium-sensing receptor and associated proteins: current treatment concepts. Eur J Endocrinol. 2016 May;174(5):R189–208. [PMID: 26646938]

Nesbit MA et al. Mutations affecting G-protein subunit α11 in hypercalcemia and hypocalcemia. N Engl J Med. 2013 Jun 27;368(26):2476–86. [PMID: 23802516]

Nesbit MA et al. Mutations in *AP2S1* cause familial hypocalciuric hypercalcemia type 3. Nat Genet. 2013 Jan;45(1):93–7. [PMID: 23222959]

Thakker RV. The calcium-sensing receptor: and its involvement in parathyroid pathology. Ann Endocrinol (Paris). 2015 May;76(2):81–3. [PMID: 25910996]

Fibroblast Growth Factor 23 & Phosphate Handling

Blau JE et al. The PTH-Vitamin D-FGF23 axis. Rev Endocr Metab Disord. 2015 Jun;16(2):165–74. [PMID: 26296372]

Christov M et al. Insights from genetic disorders of phosphate homeostasis. Semin Nephrol. 2013 Mar;33(2):143–57. [PMID: 23465501]

Hanudel M et al. Fibroblast growth factor 23: fueling the fire. Kidney Int. 2016 Nov;90(5):928–30. [PMID: 27742194]

Leaf DE et al. Fibroblast growth factor 23 levels associate with AKI and death in critical illness. J Am Soc Nephrol. 2017 Jun;28(6):1877–85. [PMID: 28028134]

Portale AA et al. Disordered FGF23 and mineral metabolism in children with CKD. Clin J Am Soc Nephrol. 2014 Feb;9(2):344–53. [PMID: 24311704]

Hypercalcemia of Malignancy & Other Forms of Hypercalcemia

Carpenter TO. *CYP24A1* loss of function: clinical phenotype of monoallelic and biallelic mutations. J Steroid Biochem Mol Biol. 2017 Oct;173:337–40. [PMID: 28093352]

Donovan PJ et al. Calcitriol-mediated hypercalcemia: causes and course in 101 patients. J Clin Endocrinol Metab. 2013 Oct;98(10):4023–9. [PMID: 23979953]

Donovan PJ et al. PTHrP-mediated hypercalcemia: causes and survival in 138 patients. J Clin Endocrinol Metab. 2015 May;100(5):2024–9. [PMID: 25719931]

Gastanaga VM et al. Prevalence of hypercalcemia among cancer patients in the United States. Cancer Med. 2016 August;5(8):2091–100. [PMID: 27263488]

Goldner W. Cancer-related hypercalcemia. J Oncol Pract 2016 May;12(8):426–32. [PMID: 27170690]

Goswamy J et al. Parathyroid carcinoma. Curr Opin Otolaryngol Head Neck Surg. 2016 Apr;24(2):155–62. [PMID: 26771263]

Maier JD et al. Hypercalcemia in the intensive care unit: a review of pathophysiology, diagnosis, and modern therapy. J Intensive Care Med. 2015 Jul;30(5):235–52. [PMID: 24130250]

Medas F et al. Controversies in the management of parathyroid carcinoma: a case series and review of the literature. Int J Surg. 2016 Apr;28(Suppl 1):S94–8. [PMID: 26708847]

Meng QH et al. Laboratory approaches for the diagnosis and assessment of hypercalcemia. Crit Rev Clin Lab Sci. 2015;52(3):107–19. [PMID: 25327435]

Mirrakhimov AE. Hypercalcemia of malignancy: an update on pathogenesis and management. North Am J Med Sci. 2015 Nov;7(11): 483–93. [PMID: 26713296]

Sternlicht H et al. Hypercalcemia of malignancy and new treatment options. Ther Clin Risk Manag. 2015 Dec 4;11:1779–88. [PMID: 26675713]

Tebben PJ et al. Vitamin D-mediated hypercalcemia: mechanisms, diagnosis, and treatment. Endocr Rev. 2016 Oct;37(5):521–47. [PMID: 27588937]

Thosani S et al. Denosumab: a new agent in the management of hypercalcemia of malignancy. Future Oncol. 2015;11(21):2865–71. [PMID: 26403973]

Wagner J et al. Oncologic metabolic emergencies. Emerg Med Clin North Am. 2014 Aug;32(3):509–25. [PMID: 25060247]

Hypoparathyroidism & Hypocalcemia

Betterle C et al. Diagnosis and classification of autoimmune parathyroid disease. Autoimmun Rev. 2014 Apr-May;13(4-5):417–22. [PMID: 24424178]

Clarke BL et al. Epidemiology and diagnosis of hypoparathyroidism. J Clin Endocrinol Metab. 2016 Jun;101(6):2284–99. [PMID: 26943720]

Hannan FM et al. Investigating hypocalcaemia. BMJ. 2013 May 9;346:f2213. [PMID: 23661111]

Jüppner H. Genetic and epigenetic defects at the *GNAS* locus cause different forms of pseudohypoparathyroidism. Ann Endocrinol (Paris). 2015 May;76(2):92–7. [PMID: 25882888]

Kakava K et al. Postsurgical hypoparathyroidism: a systematic review. In Vivo. 2016 May-Jun;30(3):171–9. [PMID: 27107072]

Lemos MC et al. *GNAS* mutations in pseudohypoparathyroidism type 1a and related disorders. Hum Mutat. 2015 Jan;36(1):11–9. [PMID: 25219572]

Mannstadt M et al. Efficacy and safety of recombinant human parathyroid hormone (1-84) in hypoparathyroidism (REPLACE): a double-blind, placebo-controlled, randomised, phase 3 study. Lancet Diabetes Endocrinol. 2013 Dec;1(4):275–83. [PMID: 24622413]

Mannstadt M et al. Germline mutations affecting Gα11 in hypoparathyroidism. N Engl J Med. 2013 Jun 27;368(26):2532–4. [PMID: 23802536]

Shaw NJ. A practical approach to hypocalcaemia in children. Endocr Dev. 2015;28:84–100. [PMID: 26138837]

Shoback D. Clinical practice. Hypoparathyroidism. N Engl J Med. 2008 Jul 24;359(4):391–403. [PMID: 18650515]

Tafaj O et al. Pseudohypoparathyroidism: one gene, several syndromes. J Endocrinol Invest. 2017 Apr;40(4):347–56. [PMID: 27995443]

Medullary Carcinoma of the Thyroid

Chernock RD et al. Molecular pathology of hereditary and sporadic medullary thyroid carcinomas. Am J Clin Pathol. 2015 Jun;143(6):768–77. [PMID: 25972318]

Frank-Raue K et al. Hereditary medullary thyroid cancer genotype-phenotype correlation. Recent Results Cancer Res. 2015;204:139–56. [PMID: 26494387]

Hadoux J et al. Management of advanced medullary thyroid cancer. Lancet Diabetes Endocrinol. 2016 Jan;4(1):64–71. [PMID: 26608066]

Moraitis AG et al. Genetics, diagnosis, and management of medullary thyroid carcinoma and pheochromocytoma/paraganglioma. Endocr Pract. 2014 Feb;20(2):176–87. [PMID: 24449662]

Moura MM et al. RAS proto-oncogene in medullary thyroid carcinoma. Endocr Relat Cancer. 2015 Oct;22(5):R235–52. [PMID: 26285815]

Raue F et al. Epidemiology and clinical presentation of medullary thyroid carcinoma. Recent Results Cancer Res. 2015;204:61–90. [PMID: 26494384]

Schmid KW. Histopathology of C cells and medullary thyroid carcinoma. Recent Results Cancer Res. 2015;204:41–60. [PMID: 26494383]

Wells SA Jr et al. Revised American Thyroid Association guidelines for the management of medullary thyroid carcinoma. Thyroid. 2015 Jun;25(6):567–610. [PMID: 25810047]

Osteoporosis

Black DM et al. Clinical practice. Postmenopausal osteoporosis. N Engl J Med. 2016 Jan 21;374(3):254–62. [PMID: 26789873]

Cosman F et al. Clinician's guide to prevention and treatment of osteoporosis. Osteoporos Int. 2014 Oct;25(10):2359–81. [PMID: 25182228]

Drake MT et al. The pathophysiology and treatment of osteoporosis. Clin Ther. 2015 Aug;37(8):1837–50. [PMID: 26163201]

Emkey GR et al. Secondary osteoporosis: pathophysiology & diagnosis. Best Pract Res Clin Endocrinol Metab. 2014 Dec;28(6):911–35. [PMID: 25432361]

Frenkel B et al. Glucocorticoid-induced osteoporosis. Adv Exp Med Biol. 2015;872:179–215. [PMID: 26215995]

Khan AA et al. Primary hyperparathyroidism: review and recommendations on evaluation, diagnosis, and management. A Canadian and international consensus. Osteoporos Int. 2017 Jan;28(1):1–19. [PMID: 27613721]

Khosla S et al. Osteoporosis treatment: recent developments and ongoing challenges. Lancet Diabetes Endocrinol. 2017 Nov;5(11):898-907. [PMID: 28689769]

Mirza F et al. Management of Endocrine Disease: Secondary osteoporosis: pathophysiology and management. Eur J Endocrinol. 2015 Sep;173(3):R131–51. [PMID: 25971649]

Shane E et al. Atypical subtrochanteric and diaphyseal femoral fractures: second report of a task force of the American Society for Bone and Mineral Research. J Bone Miner Res. 2014 Jan;29(1):1–23. [PMID: 23712442]

Siris ES et al. The clinical diagnosis of osteoporosis: a position statement from the National Bone Health Alliance Working Group. Osteoporos Int. 2014 May;25(5):1439–43. [PMID: 24577348]

Weaver CM et al. The National Osteoporosis Foundation's position statement on peak bone mass development and lifestyle factors: a systematic review and implementation recommendations. Osteoporos Int. 2016 Apr;27(4):1281–386. [PMID: 26856587]

Osteomalacia & Rickets

Allgrove J et al. A practical approach to vitamin D deficiency and rickets. Endocr Dev. 2015;28:119–33. [PMID: 26138839]

Elder CJ et al. Rickets. Lancet. 2014 May 10;383(9929):1665–76. [PMID: 24412049]

Goldsweig BK et al. Hypophosphatemic rickets: lessons from disrupted FGF23 control of phosphorus homeostasis. Curr Osteoporos Rep. 2015 Apr;13(2):88–97. [PMID: 25620749]

Hautmann AH et al. Tumor-induced osteomalacia: an up-to-date review. Curr Rheumatol Rep. 2015 Jun;17:512. [PMID: 25900190]

Munns CF et al. Global consensus recommendations on prevention and management of nutritional rickets. J Clin Endocrinol Metab. 2016 Feb;101(2):394–415. [PMID: 26745253]

Razali NN et al. Phosphate homeostasis and genetic mutations of familial hypophosphatemic rickets. J Pediatr Endocrinol Metab. 2015 Sep;28(9-10):1009–17. [PMID: 25894638]

Rosen CJ. Clinical practice. Vitamin D insufficiency. N Engl J Med. 2011 Jan 20;364(3):248–54. [PMID: 21247315]

Shaw NJ. Prevention and treatment of nutritional rickets. J Steroid Biochem Mol Biol. 2016 Nov;164:145–7. [PMID: 26493853]

Disorders of the Endocrine Pancreas

Janet L. Funk, MD

Insulin and glucagon, the two key hormones that orchestrate fuel storage and use, are produced by the islet cells in the pancreas. Islet cells are distributed in clusters throughout the exocrine pancreas. Together, they comprise the endocrine pancreas. Diabetes mellitus, a heterogeneous disorder, is the most common disease of the endocrine pancreas. Affecting

9% of the world's adult population in 2014, the prevalence of diabetes continues to increase worldwide, having already more than doubled over the past three decades. Pancreatic tumors secreting excessive amounts of specific islet cell hormones are far less common, but their clinical presentations underscore the important regulatory roles of each hormone.

NORMAL STRUCTURE & FUNCTION OF THE PANCREATIC ISLETS

ANATOMY & HISTOLOGY

The endocrine pancreas is composed of nests of cells (islets of Langerhans) that are distributed throughout the exocrine pancreas. This anatomic feature allows for their enzymatic isolation from the exocrine pancreas for islet cell transplantation. Although numbering in the millions, the multicellular islets comprise only 1% of the total pancreas. The endocrine pancreas has great reserve capacity; more than 70% of the insulin-secreting β cells must be lost before dysfunction occurs. Each of the four major islet cell types produces a different secretory product. Insulin-secreting β cells are the predominant cell type (60%). The majority of the remaining islet cells, glucagon-secreting α cells (30%) and somatostatin-secreting δ cells (<10%), secrete hormones that counter the effects of insulin. A fourth islet cell type, the pancreatic polypeptide (PP)–secreting cell (<1%), is primarily located in the posterior lobe of the head of the pancreas, an embryologically distinct region receiving a different blood supply.

The islets are much more highly vascularized than the exocrine pancreatic tissues (see Chapter 15), with at least one major arteriole supplying each islet. The majority of islet cells are closely apposed to the vasculature and to islet cells of opposing types, suggesting an important role for endocrine

(via the microcirculation) and/or intra-islet paracrine (via the interstitium) effects on hormone release (Figure 18–1). Blood from the islets then drains into the hepatic portal vein. Thus, the islet cell hormones pass directly into the liver, a major site of action of glucagon and insulin, before proceeding into the systemic circulation, allowing for much higher hepatic than systemic levels of pancreatic hormones.

The islets are also abundantly innervated. Both parasympathetic and sympathetic axons enter the islets and either directly contact cells or terminate in the interstitial space between the cells. Neural regulation of islet cell hormone release, both directly through the sympathetic fibers and indirectly through the stimulation of catecholamine release by the adrenal medulla, plays a key role in glucose homeostasis during stress.

CHECKPOINT

1. What percentage of islets must be lost before endocrine pancreatic dysfunction becomes manifest?
2. Identify the major hormone-secreting cells in an islet of Langerhans.

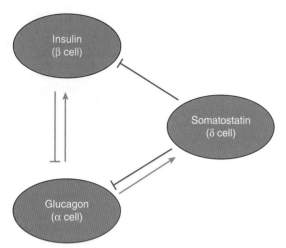

FIGURE 18–1 Schematic diagram indicating paracrine/endocrine regulation of islet cell hormones. Inhibition is indicated by a blunt line, stimulation by an arrow.

PHYSIOLOGY

1. Insulin

Synthesis and Metabolism of Insulin

Insulin is a protein composed of two peptide chains (A and B) connected by two disulfide bonds (Figure 18–2). The precursor of insulin, **preproinsulin** (MW 11,500), is synthesized in the ribosomes and enters the endoplasmic reticulum of β cells, where it is promptly cleaved by microsomal enzymes to form proinsulin (MW 9000). **Proinsulin**, consisting of A and B chains joined by a 31-amino-acid **C peptide**, is transported to the Golgi apparatus, where it is packaged into secretory vesicles. While in the secretory vesicle, proinsulin is cleaved to form insulin (51 amino acids; MW 5808) and the C peptide fragment (see Figure 18–2). Insulin secretion is, therefore, accompanied by an equimolar secretion of C peptide and also by small amounts of proinsulin that escape cleavage. In the acidic environment of the secretory granules, stored insulin forms a hexamer in association with zinc atoms, dissociating into active monomers upon secretion. Insulin has a circulatory half-life of 3–5 minutes and is catabolized in both the liver and kidney. Approximately 50% of insulin is catabolized on its first pass through the liver after it is secreted from the pancreas into the portal vein. In contrast, both C peptide and proinsulin are catabolized only by the kidney and, therefore, have half-lives three to four times longer than that of insulin itself. Recombinant human insulin or related analogs, modified either to enhance monomer formation (rapid acting) or decrease solubility and/or clearance (longer acting), are used clinically to treat diabetes.

Regulation of Secretion

Glucose is the primary physiologic stimulant of insulin release (Figure 18–3). Glucose entry into β cells is facilitated by one

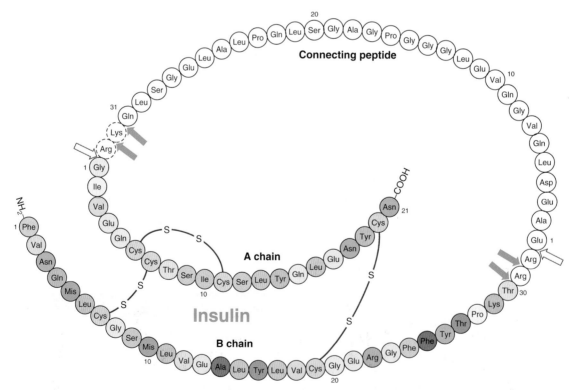

FIGURE 18–2 Amino acid sequence and covalent structure of human proinsulin. Initial cleavage by a trypsin-like enzyme (open arrows) followed by several more cleavages by a carboxypeptidase-like enzyme (solid green arrows) results in the production of the insulin molecule (AB) that consists of two polypeptide chains differing in composition in the order, number, and kind of their (colored) amino acid residues, along with the C-peptide (white) amino acid residues. (Redrawn, with permission, from Rodwell VW et al, eds. *Harper's Illustrated Biochemistry,* 30th ed. McGraw-Hill, 2015.)

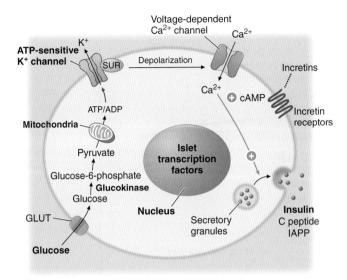

FIGURE 18–3 Schematic diagram of glucose-stimulated insulin release from a β cell. Glucose enters the β cell via GLUT–mediated diffusion. Glucose metabolism, the first step of which is controlled by glucokinase, results in ATP production. Cytosolic ATP, sensed by the sulfonylurea receptor (SUR) subunit of ATP-dependent K⁺ channels (K_{ATP}), blocks the K_{ATP} channels and thus K⁺ efflux, resulting in cell depolarization. This allows Ca^{2+} to enter via voltage-dependent calcium channels, stimulating the exocytosis of insulin-containing secretory granules. (Redrawn, with permission, from Kasper D et al, eds. *Harrison's Principles of Internal Medicine*, 19th ed. McGraw-Hill, 2015.)

TABLE 18–1   Regulation of islet cell hormone release.

	β-Cell Insulin Release	δ-Cell Somatostatin Release	α-Cell Glucagon Release
Nutrients			
Glucose	↑	↑	↓
Amino acids	↑	↑	↑
Fatty acids	—	—	↓
Ketones	—	—	↓
Hormones			
Enteric hormones			
GLP-1	↑	↓	↓
GIP	↑	↓	↑
Insulin	↓	↓?	↓
GABA	—	↓	↓
Somatostatin	↓	↓	↓
Glucagon	↑	↑	—
Cortisol	—	—	↑
Catecholamines	↓ (α-adrenergic)	—	↑ (β-adrenergic)
Neural			
Vagal	↑	—	↑
α-Adrenergic	↑	—	↑
β-Adrenergic	↓	—	↓

Key: ↑, increased; ↓, decreased; —, no effect or no known effect. (GABA, gamma aminobutyric acid; GIP gastric inhibitory peptide; GLP-1. glucagon-like peptide 1)

or more **glucose transporters** (GLUT-1, GLUT-2, and/or GLUT-3), which are in excess to glucose and allow the bidirectional transport of glucose, thereby creating an equilibrium between extracellular and intracellular glucose concentrations. Once in the cell, the metabolism of glucose—rather than glucose itself—stimulates insulin secretion.

Glucokinase, an enzyme with low affinity for glucose whose activity is regulated by glucose, controls the first and rate-limiting step in glucose metabolism: the phosphorylation of glucose to form glucose 6-phosphate. This enzyme, by determining the rate of glycolysis, functions as the β-cell **glucose sensor**. Glycolysis produces an increase in adenosine triphosphate (ATP), which is sensed by the sulfonylurea receptor subunit of ATP-dependent K⁺ channels (K_{ATP}) in the β-cell membrane, resulting in a closure of the channel. The resultant cell depolarization allows Ca^{2+} to enter, triggering the exocytosis of insulin-containing granules. Sulfonylurea drugs used to treat type 2 diabetes mellitus (DM) stimulate insulin secretion in a glucose-independent fashion by binding to the sulfonylurea receptor subunit and blocking K_{ATP}. Conversely, loss-of-function mutations in glucokinase that impair insulin release can lead to an early onset of mild diabetes (maturity-onset diabetes of the young).

Although glucose is the most potent stimulator of insulin release, other factors such as amino acids ingested with a meal or vagal stimulation also result in insulin release (Table 18–1). Up to 50% of insulin secretion in response to an oral glucose load can be attributed to enteric hormones

(**incretins**) such as **glucagon-like peptide-1** (GLP-1), which are released following the oral ingestion of nutrients and enhance the glucose-stimulated insulin secretion in β cells via activation of cAMP/PKA signaling pathways following binding to their G protein–coupled receptors (see Figure 18–3). This has led to the development of incretin-like drugs for the treatment of type 2 DM, which, unlike sulfonylureas, are less likely to induce hypoglycemia. Glucagon similarly enhances glucose-stimulated insulin secretion, a counter-regulatory effect that allows for insulin-mediated glucose disposal following glucagon-induced hepatic glucose production. Insulin secretion is inhibited by catecholamines and by somatostatin.

Mechanism of Action

Insulin exerts its effects by binding to **insulin receptors** present on the surfaces of target cells (Figure 18–4).

FIGURE 18–4 Model of insulin receptor signaling. The insulin receptor is composed of two α and two β subunits linked by disulfide bonds. Binding of insulin to the extracellular α subunits activates a tyrosine kinase present in the cytoplasmic domain of the β subunit, resulting in autophosphorylation of the β subunit. Receptor kinase activation is also the critical first step in a cascade of intracellular events that begins with the phosphorylation of multiple docking proteins (insulin receptor substrates [IRSs]). Once activated, these multifunctional proteins initiate complex intracellular signaling pathways. Binding of IRS to phosphatidylinositol 3–kinase (PI3-K) initiates a metabolic pathway by (1) stimulating glucose uptake by translocating the glucose transporter, GLUT-4, to the cell surface in skeletal muscle and adipose; (2) stimulating glucose storage by inactivating (via phosphorylation) glycogen synthase kinase 3 (GSK3) and subsequently dephosphorylating and activating glycogen synthase; and (3) increasing protein synthesis by activating the serine/threonine protein kinase, mechanistic target of rapamycin (mTOR). In contrast, the mitogenic effects of insulin are mediated by a mitogen-activated protein (MAP) kinase pathway. Additionally, important transcriptional effects occur, many of which involve inactivation (via phosphorylation) of the transcription factor, FoxO1, which is abundant in insulin-sensitive tissues. This change, in concert with the effects of other transcription factors (SREBP-1c, PPARs), allows for additional insulin-mediated effects, including increased lipogenesis vs. decreased gluconeogenesis and glycogenolysis in the liver, together with increased adipogenesis and lipid storage in adipose tissue. (PPAR, peroxisome proliferator activated receptor; SREBP-1c, sterol regulatory element-binding protein-1c.)

Insulin receptors are present in liver, muscle, and fat, the classic insulin-sensitive tissues responsible for fuel homeostasis. In addition, insulin can mediate other effects in nonclassic target tissues, such as the ovary, via interaction with insulin receptors or by cross-reactivity with **insulin-like growth factor–1** (**IGF-1**) receptors. The binding of insulin to its receptor causes the activation of a tyrosine kinase region of the receptor and the autophosphorylation of the receptor. Activation of the insulin receptor initiates a phosphorylation cascade within the cell, beginning with the phosphorylation of a network of docking proteins (**insulin receptor substrates** [**IRSs**]) that engage and amplify downstream signaling molecules, ultimately leading to the biologic effects of insulin (eg, translocation of GLUT-4

glucose transporter to the plasma membranes of muscle and fat cells and activation of hepatic glycogen synthase).

Effects

Insulin plays a major role in fuel homeostasis (Table 18–2). Insulin mediates changes in fuel metabolism through its effects on three main tissues: liver, muscle, and fat. In these tissues, insulin promotes fuel storage (anabolism) and prevents the breakdown and release of fuel that has already been stored (catabolism). The total lack of insulin is incompatible with life, and the same is true of excess insulin.

In the liver, insulin promotes fuel storage by stimulating glycogen synthesis and storage. Insulin inhibits hepatic glucose

TABLE 18-2 Hormonal regulation of fuel homeostasis.

	Insulin	Somatostatin	Glucagon	Catecholamines	Cortisol	Growth Hormone
Liver						
Fuel storage						
Glycogenesis	↑		↓			
Lipid synthesis	↑		↓			
Fuel breakdown						
Glycogenolysis	↓		↑	↑		↑
Gluconeogenesis	↓		↑	↑	↑	↑
Fatty acid oxidation or ketogenesis	↓		↑			
Kidneys						
Fuel breakdown						
Gluconeogenesis	↓			↑		
Muscle						
Fuel storage						
Glucose uptake or glycogenesis	↑			↓	↓	↓
Fuel breakdown						
Protein catabolism	↓				↑	
Adipose tissue						
Fuel storage						
Lipoprotein lipolysis	↑					
Fatty acid esterification	↑					
Fuel breakdown						
Lipolysis of stored fat	↓			↑	↑	↑
Pancreas						
Secretion of:						
Insulin (β cell)	↓	↓	↑	↓		
Glucagon (α cell)	↓	↓		↑	↑	↑
Somatostatin (δ cell)	(↓?)	↓	↑			

Key: ↑, increased; ↓, decreased.

output by inhibiting gluconeogenesis (glucose synthesis) and glycogenolysis (glycogen breakdown). By also stimulating glycolysis (the metabolism of glucose to pyruvate), insulin promotes the formation of precursors for fatty acid synthesis. Insulin stimulates lipogenesis (the biosynthesis of fatty acids from glucose) while inhibiting fatty acid oxidation and the production of ketone bodies (ketogenesis), an alternative fuel produced only in the liver that can be used by the brain when glucose is not available.

Although the hepatic uptake of glucose, occurring via low-affinity GLUT-2 transporters, is not regulated by insulin, glucose uptake in both muscle and fat is regulated by insulin, which causes the rapid translocation of an insulin-sensitive glucose transporter (GLUT-4) to the surface of these cells. Glucose uptake by muscle accounts for the vast majority (85%) of insulin-stimulated glucose disposal. In muscle, insulin promotes glucose storage by stimulating glycogen synthesis and inhibiting glycogen catabolism. Insulin also stimulates protein synthesis in muscle.

Insulin stimulates fat storage in adipose tissue by stimulating lipoprotein lipase, the enzyme that hydrolyzes the triglycerides carried in very-low-density lipoproteins (VLDLs) and other triglyceride-rich lipoproteins to fatty acids, which can then be taken up by fat cells. Increased glucose uptake caused by the upregulation of the GLUT-4 transporter also aids in fat storage because this increases the levels of glycerol phosphate, a substrate in the esterification of free fatty acids, which are then stored as triglycerides. In fat cells, insulin also inhibits lipolysis, preventing the release of fatty acids, which are potential substrates for hepatic ketone body synthesis and/or hepatic VLDL–triglyceride synthesis. Insulin exerts this effect by preventing the phosphorylation of hormone-sensitive lipase, thus inactivating the enzyme that hydrolyzes stored triglycerides to releasable fatty acids. Together, these changes result in increased fat storage in adipose tissue.

CHECKPOINT

3. What is the half-life of insulin? How is it catabolized? What percentage is extracted on first pass through the liver?

4. How do the half-lives of C peptide and proinsulin compare with that of insulin?

5. List the main substances that stimulate insulin secretion.

6. What characteristics of the β-cell glucose transporter allow intracellular glucose levels to equal those of the extracellular space?

7. What is the probable "glucose sensor" in the β cell?

8. What are the major inhibitors of insulin secretion?

9. What are the current thoughts on the mechanisms of insulin action?

10. Which tissues are insulin dependent for glucose uptake?

11. What are three ways in which insulin stimulates fat storage?

2. Glucagon

Synthesis and Metabolism

Glucagon, a 29-amino-acid peptide, is produced in α cells of the pancreas by the proteolytic processing of proglucagon, a larger precursor protein. In addition to the pancreas, proglucagon is also expressed in the intestine and brain. While glucagon is the major bioactive metabolite produced in the pancreatic α cell, tissue-specific expression of cleaving enzymes leads to the production of glucagon-like peptide (GLP)-1 (and the non-incretin GLP-2) in response to a meal by L cells in the small intestine (Figure 18–5). This tissue-specific processing results in peptides with opposing effects on carbohydrate metabolism: Pancreatic glucagon opposes the hepatic effects of insulin, whereas GLP-1 acts as an **incretin**, enhancing glucose-stimulated insulin secretion. The circulatory half-life of glucagon is 3–6 minutes. Like insulin, glucagon is metabolized in the liver and kidneys, with the kidneys, rather than the liver, playing a significant role. Long-acting analogs of GLP-1 or enzyme inhibitors that extend the half-life of endogenous GLP-1, which also slow gastric emptying and stimulate β-cell proliferation, thus increasing β-cell mass, are a newer and important class of drugs used for the treatment of type 2 DM.

Regulation of Secretion

Glucagon and insulin, consistent with their opposing actions, are reciprocally regulated by glucose. While glucose uptake and signaling pathways are similar in β and α cells (see Figure 18–3), a higher sensitivity of α-cell K_{ATP} to the inhibitory effects of ATP depolarizes the cell membrane under conditions of high glucose to the point at which calcium channels are inactive, thus inhibiting glucagon exocytosis (see Table 18–1). Direct paracrine inhibition of glucagon secretion by insulin, somatostatin

FIGURE 18–5 Organ-specific post-translational processing of proglucagon. The major peptide produced is colored orange.

and two additional β-cell secretory products, γ-**aminobutyric acid (GABA)** and **insulin-associated zinc**, also contributes to glucagon regulation. Thus, the loss of the suppressive effects of insulin in response to hyperglycemia in diabetes results in an inappropriately high level of glucagon, which contributes to the hyperglycemia of diabetes mellitus. Incretins also inhibit glucagon secretion albeit indirectly via their insulinotropic effect. Like insulin, glucagon secretion is stimulated by amino acids, an important regulatory feature in the metabolism of protein meals. In contrast, fatty acids and ketones inhibit glucagon secretion. Other counter-regulatory hormones such as catecholamines (via a predominating β–adrenergic effect) and cortisol stimulate glucagon release.

Mechanism of Action

A major biological role of glucagon is to oppose the hypoglycemic effects of insulin (hence its name deriving from "glucose agonist") by inducing hepatic glucose production. Glucagon binds to a G protein–coupled glucagon receptor present on the cell surface of hepatocytes, activating adenylyl cyclase and generating cAMP. Cyclic AMP activates protein kinase A, which activates gene transcription for the enzymes responsible for the biologic activity of glucagon in the liver, and subsequently phosphorylates and activates these same enzymes. There is also some evidence that the glucagon receptor may act via an adenylyl cyclase-independent mechanism by stimulating phospholipase C.

Effects

The actions of glucagon were first demonstrated in 1921 by Banting and Best when they observed a mild transient hyperglycemia preceding insulin-induced hypoglycemia when testing pancreatic extracts in vivo. Glucagon is a **counter-regulatory hormone**, acting in a catabolic fashion to oppose the effects of insulin. Indeed, glucagon injections are used clinically to treat severe hypoglycemia. Hepatic effects of glucagon (see Table 18–2) include the following: (1) increased hepatic glucose output via the release of glycogen stores (glycogenolysis) and, in concert with other counter-regulatory hormones, stimulation of hepatic glucose synthesis (gluconeogenesis); (2) increased hepatic uptake of amino acids, which fuels gluconeogenesis; and (3) stimulation of fatty acid oxidation and ketogenesis, thus providing an alternative fuel (**ketone bodies**) that can be used by the brain when glucose is not available. The physiologic significance of glucagon receptors in nonhepatic tissue (kidney, adipose, pancreas) is less certain. For example, glucagon, while less potent, shares with GLP-1 the ability to enhance glucose-induced β-cell insulin secretion. Evidence also supports its ability to induce satiety and increase the basal metabolic rate. These latter points suggest a potential beneficial medicinal use for glucagon in obesity, which is clearly counterbalanced by evidence that elevated glucagon levels contribute to hyperglycemia in diabetes, an effect that has raised interest in glucagon inhibition for diabetes treatment.

3. Somatostatin
Synthesis, Metabolism & Secretion Regulation

Like preproglucagon, preprosomatostatin is synthesized in the pancreas, gastrointestinal (GI) tract, and brain, where it is differentially processed in a tissue-specific fashion to produce several biologically active cyclic peptides. Somatostatin-14 (SS-14), the first somatostatin to be isolated, is a 14-amino-acid peptide that was initially discovered in the hypothalamus as the factor responsible for inhibiting growth hormone release. Only later was it appreciated that δ cells of the pancreas also secrete SS-14. In the brain and intestine, somatostatin-28 (SS-28), an amino-terminally extended peptide that includes the 14-amino-acid sequence of SS-14, is also produced from preprosomatostatin and has a range of action comparable to that of SS-14 but a potency that is somewhat greater. The half-life of somatostatin (<3 minutes) is shorter than that of insulin and glucagon. Because somatostatin has been shown to inhibit the synthesis and secretion of most peptide hormones, synthetic somatostatin analogs, such as octreotide, that have a much longer half-life (hours) have been developed for clinical use in inhibiting ectopic peptide hormone production by a variety of tumors. The same secretagogues that stimulate insulin secretion also stimulate somatostatin (see Table 18–1). These include glucose, amino acids, enteric hormones, and glucagon.

Mechanism of Action and Effects

Somatostatin exerts its effects via binding to a family of inhibitory G (G_i) protein–coupled receptors (SST1-5) that are distributed in a tissue-specific fashion. In all tissues in which somatostatin is produced, it acts primarily in an inhibitory fashion. In the endocrine pancreas, somatostatin is thought to act via paracrine effects on the other islet cells, inhibiting the release of insulin, glucagon (see Table 18–1), and PP. In addition, somatostatin acts in an autocrine fashion to inhibit its own release. In the GI tract, somatostatin retards the absorption of nutrients through multiple mechanisms, including inhibiting gut motility, inhibiting several enteric peptides, and inhibiting pancreatic exocrine function. Consistent with the multiple inhibitory effects of this peptide, the synthetic somatostatin analog octreotide has multiple clinical uses, including inhibiting hormone production by pituitary adenomas, inhibiting certain types of chronic diarrhea, inhibiting tumor growth, and inhibiting bleeding from esophageal varices.

4. Pancreatic Polypeptide

Pancreatic polypeptide (PP), a 36-amino-acid peptide produced by the PP cells (F cells) in the islets of the posterior lobe of the head of the pancreas, is released in response to a mixed meal, an effect that appears to be mediated by protein and vagal stimulation. While long known to inhibit gastrointestinal motility and pancreatic exocrine secretions, more recent evidence suggests that PP may also control satiety and weight, inhibiting food intake and stimulating energy expenditure, making it a target of interest for obesity treatment. These latter effects of PP (a member of the neuropeptide Y family of peptide hormones) are mediated centrally, via binding to an inhibitory G protein–coupled Y4 receptor and are thought to involve the inhibition of hepatic vagal nerve afferent activity.

CHECKPOINT

12. What are some important stimulators and inhibitors of glucagon secretion?

13. What is the major target organ for glucagon? What are the mechanisms of glucagon action?

14. Which metabolic pathways are sensitive to glucagon, and how are they affected?

15. Which hormone antagonizes glucagon's effect on metabolic pathways?

16. Where else in the body besides the islets of Langerhans is glucagon made?

17. By what mechanisms can GLPs enhance glucose-stimulated insulin secretion?

18. What is the role of somatostatin in the islets of Langerhans?

5. Hormonal Control of Carbohydrate Metabolism

Carbohydrate metabolism is primarily controlled by the relative amounts of insulin and glucagon produced by the endocrine pancreas (Figure 18–6; see also Table 18–2). Conversely, the dysregulation of both of these hormones contributes to hyperglycemia in diabetes. Under normal conditions, when plasma glucose levels are high, the actions of insulin predominate, including the suppression of glucagon secretion. Fuel storage is promoted by insulin stimulating glycogen storage in the liver; glucose uptake, glycogen synthesis, and protein synthesis by muscle; and fat storage by adipose tissue. Insulin inhibits the mobilization of substrates from peripheral tissues and opposes any effects of glucagon on the stimulation of hepatic glucose output.

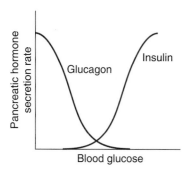

FIGURE 18–6 Pancreatic islet cell secretion of glucagon (from α cells) and insulin (from β cells), which are reciprocally regulated by glucose, plays a key role in maintaining glucose homeostasis.

In contrast, when glucose levels are low, plasma insulin levels are suppressed and the effects of glucagon predominate in the liver (ie, increased hepatic glucose output and ketone body formation). In the absence of insulin, muscle glucose uptake is markedly decreased, muscle protein is catabolized, and fat is mobilized from adipose tissue. Therefore, with insulinopenia, glucose loads cannot be cleared, and substrates for hepatic gluconeogenesis (amino acids, glycerol) and ketogenesis (fatty acids)—processes stimulated by glucagon—are increased.

Fasting State

After an overnight fast, the liver plays a primary role in maintaining blood glucose by producing glucose at the same rate at which it is used by resting tissues. Glucose uptake and use occur predominantly in tissues that do not require insulin for glucose uptake, such as the brain. Hepatic glucose output is stimulated by glucagon and is primarily a result of glycogenolysis, which can provide, on average, an 8-hour supply of glucose. The low levels of insulin present (basal secretion of 0.25–1.0 unit/h) are insufficient to block the release of fatty acids from fat, which provide fuel for muscles (fatty acid oxidation) and substrate for hepatic ketogenesis. However, these levels of insulin are sufficient to prevent excessive lipolysis, ketogenesis, and gluconeogenesis, thus preventing hyperglycemia and ketoacidosis.

With prolonged fasting (>24–60 hours), liver glycogen stores are depleted. Glucagon levels rise slightly, and insulin levels decline further. Gluconeogenesis now becomes the sole source of hepatic glucose production, using substrates such as amino acids that are mobilized from the periphery at a greater rate. With starvation, a switch occurs in the liver from gluconeogenesis to the production of ketones, an alternative fuel source that provides 90% of the energy used by the brain, a critical organ that accounts for 25% of basal metabolic energy needs. In this manner, survival is prolonged as muscle protein is conserved in favor of increased fatty acid mobilization from adipose tissue, a process made possible by increased insulinopenia. The liver then converts fatty acids to ketone bodies, a process stimulated by glucagon. With prolonged fasting or starvation, the kidney also begins to contribute significantly to gluconeogenesis.

Fed State

With the ingestion of a carbohydrate load, insulin secretion is stimulated and glucagon is suppressed. Hepatic glucose production and ketogenesis are suppressed by the high ratio of insulin to glucagon. Insulin stimulates hepatic glycogen storage. Insulin-mediated glucose uptake, which occurs primarily in muscle, is also stimulated, as is muscle glycogen synthesis. Fat storage occurs in adipose tissue.

With the ingestion of a protein meal, both insulin and glucagon are stimulated. In this way, insulin stimulates amino acid uptake and protein formation by muscle. However, the stimulation of hepatic glucose output by glucagon counterbalances the tendency of insulin to cause hypoglycemia.

Conditions of Stress

During severe stress, when fuel delivery to the brain is in jeopardy, **counter-regulatory hormones**, in addition to glucagon, act synergistically. They maintain blood glucose levels by maximizing the hepatic output of glucose and the peripheral mobilization of substrates and by minimizing fuel storage. **Glucagon** and **epinephrine** act within minutes to elevate blood glucose levels, whereas the counter-regulatory effects of **cortisol** and **growth hormone** are not seen for several hours. Epinephrine, cortisol, and growth hormone stimulate glucagon release, and epinephrine inhibits insulin, thus maximally increasing the glucagon–insulin ratio. In addition, these three hormones act directly on the liver to increase hepatic glucose production and peripherally to stimulate lipolysis and inhibit insulin-sensitive glucose uptake. During severe stress, hyperglycemia may actually result from the combined effects of counter-regulatory hormones.

Similar but less marked effects occur in response to exercise when glucagon, catecholamines, and, to a lesser extent, cortisol help meet the several-fold increase in the rate of glucose use resulting from exercising muscle by increasing hepatic glucose output and the lipolysis of fat stores, effects made possible by lowering insulin levels. Low insulin levels also allow muscles to use glycogen stores for energy.

Role of Renal Gluconeogenesis in Glucose Homeostasis

The kidneys and liver both express the enzymes required to augment the glucose pool by gluconeogenesis and the secretion of glucose stored as glycogen. While the kidney contributes little to the glucose pool during an overnight fasting, it contributes approximately 50% of endogenous glucose production during a prolonged (>40 hours) fast. Gluconeogenesis predominates in the kidney, as its glycogen stores are minimal, a process stimulated by epinephrine, inhibited by insulin, and unaffected by glucagon.

CHECKPOINT

19. In insulinopenic states, why are substrates for hepatic gluconeogenesis and ketogenesis increased?
20. What is the effect of a protein meal on insulin versus glucagon secretion?
21. What is the difference in time course of action of the various counter-regulatory hormones?

PATHOPHYSIOLOGY OF SELECTED ENDOCRINE PANCREATIC DISORDERS

DIABETES MELLITUS

Clinical Presentation

Diabetes mellitus is a heterogeneous disorder defined by the presence of hyperglycemia. Diagnostic criteria for diabetes include the following (any one of which establishes the diagnosis): (1) a fasting plasma glucose (FPG) of ≥126 mg/dL (7.0 mmol/L); (2) classic symptoms of hyperglycemia plus a random plasma glucose of ≥200 mg/dL (11.1 mmol/L); (3) a 2-hour plasma glucose level ≥200 mg/dL following a standard 75 g oral glucose load (**oral glucose tolerance test [OGTT]**); or (4) a glycated hemoglobin (**Hb$_{A1C}$**) >6.5%. While Hb$_{A1C}$ (**A1C**) values, which reflect average blood glucose levels during the previous 2–3 months (the predicted half-life of erythrocytes), have long been used to monitor therapeutic responses, their use for diagnosis is more recent now that assays are more standardized and evidence supports their correlation with risk of diabetic complications, analogous to FPG. The advantages of using A1C for screening (no need to fast, a reflection of glucose over time) are countered by its lower sensitivity, as it identifies one-third fewer cases of undiagnosed diabetes in large epidemiologic studies, leading to some controversy surrounding its appropriate use.

Hyperglycemia in all cases is due to a functional deficiency of insulin action. Deficient insulin action can result from a decrease in insulin secretion by the β cells of the pancreas, a decreased response to insulin by target tissues (**insulin resistance**), and/or an increase in the counter-regulatory hormones that oppose the effects of insulin. The relative contributions of these three factors form the basis for the classification of this disorder into subtypes and also help explain the characteristic clinical presentations of each subtype (Table 18–3).

More than 90% of diabetes cases are believed to occur in the context of a genetic predisposition and are classified as either **type 1 diabetes mellitus** or **type 2 diabetes mellitus** (Tables 18–3 and 18–4). The worldwide prevalence of both type 1 DM and type 2 DM has been increasing over the past three decades, reaching a total prevalence of 9% in 2014 in adults 20 years or older (14% in the United States). Type 1 DM is much less common than type 2 DM, accounting for 5–10% of cases of primary diabetes. Type 1 DM is characterized by the autoimmune destruction of pancreatic β cells with resultant severe insulin deficiency. In a minority of patients, because autoantibodies are not detected, the cause of type 1 DM is unclear (idiopathic). The disease commonly affects individuals younger than 30 years, peaking in incidence at puberty, but also can be diagnosed in adults older than 50 years of age. Although autoimmune destruction of the β cells does not occur acutely, clinical symptoms usually do (Figure 18–7). Patients present after only days or weeks of polyuria, polydipsia, and weight loss with markedly elevated serum glucose concentrations. **Ketone bodies** are also increased because of

TABLE 18–3   Etiologic classification of diabetes mellitus.

Classification	Description and Categories
I. Type 1 diabetes mellitus	β-cell destruction, usually leading to absolute insulin deficiency • Autoimmune • Idiopathic
II. Type 2 diabetes mellitus	Ranges from predominantly insulin resistant with relative insulin deficiency to a predominant secretory defect with insulin resistance
III. Gestational diabetes mellitus (GDM)	Defined as any degree of glucose intolerance occurring or first being recognized during pregnancy, a time when insulin resistance and β-cell hyperplasia occur normally. Women diagnosed with gestational DM have a high risk for later developing type 2 DM.
IV. Other specific types	• Genetic defects of β-cell function

For category IV, the full list of items:

• Genetic defects of β-cell function
  - Maturity-onset diabetes of the young (MODY), autosomal dominant mutations of single genes:
    • MODY 3, *HNF-1α*
    • MODY 2, *GCK* (glucokinase)
    • MODY 1, *HNF-4α*
    • MODY, other rare forms
  - Transient neonatal diabetes, most commonly imprinting defect on 6q24
  - Permanent neonatal diabetes; eg, gene encoding subunit of β-cell K_{ATP}
  - Mitochondrial DNA
  - Others

• Genetic defects in insulin action
  - Type A insulin resistance
  - Leprechaunism
  - Rabson–Mendenhall syndrome
  - Lipoatrophic diabetes
  - Others

• Diseases of the exocrine pancreas
  - Pancreatitis
  - Trauma, pancreatectomy
  - Neoplasia
  - Cystic fibrosis
  - Hemochromatosis
  - Fibrocalculous pancreatopathy
  - Others

• Endocrine disorders
  - Acromegaly
  - Cushing syndrome
  - Glucagonoma
  - Pheochromocytoma
  - Hyperthyroidism
  - Somatostatinoma
  - Aldosteronoma
  - Others

• Drug-induced
  - α-Interferon
  - β-Adrenergic agonists
  - Diazoxide
  - Glucocorticoids
  - Nicotinic acid
  - Pentamidine
  - Phenytoin
  - Thiazides
  - Thyroid hormone
  - Others

• Infections
  - Congenital rubella
  - Cytomegalovirus
  - Others

• Uncommon forms of immune-mediated diabetes
  - "Stiff-man" syndrome
  - Anti-insulin receptor antibodies
  - Others

• Other genetic syndromes sometimes associated with diabetes
  - Down syndrome
  - Klinefelter syndrome
  - Turner syndrome
  - Wolfram syndrome
  - Friedreich ataxia
  - Huntington chorea
  - Laurence–Moon–Biedl syndrome
  - Myotonic dystrophy
  - Porphyria
  - Prader–Willi syndrome
  - Others

HNF, hepatocyte nuclear factor.
Data from the American Diabetes Association. Diagnosis and classification of diabetes mellitus. Diabetes Care. 2014:37(Suppl 1):S81–90.

TABLE 18–4 **Some features distinguishing type 1 diabetes mellitus from type 2 diabetes mellitus.**

	Type 1 DM	Type 2 DM
Epidemiology		
Age at diagnosis	Childhood	Adult
		(incidence increasing with obesity in children)
Prevalence (in United States)	0.3%, age <20 years	14%, age >20 years
Phenotype		
β-Cell insulin secretion abnormal	Absolute deficiency	Impaired secretion
Insulin resistance	No	Yes
Obese	No	Yes
BMI	Usually <25	>25 in 85%; >30 in 50%
Autoimmune disease	Yes	No
Islet cell antibodies	In 90%	No
Postulated environmental triggers	Viral infections, dietary exposures (cow's milk, cereal)	Obesity (diet, exercise)
Genotype		
Concordance in monozygotic twins	30%	90%
Incidence in offspring		
Single parent affected	5%	40%
Both parents affected	10%	50%
Genetic loci associated with risk	HLA class II genes (eg, DR-DQ)	Heterogeneous sets of interacting genes

BMI, body mass index: weight (kg)/height^2 (m^2).

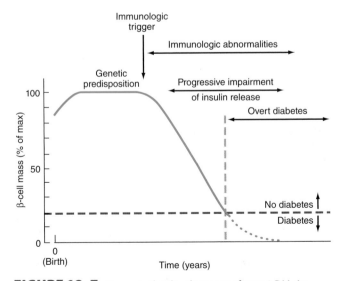

FIGURE 18–7 Stages in the development of type 1 DM. An initial asymptomatic period defined primarily by the presence of β-cell autoantibodies is followed by a stage during which antibodies persist and dysglycemia begins as β cells are destroyed. In a final stage, symptoms of severe insulin insufficiency appear, culminating in a diagnosis of type 1 DM. (Adapted from Kaufman ER: *Medical Management of Type 1 Diabetes*, 6th ed. American Diabetes Association, 2012.)

the marked lack of insulin, resulting in severe, life-threatening acidosis (**diabetic ketoacidosis [DKA]**). Patients with type 1 DM require treatment with insulin.

Type 2 DM differs from type 1 DM in several distinct ways (Table 18–4). Type 2 DM accounts for the overwhelming majority of cases of diabetes (90–95%); has a stronger genetic component; increases in prevalence with age, occurring most commonly in adults (ie, 18% of individuals older than 65 years worldwide and 33% in the United States); has increased markedly in prevalence in parallel with increases in obesity; occurs more commonly (two-fold increase) in Native American, Black, Hispanic, and Asian American populations in the United States; and is associated with increased resistance to the effects of insulin, as well as a decrease in insulin secretion by the pancreas. It is often (85% of cases) associated with obesity, a factor that increases insulin resistance. Thus, the rising prevalence of diabetes worldwide is largely attributable to the increasing prevalence of obesity (13% obese; 38% overweight). **Insulin resistance** is the hallmark of type 2 DM. Because these patients often have varying amounts of residual insulin secretion, which prevent severe hyperglycemia or ketosis, they are often asymptomatic and not diagnosed until 5–7 years after the actual onset of disease (frank hyperglycemia) by the discovery of an elevated fasting glucose on routine screening tests. Population screening surveys show that a remarkable 36% of cases of type 2 DM in the United States, and 50% of cases worldwide, remain undiagnosed. Additionally, it is estimated that almost 40% of the adult population in the United States is insulin resistant and hence in a pre-diabetic (still normoglycemic) state. Once diagnosed with type 2 DM, most individuals (70%) are managed with lifestyle modifications (eg, diet, exercise, weight management) alone or in combination with medications that (1) enhance endogenous glucose-independent insulin secretion (sulfonylureas); (2) amplify endogenous glucose-dependent insulin secretion (incretins such as GLP-1); (3) decrease insulin resistance in hepatic or peripheral tissues (eg, sulfonylureas or glitazones, respectively); (4) interfere with the intestinal absorption of carbohydrates (eg, intestinal α-glycosidase inhibitors); or (5) inhibit renal glucose reabsorption (sodium-glucose co-transporter 2 [SGLT2] inhibitors). Type 2 diabetic patients do not usually require insulin treatment for survival. However, to achieve optimal glucose control, one-third of patients with type 2 DM in the United States are treated with insulin alone or in combination with other drugs.

An epidemic of type 2 DM is occurring worldwide, particularly in non-European populations; it has been estimated that 1 in 3 children born after 2000 will develop diabetes, particularly type 2 DM, in their lifetime. Thus, while type 1 DM remains the most common cause of diabetes in children younger than 10 years (regardless of ethnicity) and in older non-Hispanic white children, type 2 DM accounts for more than 50% of diabetes diagnoses in older children of Hispanic, African American, Native American, and Asian Pacific Islander ancestry. In all age groups and ethnicities, the increased incidence of type 2 DM is associated with obesity.

Other causes of diabetes, accounting for less than 5% of cases, include processes that destroy the pancreas (eg, pancreatitis), that specifically inhibit insulin secretion (eg, the genetic β-cell defect that causes maturity-onset diabetes of the young [MODY]), that induce insulin resistance (eg, certain HIV protease inhibitors), or that increase counter-regulatory hormones (eg, Cushing syndrome) (see Table 18–3, part IV). Clinical presentations in these cases depend on the exact nature of the process and are not discussed here.

Gestational diabetes mellitus occurs in pregnant women with an incidence ranging from 9% in the general population in the United States to 30% in Native American women (see Table 18–3, part III). It tends to resolve at parturition, although it may recur with subsequent pregnancies. The prevalence of gestational diabetes mellitus in a population varies in direct proportion to the prevalence of diabetes. Up to 50% of women with gestational diabetes mellitus eventually progress to diabetes (predominantly type 2 DM). Gestational diabetes usually occurs in the second half of gestation, precipitated by the increasing levels of hormones such as chorionic somatomammotropin, progesterone, cortisol, and prolactin, which have counter-regulatory anti-insulin effects. Because of its potential adverse effects on fetal outcome, gestational diabetes in the United States is currently diagnosed or ruled out by routine screening with an oral glucose load at 24 weeks of gestation in those women at average risk or at the first prenatal visit those women at high risk due to being obese, older than 25 years of age, a member of an ethnic group with a high prevalence of diabetes, or having a family history of diabetes.

Etiology

A. Type 1 Diabetes Mellitus

Type 1 DM is an autoimmune disease caused by the selective destruction of pancreatic β cells by T lymphocytes targeting ill-defined β-cell antigens. An asymptomatic stage of β-cell autoantibody positivity, which peaks in incidence at 1–2 years of age, is followed by at least 1–2 years of dysglycemia (abnormal OGTT and A1C and loss of first-phase insulin release) attributable to gradual T-cell mediated islet dysfunction and/or destruction (see Figure 18–7). The clinical onset of symptoms, and thus diagnosis, occurs only after sufficient β-cell mass has been lost to cause extreme insulinopenia (see Figure 18–7). At the time of diagnosis, ongoing inflammation is present in some islets, whereas other islets are atrophic and consist only of glucagon-secreting α cells and somatostatin-secreting δ cells.

Islet cell antibodies (**ICAs**), while appearing early in the course of disease, are thought to serve as markers, rather than mediators, of β-cell destruction and appear in a predictable course, beginning with antibodies targeting **insulin** or **glutamic acid decarboxylase 65** (**GAD65**) and followed by antibodies directed against a **β-cell zinc transporter** (**ZnT8**) and the **tyrosine phosphatase-IA-2 protein** (**IA2**). Risk of progression to symptomatic type 1 DM correlates with the number of detectable antibodies, which are also detected more frequently in first-degree relatives (5% vs <1% in the general population). Because the appearance of autoantibodies is followed by the progressive impairment of insulin release in response to glucose (see Figure 18–7), both criteria have been used with great success to identify at-risk first-degree relatives. However, because only 15% of individuals newly diagnosed with type 1 DM have a positive family history, these targeted screening methods cannot be used to identify the vast majority of individuals developing this low-incident disease.

At least 50% of the genetic susceptibility for type 1 DM has been linked to the genes of the major histocompatibility complex (MHC) that encode **class II human leukocyte antigen** (**HLA**) **molecules** expressed on the surface of specific antigen-presenting cells such as macrophages. Class II molecules form a complex with processed foreign antigens or autoantigens, which then activates CD4 T lymphocytes via interaction with the T-cell receptor. Alleles at the HLA-DR or HLA-DQ loci have the strongest influence on the risk of type 1 DM. While 95% of individuals with type 1 DM have either DR3-DQ2 or DR4-DQ8 haplotypes, they share this genotype with 40% of the general population. In addition, only 6% of children with high-risk HLA types will develop diabetes. Thus, the identification of HLA haplotypes remains a research tool. Genome-wide association studies (GWASs) have also identified more than 50 non-HLA genetic factors, mostly related to immune function, that make smaller contributions to disease risk.

While genetic susceptibility clearly plays a role in type 1 DM, the 30% concordance rate in identical twins, as well as the continuing increase in the incidence of type 1 DM since World War II, provides additional evidence that environmental factors may also play a critical role. Evidence suggests that viral infections, such as congenital exposure to rubella, may precipitate disease, particularly in genetically susceptible individuals. It is hypothesized that an immune response to foreign antigens could incite β-cell destruction if these foreign antigens have some homology with islet cell antigens (**molecular mimicry**). For example, coxsackievirus infections are associated with the onset of type 1 DM, and one particular coxsackie viral protein shares homology with the islet cell antigen GAD. Vitamin D deficiency also correlates with a greater risk of type 1 DM, which may partially explain the increased incidence of type 1 DM at higher latitudes.

B. Type 2 Diabetes Mellitus

Given the current obesity-associated type 2 DM epidemic, environmental factors are clearly critical in the development of this disorder. And yet, the genetic components underlying type 2 DM are even stronger than those associated with type 1 DM (eg, 90% vs. 30% concordance in identical twins, respectively; see Table 18–3). However, identifying what are clearly polygenic loci contributing to type 2 DM risk remains an elusive goal, since, after decades of ongoing work, beginning with efforts targeting specific candidate genes and more recently including GWAS studies, only 10% of the heritability of type

2 DM has been explained. A small subset of monogenic type 2 DM cases has been identified. **Maturity-onset diabetes of the young** (**MODY**) is one such autosomal dominant disorder (see Table 18–3, part IV), accounting for 1–5% of type 2 DM cases. MODY is caused by mutations in glucokinase, the β-cell glucose sensor, or in five other distinct pancreatic genes, and is characterized by the onset of mild diabetes in lean individuals before the age of 25.

In contrast to the causal role of an absolute lack of insulin in type 1 DM or insufficient insulin release in MODY, in the majority of cases of type 2 DM, two metabolic defects are responsible for hyperglycemia: (1) target tissue resistance to the effects of insulin; and (2) inadequate pancreatic β-cell insulin secretion in the setting of insulin resistance. The relative importance of these two defects remains a matter of debate that will likely not be easily settled owing to the polygenic nature of the disorder. Temporally, it is clear that **insulin resistance**, a hallmark of this disorder, precedes the onset of diabetes by decades, usually occurring in association with obesity, and requires a compensatory increase in pancreatic insulin secretion to maintain euglycemia (Figure 18–8). Overt disease (ie, hyperglycemia) occurs much later, after a **progressive decline in β-cell function** (see Figure 18–8), which first manifests as an impairment in the acute insulin release that precedes sustained insulin secretion in response to a meal (**first-phase insulin release**). Indeed, while increases in β-cell mass of up to 50% have been reported in obese individuals compared to lean individuals, declines in β-cell mass of 40%

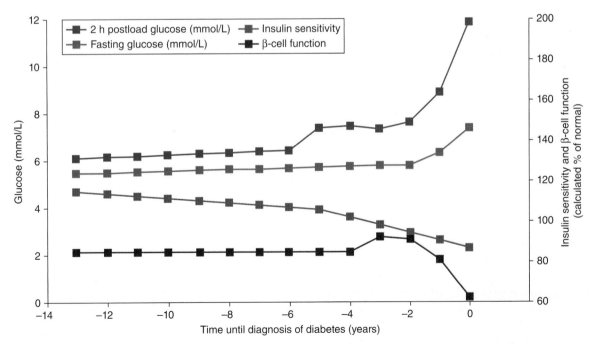

FIGURE 18–8 Stages in the development of type 2 DM from a prediabetic, insulin-resistant state. As insulin sensitivity decreases, insulin-mediated glucose disposal after a meal is impaired owing to insulin resistance in skeletal muscle despite increased pancreatic insulin secretion. With continued insulin resistance, as pancreatic insulin secretion begins to fail, fasting glucose increases because insulin activity is now insufficient to suppress hepatic glucose output. Time 0 refers to the time of diagnosis of diabetes. Data are from the British Whitehall II study of 505 diabetes cases. (Adapted from Kaufman ER: *Medical Management of Type 1 Diabetes*, 6th ed. American Diabetes Association, 2012; and Tabak AG et al. Trajectories of glycemia, insulin sensitivity and insulin secretion before diagnosis of type 2 diabetes: an analysis from the Whitehall II study. Lancet. 2009 June 27;373(9682):2215–21.)

to 60% owing to **β-cell apoptosis**, have been documented in patients with impaired fasting glucose and frank type 2 DM, respectively. In addition to possible underlying genetic defects, chronic exposure to elevated free fatty acids and/or hyperglycemia (**glucolipotoxicity**), as well as inflammatory cytokines, may contribute to impaired β-cell insulin secretion in a setting of insulin resistance. Lipid accumulation in β cells is also thought to contribute to impaired β-cell function by various mechanisms, including activation of the pro-apoptotic unfolded protein response (UPR) in the endoplasmic reticulum. These defects explain the benefits of type 2 DM pharmacologic interventions aimed at increasing β-cell insulin secretion (eg, sulphonylureas, incretins).

Obesity, a major driver of the worldwide increase in diabetes prevalence, clearly plays a critical role in disease pathogenesis. Not only are 85% of patients with type 2 DM obese, but even a 5–10% weight loss in obese individuals with type 2 DM can ameliorate or even terminate the disorder. Insulin resistance is the key factor linking obesity and type 2 DM. Nutritional excess from any source ultimately leads to increased free fatty acid (FFA) storage as triglyceride in adipose tissue. While subcutaneous tissue is the body's major site of fat storage, its inability to adequately expand to accommodate excess lipid in obesity is thought to contribute to an increase in **visceral (central) adipose tissue**. Visceral adipose tissue is the adipose site that most closely correlates with insulin resistance owing to its high lipid turnover, which can be attributed to (1) its enhanced sensitivity to the stimulatory effects of counter-regulatory hormones (increased number of β-adrenergic receptors and increased local conversion of inactive cortisone to active cortisol owing to high levels of type 1 11β-hydroxysteroid dehydrogenase); and (2) weaker suppressive effect of insulin owing to lower insulin receptor affinity. **Excess lipolysis** from visceral stores directly feeds FFAs into the liver, thus contributing to hepatic lipid accumulation (**steatosis**), insulin resistance, and increased hepatic gluconeogenesis, which raises the level of fasting glucose. Metformin, a first-line therapy for type 2 DM, is particularly effective in reversing these hepatic effects of insulin resistance.

Local deposition of excess lipids in both the liver and muscle has been postulated to block insulin receptor signaling (phosphorylation of insulin receptor substrate-1 [IRS-1]) owing to sustained activation of the theta form of protein kinase C, an effect that occurs secondary to lipid-induced increases in intracellular diacylglycerol (DAG) content. Lower rates of mitochondrial fat oxidation, which occur with aging, can also contribute to excess lipid stores and insulin resistance, an observation that may help to explain the increased prevalence of type 2 DM with age. The release of factors from visceral adipose tissue in addition to FFA also drive insulin resistance, including (1) the dysregulated secretion of fat-specific proteins (**adipokines**), such as **adiponectin**, an insulin-sensitizing hormone, and **leptin**, an anti-diabetogenic hormone that acts centrally to control satiety and enhance insulin sensitivity; and (2) the increased production of adipose-derived **inflammatory cytokines**. For example, the secretion of **tumor**

necrosis factor (TNF) from macrophages attracted into adipose tissue by other adipocyte secretory products (eg, **macrophage chemoattractant protein**-1 [**MCP-1**]) is thought to block **peroxisome proliferator–activated receptor gamma (PPARδ)**, an adipose transcription factor that enhances insulin sensitivity by altering adipokine secretion and decreasing FFA release. Glitzazones, PPARδ agonists used to treat type 2 DM, help restore insulin sensitivity by countering these effects. In skeletal muscle, decreases in insulin-stimulated GLUT-4 translocation after a meal impair insulin-stimulated glucose disposal/transport, causing postprandial hyperglycemia. Hyperglycemia may also lead to increased flux through otherwise minor glucose metabolic pathways that result in products associated with insulin resistance (eg, hexosamines). Hyperinsulinemia can itself contribute to insulin resistance by downregulating insulin receptor levels and desensitizing downstream pathways.

CHECKPOINT

22. What are the key characteristics of type 1 DM and type 2 DM?

23. What is the role of heredity versus the environment in each of the two major types of diabetes mellitus?

24. What are two possible mechanisms of insulin resistance in type 2 DM?

25. What is the role of obesity in type 2 DM?

Pathology & Pathogenesis

No matter the origin, all types of diabetes result from a relative deficiency of insulin action. In addition, glucagon levels can be inappropriately high. This high **glucagon–insulin ratio** creates a state similar to that seen in fasting and results in a superfasting milieu that is inappropriate for the maintenance of normal fuel homeostasis (see Table 18–2 and Figure 18–6).

The resulting metabolic derangements depend on the degree of loss of insulin action. Adipose tissue is most sensitive to insulin action. Therefore, low insulin activity is capable of suppressing excessive lipolysis and enhancing fat storage. Higher levels of insulin are required to oppose glucagon effects on the liver and block hepatic glucose output. In normal individuals, basal levels of insulin activity are capable of mediating both these responses. The liver in particular is exquisitely responsive to changes in pancreatic insulin secretion owing to its high sensitivity and exposure to elevated levels of insulin in the portal circulation. However, the ability of skeletal muscle to respond to a glucose load with insulin-mediated glucose uptake requires the stimulated secretion of additional insulin from the pancreas.

Mild deficiencies in insulin action are, therefore, frequently manifested by an inability of skeletal muscle, which is responsible for 85% of postprandial glucose clearance, to clear glucose loads. Clinically, this results in **postprandial hyperglycemia** (see Figure 18–8). Such individuals, most commonly type 2 diabetics with residual insulin secretion but increased insulin resistance, will have abnormal oral glucose tolerance test results and/or high nonfasting (postprandial) glucose levels. However, fasting glucose levels remain normal because sufficient insulin action is present to counterbalance the glucagon-mediated hepatic glucose output that maintains them. When a further loss of insulin action occurs, glucagon's effects on the liver are not sufficiently counterbalanced. Individuals, therefore, have both postprandial hyperglycemia and **fasting hyperglycemia** (see Figure 18–8). Interestingly, skeletal tissue remains insulin sensitive in some prediabetic individuals who may present instead with isolated increases in hepatic glucose output and fasting glucose levels. Because of the importance of excessive hepatic glucose output in the pathogenesis of type 2 DM (driven by insulin resistance and inappropriately high levels of glucagon), metformin, a drug that specifically targets hepatic glucose output, is used as a first-line treatment in these individuals.

Although type 2 diabetics usually have some degree of residual endogenous insulin action, type 1 diabetics have none. Therefore, untreated or inadequately treated type 1 diabetics manifest the most severe signs of insulin deficiency. In addition to fasting and postprandial hyperglycemia, they also develop **ketosis**, because a marked lack or absolute deficiency of insulin allows for maximal lipolysis of fat stores to supply substrates for unopposed glucagon stimulation of ketogenesis in the liver.

Fatty acids liberated from increased lipolysis, in addition to being metabolized by the liver into ketone bodies, can also be re-esterified and packaged into VLDLs. Furthermore, insulin deficiency causes a decrease in lipoprotein lipase, the enzyme responsible for the hydrolysis of VLDL triglycerides in preparation for fatty acid storage in adipose tissue, thereby slowing VLDL clearance. Therefore, both type 1 and type 2 diabetics can have **hypertriglyceridemia** as a result of both an increase in VLDL production and a decrease in VLDL clearance.

Because insulin also stimulates amino acid uptake and protein synthesis in muscle, the decrease in insulin action in diabetes results in decreased muscle protein synthesis. Marked insulinopenia, such as occurs in type 1 DM, can cause a negative nitrogen balance and marked **protein wasting**. Amino acids not taken up by muscle are instead diverted to the liver, where they are used to fuel gluconeogenesis.

In both type 1 DM and type 2 DM, the superimposition of stress-induced counter-regulatory hormones on what is already an insulinopenic state exacerbates the metabolic manifestations of deficient insulin action. The stress of infection, for example, can, therefore, induce DKA in both type 1 and some type 2 diabetics.

In addition to the metabolic derangements discussed previously, diabetes causes other chronic, progressive complications that are responsible for the high morbidity and mortality rates associated with this disease. **Diabetic complications** are largely the result of vascular disease affecting both the microvasculature (retinopathy, nephropathy, some types of neuropathy) and the macrovasculature (coronary artery disease, peripheral vascular disease).

Clinical Manifestations

A. Acute Complications

1. Hyperglycemia—When elevated glucose levels exceed the renal threshold for glucose reabsorption (approximately 200 mg/dL), **glucosuria** results. This causes an osmotic diuresis manifested clinically by **polyuria**, including **nocturia**. Dehydration results, stimulating thirst that results in **polydipsia**. A significant loss of calories can result from glucosuria, because urinary glucose losses can exceed 75 g/d (75 g × 4 kcal/g = 300 kcal/d). **Polyphagia** also accompanies uncontrolled hyperglycemia. The three "polys" of diabetes—polyuria, polydipsia, and polyphagia—are common presenting symptoms in both type 1 and symptomatic type 2 patients. Weight loss can also occur as a result of both dehydration and loss of calories in the urine. Severe weight loss is most likely to occur in patients with severe insulinopenia (type 1 DM) and is due to both caloric loss and muscle wasting. Increased protein catabolism also contributes to the growth failure seen in children with type 1 DM.

Elevated glucose levels raise plasma osmolality:

$$\text{Osmolality (mOsm/L)} = 2[Na^+(mEq/L) + K^+(mEq/L)]$$
$$+ \frac{\text{Glucose (mg/dL)}}{18} + \frac{\text{BUN (mg/dL)}}{2.8}$$

Changes in the water content of the lens of the eye in response to changes in osmolality can cause blurred vision.

In women, glucosuria can lead to an increased incidence of candidal vulvovaginitis. In some cases, this may be the only presenting symptom. In uncircumcised men, candidal balanitis (a similar infection of the glans penis) can occur.

2. Diabetic ketoacidosis—A profound loss of insulin activity leads not only to increased serum glucose levels because of increased hepatic glucose output and decreased glucose uptake by insulin-sensitive tissues, but also to ketogenesis. In the absence of insulin, lipolysis is stimulated, providing fatty acids that are preferentially converted to ketone bodies in the liver by unopposed glucagon action. Typically, profound hyperglycemia and ketosis (DKA) occur in type 1 diabetics, individuals who lack endogenous insulin. However, DKA can also occur in individuals with type 2 DM, particularly during infections, severe trauma, or other causes of stress that increase levels of counter-regulatory hormones, thus producing a state of profound inhibition of insulin action. Interestingly, the newest class of pharmacologic agents approved for type 2 DM (sodium–glucose cotransporter-2 inhibitors [SGLT2i]), which lower plasma glucose in an insulin-independent fashion by inhibiting renal glucose reabsorption, are associated with an increased risk of DKA. This increased risk may be attributed to the lower levels of insulin required to maintain euglycemia, which may be insufficient to suppress ketogenesis.

Severe hyperglycemia with glucose levels reaching an average of 500 mg/dL can occur if compensation for the osmotic diuresis associated with hyperglycemia fails. Initially, when elevated glucose levels cause an increase in osmolality, a shift of water from the intracellular to the extracellular space and increased water intake stimulated by thirst help to maintain intravascular volume. If polyuria continues and these compensatory mechanisms cannot keep pace with fluid losses—particularly decreased intake as a result of the nausea and increased losses resulting from the vomiting that accompany ketoacidosis—the depletion of intravascular volume leads to decreased renal blood flow. The kidney's ability to excrete glucose is, therefore, reduced. Hypovolemia also stimulates counter-regulatory hormones. Therefore, glucose levels rise acutely owing to the increased glucose production stimulated by these hormones and decreased clearance by the kidney, an important source of glucose clearance in the absence of insulin-mediated glucose uptake.

In DKA, coma occurs in a minority of patients (10%), with hyperosmolality (not acidosis) being causative. Profound cellular dehydration occurs in response to the marked increase in plasma osmolality. A severe loss of intracellular fluid in the brain leads to coma. Coma occurs when the effective plasma osmolality reaches 330 mOsm/L (normal: 280–295 mOsm/L). Because urea is freely diffusible across cell membranes, blood urea nitrogen is not used to calculate the effective plasma osmolality:

$$\text{Effective osmolality} = 2[\text{Na}^+(\text{mEq/L}) + \text{K}^+(\text{mEq/L})] + \frac{\text{Glucose (mEq/L)}}{18}$$

The increase in **ketogenesis** caused by a severe lack of insulin action results in increased serum levels of ketones and ketonuria. Insulinopenia is also thought to decrease the ability of tissues to use ketones, thus contributing to the maintenance of ketosis. **Acetoacetate** and **β-hydroxybutyrate**, the chief ketone bodies produced by the liver, are organic acids and therefore cause metabolic acidosis, decreasing blood pH and serum bicarbonate (Figure 18–9). Respiration is stimulated, which partially compensates for the metabolic acidosis by reducing PCO_2. The presence of unmeasured ketoacid anions in DKA causes an **increased anion gap** (the calculated difference between measured cations and anions), which

under normal circumstances is primarily a result of negatively charged proteins, such as albumin:

$$\text{Anion Gap (mEq/L)} = (\text{Na}^+ + \text{K}^+) - (\text{Cl}^- + \text{HCO}_3^-)$$

When the pH level is lower than 7.20, characteristic deep, rapid respirations occur (**Kussmaul breathing**). Although acetone is a minor product of ketogenesis (see Figure 18–9), its fruity odor can be detected on the breath during DKA. It should be noted that the ketosis of DKA is much more severe than that appropriately occurring with starvation, because in the latter case, residual insulin action can prevent excessive lipolysis and hepatic ketogenesis while still allowing for peripheral ketone use.

Na^+ is lost in addition to water during the osmotic diuresis accompanying DKA. Therefore, total body Na^+ is depleted. Serum levels of Na^+ are usually low owing to the osmotic activity of the elevated glucose, which draws water into the extracellular space and, in that way, decreases the Na^+ concentration (serum Na^+ falls approximately 1.6 mmol/L for every 100 mg/dL increase in glucose).

Total body stores of K^+ are also depleted by diuresis and vomiting. However, acidosis, insulinopenia, and elevated glucose levels cause a shift of K^+ out of cells, thus maintaining normal or even elevated serum K^+ levels until acidosis and hyperglycemia are corrected. With the administration of insulin and correction of acidosis, serum K^+ falls as K^+ moves back into cells. Without treatment, K^+ can fall to dangerously low levels, leading to potentially lethal cardiac arrhythmias. Therefore, K^+ supplementation is routinely given in the treatment of DKA. Similarly, phosphate depletion accompanies DKA, although acidosis and insulinopenia can cause serum phosphorus levels to be normal before treatment. Phosphate replacement is provided only in cases of extreme depletion given the risks of phosphate administration. (Intravenous phosphate may complex with Ca^{2+}, resulting in hypocalcemia and Ca^{2+} phosphate deposition in soft tissues.)

Marked **hypertriglyceridemia** can also accompany DKA because of the increased production and decreased clearance of VLDL that occurs in insulin-deficient states. Increased production is a result of (1) the increased hepatic flux of fatty acids, which, in addition to fueling ketogenesis, can be repackaged and secreted as VLDL; (2) increased hepatic

FIGURE 18–9 Interconversion of ketone bodies. The relative amounts of the two major ketone bodies depend on the redox state of the hepatocytes. Acetone is a minor product. The nitroprusside reaction, used for clinical testing, detects only compounds with ketone moieties (denoted in blue).

VLDL production owing to the loss of the inhibitory effects of insulin on proteins required for VLDL assembly (apoB and microsomal triglyceride transfer protein [MTP]); and (3) decreased clearance owing to decreased lipoprotein lipase activity. Although serum Na^+ levels can be decreased owing to the osmotic effects of glucose, hypertriglyceridemia can interfere with some common procedures used to measure serum Na^+. This causes pseudohyponatremia (ie, falsely low serum Na^+ values, owing to the overestimation of the actual serum volume).

Nausea and vomiting often accompany DKA, contributing to further dehydration. Abdominal pain, present in 30% of patients, may be due to gastric stasis and distention. Amylase is frequently elevated (90% of cases), in part because of elevations in salivary amylase, but is usually not associated with symptoms of pancreatitis. Leukocytosis is frequently present but does not necessarily indicate the presence of infection. However, because infections can precipitate DKA in type 1 DM and type 2 DM, other manifestations of infection should be sought, such as fever, that cannot be attributed to DKA.

DKA is treated by replacing water and electrolytes (Na^+ and K^+) and administering insulin. Both treatment modalities are of great importance, as evidenced historically by the marked decrease in mortality from DKA with the advent of insulin therapy (from 100% to 50%) and the further significant decrease (from 50% to 20%) when the importance of hydration was recognized and instituted. With fluid and electrolyte replacement, renal perfusion is increased, restoring the renal clearance of elevated blood glucose, and counter-regulatory hormone production is decreased, thus decreasing hepatic glucose production. Insulin administration also corrects hyperglycemia by restoring insulin-sensitive glucose uptake and inhibiting hepatic glucose output. Rehydration is a critical component of the treatment of hyperosmolality. If insulin is administered in the absence of fluid and electrolyte replacement, water will move from the extracellular space back into the cells with the correction of hyperglycemia, leading to vascular collapse. Insulin administration is also required to inhibit further lipolysis, thus eliminating substrates for ketogenesis, and to inhibit hepatic ketogenesis, thereby correcting ketoacidosis.

During the treatment of DKA, measured serum ketones may transiently rise instead of showing a steady decrease. This is an artifact attributable to the limitations of the nitroprusside test that is often used at the bedside to measure ketones in both serum and urine. Nitroprusside detects only acetoacetate and not β-hydroxybutyrate. During untreated DKA, accelerated fatty acid oxidation generates large quantities of nicotinamide adenine dinucleotide (reduced form) in the liver, which favors the formation of β-hydroxybutyrate over acetoacetate (see Figure 18–9). With insulin treatment, fatty acid oxidation decreases, and the redox potential of the liver shifts back in favor of acetoacetate formation. Therefore, although the absolute amount of hepatic ketone body production decreases with DKA treatment, the relative amount of acetoacetate production increases, leading to a transient increase in measured serum ketones when using nitroprusside testing.

3. Hyperosmolar coma—Severe hyperosmolar states in the absence of ketosis can occur in type 2 DM. These episodes are frequently precipitated by decreased fluid intake such as can occur during an intercurrent illness or in older, debilitated patients who lack sufficient access to water and have abnormal renal function, thus hindering the clearance of excessive glucose loads. The mechanisms underlying the development of hyperosmolality and **hyperosmolar coma** are the same as in DKA. However, because only minimal levels of insulin activity are required to suppress lipolysis, these individuals have sufficient insulin to prevent the ketogenesis that results from increased fatty acid flux. Because of the absence of ketoacidosis and its symptoms, patients often present later and, therefore, have more profound hyperglycemia and dehydration; glucose levels often range from 800 mg/dL to 2400 mg/dL. Therefore, the effective osmolality exceeds 330 mOsm/L more frequently in these patients than in those presenting with DKA, resulting in a higher incidence of coma.

Although ketosis is absent, mild ketonuria can be present if the patient has not been eating. K^+ losses are less severe than in DKA. Treatment is similar to that of DKA. Mortality is 10 times higher than in DKA, because those with type 2 diabetes who develop hyperosmolar nonketotic states are older and often have other serious precipitating or complicating illnesses. For example, myocardial infarction can precipitate hyperosmolar states or can result from the alterations in vascular blood flow or other stressors that accompany severe dehydration.

4. Hypoglycemia—Hypoglycemia, a critical factor limiting the achievement of tight glucose control, is a complication of insulin treatment in both type 1 DM and type 2 DM and can also occur with oral hypoglycemic drugs that stimulate glucose-independent insulin secretion (eg, sulfonylureas). Hypoglycemia often occurs during exercise or with fasting, states normally characterized by slight elevations in counter-regulatory hormones and depressed insulin levels. Under normal circumstances, the low insulin levels in these conditions allow the counter-regulatory hormone-mediated mobilization of fuel substrates, increased hepatic glucose output, and the inhibition of glucose disposal in insulin-sensitive tissues. In addition, the fall in insulin secretion by the pancreatic β cell in response to low glucose levels is an important stimulus for increased glucagon secretion. All these responses would normally restore blood glucose levels. However, in diabetic patients, these responses all fail when insulin is maintained at excessive levels (relative to plasma glucose) owing to excessive exogenous insulin dosing or endogenous glucose-independent insulin stimulation. When counter-regulatory mechanisms fail, initial **neurogenic symptoms** of hypoglycemia occur secondary to central nervous system (CNS)-mediated sympathoadrenal discharge. This sympathoadrenal discharge results in both **adrenergic** (shaking, palpitations, anxiety) and **cholinergic** (sweating, hunger) responses that

TABLE 18–5   Symptoms of hypoglycemia.

Autonomic	
Adrenergic	**Cholinergic**
Tremor/shakiness	Sweating
Anxiety	Hunger
Palpitations/tachycardia	
Neuroglycopenic	
Weakness/fatigue/drowsiness	Diplopia
Headache	Difficulty speaking
Behavioral changes	Seizures
Confusion	Coma
Associated with nocturnal hypoglycemia	
Night sweats	Morning headaches
Nightmares	Lassitude
Restlessness	Difficulty awakening

TABLE 18–6   Chronic complications of diabetes mellitus.

Microvascular disease
Nephropathy
Neuropathy
Sensorimotor distal symmetric neuropathy
Autonomic neuropathy
Focal and multifocal neuropathies
Vascular
Nonvascular (entrapment)
Macrovascular disease
Coronary artery disease
Cerebrovascular disease
Peripheral vascular disease
Associated complications
Foot ulcers
Infections
Skeletal fractures

encourage carbohydrate-seeking behavior (Table 18–5). However, as glucose drops further, **neuroglycopenic symptoms** also occur from the direct effects of hypoglycemia on CNS function (confusion, coma). A characteristic set of symptoms (night sweats, nightmares, morning headaches) also accompanies hypoglycemic episodes that occur during sleep (**nocturnal hypoglycemia**).

Recent, recurrent episodes of hypoglycemia reduce the adrenal epinephrine response to subsequent hypoglycemia and cause hypoglycemia unawareness by reducing the sympathoadrenal response and associated neurogenic symptoms via unknown mechanisms. This hypoglycemia-induced autonomic failure, which is distinct from diabetic autonomic neuropathy, has been described in 20% of type 1 diabetics (particularly in those experiencing more than one severe episode per year). It can be reversed by avoiding hypoglycemia but is exacerbated by exercise and sleep, both of which can similarly decrease the sympathoadrenal response to a given level of hypoglycemia.

The acute treatment of hypoglycemia in diabetic individuals consists of the rapid oral administration of glucose at the onset of warning symptoms or the intramuscular administration of exogenous glucagon by another person when neuroglycopenic symptoms preclude oral glucose self-treatment. Rebound hyperglycemia can occur after hypoglycemia because of the actions of counter-regulatory hormones (**Somogyi phenomenon**), an effect that can be aggravated by excessive glucose administration.

B. Chronic Complications

Over time, diabetes results in damage and dysfunction in multiple organ systems (Table 18–6). Vascular disease is a major cause of most of the sequelae of this disease. Both **microvascular disease** (retinopathy, nephropathy, neuropathy), which is specific to diabetes, and **macrovascular disease** (coronary artery disease, peripheral vascular disease), which occurs with increased frequency in diabetes, contribute to the high morbidity and mortality rates associated with this disease. **Neuropathy** also causes increased morbidity, particularly by virtue of its role in the pathogenesis of foot ulcers.

Although both type 1 DM and type 2 DM are associated with the complete spectrum of diabetic complications, the incidence varies with each type and with treatment. Macrovascular disease is the major cause of death in type 2 DM. With the advent of intensive glucose control strategies and the use of renin–angiotensin system inhibitors, renal failure secondary to **nephropathy** is no longer the most common cause of death in individuals with type 1 DM, who now, with increased longevity, are increasingly suffering from macrovascular complications. Although blindness can occur in both types, proliferative changes in retinal vessels (**proliferative retinopathy**) are a major cause of blindness in type 1 DM, whereas **macular edema** is the most important cause in type 2 DM. **Autonomic neuropathy**, one of the manifestations of diabetic neuropathy, occurs more commonly in type 1 DM (40%).

1. Role of glycemic control in preventing complications— A paradigm shift in diabetes treatment occurred in 1993 with the publication of the results of the Diabetes Control and

Complications Trial (**DCCT**), the first major trial to examine the effects of attempted glucose normalization (**tight** or **intensive diabetic control**) on the incidence of complications. In this study of individuals with type 1 DM, intensive (vs. conventional) treatment reduced microvascular complications (retinopathy, nephropathy, neuropathy) by 60%. A subsequent study in type 2 DM (the United Kingdom Prospective Diabetes Study [**UKPDS**]) demonstrated a 25% decrease in microvascular complications (retinopathy, nephropathy) with improved glycemic control. In contrast, the role of glycemic control in preventing macrovascular disease, the major cause of death in type 2 DM, is less clear. With the publication in 2008 of three major clinical trials demonstrating either no improvement or indeed an increase (the **ACCORD** trial) in mortality and macrovascular complications with intensive treatment in type 2 DM, discussions regarding the most appropriate treatment goals (e.g., degree of glucose normalization) and modalities (eg, therapeutics that minimize the risk of hypoglycemia and/or weight gain) in type 2 DM continue.

While the importance of glycemic control in influencing the occurrence of microvascular complications is undisputed, genetic factors also clearly play a role. For example, evidence from a variety of studies suggests that approximately 40% of type 1 diabetics are particularly susceptible to the development of severe microvascular complications. This observation suggests that not all individuals with type 1 DM achieve the same benefits from intensive control regimens, which are both inconvenient and associated with an increased risk of hypoglycemia. The identification of genetic factors associated with microvascular disease risk is the subject of ongoing investigations, which have already identified numerous candidate genes coding for the extracellular matrix, transcription factors, growth factor signaling, and/or erythropoietin.

2. Microvascular complications—Consistent with clinical evidence defining the critical role of hyperglycemia in microvascular disease, data indicate that high intracellular levels of glucose in cells that cannot down-regulate glucose entry (the endothelium, glomeruli, and nerve cells) result in microvascular damage via four distinct diabetes-specific pathways that were sequentially discovered (Figure 18–10): (1) increased polyol pathway flux; (2) increased formation of advanced glycation end-product (AGE); (3) activation of protein kinase C (PKC); and (4) increased hexosamine pathway flux. More recent information suggests that increased flux through these four pathways is induced by a common factor: the overproduction of mitochondrial-derived reactive oxygen species generated by an increased flux of glucose through the tricarboxylic acid (TCA) cycle (see Figure 18–10). The end result of these changes in the microvasculature is an increase in protein accumulation in vessel walls, endothelial cell dysfunction, loss of endothelial cells, and, ultimately, occlusion.

The **polyol pathway** has been extensively studied in diabetic nerve cells and is also present in endothelial cells (see Figure 18–10). Many cells contain aldose reductase, an enzyme that converts toxic aldehydes to their respective alcohols (polyol pathway). While aldose reductase has a low affinity for glucose, under conditions of intercellular hyperglycemia,

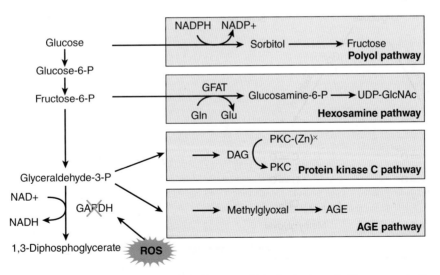

FIGURE 18–10 Mechanisms of microvascular damage initiated by intracellular hyperglycemia. The overproduction of reactive oxygen species (ROS) in response to high glucose is thought to inhibit glyceraldehyde-3-phosphate dehydrogenase (GAPDH), thus increasing the concentration of upstream glycolytic metabolites that are shunted into alternative pathways. Among these are (1) the conversion of glucose to sorbitol, which depletes NADPH, thus preventing the regeneration of ROS scavengers; (2) the conversion of fructose-6-phosphate to uridine diphosphate-N-acetylglucosamine (UDP-GLcNAc), which leads to protein modifications that alter gene expression; (3) the metabolism of glyceraldehyde-3 to form diacylglycerol (DAG), which in turn activates protein kinase C (PKC), resulting in altered vascular hemodynamics; and (4) the formation of carbonyls by multiple mechanisms, including the oxidation of glyceraldehyde-3 phosphate to form methylglyoxal, which react irreversibly with proteins to form dysfunctional products (advanced glycosylated end-products [AGEs]) that cause intracellular and extracellular vascular changes. (Redrawn, with permission, from Kronenberg H. *Williams Textbook of Endocrinology*, 11th ed. Copyright © 2008 Elsevier.)

this pathway can account for up to one-third of glucose flux, converting glucose to sorbitol. While excess **sorbitol** was originally thought to cause osmotic damage, more recent data instead suggest that the real culprit is the consumption of nicotinamide adenine dinucleotide phosphate (NADPH) during glucose reduction. As NADPH is required to regenerate reduced glutathione (GSH), a thiol that detoxifies reactive oxygen species, NADPH consumption prevents the clearance of damaging free radicals. While polyol pathway–mediated damage appears to be a prominent feature in nerve cells, its role in the vasculature is less clear.

The formation of irreversibly glycated proteins called **advanced glycosylation end-products (AGEs)** also causes microvascular damage in diabetes (see Figure 18–10). When present in high concentrations, glucose can react reversibly and nonenzymatically with protein amino groups to form an unstable intermediate, a Schiff base, which then undergoes an internal rearrangement to form a more stable glycated protein, also known as an early glycosylation product (**Amadori product**) (Figure 18–11). Such a reaction accounts for the formation of **glycated HbA**, also known as HbA$_{1c}$. In diabetics, elevated glucose leads to increased glycation of HbA within red blood cells. Because red blood cells circulate for 90 days, the measurement of HbA$_{1c}$ in diabetic patients serves as an index of glycemic control over the preceding months. Early glycosylation products can undergo a further series of chemical reactions and rearrangements, often involving the formation of reactive **carbonyl** intermediates, leading to the

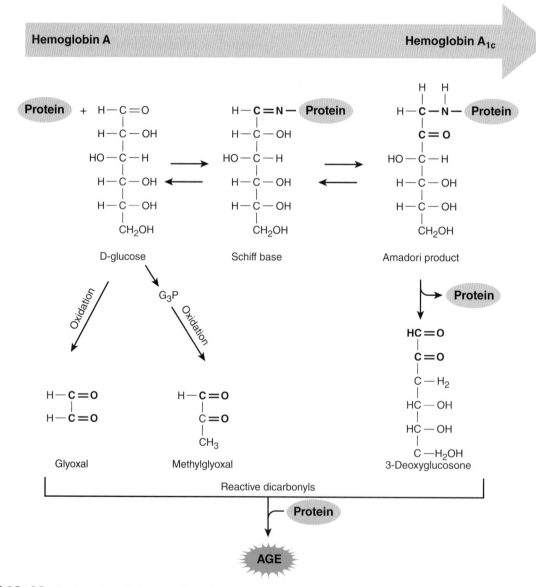

FIGURE 18–11   The formation of advanced glycosylation end-products (AGEs) occurs via multiple pathways. The reversible formation of glycated proteins (Amadori products), such as hemoglobin A$_{1c}$, through a complex series of chemical reactions, or the direct oxidation of glucose and its metabolites (eg, glyceraldehyde-3 phosphate, G$_3$P), results in the production of reactive dicarbonyls. These moieties react irreversibly with proteins to form AGEs.

irreversible formation of AGE. Dicarbonyl formation from the direct auto-oxidation of glucose also contributes to AGE formation (see Figure 18–11). AGE damage the microvasculature via three major pathways: (1) intracellular AGE formation from proteins involved in transcription alters endothelial gene expression; (2) irreversible cross-linking of AGE adducts formed from matrix proteins results in vascular thickening and stiffness; and (3) the binding of extracellular AGE adducts to AGE receptors (RAGEs) on macrophages and the endothelium stimulates NF-κB-regulated inflammatory cascades and resultant vascular dysfunction.

Intracellular endothelial hyperglycemia stimulates glycolysis and, with this, an increase in the de novo synthesis of diacylglycerol (DAG) from the glycolytic intermediate, glyceraldehyde-3-phosphate (see Figure 18–10). DAG, in turn, activates several isoforms of **protein kinase C** (**PKC**) that are present in these cells. This inappropriate activation of PKC alters blood flow, changes endothelial permeability, in part via effects on nitric oxide pathways, and also contributes to the thickening of the extracellular matrix.

Last, increased glucose shunting through the **hexosamine pathway** via diversion of the glycolytic intermediate, fructose-6-phosphate, is also postulated to play a role in microvascular disease (see Figure 18–10). The **hexosamine pathway** contributes to insulin resistance, producing substrates that, when covalently linked to transcription factors, stimulate the expression of proteins, such as transforming growth factor and plasminogen activator inhibitor, that enhance microvascular damage.

Evidence suggests that all four pathways may actually be linked by a common mechanistic element: hyperglycemia-induced **oxidative stress**. In particular, the increase in electron donors that results from shunting glucose through the TCA cycle increases the mitochondrial membrane potential by pumping proteins across the mitochondrial inner membrane. This increased potential prolongs the half-life of superoxide-generating enzymes, thus increasing the conversion of O_2 to O_2^-. These increased **reactive oxygen species** lead to the inhibition of the glycolytic enzyme, glyceraldehyde-3-phosphate dehydrogenase (GADPH), and a resultant increase in upstream metabolites that can now be preferentially diverted into the four mechanistic pathways (see Figure 18–10).

a. Retinopathy—Diabetes is a leading cause of blindness in developed countries (vs. untreated cataracts in developing nations). Diabetic retinopathy is present in one-third of all diabetics, increasing in frequency with disease duration (lifetime risk of 90% for type 1 diabetics vs. 60% for type 2 diabetics) and occuring in two distinct stages: nonproliferative and proliferative.

Nonproliferative retinopathy occurs frequently in both type 1 DM and type 2 DM and is already present at the time of diagnosis in more than 20% of individuals with type 2 DM. **Microaneurysms** of the retinal capillaries, appearing as tiny red dots, are the earliest clinically detectable sign of diabetic retinopathy (**background retinopathy**). These outpouchings in the capillary wall are due to a loss of surrounding pericytes

that support the capillary walls. Vascular permeability is increased. Fat that has leaked from excessively permeable capillary walls appears as shiny yellow spots with distinct borders (**hard exudates**) forming a ring around the area of leakage. The appearance of hard exudates in the area of the macula is often associated with **macular edema**, which can occur at any stage of retinopathy progression and is the most common cause of blindness in type 2 DM, occurring in 7% of diabetics. As retinopathy progresses, signs of ischemia appearing as background retinopathy worsen (**preproliferative stage**). Occlusion of capillaries and terminal arterioles causes areas of retinal ischemia that appear as hazy yellow areas with indistinct borders (**cotton wool spots** or **soft exudates**) because of the accumulation of axonoplasmic debris at areas of infarction. Retinal hemorrhages can also occur, and retinal veins develop segmental dilation.

Retinopathy can progress to a second, more severe stage characterized by the proliferation of new vessels (**proliferative retinopathy**). Neovascularization is more prevalent in type 1 DM than in type 2 DM (32% vs. 3%, respectively) and is a leading cause of blindness in type 1 DM. It is hypothesized that retinal ischemia stimulates the release of growth-promoting factors, such as **vascular endothelial growth factor** (**VEGF**), resulting in new vessel formation. However, these capillaries are abnormal, and traction between new fibrovascular networks and the vitreous can lead to **vitreous hemorrhage** or **retinal detachment**, two potential causes of blindness.

b. Nephropathy—Diabetes is the most common cause of end-stage renal disease (ESRD) worldwide. Although ESRD occurs more frequently in type 1 DM than in type 2 DM (35% vs. 20% after 20 years), type 2 DM accounts for more than half of the diabetic population with ESRD because of its greater prevalence. ESRD also occurs more frequently in Native Americans, African Americans, and Hispanic Americans than in non-Hispanic whites with type 2 DM in the United States.

Diabetic nephropathy results primarily from disordered glomerular function. Histologic changes in glomeruli are indistinguishable in type 1 DM and type 2 DM and occur to some degree in the majority of diabetic individuals. Basement membranes of the glomerular capillaries are thickened and can obliterate the vessels; the mesangium surrounding the glomerular vessels is increased owing to the deposition of basement membrane–like material and can encroach on the glomerular vessels; and the afferent and efferent glomerular arteries are also sclerosed. **Glomerulosclerosis** is usually diffuse but in 50% of cases is associated with nodular sclerosis. This nodular component, called **Kimmelstiel–Wilson nodules** after the investigators who first described the pathologic changes in diabetic kidneys, is pathognomonic for diabetes but is present in only 30% of patients with microalbuminuria.

In type 1 DM patients, glomerular changes are preceded by a phase of **hyperfiltration** resulting from vasodilation of both the afferent and efferent glomerular arterioles, an effect perhaps mediated by two of the counter-regulatory hormones, glucagon and growth hormone, or by hyperglycemia. It is unclear whether this early hyperfiltration phase occurs in type

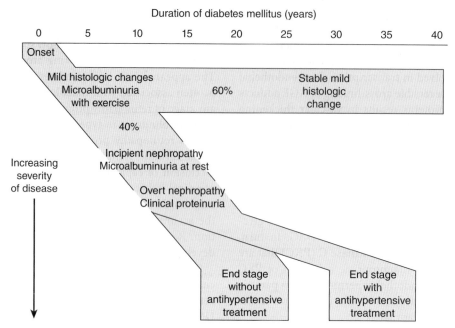

FIGURE 18–12 Development of renal failure in type 1 diabetes mellitus. (Redrawn, with permission, from Omachi R. The pathogenesis and prevention of diabetic nephropathy. West J Med. 1986;145:222. Reproduced, with permission, from the BMJ Publishing Group.)

2 DM. It has been proposed that the presence of atherosclerotic lesions in older type 2 DM patients may prevent hyperfiltration and thus account for the lower incidence of overt clinical nephropathy in these individuals.

Early in the course of the disease, the histologic changes in renal glomeruli are accompanied by **microalbuminuria**, a urinary loss of albumin that cannot be detected by routine urinalysis dipstick methods (Figure 18–12). Albuminuria is thought to be due to a decrease in the heparan sulfate content of the thickened glomerular capillary basement membrane. Heparan sulfate, a negatively charged proteoglycan, can inhibit the filtration of other negatively charged proteins, such as albumin, through the basement membrane; its loss, therefore, allows for increased albumin filtration.

If glomerular lesions worsen, **proteinuria** increases and overt nephropathy develops (see Figure 18–12). Diabetic nephropathy is defined clinically by the presence of more than 300 mg of urinary protein per day, an amount that can be detected by routine urinalysis. In diabetic nephropathy (unlike other renal diseases), proteinuria continues to increase as renal function decreases. Therefore, ESRD is preceded by massive, nephrotic-range proteinuria (>4 g/d). The presence of hypertension speeds this process. Although type 2 DM patients often already have hypertension at the time of diagnosis, type 1 DM patients usually do not develop hypertension until after the onset of nephropathy. In both cases, hypertension worsens as renal function deteriorates. Therefore, controlling hypertension is critical in preventing the progression of diabetic nephropathy.

Retinopathy, a process also worsened by the presence of hypertension, usually precedes the development of nephropathy. Therefore, other causes of proteinuria should be considered in diabetic individuals who present with proteinuria in the absence of retinopathy.

c. Neuropathy—Neuropathy (see Table 18–6) occurs in about 60% of both type 1 and type 2 DM patients and is a major cause of morbidity. Diabetic neuropathy can be divided into three major types: (1) a distal, primarily sensory, symmetric polyneuropathy that is by far the most common (50% incidence); (2) an autonomic neuropathy, occurring frequently in individuals with distal polyneuropathy (>20% incidence); and (3) much less common, transient asymmetric neuropathies involving specific nerves, nerve roots, or plexuses.

d. Symmetric distal polyneuropathy—The demyelination of peripheral nerves, a hallmark of diabetic polyneuropathy, affects distal nerves preferentially and is usually manifested clinically by a symmetric sensory loss in the distal lower extremities (**stocking distribution**) that is preceded by numbness, tingling, and paresthesias. These symptoms, which begin distally and move proximally, can also occur in the hands (**glove distribution**). Pathologic features of affected peripheral somatic nerves include the demyelination and loss of nerve fibers with reduced axonal regeneration, accompanied by microvascular lesions, including the thickening of basement membranes. The activation of the polyol pathway in nerve cells is thought to play a major role in inducing symmetric distal polyneuropathy in diabetes. In addition, the microvascular disease that accompanies these neural lesions may also contribute to nerve damage. The presence of antibodies to autoantigens in patients with neuropathy also suggests a possible immune component to this disorder. Last, defects in the production or delivery of neurotrophic factors, such as nerve growth factor (NGF), are hypothesized to play a role in the pathogenesis of symmetric distal neuropathy.

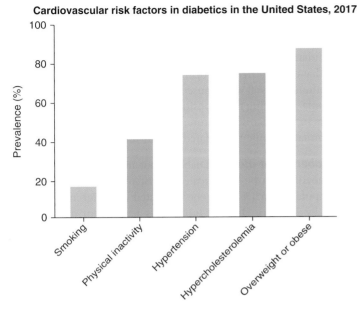

Cardiovascular risk factors in diabetics in the United States, 2017

FIGURE 18–13 Individuals with diabetes, which is itself an independent risk factor for cardiovascular disease, have a high prevalence of other modifiable cardiovascular risk factors. (Data represent risk prevalence for individuals with diabetes in the United States, as reported in the CDC National Diabetes Statistics Report, 2017).

e. Autonomic neuropathy—Autonomic neuropathy often accompanies symmetric peripheral neuropathy, occurs more frequently in type 1 DM, and can affect all aspects of autonomic functioning, most notably those involving the cardiovascular, genitourinary, and GI systems. Less information is available regarding the morphologic changes occurring in affected autonomic nerves, but similarities to somatic nerve alterations suggest a common pathogenesis.

Fixed, resting **tachycardia** and **orthostatic hypotension** are signs of cardiovascular autonomic nervous system damage that can be easily ascertained on physical examination. Orthostatic hypotension can be quite severe. **Erectile dysfunction** occurs in more than 50% of diabetic men and is due both to neurogenic (parasympathetic control of penile vasodilation) and vascular factors. Sexual dysfunction in diabetic women has not been well studied. Loss of bladder sensation and difficulty emptying the bladder (neurogenic bladder) lead to overflow **incontinence** and an increased risk of urinary tract infections as a result of residual urine. Motor disturbances can occur throughout the GI tract, resulting in delayed gastric emptying (**gastroparesis**), constipation, or diarrhea. Anhidrosis in the lower extremities can lead to excessive sweating in the upper body as a means of dissipating heat, including increased sweating in response to eating (**gustatory sweating**). Autonomic neuropathy can also result in decreased glucagon and epinephrine responses to hypoglycemia.

f. Mononeuropathy and **mononeuropathy multiplex**—The abrupt, usually painful onset of motor loss in isolated cranial or peripheral nerves (**mononeuropathy**) or in multiple isolated nerves (**mononeuropathy multiplex**) occurs much less

frequently than does symmetric polyneuropathy or autonomic neuropathy. Vascular occlusion and ischemia are thought to play a central role in the pathogenesis of these asymmetric focal neuropathies, which are usually of limited duration and occur more frequently in type 2 DM. The third cranial nerve is the most frequently involved, causing ipsilateral headache followed by ptosis and ophthalmoplegia with sparing of papillary reactivity. In contrast to the rare occurrence of these vascular neuropathies, symptomatic compression by peripheral nerve entrapment (eg, ulnar nerve at the elbow, median nerve at the wrist) occurs in 30% of diabetics and usually involves both the nerve and surrounding tissues.

3. Macrovascular complications—Atherosclerotic macrovascular disease occurs with increased frequency in diabetes, resulting in an increased incidence of myocardial infarction, stroke, and claudication and gangrene of the lower extremities. Although macrovascular disease accounts for significant morbidity and mortality in both types of diabetes, the effects of large-vessel disease are particularly devastating in type 2 DM and are responsible for approximately 75% of deaths. The protective effect of gender is lost in women with diabetes; their risk of atherosclerosis is equal to that of men (Figure 18–13).

The reasons for the increased risk of **atherosclerosis** in diabetes are threefold: (1) the incidence of traditional risk factors, such as hypertension and hyperlipidemia, is increased (50% and 30% incidence at diagnosis, respectively); (2) diabetes itself (likely due to both hyperglycemia and insulin resistance) is an independent risk factor for atherosclerosis; and (3) diabetes appears to synergize with other known risk factors to increase atherosclerosis. The elimination of other risk factors, therefore, can greatly reduce the risk of atherosclerosis in diabetes (see Figure 18–13).

Hypertension associated with increased total body extracellular Na$^+$ content and volume expansion occurs with increased frequency in type 1 DM and type 2 DM and is responsive to targeted inhibition of the renin–angiotensin system. Despite this, the epidemiology of hypertension in the two DM subtypes suggests that different pathophysiologic mechanisms may be operative. In type 1 DM, hypertension usually occurs after the onset of nephropathy (40% incidence after 40 years of type 1 DM), when renal insufficiency impairs the ability to excrete water and solutes. In type 2 DM, hypertension is often already present at the time of diagnosis (70% are hypertensive) in these older, obese, insulin-resistant individuals. Indeed, it has been proposed that insulin resistance plays a central role in both diabetes and hypertension. For example, insulin resistance is associated with activation of the renin–angiotensin system, which leads to hypertension, while renin–angiotensin system activation, in turn, decreases insulin sensitivity.

In contrast to the central role of hyperglycemia in microvascular disease, its importance as a risk factor for macrovascular disease, which occurs in 40% of 40-year-old individuals with type 1 DM (vs. <10% of controls), remains uncertain. However, **insulin resistance**, a hallmark of type 2 DM that can also develop in response to hyperglycemia in type 1 DM, is clearly an important driver of macrovascular complications in diabetes. Insulin resistance is central to the pathogenesis of two obesity-associated syndromes: (1) **prediabetes** (eg, FPG 100–125 mg/dL, A1C 5.7–6.4%); and (2) **metabolic syndrome** (a cluster of metabolic abnormalities, including central obesity [waist ≥102 cm for males or ≥88 cm for females], elevated glucose [≥100 mg/dL], elevated blood pressure [≥130/≥85 mm Hg], elevated triglycerides [≥150 mg/dL], and low high-density lipoprotein [HDL] cholesterol [<40 mg/dL]). Both syndromes are associated with increased cardiovascular risk, as well as an increased risk for the later development of diabetes. At present in the United States, one-third of the adult population is thought to fall into one or more of high-risk categories. Fortunately, an important clinical trial (the **Diabetes Prevention Program**) has demonstrated that significant risk reductions for the development of type 2 DM occur in response to lifestyle interventions in this population.

In addition to being a component of metabolic syndrome, **hypertriglyceridemia**, which is associated with an increased risk of cardiovascular disease, is the principal lipid abnormality in poorly controlled type 1 and type 2 DM. Very-low-density lipoprotein–triglyceride (VLDL-TG) levels are increased because of insufficient insulin action in the liver and adipose tissue. This results in (1) increased VLDL production due to the increased flux of fatty acids from adipose tissue to the liver (ie, increased lipolysis) and the loss of insulin suppression of hepatic proteins required for VLDL assembly (ie, loss of phosphoinositide 3-kinase [PI 3-kinase] inhibition of apolipoprotein B [apoB] production and loss of inhibition of the transcription factor FoxO1-induced expression of microsomal triglyceride transfer protein [MTP]); and (2) decreased VLDL clearance as a result of decreased lipoprotein lipase activity. Excessive VLDL levels alter the composition of LDL and HDL, transferring triglycerides to these particles while depleting them of cholesterol, creating **small, dense LDL particles** and **low HDL cholesterol levels**, both of which are independent risk factors for cardiovascular disease. LDL cholesterol may also be elevated both because of its increased production (VLDL is catabolized to LDL) and decreased clearance (insulin deficiency may reduce LDL receptor activity). Insulin treatment usually corrects lipoprotein abnormalities in type 1 DM. In contrast, treatment of hyperglycemia often does not normalize lipid profiles in obese, insulin-resistant individuals with type 2 DM unless accompanied by weight reduction (ie, by a concomitant reduction in insulin resistance).

Possible reasons why diabetes may be an independent risk factor for atherosclerosis and may also act synergistically with other risk factors include the following: (1) alterations in lipoprotein composition in diabetes that make the particles more atherogenic (eg, increased small, dense LDL; increased Lp[a] levels; enhanced lipoprotein oxidation and glycation); (2) the occurrence of a relative procoagulant state in diabetes, including an increase in certain clotting factors and increased platelet aggregation; (3) proatherogenic alterations in vessel walls caused either by the direct effects of hyperinsulinemia in type 2 DM or by boluses of exogenously administered insulin

(vs. hepatic first-pass clearance of endogenously secreted insulin) in type 1 DM, which include the promotion of smooth muscle proliferation, alteration of vasomotor tone, and enhancement of foam cell formation (cholesterol-laden cells that characterize atherogenic lesions); (4) proatherogenic alterations in vessel walls caused by the direct effects of hyperglycemia, including the deposition of glycated proteins, just as occurs in the microvasculature; and, importantly, (5) the proinflammatory milieu associated with insulin resistance.

4. Diabetic foot ulcers—Diabetic foot ulcers occur in 10% of diabetics, can be complicated by osteomyelitis, and result in amputation in 1%, an event associated with high mortality (50% by 3 years). Diabetic foot ulcers account for over 60% of nontraumatic amputations in the United States. Risk factors for ulcer development include (1) increased injuries in insensate feet owing to symmetric polyneuropathy (present in 75–90% of diabetics with foot ulcers), which can be detected clinically by decreased vibratory and cutaneous pressure sensation and the absence of ankle reflexes; (2) macrovascular disease (present in 30–40% of those with foot ulcers) and microvascular disease; (3) infections caused by alterations in neutrophil function and vascular insufficiency; and (4) faulty wound healing caused by unknown factors.

5. Infection—Neutrophil chemotaxis and phagocytosis are defective in poorly controlled diabetes. Cell-mediated immunity may also be abnormal. In addition, vascular lesions can hinder blood flow, preventing inflammatory cells from reaching wounds (eg, foot ulcers) or other possible sites of infection. Therefore, individuals with diabetes are more prone to develop infections and may have more severe infections. As a result, certain common infections (eg, **candidal infections, periodontal disease**) occur more frequently in diabetics. A number of unusual infections also are seen in diabetics (ie, **necrotizing papillitis**, **mucormycosis** of the nasal sinuses invading the orbit and cranium, and **malignant otitis externa** caused by *Pseudomonas aeruginosa*).

6. Skeletal changes in diabetes—Children with type 1 DM have a much lower bone mass, attributed to the loss of the anabolic effects of insulin on bone that stimulate the differentiation of bone-forming osteoblasts, and an associated 7-fold increased risk of fragility bone fractures. Adults with type 2 DM have a 40–70% increased fracture risk, perhaps owing to subtle micro-architectural changes (eg, increased cortical porosity), since bone mineral density in these typically obese individuals is normal or increased. Emerging evidence suggests that bone fragility in diabetes may be an additional factor attributable to microvascular disease. Also intriguing is a growing body of evidence suggesting that interactions between carbohydrate homeostasis and the skeleton may be bidirectional. For example, circulating levels of sclerostin, an osteocyte-derived factor favoring the differentiation of mesenchymal stem cells into adipocytes rather than bone-forming osteoblasts, is elevated in obesity and correlates with insulin resistance in humans, whereas the osteoblast-derived factor, osteocalcin, can enhance glucose-stimulated β-cell insulin secretion and improve insulin sensitivity in mouse models of obesity.

NEUROENDOCRINE ISLET CELL TUMORS OF THE PANCREAS

While highly prevalent in individuals with multiple endocrine neoplasia type 1 (MEN-1), neuroendocrine tumors arising from the islet cells are otherwise infrequent and account for only 5% of primary pancreatic neoplasms, most of which instead arise from cells of the exocrine pancreas. However, the clinical manifestations associated with islet cell tumor overproduction of a given hormone are illustrative of their normal physiologic functions (Table 18–7). Those tumors associated with the inappropriate secretion of hormones regulating carbohydrate metabolism (insulin, glucagon, somatostatin) are highlighted here.

Insulinoma (β-cell tumor)

A. Clinical Presentation

The occurrence of **fasting hypoglycemia** in an otherwise healthy individual is usually due to an insulin-secreting tumor of the β cells of the islets of Langerhans (**insulinoma**; see Table 18–7). Although insulinoma is the most common islet cell tumor, it is still rare. Insulinomas occur most frequently in the fourth to seventh decades, although they can occur earlier, particularly when associated with MEN-1, a neoplastic syndrome characterized by tumors of the parathyroids, pituitary, and endocrine pancreas (see Chapter 17). The diagnosis of hypoglycemia is based on the Whipple triad: (1) symptoms and signs of hypoglycemia; (2) an associated low plasma glucose level; and (3) the reversibility of symptoms on glucose administration.

B. Etiology

In the great majority of cases, insulinomas are solitary benign lesions composed of whorls of insulin-secreting β cells. Multiple tumors, although infrequent (<10%), are seen most often in patients with MEN-1. Fewer than 10% of the tumors are malignant, as determined by the presence of metastases.

C. Pathology and Pathogenesis

Inappropriately high levels of insulin in situations normally characterized by a lowering of insulin secretion (eg, fasting and exercise) result in hypoglycemia. Normally, in the postabsorptive and fasting state, insulin levels decline, leading to an increase in glucagon-stimulated hepatic glucose output and a decrease in insulin-mediated glucose disposal in the periphery, which maintains normal serum glucose levels. With exercise, low insulin levels allow muscles to use glycogen, glucagon, and other counter-regulatory hormones to increase hepatic glucose output and to use counter-regulatory hormones to mobilize fatty acids for ketogenesis and fatty acid oxidation. With an insulinoma, insulin levels remain high during fasting or exercise. In this circumstance, glucagon-mediated hepatic glucose output is suppressed while insulin-mediated peripheral glucose uptake continues, and insulin stimulates hepatic fatty acid synthesis and peripheral fatty acid storage while suppressing fatty acid mobilization and hepatic ketogenesis. The result is fasting or exercise-induced hypoglycemia in the absence of ketosis.

D. Clinical Manifestations

Individuals with insulinomas often are symptomatic for years before diagnosis and self-treat with frequent food intake. Not all patients experience fasting hypoglycemia in the morning (only 30% of insulinoma patients develop hypoglycemia after a diagnostic 12-hour fast). Often, they experience late-afternoon

TABLE 18–7   Islet cell tumor syndromes.

Tumor	Major Signs & Symptoms	Malignant (%)	Prevalence in MEN Syndrome
Insulinoma	Fasting hypoglycemia with symptoms of same	10%	10%
Glucagonoma	Diabetes, characteristic rash, anorexia, weight loss, anemia, diarrhea	60%	<2%
Somatostatinoma	Diabetes, cholelithiasis, steatorrhea, weight loss, abdominal pain and fullness	66%	<2%
PPoma	Asymptomatic (watery diarrhea)	40%	15%
Gastrinoma	Enhanced acid secretion with peptic ulcers, esophageal reflux, diarrhea (Zollinger–Ellison syndrome)	50%	40%
VIPoma	Watery diarrhea, hypokalemia, hypochlorhydria	40%	<2%

MEN, multiple endocrine neoplasia.

hypoglycemia, particularly when precipitated by exercise. Because alcohol, like insulin, inhibits gluconeogenesis, alcohol ingestion can also precipitate symptoms. A high percentage of individuals with insulinoma experience neuroglycopenic as well as autonomic symptoms (see Table 18–5). Confusion (80%), loss of consciousness (50%), and seizures (10%) often lead to misdiagnoses of psychiatric or neurologic disorders.

Fasting hypoglycemia can occur as a result of either (1) elevated insulin, as occurs in insulinoma; or (2) non–insulin-mediated effects such as the loss of counter-regulatory hormones (eg, loss of cortisol in Addison disease), severe hepatic damage that prevents hepatic glucose production, loss of peripheral stores of substrates for hepatic glucose production (eg, cachexia), or some states of markedly increased glucose use (eg, sepsis, cancer). To distinguish **insulin-mediated** from **non–insulin-mediated fasting hypoglycemia**, patients suspected of having insulinoma are subjected to a diagnostic fast during which glucose, insulin, and C-peptide levels are measured. An inappropriately elevated insulin level in the setting of hypoglycemia is diagnostic of an insulin-mediated cause of hypoglycemia. Further, because insulin and C peptide are co-secreted, documentation of a concurrent elevation in both peptides is necessary to confirm a pancreatic source of insulin (vs. **surreptitious insulin injection**). Last, because oral hypoglycemic medications that stimulate glucose-independent endogenous insulin secretion (**sulfonylureas**) can also enhance the pancreatic secretion of insulin (and, therefore, C peptide), the differentiation of insulinoma versus the inappropriate ingestion of these agents can be assessed only by an assay of plasma drug levels.

Glucagonoma (α-cell tumor)

Glucagonomas are usually diagnosed by the appearance of a characteristic rash in middle-aged individuals with mild diabetes mellitus (see Table 18–7). While rare, representing 3–7% of pancreatic neuroendocrine tumors, the early diagnosis of a glucagonoma is key given the propensity to metastasize to the liver: Metastases are present in 50–90% at the time of

diagnosis. Glucagon levels are usually increased 10-fold relative to normal values but can even be increased 100-fold.

Necrolytic migratory erythema begins as an erythematous rash on the face, abdomen, perineum, or lower extremities. After induration with central blistering develops, the lesions crust over and then resolve, leaving an area of hyperpigmentation. These lesions may be the result of nutritional deficiency, such as the hypoaminoacidemia that occurs from the excessive glucagon stimulation of hepatic amino acid uptake and use as fuel for gluconeogenesis, rather than the direct effect of glucagon on the skin. The appearance of the rash is a late manifestation of the disease.

Diabetes mellitus or glucose intolerance is present in the vast majority of patients as a result of the increased stimulation of hepatic glucose output by inappropriately high glucagon levels. Insulin levels are secondarily increased. Diabetes is therefore mild and not accompanied by glucagon-stimulated ketosis, because sufficient insulin is present to suppress lipolysis, thus limiting potential substrates for ketogenesis. Anemia and a variety of nonspecific GI symptoms related to decreased intestinal motility can also accompany glucagonomas.

Although these tumors are solitary and their growth is slow, they are usually large with accompanying metastases. Therefore, tumor burden and thus prognosis correlate with glucagon secretion and consequent plasma glucose levels. Octreotide, the synthetic somatostatin analog, can be used to visualize the tumor ([111]I-octreotide scintography) and ameliorate symptoms via its suppression of glucagon secretion.

Somatostatinoma (δ-cell tumor)

Somatostatinomas present with a variety of GI symptoms in individuals with mild diabetes (see Table 18–7). However, these extremely rare tumors are almost uniformly found incidentally during operations for cholelithiasis or other abdominal complaints because the presenting symptoms are both nonspecific and common in an adult population. Documentation of elevated somatostatin levels confirms the diagnosis.

A **classic triad** of symptoms frequently occurs with excessive somatostatin secretion: (1) **diabetes mellitus**, because of its inhibition of insulin and glucagon secretion; (2) **cholelithiasis**, because of its inhibition of gallbladder motility; and (3) **steatorrhea**, because of its inhibition of pancreatic exocrine function. Hypochlorhydria, diarrhea, and anemia can also occur.

In both types 1 and 2 DM, the effects of insulin insufficiency are aggravated by the occurrence of elevated glucagon levels. In contrast, with somatostatinomas, both insulin and glucagon are suppressed. Therefore, the hyperglycemia resulting from insulinopenia is tempered by the absence of glucagon stimulation of hepatic glucose output. Although low insulin levels are permissive for lipolysis, glucagon deficiency prevents hepatic ketogenesis. The diabetes associated with somatostatinomas is, therefore, mild and not ketosis prone.

Although the majority of somatostatinomas occur in the pancreas, a significant number are found in the duodenum or jejunum. Like glucagonomas, somatostatinomas are often solitary and large and have frequently metastasized by the time of diagnosis.

CASE STUDIES

Yeong Kwok, MD

(See Chapter 25, p. 779–80 for answers)

CASE 96

A 12-year-old girl is brought to her pediatrician for evaluation of fatigue, weight loss, bedwetting, and extreme thirst. She had been healthy with no significant past medical history until 2 weeks ago when she started exhibiting these symptoms. The physical examination is notable for a fatigued girl with dry mucous membranes. Her weight is 5 kg less than at her well child examination 5 months before. Laboratory studies show a random blood glucose of 351 mg/dL, a hemoglobin A_{1c} of 11.4%, metabolic acidosis, and an anion gap. Her urine is positive for ketones. She is diagnosed with type 1 diabetes mellitus.

Questions

A. What is the pathogenesis of type 1 diabetes mellitus?
B. What are the roles of genetic and environmental factors in the risk of developing type 1 diabetes mellitus?
C. Why do patients with type 1 diabetes mellitus develop ketoacidosis much more frequently than patients with type 2 diabetes mellitus?

CASE 97

A 58-year-old homeless man with long-standing insulin-treated type 2 diabetes has been diagnosed with right lower extremity cellulitis. He has taken a prescribed oral antibiotic for the past week but has not noticed much improvement. For the past 2 days, he has experienced intermittent fevers and chills, nausea with poor oral intake, and proximally spreading erythema over his right leg. On the evening of admission, a friend notices that he is markedly confused and calls 911. In the emergency department, he is oriented only to his name. The patient is tachypneic, breathing deeply at a rate of 24/min. He is febrile at 38.8°C. He is normotensive, but his heart rate is elevated at 112 bpm.

On examination, the patient is a delirious, unkempt man with a fruity breath odor. His right lower extremity is markedly erythematous and exquisitely tender to palpation. Serum chemistries reveal a glucose level of 488 mg/dL, potassium of 3.7 mEq/dL, and sodium of 132 mEq/L. Urine dipstick is grossly positive for ketones.

Questions

A. Describe the precipitants of ketoacidosis in this diabetic patient.
B. What is the cause of his altered mental status?
C. Describe the patient's respiratory pattern. What is the pathogenetic mechanism?
D. What issues are important to consider in replacing electrolytes in this patient?

CASE 98

A 61-year-old man recently moved to town and is establishing primary care. During a comprehensive review of systems, he reports that he has experienced a 3-year history of "hypoglycemic attacks." These short periods of lightheadedness, confusion, palpitations, and tremor occur more frequently in the late afternoon while jogging. His symptoms are relieved after drinking a sugared sports drink. He has no history of diabetes or cancer. His physical examination is unremarkable, and in the clinic, his fasting morning glucose level is 93 mg/dL. Suspecting that an insulinoma-induced hypoglycemic state may be responsible for his symptoms, his physician requests a diagnostic fast period during which glucose, insulin, and C-peptide levels are measured.

Questions

A. Describe the Whipple triad in the diagnosis of hypoglycemia.
B. What patient history clues suggest insulinoma? Discuss the pathogenesis.
C. How might the tests ordered help identify the cause of the hypoglycemia?

CASE 99

A 52-year-old woman with a 3-year history of diet-controlled diabetes presents to her primary care provider complaining of a "stubborn poison ivy rash" over her legs, which she attributed to a possible exposure to the plant during a recent hike. She presented twice to the urgent care center and received high-potency topical steroid cream for this refractory erythematous rash with central blistering. A review of systems reveals intermittent diarrhea and constipation as well as weight loss. Her serum glucagon level is measured and found to be 20 times normal.

Questions

A. What is the rash found in this disease? What is thought to be the cause?
B. Why is the diabetes found in this condition usually mild?
C. What is the typical prognosis?

CASE 100

At the time of an elective laparoscopic cholecystectomy for gallstones, a 44-year-old woman with mild diabetes mellitus and chronic diarrhea is noted to have a 3–4 cm solitary mass on the surface of her duodenum. Omental lymphadenopathy is seen. Biopsy demonstrates a high-grade somatostatinoma with lymph node metastasis.

Questions

A. Describe the triad of signs typically seen in patients with somatostatinomas.
B. Why is the diabetes found in this condition usually mild?

REFERENCES

Diabetes Mellitus

Diabetes Control and Complications Trial Research Group. The effect of intensive treatment of diabetes on the development and progression of long-term complications in insulin-dependent diabetes mellitus. N Engl J Med. 1993 Sep 30;329(14):977–86. [PMID: 8366922]

Diabetes Prevention Program Research Group. Long-term effects of lifestyle intervention or metformin on diabetes development and microvascular complications over 15-year follow-up: the Diabetes Prevention Program Outcomes Study. Lancet Diabetes Endocrinol. 2015 Nov;3(11):866–75. [PMID: 26377054]

Flannick J et al. Type 2 diabetes: genetic data sharing to advance complex disease research. Nat Rev Genet. 2016 Sep;17(9):535–49. [PMID: 27402621]

Genser L et al. Obesity, type 2 diabetes, and the metabolic syndrome: pathophysiologic relationships and guidelines for surgical intervention. Surg Clin North Am. 2016 Aug;96(4):681–701. [PMID: 27473795]

Gregg EW et al. Global health effects of overweight and obesity. N Engl J Med. 2017 Jul 6;377(1):80–1. [PMID: 28604226]

Grundy SM. Metabolic syndrome update. Trends Cardiovasc Med. 2016 May;26(4):364–73. [PMID: 26654259]

International Hypoglycaemia Study Group. Minimizing hypoglycemia in diabetes. Diabetes Care. 2015 Aug;38(8):1583–91. [PMID: 26207052]

Katsarou A et al. Type 1 diabetes mellitus. Nat Rev Dis Primers. 2017 Mar 30;3:17016. [PMID: 28358037]

Levin PA. Practical combination therapy based on pathophysiology of type 2 diabetes. Diabetes Metab Syndr Obes. 2016 Oct 31;9:355–69. [PMID: 27826204]

Menke A et al. Prevalence of and trends in diabetes among adults in the United States, 1988–2012. JAMA. 2015 Sep 8;314(10):1021–9. [PMID: 26348752]

Müller TD et al. The new biology and pharmacology of glucagon. Physiol Rev. 2017 Apr;97(2):721–66. [PMID: 28275047]

Shanbhogue VV et al. Bone disease in diabetes: another manifestation of microvascular disease? Lancet Diabetes Endocrinol. 2017 Oct;5(10):827–38. [PMID: 28546096]

Shulman GI. Ectopic fat in insulin resistance, dyslipidemia, and cardiometabolic disease. N Engl J Med. 2014 Dec 4;371(23):2237–8. [PMID: 25470706]

UK Prospective Diabetes Study (UKPDS) Group. Intensive blood glucose control with sulphonylureas or insulin compared with conventional treatment and risk of complications in patients with type 2 diabetes (UKPDS 33). Lancet. 1998 Sep 12;352(9131): 837–53. [PMID: 9742976]

Insulinoma, Glucagonoma & Somatostatinoma

Anderson CW et al. Clinical presentation and diagnosis of pancreatic neuroendocrine tumors. Surg Oncol Clin N Am. 2016 Apr;25(2):363–74. [PMID: 27013370]

Iglesias P et al. Insulinoma: a multicenter, retrospective analysis of three decades of experience (1983-2014). Endocrinol Nutr. 2015 Aug-Sep;62(7):306–13. [PMID: 26050581]

John AM et al. Glucagonoma syndrome: a review and update on treatment. J Eur Acad Dermatol Venereol. 2016 Dec;30(12):2016–22. [PMID: 27422767]

Disorders of the Hypothalamus & Pituitary Gland

Tobias Else, MD, & Gary D. Hammer, MD, PhD

The hypothalamus is the part of the brain where the activity of the autonomic nervous system and endocrine glands, which directly control various systems of the body, is integrated with input from other centers that give rise to emotions and behavior. The hypothalamus thus serves to ensure that (1) the organism responds appropriately to deviations from various internal set points (including those for temperature, volume, osmolality, satiety, and body fat content); (2) the responses to such deviations from a set point include coordinated activity of the nervous and endocrine systems; and (3) the emotions and behavior being manifested are appropriate for reflex responses being triggered to correct the deviations from internal set points. The following description outlines the integrative function of the hypothalamus in regard to the coordination of endocrine and central nervous system (CNS) responses.

Intravascular volume loss from any cause activates autonomic neural responses, mainly via the sympathetic nervous system to retain fluid and electrolytes, maintain blood pressure through vascular smooth muscle contraction, and maintain cardiac output by increasing heart rate. The effect of these immediate neural responses is reinforced by the activation of several hormonal systems. In response to a decrease in intravascular volume, the renin–angiotensin–aldosterone system (RAAS) is activated and sodium is retained. Additionally, increasing osmolarity triggers thirst and leads to the release of vasopressin (antidiuretic hormone [ADH]) from hypothalamic neurons that end in the posterior pituitary, resulting in free water absorption in the kidney. In short, the body maintains intravascular volume by regulating sodium reabsorption through aldosterone, while it regulates osmolarity by increasing fluid intake (thirst) and free water retention by vasopressin.

Emotions interplay with these systems to coordinate appropriate behavioral and hormonal responses. Fear and pain activate limbic, hypothalamic, and other centers to coordinate defensive (fight-or-flight) and recuperative behaviors, respectively. These emotional responses to various stressors (eg, perceived threat to body, fear) also activate the sympathetic nervous system and the hypothalamic–pituitary–adrenal (HPA) axis, which coordinate the mammalian stress response by preparing the body for "fight and flight" and by mobilizing energy stores. Any kind of stress (eg, physical, mental, metabolic) leads to the release of corticotropin-releasing hormone (CRH) from the hypothalamus and consequent adrenocorticotropin (ACTH; pituitary) and cortisol (adrenal cortex) secretion. For example, starvation leads to the activation of the HPA axis and ultimately a cortisol-mediated increase in gluconeogenesis to maintain basic physiologic functions.

The pituitary gland is the partner of the hypothalamus on the body side of the mind–body interface. Once viewed as the "master gland" in regulating neuroendocrine systems, the pituitary is now known to be a "middle manager" responding to input from both the brain (via the hypothalamus) and the body (via the various peripheral endocrine glands).

The basic framework for hypothalamic–pituitary function is the **neuroendocrine axis**, a cascade of interacting hormonal products from various regions of the CNS to the hypothalamus, anterior pituitary gland, peripheral endocrine end organs, and peripheral target tissues. Some neuroendocrine axes involve hormones released by the hypothalamus that stimulate cells in the anterior pituitary to secrete other hormones into the systemic circulation. Each of these anterior pituitary hormones travels to a distant endocrine gland to stimulate the secretion of yet other hormones that affect various target tissues. Thus, disorders of the hypothalamus and pituitary have important consequences for the pathophysiologic mechanisms of a wide range of disorders involving many different tissues and organs.

This chapter focuses on five clinical entities. The first four reflect the diversity of pituitary disease: pituitary adenomas, panhypopituitarism, vasopressin excess, and vasopressin deficiency. The last, obesity, is one in which the hypothalamus plays a crucial role and which has enormous implications for diseases involving many other organ systems.

NORMAL STRUCTURE & FUNCTION OF THE HYPOTHALAMUS & PITUITARY GLAND

ANATOMY, HISTOLOGY & CELL BIOLOGY

The hypothalamus is located in the floor and lateral walls of the third ventricle below the hypothalamic sulcus and comprises about 1% of the mass of the brain (Figure 19–1). Hypothalamic nuclei are clusters of neurons whose cell bodies lie in discrete regions (Figure 19–2). From these nuclei, hypothalamic neurons send projections either directly or via neuronal relay to other parts of the central and peripheral nervous systems and secrete hormones that make possible the hierarchical control of various physiologic processes (Table 19–1).

The hypothalamus is connected to the pituitary gland by a stalk consisting of the axons of some hypothalamic neurons with terminal boutons composing the posterior pituitary gland (Figure 19–3). The posterior pituitary neurons secrete the peptide hormones oxytocin and vasopressin directly into the systemic circulation. The development of the anterior pituitary from the oral ectoderm is dictated by a tight program of consecutive activation of distinct transcription factors in the differentiating pituitary cell types (Figure 19–4). The pituitary gland is encased in a tough fibrous capsule, positioned in the bony sella turcica. The pituitary gland is bounded above by the optic chiasm and laterally by the cavernous sinus and the structures that traverse it (internal carotid artery, cranial

nerves [CNs] III and IV, first and second divisions of CNs V and VI).

In circumventricular parts of the CNS, the capillaries are fenestrated, allowing neurons to sense various specific chemical stimuli in the bloodstream. These sensory neurons transmit information regarding changes in stimuli (eg, change in osmolality) to other hypothalamic neurons involved in a variety of specific types of secretory activities.

Other hypothalamic neurons secrete peptide hormones into a specialized capillary bed termed the **pituitary portal system**. Blood in this capillary system flows directly from the median eminence to the anterior pituitary gland, where specific cells that display receptors for the various hypothalamic releasing hormones are found. The binding of hypothalamic hormones to their receptors on cells of the anterior pituitary in turn stimulates the secretion of specific anterior pituitary hormones into the systemic circulation. The portal system allows the cells of the anterior pituitary to be bathed in blood rich in hypothalamic hormones without the dilution that would have occurred in the systemic circulation. This intimate connection between the hypothalamus and pituitary has important pathophysiologic consequences (see later).

Once secreted, the anterior pituitary hormones travel via the general bloodstream throughout the body and trigger the release of other hormones from particular endocrine glands. These hormones, in turn, have effects on target tissues that

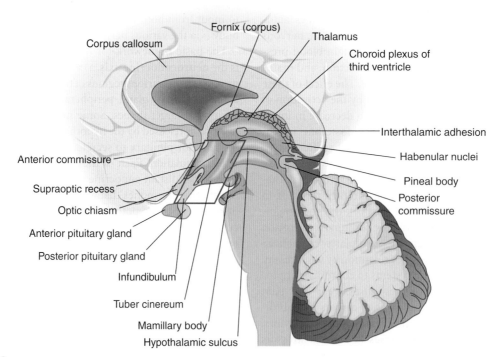

FIGURE 19–1 Sagittal section through the brain showing the diencephalon. (Redrawn, with permission, from Chusid JG. *Correlative Neuroanatomy and Functional Neurology*, 19th ed. Originally published by Lange Medical Publications. Copyright © 1985 by The McGraw-Hill Companies, Inc.)

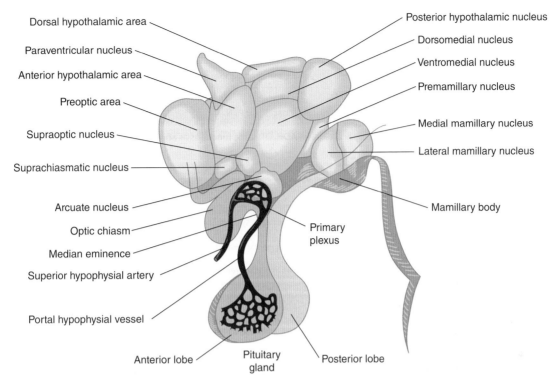

FIGURE 19–2 Human hypothalamus, with a superimposed diagrammatic representation of the portal hypophyseal vessels. (Redrawn, with permission, from Kibble JD et al, eds. *Medical Physiology: The Big Picture.* McGraw-Hill, 2009; and Barrett KE et al, eds. *Ganong's Review of Medical Physiology*, 25th ed. McGraw-Hill, 2016.)

influence growth, reproduction, metabolism, and responses to stress. In addition to their effects on target tissues, hormones secreted in response to stimulation by pituitary hormones also feed back and inhibit secretion of the corresponding pituitary and hypothalamic hormones.

The posterior pituitary hormones are involved in a very different type of neuroendocrine axis, one that bypasses secondary endocrine glands and affects peripheral target tissues directly.

Although most peptide factors secreted by the hypothalamus cause the release of a pituitary hormone, some are inhibitory factors that block or diminish the secretion of particular hormones. There are five main cell types in the anterior pituitary, each of which produces and secretes one of five hormone families: pro-opiomelanocortin and adrenocorticotropic hormone (ACTH); thyrotropin (TSH); growth hormone (GH); prolactin (PRL); and the gonadotropins, luteinizing hormone (LH) and follicle-stimulating hormone (FSH) (Table 19–2).

In addition to their roles in regulating the neuroendocrine axes, some hypothalamic and pituitary hormones are important, but poorly understood, regulators of immune functions and the inflammatory response. Furthermore, the secretion of hypothalamic and pituitary hormones can be significantly influenced by cytokines that regulate the immune response.

CHECKPOINT

1. What is the role of the hypothalamus?
2. What are the neuroendocrine axes, and how do they work?
3. What structures surround the pituitary?
4. Where do the neurons whose axons compose the posterior pituitary originate?

PHYSIOLOGY OF THE HYPOTHALAMUS & PITUITARY GLAND

ANTERIOR PITUITARY HORMONES

Pro-opiomelanocortin & ACTH

The HPA axis is a major part of the physiologic stress system. A variety of stressors (eg, metabolic, physical, mental) result in the activation of the HPA axis. The major hypothalamic regulators are the peptide CRH and, to a lesser extent, arginine vasopressin (AVP), which are produced in the paraventricular and supraoptic nuclei of the hypothalamus and released into the hypothalamic–pituitary portal system. These hormones trigger the synthesis and intracellular transport of a large protein

TABLE 19–1   The hypothalamic nuclei and their main functions.

Nucleus	Location	Major Neurohormones and/or Functions
Supraoptic (SON)	Anterolateral, above the optic tract	ADH: osmoregulation, regulation of ECF volume; OT: regulation of uterine contractions and milk ejection
Paraventricular (PVN)	Dorsal anterior periventricular	Magnacellular PVN
		ADH, OT: same functions as above
		Parvocellular PVN
		TRH: regulation of thyroid function
		CRH: regulation of adrenocortical function, regulation of the sympathetic nervous system and adrenal medulla, regulation of appetite
		ADH: co-expressed with CRH, regulation of adrenocortical function
		VIP: Prolactin-releasing factor (?)
Suprachiasmatic (SCN)	Above the optic chiasm, anteroventral periventricular zone	Regulator of circadian rhythms and pineal function ("Zeitgeber" [pacemaker]): VIP, ADH neurons project mainly to the PVN
Arcuate (ARCN)	Medial basal hypothalamus close to the third ventricle	GHRH: Stimulation of growth hormone
		GnRH: Regulation of pituitary gonadotropins (FSH and LH)
		Dopamine: functions as PIH
		SRIF: Inhibition of GHRH release
		Regulation of appetite (NPY, ART, α-MSH, CART)
Periventricular	Anteroventral	SRIF: Inhibition of growth hormone secretion by direct pituitary action; most abundant SRIF location
Ventromedial (VMN)		GHRH (as above)
		SRIF: Inhibition of GHRH release
		Functions as a satiety center
Dorsomedial (DMN)		Focal point of information processing: receives input from VMN and lateral hypothalamus and projects to the PVN
Lateral hypothalamus		Functions as a hunger center (MCH, orexins)
Preoptic area (POA)		Main regulator of ovulation in rodents. Only a few GnRH neurons in primates
Anterior hypothalamus		Thermoregulation: "cooling center"
		AVOV region: regulation of thirst
Posterior hypothalamus		Thermoregulation: "heating center"

α-MSH, α-melanocyte–stimulating hormone; ADH, antidiuretic hormone; ART, agouti-released transcript; CART, cocaine- and amphetamine-regulated transcript; CRH, corticotropin-releasing hormone; ECF, extracellular fluid; FSH, follicle-stimulating hormone; GHRH, growth hormone–releasing hormone; GnRH, gonadotropin-releasing hormone; LH, luteinizing hormone; MCH, melanin-concentrating hormone; NPY, neuropeptide Y; OT, oxytocin; PIH, prolactin-inhibiting hormone; SRIF, somatotropin release–inhibiting factor; TRH, thyrotropin-releasing hormone; VIP, vasoactive intestinal polypeptide.

termed pro-opiomelanocortin (POMC). POMC is further processed by proteases (prohormone convertases) to release smaller peptides, including a 39-amino-acid-residue peptide, ACTH (Figure 19–5). Although ACTH is the major pituitary hormone that stimulates adrenocortical endocrine function, the amino-terminal part of the POMC peptide (N-POMC) seems to harbor an adrenal growth-promoting function.

ACTH released into the systemic circulation triggers the synthesis and secretion of corticosteroids and adrenal androgens. The effect of ACTH on mineralocorticoid synthesis and

FIGURE 19–3 The component parts of the pituitary and their relationship to the hypothalamus. The pars tuberalis, pars intermedia, and pars distalis, which are rudimentary in humans, form the anterior pituitary, or adenohypophysis. The infundibulum (including the infundibular stalk) and pars nervosa form the posterior pituitary, or neurohypophysis.

release is much less pronounced, as it is mainly regulated by the RAAS.

These steroid hormones, in turn, have complex effects on many tissues to protect the individual from stress; for example, they raise blood pressure and blood glucose and alter the responsiveness of the immune system. Glucocorticoids also feed back to the hypothalamus, where they inhibit CRH secretion, and to the pituitary, where they further inhibit ACTH secretion. In the absence of unusual stress, there is a daily diurnal rhythm of CRH, ACTH, and adrenal steroid release.

Pituitary factors (ie, N-POMC, ACTH) are involved in regulating the proliferation of adrenal cells and the growth of the adrenal layers involved in glucocorticoid and androgen secretion. As a result of chronic activation of the HPA axis, hypertrophy of the target organ (adrenal cortex) occurs. Conversely, conditions that downregulate the HPA axis (eg, the use of exogenous glucocorticoids) result in atrophy of the adrenal cortex. On the other hand, the overall tone of the HPA axis has little or no effect on the growth of the mineralocorticoid-secreting tissues, despite the fact that acute ACTH stimulation triggers the release of mineralocorticoids.

FIGURE 19–4 Diagram of the transcription factors involved in anterior pituitary development. The factors on the left are mainly responsible for Rathke pouch formation and early pituitary development. On the right side are factors inducing differentiation into the five major pituitary cell types. Mutations of some of the genes encoding these transcription factors have been shown to result in hypopituitarism.

TABLE 19–2   Pituitary hormones.

	ACTH	GH	Prolactin	TSH	LH	FSH
Peptides	Derived from POMC precursor	Single-chain polypeptide	Single-chain polypeptide	α: α1 β: TSH-β	α: α1 β: LH-β	α: α1 β: FSH-β
Receptor	ACTH-receptor (melanocortin-2-receptor)	GH receptor	Prolactin receptor	TSH receptor	LH receptor	FSH receptor
Source	Corticotropes (pituitary)	Somatotropes (pituitary)	Lactotropes (pituitary)	Thyrotropes (pituitary)	Gonadotropes (pituitary)	Gonadotropes (pituitary)
Hypothalamic releasing hormone	CRH, AVP	GHRH (ghrelin)	TRH	TRH	GnRH	GnRH
Hypothalamic inhibiting factors		Somatostatin	Dopamine	Somatostatin, dopamine		
Target	Adrenal gland	Liver (production of IGF-1), peripheral tissue	Mammary gland	Thyroid gland	Ovary (theca cell, granulosa cell, luteal cell)/testis (Leydig cell)	Ovary (granulosa cell)/testis (Sertoli cell)
Function	Stimulating cortisol and adrenal androgen release	Stimulating growth (direct and indirect effect via IGF-1)	Stimulating lactation	Stimulating thyroid hormone release	Stimulating estrogen/ testosterone production	Regulating granulosa and Sertoli cell function

ACTH, adrenocorticotropic hormone (corticotropin); AVP, arginine-vasopressin; CRH, corticotropin-releasing hormone; FSH, follicle-stimulating hormone; GH, growth hormone; GHRH, growth hormone–releasing hormone; GnRH, gonadotropin-releasing hormone; IGF, insulin-like growth factor; LH, luteinizing hormone; POMC, pro-opiomelanocortin; TRH, thyrotropin-releasing hormone; TSH, thyroid-stimulating hormone.

FIGURE 19–5 Schematic representation of the prepro-opiomelanocortin molecule formed in pituitary cells, neurons, and other tissues. The numbers in parentheses identify the amino acid sequences in each of the polypeptide fragments. For convenience, the amino acid sequences are numbered from the amino terminal of corticotrope (ACTH) and read toward the carboxyl terminal portion of the parent molecule, whereas the amino acid sequences in the other portion of the molecule read to the left to –131, the amino terminal of the parent molecule. The locations of Lys-Arg and other pairs of basic amino acid residues are also indicated; these are the sites of proteolytic cleavage in the formation of the smaller fragments of the parent molecule. (AL, anterior lobe; IL, intermediate lobe.) (Redrawn, with permission, from Barrett KE et al, eds. *Ganong's Review of Medical Physiology*, 25th ed. McGraw-Hill, 2016.)

The Glycoprotein Hormones

TSH and the gonadotropins belong to the family of glycoprotein hormones (see Table 19–2). The classic glycoprotein hormone family members, TSH and the gonadotropins (FSH, LH), as well as the placenta-derived pregnancy hormone human chorionic gonadotropin (hCG), are composed of a common α-glycoprotein subunit (α-GSU) and an individual β-subunit (eg, TSH-β, LH-β). The unique β-subunit of the glycoprotein hormones is responsible for the biologic differences of these hormones. Another member of this family is thyrostimulin, which shares the composition of an α- and β-subunit (α-2, β-5). The physiologic role of this hormone has yet to be determined.

A. Thyrotropin (Thyroid-Stimulating Hormone)

Thyrotropin (thyroid-stimulating hormone [TSH]) is released from specific cells in the pituitary when stimulated by thyrotropin-releasing hormone (TRH) from the hypothalamus. A hypothalamic factor negatively regulating TSH release is somatostatin. TSH, in turn, travels via the systemic bloodstream to the thyroid gland, where it stimulates the synthesis and secretion of the thyroid hormones thyroxine and triiodothyronine. Thyroid hormones have effects on nearly every tissue in the body but especially the cardiovascular, respiratory, skeletal, and central nervous systems. Thyroid hormones are critical at key points in development, and their deficiency during development has effects (eg, severe mental retardation, short stature) that are not fully reversible by subsequent thyroid hormone administration (see Chapter 20).

Besides its target tissue effects, thyroid hormone feeds back to the pituitary and hypothalamus to inhibit the secretion of TSH and TRH. TSH also triggers the growth of thyroid tissue, resulting in goiter under conditions of chronic TSH stimulation such as iodine deficiency (see Chapter 20).

B. Gonadotropin

The role of the gonadotropins is to regulate the reproductive system's neuroendocrine axis. Thus, a releasing factor from the hypothalamus termed gonadotropin-releasing hormone (GnRH) stimulates LH and FSH secretion, which stimulates steroidogenesis within the ovaries and testes. Furthermore, the gonadotropins promote Sertoli and theca cell function and gametogenesis. The steroids produced by the ovaries (estrogens) and by the testes (testosterone) inhibit GnRH, LH, and FSH production and have target tissue effects on developing follicles within the ovary itself, on the uterus (controlling the menstrual cycle), on breast development, on spermatogenesis, and on many other tissues and physiologic processes (see Chapters 22 and 23).

As is the case with all neuroendocrine axes, the simple feedback loop is complicated by other inputs (eg, from the CNS) that modify responsiveness (see Chapter 7). The discovery that KiSS1-derived peptides (eg, metastin) induce hypothalamic GnRH release via signaling through a G protein–coupled receptor (GPR54) illustrates this point. Mutations in either of these can result in the failure of puberty to develop. Notable features for many hypothalamic releasing factors, but particularly GnRH, are that secretion occurs in a pulsatile fashion and that changes in the rate and amplitude of secretion result in altered pituitary responsiveness because of downregulation or upregulation of the receptors for the hypothalamic releasing factors found on the surface of the pituitary cells. Not only is the secretion of GnRH episodic, but the secretion of FSH and LH is as well, with a secretory burst every 60 minutes. The gonadotropins follow a typical secretion pattern during the estrus cycle with a midcycle LH surge initiating ovulation.

Growth Hormone & Prolactin

Growth hormone and prolactin are structurally related single-chain polypeptides with different spectrums of action.

A. Growth Hormone

Growth hormone (GH), positively regulated by hypothalamic growth hormone–releasing hormone (GHRH) and inhibited by somatostatin, triggers growth-promoting effects in a wide range of tissues (Figure 19–6). GH has both direct (eg, stimulating the growth of cartilage) and indirect (eg, via insulin-like growth factor-1 [IGF-1], a polypeptide secreted by the liver and other tissues) actions (Figure 19–7). IGF-1 has the insulin-like

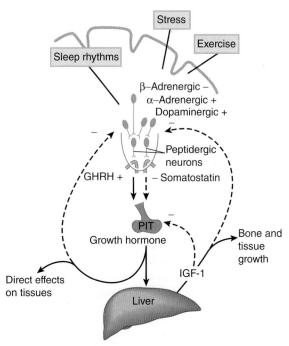

FIGURE 19–6 Schematic diagram of the hypothalamic control of growth hormone secretion. Inhibitory arrows are dashed; stimulating arrows are solid. (GHRH, growth hormone–releasing hormone; IGF, insulin-like growth factor.) (Redrawn from Cone RD. Neuroendocrinology. In: Larsen PR et al, eds. *Williams Textbook of Endocrinology*, 10th ed. Saunders, 2003.)

FIGURE 19–7 Schematic representation of multiple sites of growth hormone (GH) action. (GHRH, growth hormone–releasing hormone; GHRP, growth hormone–releasing peptide; IGF-1, insulin-like growth factor 1. (Redrawn, with permission, from Thorner MO et al. The anterior pituitary. In: Wilson JD et al, eds. *Williams Textbook of Endocrinology*, 9th ed. Saunders, 1998. Copyright © Elsevier.)

effects of promoting fuel storage in various tissues. IGF-1 in turn inhibits GHRH and GH secretion. As in the other neuroendocrine feedback axes, the CNS and other factors can significantly influence the simple regulatory axis (Table 19–3). One of these factors is the gastrointestinal peptide hormone ghrelin, which acts through the growth hormone–secretagogue receptor to induce GH release. The physiological significance of this process has yet to be determined. Somatostatin inhibits GH release; therefore, somatostatin analogs are used to inhibit GH secretion from GH-secreting pituitary tumors.

Some of the actions of GH appear to have a counter-regulatory character in that they raise blood glucose levels and antagonize the action of insulin. In contrast, other actions of GH via IGF-1 are insulin-like. This apparent contradiction makes sense when one considers that promoting growth requires first raising the blood levels of substrates and then using them for synthesis. To do the latter without the former would simply make the individual hypoglycemic without promoting long-term growth.

B. Prolactin

The primary role of prolactin in humans is to stimulate breast development and milk synthesis. It is discussed in greater detail in Chapter 22. Prolactin secretion is mainly negatively regulated by the neurotransmitter dopamine from the hypothalamus rather than by a peptide. That is, dopamine acts to inhibit rather than stimulate prolactin secretion. Pathologic processes that result in the separation of the pituitary gland from the hypothalamus cause the loss of all pituitary hormones except prolactin (**panhypopituitarism** from lack of the hypothalamic releasing hormones). Loss of dopamine results instead in an increase in prolactin secretion from specific anterior pituitary cells now freed of inhibition by dopamine. Primary hypothyroidism is often accompanied by hyperprolactinemia because increased levels of TRH can exhibit prolactin–releasing factor properties.

POSTERIOR PITUITARY HORMONES

Vasopressin & Oxytocin

The peptide hormones vasopressin and oxytocin are synthesized in the supraoptic and paraventricular nuclei of the hypothalamus. The axons of the neurons in these nuclei form the posterior pituitary, where these peptide hormones are stored. Thus, there is no need for a separate set of hypothalamic releasing factors to trigger vasopressin or oxytocin release.

A. Vasopressin

In response to a small increase in blood osmolality, the hypothalamic "osmostat" responds by triggering the subjective sense of thirst and, at the same time, the release of vasopressin. Vasopressin increases the number of active water channels in the cell membranes of renal collecting duct cells, allowing the conservation of free water. This increases the concentration of the urine. The conservation of free water and stimulation of thirst have the net effect of correcting the small change in blood osmolality.

Vasopressin binds to at least three classes of receptors. One of these classes of vasopressin receptor (V_{1A}) is found on smooth muscle. Its major effect is to trigger vasoconstriction. V_{1B} receptors are found on corticotropes, and they contribute to increased ACTH secretion. The other class of receptor (V_2) is found in the distal nephrons in the kidneys; its major action is to mediate vasopressin's effects on osmolality. Because of its V_2-mediated actions, vasopressin is also known as **antidiuretic hormone** (**ADH**). Figure 19–8 illustrates the relationship among osmotic forces, volume, and vasopressin secretion. Although the minute-to-minute function of vasopressin is to maintain blood osmolality, its secretion is also increased by large decreases in intravascular volume. This assists aldosterone in raising intravascular volume, albeit at the expense of lowered osmolality. The combination of ADH-mediated peripheral vasoconstriction and water retention (in the setting of hypotension, even with lower or normal osmolarity) can be understood as a way of helping maintain perfusion in the face of major intravascular volume deficits (eg, with hemorrhage), even if the volume and osmolar composition of the perfusing blood are not ideal. In pharmacologic doses, vasopressin can be used as an adjunct in the treatment of severe hypotensive crises.

TABLE 19–3   Factors influencing normal growth hormone secretion.

Factor	Augmented Secretion	Inhibited Secretion
Neurogenic	Stage III and stage IV sleep	REM sleep
	Stress (traumatic, surgical, inflammatory, psychic, exercise)	Alpha-adrenergic antagonists
	Alpha-adrenergic agonists	Beta-adrenergic agonists
	Beta-adrenergic antagonists	Acetylcholine antagonists
	Dopamine agonists	H1-histamine antagonists
	Acetylcholine agonists	Serotonin antagonists
		Nicotinic cholinergic agonists
Metabolic	Hypoglycemia	Postprandial, glucose-infusion-related hyperglycemia
	Fasting, postprandial glucose decline	Rising fatty acid level
	Falling fatty acid level	Obesity
	Amino acids	Aging, senescence
	Uncontrolled diabetes mellitus	
	Uremia	
	Hepatic cirrhosis	
	Anorexia nervosa, protein depletion	
Hormonal	GHRH	Somatostatin
	Glucagon	Calcitonin
	Low insulin-like growth factor	High insulin-like growth factor
	(IGF-1)	(IGF-1) (pituitary)
	Estrogens, tesosterone	Hypothyroidism, hyperthyroidism
	Glucocorticoids (acute)	High glucocorticoid levels
	Opioids	Glucocorticoids (chronic)
	Arginine vasopressin	Neuropeptide Y
	Ghrelin, GNRH, galanin (via interaction with hypothalamic somatostatin and via GHRH)	Corticotropin-releasing hormone
		Acromegaly (L-Dopa, dopamine receptor D2 agonists, phentermine)
	Acromegaly (TRH, LHRH, glucose, arginine)	
	Type 1 diabetes mellitus	

GHRH, growth hormone–releasing hormone; GNRH, gonadotropin-releasing hormone; LHRH, luteinizing hormone releasing hormone; REM, rapid eye movement; TRH, thyrotropin-releasing hormone.

Reproduced, with permission, from Cone RD et al. Neuroendocrinology. In: Larsen PR et al, eds. *Williams Textbook of Endocrinology*, 10h ed. Saunders, 2003. Copyright © Elsevier.

B. Oxytocin

Like vasopressin, the peptide oxytocin is stored in the nerve terminals of hypothalamic neurons in the posterior pituitary. It plays an important role in breast and uterine smooth muscle contraction both on a minute-to-minute basis during breastfeeding and in contraction of the uterus during parturition. Besides its function in lactation and parturition, recent research suggests a significant role for oxytocin in the neuropsychological regulation of behavior, such as trust formation and interpersonal bonding (eg, pair and parental attachment).

CHECKPOINT

5. How do the neuroendocrine feedback loops of the anterior and posterior pituitary differ?
6. How can two polypeptide hormones whose mature forms have no sequence in common be derived from the same precursor?
7. Describe the distinguishing features of each pituitary neuroendocrine feedback axis.
8. What is the significance of receptor downregulation for hypothalamic control of pituitary function?

PHYSIOLOGY OF THE NEUROENDOCRINE AXIS

A number of features of neuroendocrine axis physiology have important implications for the pathophysiology of disease.

First, the hypothalamic hormones that traverse the pituitary portal system are short-lived. They also have relatively

FIGURE 19–8 The influence of hemodynamic status on the osmoregulation of vasopressin in otherwise healthy humans. The numbers in the circles refer to the percentage change in volume or pressure; N refers to the normovolemic normotensive subject. Note that hemodynamic status affects both the slope of the relationship between plasma vasopressin and osmolality and the osmotic threshold for vasopressin release. (Redrawn and adapted from Robertson GL et al. The osmoregulation of vasopressin. Kidney Int. 1976;10:25. Adapted by Rose BD in: *Clinical Physiology of Acid–Base and Electrolyte Disorders*, 3rd ed. McGraw-Hill, 1989. Reprinted, with permission, from Kidney International.)

low affinity for their receptors. These properties are generally more characteristic of neurotransmitters in the nervous system than of hormones in the bloodstream. Some of these hormones, and the receptor systems with which they interact,

have evolved in ways that take advantage of the unique features of a neuroendocrine axis. For example, in the case of GnRH, secretion is markedly pulsatile in character; a particular rate and amplitude of hypothalamic hormone secretion are crucial for a proper response by the receptor-bearing gonadotropes. If the pulse rate or amplitude is too high, the receptors are downregulated.

Second, for some of the neuroendocrine axes, measuring a random blood level of the end-organ hormone is not generally clinically useful. A more reliable approach to assess neuroendocrine axis function is often to assess the secretory response to a provocative stimulus: a **challenge test**. Thus, an adequate increase in blood cortisol 1 hour after an intravenous injection of ACTH provides far more compelling evidence for an intact adrenal gland than does a randomly drawn, unprovoked normal blood level of cortisol.

Finally, besides stimulating end-organ hormone secretion, most pituitary hormones exert trophic effects on the hormone-secreting cells of the end organ. Thus, an excess of pituitary hormone results in end-organ hypertrophy, and a lack of pituitary hormone results in end-organ atrophy.

PHYSIOLOGY OF BODY WEIGHT CONTROL

Various physiologic control mechanisms integrated by the hypothalamus work to maintain body weight over the short and the long term (Figure 19–9).

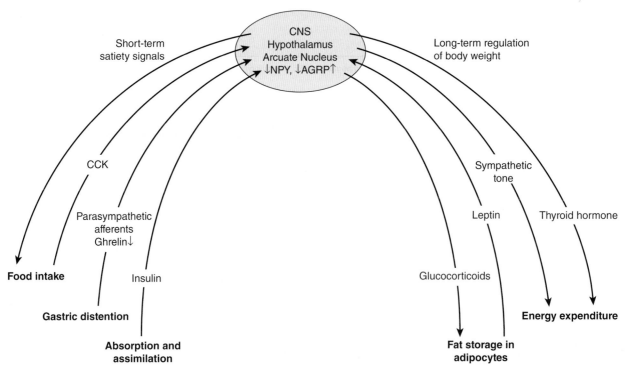

FIGURE 19–9 Physiologic control mechanisms regulating body weight. (AGRP, agouti-related peptide; CCK, cholecystokinin; NPY, neuropeptide Y.)

The key parameters of the short-term regulation of body weight are (1) the amount and composition of food; (2) nutrient absorption and assimilation; and (3) satiety, the sense of having eaten enough food. Satiety is a complex response to food intake that has mechanical, neural, and hormonal components.

A main mechanism by which short-term food intake and satiety are regulated is communication via the "gut–brain axis." The gut–brain cross-talk uses two main routes of communication, including both neural (mainly afferent vagal fibers) and hormonal components. Thus, we feel a sense of fullness in response to the mechanical distention of the stomach, which triggers afferent neural pathways to the hypothalamus, or via brainstem centers (eg, nucleus of the solitary tract). In addition, hormones are secreted in response to food ingestion and absorption and have direct effects on the hypothalamus to induce satiety. These hormonal signals mainly include anorexigenic satiety signals, such as glucagon-like peptide-1 (GLP-1), which are released in the gut and directly impact gastrointestinal mobility and function but also stimulate gastrointestinal neural signaling to the hypothalamus. Some of these hormones travel directly to the brain and bind to receptors in the hypothalamus or in areas of the blood–brain barrier that are regulated "open." The only known orexigenic signal arising from the gut is the peptide hormone ghrelin, suggesting that satiety is more abundantly regulated by the gastrointestinal system than is hunger.

In contrast to the short-term control of body weight, long-term regulation is largely influenced by the degree of obesity. Fat cells secrete the hormone leptin in proportion to the amount of triglyceride they have stored. Thus, over the long term, an excess ingestion of calories resulting in increased fat deposition triggers an increase in leptin secretion. Leptin impinges on its receptors in the hypothalamus so that the individual eats less and, therefore, assimilates fewer calories. Another response to leptin is to increase sympathetic nervous system activity so that more calories are burned.

Conversely, when caloric intake is insufficient to maintain body weight, fat is mobilized, leptin secretion decreases, and set points in the hypothalamus are changed in ways that promote food-seeking behavior, diminish sympathetic neural activity, and generally conserve calories to offset the tendency toward weight loss. As a result of this feedback loop, a further decrease in body weight is resisted. It is likely that this system evolved primarily as a defense against starvation, but it also serves to defend against obesity.

How these signals are normally integrated in the hypothalamus to achieve satiety in the short term and maintain normal body weight in the long term is less clear. The arcuate nucleus of the hypothalamus is the best understood integrator of the regulation of food intake (Figure 19–10). However, several other hypothalamic nuclei appear to be involved in the control of energy homeostasis and food intake. For example, lesions in the ventromedial region result in obesity, and lesions in the lateral hypothalamus result in weight loss. One hypothesis

attempting to integrate current information on the regulation of fuel homeostasis proposes different responses by the body to falling versus rising leptin concentrations, as would be seen in weight loss versus weight gain, respectively. Thus, in response to falling leptin levels, neuropeptide Y is secreted from leptin receptor–bearing cells of the arcuate nucleus in the ventromedial hypothalamus. Neuropeptide Y is believed to mediate hypothalamic responses to starvation.

Another well-described system regulating satiety and food intake within the arcuate nucleus of the hypothalamus is the POMC system. Although the hypothalamic POMC system uses the same peptides for signaling mediators as the pituitary POMC system, they are very different in POMC expression, processing, and receptors. In particular, the main receptor mediating satiety and food intake is a special subtype of melanocortin receptors (MC4R). In the state of caloric excess, hypothalamic-derived POMC peptides, such as melanocyte-stimulating hormone (α-MSH), keep these MC4R in a tonic activated state. In addition, hypothalamic POMC neurons are leptin responsive; therefore, these neurons represent an interface between leptin and the POMC system. As circulating leptin levels parallel the total quantity of fat storage, it makes sense that the activation of POMC neurons leads to the inhibition of food intake. In the event of caloric restriction, the tonic activation of the MC4R is reduced by two mechanisms: a decrease in agonists (MSH) and, even more important, an increase in the availability of antagonists, namely agouti-related peptide (AGRP). These antagonists downregulate not only MSH (agonist driven) but also an intrinsic constitutive activity of the MC4R. The mode of action of the MC4R antagonism by AGRP has been termed "inverse agonism." Furthermore, it is believed that many other neuropeptides, including bombesin, insulin, and a group of peptides termed orexins, have complex effects on the hypothalamus that affect feeding, satiety, energy balance, and other parameters relevant for weight control (Table 19–4). The orexins appear to be ligands for previously "orphan" G protein–coupled receptors in the brain. How the effects of these peptides are integrated with those of leptin and neuropeptide Y is a current focus of research. Finally, research strongly implicates leptin in other physiologic functions such as regulating reproductive and immune function as well as bone density.

CHECKPOINT

9. What are the short- and long-term factors involved in the normal control of body weight?
10. What is the significance of the short half-life, low affinity, and restricted circulation of most hypothalamic hormones?
11. Why are challenge tests particularly important in assessing the function of a neuroendocrine axis?
12. What happens to an end organ in the absence of the pituitary hormone that normally triggers its secretion?

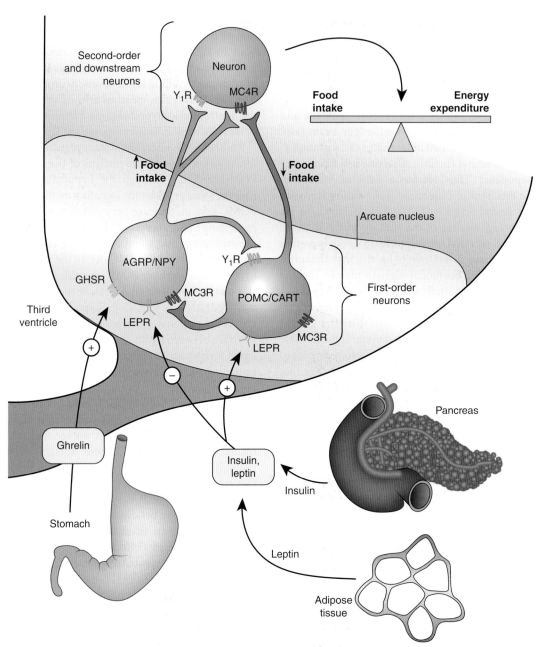

FIGURE 19–10 Control of energy homeostasis by arcuate nucleus neurons. The arcuate neurons contain stimulatory and inhibitory neurons related to food intake. Agouti-related protein (AGRP) and neuropeptide Y (NPY) stimulate food intake and decrease energy expenditure, whereas α-melanocyte-stimulating hormone and cocaine- and amphetamine-regulated transcript (CART) inhibit food intake and increase energy expenditure. Additionally, the core neurons within the arcuate nucleus receive input from circulating hormones as well as projections from other neurons. (GHSR, growth hormone secretagogue receptor; LEPR, leptin receptor; MC3R, melanocortin receptor type 3; MC4R, melanocortin receptor type 4; POMC, proopiomelanocortin; Y_1R, neuropeptide Y receptor Y1.) (Redrawn, with permission, from Barsh GS et al. Genetic approaches to studying energy balance: perception and integration. Nat Rev Genetics 2002 Aug;3:589–600. By permission from Springer Nature.)

PATHOPHYSIOLOGY OF SELECTED HYPOTHALAMIC & PITUITARY DISEASES

The hypothalamus and pituitary are implicated in the pathophysiology of a variety of complex diseases. These include anxiety disorders, in which abnormalities of the hypothalamic–pituitary–growth hormone axis appear to be a specific pathologic marker; alcoholism, in which neuropeptide Y has been implicated in mouse models of this condition; and obesity, in which a host of hypothalamic neuropeptides are affected and, in turn, affect parameters of fuel homeostasis.

TABLE 19–4   Peptides regulating food intake (mainly on the level of the hypothalamus).

Inhibitory	Stimulatory
α-MSH (a product of POMC)	Agouti-related peptide (AGRP)
Leptin	Ghrelin
Cocaine- and amphetamine-related peptide (CART)	Neuropeptide Y
Insulin	Melanin-concentrating hormone (MCH)
Peptide YY3–36	Orexins
Corticotropin releasing hormone (CRH)	Galanin
Cholecystokinin (CCK)	Endocannabinoids
Glucagon-like peptide-1 (GLP-1)	
Prolactin-releasing peptide	
Insulin-like growth factors I and II	
Calcitonin gene–related peptide (CGRP)	
Somatostatin	
Neuromedin U	
Serotonin	
Bombesin	

In most of these disorders, it remains unclear whether hypothalamic and endocrine dysregulation are important causative factors in pathogenesis or epiphenomena mirroring central nervous dysfunction, or likely both.

OBESITY

Changes in body weight can occur through alteration of several variables, including (1) the amount and type of food ingested; (2) central control of satiety; (3) hormonal control of assimilation or storage; and (4) physical activity or metabolic rate.

Clinical Presentation & Etiology

Obesity can be defined as excess body weight sufficient to increase overall morbidity and mortality. Although extreme obesity is associated with dramatically increased mortality, the risks of mild to moderate obesity are less clear. An index of "fatness" is the body mass index (BMI), which equals weight (in kilograms) divided by height (in meters squared). The normal range is 18.5–25 kg/m², with clinically significant obesity defined as a BMI >30 kg/m². More than 20% of the U.S. population is obese by this criterion. Individuals with a BMI of 150% of normal have an overall 2-fold risk of premature death, whereas those with a BMI 200% of normal have a 10-fold risk. Table 19–5 lists some important causes of morbidity and mortality

TABLE 19–5   Some disorders associated with obesity.

Hypertension
Diabetes mellitus
Coronary artery disease
Gallstones
Sudden death
Cardiomyopathy
Sleep apnea
Hirsutism
Osteoarthritis
Gout
Stroke
Cancer (breast, endometrial, ovarian, cervical, gallbladder in women; prostatic, colorectal in men)

associated with obesity, and Figure 19–11 shows possible pathophysiologic mechanisms involved in their production.

Pathophysiology

The recognition that obesity plays a role in the pathophysiology of disease comes from epidemiologic studies identifying obesity as a risk factor without providing insight into the mechanism of the risk.

Although growing, only a very small number of cases of monogenetic disorders result in obesity in humans. These syndromes highlight the importance of the aforementioned hypothalamic regulatory systems of body weight control. Several mutations in leptin or the leptin receptor, both resulting in the lack of a sufficient leptin effect on the hypothalamus, have been described as a cause of both human and murine obesity. Most strikingly, leptin replacement therapy in cases of leptin deficiency leads to the complete normalization of body weight. Other mutations have been described in the hypothalamic POMC system. Mutations in the *MC4R* or *POMC* gene or in POMC-processing proteases, all of which result in reduced MSH levels, lead to severe childhood obesity. Consistent with data describing the involvement of the POMC system in hypothalamic body weight regulation, all mutations within this system result in decreased signaling through the MC4R and, therefore, increased food intake.

Aside from the monogenic disorders mentioned previously, obesity appears to be the result of multiple mechanisms, and many studies have established an imbalance in the neuroendocrine hypothalamic and brain–gut systems. Thus, obesity may be either a cause or a consequence of disease, depending on the disorder. For example, type 2 diabetes mellitus is sometimes first manifested clinically by sudden weight gain, and

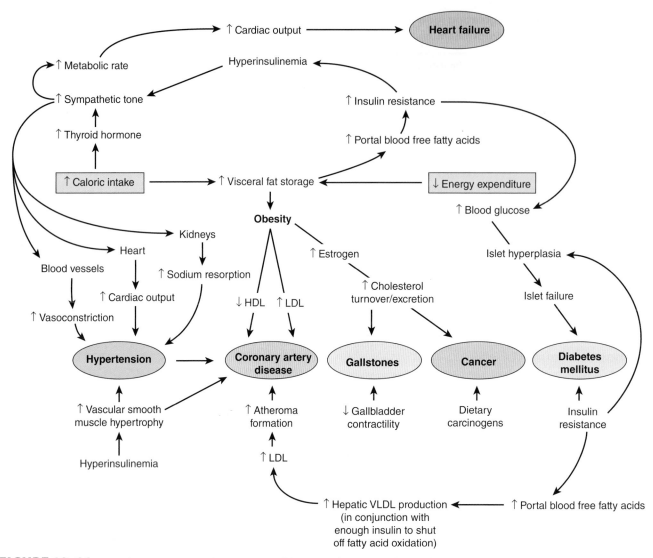

FIGURE 19–11 Role of obesity in the pathophysiology of disease and some ways by which obesity contributes to disease. Short arrows refer to a change in the indicated parameter, and long arrows indicate a consequence of that change. In some cases, evidence is epidemiologic; in others, it is experimental. (HDL, high-density lipoprotein; LDL, low-density lipoprotein; VLDL, very-low-density lipoprotein.) (Redrawn, with permission, from Bray GA. Pathophysiology of obesity. Am J Clin Nutr. 1992;55:488S.)

this disorder can be difficult to control without weight loss, reflecting the insulin-resistant character of the obese state. Moreover, if the weight can be lost, the diabetes may once again become latent, controlled by diet and exercise alone. In such cases, obesity seems clearly to be an etiologic factor in the development of diabetes mellitus. Yet insulin injections, which may be necessary to control the symptoms of diabetes in such a patient, further exacerbate the weight gain that precipitated the disorder in the first place. Such "chicken-or-egg" relationships make the pathophysiology of obesity particularly difficult to dissect. Nevertheless, important progress has been made toward developing a coherent framework in which to view obesity as both cause and consequence of disease. Some of these observations are noted next.

The number of fat cells in the body is probably established during infancy. One hypothesis is that obesity appearing during adulthood results from an enlargement of individual fat cells (hypertrophy) rather than an increased number of fat cells (hyperplasia). Obesity from fat cell hypertrophy appears to be much more easily controlled than obesity from fat cell hyperplasia. Perhaps feedback signals in response to the degree of fat cell hypertrophy are important to the hypothalamic "lipostat."

It now appears that *where* fat is deposited is more important than *how much* is deposited. Thus, so-called visceral or central obesity (omental fat in the distribution of blood flow draining into the portal vein) seems far more important as a risk factor for obesity-related morbidity and mortality than so-called subcutaneous (gynecoid, lower body) or peripheral fat. It appears that visceral fat is more sensitive to catecholamines and less sensitive to insulin, making it a marker of insulin resistance. Consistent with these findings is the observation that obese individuals who engage in vigorous physical activity and whose obesity is largely due to high caloric intake (eg, sumo wrestlers) have subcutaneous rather than visceral fat and do not demonstrate substantially increased insulin resistance. In contrast, the obesity associated with a sedentary lifestyle is believed to be largely visceral obesity and is associated with a greater degree of insulin resistance in patients both with and without a diagnosis of diabetes mellitus. A parameter reflecting the different kinds of fat distribution is the waist-to-hip ratio, which has been shown to correlate with morbidity.

As mentioned, leptin mutations are also associated with obesity in some humans. However, in the vast majority of obese humans, excessive rather than deficient leptin levels are observed. Thus, it appears that the most common form of human obesity involves leptin resistance in the face of high endogenous leptin levels rather than defective leptin secretion as observed in *ob/ob* mice. An animal model for this condition is the obese *db/db* mouse, in which there is a defective leptin receptor. A variety of mechanisms, including diminished signaling through the leptin receptor and diminished transport across the blood–brain barrier, could account for leptin resistance in different individuals.

Psychologic factors also make an important contribution to the development of obesity. For example, obese individuals appear to regulate their desire for food by greater reliance on external cues (eg, time of day, appeal of the food) rather than endogenous signals (eg, feeling hungry).

Last, there is great interest in the development of drugs that alter these pathways (eg, neuropeptide Y and endocannabinoid antagonists) in ways that would promote weight loss as a treatment for obesity. On the contrary, endocannabinoid agonists are used to promote appetite and weight gain in the setting of severe wasting syndrome.

CHECKPOINT

13. Define obesity.
14. What diseases are associated with obesity?
15. Outline several pathophysiologic mechanisms by which obesity contributes to disease.

PITUITARY ADENOMA

An adenoma is a benign tumor of epithelial cell origin. Pituitary adenomas are of particular significance because (1) the pituitary is in an enclosed space with very limited capacity to accommodate an expanding mass; and (2) pituitary adenomas may arise from cells that secrete hormones, giving rise to hormone overproduction syndromes.

Clinical Presentation

Pituitary adenomas are extremely common and are observed in about one in six autopsies. The majority of pituitary adenomas are clinically inapparent, either because they are nonfunctional, because hormone processing and secretion are inefficient, or because hormone production does not reach the critical threshold to elicit clinical symptoms. If pituitary adenomas come to medical attention, symptoms and signs are related either to an expanding intracranial mass (headaches, diabetes insipidus, vision changes) or to manifestations of an excess or deficiency of one or more pituitary hormones. Hormone deficiency results from the destruction of the normal pituitary by the expanding adenoma. Hormone excess occurs when the adenoma secretes a particular hormone. **Microadenomas** (<10 mm in diameter) are more likely to present with complaints related to hormone excess than to local mass effects because they are small. Conversely, whether or not they secrete hormones, **macroadenomas** (>10 mm in diameter) can impinge on the optic chiasm above the sella turcica or the cavernous sinuses laterally.

Etiology

Any cell type in the pituitary gland can undergo hyperplasia or give rise to a tumor. Whether the patient with a pituitary tumor presents with a mass effect or symptoms referable to pituitary hormones depends on the size, growth rate, and secretory characteristics of the tumor. Which, if any, hormones the tumor secretes is generally a reflection of the cell type from which the tumor originated. **Gigantism** and **acromegaly** are due to the oversecretion of growth hormone. **Cushing disease** is the condition of glucocorticoid excess resulting from the oversecretion of pituitary ACTH. **Galactorrhea** occurs in patients with prolactin-secreting tumors. Tumors secreting TSH, LH, and FSH are extremely rare and (in accordance with their physiological function) can cause secondary hyperthyroidism, precocious puberty, or ovarian hyperstimulation, respectively.

Pathophysiology

Most pituitary adenomas are clonal in origin: A single cell with altered growth control and feedback regulation gives rise to the adenoma. Evidence for the involvement of genetic mutations in the cause of pituitary adenomas comes from the occurrence of familial pituitary tumor syndromes. At least four different syndromes caused by defined genetic mutations are known to significantly increase the incidence of pituitary tumor formation: multiple endocrine neoplasia type 1 (MEN-1), Carney complex (CNC), McCune–Albright syndrome, and aryl hydrocarbon receptor–interacting protein (AIP)-related predisposition to pituitary adenoma. Mutation of the *MENIN* tumor suppressor gene is the underlying cause of MEN-1. As is typical for tumor suppressor genes, the loss of heterozygosity results in tumor formation. Pituitary tumors, as well as tumors of the pancreas and hyperplasia of the parathyroid glands, are typical manifestations in MEN-1 patients. Pituitary hyperplasia and microadenomas are also part of CNC. A subgroup of these patients harbors a mutation in the gene encoding for a protein A kinase subunit, resulting in an altered response to growth regulatory factors. In McCune–Albright syndrome, the *GNAS1* gene, which encodes a G-protein stimulatory subunit, is mutated and renders the protein product constitutively active. Thus, cyclic adenosine monophosphate levels are chronically elevated in these cells, resulting in constitutive hormone gene activation and cell hyperplasia. Patients with *AIP* mutations are mainly predisposed to the development of growth hormone–secreting tumors.

Aside from these rare syndromes, the pathogenesis of pituitary adenomas is believed to be a multistep process analogous to the well-described consecutive mutations necessary for the induction of colon carcinomas. Several known or proposed factors have been shown to contribute to the transformation of pituitary cells (eg, *GNAS1, PTTG*).

Clinical Manifestations

Figure 19–12 summarizes the clinical manifestations related to mass effects. Bitemporal hemianopia is the classic visual field defect in a patient with an expanding pituitary mass (see Figure 19–12, panel C). It occurs because the crossing fibers of the optic tract, which lie directly above the pituitary gland and innervate the part of the retina responsible for temporal vision, are compressed by the tumor. However, in practice, a wide variety of visual field defects is seen, reflecting the unpredictable nature of the direction and extent of tumor growth, as well as anatomic variability. The clinical manifestations of hormone excess are discussed next.

Regardless of whether a pituitary tumor is producing hormones, infarction of or hemorrhage into the expanding mass can destroy the normal pituitary gland. This leaves the patient without one or more pituitary hormones. The resulting clinical manifestations are considered later in the discussion of panhypopituitarism.

A. Prolactinoma

Hyperprolactinemia is the most common anterior pituitary disorder and has many causes (Table 19–6). Pathologic hyperprolactinemia, caused by prolactin-secreting adenomas (prolactinomas) or other clinical states that result in elevated prolactin levels, such as primary hypothyroidism or dopamine receptor–blocking drug therapy, must be distinguished from the physiologic hyperprolactinemia of pregnancy and lactation. Roughly 40% of pituitary adenomas found in autopsies are prolactinomas. Most patients had no symptoms from microadenomas and died of unrelated causes.

Patients with prolactin-secreting macroadenomas generally present with mass effect symptoms, whereas those with microadenomas may develop symptoms related to hormonal effects, from either the direct actions of prolactin (galactorrhea in 30–80% of women and up to 33% of men) or prolactin's inhibitory effects on the hypothalamic–pituitary–gonadal axis. The resulting reproductive dysfunction presents variably: amenorrhea, irregular menses, or menses with infertility in women and decreased libido and partial or complete impotence or infertility in men.

Decreased bone density is another common consequence of hyperprolactinemia resulting from hypogonadism and perhaps also poorly understood direct effects of prolactin on bone.

Headaches

A. Stretching of dura by tumor

B. Hydrocephalus (rare)

Visual field defects

C. Nasal retinal fibers compressed by tumor

Cranial nerve palsies and temporal lobe epilepsy

D. Lateral extension of tumor

Cerebrospinal fluid rhinorrhea

E. Downward extension of tumor

FIGURE 19–12 Various symptoms of pituitary tumor. Headaches are rarely caused by hydrocephalus. Visual field defects caused by extension of the tumor are plotted with the Goldmann perimeter. (Redrawn, with permission, from Wass JAH. Hypopituitarism. In: Besser GM et al, eds. *Clinical Endocrinology: An Illustrated Text.* Gower, 1987.)

B. Growth Hormone–Secreting Adenoma

GH-secreting tumors give rise to the syndromes of **gigantism** or **acromegaly** depending on whether they develop before or after closure of the epiphyses. Clinical findings in gigantism and acromegaly are summarized in Table 19–7 and reflect a combination of the insulin-like effects of the hormone, promoting visceromegaly, and the counter-regulatory effects, promoting glucose intolerance.

TABLE 19–6   Causes of hyperprolactinemia.

Physiologic causes
Pregnancy
Lactation, suckling
Stress (eg, physical, psychologic)
Sleep
Exercise
Coitus
Hypothalamic disease
Tumor (eg, metastases, craniopharyngioma, dysgerminoma, meningioma, Rathke's cyst, glioma, hamartoma, suprasellar pituitary mass extension)
Infiltrative disease (eg, sarcoidosis, tuberculosis, histiocytosis X, granuloma)
Pseudotumor cerebri
Cranial radiation
Trauma (pituitary stalk section, sellar surgery, head trauma)
Pituitary disease
Prolactinoma, macroadenoma (compressive), parasellar mass, macroprolactinemia
Acromegaly
Cushing disease
Empty sella syndrome
Other tumors (eg, metastases, nonfunctioning adenoma, gonadotrope adenoma, meningioma)
Infiltrative disease (eg, sarcoidosis, giant cell granuloma, tuberculosis)
Lymphocytic hypophysitis
Drugs
Dopamine receptor antagonists (eg, neuroleptics such as chlorpromazine, fluphenazine, haloperidol, metoclopramide, perphenazine, promazine, promethazine, risperidone, thioridazine, thioxanthenes, trifluoperazine)
Other drugs
Anticonvulsants (eg, phenytoin)
Antidepressants (tricyclics [eg, amitriptyline, chlorimipramine], selective serotonin reuptake inhibitors [eg, fluoxetine]
Antihypertensives (eg, labetolol, methyldopa, reserpine, verapamil)
Opioids (eg, heroin, methadone, morphine, apomorphine)
H2 antihistamines (cimetidine, ranitidine)
Systemic disorders
Chronic kidney disease
Cirrhosis
Chest (eg, breast manipulation, chest wall lesions, neurogenic [herpes zoster], spinal cord lesions, surgery, trauma)
Epileptic seizures
Polycystic ovarian syndrome
Pseudocyesis
Idiopathic
Genetic
Inactivating prolactin receptor mutation

Data from Kaiser U et al. Pituitary physiology and diagnostic evaluation. In: Melmed S et al, eds. *Williams Textbook of Endocrinology*, 13th ed. Elsevier, 2016.

TABLE 19–7   Clinical and laboratory findings in patients with acromegaly.

Clinical Finding
Recent acral growth, acral enlargement
Typical facial changes
Soft tissue swelling (heal pad, hands, subcutaneous scalp tissue)
Excessive sweating
Carpal tunnel syndrome
Malocclusion
New skin tags
Hypertension
Headache
Visual field defects with large tumors
Goiter
Symptoms of other secondary hormone deficiencies (tiredness, lethargy, weakness, decreased libido, oligomenorrhea)
Laboratory and Imaging Findings
Increased fasting blood glucose, abnormal glucose tolerance, diabetes
Hyperprolactinemia
Hyperphosphatemia
Increased sella volume, pituitary tumor
Other secondary hormone deficiency with large tumors (low testosterone, cortisol, thyroid hormone)

C. ACTH-Secreting Pituitary Adenoma (Cushing Disease)

The secretion of excess cortisol as a result of ACTH overproduction by a pituitary adenoma (termed Cushing disease) is the most common cause of spontaneous Cushing syndrome (see Chapter 21). ACTH-secreting pituitary adenomas are eight times more common in women than in men and must be distinguished from the effects of CRH or ACTH arising from outside the hypothalamus and pituitary gland, respectively, and from hypercortisolism due to adrenal adenomas and carcinomas.

The symptoms and signs of ACTH-secreting pituitary adenomas are a consequence of both local mass effects, similar to those discussed previously for other types of pituitary tumors, and effects of the overproduction of cortisol by the adrenal gland, as discussed in Chapter 21. **Nelson syndrome** is the rapid progression of an ACTH-secreting pituitary adenoma, which is often observed after bilateral adrenalectomy to control the symptoms of cortisol excess. With the advent of vigorous glucocorticoid substitution regimens, transsphenoidal pituitary surgery, and radiation therapy, the incidence of this complication has greatly diminished.

HYPOPITUITARISM

Panhypopituitarism is the syndrome resulting from the complete loss of all hormones secreted by the pituitary gland. Hypopituitarism refers to the loss of one or more pituitary hormones. Table 19–8 lists the causes of hypopituitarism.

Clinical Presentation

The complex of symptoms in hypopituitarism varies depending on the extent and duration of disease. Regardless of the underlying cause, in noncongenital forms of hypopituitarism, GH deficiency often occurs as the earliest hormonal deviance, followed by ACTH and gonadotropin (LH and FSH) deficiencies, and finally, TSH deficiency. In some cases, panhypopituitarism is of sudden onset (eg, caused by pituitary infarction or trauma). These patients may rapidly develop two potentially life-threatening situations as a consequence of the loss of ACTH and vasopressin. First, since the patient is unable to mount a stress response because of a lack of ACTH-stimulated glucocorticoid secretion, even relatively mild stress may be lethal. Second, a patient unable to maintain water intake will be unable to compensate for the massive diuresis associated with vasopressin deficiency (**diabetes insipidus**). Thus, the patient will quickly become comatose as a result of profound water loss and the complications of dehydration and hyperosmolarity. However, most patients with diabetes insipidus manage to compensate for the volume loss by increased fluid intake, unless there is a concomitant disturbance of the hypothalamic thirst centers.

In other cases, pituitary insufficiency develops more insidiously (eg, from progressive destruction of the pituitary gland by a nonsecreting tumor or subsequent to pituitary radiation therapy). In many of these slowly developing cases of panhypopituitarism, the patient comes to medical attention with complaints related to reproductive functions (amenorrhea in women; infertility or erectile dysfunction in men) caused by LH and FSH deficiency. Other patients have nonspecific complaints (eg, lethargy or altered bowel habits), perhaps related to the gradual development of hypothyroidism (from TSH deficiency). Panhypopituitarism may be unmasked only when the patient responds poorly during some other unrelated medical emergency because of an inability to mount a protective stress response because of an ACTH and consequent glucocorticoid deficiency.

Etiology

Panhypopituitarism of sudden onset is usually due to traumatic disruption of the pituitary stalk, infarction and hemorrhage

TABLE 19–8   Causes of hypopituitarism.

Ischemic necrosis of the pituitary
Postpartum necrosis (Sheehan syndrome)
Head injury
Vascular disease, commonly associated with diabetes mellitus
Neoplasms involving the sella turcica
Nonfunctioning adenoma
Craniopharyngioma
Suprasellar chordoma
Histiocytosis X (eosinophilic granuloma; Hand–Schüller–Christian disease)
Intrasellar cysts
Chronic inflammatory lesions
Tuberculosis, syphilis, sarcoidosis
Hypophysitis related to cancer immunotherapy
Infiltrative diseases
Amyloidosis
Hemochromatosis
Mucopolysaccharidoses
Genetic mutations
Part of a syndrome
PITX2, HESX1, LHX3, LHX4
Resulting in combined or isolated hormone deficiency
PROP1, PIT1 (combined pituitary hormone deficiency)
TPIT (ACTH deficiency), *DAX1* (hypogonadotropic hypogonadism)
Hormone genes (eg, *POMC* for proopiomelanocortin, and *TSHB* for TSH β subunit)
Prohormone convertases (*PC1*)
Releasing hormone receptor genes (eg, *TRH-R, GnRH-R*)

into a pituitary tumor, or ischemic destruction of the pituitary after systemic hypotension (eg, **Sheehan syndrome**, postpartum hypopituitarism after massive blood loss in childbirth). A number of rare genetic causes have also been reported (see Table 19–8 and Figure 19–4). Hypopituitarism has followed immunotherapy for cancer, which can lead to hypophysitis and loss of several anterior pituitary hormone functions. As opposed to sporadic hypophysitis, diabetes insipidus is never seen in these patients. Gradually acquired hypopituitarism is most often due to the extension of pituitary tumors or occurs as a complication of radiation therapy for brain tumors.

Pathophysiology

The biochemical hallmark of hypopituitarism is low levels of pituitary hormones in the face of low end-organ products of one or more components of the neuroendocrine axes involving the pituitary. By contrast, primary end-organ failure results in compensatory high levels of the relevant pituitary hormones.

Another biochemical difference between primary end-organ failure and end-organ failure secondary to hypopituitarism is that not all end-organ functions are equally controlled by the pituitary. In the case of the adrenal cortex, for example, although mineralocorticoid secretion can be stimulated by ACTH, it is not dependent on it.

Both biochemical distinctions between primary end-organ failure and pituitary failure have important clinical implications. For example, hyperpigmentation occurs in primary adrenal insufficiency because several POMC-derived peptides (MSHs, ACTH) stimulate skin pigmentation via binding to the melanocortin-1 receptor (MC1R). Because levels of POMC-derived peptides are not elevated in pituitary and hypothalamic insufficiency, hyperpigmentation does not occur. Similarly, the symptoms of adrenal insufficiency secondary to pituitary disease may be subtler than in the case of primary adrenal failure, because a significant fraction of mineralocorticoid production is preserved even in the absence of ACTH (see Chapter 21).

In the case of trauma and pituitary stalk transection, it is notable that hypopituitarism may improve over time as local edema diminishes and some degree of integrity of the pituitary stalk with its connection to the hypothalamus is re-established. Sometimes, however, these symptoms and signs may worsen over time as the few residual intact cells or connections are lost.

Notably, injuries disconnecting the pituitary from the hypothalamus result in deficiencies of most of the anterior pituitary hormones except prolactin. Indeed, prolactin secretion is usually preserved or elevated because it is the only pituitary hormone regulated by tonic hypothalamic inhibition.

Clinical Manifestations

The symptoms and signs of hypopituitarism depend on the extent and duration of specific pituitary hormone deficiencies and the patient's overall clinical status. Thus, a relative deficiency of vasopressin can be compensated for by increasing water intake; adrenal insufficiency may not be manifest until the patient needs to mount a stress response. Hypothyroidism may become manifest gradually over months because of the relatively long half-life and large reservoir of thyroid hormone normally available in the gland.

The clinical manifestations of hypopituitarism are those of the end-organ deficiency syndromes. Most important are adrenal insufficiency, hypothyroidism, and diabetes insipidus. Less crucial, but often the most sensitive clues to the presence of pituitary disease, are amenorrhea in women and infertility or impotence in men.

CHECKPOINT

20. What are the most common causes of panhypopituitarism?
21. How do patients with panhypopituitarism come to medical attention?
22. How would you determine what replacement therapy is required for a patient with panhypopituitarism?

DIABETES INSIPIDUS

Diabetes insipidus is a syndrome of polyuria resulting from the inability to concentrate urine and, therefore, to conserve water as a result of a lack of vasopressin action.

Clinical Presentation

The initial clinical presentation of diabetes insipidus is polyuria that persists in circumstances that would normally lead to diminished urine output (eg, dehydration), accompanied by thirst. Adults may complain of frequent urination at night (nocturia), and children may present with bedwetting (enuresis). No further symptoms develop if the patient is able to maintain a water intake commensurate with water loss. The volume of urine produced in the total absence of vasopressin may reach 10–20 L/d. Thus, should the patient's ability to maintain this degree of fluid intake be compromised (eg, damage to hypothalamic thirst regulating centers), dehydration can develop and may rapidly progress to coma.

Etiology

Diabetes insipidus can result from (1) diseases of the CNS (**central diabetes insipidus**), affecting the synthesis or secretion of vasopressin; (2) diseases of the kidney (**nephrogenic diabetes insipidus**), with a loss of the kidney's ability to respond to circulating vasopressin by retaining water; or (3) pregnancy, with a probable increased metabolic clearance of vasopressin. In both central and nephrogenic diabetes insipidus, urine is hypotonic. The most common central causes are accidental head trauma, intracranial tumor (eg, craniopharyngioma), and the postintracranial surgery state. Table 19–9 lists less common causes. Nephrogenic diabetes insipidus may be familial or caused by renal damage from a variety of drugs. Diabetes insipidus–like syndromes may result from pregnancy or from other causes. True nephrogenic diabetes insipidus must be distinguished from an osmotic (and hence vasopressin-resistant) diuresis. Likewise, washout of the medullary interstitial osmotic gradient, which is necessary for the concentration of urine, may occur with prolonged diuresis resulting from any cause and may be confused with true diabetes insipidus. In both cases (osmotic diuresis and medullary washout), the urine is hypertonic or isotonic rather than hypotonic. Finally, extreme primary polydipsia (drinking excessive amounts of water, often because of a psychiatric disorder)

TABLE 19–9   Causes of central and nephrogenic diabetes insipidus.

Central (pituitary) diabetes insipidus
Acquired
Head trauma, pituitary surgery
Neoplasms (craniopharyngioma, suprasellar pituitary adenoma, dysgerminoma, meningioma, metastatic lung or breast cancer, lymphoma, leukemia)
Granulomas (sarcoidosis, histiocytosis)
Infections (chronic meningitis, viral encephalitis, toxoplasmosis)
Inflammation (lymphocytic hypophysitis, granulomatosis with polyangiitis, systemic lupus erythematosus [SLE], scleroderma)
Vascular (Sheehan syndrome, aneurysm, hypoxic encephalopathy)
Gestational (second and third trimesters of pregnancy)
Toxins
Idiopathic
Congenital malformation
Genetic disorders (eg, mutation in the vasopressin gene [autosomal dominant], Wolfram syndrome)
Nephrogenic diabetes insipidus
Acquired
Drugs (eg, aminoglycosides, amphotericin B, cisplatin, demeclocycline, foscarnet, lithium, rifampin)
Metabolic (hypercalcemia, hypercalciuria, hypokalemia)
Obstruction (ureter or urethra)
Vascular
Sickle cell disease and trait
Ischemia (acute tubular necrosis)
Granulomas (eg, sarcoidosis)
Neoplasms (eg, sarcoma)
Infiltration (eg, amyloidosis)
Genetic disorders
Idiopathic

Modified, with permission, from Robertson GL. Disorders of the neurohypophysis. In: Kasper D et al, eds. *Harrison's Principles of Internal Medicine*, 19th ed. McGraw-Hill, 2015.

results in an appropriately large volume of dilute urine and a low plasma vasopressin level, thus mimicking true central diabetes insipidus.

Pathophysiology

A. Central Diabetes Insipidus

Central diabetes insipidus can be either permanent or transient, reflecting the natural history of the underlying disorder (see Table 19–9). Only about 15% of the vasopressin-secreting cells of the hypothalamus need to be intact to maintain fluid balance under normal conditions. Simple destruction of the posterior pituitary does not cause sufficient neuronal loss

to result in permanent diabetes insipidus. Rather, destruction of the hypothalamus or at least some of the supraoptic-hypophysial tract must also occur.

A more common finding is transient disease resulting from acute injury with neuronal shock and edema (eg, post-infarction or post-trauma), leading to the cessation of vasopressin secretion with a subsequent resumption of sufficient vasopressin secretion to resolve symptoms, because of either neuronal recovery or the resolution of edema with the re-establishment of hypothalamic–pituitary neurovascular integrity.

B. Nephrogenic Diabetes Insipidus

Familial nephrogenic diabetes insipidus is the result of a generalized defect in either the V_2 class of vasopressin receptors or the aquaporin-2 water channel of the renal collecting ducts.

Drug-induced nephrogenic diabetes insipidus appears to result from sensitivity of the vasopressin receptor to lithium, fluoride, and other salts. This occurs in 12–30% of patients treated with these drugs. It is generally reversible on termination of exposure to the offending drug (see Table 19–9).

C. Diabetes Insipidus–Like Syndromes

There are several diabetes insipidus–like syndromes. As an example, diabetes insipidus is a rare complication of pregnancy that appears to result from excessive vasopressinase in plasma. This enzyme, which selectively degrades vasopressin, is presumably released from the placenta. A hallmark of this entity is that it is reversed by the administration of the vasopressin analog desmopressin acetate, which is resistant to degradation by the enzyme.

Clinical Manifestations

Diabetes insipidus must be distinguished from other causes of polyuria and hypernatremia (Table 19–10). The hallmark of diabetes insipidus is dilute urine, even in the face of hypernatremia. Dipstick testing of the urine for glucose distinguishes diabetes mellitus. Conditions in which **osmotic diuresis** is responsible for polyuria can be distinguished from diabetes insipidus by their normal or elevated urine osmolality. Primary polydipsia is distinguished by the presence of hyponatremia, whereas in diabetes insipidus, the serum sodium should be normal or elevated. In primary polydipsia, uncontrolled excess water ingestion drives the polyuria, whereas in diabetes insipidus, hypertonicity stimulates thirst.

Distinguishing central from nephrogenic diabetes insipidus ultimately depends on a determination of responsiveness to injected vasopressin, with a dramatic decrease in urine volume and increase in urine osmolality in the former and little or no change in the latter. In central diabetes insipidus, circulating vasopressin levels are low for a given plasma osmolality, whereas in nephrogenic diabetes insipidus, they are high.

Polyuria in nephrogenic diabetes insipidus results from an inability to conserve water in the distal nephron because of a lack of vasopressin-dependent water channels. These

TABLE 19–10   Major causes of hypernatremia: classification and clinical conditions.

Classification	Clinical Conditions
Hypervolemic hypernatremia	Cushing syndrome
	Primary hyperaldosteronism
	Salt water intake
	Iatrogenic (hypertonic saline or hypertonic sodium bicarbonate administration)
Normovolemic hypernatremia	Diabetes insipidus (DI)
	Central DI
	Gestational DI
	Nephrogenic DI
	Impaired medullary hypertonicity
Renal hypovolemic hypernatremia	Solute diuresis
	Diabetic ketoacidosis
	Nonketotic hyperosmolar coma
	Osmotic diuretics (eg, mannitol or glycerol administration)
	Loop diuretics
	Postobstructive diuresis
Extrarenal hypovolemic hypernatremia	Vomiting
	Osmotic diarrhea
	Gastrointestinal fistulas
	Sweating
	Burn
	Impaired thirst (eg, coma, essential hypodipsia)

Modified, with permission, from Petrina R et al. Fluids and electrolytes. In: Tintinalli JE et al, eds. *Tintinalli's Emergency Medicine: A Comprehensive Study Guide,* 8th ed. McGraw-Hill, 2016.

channels, which reside within vesicles in the cytoplasm of collecting duct cells, are normally inserted into the apical plasma membrane in response to vasopressin stimulation, permitting increased reabsorption of water. Up to 13% of the volume of the glomerular filtrate can be reclaimed in this manner.

In diabetes insipidus of either central or nephrogenic origin, if the patient is unable to maintain sufficient water intake to offset polyuria, dehydration with consequent hypernatremia develops. Hypernatremia leads to a number of neurologic manifestations, including progressive obtundation (decreased responsiveness to verbal and physical stimuli), myoclonus, seizures, focal deficits, and coma. These neurologic manifestations result from cell shrinkage and volume loss as a result of osmotic forces, sometimes complicated by intracranial hemorrhage because of the stretching and rupture of small blood vessels. Barring structural changes such as those leading to hemorrhage, the neurologic consequences of hypernatremia are reversible on resolution of the underlying metabolic disorder.

The time course of hypernatremia is an important variable in the development of neurologic symptoms in that, over time, neurons generate "idiogenic osmoles" (ie, amino acids and other metabolites that serve to raise intracellular osmolality to the level in the blood and thereby minimize fluid shifts out of the cells of the brain). Thus, the more slowly hypernatremia develops, the less likely are neurologic complications resulting from fluid shifts in the brain or from a vascular catastrophe to occur.

CHECKPOINT

23. What clues would suggest diabetes insipidus in a new patient?
24. How would you make a definitive diagnosis of diabetes insipidus?
25. What are the pathophysiologic differences between central and nephrogenic diabetes insipidus?

SYNDROME OF INAPPROPRIATE VASOPRESSIN SECRETION (SIADH)

The syndrome of inappropriate ADH (vasopressin) secretion (SIADH) is one of several causes of a hypotonic state (Table 19–11). SIADH is due to the secretion of vasopressin in

TABLE 19–11   The hypotonic syndromes.

Excessive water ingestion
Decreased water excretion
Decreased solute delivery to diluting segments
Starvation
Beer potomania
Vasopressin excess
Syndrome of inappropriate antidiuretic hormone (SIADH)
Drug-induced vasopressin secretion
Vasopressin excess with decreased distal solute delivery
Heart failure
Cirrhosis of the liver
Nephrotic syndrome
Cortisol deficiency
Hypothyroidism
Diuretic use
Renal failure

Modified and reproduced, with permission, from Reeves BW et al. The posterior pituitary and water metabolism. In: Wilson JD et al, eds. *Williams Textbook of Endocrinology,* 9th ed. Saunders, 1998. Copyright © Elsevier.

excess of what is appropriate for hyperosmolality or intravascular volume depletion.

CLINICAL PRESENTATION

The cardinal clinical presentation of SIADH is hyponatremia without edema. Depending on the rapidity of onset and the severity, the neurologic consequences of hyponatremia include confusion, lethargy and weakness, myoclonus, asterixis, generalized seizures, and coma.

ETIOLOGY

A variety of vasopressin-secreting tumors, CNS disorders, pulmonary disorders, and drugs have been associated with SIADH (Table 19–12). Therefore, it is worth mentioning that the hypothalamic neurons and the posterior pituitary are not always the source of vasopressin secretion. In fact, the hypothalamus and pituitary account for elevated vasopressin levels in only one-third of patients with SIADH, and it is important to regard SIADH not necessarily as a disorder of the hypothalamic–pituitary system. Several metabolic disorders can produce hyponatremia and must be investigated and ruled out before the diagnosis of true SIADH can be made. In particular, adrenal insufficiency and hypothyroidism are often associated with hyponatremia. In these conditions, sodium deficiency and subsequent volume depletion trigger vasopressin secretion. Hyponatremia accompanying CNS disorders is caused either by SIADH or by cerebral salt wasting (CSW) with an increased release of natriuretic peptides (eg, BNP, ANP). A major difference between these two disorders is in the total extracellular volume, which is increased in SIADH and reduced in CSW.

PATHOPHYSIOLOGY

The serum sodium concentration (and hence osmolarity) is normally determined by the balance of water intake, renal solute delivery (a necessary step in water excretion), and vasopressin-mediated distal renal tubular water retention. Disorders in any one of these features of normal sodium balance, or factors controlling them, can result in hyponatremia. Hyponatremia occurs when the magnitude of the disorder exceeds the capacity of homeostatic mechanisms to compensate for dysfunction. Thus, simple excess water ingestion is generally compensated for by renal water diuresis. The exceptions are (1) when water ingestion is extreme (greater than the approximately 18 L daily that can be excreted via the kidney); or (2) when renal solute delivery is limited (eg, in salt depletion), thereby limiting the ability of the kidney to excrete free water.

In hypoadrenal states, renal sodium loss resulting from a lack of aldosterone has two consequences. Most importantly, volume depletion as a consequence of renal sodium loss results in the release of vasopressin; although the primary

TABLE 19–12   Causes of SIADH

Tumors
Lung carcinoma (particularly small-cell type)
Other carcinomas: duodenum, pancreas, bladder, ureter, prostate, ovary
Leukemia, lymphoma
Thymoma, mesothelioma, bronchial adenoma, carcinoid, Ewing sarcoma
CNS disorders
Mass lesions: tumors, brain abscess, hematoma, congenital malformations
Infections: encephalitis, meningitis (bacterial or viral), AIDS-related CNS opportunistic infection
Cerebrovascular occlusions, hemorrhage, cavernous sinus thrombosis
Senile cerebral atrophy
Hydrocephalus
Head trauma
Delirium tremens
Acute psychosis
Demyelinating and degenerative disease (multiple sclerosis, amyotrophic lateral sclerosis)
Inflammatory disease (Guillain–Barré syndrome, peripheral neuropathy)
Pulmonary disorders
Infections: tuberculosis, pneumonia (bacterial or viral), abscess, cavitation (eg, aspergillosis)
Acute respiratory failure
Positive pressure ventilation
Drugs
Vasopressin, desmopressin acetate
Chlorpropamide
Clofibrate
Carbamazepine
Antidepressants: tricyclics, monoamine oxidase inhibitors, serotonin reuptake inhibitors
Others: vincristine, vinblastine, cyclophosphamide, phenothiazines, nicotine, oxytocin (high dose)
Metabolic
Acute intermittent porphyria
Idiopathic

Modified, with permission, from Robertson GL. Disorders of the neurohypophysis. In: Kasper D et al, eds. *Harrison's Principles of Internal Medicine*, 19th ed. McGraw-Hill, 2015.

TABLE 19–13   Causes of pseudohyponatremia.

Hyponatremia with elevated plasma osmolality
Hyperglycemia
Mannitol administration
Glycerol administration
Hyponatremia with normal plasma osmolality
Marked hyperproteinemia (eg, plasma cell myeloma)
Marked hyperlipidemia
Prostate surgery, with use of irrigant fluid containing glycine or sorbitol

Modified and reproduced, with permission, from Butterworth JF et al. Management of patients with fluid & electrolyte disturbances. In: *Morgan & Mikhail's Clinical Anesthesiology*, 5th ed. McGraw-Hill, 2013.

stimulus for ADH secretion is an elevated plasma osmolarity, ADH release is also stimulated by low intravascular volume. Second, diminished renal solute delivery impairs the ability of the kidney to excrete a water load when the ingestion of water exceeds nonrenal water loss.

In hypothyroidism, both renal solute delivery and the function of the osmostat to which vasopressin secretion is coupled appear to be impaired, resulting in hyponatremia.

True causes of hyponatremia, including SIADH, must also be distinguished from so-called pseudohyponatremia. **Pseudohyponatremia** occurs in two groups of conditions (Table 19–13). First, there are those in which the infusion of hyperosmolar solutions (eg, glucose) pulls water out of cells, thereby diluting the sodium. The key feature of these conditions is hyponatremia without hypo-osmolality. Second, pseudohyponatremia occurs when the nonaqueous fraction of plasma is larger than normal. Sodium equilibrates only with, and is regulated in, the aqueous fraction of plasma, and calculations of serum sodium concentration typically correct for total plasma volume because the nonaqueous fraction of plasma volume is normally negligible. In those relatively rare conditions in which the nonaqueous fraction is significant (eg, severe hyperlipidemic states, plasma cell myeloma, and other conditions with higher than normal serum lipid or protein concentrations), the calculated sodium concentration will, therefore, be misleadingly low.

The pathophysiologic mechanisms behind most cases of SIADH are not well understood. It has been proposed that baroreceptor input from the lung is impaired in those pulmonary disorders that result in SIADH. CNS lesions causing SIADH are presumed to interrupt the vasopressin-inhibiting neural pathways. Regardless of the mechanism, in most cases the hyponatremia of SIADH is partially limited by the secretion of atrial natriuretic peptide. Thus, severe hyponatremia develops only when water intake is relatively increased, and edema formation is rare. The simplest therapy is the restriction of free water intake and, in the case of CNS or pulmonary lesions, treatment of the underlying disease.

CLINICAL MANIFESTATIONS

The clinical manifestations of SIADH are in part determined by the nature and course of any underlying disorder (eg, CNS or pulmonary disease), by the severity of hyponatremia, and by the rapidity with which hyponatremia develops. Regardless of its cause, SIADH can have neurologic manifestations, including confusion, asterixis, myoclonus, generalized seizures, and coma. These occur as a result of osmotic fluid shifts and resulting brain edema and elevated intracranial pressures; brain swelling is limited by the size of the skull. Physiologic mechanisms to counter this swelling include the depletion of intracellular osmoles, especially potassium ions. The more rapid the progression of hyponatremia, the more likely it is that brain edema and increased intracranial pressure will develop and that the neurologic complications and herniation will lead to permanent damage. However, even when hyponatremia develops slowly, it can in extreme cases (eg, serum sodium <110 mEq/L) result in seizures and altered mental status. Central pontine myelinolysis can develop and cause permanent neurologic damage in patients whose hyponatremia is corrected too rapidly.

CHECKPOINT

26. What conditions are associated with SIADH?
27. How would you distinguish SIADH from other causes of hyponatremia?
28. What are the neurologic consequences of SIADH, and how may they be prevented?

CASE STUDIES

Yeong Kwok, MD

(See Chapter 25, p. 780–82 for answers)

CASE 101

A 53-year-old woman came to the clinic to get help managing her weight. She has been overweight since childhood and has continued to gain weight throughout her adult life. She has tried numerous diets without lasting success. She initially loses weight but then regains it after a few months. She is otherwise healthy and is not taking any medications. Other family members are also overweight or obese. She does not do any regular exercise and has a sedentary office job. On examination, she is 5 feet 3 inches tall and weighs 260 pounds, with a body mass index (BMI) of 46.2 (normal <25).

Questions

A. How is body weight controlled?
B. How is obesity defined?
C. What medical conditions is this patient at increased risk for as a result of her obesity?

CASE 102

A 30-year-old woman presents to the emergency department after sideswiping a parked car. She reports that she never saw the car until after she hit it. She denies any trauma to herself but complains of headache. She states that she has had headaches every day for the past 3 months, and this one is similar to her other headaches. She describes the headache as a frontal throbbing pain that is worse when she lies down, and she states that it occasionally wakes her from sleep. She has no significant medical history, takes no medications, and denies alcohol, tobacco, and drug use. On review of systems, she notes irregular menses but denies other complaints. On examination, she appears to be well, with normal vital signs. Her neurologic examination is notable for bitemporal hemianopia. On breast examination, galactorrhea is present but with no masses. The remainder of the examination is unremarkable.

Questions

A. What is the likely diagnosis?
B. How did this condition arise?
C. What is the pathogenetic mechanism of this patient's bitemporal hemianopia? Her headaches?
D. What is the cause of her irregular menses? Her galactorrhea?

CASE 103

A 31-year-old woman with a medical history significant for pituitary macroadenoma status post–radiation therapy presents to the clinic with a complaint of amenorrhea. Before the diagnosis of pituitary adenoma, she had irregular menses. This irregularity had persisted, with menses lasting approximately 3 days and occurring about once every 1.5–2 months. However, for the past 4 months, she has had no menses. She denies sexual activity. On review of systems, she notes progressive fatigue and 10 pounds of weight gain over several months.

The pituitary macroadenoma was treated with radiation therapy 1 year ago. She has been without medical care since completing therapy because she moved and has not yet found a physician. She is taking no medications. On examination, her blood pressure is 100/60 mm Hg, and her heart rate is 80 bpm. Her neurologic examination is normal except for a slight delay in the relaxation phase of her deep tendon reflexes. On head–neck examination, she has somewhat coarse, brittle brown hair. The neck examination discloses no goiter or masses. The lung, cardiac, and abdominal examinations show no abnormalities. The pelvic examination reveals normal female genitalia without uterine or ovarian masses. A urine pregnancy test is negative.

Questions

A. What is the likely cause of this, and why?

B. On the basis of this patient's history and physical examination, do you suspect any other hormone deficiencies? If so, why?

C. What other hormonal deficiencies should you be concerned about in this patient? Why might they be asymptomatic currently?

CASE 104

A 54-year-old man with a medical history significant for bipolar disease presents to his physician with complaints of polyuria. He states that he must get up three or four times each night to urinate. He also notes frequent thirst. He denies polyphagia, urinary urgency, difficulty initiating urination, and postvoid dribbling. His medical history is notable only for bipolar disease. He has a longstanding history of noncompliance with medications for the disease, with frequent hospitalizations for both mania and depression, but has been stable on lithium for the past 6 months. He denies any symptoms of mania or depression at this time. He takes no other medications. His family history is notable for depression and substance abuse but is otherwise negative. The patient has a history of polysubstance abuse but has been "clean and sober" for the past 6 months.

On examination, the patient's vital signs are within normal limits. The head–neck examination reveals slightly dry mucous membranes. The rectal examination reveals a normal prostate without masses. The remainder of his examination is unremarkable. Urinalysis reveals dilute urine without glucose or other abnormalities. Serum electrolytes reveal a mildly increased sodium level. A diagnosis of diabetes insipidus is entertained.

Questions

A. Do you suspect central or nephrogenic diabetes insipidus? Why? How would you confirm the diagnosis?

B. How does lithium cause diabetes insipidus?

C. What is the cause of this patient's polyuria? His thirst?

D. What might occur if this patient were unable to maintain sufficient water intake?

CASE 105

A 75-year-old man with terminal small-cell carcinoma of the lung presents to the emergency department with altered mental status. The patient's wife, who cares for him at home, states that he is quite weak at baseline, requiring assistance with all activities of daily living. Over the past few days, he has become progressively more lethargic. She has been careful to adequately hydrate him, waking him every 2 hours to give him water to drink. His appetite has been poor, but he willingly ingests the water, consuming 2–3 quarts per day. He is taking morphine for pain and dyspnea.

On examination, the patient is a cachectic white man in mild respiratory distress. He is lethargic but arousable. He is oriented to person only. Vital signs reveal a temperature of 38 °C, blood pressure of 110/60 mm Hg, heart rate of 88 bpm, respiratory rate of 18/min, and oxygen saturation of 96% on 3 L of oxygen. On head–neck examination, pupils are 3 mm and reactive, scleras are anicteric, and conjunctivas are pink. Mucous membranes are moist. The neck is supple. There are decreased breath sounds in the left lower posterior lung field and rales in the upper half. The cardiac examination shows a regular heartbeat without murmur, gallop, or rub. The abdomen is benign without masses. The extremities are without edema, cyanosis, or clubbing. The neurologic examination shows only bilateral positive Babinski reflexes and asterixis. Laboratory studies reveal a serum sodium level of 118 mEq/L.

Questions

A. What conditions are associated with SIADH? Which are present in this patient?
B. What pathophysiologic mechanism produces SIADH?
C. What is the cause of this patient's lethargy, confusion, and asterixis?
D. How would you treat this patient's hyponatremia?

REFERENCES

General

Javorsky BR et al. Hypothalamus and pituitary gland. In: Gardner DG et al, eds. *Greenspan's Basic & Clinical Endocrinology*, 10th ed. McGraw-Hill, 2017.

Obesity

Cornejo MP et al. Neuroendocrine regulation of metabolism. J Neuroendocrinol. 2016 Jul;28(7). [PMID: 27114114]

Ramachandrappa S et al. Genetic approaches to understanding human obesity. J Clin Invest. 2011 Jun;121(6):2080–6. [PMID: 21633175]

Wilson JL et al. A talk between fat tissue, gut, pancreas and brain to control body weight. Mol Cell Endocrinol. 2015 Dec 15;418 (Pt 2):108–19. [PMID: 26316427]

Pituitary Adenoma

Melmed S et al. Diagnosis and treatment of hyperprolactinemia: an Endocrine Society clinical practice guideline. J Clin Endocrinol Metab. 2011 Feb;96(2):273–88. [PMID: 21296991]

Molitch ME. Diagnosis and treatment of pituitary adenomas: a review. JAMA. 2017 Feb 7;317(5):516–24. [PMID: 28170483]

Hypopituitarism

Fernandez-Rodriguez E et al. Subclinical hypopituitarism. Best Pract Res Clin Endocrinol Metab. 2012 Aug;26(4):461–9. [PMID: 22863388]

Giordano M. Genetic causes of isolated and combined pituitary hormone deficiency. Best Pract Res Clin Endocrinol Metab. 2016 Dec;30(6):679–91. [PMID: 27974184]

Higham CE et al. Hypopituitarism. Lancet. 2016 Nov 12;388(10058):2403–15. [PMID: 27041067]

Diabetes Insipidus/Oxytocin

Fenske W et al. Clinical review: current state and future perspectives in the diagnosis of diabetes insipidus: a clinical review. J Clin Endocrinol Metab. 2012 Oct;97(10):3426–37. [PMID: 22855338]

Robertson GL. Diabetes insipidus: differential diagnosis and management. Best Pract Res Clin Endocrinol Metab. 2016 Mar;30(2):205–18. [PMID: 27156759]

Syndrome of Inappropriate ADH Secretion

Cuesta M et al. The syndrome of inappropriate antidiuresis (SIAD). Best Pract Res Clin Endocrinol Metab. 2016 Mar;30(2):175–87. [PMID: 27156757]

Verbalis JG et al. Diagnosis, evaluation, and treatment of hyponatremia: expert panel recommendations. Am J Med. 2013 Oct;126 (10 Suppl 1):S1–42. [PMID: 24074529]

Thyroid Disease

Nazanene H. Esfandiari, MD, &
Stephen J. McPhee, MD

The thyroid gland synthesizes the hormones **thyroxine** (T_4) (prohormone) and **triiodothyronine** (T_3) (active hormone), iodine-containing amino acids that regulate the body's metabolic rate. Adequate levels of thyroid hormone are necessary in infants for normal central nervous system (CNS) development, in children for normal skeletal growth and maturation, and in adults for the normal function of multiple organ systems. Thyroid dysfunction is one of the most common endocrine disorders encountered in clinical practice. Although abnormally high or low levels of thyroid hormones may be tolerated for long periods of time, there are usually symptoms and signs of overt thyroid dysfunction.

NORMAL STRUCTURE & FUNCTION

ANATOMY

The normal thyroid gland is a firm, reddish brown, smooth gland consisting of two lateral lobes and a connecting central isthmus, located in front of the trachea (Figure 20–1). A pyramidal lobe of variable size may extend upward from the isthmus. The normal weight of the thyroid ranges from 10 g to 20 g. It is surrounded by an adherent fibrous capsule from which multiple fibrous projections extend deeply into its structure, dividing it into many small lobules. The thyroid is highly vascular and has one of the highest rates of blood flow per gram of tissue of any organ.

HISTOLOGY

Histologically, the thyroid gland consists of many closely packed acini, called **follicles**, each surrounded by capillaries and stroma. Each follicle is roughly spherical, lined by a single layer of cuboidal epithelial cells and filled with **colloid**, a proteinaceous material composed mainly of **thyroglobulin** and stored thyroid hormones. When the gland is inactive, the follicles are large, the lining cells are flat, and the colloid is abundant. When the gland is active, the follicles are small, the lining cells are cuboidal or columnar, the colloid is scanty, and its edges are scalloped, forming **reabsorption lacunae** (Figure 20–2).

Scattered between follicles are the **parafollicular cells** (**C cells**), which secrete **calcitonin**, a hormone that inhibits bone resorption though its function is usually not significant in the regulation of normal calcium homeostasis (see Chapter 17).

Figure 20–3 diagrams the ultrastructure of a follicular epithelial cell. The cells vary in appearance with the degree of gland activity. The follicular cell rests on a basal lamina. The nucleus is round and centrally located. The cytoplasm contains mitochondria, rough endoplasmic reticulum, and ribosomes. The apex has a discrete Golgi apparatus, small secretory granules containing thyroglobulin, and abundant lysosomes and phagosomes. At the apex, the cell membrane is folded into microvilli.

PHYSIOLOGY

Formation & Secretion of Thyroid Hormones

A. T_4, T_3, and Thyroglobulin

Thyroid follicular cells have three functions: (1) to collect and transport iodine to the colloid; (2) to synthesize **thyroglobulin**, a 660,000-Da glycoprotein made up of two subunits and containing many tyrosine residues, and secrete it into the colloid; and (3) to release thyroid hormones from thyroglobulin

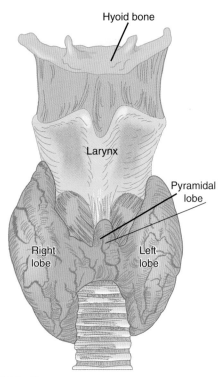

FIGURE 20-1 The human thyroid. (Redrawn, with permission, from Barrett KE et al, eds. *Ganong's Review of Medical Physiology*, 25th ed. McGraw-Hill, 2016.)

and secrete them into the circulation. Figure 20–4 illustrates the structures of the two thyroid hormones, T_3 and T_4. T_3 and T_4 are synthesized in the colloid by the iodination and condensation of tyrosine molecules bound together in thyroglobulin.

B. Iodine Metabolism and Trapping

For normal thyroid hormone synthesis, an adult requires a minimum daily intake of 150 μg of iodine. In the United States, the average intake is about 500 μg/d. Iodine ingested in food is first converted to **iodide**, which is absorbed and taken up by the thyroid. The follicular cells transport iodide from the circulation to the colloid ("iodide trapping" or "iodide pump"). The sodium–iodide symporter is a 65-kDa cell membrane protein. This iodide transport is an example of secondary active transport dependent on Na^+-K^+ adenosine triphosphatase (ATPase) for energy; it is stimulated by **thyroid-stimulating hormone** (**TSH, thyrotropin**). At the normal rate of thyroid hormone synthesis, about 120 μg/d of iodide enters the thyroid. About 80 μg/d is secreted in T_3 and T_4, and the rest diffuses into the extracellular fluid and is excreted in the urine.

C. Thyroid Hormone Synthesis and Secretion

Thyroid hormones are synthesized in the colloid, near the apical cell membrane of the follicular cells. Catalyzed by the enzyme thyroidal peroxidase, iodide in the thyroid cell is oxidized to iodine. The iodine enters the colloid and is rapidly

FIGURE 20-2 Normal and abnormal thyroid histology. (Redrawn, with permission, from Barrett KE et al, eds. *Ganong's Review of Medical Physiology*, 25th ed. McGraw-Hill, 2016; Chandrasoma P et al, eds. *Concise Pathology*, 3rd ed. Originally published by Appleton & Lange. Copyright © by The McGraw-Hill Companies, Inc.; Gardner DG et al, eds. *Greenspan's Basic and Clinical Endocrinology*, 10th ed. McGraw-Hill, 2017.)

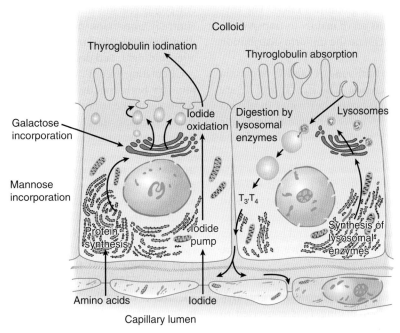

FIGURE 20–3 Thyroid cell ultrastructure (schematic). The processes of thyroglobulin synthesis and iodination are shown on the left and its reabsorption and digestion on the right. (Redrawn, with permission, from Junqueira LC et al, eds. *Basic Histology*, 9th ed. Originally published by Appleton & Lange. Copyright © 1998 by The McGraw-Hill Companies, Inc.)

bound at the 3 position (see Figure 20–4) to tyrosine molecules attached to thyroglobulin, forming **monoiodotyrosine** (**MIT**). MIT is next iodinated at the 5 position, forming **diiodotyrosine** (**DIT**). Two DIT molecules then condense in an oxidative process ("coupling reaction") catalyzed by thyroperoxidase to form one **thyroxine** (**T₄**) molecule. Some **T₃** is probably formed within the thyroid gland by the condensation of MIT with DIT. A small amount of reverse T₃ (rT₃) is also formed. (Figure 20–4 shows the structures of MIT, DIT, T₄, T₃, and rT₃). In the normal thyroid, the average distribution of iodinated compounds is 23% MIT, 33% DIT, 35% T₄, 7% T₃, and 2% rT₃.

The thyroid secretes about 80 μg (103 nmol) of T₄ and 4 μg (7 nmol) of T₃ per day. The folds of the apical cell membrane (lamellipodia) encircle bits of colloid and bring them into the cytoplasm by endocytosis, forming **endosomes**. This process is accelerated by TSH. The endosomes fuse with lysosomes containing proteases that break peptide bonds between the iodinated residues and thyroglobulin, releasing T₄, T₃, DIT, and MIT into the cytoplasm. The free T₄ and T₃ then cross the cell membrane and enter adjacent capillaries. The MIT and DIT are enzymatically degraded in the cell by thyroid deiodinase (iodotyrosine dehalogenase) to iodine and tyrosine, which are reused in colloid synthesis.

D. Thyroid Hormone Transport and Metabolism

The normal plasma level of T₄ is approximately 8 μg/dL (103 nmol/L) (range: 5–12 μg/dL or 65–156 nmol/L), and the normal plasma level of T₃ is approximately 0.15 μg/dL (2.3 nmol/L) (range: 0.08–0.22 μg/dL or 1.2–3.3 nmol/L). Both hormones are bound to plasma proteins, including albumin, **transthyretin** (formerly called thyroxine-binding prealbumin

3-Monoiodotyrosine (MIT)

3,5-Diiodotyrosine (DIT)

3,3',5'-Triiodothyronine (rT₃)

3,5,3'-Triiodothyronine (T₃)

3,5,3',5'-Tetraiodothyronine (T₄, thyroxine)

FIGURE 20–4 MIT, DIT, T₃, T₄, and rT₃.

[TBPA]), and **thyroxine-binding globulin (TBG)**. The thyroid hormone–binding proteins serve mainly to transport T_4 and T_3 in the serum and to facilitate the uniform distribution of hormones within tissues.

Physiologically, it is the free (unbound) T_4 and T_3 in plasma that inhibit pituitary TSH secretion. The free T_4 and T_3 are in equilibrium with the protein-bound hormones in plasma and tissue and circulate in much lower concentrations. Tissue uptake of the free hormones is proportionate to their plasma concentrations.

Almost all (99.98%) of the circulating T_4 is bound to TBG and other plasma proteins, so that the free T_4 level is approximately 2 ng/dL. The biologic half-life of T_4 is long (about 6–7 days). Somewhat less T_3 (99.8%) is protein bound. Therefore, compared with T_4, T_3 acts more rapidly and has a shorter half-life (about 24 hours). It is also three to five times more potent on a molar basis.

T_4 and T_3 are metabolized in the liver, kidneys, and many other tissues by **deiodination** and by **conjugation to glucuronides**. Normally, one-third of circulating T_4 is converted to T_3 by 5′-deiodination, and 45% is converted to the metabolically inert **reverse triiodothyronine (rT$_3$)** by 5-deiodination. About 80% of circulating T_3 derives from the peripheral conversion of T_4 to T_3, with the remaining 20% deriving from thyroid secretion. Both T_4 and T_3 are conjugated to glucuronides in the liver and excreted into the bile. On passage into the intestine, the conjugates are hydrolyzed, and small amounts of T_4 and T_3 are reabsorbed (enterohepatic circulation). The rest is excreted in the stool.

Regulation of Thyroid Secretion

Thyroid hormone secretion is stimulated by pituitary **thyroid-stimulating hormone (TSH, thyrotropin)**. Pituitary TSH secretion is, in turn, stimulated by **thyrotropin-releasing hormone (TRH)**, a tripeptide secreted by the hypothalamus that also increases the biologic activity of TSH, by altering its glycosylation.

TSH is a two-subunit glycoprotein containing 211 amino acids. The α-subunit is identical to that of pituitary follicle-stimulating hormone (FSH), luteinizing hormone (LH), and placental human chorionic gonadotropin (hCG). The β-subunit confers the specific binding properties and biologic activity of TSH. The gene encoding the α-subunit is located on chromosome 6, and the gene for the β-subunit is on chromosome 1.

TSH has a biologic half-life of about 60 minutes. The average plasma level of TSH is 2 mU/L (normal range: 0.45–4.12 mU/L). When individuals with thyroid autoantibodies, goiter, or a family history of thyroid disease are excluded, the upper limit is somewhat lower, between 2.5 mU/L and 3.0 mU/L. Controversy exists over the effects of advanced age on the normal range for TSH. Several population-based studies have found that the upper limit of normal in healthy older individuals (older than 80 years) might be as high as 7.5 mU/L, but the clinical significance of using age-specific upper limit

cut-points remains unclear. Although the phenomenon is not clinically important, normal TSH secretion exhibits a circadian pattern, rising in the afternoon and evening, peaking after midnight, and declining during the day.

Circulating free T_4 and T_3 inhibit TSH secretion by the pituitary both directly and indirectly by regulating TRH biosynthesis in the hypothalamus. TSH secretion is inhibited by stress, perhaps via glucocorticoid inhibition of TRH secretion. In infants, but not in adults, TSH secretion is increased by cold and inhibited by warmth. Dopamine and somatostatin also inhibit pituitary TSH secretion. In animals, there is a pituitary-specific form of the thyroid hormone receptor that may be selectively regulated by thyroid hormone. Figure 20–5 illustrates the hypothalamic–pituitary–thyroid axis and various stimulatory and inhibitory factors.

When TSH is secreted or administered, it binds to a specific **TSH receptor (TSH-R)** in the thyroid cell membrane, activating the GTP-binding (G_s) protein–adenylyl cyclase–cyclic adenosine monophosphate (cAMP) cascade. The increase in intracellular cAMP mediates the immediate increases in iodide uptake and transport, thyroglobulin iodination, and iodotyrosine T_3 and T_4 synthesis. Within a few hours, there is an increase in mRNA for thyroglobulin and thyroidal peroxidase, enhanced lysosomal activity, increased secretion of thyroglobulin into colloid, more endocytosis of colloid, and increased secretion of T_4 and T_3 from the gland. TSH-R is also expressed in lymphocytes and other tissues, including the pituitary, thymus, kidney, testis, brain, adipocytes, and fibroblasts.

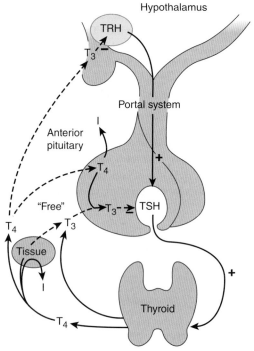

FIGURE 20–5 Hypothalamic–pituitary–thyroid axis. (T_3, triiodothyronine; T_4, thyroxine; TRH, thyrotropin-releasing hormone; TSH, thyroid-stimulating hormone.) (Redrawn and modified, with permission, from Gardner DG et al, eds. *Greenspan's Basic and Clinical Endocrinology*, 10th ed. McGraw-Hill, 2017.)

TSH-R has also been detected on osteoblast precursors, suggesting that TSH may have a direct effect on bone resorption.

TSH binding to TSH-R also stimulates membrane phospholipase C, which leads to thyroid cell hypertrophy. With chronic TSH stimulation, the entire gland hypertrophies, increases in vascularity, and becomes a **goiter**.

TSH-R has been cloned. It is a single-chain glycoprotein composed of 744 amino acids. Two specific amino acid sequences are thought to represent different binding sites for TSH and for the **TSH-R–stimulating antibody (TSH-R [stim] Ab)** (also called **thyroid stimulating immunoglobulin [TSI]** in Graves disease [see later]).

The amount of thyroid hormone needed to maintain normal organ system function in thyroidectomized individuals is defined as the amount necessary to maintain the plasma TSH within the normal range (0.45–4.12 mU/L). About 80% of orally administered levothyroxine is absorbed from the gastrointestinal (GI) tract (in the jejunum and ileum), and 100–125 μg/d usually maintains a normal plasma TSH in individuals of average size.

Mechanism of Action of Thyroid Hormones

Thyroid hormones exert their actions by two mechanisms: (1) genomic actions mediated by T_3 interactions with its nuclear receptors, regulating gene activity; and (2) nongenomic actions effected by T_3 and T_4 interactions with specific enzymes (eg, pyruvate kinase, adenylate cyclase, calcium ATPase), mitochondrial proteins, and glucose transporters. Thyroid hormones enter target tissue cells either by passive diffusion or specific transport carriers through the cell membrane and cytoplasm. Within the cell cytoplasm, most of the T_4 is converted to T_3. The nuclear receptor for T_3 has been cloned and found to be similar to the nuclear receptors for glucocorticoids, mineralocorticoids, estrogens, progestins, vitamin D_3, and retinoic acid. For reasons that are unclear, there are two different receptor (TR) genes in humans. Each gene (hTR-α and hTR-β) yields at least two differently spliced proteins: hTR-α (hTR-α1 and hTR α2) and hTR-β (hTR-β1 and hTR-β1). hTR-α2 may be biologically inactive. The TR gene for the alpha form is on chromosome 17 and for the beta form, on chromosome 3. The two different receptor forms may help explain both the normal variation in the thyroid hormone responsiveness of various organs and the selective tissue abnormalities found in various thyroid resistance syndromes. For example, the brain contains mostly α receptors, the liver contains mostly β receptors, and the heart contains both. Point mutations in the *hTR-β1* gene result in abnormal T_3 receptors and the syndrome of **generalized resistance to thyroid hormone (Refetoff syndrome)**.

When the T_3 receptor complex binds to DNA, it increases the expression of specific genes, with the induction of related messenger RNAs. A wide variety of enzymes must be produced to account for the many effects of thyroid hormones on cell function.

Effects of Thyroid Hormones

Table 20–1 summarizes the effects of thyroid hormones in various organs. Thyroid hormones increase the activity of

TABLE 20–1 **Physiologic effects of thyroid hormones.**

Target Tissue	Effect	Mechanism
Heart	Chronotropic	Increase number and affinity of β-adrenergic receptors
	Inotropic	Enhance responses to circulating catecholamines
		Increase proportion of alpha-myosin heavy chain (with higher ATPase activity)
Lung	Metabolic	Maintenance of ventilator responses to hypoxia and hypercapnia
Adipose tissue	Catabolic	Stimulate lipolysis
Muscle	Catabolic	Increase protein breakdown
Bone	Developmental and metabolic	Promote normal growth and skeletal development; accelerate bone turnover
Nervous system	Developmental	Promote normal brain development
Gut	Metabolic	Increase rate of carbohydrate absorption, increased gut motility
Lipoprotein	Metabolic	Stimulate formation of hepatic LDL receptors
Endocrine	Metabolic	Alterations in production, responsiveness, and metabolic clearance
Other	Calorigenic	Stimulate oxygen consumption by metabolically active tissues (exceptions: adult brain, testes, uterus, lymph nodes, spleen, anterior pituitary)
		Increase metabolic rate

ATPase, adenosine triphosphatase; LDL, low-density lipoprotein.

membrane-bound Na$^+$-K$^+$ ATPase, increase heat production, and stimulate oxygen consumption (calorigenesis). Thyroid hormones also affect tissue growth and maturation, help regulate lipid metabolism, increase cardiac contractility by stimulating the expression of myosin protein, and increase intestinal carbohydrate absorption.

The effects of the thyroid hormones, T$_4$ and T$_3$, and the catecholamines, epinephrine and norepinephrine, are closely interrelated. All of these increase the metabolic rate and stimulate the nervous system and heart. In humans, the transcriptional effects of T$_3$ include the production of increased numbers of (and perhaps sensitivity to) β-adrenergic receptors in the heart, skeletal muscle, adipose tissue, and lymphocytes.

CHECKPOINT

1. Describe a thyroid follicle and how it changes with gland activity versus inactivity.
2. Which forms of thyroid hormone does the thyroid gland secrete? What are the normal proportions of the different forms? What are the relative potencies of each hormone?
3. To what is thyroid hormone bound during its transport in plasma?
4. How are thyroid hormone levels regulated?
5. What is the mechanism of action of thyroid hormone?
6. What are the most prominent organ system–specific effects of thyroid hormone?

OVERVIEW OF THYROID DISEASE

The symptoms and signs of thyroid disease in humans are predictable consequences of the physiologic effects of thyroid hormones discussed previously. The clinician commonly encounters patients with one of five types of thyroid dysfunction: (1) **hyperthyroidism** (thyrotoxicosis), caused by an excess of thyroid hormones; (2) **hypothyroidism** (myxedema), caused by a deficiency of thyroid hormones; (3) **goiter**, a diffuse enlargement of the thyroid gland, caused by a prolonged elevation of TSH; (4) **thyroid nodule**, a focal enlargement of a portion of the gland, caused by a benign or malignant neoplasm; and (5) **abnormal thyroid function tests** in a clinically euthyroid patient.

Several laboratory tests are useful in the initial evaluation of patients suspected of having thyroid dysfunction. The first is plasma TSH measured by a sensitive assay (usually defined by a lower detection limit of 0.01 mU/L on the third-generation assay). TSH is below normal range in hyperthyroidism and above normal range in hypothyroidism (except in the rare instances of pituitary or hypothalamic disease). The second useful laboratory test is a measurement of non-protein-bound thyroxine. Most clinical laboratories are now able to accurately measure free thyroxine (FT$_4$) directly. Although rarely used today, an estimate of non-protein-bound thyroxine is provided by the free thyroxine index (FT$_4$I): the product of the total plasma thyroxine (TT$_4$) and the T$_4$ resin uptake (RT$_4$U)

(ie, FT$_4$I = TT$_4$ × RT$_4$U). The TT$_4$ by itself often reflects the functional state of the thyroid hormone–binding proteins. The RT$_4$U is an indicator of thyroid-binding globulin and serves to correct for alterations in the concentration of binding protein. Some laboratories instead measure T$_3$ resin uptake (RT$_3$U).

Although total and free T$_3$ levels can be measured, they have a short half-life and are technically difficult assays. Under most circumstances, circulating levels of T$_3$ correlate less well with clinical hyperthyroidism or hypothyroidism.

A variety of thyroid autoantibodies are detectable in patients with thyroid dysfunction, including (1) **thyroidal peroxidase antibody (TPO Ab)**, formerly termed antimicrosomal antibody; (2) **thyroglobulin antibody (Tg Ab)**; and (3) **TSH-receptor antibody**, either **stimulating (TSH-R [stim] Ab or TSI)** or **blocking (TSH-R [block] Ab)**. Thyroglobulin and thyroidal peroxidase antibodies are commonly found in hypothyroidism resulting from Hashimoto thyroiditis and occasionally in hyperthyroidism from Graves disease (see later). TSH-R [stim] Ab (TSI) is present in individuals with hyperthyroidism caused by Graves disease. Detection of TSH-R [block] Ab in maternal serum is predictive of congenital hypothyroidism in newborns of mothers with autoimmune thyroid disease.

Other procedures such as thyroid scans and the thyrotropin-releasing hormone (TRH) test are discussed later.

PATHOPHYSIOLOGY OF SELECTED THYROID DISEASES

The pathogenesis of the most common thyroid diseases probably involves an autoimmune process with sensitization of the host's lymphocytes to various thyroidal antigens. Three major thyroidal antigens have been documented: thyroglobulin (Tg), thyroidal peroxidase (TPO), and the TSH receptor. Both environmental factors (eg, viral or bacterial infection or high iodine intake) and genetic factors (eg, a defect in suppressor T lymphocytes) may be responsible for initiating autoimmune thyroid disease.

HYPERTHYROIDISM

Etiology

Table 20–2 lists the causes of hyperthyroidism. Most commonly, thyroid hormone overproduction is due to Graves disease. In Graves disease, the TSH receptor autoantibody TSH-R [stim] Ab (TSI) stimulates the thyroid follicular cells to produce excessive amounts of T_4 and T_3. Less commonly, patients with multinodular goiter may become thyrotoxic without circulating antibodies if given inorganic iodine (eg, potassium iodide) or organic iodine compounds (eg, the antiarrhythmic drug amiodarone, which contains 37% iodine by weight). Multinodular goiters may also develop one or more nodules that become autonomous from TSH regulation and

TABLE 20–2 Hyperthyroidism: causes and pathogenetic mechanisms.

Etiologic Classification	Pathogenetic Mechanism
Thyroid hormone overproduction	
Graves disease	Thyroid-stimulating hormone receptor–stimulating antibody (TSH-R [stim] Ab)
Toxic multinodular goiter	Autonomous hyperfunction
Follicular adenoma	Autonomous hyperfunction
Pituitary adenoma	TSH hypersecretion (rare)
Pituitary insensitivity	Resistance to thyroid hormone (rare)
Hypothalamic disease	Excess TRH production
Germ cell tumors: choriocarcinoma, hydatidiform mole	Human chorionic gonadotropin stimulation
Struma ovarii (ovarian teratoma)	Functioning thyroid elements
Metastatic follicular thyroid carcinoma	Functioning metastases
Thyroid gland destruction	
Lymphocytic thyroiditis	Release of stored hormone
Granulomatous (subacute) thyroiditis	Release of stored hormone
Hashimoto thyroiditis	Transient release of stored hormone
Drug effect	
Thyrotoxicosis medicamentosa, thyrotoxicosis factitia	Ingestion of excessive exogenous thyroid hormone
Amiodarone	Excess iodine and/or thyroiditis
Interferon alpha	Thyroiditis

secrete excessive quantities of T_4 or T_3. Patients from regions where goiter is endemic may develop thyrotoxicosis when given iodine supplementation (Jod-Basedow phenomenon). Large follicular adenomas (>3 cm in diameter) may produce excessive thyroid hormone.

Occasionally, TSH overproduction (eg, from a pituitary adenoma) or hypothalamic disease may cause excessive thyroid hormone production. The diagnosis is suggested by clinically evident hyperthyroidism with elevated serum T_4 and T_3 and *elevated* serum TSH levels. Neuroradiologic imaging such as computed tomography (CT) scans or magnetic resonance imaging (MRI) of the sella turcica confirm the presence of a pituitary tumor. Even more rarely, hyperthyroidism results from TSH overproduction caused by pituitary (but not peripheral tissue) resistance to the suppressive effects of T_4 and T_3. The diagnosis is suggested by finding elevated serum T_4 and T_3 levels with an inappropriately normal serum TSH level.

Hyperthyroidism may be precipitated by germ cell tumors (choriocarcinoma and hydatidiform mole), which secrete large quantities of human chorionic gonadotropin (hCG). The large quantities of hCG secreted by these tumors bind to the follicular cell TSH receptor and stimulate overproduction of thyroid hormone. Rarely, hyperthyroidism can be produced by ovarian teratomas containing thyroid tissue (struma ovarii). Hyperthyroidism results when this ectopic thyroid tissue begins to function autonomously. Struma ovarii is diagnosed when an ovarian tumor contains 50% or more thyroid tissue; clinical signs of thyrotoxicosis are reported in only about 5–8% of cases of struma ovarii. Patients with large metastases from follicular thyroid carcinomas may produce excess thyroid hormone, particularly after iodide administration.

Transient hyperthyroidism is occasionally observed in patients with lymphocytic or granulomatous (subacute) thyroiditis (Hashimoto thyroiditis). In such cases, the hyperthyroidism is due to the destruction of the thyroid with the release of stored hormone.

Finally, patients who consume excessive amounts of exogenous thyroid hormone (accidentally or deliberately) and those treated with amiodarone or interferon alpha may present with symptoms, signs, and laboratory findings of hyperthyroidism.

Pathogenesis

Whatever the cause of hyperthyroidism, serum thyroid hormones are elevated. Both the free thyroxine (FT_4) and the free thyroxine index (FT_4I) are elevated. In 5–10% of patients, T_4 secretion is normal while T_3 levels are high (so-called **T_3 toxicosis**). Total serum T_4 and T_3 levels are not always definitive because of variations in concentrations of thyroid hormone–binding proteins.

Hyperthyroidism resulting from Graves disease is characterized by a suppressed serum TSH level as determined by sensitive immunoenzymometric or immunoradiometric assays. However, TSH levels may also be suppressed in some acute psychiatric and other nonthyroidal illnesses. In the rare TSH-secreting pituitary adenomas (so-called **secondary hyperthyroidism**) and in hypothalamic disease with excessive TRH production (so-called **tertiary hyperthyroidism**), hyperthyroidism is accompanied by a high or high normal plasma TSH level.

The radioactive iodine (RAI) uptake of the thyroid gland at 4 or 24 hours is increased when the gland produces an excess of hormone (eg, Graves disease); it is decreased when the gland is leaking stored hormone (eg, thyroiditis), when hormone is produced elsewhere (eg, struma ovarii), and when excessive exogenous thyroid hormone is being ingested (eg, factitious hyperthyroidism). Technetium 99m scanning can provide information similar to that obtained with RAI and is quicker and entails less radiation exposure.

The TRH test is sometimes helpful in diagnosis when patients have confusing thyroid function test results. In normal individuals, TRH administration (500 µg intravenously) produces an increase in serum TSH of at least 6 mU/L within 15–30 minutes. In primary hyperthyroidism, TSH levels are low and TRH administration induces little or no increase in the TSH level.

Graves Disease

A. Pathology

Graves disease is the most common cause of hyperthyroidism among individuals in their third and fourth decades but can occur at any age. In this condition, the thyroid gland is symmetrically enlarged and its vascularity markedly increased. The gland may double or triple in weight. Microscopically, the follicular epithelial cells are columnar in appearance and increased in number and size (see Figure 20–2). The follicles are small and closely packed together. The colloid is scanty, and the edges are scalloped in appearance secondary to the rapid proteolysis of thyroglobulin. The gland's interstitium is diffusely infiltrated with lymphocytes and may contain lymphoid follicles with germinal centers.

B. Pathogenesis

The serum of more than 90% of patients with Graves disease contains **TSH-R [stim] antibody**, directed against the TSH receptor site in the thyroid follicular epithelial membrane. This antibody, formerly called long-acting thyroid stimulator (LATS), is now also called **thyroid-stimulating immunoglobulin (TSI)**. When it binds to the cell membrane TSH receptors, TSH-R [stim] Ab (TSI) stimulates hormone synthesis and secretion in somewhat the same way as TSH. Although serum levels of TSH-R [stim] Ab (TSI) correlate poorly with disease severity, its presence can be helpful diagnostically and perhaps prognostically. After discontinuing antithyroid drug treatment, about 30–50% of patients with Graves hyperthyroidism relapse. There seems to be a greatly increased recurrence risk if the TSH-R [stim] Ab (TSI) is still found in plasma at the time of discontinuing antithyroid drug treatment, so this test can perhaps be used to predict likely relapse.

TABLE 20–3   Autoimmune disorders associated with Graves disease and Hashimoto thyroiditis.

Endocrine disorders
Type 1 diabetes mellitus
Primary hypoadrenalism, autoimmune (Addison disease)
Orchitis or oophoritis, autoimmune
Hypoparathyroidism, idiopathic
Nonendocrine disorders
Pernicious anemia
Vitiligo
Systemic lupus erythematosus
Rheumatoid arthritis
Immune thrombocytopenic purpura
Myasthenia gravis
Sjögren syndrome
Primary biliary cholangitis
Chronic active hepatitis

The genesis of TSH-R [stim] Ab (TSI) in patients with Graves disease is uncertain. However, Graves disease is familial. A genetic contribution to the development of Graves disease is suggested by the finding of much higher concordance rates in monozygotic same-sex twin pairs (0.35) than in dizygotic pairs (0.03). In Caucasians, it is associated with the HLA-B8 and HLA-DR3 histocompatibility antigens; in Asians, with HLA-Bw46 and HLA-B5; and in blacks, with HLA-B17. Furthermore, patients with Graves disease frequently suffer from other autoimmune disorders (Table 20–3). The precipitating cause of this antibody production is unknown, but an immune response against a viral antigen that shares homology with TSH-R may be responsible. Another theory of the pathogenesis of Graves disease is a defect of suppressor T lymphocytes, which allows helper T lymphocytes to stimulate B lymphocytes to secrete antibodies directed against follicular cell membrane antigens, including TSH-R (Figure 20–6).

Moderate titers of other autoantibodies (thyroidal peroxidase antibody and TSH-R [block] Ab) can be found in patients with Graves disease. Their significance is uncertain. In some cases, TSH-R [block] Ab appears after ^{131}I radioiodine therapy for Graves disease.

Patients with hyperthyroidism from Graves disease may later develop hypothyroidism by one of several mechanisms: (1) thyroid ablation by surgery or ^{131}I radiation treatment; (2) autoimmune thyroiditis, leading to thyroid destruction; or (3) the development of antibodies that block TSH stimulation (TSH-R [block] Ab).

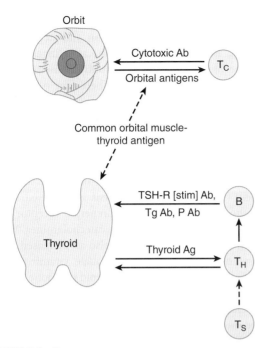

FIGURE 20–6 Proposed pathogenesis of Graves disease. A defect in suppressor T lymphocytes (T$_s$) allows helper T lymphocytes (T$_H$) to stimulate B lymphocytes (B) to synthesize thyroid autoantibodies. The thyroid receptor–stimulating antibody (TSH-R [stim] Ab or TSI) is the driving force for thyrotoxicosis. Inflammation of the orbital muscles may be due to the sensitization of cytotoxic T lymphocytes (T$_c$) or to the sensitization of killer cells to a common antigen, the TSH-R, found in both orbital fibroblasts and thyroid follicular cells. What triggers this immunologic cascade is not known. (Ag, antigen; P Ab, peroxidase or microsomal antibody; Tg Ab, thyroglobulin antibody.) (Redrawn, with permission, from Gardner DG et al, eds. *Greenspan's Basic and Clinical Endocrinology*, 10th ed. McGraw-Hill, 2017.)

After radioactive iodine therapy, there is often a lag in the recovery of thyrotropin (TSH) responsiveness that may last 60–90 days or longer. During this period, decisions regarding further therapy must be based on the patient's clinical status as well as on the serum levels of TSH and thyroid hormones.

CHECKPOINT

7. What are the five categories of thyroid dysfunction most commonly observed in patients?

8. What are seven different pathophysiologic mechanisms by which a patient might develop hyperthyroidism?

9. What is the most useful initial test of thyroid function in hyperthyroidism? What results would you expect compared with normal?

10. How can thyroid scanning help confirm the suspected cause of hyperthyroidism?

11. Describe the mechanism of hyperthyroidism in Graves disease.

Clinical Manifestations

The clinical consequences of thyroid hormone excess (Table 20–4) are exaggerated expressions of the physiologic activity of T$_3$ and T$_4$.

An excess of thyroid hormone causes enough extra heat production to result in a slight increase in body temperature and to activate heat-dissipating mechanisms, including cutaneous vasodilation, a decrease in peripheral vascular resistance, and increased sweating. The increased basal metabolic rate leads to weight loss, especially in older patients with poor appetite. In younger patients, food intake typically increases, and some patients have seemingly insatiable appetites.

The apparent increased catecholamine effect of hyperthyroidism is probably multifactorial in origin. Thyroid hormones increase β-adrenergic receptors in many tissues, including heart muscle, skeletal muscle, adipose tissue, and lymphocytes. They also decrease α-adrenergic receptors in heart muscle and may amplify catecholamine action at a postreceptor site. Thus, thyrotoxicosis is characterized by an

TABLE 20–4   Clinical findings in hyperthyroidism (thyrotoxicosis).

Symptoms
Alertness, emotional lability, nervousness, irritability
Poor concentration
Muscular weakness, fatigability
Palpitations
Voracious appetite, weight loss
Hyperdefecation (increased frequency of bowel movements)
Heat intolerance
Signs
Hyperkinesia, rapid speech
Proximal muscle (quadriceps) weakness, fine tremor
Fine, moist skin; fine, abundant hair; onycholysis
Lid lag, stare, chemosis, periorbital edema, proptosis
Accentuated first heart sound, tachycardia, atrial fibrillation (resistant to digitalis), widened pulse pressure, dyspnea
Laboratory findings
Suppressed serum TSH level
Elevated serum free thyroxine, elevated serum total T$_4$, elevated resin T$_3$ or T$_4$ uptake, elevated free thyroxine index
Increased radioiodine uptake by thyroid gland (some causes)
Increased basal metabolic rate
Decreased serum cholesterol level

increased metabolic and hemodynamic sensitivity of the tissues to catecholamines. However, circulating catecholamine levels are normal. Drugs that block β-adrenergic receptors reduce or eliminate the tachycardia, arrhythmias, sweating, and tremor of hyperthyroidism. When β blockers are used in the treatment of hyperthyroidism, it appears that "nonselective" β blockers (such as propranolol), which block both β_1 and β_2 receptors, have an advantage over "selective" β_1 blockers (such as metoprolol). The "nonselective" agents appear to reduce the metabolic rate significantly, whereas the "selective" β_1 blockers do not reduce oxygen consumption and provide only symptomatic relief related to heart rate normalization.

Thyroid hormone excess causes rapid mentation, nervousness, irritability, emotional lability, restlessness, and even mania and psychosis. Patients complain of poor concentration and reduced performance at work or in school. Tremor is common, and deep tendon reflexes are brisk, with a rapid relaxation phase. Muscle weakness and atrophy (**thyrotoxic myopathy**) commonly develop in hyperthyroidism, particularly if severe and prolonged. Proximal muscle weakness may interfere with walking, climbing, rising from a deep knee bend, or weight lifting. Such muscle weakness may be due to increased protein catabolism and muscle wasting, decreased muscle efficiency, or changes in myosin. Despite an increased number of β-adrenergic receptors in muscle, the increased proteolysis is apparently not mediated by β receptors, and muscle weakness and wasting are not affected by β-adrenergic blockers. Myasthenia gravis or periodic paralysis may accompany hyperthyroidism.

Vital capacity and respiratory muscle strength are reduced. Extreme muscle weakness may cause respiratory failure.

In hyperthyroidism, cardiac output is increased as a result of increased heart rate and contractility and reduced peripheral vascular resistance. Pulse pressure is increased, and circulation time is shortened. Tachycardia, usually supraventricular, is frequent and thought to be related to the direct effects of thyroid hormone on the cardiac conducting system. Atrial fibrillation may occur, particularly in elderly patients. Continuous 24-hour electrocardiographic monitoring of thyrotoxic patients shows persistent tachycardia but preservation of the normal circadian rhythm of the heart rate, suggesting that normal adrenergic responsiveness persists. Myocardial calcium uptake is increased in thyrotoxic rats; in humans, calcium channel–blocking agents (eg, diltiazem) can decrease heart rate; the number of premature ventricular beats' and the number of bouts of supraventricular tachycardia, paroxysmal atrial fibrillation, and ventricular tachycardia. Patients with hyperthyroidism may manifest acute heart failure as a result of left ventricular dysfunction with segmental wall motion abnormalities; its rapid reversibility with treatment suggests that it may be due to myocardial "stunning." Long-standing hyperthyroidism may lead to cardiomegaly and a "high-output" heart failure. Flow murmurs are common, and extracardiac sounds occur, generated by the hyperdynamic heart.

Hyperthyroidism leads to increased hepatic gluconeogenesis, enhanced carbohydrate absorption, and increased insulin degradation. In nondiabetic patients, after ingesting carbohydrate, the blood glucose rises rapidly, sometimes causing glycosuria, and then falls rapidly. There may be an adaptive increase in insulin secretion, perhaps explaining the normal glycemic, glycogenolytic, glycolytic, and ketogenic sensitivity to epinephrine. Diabetic patients have an increased insulin requirement in the hyperthyroid state.

Metabolically, total plasma cholesterol is usually low, related to an increase in the number of hepatic low-density lipoprotein (LDL) receptors. Lipolysis is increased, and adipocytes show an increase in β-adrenergic receptor density and an increased responsiveness to catecholamines. With the increase in metabolic rate, there is also an increased need for vitamins; if dietary sources are inadequate, vitamin deficiency syndromes may occur. Normally, thyroid hormone stimulates the osteoblastic production of insulin-like growth factor 1 (IGF-1), clearly important for the anabolic effects of thyroid hormone on bone. In hyperthyroid patients, levels of serum IGF-1 and several binding proteins (IGFBP-3 and IGFBP-4) are significantly increased before treatment and return to normal after antithyroid drug treatment. In addition, because of enhanced osteoblastic and osteoclastic activity, overtly hyperthyroid patients frequently exhibit accelerated bone turnover and a negative calcium and phosphorus balance, resulting in low bone mineral density and increased skeletal fragility. Hypercalciuria and sometimes hypercalcemia can occur. Normalization of thyroid function is associated with a significant attenuation of increased bone turnover, followed by an increase in bone mineral density.

There is an increase in frequency of bowel movements (hyperdefecation) as a result of increased GI motility. Accelerated small bowel transit may be caused by an increased frequency of bowel contractions and giant migrating contractions. In severe thyrotoxicosis, abnormal liver function tests may be observed, reflecting malnutrition. Anorexia in untreated hyperthyroidism is associated with older age, anxiety, and abnormal liver function, but not with hypercalcemia.

In women, hyperthyroidism may lead to oligomenorrhea and decreased fertility. In the follicular phase of the menstrual cycle, there is an increased basal plasma LH level and an increased LH and FSH response to GnRH (see Chapter 22). There is an increase in sex hormone–binding globulin, leading to increased levels of total estradiol. In men, hyperthyroidism may cause decreased fertility and impotence from altered steroid hormone metabolism. Serum levels of total testosterone, total estradiol, sex hormone–binding globulin, LH, and FSH, and the response of gonadotropin to GnRH are significantly greater than normal. However, the ratio of free testosterone to free estradiol is lower than normal. Mean sperm counts are normal, but the percentage of forward progressive sperm motility is lower than normal. These hormone and semen abnormalities are reversible with successful treatment of the hyperthyroidism. Gynecomastia may occur despite high normal serum testosterone levels secondary to the increased peripheral conversion of androgens to estrogens (see Chapter 23).

There is an increased plasma concentration of atrial natriuretic peptide (ANP) and its precursors. The plasma ANP concentration correlates with the serum thyroxine level and heart rate and decreases to normal with successful antithyroid therapy.

The wide-eyed stare of hyperthyroid patients may be due to increased sympathetic tone. In addition, proptosis develops in 25–50% of patients with Graves disease as a result of the infiltration of orbital soft tissues and extraocular muscles with lymphocytes, mucopolysaccharides, and edema fluid (Figure 20–7). This may lead to fibrosis of the extraocular muscles, restricted ocular motility, and diplopia. In severe Graves ophthalmopathy, pressure on the optic nerve or keratitis from corneal exposure may lead to blindness. In patients with Graves disease, it is clear that TSH-R [stim] Ab (TSI) is related to Graves ophthalmopathy. In addition, autoantibodies against G2s, a 55-kDa protein found in both thyroid and eye muscle tissue, are definitely associated with Graves ophthalmopathy. For instance, antibodies reactive with G2s are identified in significantly more patients with active thyroid ophthalmopathy than in patients with Graves disease without ophthalmopathy, those with Hashimoto thyroiditis or nonimmunologic thyroid disorders, and those without

thyroid disease. The pathogenesis of Graves ophthalmopathy may involve cytotoxic lymphocytes (killer cells) and cytotoxic antibodies to an antigen common to orbital fibroblasts, orbital muscle, and thyroid tissue (see Figure 20–6). It is postulated that cytokines released from these sensitized lymphocytes cause orbital tissue inflammation, resulting in the proptosis, diplopia, and edema. Furthermore, involvement of the insulin–like growth factor 1 receptor in ophthalmopathy is suggested by its overexpression by orbital fibroblasts, T cells, and B cells in Graves disease. For unknown reasons, Graves ophthalmopathy is worse in smokers and may be exacerbated by radioiodine therapy.

The skin is warm, sweaty, and velvety in texture. Hyperpigmentation can be seen on the lower extremities, most strikingly on the shins, the backs of the feet, and the nail beds. The hyperpigmentation is due to basal melanosis and heavy deposition of hemosiderin around dermal capillaries and sweat glands. Its distribution, hemosiderin deposition, and poor response to treatment distinguish it from the hyperpigmentation seen with Addison disease. There may be onycholysis (ie, retraction of the nail from the nail plate). In Graves disease, the pretibial skin may become thickened, resembling an orange peel (**pretibial myxedema** or **thyrotoxic dermopathy**). The dermopathy is usually a late manifestation of Graves disease, and affected patients invariably have ophthalmopathy. The most common form of the dermopathy is nonpitting edema, but nodular, plaque-like, and even polypoid forms also occur. The pathogenesis of thyroid dermopathy may also involve lymphocyte cytokine stimulation of fibroblasts. Thyroid dermopathy is associated with a very high serum titer of TSH-R [stim] Ab (TSI).

Untreated hyperthyroidism may decompensate into a state called **thyroid storm**. Patients so affected have tachycardia, fever, agitation, nausea, vomiting, diarrhea, and restlessness or psychosis. The condition is usually precipitated by an intercurrent illness or by a surgical emergency. Thyroid storm should be treated aggressively since its mortality rate is high (8–25%).

FIGURE 20–7 Graves disease. (Reproduced with the permission of PH Forsham.)

CHECKPOINT

12. Describe the physiologic consequences of hyperthyroidism, and identify their mechanism (as is best known) on the following systems:
    Heart
    Liver
    Lungs
    GI tract
    Kidneys
    Eyes
    Skin
    Brain
    Bone
    Reproductive system

HYPOTHYROIDISM

Etiology

Table 20–5 lists the causes of hypothyroidism. The most common cause is Hashimoto thyroiditis, which results from an autoimmune destruction of the thyroid, although the precipitating cause and exact mechanism of the autoimmunity and subsequent destruction are unknown. Hypothyroidism may also be caused by lymphocytic thyroiditis after a transient period of hyperthyroidism. Thyroid ablation, whether by surgical resection or by therapeutic radiation, commonly results in hypothyroidism.

Congenital hypothyroidism, a preventable cause of mental retardation, occurs in approximately 1 in 4000 births; girls are affected about twice as often as boys. Most cases (85%) are sporadic in distribution, but 15% are hereditary. The most common cause of sporadic congenital hypothyroidism is thyroid dysgenesis, in which hypofunctioning ectopic thyroid tissue is more common than thyroid hypoplasia or aplasia. Although the pathogenesis of thyroid dysgenesis is largely unknown, some cases have been described as resulting from mutations in the transcription factors PAX-8 and TTF-2. The most common problems causing hereditary congenital hypothyroidism are inborn errors of thyroxine (T_4) synthesis. Mutations have been described in the genes coding for the sodium iodide transporter, thyroid peroxidase (TPO), and thyroglobulin. Other cases of congenital hypothyroidism are caused by loss-of-function TSH-R mutations. Finally, a transient form of familial congenital hypothyroidism is caused by transplacental passage of a maternal TSH receptor–blocking antibody (**TSH-R [block] Ab**).

Central hypothyroidism, characterized by insufficient TSH secretion in the presence of low levels of thyroid hormones, is a rare disorder. It is caused by diseases of the pituitary or hypothalamus that result in diminished or abnormal TSH secretion, such as tumors or infiltrative diseases of the hypothalamopituitary area, pituitary atrophy, and inactivating mutations in genes that code for the various proteins involved in regulating the hypothalamic–pituitary–thyroid axis (see Figure 20–5). For example, mutations have been identified in the genes for the TRH receptor, the transcription factors Pit-1 and PROP1, and the TSH β-subunit. Pituitary ("secondary") hypothyroidism is characterized by a diminished number of functioning thyrotropes in the pituitary gland, accounting for a quantitative impairment of TSH secretion. Hypothalamic ("tertiary") hypothyroidism is characterized by normal or sometimes even increased TSH concentrations but qualitative abnormalities of the TSH secreted. These abnormalities cause the circulating TSH to lack biologic activity and to exhibit impaired binding to its receptor. This defect can be reversed by administering TRH. Thus, TRH may regulate not only the secretion of TSH but also the specific molecular and conformational features that enable it to act at its receptor.

Finally, a variety of drugs, including the thioamide antithyroid medications propylthiouracil and methimazole, may produce hypothyroidism. The thioamides inhibit thyroid peroxidase and block the synthesis of thyroid hormone. In addition, propylthiouracil, but not methimazole, blocks the peripheral conversion of T_4 to T_3. Deiodination of iodine-containing compounds such as amiodarone, releasing large amounts of iodide, may also cause hypothyroidism by blocking iodide organification, referred to as the Wolff–Chaikoff effect. Lithium is concentrated by the thyroid and inhibits the release of hormone from the gland. Most patients treated with lithium compensate by increasing TSH secretion, but some become hypothyroid. Lithium-associated clinical hypothyroidism

TABLE 20–5 Hypothyroidism: causes and pathogenetic mechanisms.

Cause	Pathogenetic Mechanism
Congenital	Aplasia or hypoplasia of thyroid gland
	Defects in hormone biosynthesis or action
Acquired	
Hashimoto thyroiditis	Autoimmune destruction
Severe iodine deficiency	Diminished hormone synthesis, release
Lymphocytic thyroiditis	Diminished hormone synthesis, release
Thyroid ablation	Diminished hormone synthesis, release
Thyroid surgery	
[131]I radiation treatment of hyperthyroidism	
External beam radiation therapy of head and neck cancer	
Drugs	Diminished hormone synthesis, release
Iodine, inorganic	
Iodine, organic (amiodarone)	
Thioamides (propylthiouracil,[1] methimazole)	
Potassium perchlorate	
Thiocyanate	
Lithium	
Amiodarone	
Sunitinib	
Hypopituitarism	Deficient TSH secretion
Hypothalamic disease	Deficient TRH secretion

[1]Also blocks peripheral conversion of T_4 to T_3.

occurs in about 10% of patients receiving the drug. It occurs more commonly in middle-aged women, particularly during the first 2 years of lithium treatment. Another rare cause of hypothyroidism is consumptive hypothyroidism. This paraneoplastic syndrome is the result of an elevated D3 enzyme, which inactivates (consumes) the bioactive T_4. Directly proportional to (1) the size of the tumor expressing D3; and (2) the specific activity of the D3 enzyme, consumptive hypothyroidism was first identified in newborns with infantile hepatic hemangiomatosis but has since been reported in adults as well.

Pathogenesis

Hypothyroidism is characterized by abnormally low serum T_4 and T_3 levels. Free thyroxine levels are always depressed. The serum TSH level is elevated in hypothyroidism (except in cases of pituitary or hypothalamic disease). TSH is the most sensitive test for early hypothyroidism, and marked elevations of serum TSH (>20 mU/L) are found in frank hypothyroidism. Modest TSH elevations (5–20 mU/L) may be found in euthyroid individuals with normal serum T_4 and T_3 levels and indicate impaired thyroid reserve and incipient hypothyroidism (see Subclinical Thyroid Dysfunction, below). In patients with primary hypothyroidism (end-organ failure), the nocturnal TSH surge is intact. In patients with central (pituitary or hypothalamic) hypothyroidism, the serum TSH level is low and the normal nocturnal TSH surge is absent.

In hypothyroidism resulting from thyroid gland failure, administering TRH produces a prompt increase in the TSH level, the magnitude of which is proportionate to the baseline serum TSH level. The hypernormal response is caused by an absence of feedback inhibition by T_4 and T_3. However, the TRH stimulation test is not usually performed in patients with primary hypothyroidism because the elevated basal serum TSH level suffices to make the diagnosis. This test may be useful in the clinically hypothyroid patient with an unexpectedly low serum TSH level in establishing a central (pituitary or hypothalamic) origin. Pituitary disease is suggested by the failure of TSH to rise after TRH administration; hypothalamic disease is suggested by a delayed TSH response (at 60–120 minutes rather than 15–30 minutes) with a normal increment.

Hashimoto Thyroiditis

A. Pathology

In the early stages of Hashimoto thyroiditis, the gland is diffusely enlarged, firm, rubbery, and nodular. As the disease progresses, the gland becomes smaller. In the late stages, the gland is atrophic and fibrotic, weighing as little as 5–10 g. Microscopically, there is a destruction of thyroid follicles and lymphocytic infiltration with lymphoid follicles. The surviving thyroid follicular epithelial cells are large, with abundant pink cytoplasm (Hürthle cells). As the disease progresses, there is an increasing amount of fibrosis.

B. Pathogenesis

The pathogenesis of Hashimoto thyroiditis is unclear. Again, it is possible that a defect in suppressor T lymphocytes allows helper T lymphocytes to interact with specific antigens on the thyroid follicular cell membrane. Once these lymphocytes become sensitized to thyroidal antigens, autoantibodies are formed that react with these antigens. Cytokine release and inflammation then cause glandular destruction. The most important thyroid autoantibodies in Hashimoto thyroiditis are thyroglobulin antibody (Tg Ab), thyroidal peroxidase antibody (TPO Ab; formerly termed antimicrosomal antibody), and the TSH receptor–blocking antibody (TSH-R [block] Ab). During the early phases, Tg Ab is markedly elevated and TPO Ab only slightly elevated. Later, Tg Ab may disappear, but TPO Ab persists for many years. TSH-R [block] Ab is found in patients with atrophic thyroiditis and myxedema and in mothers who give birth to mentally impaired infants with no detectable thyroid tissue (**athyreotic cretins**). Serum levels of these antibodies do not correlate with the severity of the hypothyroidism, but their presence is helpful in diagnosis. In general, high antibody titers are diagnostic of Hashimoto thyroiditis; moderate titers are seen in Graves disease, multinodular goiter, and thyroid neoplasm; and low titers are found in the elderly.

Patients with Hashimoto thyroiditis have an increased frequency of the HLA-DR5 histocompatibility antigen, and the disease is associated with a host of other autoimmune diseases (see Table 20–3). A **polyglandular failure syndrome** has been defined in which two or more endocrine disorders mediated by autoimmune mechanisms occur (see Chapter 17). Affected patients frequently have circulating organ- and cell-specific autoantibodies that lead to organ hypofunction.

CHECKPOINT

13. What are some drugs that cause hypothyroidism?
14. What are the most useful initial tests of thyroid function in hypothyroidism? What results would you expect compared with normal?
15. What are the key pathophysiologic findings in Hashimoto thyroiditis?

Clinical Manifestations

Table 20–6 summarizes the clinical consequences of thyroid hormone deficiency in the adult.

Hypothermia is common, and the patient may complain of cold intolerance. The decreased basal metabolic rate leads to weight gain despite reduced food intake.

Thyroid hormones are required for the normal development of the nervous system. In hypothyroid infants, synapses develop abnormally, myelination is defective, and mental retardation occurs. Hypothyroid adults have several reversible neurologic abnormalities, including slowed mentation, forgetfulness, decreased hearing, and ataxia. Some patients have severe mental symptoms, including reversible dementia

TABLE 20–6   Clinical findings in adult hypothyroidism (myxedema).

Symptoms
Slow thinking
Lethargy, decreased vigor
Dry skin, thickened hair, hair loss, broken nails
Diminished food intake, weight gain
Constipation
Menorrhagia, diminished libido
Cold intolerance
Signs
Round, puffy face; slow speech; hoarseness
Hypokinesia, generalized muscle weakness, delayed relaxation of deep tendon reflexes
Cold, dry, thick, scaling skin; dry, coarse, brittle hair; dry, longitudinally ridged nails
Periorbital edema
Normal or faint cardiac impulse, indistinct heart sounds, cardiac enlargement, bradycardia
Ascites, pericardial effusion, ankle edema
Mental clouding, depression
Laboratory findings
Increased serum TSH level
Decreased serum free thyroxine, decreased serum total T_4 and T_3, decreased resin T_3 or T_4 uptake, decreased free thyroxine index
Decreased radioiodine uptake by thyroid gland
Diminished basal metabolic rate
Macrocytic anemia
Elevated serum cholesterol level
Elevated serum creatine kinase level
Hyponatremia (from excess secretion of antidiuretic hormone)
Decreased circulation time, low voltage of QRS complex on ECG

or overt psychosis ("myxedema madness"). The cerebrospinal fluid protein level is abnormally high. However, total cerebral blood flow and oxygen consumption are normal. Deep tendon reflexes are sluggish, with a slowed ("hung-up") relaxation phase. Paresthesias are common, often caused by compression neuropathies resulting from an accumulation of myxedema (carpal tunnel syndrome and tarsal tunnel syndrome).

Hypothyroidism is associated with muscle weakness, cramps, and stiffness. The serum creatine kinase (CK) level

may be elevated. The pathophysiology of the muscle disease in hypothyroidism is poorly understood. Study of the bioenergetic abnormalities in hypothyroid muscle suggests a hormone-dependent, reversible mitochondrial impairment. Changes in energy metabolism are not found in hyperthyroid muscle.

Patients rendered acutely hypothyroid by total thyroidectomy exhibit a decreased cardiac output, decreased stroke volume, decreased diastolic volume at rest, and increased peripheral resistance. However, the pulmonary capillary wedge pressure, right atrial pressure, heart rate, left ventricular ejection fraction, and left ventricular systolic pressure–volume relation (a measure of contractility) are not significantly different from the euthyroid state. Thus, in early hypothyroidism, alterations in cardiac performance are probably primarily related to changes in loading conditions and exercise-related heart rate rather than to changes in myocardial contractility.

In chronic hypothyroidism, echocardiography shows bradycardia and features that suggest cardiomyopathy, including an increased thickening of the intraventricular septum and ventricular wall, decreased regional wall motion, and decreased systolic and diastolic global left ventricular function. These changes may be due to deposition of excessive mucopolysaccharides in the interstitium between myocardial fibers, leading to fiber degeneration, decreased contractility, low cardiac output, cardiac enlargement, and heart failure. Pericardial effusion (with high protein content) may lead to findings of decreased electrocardiographic voltage and flattened T waves, but cardiac tamponade is rare.

Hypothyroid patients exhibit decreased ventilatory responses to hypercapnia and hypoxia. There is a high incidence of sleep apnea in untreated hypothyroidism; such patients sometimes demonstrate myopathy of the upper airway muscles. Weakness of the diaphragm also occurs frequently and, when severe, can cause chronic alveolar hypoventilation (CO_2 retention). Pleural effusions (with high protein content) may occur.

In hypothyroidism, the plasma cholesterol and triglyceride levels increase, related to decreased lipoprotein lipase activity and decreased formation of hepatic LDL receptors. In hypothyroid children, bone growth is slowed and skeletal maturation (closure of epiphyses) is delayed. Pituitary secretion of growth hormone may also be depressed because thyroid hormone is needed for its synthesis. Hypothyroid animals demonstrate a decreased width of the epiphysial growth plate and articular cartilage and a decreased volume of epiphyseal and metaphyseal trabecular bone. These changes are not solely due to the lack of pituitary growth hormone, because administering exogenous growth hormone does not restore normal cartilage morphology or bone remodeling, whereas administering T_4 does. If unrecognized, prolonged juvenile hypothyroidism results in a permanent height deficit.

A normochromic, normocytic anemia may occur as a result of decreased erythropoiesis. Alternatively, a moderate macrocytic anemia can occur as a result of decreased cyanocobalamin (vitamin B_{12}) absorption from the intestine and diminished bone marrow metabolism. Frank megaloblastic anemia suggests coexistent pernicious anemia.

Constipation is common and reflects decreased GI motility. Achlorhydria occurs when hypothyroidism is associated with pernicious anemia. Ascitic fluid with high protein content may accumulate.

The skin in hypothyroidism is dry and cool. Normally, the skin contains a variety of proteins complexed with polysaccharides, chondroitin sulfate, and hyaluronic acid. In hypothyroidism, these complexes accumulate, promoting sodium and water retention and producing a characteristic diffuse, nonpitting puffiness of the skin (myxedema). The patient's face appears puffy, with coarse features (Figure 20–8). A similar accumulation of mucopolysaccharides in the larynx may lead to hoarseness. The hair is brittle and lacking in luster, and there is frequently a loss of body hair, particularly over the scalp and lateral eyebrows. If thyroid hormone is administered, the protein complexes are mobilized, a diuresis ensues, and myxedema resolves.

Carotenemia (manifested as a yellow-orange discoloration of the skin) may occur in hypothyroidism because thyroid hormones are needed for the hepatic conversion of carotene to vitamin A. In the absence of sufficient hormone, carotene accumulates in the bloodstream and skin.

In women, hypothyroidism may lead to menorrhagia from anovulatory cycles. Alternatively, menses may become scanty or disappear secondary to the diminished secretion of gonadotropins. Because thyroid hormone normally has an inhibitory effect on prolactin secretion, hypothyroid patients may exhibit hyperprolactinemia, with galactorrhea and amenorrhea. In men, hypothyroidism can cause infertility and gynecomastia

from an enhanced release of prolactin. Hyperprolactinemia occurs because TRH also stimulates prolactin release.

There is reduced renal blood flow and a decreased glomerular filtration rate. The vasoconstriction may be due to decreased concentrations of plasma ANP. The consequent reduced ability to excrete a water load may cause hyponatremia. However, the serum creatinine level is usually normal.

Long-standing, severe untreated hypothyroidism may lead to a state called **myxedema coma**. Affected patients have typical myxedematous facies and skin, bradycardia, hypothermia, alveolar hypoventilation, and severe obtundation or coma. This condition is usually precipitated by an intercurrent illness, such as an infection or stroke, or by a medication, such as a sedative-hypnotic. The mortality rate approaches 100% unless myxedema coma is recognized and treated promptly.

Levothyroxine therapy is the mainstay of treatment in patients with hypothyroidism. The correct dose is the amount required to keep the serum TSH within the normal range in primary hypothyroidism. However, keeping the serum T_4 level within the normal range is the aim when treating a patient with central (pituitary or hypothalamic) hypothyroidism.

CHECKPOINT

16. Describe and explain the physiologic consequence of hypothyroidism (as is best known) on the following:
    Nervous system
    Muscle
    Cardiovascular system
    Lungs
    Liver
    Blood
    GI tract
    Skin
    Reproductive system
    Kidneys

GOITER

Etiology

Diffuse thyroid enlargement most commonly results from prolonged stimulation by TSH (or a TSH-like agent). Such stimulation may be the result of one of the causes of hypothyroidism (eg, TSH in Hashimoto thyroiditis) or hyperthyroidism (eg, TSH-R [stim] Ab in Graves disease, hCG in germ cell tumors, or TSH in pituitary adenoma). Alternatively, goiter may occur in a clinically euthyroid patient. Table 20–7 lists the causes and pathogenetic mechanisms of goiter.

Iodine deficiency is the most common cause of goiter in developing nations. A diet that contains less than 10 μg/d of iodine hinders the synthesis of thyroid hormone, resulting in an elevated TSH level and thyroid hypertrophy. The iodination of salt has eliminated this problem in much of the developed world.

FIGURE 20–8 Myxedema. (Reproduced, with permission, from Greenspan FS et al, eds. *Basic and Clinical Endocrinology*, 7th ed. McGraw-Hill, 2004.)

TABLE 20–7   Goiter: causes and pathogenetic mechanisms.

Causes	Pathogenetic Mechanism
I. Goiter associated with hypothyroidism or euthyroidism	
Iodine deficiency	Interferes with hormone biosynthesis
Iodine excess	Blocks hormone secretion
Goitrogen in diet or drinking water	Interferes with hormone biosynthesis
Goitrogenic medication	Interferes with hormone biosynthesis
Thioamides: propylthiouracil, methimazole, carbimazole	
Thiocyanates: nitroprusside	
Aniline derivatives: sulfonylureas, sulfonamides, aminosalicylic acid, aminoglutethimide	
Lithium	Blocks hormone secretion
Congenital disorders	Various defects in hormone biosynthesis
Defective iodide transport	
Defective iodide organification due to absence or reduction of peroxidase or production of an abnormal peroxidase	
Synthesis of an abnormal thyroglobulin	
Abnormal interrelationships of iodotyrosine	
Impaired thyroglobulin proteolysis	
Defective iodotyrosine deiodination	
Pituitary and peripheral resistance to thyroid hormone	? Receptor defects
II. Goiter associated with hyperthyroidism	
Graves disease	TSH-R [stim] Ab or TSI gland stimulation
Toxic multinodular goiter	Autonomous hyperfunction
Germ cell tumor	hCG gland stimulation
Pituitary adenoma	TSH overproduction
Thyroiditis	Enlargement due to "injury," infiltration, or edema

A goiter may also develop from the ingestion of **goitrogens** (factors that block thyroid hormone synthesis) either in food or in medication. Dietary goitrogens are found in vegetables of the Brassicaceae family (eg, rutabagas, cabbage, turnips, cassava). A goitrogenic hydrocarbon has also been found in the water supply in some locations. Medications that act as goitrogens include thioamides and thiocyanates (eg, propylthiouracil, methimazole, nitroprusside), sulfonylureas, and lithium. Lithium inhibits thyroid hormone release and perhaps also iodide organification. Most patients remain clinically euthyroid because TSH production increases.

A congenital goiter associated with hypothyroidism (**sporadic cretinism**) may occur as a result of a defect in any of the steps of thyroid hormone synthesis (see Table 20–5). All of these defects are rare.

Goiter with hyperthyroidism is usually due to Graves disease. In Graves disease, the gland is diffusely enlarged because of stimulation by TSH-R [stim] Ab (TSI) and other antibodies rather than by TSH.

Pathogenesis & Pathology

In goiter resulting from impaired thyroid hormone synthesis, there is a progressive fall in serum T_4 and a progressive rise in serum TSH. As TSH increases, iodine turnover by the gland is accelerated, and the ratio of T_3 secretion relative to T_4 secretion is increased. Consequently, the serum T_3 may be normal or increased, and the patient may remain clinically euthyroid. If there is a more marked impairment of hormone synthesis, goiter formation is associated with a low T_4, low T_3, and elevated TSH, and the patient becomes clinically hypothyroid.

In the early stages of goiter, there is diffuse enlargement of the gland, with cellular hyperplasia caused by the TSH stimulation. Later, there are enlarged follicles with flattened follicular epithelial cells and an accumulation of thyroglobulin. This accumulation occurs particularly in iodine deficiency goiter, perhaps because poorly iodinated thyroglobulin is less easily digested by proteases. As TSH stimulation continues, multiple nodules may develop in some areas and atrophy and fibrosis in others, producing a multinodular goiter (Figure 20–9).

In patients with severe iodine deficiency or inherited metabolic defects, a nontoxic goiter develops because impaired hormone secretion leads to an increase in TSH secretion. The elevation in serum TSH level results in diffuse thyroid hyperplasia. If TSH stimulation is prolonged, the diffuse hyperplasia is followed by focal hyperplasia with necrosis, hemorrhage, and nodule formation. These nodules often vary from "hot" nodules that can trap iodine and synthesize thyroglobulin to "cold" ones that cannot. In early goiters, the hyperplasia is TSH dependent, but in later stages the nodules become TSH-independent **autonomous nodules**. Thus, over a period of time, there may be a transition from a nontoxic, TSH-dependent, diffuse hyperplasia to a toxic or nontoxic, TSH-independent, multinodular goiter.

The exact mechanism underlying the transition to autonomous growth and function is unknown. However, mutations

FIGURE 20–9 Large multinodular goiter (arrow) with substernal extension producing tracheal narrowing and rightward deviation. (Reproduced, with permission, from Gardner DG et al, eds. *Greenspan's Basic and Clinical Endocrinology*, 10th ed. McGraw-Hill, 2017.)

of the *gsp* oncogene have been found in nodules from many patients with multinodular goiter. Such mutations presumably occur during TSH-induced cell division. The *gsp* oncogene is responsible for activating the regulatory GTP-binding (G$_s$) protein in the follicular cell membrane. Chronic activation of this protein and its effector, adenylyl cyclase, is postulated to result in thyroid cell proliferation, hyperfunction, and independence from TSH.

Clinical Manifestations

With decades of TSH stimulation, considerable hypertrophy and gland enlargement can occur. In one pathologic study of 200 goiters removed surgically, the mean specimen size was 10.5 ± 4.8 cm, and the mean weight was 142.9 ± 113.3 g. Very large goiters may produce respiratory difficulties secondary to obstruction of the trachea, dysphagia secondary to obstruction of the esophagus, or neck vein compression producing superior vena cava syndrome (Pemberton sign). More modest enlargements pose cosmetic problems.

Some patients with multinodular goiter also develop hyperthyroidism late in life (**Plummer disease**), particularly after the administration of iodide or iodine-containing drugs.

THYROID NODULES & NEOPLASMS

Tumors of the thyroid usually present as a solitary mass in the neck. The most common neoplasm, accounting for 30% of all solitary thyroid nodules, is the **follicular adenoma** (benign thyroid nodule). It is a solitary, firm, gray or red nodule, up to 5 cm in diameter, completely surrounded by a fibrous capsule.

The surrounding normal thyroid tissue is compressed by the adenoma. Microscopically, the adenoma consists of normal-appearing follicles of varying size, sometimes associated with hemorrhage, fibrosis, calcification, and cystic degeneration. Occasionally, only ribbons of follicular cells are present, without true follicles. Malignant change probably occurs in less than 10% of follicular adenomas. Fine-needle aspiration (FNA) biopsy of a thyroid nodule is the gold standard test to differentiate between a benign and malignant thyroid mass. Despite the high sensitivity and specificity of this test, approximately 20% of FNA biopsy specimens are reported as having an indeterminate cytology. Further evaluation using an mRNA classifier system (gene expresser classifier), mutational analysis (using a broad next-generation sequencing assay with an expanded panel of point mutations and gene fusions), or a combination of tests has been suggested. An mRNA classifier has a negative predictive value of 98%, helping patients with benign lesions avoid unnecessary surgeries. Mutational analysis, on the other hand, predicts which nodules are most likely to be malignant. These tests help the clinician decide if the patient with an indeterminate thyroid nodule cytology can be followed or needs thyroid surgery.

Thyroid cancers are not common, but the incidence of thyroid cancer is rising. Most are derived from the follicular epithelium and, depending on their microscopic appearance, are classified as **papillary** or **follicular carcinoma**. The major risk factor predisposing to epithelial thyroid carcinoma is exposure to radiation, but genetic factors have also been recognized. Most papillary and follicular cancers pursue a prolonged clinical course (15–20 years). Papillary carcinoma typically metastasizes to regional lymph nodes in the neck, whereas follicular cancer tends to spread via the bloodstream to distant sites such as bone or lung. **Medullary carcinoma** is an uncommon neoplasm of the C cells (parafollicular cells) of the thyroid that produce calcitonin (see Chapter 17). Approximately 30% of all medullary thyroid carcinomas are a manifestation of multiple endocrine neoplasia type 2 (MEN-2), inherited in an autosomal dominant fashion. Thyroid lymphoma and anaplastic thyroid cancer are extremely rare. Thyroid lymphoma is usually seen in a patient with longstanding Hashimoto thyroiditis and a sudden onset of thyroid growth. Anaplastic thyroid cancer refers to a dedifferentiated aggressive thyroid cancer, often derived from a pre-existing differentiated thyroid cancer. At the time of the diagnosis of anaplastic thyroid cancer, the prognosis remains very poor.

THYROID DISORDERS IN PREGNANCY

The diagnosis of thyroid disorders during pregnancy requires an understanding of the changes in thyroid physiology and thyroid function tests that accompany normal pregnancy. The major changes are an increase in serum thyroxine-binding globulin (TBG) and the stimulation of the thyrotropin receptor by human chorionic gonadotropin (hCG). The fetus depends on maternal thyroid hormones until the tenth week of gestation when the fetal thyroid is capable of concentrating iodine and synthesizing iodothyronines. Pregnant women can develop hyperthyroidism, hypothyroidism, thyroid nodule, goiter, and thyroid cancer. Overt hyperthyroidism and hypothyroidism during pregnancy are responsible for adverse obstetric and neonatal events and must be promptly treated. After pregnancy, postpartum thyroiditis can develop during the first 6 to 12 months after delivery in women who were euthyroid during pregnancy.

ABNORMAL THYROID FUNCTION TESTS IN CLINICALLY EUTHYROID INDIVIDUALS

Increases & Decreases in Hormone-Binding Proteins

Sustained increases or decreases in the concentration of TBG and other thyroid-binding proteins in the plasma are produced by several normal and disordered physiologic states and by medications (Table 20–8). For example, TBG levels are elevated during pregnancy and by estrogen and oral contraceptive therapy. TBG levels are depressed in nephrotic syndrome and by glucocorticoid or androgen therapy.

When a sustained increase in the concentration of TBG and other binding proteins occurs, the concentration of free thyroid hormones falls temporarily. This fall stimulates TSH secretion, which then results in an increase in the production of free hormone. Eventually, a new equilibrium is reached in which the levels of total plasma T_4 and T_3 are elevated, but the concentrations of free hormones, the rate of hormone degradation, and the rate of TSH secretion are normal. Therefore, individuals manifesting sustained increases in TBG and other binding proteins remain euthyroid. When a sustained decrease in the concentration of TBG and other binding proteins occurs, equivalent changes occur in the opposite direction, and again the individuals remain euthyroid.

Abnormal Hormone-Binding Proteins

Changes in serum concentrations of the hormone-binding proteins transthyretin or albumin alone usually do not cause significant changes in thyroid hormone levels. However, several unusual syndromes of **familial euthyroid hyperthyroxinemia** have been described. In the first, a familial syndrome called **euthyroid dysalbuminemic hyperthyroxinemia**, there is abnormal binding of T_4 (but not T_3) to albumin. In the second, there is an increased serum level of transthyretin, a tetrameric protein that transports 15–20% of circulating T_4. In the third, there are alterations in transthyretin structure produced by different point mutations that can markedly increase its affinity for T_4. In some families, these mutations in transthyretin are transmitted by autosomal dominant inheritance. In all three syndromes, total T_4 is elevated, but free T_4 is normal and patients are euthyroid. A fourth syndrome has also been described in which there is both pituitary and peripheral resistance to thyroid hormone. This condition may be due to point mutations in the human thyroid receptor (hTR-$\beta1$) gene, resulting in abnormal nuclear T_3 receptors.

Effects of Nonthyroidal Illness & Drugs

Several nonthyroidal illnesses and various drugs inhibit the 5′-deiodinase that converts T_4 to T_3, resulting in a fall in plasma T_3. Conditions or illnesses that depress 5′-deiodinase include severe burns or trauma, surgery, advanced cancer, cirrhosis, renal failure, myocardial infarction, prolonged fever, caloric deprivation (fasting, anorexia nervosa, malnutrition), and selenium deficiency. The decreased serum T_3 in nonthyroidal illnesses is thought to be an adaptive physiologic change, enabling the sick patient to conserve energy and protein. Drugs that depress 5′-deiodinase include glucocorticoids, propranolol, amiodarone, propylthiouracil, and cholecystography dyes (eg, ipodate, iopanoic acid).

Because T_3 is the major active thyroid hormone at the tissue level, it is surprising that patients with mild to moderate nonthyroidal illness exhibit normal TSH levels despite low T_3

TABLE 20–8   **Effects of normal and disordered physiologic states and medications on plasma thyroid-binding proteins and thyroid hormone levels.**

Condition	Concentrations of Binding Proteins	Total Plasma T_4, T_3, RT	Free Plasma T_4, T_3, RT	Plasma TSH
Primary hyperthyroidism	Normal	High	High	Low
Primary hypothyroidism	Normal	Low	Low	High
Drugs (estrogens, methadone, heroin, perphenazine, clofibrate), pregnancy, acute and chronic hepatitis, acute intermittent porphyria, estrogen-producing tumors, idiopathic, hereditary	High	High	Normal	Normal
Drugs (glucocorticoids, androgens, danazol, asparaginase), acromegaly, nephrotic syndrome, hypoproteinemia, chronic liver disease (cirrhosis), testosterone-producing tumors, hereditary	Low	Low	Normal	Normal

RT, reverse T_3.

Modified and reproduced, with permission, from Barrett KE et al, eds. *Ganong's Review of Medical Physiology*, 24th ed. McGraw-Hill, 2012.

levels and do not appear hypothyroid. However, such patients retain the ability to respond to a further reduction (or to an increase) in serum T_3 by increasing (or decreasing) pituitary TSH secretion. Patients with severe illnesses (eg, those undergoing bone marrow transplantation for leukemia) may manifest impaired TSH secretion.

Most patients with nonthyroidal illnesses have low serum T_3 levels related to the decreased peripheral conversion of T_4 to T_3. However, in some patients, the primary cause of the low serum T_3 is a reduced secretion of T_4 by the gland. In others, the binding of T_4 and T_3 by serum thyroid-binding proteins is impaired because of the decreased concentrations of thyroid-binding proteins (see Table 20–8) and the presence of circulating binding inhibitors.

The low T_3 state generally disappears with recovery from the illness or cessation of the drug. Among critically ill patients with low T_3 levels, clinical trials have not demonstrated a benefit from T_3 replacement. Because low T_3 levels are difficult to interpret during acute illness, the diagnostic approach should be based primarily on serum TSH levels.

Subclinical Thyroid Dysfunction

With the development of more sensitive laboratory tests of thyroid function, it is increasingly recognized that some clinically euthyroid individuals have subclinical thyroid dysfunction, defined by low or high TSH levels but normal circulating T_4 and T_3 levels. Many individuals with subclinical thyroid disease have abnormal TRH stimulation tests, but the clinical significance of these biochemical abnormalities continues to be debated. **Subclinical hypothyroidism** is defined as an elevated TSH level (above the normal reference range) but with normal circulating thyroid hormone levels. Subclinical hypothyroidism is more common among women and among individuals older than 65 years, in whom the prevalence is as high as 10–12%. Importantly, the typical symptoms and signs of overt hypothyroidism, including weight gain, fatigue, and cold intolerance, are not consistently associated with subclinical dysfunction. The underlying causes of subclinical hypothyroidism are similar to those associated with overt hypothyroidism, particularly Hashimoto thyroiditis, but a substantial proportion have no obvious etiology. In the presence of circulating thyroid (anti-TPO) autoantibodies, approximately 5% of individuals with subclinical hypothyroidism progress to overt hypothyroidism each year, compared with 2% per year or less among those without thyroid autoantibodies.

Pooled data analyses from multiple prospective studies suggest that subclinical hypothyroidism is associated with an increased risk of atherosclerotic heart disease and heart failure, particularly in individuals whose TSH levels are greater than 10 mU/L. Other studies suggest the risk of cardiovascular complications may be limited to younger individuals (those younger than 55 years). Some, but not all, studies suggest subtle neurocognitive abnormalities, particularly related to executive functions.

Unfortunately, there are no large randomized trials of subclinical hypothyroidism treatment with clinical endpoints such as heart disease or heart failure. Some individuals report improved exercise tolerance and an improved sense of well-being when given sufficient thyroxine to normalize serum TSH, but there is insufficient evidence to recommend the routine treatment of individuals with persistent subclinical hypothyroidism that does not progress to overt hypothyroidism. A large multicenter placebo-controlled trial in Europe (TRUST) has been designed to address this issue, and published results have revealed that levothyroxine provided no symptomatic benefits for elderly patients with subclinical hypothyroidism.

Subclinical hyperthyroidism is defined as a low TSH level (below the normal reference range) but with normal circulating thyroid hormone levels. Autonomous thyroid nodules or early Graves disease is believed to account for the majority of cases. The prevalence of subclinical hyperthyroidism is considerably lower than that of subclinical hypothyroidism at 1–3% but also increases with age. The classic symptoms and signs of hyperthyroidism are typically absent among individuals with subclinical hyperthyroidism. The natural history of subclinical hyperthyroidism is not well known, but one study of postmenopausal women with endogenous subclinical hyperthyroidism found that more than 50% had normal TSH levels after 1 year of follow-up.

Prospective studies have demonstrated subtle abnormalities of cardiac contractility in individuals with subclinical hyperthyroidism, and one prospective study found that individuals older than 65 years with TSH levels of less than 0.1 mU/L had a threefold greater risk of developing atrial fibrillation than those with normal TSH levels. Subclinical hyperthyroidism may also be associated with bone loss and fracture in postmenopausal women. In a prospective study of women older than 65 years, the risks of hip and spine fracture were two to three times higher among those with TSH levels of less than 0.1 mU/L (mostly from thyroid hormone over-replacement) compared with those with normal TSH levels.

CHECKPOINT

17. What is a goiter?
18. What are the causes and mechanisms of goiter formation?
19. What is the basis for the transition from nontoxic, TSH-dependent, diffuse hyperplasia to a toxic or nontoxic, TSH-independent, multinodular goiter?
20. How large can the thyroid gland become with decades of stimulation?
21. What are the different types of thyroid cancer and their characteristics?
22. What are some physiologic and pathophysiologic conditions in which thyroid metabolism is altered? How, and with what effects?
23. What is the overall thyroid status of a patient with a sustained decrease in thyroid-binding globulin?
24. What are some of the factors that depress 5'-deiodinase activity?
25. How do pregnancy and nonthyroidal illness typically affect thyroid hormone levels?

CASE STUDIES

Yeong Kwok, MD

(See Chapter 25, p. 782–84 for answers)

CASE 106

A 25-year-old woman presents with a complaint of rapid weight loss despite a voracious appetite. Physical examination reveals tachycardia (pulse rate 110 bpm at rest), fine moist skin, a symmetrically enlarged thyroid, mild bilateral quadriceps muscle weakness, and fine tremor. These findings strongly suggest hyperthyroidism.

Questions

A. What other features of the history should be elicited?
B. What other physical findings should be sought?
C. Serum TSH and free thyroxine level are ordered. What results should be anticipated?
D. What are the possible causes of this patient's condition?
E. What is the most common cause of this patient's condition, and what is the pathogenesis of this disorder?
F. What is the pathogenesis of this patient's tachycardia, weight loss, skin changes, goiter, and muscle weakness?

CASE 107

A 45-year-old woman presents complaining of fatigue, 30 pounds of weight gain despite dieting, constipation, and menorrhagia. On physical examination, the thyroid is not palpable; the skin is cool, dry, and rough; the heart sounds are quiet; and the pulse rate is 50 bpm. The rectal and pelvic examinations show no abnormalities, and the stool is negative for occult blood. The clinical findings suggest hypothyroidism.

Questions

A. What other features of the history should be elicited? What other findings should be sought on physical examination?
B. What is the pathogenesis of this patient's symptoms?
C. What laboratory tests should be ordered, and what results should be anticipated?
D. What are the possible causes of this patient's condition? Which is most likely?
E. What other conditions may be associated with this disorder?

CASE 108

A 40-year-old woman who has recently emigrated from Afghanistan comes to a practice office to establish medical care. She complains only of mild fatigue and depression. The physical examination reveals a prominent, symmetrically enlarged thyroid about twice the normal size. The remainder of the examination is unremarkable.

Questions

A. What other features of the history should be elicited?
B. What is the most likely cause of the patient's thyroid enlargement? What is the pathogenetic mechanism of goiter formation in this disease?
C. What laboratory test(s) should be ordered, and why?

CASE 109

A 47-year-old man presents complaining of nervousness, difficulty concentrating, restlessness, and insomnia. He has lost 25 pounds over the past 6 weeks and complains of heat intolerance. Physical examination reveals a 1 cm nodule in the left lobe of the thyroid gland.

Questions

A. What is the most likely explanation for the patient's condition?
B. What laboratory tests should be ordered to confirm the diagnosis? What would you expect the results to be?
C. What further evaluation of the nodule could be undertaken?
D. If a biopsy is done, what can be expected in the pathologist's report?

CASE 110

A 28-year-old woman returns for follow-up after routine laboratory tests show a markedly elevated total T_4 level. The patient is totally asymptomatic, and the physical examination is unremarkable.

Questions

A. What conditions and medications could be responsible for this presentation?
B. What further laboratory tests should be ordered?
C. If the patient is pregnant, how can the elevated total plasma T_4 level be explained?
D. If several asymptomatic family members have been told of similar laboratory test results, what is the most likely explanation of the patient's disorder?

CASE 111

A 41-year-old woman with a family history of hypothyroidism has her TSH checked during a routine physical examination. Her TSH is 7.8 mU/L (normal: ≤4.5 mU/L). She feels fine and denies any weight gain, fatigue, cold intolerance, and dry skin. Further testing reveals normal circulating T_4 and T_3 levels but positive thyroid peroxidase (anti-TPO) autoantibodies.

Questions

A. What is the patient's risk of progressing to overt hypothyroidism?
B. What are possible consequences of subclinical hypothyroidism?
C. If her laboratory test values remain stable, and she develops no new symptoms, should she be treated?

CASE 112

A 67-year-old woman brings in the results of blood tests that she obtained while applying for a life insurance policy. Her laboratory test values are normal except for a TSH of 0.1 mU/L. (normal: >0.5 mU/L). She feels fine and denies palpitations, weight loss, heat intolerance, and change in bowel movements. Further testing reveals normal circulating T_4 and T_3 levels.

Questions

A. What are some possible complications of subclinical hyperthyroidism?
B. What two conditions account for the majority of cases of subclinical hyperthyroidism?
C. Is treatment for this condition always necessary?

REFERENCES

General

Barbesino G et al. Clinical review: clinical utility of TSH receptor antibodies. J Clin Endocrinol Metab. 2013 Jun;98(6):2247–55. [PMID: 23539719]

Cooper DS et al. The thyroid gland. Chapter 7. In: Gardner DG et al, eds. *Greenspan's Basic and Clinical Endocrinology*, 10th ed. McGraw-Hill, 2017.

Grais IM et al. Thyroid and the heart. Am J Med. 2014 Aug;127(8): 691–8. [PMID: 24662620]

Ladenson PW. Precision medicine comes to thyroidology. J Clin Endocrinol Metab. 2016 Mar;101(3):799–803. [PMID: 26908108]

Leung AM et al. Iodine-induced thyroid dysfunction. Curr Opin Endocrinol Diabetes Obes. 2012 Oct;19(5):414–9. [PMID: 22820214]

Rugge JB et al. Screening and treatment of thyroid dysfunction: an evidence review for the U.S. Preventive Services Task Force. Ann Intern Med. 2015 Jan 6;162(1):35–45. [PMID: 25347444]

Taylor PN et al. Clinical review: A review of the clinical consequences of variation in thyroid function within the reference range. J Clin Endocrinol Metab. 2013 Sep;98(9):3562–71. [PMID: 23824418]

Hyperthyroidism

Bahn RS. Autoimmunity and Graves' disease. Clin Pharmacol Ther. 2012 Apr;91(4):577–9. [PMID: 22434030]

Burch HB et al. Management of Graves disease: a review. JAMA. 2015;314(23):2544–54. [PMID:26670972]

De Leo S et al. Hyperthyroidism. Lancet. 2016;388:306–18. [PMID: 27038492]

Hampton J. Thyroid gland disorder emergencies: thyroid storm and myxedema coma. AACN Adv Crit Care. 2013 Jul-Sep;24(3):325–32. [PMID: 23880755]

Khong JJ et al. Pathogenesis of thyroid eye disease: review and update on molecular mechanisms. Br J Ophthalmol. 2016 Jan;100(1): 142–50. [PMID: 26567024]

Sahli E et al. Thyroid-associated ophthalmopathy. Turk J Ophthalmol. 2017;47:94–105. [PMID: 28405484]

Smith TJ et al. Graves' disease. N Engl J Med. 2016;375:1552–65. [PMID: 27797318]

Wirth CD et al. Subclinical thyroid dysfunction and the risk for fractures: a systematic review and meta-analysis. Ann Intern Med. 2014 Aug 5;161(3):189–99. [PMID: 25089863]

Hypothyroidism

Antonelli A et al. Autoimmune thyroid disorders. Autoimmun Rev. 2015 (14):174–80. [PMID: 25461470]

Caturegli P et al. Hashimoto thyroiditis: clinical and diagnostic criteria. Autoimmun Rev. 2014 (13):391–7. [PMID 24434360]

Hampton J. Thyroid gland disorder emergencies: thyroid storm and myxedema coma. AACN Adv Crit Care. 2013 Jul-Sep;24(3):325–32. [PMID: 23880755]

Szinnai G. Clinical genetics of congenital hypothyroidism. Endocr Dev. 2014;26:60–78. [PMID: 25231445]

Zimmermann MB et al. Iodine deficiency and thyroid disorders. Lancet Diabetes Endocrinol. 2015;4:286–95. [PMID: 25591468]

Goiter

Knobel M. Epidemiology, clinical features, and treatment of diffuse and multinodular nontoxic goiters. J Endocrinol Invest. 2016;4:357–73. [PMID 26392367]

Sørensen JR et al. The impact of goitre and its treatment on the trachea, airflow, oesophagus and swallowing function. A systematic review. Best Pract Res Clin Endocrinol Metab. 2014 Aug;28(4):481–94. [PMID: 25047200]

Thyroid Nodules & Neoplasms

Bhatia P et al. Diagnostic potential of ancillary molecular testing in differentiation of benign and malignant thyroid nodules. Anticancer Res. 2015 Mar;35(3):1237–41. [PMID: 25750270]

Ferris RL et al. American Thyroid Association statement on surgical application of molecular profiling of thyroid nodules: current impact on perioperative decision making. Thyroid. 2015 Jul;25(7):760–8. [PMID: 26058403]

Krátký J et al. Thyroid nodules: pathophysiological insight on oncogenesis and novel diagnostic techniques. Physiol Res. 2014;63(Suppl 2):S263–75. [PMID: 24908232]

Kuo LE et al. Management of thyroid nodular disease: current cytopathology classifications and genetic testing. Surg Oncol Clin N Am. 2016 Jan;25(1):1–16. [PubMed PMID: 26610771

Niedziela M. Thyroid nodules. Best Pract Res Clin Endocrinol Metab. 2014 Mar;28(2):245–77. [PMID: 24629865]

Trimboli P et al. *BRAF*-mutated carcinomas among thyroid nodules with prior indeterminate FNA report: a systematic review and meta-analysis. Clin Endocrinol (Oxf). 2016 Mar;84(3):315–20. [PMID: 25920006]

Tuluc M et al. Thyroid cytology. Otolaryngol Clin North Am. 2014 Aug;47(4):475–89. [PMID: 25041952]

Yip L. Molecular markers for thyroid cancer diagnosis, prognosis, and targeted therapy. J Surg Oncol. 2015 Jan;111(1):43–50. [PMID: 25155423]

Zhang M et al. Molecular testing of thyroid nodules: a review of current available tests for fine-needle aspiration specimens. Arch Pathol Lab Med. 2016 Dec;140(12):1338–44. [PMID: 27557410]

Thyroid Disorders in Pregnancy

Carney LA et al. Thyroid disease in pregnancy. Am Fam Physician. 2014 Feb 15;89(4):273–8. Erratum in: Am Fam Physician. 2014 Jul 1;90(1):8. [PMID: 24695447]

Casey BM et al. Treatment of subclinical hypothyroidism or hypothyroxinemia in pregnancy. N Engl J Med. 2017;376 (9):815–25. [PMID: 28249134]

Negro R et al. Diagnosis and management of subclinical hypothyroidism in pregnancy. BMJ. 2014 Oct 6;349:g4929. [PMID: 25288580]

Pearce EN. Thyroid disorders during pregnancy and postpartum. Best Pract Res Clin Obstet Gynaecol. 2015 Jul;29(5):700–6. [PMID: 26028555]

Tong Z et al. The effect of subclinical maternal thyroid dysfunction and autoimmunity on intrauterine growth restriction: a systematic review and meta-analysis. Medicine (Baltimore). 2016 May;95(19):e3677. [PMID: 27175703]

Yalamanchi S et al. Thyroid disorders in pregnancy. Curr Opinion Obstet Gynecol. 2015 Dec;27(6):406–15. [PMID: 26485458]

Abnormal Thyroid Function Tests in Clinically Euthyroid Individuals, Subclinical Hypothyroidism & Subclinical Hyperthyroidism

Carlé A et al. Management of endocrine disease: subclinical thyrotoxicosis: prevalence, causes and choice of therapy. Eur J Endocrinol. 2017 Jun;176(6):R325–37. [PMID: 28274949]

Carpi A et al. Subclinical hyperthyroidism and cardiovascular manifestations: a reevaluation of the association. Intern Emerg Med. 2013 Apr;8(Suppl 1):S75–7. [PMID: 2346289]

Guo QH et al. Thyroid hormone resistance syndrome caused by heterozygous A317T mutation in thyroid hormone receptor β gene: report of one Chinese pedigree and review of the literature. Medicine (Baltimore). 2016 Aug;95(33):e4415. [PMID: 27537566]

Onigata K et al. Resistance to thyroid hormone. Endocr Dev. 2014;26:118–29. [PMID: 25231448]

Ortiga-Carvalho TM et al. Thyroid hormone receptors and resistance to thyroid hormone disorders. Nat Rev Endocrinol. 2014 Oct;10(10):582–91. [PMID: 25135573]

Palmeiro C et al. Subclinical hyperthyroidism and cardiovascular risk: recommendations for treatment. Cardiol Rev. 2013 Nov-Dec;21(6):300–8. [PMID: 23563523]

Stott DJ et al. Thyroid hormone therapy for older adults with subclinical hypothyroidism. N Engl J Med. 2017 Jun 29;376(26):2534–44. [PMID: 28402245]

Disorders of the Adrenal Cortex

Tobias Else, MD, & Gary D. Hammer, MD, PhD

The adrenal gland is actually two endocrine organs, one wrapped around the other. The outer **adrenal cortex** secretes many different steroid hormones, including glucocorticoids such as cortisol, mineralocorticoids such as aldosterone, and steroids related to androgens, chiefly dehydroepiandrosterone (DHEA) and DHEA sulfate (DHEAS). The glucocorticoids help regulate carbohydrate, protein, and fat metabolism. The mineralocorticoids help to regulate Na^+ and K^+ balance and extracellular fluid volume. The glucocorticoids and mineralocorticoids are essential for survival, but no essential role has been determined for adrenal androgens. The inner **adrenal medulla**, discussed in Chapter 12, secretes catecholamines (epinephrine, norepinephrine, and dopamine).

Mainly because of their potent immunosuppressive and anti-inflammatory effects, glucocorticoids are commonly used in pharmacologic doses to treat diseases such as auto-immune disorders. Interestingly, although the deleterious effects of glucocorticoids in states of hypercortisolism and the beneficial effects of their use in pharmacotherapy are well understood, the actual role of endogenous glucocorticoids in metabolic homeostasis during times of minimal stress remains somewhat enigmatic.

The major disorders of the adrenal cortex (Table 21–1) are characterized by an excessive or deficient secretion of each type of adrenocortical hormone: **hypercortisolism (Cushing syndrome), adrenal insufficiency (Addison disease), hyperaldosteronism (aldosteronism), hypoaldosteronism,** and **androgen excess**.

NORMAL STRUCTURE & FUNCTION OF THE ADRENAL CORTEX

ANATOMY

The adrenal glands are paired organs located in the retroperitoneal area near the superior poles of the kidneys (Figure 21–1). They are flattened, crescent-shaped structures, which together normally weigh about 8–10 g. Each is covered by a tight fibrous capsule and surrounded by fat. The blood flow to the adrenals is copious.

Grossly, each gland consists of two concentric layers: The yellow peripheral layer is the **adrenal cortex**, and the reddish-brown central layer is the **adrenal medulla**. Adrenal cortical tissue is sometimes found at other sites, usually near the kidney or along the path taken by the gonads during their embryonic descent (see Figure 21–1).

HISTOLOGY

The adrenal cortex can be subdivided into three concentric layers: the zona glomerulosa, zona fasciculata, and zona reticularis (Figure 21–2). The **zona glomerulosa** is the outermost layer, situated immediately beneath the capsule. Zona glomerulosa cells are arranged in closely packed, rounded, or arched clusters surrounded by capillaries. They secrete **mineralocorticoids**, primarily **aldosterone**. The **zona fasciculata** is the middle layer of the cortex. Zona fasciculata cells are polyhedral in shape and arranged in straight cords or columns, one or two cells thick, running at right angles to the capsule with capillaries between them. The **zona reticularis**, the innermost layer of the cortex, lies between the zona fasciculata and the

TABLE 21–1   Principal diseases of the adrenal glands.

Cortex Hyperfunction
Bilateral hyperplasia
ACTH excess (mainly affects zona fasciculata and zona reticularis)
Enzyme deficiencies (with ACTH excess) (with androgen excess and cortisol deficiency)
ACTH-independent macronodular hyperplasia (eg, ectopic receptor expression)
Adenoma
Primary aldosteronism
Hypercortisolism (Cushing syndrome)
Hyperandrogenism (virilization) (rare)
Carcinoma
Cushing syndrome
Virilization
Feminization (rare)
Cortex Hypofunction
Bilateral adrenal gland destruction (Addison disease)
Congenital adrenal hyperplasia (eg, 21-hydroxylase deficiency)
Autoimmune
Infection
Ischemia, shock
Hemorrhage, anticoagulation
Metastatic cancer
Hemochromatosis
Congenital (eg, cytomegalic adrenocortical hypoplasia, *DAX1* mutation)
Medulla Hyperfunction
Pheochromocytoma
Hyperplasia (rare)
Other: ganglioneuroma, neuroblastoma
Medulla Hypofunction

adrenal medulla, accounting for only 7% of the mass of the adrenal gland. Zona reticularis cells are smaller than the other two types and are arranged in irregular cords interlaced in a network. Zona fasciculata cells secrete **glucocorticoids**, primarily **cortisol**, and zona reticularis cells secrete steroid hormones related to **androgens** such as **dehydroepiandrosterone (DHEA)**. These steroid hormones are low-molecular-weight lipid-soluble molecules, derived from cholesterol, and are able to diffuse freely across cell membranes.

FIGURE 21–1   Human adrenal glands. Note the location of the adrenal at the superior pole of each kidney. Adrenocortical tissue is stippled; adrenal medullary tissue is gray. Also shown (turquoise) are extra-adrenal sites at which cortical and medullary tissues are sometimes found. (Redrawn, with permission, from Forsham PH. The adrenal cortex. In: Williams RH, ed. *Textbook of Endocrinology*, 4th ed. Saunders, 1968. Copyright © Elsevier.)

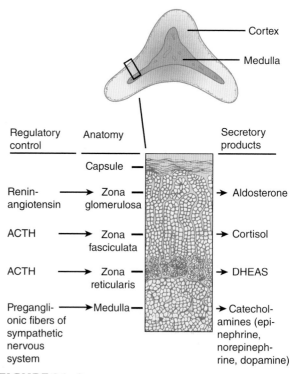

FIGURE 21–2   Anatomy, regulatory control, and secretory products of the adrenal gland. (Redrawn and modified, with permission, from Chandrasoma P et al, eds. *Concise Pathology*, 3rd ed. Originally published by Appleton & Lange. Copyright © 1998 by The McGraw-Hill Companies, Inc.)

PHYSIOLOGY OF THE NORMAL ADRENAL CORTEX

1. Glucocorticoids

Glucocorticoid Synthesis, Protein Binding & Metabolism

Cortisol and corticosterone are referred to as glucocorticoids because they increase hepatic glucose output by stimulating the catabolism of peripheral fat and protein to provide substrate for hepatic gluconeogenesis. The glucocorticoids help regulate the metabolism of carbohydrates, proteins, and fat. They act on virtually all cells of the body.

A. Synthesis and Binding to Plasma Proteins—The major glucocorticoid secreted by the adrenal cortex is cortisol. Figure 21–3 illustrates the biosynthetic pathways for this hormone.

FIGURE 21–3 A: Simplified pathways of steroid synthesis in the different zones of the adrenal cortex. Note the differences in the types of enzyme necessary and the different order of enzymatic reactions in the different zones. **B:** Enzymes involved in steroid synthesis. Four of the five enzymes involved are cytochrome P450s, which are commonly known by their cytochrome (CYP) numbers, as shown.

Cortisol is secreted in an unbound state but circulates bound to plasma proteins. It binds mainly to **corticosteroid-binding globulin (CBG)** (or **transcortin**) and to a lesser extent to albumin. Protein binding serves mainly to distribute and deliver the hormone to target tissues, but it also delays its metabolic clearance and prevents marked fluctuations in the cortisol level during episodic secretion by the gland.

B. Corticosteroid-Binding Globulin

CBG (molecular weight ~50,000 Da) is an α-globulin synthesized in the liver. Its production is increased by pregnancy, estrogen or oral contraceptive therapy, hyperthyroidism, diabetes mellitus, certain hematologic disorders, and familial CBG excess. When the CBG level rises, more cortisol is bound, and the free cortisol level falls temporarily. This fall stimulates pituitary adrenocorticotropic hormone (ACTH) secretion and more adrenal cortisol production. Eventually, the free cortisol level and the ACTH secretion return to normal but with an elevated level of protein-bound cortisol, and therefore increased total cortisol. Similarly, when the CBG level falls, the free cortisol level rises. CBG production is decreased in cirrhosis, nephrotic syndrome, hypothyroidism, multiple myeloma, and familial CBG deficiency.

C. Free and Bound Glucocorticoid

Normally, about 96% of the circulating cortisol is bound to CBG, and 4% is free (unbound). The bound hormone is inactive. The free hormone is physiologically active. The normal morning total plasma cortisol level is 5–20 μg/dL (140–550 nmol/L). Because cortisol is protein bound to a greater degree than corticosterone, its half-life in the circulation is longer (~60–90 minutes) than that of corticosterone (~50 minutes).

D. Metabolism

Glucocorticoids are metabolized in the liver and conjugated to glucuronide or sulfate groups. The inactive conjugated metabolites are excreted in the urine and stool. Cortisol metabolism is decreased in infancy, old age, pregnancy, chronic liver disease, hypothyroidism, anorexia nervosa, surgery, starvation, and other instances of major physiologic stress. Cortisol catabolism is increased in thyrotoxicosis. Because of its avid protein binding and extensive metabolism before excretion, less than 1% of secreted cortisol appears in the urine as free cortisol.

Regulation of Secretion

A. Adrenocorticotropic Hormone and Corticotropin-Releasing Hormone

Glucocorticoid secretion is regulated primarily by ACTH, a 39-amino-acid polypeptide secreted by the anterior pituitary. Its half-life in the circulation is very short (~10 minutes). The site of its catabolism is unknown. ACTH regulates both the basal secretion of glucocorticoids and their increased secretion provoked by stress.

ACTH, in turn, is regulated by hypothalamic corticotropin-releasing hormone (CRH), a 41-amino-acid polypeptide secreted into the median eminence of the hypothalamus. CRH

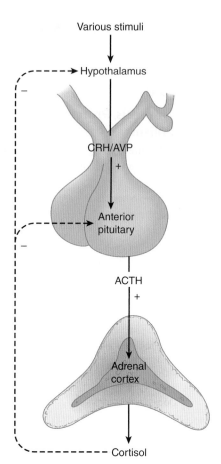

FIGURE 21–4 Feedback mechanism of ACTH-glucocorticoid secretion. Solid arrows indicate stimulation; dashed arrows, inhibition. (Redrawn, with permission, from Junqueira LC et al, eds. *Basic Histology*, 10th ed. McGraw-Hill, 2003.)

secretion by the hypothalamus is regulated by a variety of neurotransmitters (Figure 21–4) in response to physical and emotional stressors. The hypothalamus is subject to regulatory influences from other parts of the brain, including the limbic system. CRH is transported in the portal-hypophysial vessels to the anterior pituitary (see Chapter 19). There, CRH causes a prompt increase in ACTH secretion. This, in turn, leads to a transient increase in cortisol secretion by the adrenal. Arginine-vasopressin (AVP) is an additional hypothalamic peptide that regulates ACTH release.

The control of ACTH and CRH/AVP secretion involves three components: the episodic secretion and diurnal rhythm of ACTH, stress responses of the hypothalamic–pituitary–adrenal axis, and negative feedback inhibition of ACTH secretion by cortisol (see Figure 21–4).

B. Episodic and Diurnal Rhythm of ACTH Secretion

ACTH is secreted in episodic bursts throughout the day, following a diurnal (circadian) rhythm, with bursts most frequent in the early morning and least frequent in the evening (Figure 21–5). The peak level of cortisol in the plasma normally occurs between 6:00 and 8:00 AM (during sleep, just before awakening) and the nadir at around 12:00 AM.

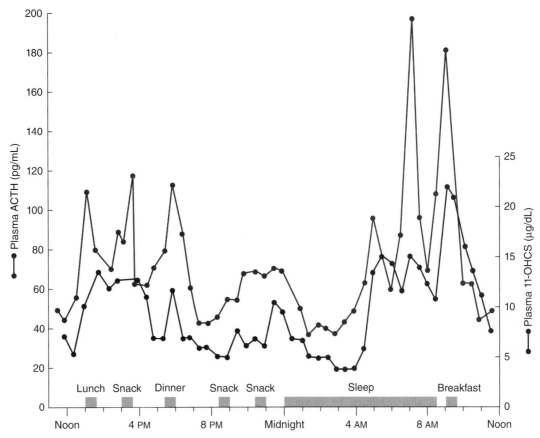

FIGURE 21–5 Fluctuations in plasma ACTH and glucocorticoids (11-OHCS) throughout the day. Note the greater ACTH and glucocorticoid rises in the morning before awakening. (Redrawn, with permission, from Krieger DT et al. Characterization of the normal temporal pattern of plasma corticosteroid levels. J Clin Endocrinol Metab. 1971;32:266. By permission of Oxford University Press on behalf of the Endocrine Society.)

The diurnal rhythm of ACTH secretion persists in patients with adrenal insufficiency who are receiving maintenance doses of glucocorticoids but is lost in Cushing syndrome. The diurnal rhythm is altered also by changes in patterns of sleep (eg, shift work), light–dark exposure, or food intake; physical stress such as major illness, surgery, trauma, or starvation; psychologic stress, including severe anxiety, depression, and mania; central nervous system (CNS) and pituitary disorders; liver disease and other conditions that affect cortisol metabolism; chronic kidney disease; alcoholism; and antiserotonergic drugs such as cyproheptadine.

Normally, the morning plasma ACTH concentration is about 25 pg/mL (5.5 pmol/L). Figure 21–6 shows plasma ACTH and cortisol values in various normal and abnormal states.

C. Stress Response—Plasma ACTH and cortisol secretion are also triggered by various forms of stress. Emotional stress (eg, fear, anxiety) and bodily injury (eg, surgery, hypoglycemia) release CRH from the hypothalamus. Similarly, vasopressin is released in response to volume depletion. ACTH secretion induced by these hormones, in turn, stimulates a transient increase in cortisol secretion (Figure 21–7). If the stress is prolonged, it may abolish the normal diurnal rhythm of ACTH and cortisol secretion.

D. Negative Feedback—A rising level of plasma cortisol inhibits the release of ACTH from the pituitary by both inhibiting CRH release from the hypothalamus and interfering with the stimulatory action of CRH on the pituitary (see Figure 21–4). The fall in plasma ACTH leads to a decline in the

FIGURE 21–6 Plasma concentrations of ACTH and cortisol in various clinical states. (Redrawn, with permission, from Liddle G. The adrenal cortex. In: Williams RH, ed. *Textbook of Endocrinology*, 5th ed. Saunders, 1974.)

FIGURE 21–7 Plasma cortisol responses to major surgery (continuous line) and minor surgery (broken line) in normal subjects. Mean values and standard errors for 20 patients are shown in each case. (Redrawn, with permission, from Plumpton FS et al. Anaesthesia. 1969;24:3. Copyright © 2007 John Wiley and Sons.)

adrenal secretion of cortisol. Conversely, the loss of negative feedback resulting from a drop in plasma cortisol induces a net increase in ACTH secretion. In untreated chronic adrenal insufficiency, there is a marked increase in the rate of ACTH synthesis and secretion.

ACTH and CRH secretion is also inhibited by chronic pharmacologic treatment with exogenous corticosteroids in proportion to their glucocorticoid potency. When prolonged corticosteroid treatment is stopped, the adrenal is atrophic and unresponsive, and the patient is at risk for acute adrenal insufficiency. The chronic suppression of the HPA axis by exogenous glucocorticoids also impacts on hypothalamic CRH and pituitary ACTH secretion, and it may take some time to recover after stopping glucocorticoid treatment. The time it takes to recover the full physiological function of the HPA axis depends on the duration and dose of glucocorticoid treatment. Moreover, there are significant inter-individual differences in these parameters. While there are no useful predictors to facilitate determining which patients are at risk for prolonged adrenal insufficiency, there is some evidence that alternate-day glucocorticoid treatment tends to preserve some adrenal function. Another well-accepted method of preventing adrenal insufficiency following glucocorticoid therapy is to slowly taper the dosage of exogenous glucocorticoids. Tapering exogenous glucocorticoid has a dual function. A short-term taper (days to a few weeks) of pharmacologic doses of glucocorticoids prevents a rebound flare of the underlying treated disease (eg, autoimmune disorder). A slow taper of exogenous glucocorticoid from physiologic replacement doses to complete discontinuation serves the purpose of allowing the endogenous HPA axis to recover. Such tapering only supports the recovery of HPA-axis function if it is done slowly (weeks to months) with doses below the daily physiologic glucocorticoid equivalent (eg, 5.0–7.5 mg of prednisone or 15–25 mg of hydrocortisone).

E. Effects of ACTH on the Adrenal—Circulating ACTH binds to high-affinity receptors (ACTH receptor or melanocortin (MC) 2 receptor) on adrenocortical cell membranes, activating adenylyl cyclase and increasing intracellular cyclic adenosine monophosphate (cAMP). There is a dual response to ACTH stimulation: (1) the immediate production and release of cortisol; and (2) the induction of steroidogenic enzyme synthesis.

The prolonged hypersecretion or administration of ACTH initially causes hypertrophy, followed by hyperplasia of the zona fasciculata and zona reticularis. Growth factors such as additional proopiomelanocortin (POMC) peptides and insulin-like growth factors play important roles in this process. Conversely, prolonged ACTH deficiency results in adrenocortical atrophy.

Mechanism of Action

The physiologic effects of glucocorticoids in various tissues are the result of their binding to the ubiquitous cytosolic glucocorticoid receptors (GRs) (Figure 21–8). The hormone–GR complexes then enter the nucleus and can act by two main mechanisms: (1) **transactivation**, in which the GRs bind to nuclear DNA and promote DNA transcription, mRNA production, and hence protein synthesis; or (2) **transrepression**, in which gene transcription is inhibited through interference with other transcription factors.

Effects

Table 21–2 summarizes the effects of glucocorticoids on target tissues. Under physiologic circumstances, the effects of glucocorticoid are not very well understood but appear to be mainly permissive. The effects of glucocorticoids secreted at supraphysiologic levels, however, are well described. In most tissues, glucocorticoids have a catabolic effect, promoting the degradation of protein and fat to provide substrate for intermediary metabolism. In the liver, however, glucocorticoids have a synthetic effect, promoting the uptake and use of carbohydrates (in glucose and glycogen synthesis), amino acids (in RNA and protein enzyme synthesis), and fatty acids (as an energy source).

During fasting, glucocorticoids help maintain plasma glucose levels by several mechanisms (see Table 21–2). In peripheral tissues, glucocorticoids antagonize the effects of insulin. Glucocorticoids inhibit glucose uptake in muscle and adipose tissue. The brain and heart are spared from this antagonism, and the extra supply of glucose helps these vital organs cope with stress. In diabetics, the insulin antagonism may worsen the control of blood sugar levels, raise plasma lipid levels, and increase the formation of ketone bodies. However, in nondiabetics, the rise in blood glucose levels stimulates a compensatory increase in insulin secretion that prevents these sequelae.

Small amounts of glucocorticoids must be present for other metabolic processes to occur (**permissive action**). For example, glucocorticoids must be present for catecholamines to produce their calorigenic, lipolytic, pressor, and bronchodilator effects, and for glucagon to increase hepatic gluconeogenesis.

Glucocorticoids are also required to resist various stresses. Indeed, the increased secretion of pituitary ACTH and

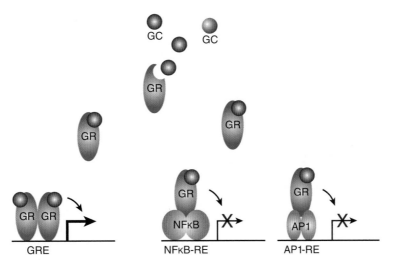

FIGURE 21–8 Mechanism of glucocorticoid action. Glucocorticoid (GC) hormone binds to the cytosolic intracellular glucocorticoid receptor (GR), which dimerizes and then translocates to the nucleus and increases the transcription of glucocorticoid-responsive target genes (eg, PEPCK, transactivation) or inhibits gene transcription (eg, collagenase, interleukin-2, transrepression) by interference with other transcription factors (eg, nuclear factor kappa-B [NFκB] or activator protein 1 [AP1]). (Arrows depict gene transcription; crossed-out arrows depict inhibited gene transcription.) (RE, response element.)

TABLE 21–2   **Effects of glucocorticoids.**

Target Tissue	Effect	Mechanism
Muscle	Catabolic	Inhibit glucose uptake and metabolism
		Decrease protein synthesis
		Increase release of amino acids, lactate
Fat	Lipolytic	Stimulate lipolysis
		Increase release of FFAs and glycerol
Liver	Synthetic	Increase gluconeogenesis
		Increase glycogen synthesis and storage
		Increase glucose-6-phosphatase activity
		Increase blood glucose
Immune system	Suppression	Reduce number of circulating lymphocytes, monocytes, eosinophils, basophils
		Inhibit T-lymphocyte production of interleukin-2
		Interfere with antigen processing, antibody production and clearance
	Anti-inflammatory	Decrease migration of neutrophils, monocytes, lymphocytes to sites of injury
	Other	Stimulate release of neutrophils from marrow
		Interfere with neutrophil migration out of vascular compartment (produces a relative neutrophilia during glucocorticoid therapy)
Cardiovascular	Increase cardiac output	
	Increase peripheral vascular tone	
Renal	Increase glomerular filtration rate	
	Aid in regulating water, electrolyte balance	

consequent increase in circulating glucocorticoids after injury are essential to survival. Hypophysectomized or adrenalectomized individuals treated with only maintenance doses of glucocorticoids may die when exposed to such stress. Hence, steroid replacement doses need to be increased in times of stress. This underscores the crucial role of glucocorticoids as stress hormones.

CHECKPOINT

1. What are the histologic layers of the adrenal cortex, and what steroids does each secrete?
2. What three roles are proposed for steroid-binding proteins?
3. In what conditions is corticosteroid-binding globulin increased? Decreased?
4. In what conditions is cortisol metabolism increased? Decreased?
5. Describe the diurnal rhythm of ACTH secretion, and name the conditions in which it is altered.
6. What stress responses trigger ACTH secretion?
7. Describe the negative feedback control of the hypothalamic–pituitary–adrenal axis.
8. Describe the major physiologic effects of glucocorticoids.

2. Mineralocorticoids

Synthesis, Protein Binding & Metabolism

The primary function of mineralocorticoids is to induce the retention of Na^+ in order to maintain a normal intravascular volume. However, other factors affect Na^+ excretion besides the mineralocorticoids, such as the glomerular filtration rate, atrial natriuretic peptide, the presence of an osmotic diuretic, and changes in the tubular reabsorption of Na^+ that are not regulated by mineralocorticoid.

A. Synthesis—Aldosterone is the principal mineralocorticoid secreted by the adrenal. Deoxycorticosterone also has minor mineralocorticoid activity.

B. Protein Binding—Aldosterone is bound to plasma proteins (albumin and corticosteroid-binding globulin) to a lesser extent than glucocorticoids. The amount of aldosterone secreted under normal circumstances is small (~0.15 mg/24 h). The normal average plasma concentration of (free and bound) aldosterone is 0.006 µg/dL (0.17 nmol/L). Free (unbound) aldosterone makes up 30–40% of the total.

C. Metabolism—The half-life of aldosterone is short (~20–30 minutes). Aldosterone is catabolized principally in the liver, and its metabolites are excreted in the urine. Less than 1% of secreted aldosterone is excreted in urine in the free form.

Regulation

Aldosterone secretion is regulated primarily by the renin–angiotensin system but also by pituitary ACTH and by the plasma electrolyte, K^+.

A. Regulation by the Renin–Angiotensin System—The **renin–angiotensin system** regulates aldosterone secretion in a feedback fashion (Figure 21–9). **Renin** is a proteolytic enzyme produced from a larger protein, **prorenin**. Renin is excreted by the juxtaglomerular cells of the kidney in response to decreases in renal perfusion pressure and reflex increases in renal nerve discharge. Once in the circulation, renin acts on **angiotensinogen** to form **angiotensin I**, a decapeptide. In the lung and elsewhere, angiotensin I is converted by **angiotensin-converting enzyme** (**ACE**) to **angiotensin II**, an octapeptide. Angiotensin II binds to zona glomerulosa cell membrane receptors and stimulates the synthesis and secretion of aldosterone. Aldosterone promotes Na^+ and therefore water retention, causing plasma volume expansion, which

FIGURE 21–9 Feedback mechanism regulating aldosterone secretion. The dashed arrow indicates inhibition. (Redrawn, with permission, from Ganong WF. *Review of Medical Physiology*, 22nd ed. McGraw-Hill, 2005.)

then shuts off renin secretion. In the supine state, there is a diurnal rhythm of aldosterone and renin secretion; the highest values are in the early morning before awakening.

The physiologic stimuli for the renin–angiotensin system to increase aldosterone secretion include factors that reduce renal perfusion, such as extracellular fluid volume depletion, dietary Na$^+$ restriction, and decreases in intra-arterial vascular pressure (eg, resulting from hemorrhage or upright posture). Other disease states that cause reduced renal perfusion include renal artery stenosis, salt-losing disorders, heart failure, and hypoproteinemic states (cirrhosis of the liver, nephrotic syndrome). These disorders increase renin secretion, producing **secondary hyperaldosteronism**.

B. Regulation by ACTH—ACTH also stimulates mineralocorticoid output. More ACTH is needed to stimulate mineralocorticoid than glucocorticoid secretion, but the amount required is still within the range of normal ACTH secretion. The effect of ACTH on aldosterone secretion is transient, however. Even if ACTH secretion remains elevated, aldosterone production declines to normal within 48 hours, perhaps because renin secretion decreases in response to hypervolemia.

C. Regulation by Plasma Electrolytes—An increase in plasma K$^+$ concentration—or a fall in plasma Na$^+$—stimulates aldosterone release. Although minor changes of plasma K$^+$ (≤1 mEq/L) have an effect, major changes in plasma Na$^+$ (drops of about 20 mEq/L) are needed to stimulate aldosterone secretion. Na$^+$ depletion increases the affinity and number of angiotensin II receptors on adrenocortical cells.

Mechanism of Action

Aldosterone, like other steroid hormones, acts by binding to a mineralocorticoid receptor (MR) in the cytosol. The expression of the MR is restricted to a small number of tissues, including the kidney. Interestingly, glucocorticoids also have a high affinity to the MR, but usually do not exert mineralocorticoid effects because mineralocorticoid-sensitive tissues express the enzyme 11-hydroxysteroid dehydrogenase type 2, which metabolizes and inactivates cortisol to the inactive metabolite, cortisone, before it can bind to the MR. The aldosterone–MR complex moves into the nucleus of the target cell and increases DNA transcription, mRNA induction, and protein synthesis stimulation by ribosomes. The aldosterone-stimulated proteins have two effects: a rapid effect to increase the activity of epithelial sodium channels (ENaCs) by increasing the insertion of ENaCs into the cell membrane from a cytosolic pool, and a slower effect to increase the synthesis of ENaCs. One of the genes activated by aldosterone is the gene for serum- and glucocorticoid-regulated kinase (sgk), a serine–threonine protein kinase. The *sgk* gene product increases ENaC activity (Figure 21–10). Aldosterone also increases the mRNAs for the three subunits that make up the ENaCs.

The fact that the principal effect of aldosterone on Na$^+$ transport takes 10–30 minutes to develop and even longer to

FIGURE 21–10 Mechanism of action of aldosterone in an epithelial cell of the renal tubule's collecting duct. In the kidney, aldosterone acts primarily on the principal cell of the collecting ducts. Under the influence of aldosterone, increased amounts of Na$^+$ are exchanged for K$^+$ and H$^+$ in the renal tubules, producing a K$^+$ diuresis and an increase in urine acidity. Na$^+$ enters via the epithelial sodium channels (ENaCs) in the apical membrane and is pumped into the interstitial fluid by Na$^+$-K$^+$ ATPases in the basolateral membrane. Aldosterone activates the genome to produce sgk and other proteins, and the number of active ENaCs is increased. (Redrawn and modified, with permission, from Ganong WF. *Review of Medical Physiology*, 22nd ed. McGraw-Hill, 2005.)

peak indicates that it depends on the synthesis of new proteins by the genomic mechanism.

Effects

The target organs for the mineralocorticoids include the kidney, colon, duodenum, salivary glands, and sweat glands. In the distal renal tubules and collecting ducts, aldosterone acts to promote the exchange of Na$^+$ for K$^+$ and H$^+$, causing Na$^+$ retention, K$^+$ diuresis, and increased urine acidity. Elsewhere, it acts to increase the reabsorption of Na$^+$ from the colonic fluid, saliva, and sweat. The mineralocorticoids may also increase K$^+$ and decrease Na$^+$ concentrations in muscle and brain cells. The action of aldosterone on epithelial cells of the choroid plexus alters the composition of cerebrospinal fluid in a fashion thought to contribute to blood-pressure regulation. In the heart, aldosterone has been shown to induce heart remodeling and interstitial and perivascular fibrosis of the myocardium.

CHECKPOINT

9. How is aldosterone secretion regulated?
10. How does the effect of ACTH on aldosterone secretion differ from its effect on glucocorticoid secretion?
11. What are the overall effects of aldosterone?

PATHOPHYSIOLOGY OF SELECTED ADRENOCORTICAL DISORDERS

Characteristic syndromes are produced by the excessive or deficient secretion of each type of adrenal hormone. Excessive glucocorticoid secretion (**Cushing syndrome**) results in a moon-faced, plethoric appearance, with truncal obesity, purple abdominal striae, hypertension, osteoporosis, mental aberrations, protein depletion, and glucose intolerance or frank diabetes mellitus.

Excessive mineralocorticoid secretion in **hyperaldosteronism** leads to excessive Na^+ retention, usually without edema, and K^+ depletion, resulting in hypertension, muscle weakness, polyuria, hypokalemia, metabolic alkalosis, and sometimes hypocalcemia and tetany.

Excessive androgen secretion causes virilization or hirsutism and precocious pseudopuberty or a disorder of sexual development (46,XX disorder of sexual development [DSD], formerly known as female pseudohermaphroditism).

Deficient glucocorticoid secretion resulting from autoimmune or other destruction of the adrenal glands (**Addison disease**) causes symptoms of weakness, fatigue, malaise, anorexia, nausea and vomiting, weight loss, hypotension, hypoglycemia, and marked intolerance of physiologic stress (eg, infection).

In this setting, ACTH levels become elevated due to the loss of negative feedback. Co-secreted with ACTH, the POMC peptide melanocyte-stimulating hormone (MSH) may produce hyperpigmentation.

The associated mineralocorticoid deficiency leads to renal Na^+ wasting and K^+ retention and can produce manifestations of severe dehydration, hypotension, decreased cardiac size, hyponatremia, hyperkalemia, and metabolic acidosis. Deficient mineralocorticoid secretion also occurs in patients with renal disease and low circulating renin levels (**hyporeninemic hypoaldosteronism**).

CUSHING SYNDROME

Cushing syndrome is the clinical condition resulting from chronic exposure to excessive circulating levels of glucocorticoids (Figure 21–11). It is also called **hypercortisolism**. The most common cause of the syndrome is an excess secretion of ACTH from the anterior pituitary gland (**Cushing disease**).

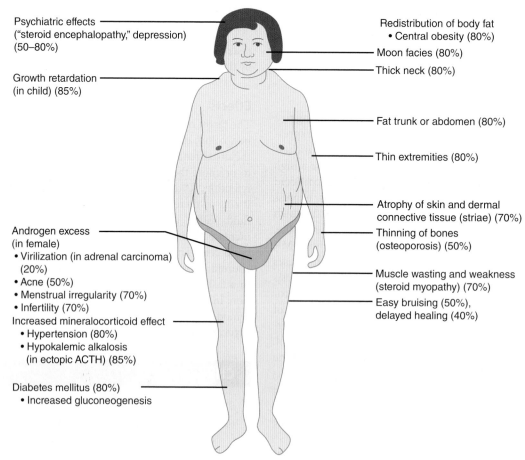

Psychiatric effects
("steroid encephalopathy," depression)
(50–80%)

Growth retardation
(in child) (85%)

Androgen excess
(in female)
• Virilization (in adrenal carcinoma)
(20%)
• Acne (50%)
• Menstrual irregularity (70%)
• Infertility (70%)
Increased mineralocorticoid effect
• Hypertension (80%)
• Hypokalemic alkalosis
(in ectopic ACTH) (85%)

Diabetes mellitus (80%)
• Increased gluconeogenesis

Redistribution of body fat
• Central obesity (80%)
Moon facies (80%)
Thick neck (80%)

Fat trunk or abdomen (80%)

Thin extremities (80%)

Atrophy of skin and dermal
connective tissue (striae) (70%)
Thinning of bones
(osteoporosis) (50%)

Muscle wasting and weakness
(steroid myopathy) (70%)
Easy bruising (50%),
delayed healing (40%)

FIGURE 21–11 Typical findings in Cushing syndrome.

Etiology

Cushing syndrome may occur either spontaneously or as the result of chronic glucocorticoid administration (iatrogenic Cushing syndrome). The overall incidence of spontaneous Cushing syndrome is approximately two to four cases per million population per year. It is nine times more common in women than in men. Table 21–3 summarizes the major causes of Cushing syndrome.

A. Hypothalamic CRH Hypersecretion

In rare cases of Cushing syndrome, a **diffuse hyperplasia of pituitary corticotroph cells** is responsible for ACTH hypersecretion. The hyperplasia is probably due to the hypersecretion of CRH by the hypothalamus or nonhypothalamic tumors that secret ectopic CRH. Chronic CRH hypersecretion does not cause pituitary adenomas.

B. Pituitary Cushing Disease

Cushing disease is the most common cause of noniatrogenic hypercortisolism. It is eight times more prevalent in women than in men. Patients with Cushing disease have a pituitary adenoma causing excessive ACTH secretion (Figure 21–12). Such adenomas are located in the anterior pituitary, are usually less than 10 mm in diameter (**microadenomas**), and are composed of basophilic corticotroph cells containing ACTH in secretory granules. **Macroadenomas** are less common and carcinomas extremely rare. The use of molecular biology techniques to determine the clonal origin of corticotroph tumors has shown that ACTH-secreting pituitary adenomas are monoclonal, arising from a single progenitor cell. Presumably, somatic mutations are required for tumorigenesis.

In Cushing disease, the chronic ACTH hypersecretion causes bilateral hyperplasia of the adrenal cortex. Combined

TABLE 21–3 Major causes of Cushing syndrome.

NONIATROGENIC
ACTH dependent
1. Cushing disease (ACTH-secreting pituitary adenomas)
• *Epidemiology:* 68% of cases of noniatrogenic Cushing syndrome. More common in women (F–M ratio of approximately 8:1). Age at diagnosis usually 20–40 years.
• *Clinical features:* Hyperpigmentation and hypokalemic alkalosis are rare; androgenic manifestations limited to acne and hirsutism. Secretion of cortisol and adrenal androgens is only moderately increased.
• *Course:* Slow progression over several years.
2. Ectopic ACTH syndrome
• *Epidemiology:* 15% of cases of spontaneous Cushing syndrome. More common in men (M–F ratio of approximately 3:1). Age at diagnosis usually 40–60 years. Occurs most commonly in patients with small cell carcinoma of lung and bronchial carcinoid tumors. Rarely, other tumors secrete ACTH; these include carcinoid tumors of the thymus, gut, pancreas, or ovary; pancreatic islet cell tumors; medullary thyroid carcinomas; and pheochromocytomas.
• *Clinical features:* Frequently limited to weakness, hypertension, and glucose intolerance resulting from the rapid onset of hypercortisolism. Weight loss and anemia are common effects of malignancy. Primary tumor usually apparent. Hyperpigmentation, hypokalemia, and alkalosis may occur from the mineralocorticoid effects of cortisol and other steroids secreted.
• *Course:* With underlying carcinomas, hypercortisolism is of rapid onset and steroid hypersecretion is frequently severe, with equally elevated levels of glucocorticoids, androgens, and deoxycorticosterone. With underlying benign tumors, more slowly progressive course.
ACTH independent
3. Functioning adrenocortical tumors
• *Epidemiology:* 20% of cases of Cushing syndrome. Adrenal adenomas in the vast majority, only rarely adrenal carcinomas. More common in women. Adrenal carcinoma occurs in about 1–2 per 1 million population per year. Age at diagnosis usually 35–40 years.
• *Clinical features and course:* Adenomas: Onset is gradual. Usually secretes only cortisol. Hypercortisolism is mild to moderate. Androgenic effects absent. Carcinomas: Rapid onset, rapidly progressive. Marked elevations of glucocorticoids, androgens, and mineralocorticoids. Hypokalemia, abdominal pain, abdominal masses, hepatic and pulmonary metastases.
IATROGENIC
4. Exogenous glucocorticoid administration
• Glucocorticoid administered in high doses in the treatment of nonendocrine disorders.

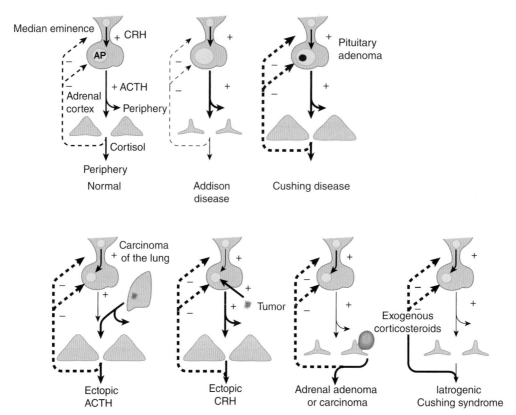

FIGURE 21–12 Hypothalamic, pituitary, and adrenal cortical relationships. Solid arrows indicate stimulation; dashed arrows, inhibition. **Normal:** Corticotropin-releasing hormone (CRH) elaborated by the median eminence of the hypothalamus stimulates secretion of adrenocorticotropic hormone (ACTH) by the anterior pituitary (AP). ACTH triggers the synthesis and release of cortisol, the principal glucocorticoid of the adrenal cortex. A rising level of cortisol inhibits the stimulatory action of CRH on ACTH release (or cortisol may inhibit CRH release), completing a negative feedback loop. **Addison disease:** In primary destructive disease of the adrenal cortex, the level of plasma cortisol is very low, and the effect of CRH on the anterior pituitary proceeds without inhibition, causing a marked increase in the secretion of ACTH. High levels of ACTH produce characteristic skin pigmentation changes. **Cushing disease:** The primary lesion may be at the level of the pituitary or hypothalamus. In either case, the production of ACTH and cortisol is excessive. The former causes bilateral adrenal hyperplasia, and the latter causes clinical manifestations of hypercortisolism. Cells of the anterior pituitary are relatively resistant to the high levels of circulating cortisol. **Ectopic ACTH:** In this syndrome, ACTH or an ACTH-like peptide is elaborated by a tumor such as carcinoma of the lung. The adrenals are stimulated, circulating cortisol is increased, and pituitary ACTH secretion is inhibited. **Ectopic CRH:** In this rare syndrome, CRH is elaborated by a tumor such as a bronchial carcinoid. The pituitary is stimulated, and there is an elaboration of excess ACTH. The adrenals are stimulated, and circulating cortisol is increased. The hypercortisolism causes diminished hypothalamic CRH production; however, the negative feedback on the pituitary production of ACTH is overcome by the ectopic CRH. **Adrenal adenoma or carcinoma:** An adenoma or carcinoma of the adrenal cortex may produce cortisol autonomously. When the rate of production exceeds physiologic quantities, Cushing syndrome results; the effect of CRH on the anterior pituitary is inhibited by the high levels of circulating cortisol, with resultant diminished ACTH secretion and atrophy of normal adrenal tissue. **Iatrogenic Cushing syndrome:** An exogenous corticosteroid administration in excess of physiologic quantities of cortisol leads directly to peripheral manifestations of hypercortisolism and inhibits the effect of CRH on the anterior pituitary, with resultant diminished ACTH secretion, diminished cortisol production, and atrophy of normal adrenal tissue. (Redrawn and modified, with permission, from Burns TW, Carlson HE. Endocrinology. In: Sodeman WA et al, eds. *Pathologic Physiology: Mechanisms of Disease.* Saunders, 1985. Copyright © Elsevier.)

adrenal weights (normal: 8–10 g) range from 12 g to 24 g. The adrenal hyperplasia is most typically micronodular, but in some patients, particularly those with long-standing Cushing disease, macronodular hyperplasia develops.

C. Ectopic ACTH Syndrome

In **ectopic ACTH syndrome**, a nonpituitary tumor synthesizes and secretes biologically active ACTH or an ACTH-like peptide (see Figure 21–12). The neoplasms most frequently responsible are small cell carcinomas of the lung and bronchial

carcinoid tumors. Ectopic ACTH hypersecretion is more common in men, largely owing to the more frequent occurrence of these lung tumors in men. Table 21–3 lists other associated tumors. Chronic ACTH hypersecretion causes marked bilateral adrenocortical hyperplasia, with combined adrenal weights ranging from 24 g to 50 g or more. The ACTH secreted by the nonpituitary tumor causes adrenal hyperfunction, and the high circulating cortisol levels suppress hypothalamic CRH secretion and pituitary ACTH secretion. Pituitary corticotroph cells have a decreased ACTH content.

D. Ectopic CRH Syndrome

Ectopic CRH syndrome is a rare cause of Cushing syndrome (see Figure 21–12). Most cases have been associated with bronchial carcinoid tumors.

E. Functioning Adrenocortical Tumors

Both **adrenocortical adenomas** and **carcinomas** may cause Cushing syndrome (see Figure 21–12). Adenomas are usually 3–6 cm in diameter, weigh 10–70 g, are encapsulated, and consist predominantly of zona fasciculata cells. They are relatively inefficient in cortisol synthesis. Adrenocortical carcinomas are usually large, weighing 100 g to several kilograms, but often cannot be palpable as an abdominal mass even at the time Cushing syndrome becomes clinically manifest. Grossly, they are highly vascular, with areas of necrosis, hemorrhage, cystic degeneration, and calcification. They are highly malignant lesions, tending to invade the adrenal capsule and neighboring organs and blood vessels and to metastasize to the liver and lungs.

F. Adrenal Micronodular Hyperplasia

ACTH-independent adrenal micronodular hyperplasia is a rare cause of Cushing syndrome (also termed primary pigmented nodular adrenocortical disease). Pathologically, it is characterized by multiple small, pigmented, usually bilateral cortisol-secreting nodules. About half of cases occur sporadically in children and young adults. The remainder occur as an autosomal dominant disorder in association with pigmented lentigines (freckles) of the skin and mucosal surfaces of the head and face; cutaneous, mammary, and atrial myxomas; pituitary somatotroph adenomas; and tumors of peripheral nerves, testes, and other endocrine glands (Carney complex).

G. Adrenal Macronodular Hyperplasia

Another rare cause of Cushing syndrome is bilateral adrenal macronodular hyperplasia. In this condition, both glands are markedly enlarged, with bulging nodules found in cut sections of surgical specimens. Microscopically, the nodules reveal a variegated histologic pattern characterized by trabecular, adenoid, and zona glomerulosa–like structures. Occasionally, the hyperplasia may be unilateral. Some patients with macronodular hyperplasia do not show typical cushingoid features. In these cases, the macronodular hyperplasia is most often discovered incidentally on ultrasound or computed tomography (CT) examination of the abdomen and can be considered benign.

Pathophysiology

The various causes of Cushing syndrome can be divided into two categories: ACTH dependent and ACTH independent. The causes of ACTH-dependent Cushing syndrome include Cushing disease (95% of ACTH-dependent cases), ectopic ACTH hypersecretion (5%), and ectopic CRH secretion (rare), all of which are characterized by chronic ACTH hypersecretion and increased cortisol secretion. Causes of ACTH-independent Cushing syndrome include glucocorticoid-secreting adrenocortical adenomas and carcinomas and adrenal micronodular and macronodular hyperplasia, all of which are characterized by autonomous cortisol secretion and pituitary ACTH suppression (Figures 21–12 and 21–13).

A. Cushing Disease

In Cushing disease, there is a persistent overproduction of ACTH by the pituitary adenoma. The ACTH hypersecretion is disorderly, episodic, and random; the normal diurnal rhythm of ACTH and cortisol secretion is usually absent, and midnight values of cortisol are elevated and can be used in diagnostic procedures. Plasma levels of ACTH and cortisol vary and may at times be within the normal range (Figure 21–13). However, a **24-hour urine free cortisol**

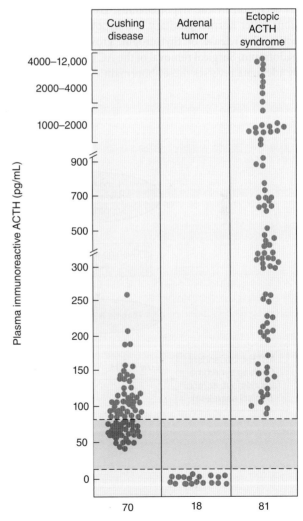

FIGURE 21–13 Basal plasma ACTH concentrations in patients with various types of noniatrogenic Cushing syndrome. The green zone represents the normal range. (Redrawn, with permission, from Scott AP et al. Pituitary adrenocorticotropin and the melanocyte stimulating hormones. In: Parsons JA, ed. *Peptide Hormones*. University Park Press, 1979.)

measurement confirms hypercortisolism. The excessive cortisol does not suppress ACTH secretion by the pituitary adenoma.

Most (90%) patients with Cushing disease have exaggerated plasma ACTH and cortisol responses to CRH stimulation and incompletely suppressed secretion of ACTH and cortisol by exogenous glucocorticoids (eg, 1 mg dexamethasone suppression test). Although these findings suggest that the pituitary adenoma cells are unusually sensitive to CRH and relatively resistant to glucocorticoids, the findings may simply be due to the increased number of ACTH-secreting cells. About 10% of patients with pituitary microadenomas do not exhibit major increases in plasma ACTH in response to CRH. Presumably, the clonal cells of such patients have a receptor or postreceptor defect.

Despite ACTH hypersecretion, the pituitary and adrenals fail to respond normally to stress. Stimuli such as hypoglycemia or surgery fail to increase ACTH and cortisol secretion, probably because chronic hypercortisolism has suppressed CRH secretion by the hypothalamus. Hypercortisolism also inhibits other normal pituitary and hypothalamic functions, affecting the release of thyrotropin, growth hormone, and gonadotropin. Surgical removal of the ACTH-producing pituitary adenoma reverses these abnormalities.

B. Ectopic ACTH Syndrome

In ectopic ACTH syndrome, the hypersecretion of ACTH and cortisol is random and episodic and quantitatively greater than in patients with Cushing disease (see Figure 21–13). Indeed, plasma levels and urinary excretion of cortisol, adrenal androgens, and other steroids are often markedly elevated. Ectopic ACTH secretion by tumors is usually not suppressible by exogenous glucocorticoids such as dexamethasone (Figure 21–14).

C. Ectopic CRH Syndrome

Clinically, ectopic CRH syndrome is indistinguishable from ectopic ACTH syndrome. Biochemically, however, plasma CRH concentrations are elevated (not suppressed), and the CRH-stimulated secretion of ACTH is suppressible with high doses of dexamethasone (not so in ectopic ACTH syndrome). Sometimes, nonpituitary tumors produce both CRH and ACTH ectopically.

D. Adrenal Tumors

Primary adrenal adenomas and carcinomas are not under hypothalamic–pituitary control and thus autonomously secrete cortisol. The hypercortisolism suppresses pituitary ACTH production, resulting in atrophy of the uninvolved

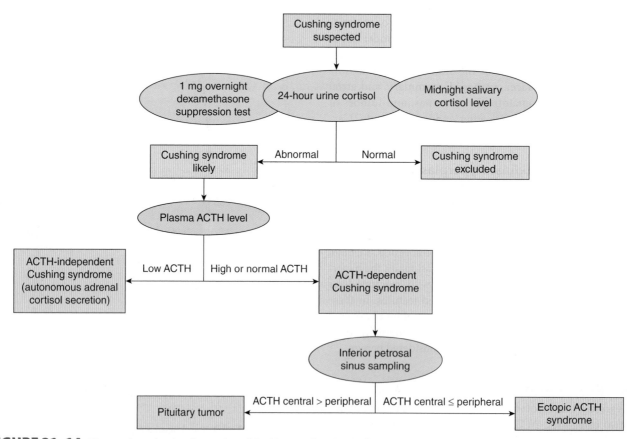

FIGURE 21–14 Diagnostic evaluation for suspected Cushing syndrome. Initial tests (1 mg overnight dexamethasone suppression test, 24-hour urine cortisol, or midnight salivary cortisol level) will confirm or exclude hypercortisolism. Then, the plasma ACTH level will differentiate adrenal (ACTH-independent) from ACTH-dependent causes. In the case of elevated or normal ACTH levels, localization by inferior petrosal sinus sampling will identify or exclude a pituitary origin. Boxes enclose clinical diagnoses; ovals indicate diagnostic tests.

adrenal cortex (see Figure 21–12). Steroid secretion is random and episodic and not usually suppressible by dexamethasone. With adrenocortical carcinomas, the overproduction of androgenic precursors is common, resulting in hirsutism or virilization in female patients or precocious puberty in children. On the other hand, with adrenal adenomas, the production of androgenic precursors is very rare. Thus, their clinical manifestations are chiefly those of cortisol excess.

E. Bilateral Micronodular Hyperplasia

ACTH levels are low, and cortisol is not suppressed by high doses of dexamethasone. This is different from classic primary pigmented nodular adrenocortical disease, in which a paradoxical increase in cortisol levels can be observed.

F. Bilateral Macronodular Hyperplasia

Again, hypercortisolism, low plasma ACTH, loss of the diurnal rhythm of ACTH, and lack of suppression with high doses of dexamethasone are found. A subset of patients with bilateral ACTH-independent macronodular adrenal hyperplasia has been found to have abnormal adrenal receptors, including those for gastric inhibitory polypeptide (food-induced hypercortisolism), vasopressin, β-adrenergic agonists, luteinizing hormone/human chorionic gonadotropin (LH/hCG) (hypertension during pregnancy and after menopause), or serotonin (5-HT). Another subset of patients has been found to carry a germline mutation in *ARMC5*, causing a hereditary predisposition to bilateral adrenal hyperplasia.

G. Subclinical Cushing Syndrome

With the routine use of ultrasound and CT imaging studies, adrenal masses are being detected with increased frequency in asymptomatic patients. Termed "incidentalomas" (see later discussion), a substantial percentage are hormonally active. Up to 20% produce glucocorticoids. Such autonomous glucocorticoid production without specific symptoms and signs of Cushing syndrome is termed subclinical Cushing syndrome. With an estimated prevalence of 79 cases per 100,000 persons, subclinical Cushing syndrome is much more common than classic Cushing syndrome. Depending on the amount of glucocorticoid secreted by the tumor, the clinical spectrum ranges from a slightly attenuated diurnal cortisol rhythm to complete atrophy of the contralateral adrenal gland with lasting adrenal insufficiency after unilateral adrenalectomy.

Clinical Manifestations

Glucocorticoid excess leads to glucose intolerance in several ways. First, cortisol excess promotes the synthesis of glucose in the liver from amino acids liberated by protein catabolism. The increased hepatic gluconeogenesis occurs via stimulation of the enzymes glucose-6-phosphatase and phosphoenolpyruvate carboxykinase. Second, there is an increase in the hepatic synthesis of glycogen and ketone bodies. Third, cortisol antagonizes the action of insulin in peripheral glucose use, perhaps by inhibiting glucose phosphorylation. The glucose intolerance and hyperglycemia are clinically manifested as thirst and polyuria. Overt diabetes mellitus occurs in 10–15% of patients with Cushing syndrome. The diabetes is characterized by insulin resistance, ketosis, and hyperlipidemia, but acidosis and microvascular complications are rare.

With chronic cortisol excess, muscle wasting occurs as a result of excess protein catabolism, decreased muscle protein synthesis, and the induction of insulin resistance in muscle via a postinsulin receptor defect. Proximal muscle weakness occurs in about 60% of cases. It is usually manifested by difficulty in climbing stairs or rising from a chair or bed without using the arms. Fatigue when combing or drying the hair is also seen.

Obesity and redistribution of body fat are probably the most recognizable features of Cushing syndrome. Weight gain is often the initial symptom. The obesity is centralized, with relative sparing of the extremities. The redistribution of adipose tissue mainly affects the face, neck, trunk, and abdomen. Thickening of facial fat rounds the facial contour, producing "moon facies." An enlarged dorsocervical fat pad ("buffalo hump") can occur with weight gain from any cause; increased fat pads that fill and bulge above the supraclavicular fossae are more specific for Cushing syndrome. Abdominal fat deposition results in centripetal obesity, with an elevated waist-to-hip circumference ratio (>1.0 in men and >0.8 in women) in 50% of patients with Cushing syndrome. This fat deposition occurs both subcutaneously and intra-abdominally, most prominently around the viscera, perhaps because intra-abdominal fat appears to have a higher density of glucocorticoid receptors than other fat tissue.

The reason for the abnormal fat distribution is unknown. However, plasma leptin levels are significantly elevated in patients with Cushing syndrome compared with both nonobese healthy individuals and obese individuals with a similar percentage of body fat but no endocrine or metabolic disorder. Leptin is an adipocyte-derived satiety factor that helps regulate appetite and body weight. The elevated leptin in patients with Cushing syndrome is probably a result of visceral obesity. Glucocorticoids may act, at least in part directly, on adipose tissue to increase leptin synthesis and secretion. Chronic hypercortisolism may also have an indirect effect via the associated hyperinsulinemia or insulin resistance.

Given the known lipolytic effects of glucocorticoids, the increased fat deposition caused by glucocorticoid excess seems paradoxical. It may be explained by the increase in appetite or by the lipogenic effects of the hyperinsulinemia that the cortisol excess causes.

Glucocorticoid excess inhibits fibroblasts, leading to a loss of collagen and connective tissue. Thinning of the skin, abdominal striae, easy bruisability, poor wound healing, and frequent skin infections are the result. Atrophy leads to a translucent appearance of the skin. Cutaneous atrophy is best appreciated as a fine "cigarette paper" wrinkling or tenting of the skin over the dorsum of the hand or over the elbow.

On the face, corticosteroid excess causes perioral dermatitis, characterized by small follicular papules on an erythematous base around the mouth, and a rosacea-like eruption, characterized by central facial erythema. Facial telangiectases and plethora over the cheeks may result from the loss of subcutaneous tissue with hypercortisolism. Steroid acne, characterized by numerous pustular lesions reflecting androgenic effects or papular lesions reflecting glucocorticoid effects, sometimes occurs on the face, chest, or back. **Acanthosis nigricans**, a dark, soft, velvety skin with fine folds and papillae, may occur in intertriginous areas, such as under the breasts or in the groin, or at sites of friction, such as the neck or belt line. Acanthosis nigricans is thought to result from two changes in the skin's extracellular matrix: decreased viscosity caused by altered glycosaminoglycan formation and abnormal deposition of the extracellular matrix in papillae that protrude from the dermis.

Prominent reddish-purple **striae** occur in 50–70% of patients, most commonly over the abdominal wall, breasts, hips, buttocks, thighs, and axillae. The striae result from increased subcutaneous fat deposition, which stretches the thin skin and ruptures the subdermal tissues. These striae are depressed below the skin surface because of the loss of underlying connective tissue and are wider (not infrequently 0.5–2.0 cm) than the pinkish-white striae of pregnancy or rapid weight gain. Easy bruisability occurs in about 40% of cases. Ecchymoses occur after minimal trauma, resulting in purpura. Wound healing is delayed, and surgical incisions sometimes undergo dehiscence. Fungal infections of the skin and mucous membranes are frequent, including tinea versicolor, seborrheic dermatitis, onychomycosis, and oral candidiasis.

In ectopic ACTH syndrome, skin hyperpigmentation may occur owing to the concomitant markedly elevated levels of circulating MSH and ACTH (which has some MSH-like activity). However, hyperpigmentation is rare in Cushing disease and is absent in adrenal tumors except after total adrenalectomy (Nelson syndrome).

In about 80% of female patients, hirsutism from the increased secretion of adrenal androgens occurs over the face, abdomen, breasts, chest, and upper thighs. Acne often accompanies the hirsutism.

Although the physiologic role of glucocorticoids in bone and Ca^{2+} metabolism is not well understood, excessive glucocorticoid production inhibits bone formation and accelerates bone resorption (see Chapter 17). Glucocorticoids exert direct effects on the main cell types that regulate bone metabolism. They inhibit osteoblast differentiation, inducing osteoblast and osteocyte apoptosis while at the same time prolonging osteoclast survival. As mentioned earlier, hypercortisolism also leads to a state of hypogonadism (due to the inhibition of hypothalamic GnRH) in both males and females and therefore reduces the beneficial effect of sex hormones on bone strength.

Furthermore, glucocorticoid excess decreases intestinal Ca^{2+} absorption and increases urinary Ca^{2+} excretion (hypercalciuria), resulting in a negative Ca^{2+} balance. Glucocorticoids impair the intestinal absorption and renal tubular reabsorption of Ca^{2+} by inhibiting the effects of vitamin D on the intestine and renal tubules, as well as the hydroxylation of vitamin D

in the liver. There is a secondary increase in PTH secretion, accelerating bone resorption.

As a result of the hypercalciuria, kidney stones occur in about 15% of patients. Such patients may present with renal colic. Glucocorticoids also reduce the renal tubular reabsorption of phosphate, leading to phosphaturia and reduced serum phosphorus concentrations.

The combination of decreased bone formation and increased bone resorption ultimately leads to a generalized loss of bone mass (**osteoporosis**) and an increased risk of bony fracture. The fracture risk is potentiated by an accompanying myopathy that predisposes to falls. Osteoporosis is present in most patients; back pain is an initial complaint in 58% of cases. X-ray films frequently reveal vertebral compression fractures (16–22% of cases), rib fractures, and sometimes multiple stress fractures. For unknown reasons, avascular (aseptic) bone necrosis (usually of the femur or humerus) sometimes occurs with exogenous (iatrogenic) corticosteroids but is rare with endogenous hypercortisolemia.

Glucocorticoid excess alters the normal inflammatory response to infection or injury by several mechanisms. On the molecular level, glucocorticoids exert their effect by activating the GR, which in turn interferes with other transcription factors (eg, nuclear factor kappa-B [NFκB], activator protein [AP1]) necessary for the transcription of pro-inflammatory genes and immune mediators. Generally, glucocorticoids decrease the number of CD_4 T lymphocytes and more potently inhibit T_H1-associated cytokines (eg, interleukin 2). They also inhibit fibroblastic activity, preventing the walling off of bacterial and other infections. Therefore, patients with hypercortisolism are more prone to diseases that require a cell-mediated immune response, such as tuberculosis, fungal, and *Pneumocystis* infections.

Glucocorticoid excess also suppresses manifestations of allergic disorders that are due to the release of histamine from tissues.

Hypertension occurs in 75–85% of patients with spontaneous Cushing syndrome, the exact pathogenesis of which is unclear. It may be related to salt and water retention from the mineralocorticoid effects of the excess glucocorticoid, which in high concentrations escape the inactivation by 11β-hydroxysteroid dehydrogenase type 2. Alternatively, it may be due to the increased secretion of angiotensinogen. Whereas plasma renin activity and concentrations are generally normal or suppressed in Cushing syndrome, angiotensinogen levels are elevated to approximately twice normal because of a direct effect of glucocorticoids on its hepatic synthesis, and angiotensin II levels are increased by about 40%. Administering the angiotensin II antagonist saralasin to patients with Cushing syndrome causes a prompt 8 to 10 mm Hg drop in systolic and diastolic blood pressure. Studies in experimental animals have demonstrated that glucocorticoids exert permissive effects on vascular tone by a variety of mechanisms. Some involve vascular smooth muscle cells, including an increased secretion of the vasoconstrictor endothelin, an increase in Ca^{2+} uptake and Ca^{2+} channel antagonist binding, and an increase of α_{1B}-adrenergic receptors. In addition, glucocorticoids cause a decrease in atrial natriuretic peptide (ANP)-mediated cyclic guanosine monophosphate formation, leading to decreased vasodilation by ANP. Glucocorticoids inhibit nitric oxide synthase in vascular endothelial cells, predisposing to vasoconstriction. Glucocorticoids also sensitize arterioles to the pressor effects of catecholamines.

Gonadal dysfunction occurs commonly in Cushing syndrome and is the result of the increased secretion of adrenal androgens (in females) and cortisol (in males and females) from the adrenal cortex. In premenopausal women, the androgens may cause hirsutism, acne, amenorrhea, and infertility. Hypercortisolism appears to affect the hypothalamic gonadotropin-releasing hormone (GnRH) pulse generator to inhibit normal LH and follicle-stimulating hormone (FSH) pulsatility and pituitary responsiveness to GnRH. The high levels of cortisol can thus suppress pituitary LH secretion. In women, this results in menstrual irregularities, including amenorrhea, oligomenorrhea, and polymenorrhea. In men, this results in decreased testosterone secretion by the testis, for which the increased adrenal secretion of weak androgens does not compensate. Decreased libido, loss of body hair, small and soft testes, and impotence ensue.

Excess glucocorticoids frequently produce mental symptoms, including euphoria, increased appetite, irritability, emotional lability, and decreased libido. Many patients experience impaired cognitive function, with poor concentration and poor memory, and disordered sleep, with decreased rapid eye movement sleep and early morning awakening. Glucocorticoid excess also accelerates the basic electroencephalographic rhythm. Significant psychiatric illness—mainly depression but also anxiety, psychosis with delusions or hallucinations, paranoia, or hyperkinetic (even manic) behavior—occurs in 51–81% of patients with Cushing syndrome. The pathogenesis of these CNS effects is not well understood.

Glucocorticoid excess inhibits growth in children, in part by directly inhibiting bone cells and by decreasing growth hormone and thyroid-stimulating hormone (TSH) secretion and insulin-like growth factor-1 (IGF-1) generation. Glucocorticoids also suppress growth by exerting direct effects on the growth plate, including inhibiting mucopolysaccharide production, resulting in reduced cartilaginous bone matrix and epiphyseal proliferation.

With long-standing hypercortisolism, there may be mild to moderate elevations in intraocular pressure and glaucoma, perhaps related to collagen strand swelling in the trabecular meshwork, which interferes with aqueous humor drainage. Posterior subcapsular cataracts may develop. About half of patients will develop exophthalmos, which is often asymptomatic. Visual field defects occur in 40% of patients with pituitary macroadenomas related to pressure on the optic chiasm; field defects do not occur with microadenomas.

Routine laboratory tests in Cushing syndrome usually demonstrate a high normal hemoglobin, hematocrit, and red blood cell number. Polycythemia occurs rarely, secondary to androgen excess. The total white blood cell count is usually normal or might be elevated; however, the percentages of lymphocytes and eosinophils and the total lymphocyte and eosinophil counts are frequently subnormal. Neutrophil counts may be elevated due to decreased capillary neutrophil margination and extravasation.

Serum electrolytes are usually normal. In patients with ectopic ACTH syndrome or adrenocortical carcinoma, hypokalemic metabolic alkalosis sometimes occurs because of the hypersecretion of mineralocorticoids or because of an overwhelming of the 11-βHSD system by the markedly elevated cortisol levels. Fasting hyperglycemia occurs in about 10–15% of patients; postprandial hyperglycemia and glucosuria are more common. Most patients with Cushing syndrome have secondary hyperinsulinemia and abnormal glucose tolerance tests. The serum Ca^{2+} is generally normal; the serum phosphorus is low normal or slightly low. Hypercalciuria can be demonstrated in 40% of cases.

Patients with subclinical Cushing syndrome lack the classic stigmas of hypercortisolism but frequently have obesity, hypertension, and type 2 diabetes mellitus.

Diagnosis

Suspected hypercortisolism can be investigated by several approaches (see Figure 21–14). Current recommendations involve a stepwise approach to diagnostic evaluation. The first step is to demonstrate pathologic hypercortisolemia and confirm the diagnosis of Cushing syndrome. The second step is to distinguish ACTH-independent disease from ACTH-dependent disease, followed by either adrenal or pituitary imaging. For patients with ACTH-dependent disease, the final step is to determine the anatomic localization of the ACTH source, by MRI or, if equivocal, by inferior petrosal sinus sampling (IPSS) or cavernous sinus sampling (CSS).

Measurement of free cortisol in a 24-hour urine specimen collected on an outpatient basis demonstrates excessive cortisol excretion (24-hour urinary free cortisol levels >100 μg/24 h). Urinary free cortisol values are rarely normal in Cushing syndrome. Urinary free cortisol measurement is the most specific test to screen for and confirm the presence of Cushing syndrome.

Performing an overnight 1 mg dexamethasone suppression test will demonstrate a lack of the normal suppression of adrenal cortisol production by exogenous corticosteroid (dexamethasone). The overnight dexamethasone suppression test is accomplished by prescribing 1 mg of dexamethasone at 11:00 PM, and then obtaining a plasma cortisol level the next morning at 8:00 AM. In normal individuals, the dexamethasone suppresses the early morning surge in cortisol, resulting in plasma cortisol levels of less than 1.8 μg/dL (50 nmol/L). This cut-off provides high test sensitivity. In Cushing syndrome, cortisol secretion is not suppressed to as great a degree, and values are often more than 5 μg/dL (140 nmol/L).

If the overnight dexamethasone suppression test is normal, the diagnosis is very unlikely; if the urine free cortisol is also normal, Cushing syndrome is excluded. If the results of both tests are abnormal, hypercortisolism is present, and the diagnosis of Cushing syndrome can be considered to be established if conditions causing false-positive results (pseudo-Cushing syndrome) are excluded (acute or chronic illness, obesity, high-estrogen states, drugs, alcoholism, and depression). The CRH test is a useful adjunct in patients with borderline elevated urinary cortisol levels resulting from a probable pseudo-Cushing state.

In patients with equivocal or borderline results, a 2-day low-dose dexamethasone suppression test is often performed (0.5 mg every 6 hours for eight doses). Normal responses to this test exclude the diagnosis of Cushing syndrome. Normal responses are an 8:00 AM plasma cortisol level of less than 2 μg/dL (56 nmol/L); a 24-hour urinary free cortisol level of less than 10 μg/24 h (<28 μmol/24 h); and a 24-hour urinary 17-hydroxycorticosteroid level of less than 2.5 mg/24 h (6.9 μmol/24 h) or 1 mg/g creatinine (0.3 mmol/mol creatinine).

Confirmation of the diagnosis of Cushing syndrome entails measuring the plasma ACTH level (see Figure 21–14). An assay of the plasma ACTH level helps differentiate ACTH-dependent from ACTH-independent causes of Cushing syndrome. These tests are then followed by imaging procedures (eg, thin-section CT scan or MRI) to determine the location of a suspected pituitary, adrenal, lung, or other tumor.

With adrenal carcinomas, CT typically demonstrates an inhomogeneous large adrenal mass with irregular margins and variable contrast enhancement of solid components. MRI can also detect these tumors and can assess invasion into large vessels.

CLINICALLY INAPPARENT ADRENAL MASS (INCIDENTALOMA)

Adrenal masses are common. Routine autopsy studies find an adrenal mass in at least 3% of persons older than 50 years. Most of these pose no threat to health, but a small proportion cause endocrinologic problems and approximately 1 in 4000 of such adrenal tumors is malignant.

Incidentalomas are clinically inapparent masses discovered incidentally in the course of diagnostic testing or treatment for other clinical conditions. The estimated prevalence of incidentalomas ranges from about 1–2% in patients undergoing routine ultrasonography for nonendocrinologic complaints to 4.3% of patients with a previous diagnosis of cancer. The prevalence rises with age from less than 1% in persons younger than 30 years to 7% in those age 70 years or older.

Pathologically, clinically inapparent adrenal masses can be either benign (adenomas, some pheochromocytomas, myelolipomas, ganglioneuromas, adrenal cysts, hematomas) or malignant (adrenocortical carcinomas, some pheochromocytomas, metastases from other cancers). Adrenocortical carcinoma occurs with an estimated incidence of 1–2 per 1 million persons per year. Adrenocortical carcinoma is more likely if the adrenal tumor is large (>4 cm).

Diagnostic evaluation is typically performed to determine whether the lesion is hormonally active or nonfunctioning and whether it is likely to be malignant or benign.

In unselected patients and those without endocrinologic symptoms, most adrenal incidentalomas (>70%) are nonfunctioning tumors. However, up to 20% of patients experience subclinical hormonal overproduction; such patients may be at risk for metabolic or cardiovascular disorders. Most common (~5–10%) is cortisol overproduction, sometimes termed subclinical Cushing syndrome. Less common are catecholamine excess from pheochromocytomas and aldosterone excess from adrenal adenomas. Sex hormone excess from virilizing or feminizing tumors is only very rarely observed in benign adenomas. Experts recommend that all patients with incidentalomas undergo a 1 mg dexamethasone suppression test and a measurement of plasma (or urinary) free metanephrines, and hypertensive patients undergo determinations of serum potassium and plasma aldosterone concentration and plasma renin activity.

Patients with subclinical autonomous glucocorticoid hypersecretion may progress to develop metabolic disorders, such as insulin resistance, but very rarely develop full-blown Cushing syndrome.

The size and appearance of the mass on CT or MRI can help distinguish malignant from benign tumors. For example, more than 60% of incidentalomas smaller than 4 cm are benign adenomas, and less than 1% are adrenocortical carcinomas. By contrast, for lesions larger than 6 cm, up to 25% are carcinomas, and less than 15% are benign adenomas. In addition, if a CT scan reveals a smooth-bordered, homogeneous mass with a low value on a standardized measure of x-ray absorption (CT attenuation value of <10 Hounsfield units), the mass is likely a benign adenoma. CT-guided fine-needle aspiration biopsy of the adrenal is reserved only for patients with a pre-existing nonadrenal cancer who then develop a new heterogeneous adrenal mass exhibiting a high CT attenuation value (>20 Hounsfield units). In this setting, an adrenal biopsy can help determine whether the new adrenal mass is a metastasis of the pre-existing nonadrenal cancer to the adrenal or represents a new primary adrenal neoplasm.

Surgery is usually recommended for patients with unilateral incidentalomas found on history, physical examination, and laboratory studies to have symptoms, signs, and biochemical evidence of any adrenal hormone excess. Surgery is also recommended for all patients with biochemical evidence of pheochromocytomas, whether symptomatic or not. The management of patients with subclinical hyperfunctioning adrenal cortical adenomas is more controversial; both surgical and nonsurgical approaches are used.

Recommended monitoring for patients in whom a benign nature cannot be established on the first evaluation consists of a second imaging study 6–12 months later and follow-up endocrinologic studies to exclude hormonal hypersecretion. No further monitoring is recommended for patients with nonsecreting tumors that remain stable in size. Follow-up of patients with nonfunctioning masses shows that the vast majority of incidentalomas remain stable in size: About 5–25% increase in size by 1 cm or more, and 3–4% decrease in size. Overall, when monitored for up to 10 years, nonfunctioning tumors rarely develop hormone overproduction (usually cortisol, rarely catecholamine or aldosterone, hypersecretion). Tumors 3 cm or larger are more likely to develop hyperfunction than smaller masses.

CHECKPOINT

12. What are the symptoms and signs of excess of each class of adrenal steroid?

13. What are the major causes of Cushing syndrome?

14. How is the regulation of glucocorticoid secretion altered in patients with Cushing disease? With ectopic ACTH secretion? With autonomous adrenal tumors?

15. What are the symptoms and signs of glucocorticoid excess?

16. Name some different ways to make the diagnosis of Cushing disease in a patient with suggestive symptoms and signs.

ADRENOCORTICAL INSUFFICIENCY

Adrenocortical insufficiency generally occurs because of either destruction or dysfunction of the adrenal cortex (**primary adrenocortical insufficiency**) or deficient pituitary ACTH or hypothalamic CRH secretion (**secondary adrenocortical insufficiency**). However, congenital defects in any one of several enzymes occurring as "inborn errors of metabolism" can lead to deficient cortisol secretion. Enzyme deficiencies can also result from treatment with various drugs, such as metyrapone and mitotane.

Table 21–4 lists the causes of adrenocortical insufficiency. No matter the origin, the clinical manifestations of primary adrenocortical insufficiency are a consequence of deficiencies of cortisol, aldosterone, and androgenic steroids. Secondary adrenal insufficiency results in a selective cortisol (and androgen) deficiency.

Etiology

A. Primary Adrenocortical Insufficiency

Primary adrenocortical insufficiency (Addison disease) is most often due to autoimmune destruction of the adrenal cortex (~80% of cases). In the past, tuberculosis involving the adrenals was the most common cause, but it has now become uncommon. Other less common causes include histoplasmosis, adrenal hemorrhage or infarction, genetic diseases, metastatic carcinoma, and AIDS-related (cytomegalovirus) adrenalitis.

Primary adrenal insufficiency is rare, with reported prevalence rates of 39–60 cases per 1 million population. Addison disease is somewhat more common in women, with a

TABLE 21–4 Causes of adrenocortical insufficiency.

Primary adrenocortical insufficiency (Addison disease)
Autoimmune (~80%)
Tuberculosis
Adrenal hemorrhage and infarction
Histoplasmosis, coccidioidomycosis, and other granulomatous infections
Metastatic carcinoma and lymphoma (non-Hodgkin)
HIV, AIDS-related opportunistic infection (eg, cytomegalovirus)
Amyloidosis
Sarcoidosis
Hemochromatosis
Radiation therapy
Antiphospholipid syndrome
Surgical adrenalectomy
Enzyme inhibitor drugs (metyrapone, aminoglutethimide, trilostane, ketoconazole, suramin, etomidate)
Cytotoxic and chemotherapeutic agents (mitotane, megestrol, mifepristone)
Congenital defects (X-linked adrenoleukodystrophy, enzyme defects, adrenal hypoplasia, familial glucocorticoid deficiency)
Secondary adrenocortical insufficiency
Chronic exogenous glucocorticoid therapy
Pituitary tumor
Hypothalamic tumor
Acquired hypothalamic isolated CRH deficiency

Data from Carroll TB et al. Glucocorticoids and adrenal androgens. In: Gardner DB et al, eds. *Greenspan's Basic and Clinical Endocrinology*, 10th ed. McGraw-Hill Companies, Inc., 2017.

female-to-male ratio of 1.25:1. It usually occurs in the third to fifth decades.

1. Autoimmune Adrenocortical Insufficiency—Autoimmune destruction of the adrenal glands is accompanied by the generation of **antiadrenal antibodies**. Circulating adrenal autoantibodies can be detected in more than 80% of patients with autoimmune adrenal insufficiency, either isolated or associated with autoimmune polyglandular syndrome type 1 or type 2 (see later discussion). These adrenal autoantibodies are of at least two types: adrenal cortex antibodies (ACAs) and antibodies to the steroid 21-hydroxylase enzyme (cytochrome P450c21). The 21-hydroxylase antibodies are highly specific for Addison disease. In asymptomatic patients, these antibodies may also be important predictors for the subsequent development of adrenal insufficiency. When adrenal autoantibodies are present, 41% of patients develop adrenal insufficiency within 3 years. In adults with other organ-specific autoimmune disorders (eg, premature ovarian failure), detection of adrenal cortex or 21-hydroxylase antibodies was associated with progression to overt Addison disease in 21% and to subclinical hypoadrenalism in 29%. In children, the risk was even higher: In those with other organ-specific autoimmune diseases (eg, hypoparathyroidism), detection of adrenal autoantibodies was associated with a 90% risk of overt Addison disease and a 10% risk of subclinical hypoadrenalism.

Autoantibodies to other tissue antigens are frequently found in patients with autoimmune adrenocortical insufficiency as well. Thyroid antibodies have been found in 45%, gastric parietal cell antibodies in 30%, intrinsic factor antibodies in 9%, parathyroid antibodies in 26%, gonadal antibodies in 17%, and islet cell antibodies in 8%.

It is not surprising, therefore, that autoimmune adrenal insufficiency is frequently associated with other autoimmune endocrine disorders. Two distinct polyglandular syndromes involving the adrenal glands have been described. **Autoimmune polyendocrine syndrome type 1 (APS1)** is a rare autosomal recessive disorder caused by a mutation in the autoimmune regulator (*AIRE*) with onset in childhood. The diagnosis requires at least two of the following: adrenal insufficiency, hypoparathyroidism, and mucocutaneous candidiasis. Other endocrine disorders are sometimes associated, including gonadal failure and type 1 diabetes mellitus. There is also an increased incidence of other nonendocrine immunologic disorders, including alopecia, vitiligo, pernicious anemia, chronic hepatitis, and gastrointestinal (GI) malabsorption. The autoimmune pathogenesis of this condition involves the formation of antibodies against the cytochrome P450 cholesterol–side chain cleavage enzyme (P450scc). This enzyme converts cholesterol to pregnenolone, an initial step in cortisol synthesis (see Figure 21–3). P450scc is found in both the adrenal glands and gonads, but not in other tissues involved in APS1.

Autoimmune polyendocrine syndrome type 2 (APS-2) consists of adrenal insufficiency, Hashimoto thyroiditis, and type 1 diabetes mellitus. It is associated with the haplotypes HLA-B8 (DW3) and DR3. Its pathogenesis involves the formation of antibodies against the 21-OH enzyme mentioned previously. Other autoimmune complications, such as vitiligo (4–17%), pernicious anemia, celiac disease, and myasthenia gravis, are present in a subset of patients.

Pathologically, the adrenal glands are small and atrophic, and the capsule is thickened. There is an intense lymphocytic infiltration of the adrenal cortex. Cortical cells are absent or degenerating, surrounded by fibrous stroma and lymphocytes. The adrenal medulla is preserved.

2. Adrenal Tuberculosis—Tuberculosis causes adrenal failure by total or near-total destruction of both glands. Such destruction usually occurs gradually and produces a picture of chronic adrenal insufficiency. Adrenal tuberculosis usually results from the hematogenous spread of systemic tuberculous infection (lung, GI tract, or kidney) to the adrenal cortex. Pathologically, the adrenal is enlarged in the acute phase and is later replaced with caseous necrosis; both cortical and medullary tissue is destroyed. Calcification of the adrenals can be detected radiographically in about 50% of cases.

3. Bilateral Adrenal Hemorrhage—Bilateral adrenal hemorrhage leads to rapid destruction of the adrenals and precipitates acute adrenal insufficiency. In children, hemorrhage is usually related to fulminant meningococcal septicemia (**Waterhouse–Friderichsen syndrome**) or pseudomonas septicemia. In adults, hemorrhage is related to anticoagulant therapy of other disorders in one-third of cases. Other causes in adults include sepsis, coagulation disorders (eg, antiphospholipid syndrome), adrenal vein thrombosis, adrenal metastases, traumatic shock, severe burns, abdominal surgery, and obstetric complications.

Pathologically, the adrenal glands are often massively enlarged. The inner cortex and medulla are almost entirely replaced by hematomas. There is ischemic necrosis of the outer cortex, and only a thin rim of subcapsular cortical cells survives. There is often thrombosis of the adrenal veins.

The pathogenesis of such acute adrenal insufficiency is thought to be related to a stress-induced increase in ACTH levels, which markedly increases adrenal blood flow to such a degree that it exceeds the capacity for adrenal venous drainage. Thrombosis may then lead to hemorrhage. In surviving patients, the hematomas may later calcify. Additionally, patients on long-term anticoagulation are more prone to develop adrenal hemorrhage.

4. Adrenal Metastases—Metastases to the adrenals occur frequently from lung and breast carcinomas, melanoma, lymphoma, and many other malignancies. However, metastatic disease seldom produces adrenal insufficiency because more than 90% of both adrenals must be destroyed before overt adrenal insufficiency develops. On pathologic examination, the adrenal glands are often massively enlarged.

5. AIDS-Related Adrenal Insufficiency—Adrenal insufficiency in AIDS usually occurs in the late stages of HIV infection. The adrenal gland is commonly affected by opportunistic infection (especially cytomegalovirus, disseminated *Mycobacterium avium-intracellulare*, *M tuberculosis*, *Cryptococcus neoformans*, *Pneumocystis jirovecii*, and *Toxoplasma gondii*) or by neoplasms such as Kaposi sarcoma. Although pathologic involvement of the adrenal glands is frequent, clinical adrenal insufficiency is uncommon. More than half of patients with AIDS have necrotizing adrenalitis (most commonly resulting from cytomegalovirus infection), but it is usually limited in extent to less than 50–70% of the gland. Because adrenal insufficiency does not occur until more than 90% of the gland is destroyed, clinical adrenal insufficiency occurs in less than 5% of patients with AIDS. Since antiretroviral therapy has improved and fewer patients progress to

AIDS, adrenal insufficiency is less often encountered in HIV-positive patients.

However, medications used by AIDS patients can alter steroid secretion and metabolism. Ketoconazole interferes with steroid synthesis by the adrenals and gonads. Rifampin, phenytoin, and opioids increase steroid metabolism.

6. Genetic Disorders of Adrenal Insufficiency—These disorders can be subclassified into four categories: (1) congenital adrenal hyperplasia (see discussion of disorders of adrenal androgen synthesis, below); (2) adrenal hypoplasia congenita with cytomegaly; (3) adrenal hypoplasia congenita without cytomegaly; and (4) degenerative and metabolic diseases affecting adrenal function.

Mutation of the *DAX1* gene causes X-linked adrenal hypoplasia congenita with delayed-onset adrenal insufficiency and hypogonadotropic hypogonadism. The adrenal cortex in this disorder consists of peculiarly shaped, large adrenal cells with large nuclei, which leads to the name "cytomegaly."

Adrenal hypoplasia congenita without cytomegaly mainly comprises the **ACTH insensitivity syndromes**, a group of rare diseases in which resistance to ACTH is either the sole feature or associated with other symptoms. In **familial glucocorticoid deficiency (FGD)**, adrenocortical unresponsiveness to ACTH causes both decreases in the adrenal secretion of glucocorticoids and androgens and the increased pituitary secretion of ACTH. Responsiveness to angiotensin II is normal. Affected infants and young children come to medical attention because of symptoms of cortisol deficiency, especially cutaneous hyperpigmentation, growth retardation, recurrent hypoglycemia, and recurrent infections. Older children may later manifest tall stature related to advanced bone age. The diagnosis is suggested when cortisol secretion does not respond to either endogenous or exogenous ACTH stimulation. On histologic examination, the zona glomerulosa is preserved, but the zona fasciculata and zona reticularis show degeneration.

To date, there are several genes known to cause the classical disorder of FGD. In FGD type 1, the resistance to ACTH is caused by one of several missense mutations within the coding region of the ACTH receptor (*MC2R*). In FGD type 2, the ACTH receptor accessory protein (*MRAP*), which ensures localization of the ACTH receptor in the plasma membrane, has been shown to be mutated and dysfunctional. So-called FGD type 4 is caused by mutations in nicotinamide nucleotide transhydrogenase (*NNT*).

Adrenal insufficiency also occurs both in the **alacrima, achalasia, and adrenal insufficiency ("triple A") syndrome** and in **adrenoleukodystrophy**. In both cases, adrenal insufficiency results from progressive gland destruction, resulting in deficiencies of androgens, glucocorticoids, and mineralocorticoids (usually in this order).

B. Secondary Adrenocortical Insufficiency

Secondary adrenocortical insufficiency most commonly results from ACTH deficiency caused by chronic exogenous glucocorticoid therapy. Rarely, ACTH deficiency results from pituitary or hypothalamic tumors or from isolated CRH deficiency. Genetic disorders leading to secondary adrenal insufficiency have also been described (eg, *TPIT* and *POMC* mutations; see Chapter 19).

Pathophysiology

A. Primary Adrenocortical Insufficiency

Gradual adrenocortical destruction, such as occurs in the autoimmune, tuberculous, and other infiltrative diseases, results initially in a decreased adrenal glucocorticoid reserve. Basal glucocorticoid secretion is normal but does not increase in response to stress or surgery; trauma or infection can precipitate acute adrenal crisis. With further loss of cortical tissue, even basal secretion of glucocorticoids and mineralocorticoids becomes deficient, leading to the clinical manifestations of chronic adrenal insufficiency. The fall in plasma cortisol reduces the feedback inhibition of pituitary ACTH secretion (see Figure 21–12), and the plasma level of ACTH rises (Figure 21–15).

Rapid adrenocortical destruction, such as occurs in septicemia and adrenal hemorrhage, results in the sudden loss of both glucocorticoid and mineralocorticoid secretion, leading to acute adrenal crisis.

B. Secondary Adrenocortical Insufficiency

Secondary adrenal insufficiency is characterized by inadequate ACTH secretion from the pituitary or inadequate CRH

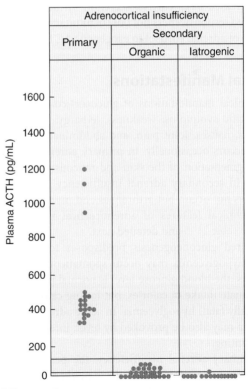

FIGURE 21–15 Basal plasma ACTH levels in primary and secondary adrenocortical insufficiency. (Data from Besser GM et al. Immunoreactive corticotropin levels in adrenocortical insufficiency. Br Med J. 1971;1:374–76.)

secretion from the hypothalamus. Most commonly, secondary adrenocortical insufficiency occurs when large doses of glucocorticoids are given for their anti-inflammatory and immunosuppressive effects in the treatment of asthma, rheumatoid arthritis, ulcerative colitis, and other diseases. If such treatment is extended beyond 4–5 weeks, it produces the prolonged suppression of CRH, ACTH, and endogenous cortisol secretion (see Figure 21–12). Should the exogenous steroid treatment be abruptly discontinued, the hypothalamus and pituitary are unable to respond normally to the reduction in level of circulating glucocorticoid. The patient may develop symptoms and signs of chronic adrenocortical insufficiency or, if subjected to stress, acute adrenal crisis. Prolonged suppression of the hypothalamic–pituitary–adrenal axis can be avoided by using alternate-day steroid regimens whenever possible.

ACTH deficiency is the primary problem in secondary adrenocortical insufficiency. It can be caused by infiltrative or inflammatory processes involving the pituitary (eg, metastasis or lymphocytic hypophysitis), or by a congenital defect; for example, due to mutations in the *POMC* gene or in transcription factors important for pituitary development (eg, *PROP*) or for *POMC* transcription (eg, *TPIT*). ACTH deficiency leads to diminished cortisol and adrenal androgen secretion, but aldosterone secretion generally remains normal. In the early stages, there is a decreased pituitary ACTH reserve. Basal ACTH and cortisol secretions may be normal but do not increase in response to stress. With progression, there is a further loss of ACTH secretion, atrophy of the adrenal cortex, and decreased basal cortisol secretion. At this stage, there is decreased responsiveness not only of pituitary ACTH to stress, but also of adrenal cortisol to exogenous ACTH stimulation.

Clinical Manifestations

The clinical manifestations of glucocorticoid deficiency are nonspecific symptoms: weakness, lethargy, easy fatigability, anorexia, nausea, joint pain, and abdominal pain. Hypoglycemia occurs occasionally. In primary adrenal insufficiency, hyperpigmentation of the skin and mucous membranes also occurs. In secondary adrenal insufficiency, hyperpigmentation does not occur, but arthralgias and myalgias may occur. Other clinical features of adrenocortical insufficiency are listed in Table 21–5 and detailed next.

Impaired gluconeogenesis predisposes to hypoglycemia. Severe hypoglycemia may occur spontaneously in children. In adults, the blood glucose level is normal provided there is an adequate intake of calories, but fasting causes severe (and potentially fatal) hypoglycemia. In acute adrenal crisis, hypoglycemia may also be provoked by fever, infection, or nausea and vomiting.

In primary adrenal insufficiency, the persistently low or absent plasma cortisol level results in marked pituitary ACTH hypersecretion. Because ACTH has intrinsic MSH activity, a variety of pigmentation changes can occur. These include generalized hyperpigmentation (diffuse darkening of the skin); increased pigmentation of skin creases, nail beds, nipples,

TABLE 21–5   Clinical features of adrenocortical insufficiency.

Primary and secondary adrenal insufficiency	Primary adrenal insufficiency	Secondary adrenal insufficiency
Tiredness, weakness, mental depression	Hyperpigmentation of skin, mucosa	Pallor
Anorexia, weight loss	Salt craving	Amenorrhea, decreased libido, impotence
Dizziness, orthostatic hypotension	Hyperkalemia	Scanty axillary and pubic hair
Nausea, vomiting, abdominal cramps, diarrhea		Small testes
Hyponatremia		Prepubertal growth deficit, delayed puberty
Hypoglycemia		Headache, visual symptoms
Normocytic anemia, lymphocytosis, eosinophilia		

Data from Oelkers W. Current concepts: Adrenal insufficiency. N Engl J Med. 1996;335:1206.

areolae, pressure points (eg, knuckles, toes, elbows, knees), and scars formed after the onset of ACTH excess; increased tanning and freckling of sun-exposed areas; and hyperpigmentation of the buccal mucosa, gums, and perivaginal and perianal areas. These changes do not occur in secondary adrenal insufficiency because ACTH secretion is low, not high, in this condition.

In primary adrenal insufficiency, aldosterone deficiency results in the renal loss of Na^+ and renal retention of K^+, causing hypovolemia and hyperkalemia. The hypovolemia, in turn, leads to prerenal azotemia and hypotension. Salt craving has been documented in about 20% of patients with adrenal insufficiency.

Patients may also be unable to excrete a water load. Hyponatremia may develop, reflecting water retention in excess of Na^+. The defective water excretion is probably related to an increase in posterior pituitary vasopressin secretion, disinhibited by low cortisol levels and increased by the perception of nausea; this can be reduced by glucocorticoid administration. In addition, the glomerular filtration rate (GFR) is low. Treatment with mineralocorticoids raises the GFR by restoring plasma volume, and treatment with glucocorticoids improves the GFR even further.

In secondary adrenal insufficiency, aldosterone secretion by the zona glomerulosa is preserved. Thus, clinical manifestations of mineralocorticoid deficiency, such as volume depletion, dehydration, hypotension, and electrolyte abnormalities, generally do not occur. Hyponatremia may occur as a result of the inability to excrete a water load and increased vasopressin release due to nausea, but it is not accompanied by hyperkalemia.

Hypotension occurs in about 90% of patients. It frequently causes orthostatic symptoms and occasionally syncope or recumbent hypotension. Hyperkalemia may cause cardiac arrhythmias, which are sometimes lethal. Refractory shock may occur in glucocorticoid-deficient individuals who are subjected to stress. Vascular smooth muscle becomes less responsive to circulating catecholamines, and capillaries dilate and become permeable. These effects impair vascular compensation for hypovolemia and promote vascular collapse. A reversible cardiomyopathy has also been described.

Cortisol deficiency commonly results in loss of appetite, weight loss, and GI disturbances. Weight loss is common and, in chronic cases, may be profound (15 kg or more). Nausea and vomiting occur in most patients; diarrhea is less frequent. Such GI symptoms often intensify during acute adrenal crisis.

In women with adrenal insufficiency, loss of pubic and axillary hair may occur as a result of decreased secretion of adrenal androgens. Amenorrhea occurs commonly, in most cases related to weight loss and chronic illness but sometimes as a result of ovarian failure.

CNS consequences of adrenal insufficiency include personality changes (irritability, apprehension, inability to concentrate, and emotional lability), increased sensitivity to olfactory and gustatory stimuli, and the appearance of electroencephalographic waves slower than the normal alpha rhythm.

Patients with **acute adrenal crisis** experience symptoms of fever, weakness, apathy, and confusion. Anorexia, nausea, and vomiting may lead to volume depletion and dehydration. Abdominal pain may mimic that of an acute abdominal process. Evidence suggests that the symptoms of acute glucocorticoid deficiency are mediated by significantly elevated plasma levels of cytokines, particularly IL-6 and, to a lesser extent, IL-1 and TNF. Hyponatremia, hyperkalemia, lymphocytosis, eosinophilia, and hypoglycemia occur frequently. Acute adrenal crisis can occur in patients with undiagnosed ACTH deficiency and in patients receiving corticosteroids who are not given an increased steroid dosage during periods of stress. Precipitants include infection, trauma, surgery, and dehydration. Gastrointestinal infections are particularly challenging because of the associated inability to ingest and absorb oral hydrocortisone replacement, which can lead to adrenal crisis despite other treatments. If unrecognized and untreated, coma, severe hypotension, or shock unresponsive to vasopressors may rapidly lead to death.

Laboratory findings in primary adrenocortical insufficiency include hyponatremia, hyperkalemia, occasional hypoglycemia, and mild azotemia (Table 21–6). The hyponatremia and hyperkalemia are manifestations of mineralocorticoid deficiency. The azotemia, with elevations of blood urea nitrogen (BUN) and serum creatinine, is due to volume depletion and dehydration. Mild acidosis is frequently present. Hypercalcemia of mild to moderate degree occurs infrequently.

TABLE 21–6 Typical plasma electrolyte levels in normal individuals and in patients with adrenocortical diseases.

	Na^+ (mEq/L)	K^+ (mEq/L)	Cl^- (mEq/L)	HCO_3^- (mEq/L)
Normal	142	4.5	105	25
Adrenal insufficiency	120	6.7	85	45
Primary aldosteronism	145	2.4	96	41
Hypoaldosteronism	145	6.7	105	25

Modified and reproduced, with permission, from Barrett KE et al, eds. *Ganong's Review of Medical Physiology*, 25th ed. McGraw-Hill, 2016.

Hematologic manifestations of adrenal insufficiency include normocytic, normochromic anemia, neutropenia, lymphocytosis, monocytosis, and eosinophilia. Abdominal x-ray films demonstrate adrenal calcification in about 50% of patients with Addison disease caused by adrenal tuberculosis and in a smaller percentage of patients with bilateral adrenal hemorrhage. CT scans detect adrenal calcification even more frequently in such cases and may also reveal bilateral adrenal enlargement in cases of adrenal hemorrhage; tuberculous, fungal, or cytomegalovirus infection; metastases; and other infiltrative diseases. Electrocardiographic findings include low voltage, a vertical QRS axis, and nonspecific ST wave changes related to electrolyte abnormalities (eg, peak T waves from hyperkalemia).

Diagnosis

A. Primary Adrenal Insufficiency

To establish the diagnosis of fully developed primary adrenal insufficiency, the physician must demonstrate an inability of the adrenal glands to respond normally to ACTH stimulation. This is usually done by performing an ACTH stimulation test (Figure 21–16). To do so, the physician obtains an 8:00 AM plasma cortisol level, then administers 250 μg of synthetic ACTH (cosyntropin) intravenously or intramuscularly. Repeat plasma cortisol levels are obtained 30 and 60 minutes later. Normal individuals demonstrate a rise in plasma cortisol levels to more than 18 μg/dL. Patients with Addison disease have a low 8:00 AM plasma cortisol (and high ACTH) and virtually no increase in plasma cortisol after cosyntropin.

B. Secondary Adrenocortical Insufficiency

The diagnosis of ACTH deficiency from exogenous glucocorticoids is suggested by obtaining a history of chronic glucocorticoid therapy or by finding cushingoid features on physical examination. Hypothalamic or pituitary tumors leading to ACTH deficiency usually produce symptoms and signs of other endocrinopathies. Deficient secretion of other pituitary hormones such as LH and FSH or TSH may produce hypogonadism or hypothyroidism (see Chapter 19). Excessive secretion of growth hormone or prolactin from a pituitary adenoma may

FIGURE 21–16 Diagnostic evaluation for suspected adrenal insufficiency. The first step is to perform a rapid ACTH stimulation test to ascertain whether there is adrenal insufficiency. Then, the plasma ACTH level differentiates between primary and secondary adrenal insufficiency. In cases in which the serum cortisol is normal after ACTH stimulation, but there is a high suspicion of adrenal insufficiency, or in which it may be of recent onset (eg, with pituitary apoplexy), an insulin tolerance test is conducted. Alternatively, a measurement of DHEAS, which, like cortisol, is dependent on the action of ACTH, or a metyrapone test can be helpful. Boxes enclose clinical diagnoses; ovals indicate diagnostic tests.

produce acromegaly or amenorrhea and galactorrhea. Unfortunately, the conventional ACTH stimulation test uses a dose (250 µg ACTH) that is supraphysiologic and capable of transiently stimulating the adrenal cortex in some patients with secondary (pituitary or hypothalamic) adrenal insufficiency. The "gold standard" test for diagnosing secondary adrenal insufficiency is the insulin tolerance test. An injection of insulin leads to hypoglycemia, which is detected by the hypothalamus, subsequently activating the entire hypothalamic–pituitary–adrenal cortex axis, provided that all axis components are intact. At the nadir of glucose levels, the patient must exhibit symptoms of hypoglycemia. A rise of plasma cortisol to more than 18 µg/dL as a response to symptomatic hypoglycemia excludes the diagnosis of secondary adrenal insufficiency.

CHECKPOINT

17. What are the major causes of glucocorticoid deficiency?
18. With what other autoimmune disorders is autoimmune adrenal failure associated?
19. What are the major causes of adrenal hemorrhage?
20. What are the clinical symptoms and signs of adrenal failure?
21. Name some different ways to diagnose adrenal insufficiency in a patient with suggestive symptoms and signs.

HYPERALDOSTERONISM (EXCESSIVE MINERALOCORTICOID PRODUCTION)

Primary aldosteronism occurs because of excessive unregulated aldosterone secretion by the adrenal cortex. It is now thought to be the most common potentially curable and specifically treatable cause of hypertension. **Secondary hyperaldosteronism** occurs when aldosterone secretion is stimulated by excessive renin secretion by the juxtaglomerular apparatus of the kidney.

The clinical features of hyperaldosteronism may also be due to non-aldosterone-mediated mineralocorticoid excess. Causes include Cushing syndrome, congenital adrenal hyperplasia resulting from 11β-hydroxylase deficiency or 17α-hydroxylase deficiency, the syndrome of apparent mineralocorticoid excess resulting from 11β-hydroxysteroid dehydrogenase (11β-HSD) deficiency, primary glucocorticoid resistance, and Liddle syndrome resulting from activating mutations of the gene encoding for β- and γ-subunits of the renal epithelial sodium channel.

Etiology

Table 21–7 lists the causes of hyperaldosteronism.

A. Primary Aldosteronism

Primary aldosteronism usually results from an aldosterone-secreting **adenoma** of the adrenal cortex (Figure 21–17) or

TABLE 21-7 Causes of hyperaldosteronism.

Primary aldosteronism
Aldosterone-secreting adrenocortical adenoma
Bilateral hyperplasia of zona glomerulosa
Glucocorticoid-remediable hyperaldosteronism
Aldosterone-secreting adrenocortical carcinoma (rare)
Idiopathic
Secondary hyperaldosteronism
Renal ischemia
Renal artery stenosis
Malignant hypertension
Decreased intravascular volume
Heart failure
Chronic diuretic or laxative use
Hypoproteinemic states (cirrhosis, nephrotic syndrome)
Sodium-wasting disorders
Chronic kidney diseases
Renal tubular acidosis
Juxtaglomerular cell hyperplasia (Bartter syndrome)
Surreptitious vomiting or diuretic ingestion (pseudo–Bartter syndrome)
Oral contraceptives
Renin-secreting tumors (rare)

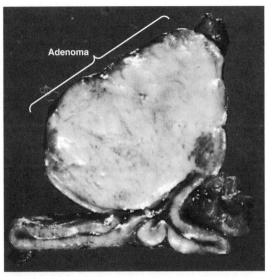

FIGURE 21-17 Cross-section of the adrenal, showing an adrenocortical adenoma in a patient with primary aldosteronism. The gross and microscopic features do not permit differentiation of aldosterone- and cortisol-secreting adenomas in most cases. (Reproduced, with permission, from Chandrasoma P et al, eds. *Concise Pathology*, 3rd ed. Originally published by Appleton & Lange. Copyright © 1998 by The McGraw-Hill Companies, Inc.)

bilateral hyperplasia of its zona glomerulosa. Adenomas are readily identified by their characteristic golden-yellow color. The adjacent adrenal cortex may be compressed. Adenomas producing excessive aldosterone are indistinguishable from those producing excessive cortisol, except that they tend to be smaller (usually <2 cm in diameter). Primary hyperaldosteronism was traditionally regarded as a rare cause of hypertension and not worth looking for in the absence of hypokalemia. However, the development and application of the ratio of plasma aldosterone concentration to plasma renin activity as a screening test for the population of hypertensives has resulted in a marked increase in detection rate, suggesting that primary aldosteronism is actually quite common in patients with hypertension; most have normal serum potassium levels. Up to 20% of patients diagnosed as having essential hypertension have primary aldosteronism. Aldosterone-producing adenomas often carry mutations in genes that impact electrophysiological properties of the cell membrane and ultimately lead to elevated intracellular calcium levels (eg, *KCNJ5*, *ATP2B3*, *CACNA1D*).

Bilateral adrenal hyperplasia accounts for 70% of cases of idiopathic (non-adenoma-related) primary aldosteronism. Affected patients have bilateral nonadenomatous hyperplasia of the zona glomerulosa. Selective adrenal vein sampling looking for lateralized aldosterone secretion is the most reliable means of differentiating a unilateral aldosterone-producing adenoma or hyperplasia from bilateral adrenal hyperplasia. For this procedure, both adrenal veins are cannulated and blood is drawn for aldosterone and cortisol (for normalization of relative aldosterone production). The ratio of aldosterone to cortisol on the side with the adenoma or hyperplasia will usually exceed the contralateral ratio by four times.

Unilateral adrenal hyperplasia is a rare cause of primary aldosteronism. Selective adrenal-vein sampling to determine plasma aldosterone concentrations can help define unilaterality of disease.

Adrenocortical carcinomas producing only aldosterone are extremely rare. Such tumors are generally large.

Three different forms of genetic primary aldosteronism have been described. All are inherited in an autosomal dominant fashion.

Type 1 primary aldosteronism is **glucocorticoid-remediable aldosteronism**. As noted in Chapter 11, affected patients have a "hybrid" 11β-hydroxylase-aldosterone synthase gene in which the 11β-hydroxylase gene's regulatory elements are fused to the coding region of the aldosterone synthase gene. Therefore, ACTH stimulates aldosterone synthase activity. The hybrid *CYP11B1/CYP11B2* gene arises from an unequal crossing-over between the two *CYP11B* genes during meiosis. The hybrid gene can be detected in peripheral blood leukocyte DNA. The clinical phenotype varies from mild blood pressure elevation to severe early-onset hypertension; hypokalemia is usually mild. Affected individuals apparently have an increased risk of premature stroke. Because expression of the hybrid gene is stimulated by ACTH, leading to an increased production of aldosterone and other steroids, the hyperaldosteronism is glucocorticoid suppressible. Treatment with low doses of dexamethasone inhibits ACTH. **Type 2 primary aldosteronism** has been linked to a locus on chromosome 7p22, but the underlying defect has not been elucidated. **Type 3 primary aldosteronism** is caused by mutations in *KCNJ5*, an inward rectifying potassium channel, leading to a loss of cation specificity.

B. Secondary Hyperaldosteronism

Secondary hyperaldosteronism is common. It results from excessive renin production by the juxtaglomerular apparatus of the kidney. The high renin output occurs in response to (1) renal ischemia (eg, renal artery stenosis or malignant hypertension); (2) decreased intravascular volume (eg, heart failure, cirrhosis, nephrotic syndrome, laxative or diuretic abuse); (3) Na^+-wasting disorders (eg, chronic kidney disease, renal tubular acidosis); (4) hyperplasia of the juxtaglomerular apparatus (Bartter syndrome); or (5) renin-secreting tumors. In these states, stimulation of the zona glomerulosa by the renin–angiotensin system leads to increased aldosterone production.

Pathologically, in secondary hyperaldosteronism, the adrenals may appear grossly normal, but microscopically there may be hyperplasia of the zona glomerulosa.

Pathophysiology

In primary aldosteronism, there is a primary (autonomous) increase in aldosterone production by the abnormal zona glomerulosa tissue (adenoma or hyperplasia). However, circulating levels of aldosterone are still modulated to some extent by variations in ACTH secretion. The chronic aldosterone excess results in expansion of the extracellular fluid volume and plasma volume. In turn, this expansion is registered by stretch receptors of the juxtaglomerular apparatus and Na^+ flux at the macula densa, leading to the suppression of renin production and low circulating plasma renin activity.

Patients with secondary hyperaldosteronism also produce excessively large amounts of aldosterone, but, in contrast to patients with primary hyperaldosteronism, plasma renin activity is not suppressed.

Clinical Consequences of Mineralocorticoid Excess

The major consequences of chronic aldosterone excess are Na^+ retention and K^+ and H^+ wasting by the kidney.

The excess aldosterone initially stimulates Na^+ reabsorption by the renal collecting and distal tubules, causing the extracellular fluid volume to expand and the blood pressure to rise. When the extracellular fluid expansion reaches a certain point, however, Na^+ excretion resumes despite the continued action of aldosterone on the renal tubule. This **"escape" phenomenon** is probably due to the increased secretion of **atrial natriuretic peptide**. Because the escape phenomenon causes the excretion of excess salt, affected patients are not edematous. Such escape from the action of aldosterone does not occur in the distal tubules. There, the elevated aldosterone levels promote continued exchange of Na^+ for K^+ and H^+, causing K^+ depletion and alkalosis. Affected patients are not markedly hypernatremic, because water is retained along with the Na^+.

The chronic aldosterone excess also produces a prolonged K^+ diuresis. Total body K^+ stores are depleted, and hypokalemia develops. Patients may complain of tiredness, loss of stamina, weakness, nocturia, and lassitude, all symptoms of K^+ depletion. Prolonged K^+ depletion damages the kidneys (**hypokalemic nephropathy**), causing ADH (vasopressin) resistance. The resultant loss of concentrating ability causes thirst and polyuria (especially nocturnal).

When the K^+ loss is marked, intracellular K^+ is replaced by Na^+ and H^+. The intracellular movement of H^+, along with the increased renal secretion of H^+, causes metabolic alkalosis to develop.

Hypertension—related to Na^+ retention and plasma volume expansion—is a characteristic finding. Hypertension can range from borderline to severe but is usually mild or moderate. Accelerated (malignant) hypertension is extremely rare. Because the hypertension is sustained, however, it may produce retinopathy, renal damage, or left ventricular hypertrophy. For example, patients with primary aldosteronism resulting from aldosterone-producing adenomas have increased wall thickness and mass and decreased early diastolic filling of the left ventricle compared with patients who have essential hypertension. Thus, the chance of curing hypertension with resection of an adrenal adenoma is less predictable than the likelihood of correcting the related biochemical abnormalities. Only 50% of patients with adenomas are normotensive 5 years after adrenalectomy; old patients in particular are more likely to require postoperative antihypertensive medications. Patients with no family history of hypertension and who required two or fewer antihypertensive agents preoperatively are more likely to resolve their hypertension after the removal of an adrenal tumor.

The heart may be mildly enlarged as a result of plasma volume expansion and left ventricular hypertrophy. Severely K^+-depleted patients may develop baroreceptor function blunting, manifested by postural falls in blood pressure without reflex tachycardia, or even malignant arrhythmias and sudden cardiac death.

The K^+ depletion causes a minor but detectable degree of carbohydrate intolerance (demonstrated by an abnormal glucose tolerance test). This may be due to impaired pancreatic insulin release and reduced insulin sensitivity related to the hypokalemia. The decrease in glucose tolerance is corrected after K^+ repletion.

In addition, the alkalosis accompanying severe K^+ depletion may lower the plasma Ca^{2+} to the point at which latent or frank tetany occurs (see Chapter 17). The hypokalemia may cause severe muscle weakness, muscle cramps, and intestinal atony. Paresthesias may develop as a result of the hypokalemia and alkalosis. A positive Trousseau or Chvostek sign is suggestive of alkalosis and hypocalcemia (see Chapter 17).

Laboratory findings in hyperaldosteronism include hypokalemia and alkalosis (see Table 21–6). Typically, the serum K^+ is below 3.6 mEq/L (3.6 mmol/L), serum Na^+ is normal or slightly elevated, serum HCO_3^- is increased, and serum Cl^- is decreased (hypokalemic, hypochloremic metabolic alkalosis). There is an inappropriately large amount of K^+ in the urine.

The hematocrit may be reduced because of hemodilution by the expanded plasma volume. Affected patients may fail to concentrate urine and may have abnormal glucose tolerance tests.

The plasma renin level is suppressed in primary aldosteronism and elevated in secondary hyperaldosteronism. Adrenal cortisol production is usually unaffected.

The ECG may show changes of modest left ventricular hypertrophy and K^+ depletion (a flattening of T waves and the appearance of U waves).

Diagnosis of Hyperaldosteronism

A. Primary Aldosteronism

In the past, the diagnosis of primary aldosteronism was usually suggested by finding hypokalemia in an untreated patient with hypertension (ie, one not taking diuretics) (see Table 21–6). However, a low Na^+ intake, by diminishing renal K^+ loss, may mask total body K^+ depletion. In patients with normal renal function, dietary salt loading will unmask hypokalemia as a manifestation of total body K^+ depletion. Thus, finding a low serum K^+ in a hypertensive patient with a high salt intake and not receiving diuretics warrants further evaluation for hyperaldosteronism. Currently, the best screening test for primary aldosteronism involves determining the plasma aldosterone concentration (normal: 1–14 ng/dL) and plasma renin activity (normal: >1 ng/mL/h) and calculating the plasma aldosterone–renin ratio (normal: <30). Patients with aldosterone–renin ratios of 30 or more require further evaluation. However, a prerequisite for hyperaldosteronism is an increased aldosterone level of at least 14 ng/dL.

Subsequent workup entails measuring the 24-hour urinary aldosterone excretion and the plasma aldosterone level with the patient on a diet containing more than 120 mEq of Na^+ per day. On a high-sodium diet in primary aldosteronism, the urinary aldosterone excretion exceeds 14 μg/24 h, and the supine plasma aldosterone is usually greater than 14 ng/dL. Alternatively, patients can either be challenged by infusing saline or fludrocortisone, a synthetic mineralocorticoid. In both cases, the normal physiological response is a decrease in plasma aldosterone level. Patients with autonomous aldosterone production exhibit elevated or inappropriately "normal" plasma aldosterone levels (ie, "normal" despite suppressed renin levels, which should result in the physiologic suppression of aldosterone).

High-resolution CT or MRI of the adrenal glands may help to differentiate between **adrenal adenoma** and bilateral **adrenal hyperplasia**. However, the gold standard for diagnosing a unilateral cause of primary aldosteronism is bilateral adrenal venous sampling, which is more sensitive and specific than imaging.

B. Secondary Hyperaldosteronism

Patients with secondary hyperaldosteronism due to malignant hypertension, renal artery stenosis, or chronic renal disease also excrete large amounts of aldosterone but, in contrast to patients with primary aldosteronism, demonstrate elevated plasma renin activity.

HYPOALDOSTERONISM: DEFICIENT MINERALOCORTICOID PRODUCTION OR ACTION

Primary mineralocorticoid deficiency (hypoaldosteronism) may result from the destruction of adrenocortical tissue, which invariably results in both androgen and glucocorticoid deficiency. It can also be caused by defects in the adrenal synthesis of aldosterone or the inadequate stimulation of aldosterone secretion (hyporeninemic hypoaldosteronism). Resistance to the downstream effectors of aldosterone, such as are seen in pseudohypoaldosteronism, cause increased aldosterone levels but decreased aldosterone action. Hypoaldosteronism is characterized by Na^+ loss, with hyponatremia, hypovolemia, and hypotension, and impaired secretion of both K^+ and H^+ in the renal tubules, resulting in hyperkalemia and metabolic acidosis. Renin activity is typically increased.

A **secondary deficiency** of endogenous mineralocorticoids may occur when renin production is suppressed or deficient. Renin production may be suppressed by the Na^+ retention and volume expansion resulting from exogenous mineralocorticoids (fludrocortisone acetate) or substances causing mineralocorticoid-like effects (licorice, carbenoxolone). When this happens, hypertension, hypokalemia, and metabolic alkalosis result. When renin production is deficient and unable to stimulate mineralocorticoid production, Na^+ loss, hyperkalemia, and metabolic acidosis occur.

Etiology

Acute and chronic adrenocortical insufficiency were discussed previously. In long-standing **hypopituitarism**, some atrophy of the zona glomerulosa may occur, and the increase in aldosterone secretion normally produced by surgery or other stress is absent. **Hyporeninemic hypoaldosteronism (type IV renal tubular acidosis)** is a disorder characterized by hyperkalemia and acidosis in association with (usually mild) chronic renal insufficiency. Typically, affected individuals are men in the fifth to seventh decades of life who have underlying pyelonephritis, diabetes mellitus, gout, or nephrotic syndrome. The chronic renal insufficiency is usually not severe enough to account for the hyperkalemia. Plasma and urinary aldosterone levels and plasma renin activity are consistently low and unresponsive to stimulation by upright posture, dietary Na^+ restriction, and furosemide administration. The syndrome is thought to be due to an impairment of the juxtaglomerular apparatus associated with the underlying renal disease. Hyporeninemic hypoaldosteronism has also been described transiently in critically ill patients, such as those with septic shock.

Two genetic disorders may produce the symptoms and signs of hypoaldosteronism. In **congenital adrenal hyperplasia**, there are enzymatic abnormalities in mineralocorticoid biosynthesis (see below). Mutations in the *CYP11B2* gene for 11-hydroxylase cause **aldosterone synthase deficiency**, an isolated defect of aldosterone biosynthesis. Aldosterone levels are low. In **pseudohypoaldosteronism**, there is renal tubular resistance to mineralocorticoid hormones. Affected patients manifest symptoms and signs of hypoaldosteronism, but aldosterone levels are high. **Pseudohypoaldosteronism type 1** is frequently due to mutations involving the amiloride-sensitive epithelial sodium channel. Gordon syndrome (**pseudohypoaldosteronism type 2**), characterized by hypertension, hyperchloremic acidemia, hyperkalemia, and intact renal function, is due to resistance to the kaliuretic but not sodium reabsorptive effects of aldosterone. The genetic basis of this condition is still unknown.

Clinical Consequences of Mineralocorticoid Deficiency

Patients undergoing bilateral adrenalectomy, if not given mineralocorticoid replacement therapy, will develop profound urinary Na^+ losses resulting in hypovolemia, hypotension, and, eventually, shock and death. In adrenal insufficiency, these changes can be delayed by increasing the dietary salt intake. However, the amount of dietary salt needed to prevent them entirely is so large that collapse and death are inevitable unless mineralocorticoid treatment with fludrocortisone acetate is also initiated. Secretion of both K^+ and H^+ is impaired in the renal tubule, resulting in hyperkalemia and metabolic acidosis.

CONGENITAL ADRENAL HYPERPLASIA

The adrenal cortex also secretes androgen-related steroids, principally **androstenedione, dehydroepiandrosterone (DHEA)**, and **dehydroepiandrosterone sulfate (DHEAS)**. In general, the secretion of adrenal androgens parallels that of cortisol. ACTH is the major factor regulating androgen production by the adrenal cortex. The adrenal androgens are secreted in an unbound state but circulate weakly bound to plasma proteins, chiefly albumin. They are metabolized either by degradation and inactivation or by peripheral conversion to the more potent androgens testosterone and dihydrotestosterone. The androgen metabolites are conjugated either as glucuronides or sulfates and excreted in the urine.

DHEA has both masculinizing and anabolic effects. However, it is less than one-fifth as potent as the androgens produced by the testis. Consequently, it has very little physiologic effect under normal conditions. In women, the androgenic steroids (adrenal and ovarian) are thought to be required for the maintenance of libido and the capacity to achieve orgasm.

In **congenital adrenal hyperplasia**, excessive secretion of adrenal androgens results from one of several enzymatic defects in steroid metabolism. This disorder occurs in both sexes, and it is the most common cause of ambiguous genitalia. It is a relatively common disease, occurring in 1 in 5000 to 1 in 15,000 births.

Congenital adrenal hyperplasia is actually a group of autosomal recessive disorders, in each of which, because of an enzyme defect, the bulk of steroid hormone production by the adrenal cortex shifts from corticosteroids to androgens. Congenital adrenal hyperplasia is caused by mutations in the *CYP21*, *CYP11B1*, *CYP17*, and *3βHSD* genes that encode steroidogenic enzymes, and by mutations in the gene encoding the intracellular cholesterol transport protein, steroidogenic acute regulatory protein (StAR). Each of these defects causes different biochemical and clinical consequences. The name of the syndrome derives from the fact that all the biochemical defects lead to impaired cortisol secretion, resulting in compensatory ACTH hypersecretion and consequent adrenal cortex hyperplasia. By far, the most frequent cause of congenital adrenal hyperplasia is 21β-hydroxylase deficiency, followed by 11β-hydroxylase deficiency (see Figure 21–3). More than 90% of cases are due to a deficiency in the enzyme steroid 21β-hydroxylase. The 21β-hydroxylase enzyme (cytochrome P450c21) is encoded by the gene *CYP21A2*. More than 50 different *CYP21A2* mutations have been reported, perhaps accounting for a wide range of congenital adrenal hyperplasia phenotypes. The 15 most common mutations, which constitute 90–95% of alleles, derive from intergenic recombination of DNA sequences between the *CYP21A2* gene and a neighboring pseudogene (an inactive gene that is transcribed but not translated). These intergenic *CYP21A2* mutations are caused by the conversion of a portion of the active *CYP21A2* gene sequence into a pseudogene sequence, resulting in a less active or inactive gene (gene conversion).

Other cases of congenital adrenal hyperplasia are related to steroid 11β-hydroxylase (cytochrome P450c11) deficiency. This form of congenital adrenal hyperplasia is associated with so-called deletion hybrid genes, because of an unequal crossing-over between *CYP11B1* (11β-hydroxylase) and *CYP11B2* (aldosterone synthase). *CYP11B1*, the gene encoding 11β-hydroxylase, is expressed in high levels in the zona fasciculata and is regulated by ACTH. *CYP11B2*, the gene encoding aldosterone synthase, is expressed in the zona glomerulosa and is primarily regulated by the renin–angiotensin system.

Impaired *CYP21A2* or *CYP11B1* activity causes deficient production of both cortisol and aldosterone. The low serum cortisol stimulates ACTH production; adrenal hyperplasia occurs, and precursor steroids—in particular 17-hydroxyprogesterone—accumulate. The accumulated precursors cannot enter the cortisol synthesis pathway and thus spill over into the androgen synthesis pathway, forming androstenedione and DHEA/DHEAS. Prenatal exposure to excessive androgens results in masculinization of the female fetus, leading to ambiguous genitalia at birth. Newborn males have normal genitalia.

During the newborn period, there are two classic presentations of congenital adrenal hyperplasia resulting from classic 21β-hydroxylase deficiency: salt wasting and non–salt wasting (also called "simple virilizing"). Neonates with the salt-wasting form have severe cortisol and aldosterone deficiencies and, if undiagnosed and untreated, will develop potentially lethal adrenal crisis and salt wasting at 2–3 weeks of age. Those with the simple virilizing form have sufficient cortisol and aldosterone production to avoid both adrenal crisis and salt wasting and are usually diagnosed because of virilization between birth and 5 years of age. Postnatally, both sexes present with virilization, reflecting the continuing androgen excess. The excess androgens during childhood can produce pseudoprecocious puberty, premature growth acceleration, early epiphyseal fusion, and adult short stature. Variability in the phenotype occurs, depending on the severity of the 21β-hydroxylase deficiency.

The diagnosis of 21β-hydroxylase-deficient nonclassic adrenal hyperplasia is suggested by finding a morning plasma level of the cortisol precursor 17-hydroxyprogesterone more than 200 ng/dL (12.0 nmol/L) (obtained in women during the follicular phase) or more than 10,000 ng/dL (30.3 nmol/L) after ACTH stimulation (see Figure 21–3). The diagnosis of specific defects is confirmed by genotyping the relevant genes.

After birth, lifelong hormonal replacement with hydrocortisone (glucocorticoid) and fludrocortisone (mineralocorticoid) can ensure normal puberty and fertility. Antiandrogen therapy (with flutamide) might permit a reduction in the dose of hydrocortisone sometimes required to suppress androgen levels.

CHECKPOINT

25. What are the causes of hypoaldosteronism?
26. What are the clinical manifestations of hypoaldosteronism?
27. What is the effect of adrenal androgen excess or deficiency on otherwise normal adult men and women (ie, individuals with normal gonads)?

CASE STUDIES

Yeong Kwok, MD

(See Chapter 25, p. 784–86 for answers)

CASE 113

A 35-year-old woman has hypertension of recent onset. The review of systems reveals several months of weight gain and menstrual irregularity. On examination, she is obese, with a plethoric appearance. The blood pressure is 165/98 mm Hg. There are prominent purplish striae over the abdomen and multiple bruises over both lower legs. The patient's physician entertains a diagnosis of hypercortisolism (Cushing syndrome).

Questions

A. What other features of the history and physical examination should be sought?
B. Assuming that the diagnosis of hypercortisolism is correct, what is the underlying pathogenesis of this patient's hypertension, weight gain, and skin striae?
C. List four causes of Cushing syndrome, and discuss the relationships among the hypothalamus, pituitary, and adrenal in each. Which is the most likely cause in this patient?
D. How can the diagnosis of hypercortisolism be established in this patient?

CASE 114

A 56-year-old man undergoes an abdominal CT scan in the evaluation of abdominal pain. The scan is unremarkable except for the finding of a 3 cm mass in the right adrenal gland. The mass is homogeneous and smooth, and it has low x-ray absorption on the CT scan. The patient has a normal examination and feels well otherwise.

Questions

A. What other features of the history and physical examination should be sought?
B. What follow-up needs to be pursued, and why?

CASE 115

A 38-year-old woman presents for an annual follow-up of previously diagnosed Hashimoto (autoimmune) thyroiditis, for which she has been receiving thyroid replacement therapy (levothyroxine, 0.15 mg/d). She reports a gradual onset of weakness, lethargy, and easy fatigability over the last 3 months. The review of systems reveals only recent menstrual irregularity, with no menses in 2.5 months. Her blood pressure is 90/50 mm Hg (compared with previous readings of 110/75 and 120/80 mm Hg), and her weight is down 13 pounds since her last visit 11 months ago. Her skin appears to be tanned, but the patient denies sun exposure. The physician seeing her wonders whether she has now developed autoimmune adrenal insufficiency (Addison disease).

Questions

A. What other features of the history and physical examination should be sought?
B. If Addison disease has developed, what should the serum electrolytes show, and why?
C. How can the diagnosis of adrenal insufficiency be established in this patient?
D. What is the pathogenesis of this patient's hypotension, weight loss, and skin hyperpigmentation?

CASE 116

A 42-year-old man presents for an evaluation of newly diagnosed hypertension. He is currently taking no medications and offers no complaints. A careful review of systems reveals symptoms of fatigue, loss of stamina, and frequent urination, particularly at night. The physical examination is normal except for a blood pressure of 168/100 mm Hg. Serum electrolytes are reported as follows: sodium, 152 mEq/L; potassium, 3.2 mEq/L; bicarbonate, 32 mEq/L; chloride, 112 mEq/L. The clinical picture is consistent with a diagnosis of primary aldosteronism.

Questions

A. What is the mechanism by which primary aldosteronism causes the history, physical examination, and laboratory findings in this patient?
B. What should the urinalysis and measurement of urine electrolytes show, and why?
C. How can the diagnosis of primary aldosteronism be established in this patient?

CASE 117

A 64-year-old man with a long history of gout and type 2 diabetes mellitus comes in for a routine check-up. Serum chemistries are as follows: sodium, 140 mEq/L; potassium, 6.3 mEq/L; bicarbonate, 18 mEq/L; BUN, 43 mg/dL; creatinine, 2.9 mg/dL; glucose, 198 mg/dL. A chart review shows previous potassium values of 5.3 mEq/L and 5.7 mEq/L. The patient is currently taking only colchicine, 0.5 mg orally once daily, and glyburide, 5 mg orally twice daily.

Questions

A. What is the most likely cause of this patient's hyperkalemia, and what is its pathogenesis?
B. What are other possible causes of hypoaldosteronism?
C. Plasma renin activity and aldosterone levels are sent to the laboratory. What results should be anticipated?

CASE 118

A newborn full-term male infant is screened for 21-hydroxylase deficiency at birth and is noted to have a high 17-hydroxyprogesterone level on a heel stick blood sample. Both parents are healthy, and there is no history of hormonal problems in the family. The baby appears normal with normal vital signs and physical examination. He is brought back for a repeat examination at 2 weeks, and repeat blood tests show a still elevated 17-hydroxyprogesterone level. In addition, he now has a serum sodium of 125 mEq/L, a potassium of 5.6 mEq/L, and a glucose of 60 mg/dL. He is suspected of having the salt wasting form of congenital adrenal hyperplasia.

Questions

A. Why do most newborns undergo screening for this condition?
B. What are the genetic abnormalities in this condition?
C. How does this disorder lead to ambiguous genitalia in female infants?

REFERENCES

General

Carroll TB et al. Glucocorticoids and adrenal androgens. In: Gardner DG et al, eds. *Greenspan's Basic & Clinical Endocrinology*, 10th ed. McGraw-Hill, 2017.

Hammer GD et al. *Adrenocortical Carcinoma: Basic Science and Clinical Concepts*. Springer, 2010.

Cushing Syndrome

Carroll TB et al. Cushing's syndrome of nonpituitary causes. Curr Opin Endocrinol Diabetes Obes. 2009 Aug;16(4):308–15. [PMID: 19491665]

Carroll TB et al. The diagnosis of Cushing's syndrome. Rev Endocr Metab Disord. 2010 Jun;11(2):147–53. [PMID: 20821267]

Di Dalmazi G et al. Subclinical hypercortisolism: a state, a syndrome, or a disease? Eur J Endocrinol. 2015 Oct;173(4):M61–71. [PMID: 26282599]

Else T et al. Adrenocortical carcinoma. Endocr Rev. 2014 Apr;35(2):282–326. [PMID: 24423978]

Espiard S et al. The genetics of adrenocortical tumors. Endocrinol Metab Clin North Am. 2015 Jun;44(2):311–34. [PMID: 26038203]

Lacroix A et al. Cushing's syndrome. Lancet. 2015 Aug 29;386(9996):913–27. [PMID: 26004339]

Lodish M et al. A genetic and molecular update on adrenocortical causes of Cushing syndrome. Nat Rev Endocrinol. 2016 May;12(5):255–62. [PMID: 26965378]

Loriaux DL. Diagnosis and differential diagnosis of Cushing's syndrome. N Engl J Med. 2017 Apr 13;376(15):1451–9. [PMID: 28402781]

Patel J et al. Nelson's syndrome: a review of the clinical manifestations, pathophysiology, and treatment strategies. Neurosurg Focus. 2015 Feb;38(2):E14. [PMID: 25639316]

Raff H et al. Cushing's syndrome: from physiological principles to diagnosis and clinical care. J Physiol. 2015 Feb 1;593(3):493–506. [PMID: 25480800]

Raff H et al. Physiological basis for the etiology, diagnosis, and treatment of adrenal disorders: Cushing's syndrome, adrenal insufficiency, and congenital adrenal hyperplasia. Compr Physiol. 2014 Apr;4(2):739–69. [PMID: 24715566]

Valassi E et al. Clinical consequences of Cushing's syndrome. Pituitary. 2012 Sep;15(3):319–29. [PMID: 22527617]

Clinically Inapparent Adrenal Mass ("Incidentaloma")

Debono M et al. Subclinical hypercortisolism in adrenal incidentaloma. Curr Opin Endocrinol Diabetes Obes. 2015 Jun;22(3):185–92. [PMID: 25871961]

Fassnacht M et al. Management of adrenal incidentalomas: European Society of Endocrinology Clinical Practice Guideline in collaboration with the European Network for the Study of Adrenal Tumors. Eur J Endocrinol. 2016 Aug;175(2):G1–34. [PMID: 27390021]

Ioachimescu AG et al. Adrenal incidentalomas: a disease of modern technology offering opportunities for improved patient care. Endocrinol Metab Clin North Am. 2015 Jun;44(2):335–54. [PMID: 26038204]

Paschou SA et al. Subclinical Cushing's syndrome in patients with bilateral compared to unilateral adrenal incidentalomas: a systematic review and meta-analysis. Endocrine. 2016 Feb;51(2):225–35. [PMID: 26498946]

Sabet FA et al. Likelihood ratio of computed tomography characteristics for diagnosis of malignancy in adrenal incidentaloma: systematic review and meta-analysis. J Diabetes Metab Disord. 2016 Apr 21;15:12. [PMID: 27104171]

Adrenocortical Insufficiency

Bornstein SR et al. Diagnosis and treatment of primary adrenal insufficiency: an Endocrine Society Clinical Practice Guideline. J Clin Endocrinol Metab. 2016 Feb;101(2):364–89. [PMID: 26760044]

Crowley RK et al. Central hypoadrenalism. J Clin Endocrinol Metab. 2014 Nov;99(11):4027–36. [PMID: 25140404]

Grossman AB. Clinical review: the diagnosis and management of central hypoadrenalism. J Clin Endocrinol Metab. 2010 Nov;95(11):4855–63. [PMID: 20719838]

Hannah-Shmouni F et al. Cortisol in the evaluation of adrenal insufficiency. JAMA. 2016 Aug 2;316(5):535–6. [PMID: 27483068]

Ospina NS et al. ACTH stimulation tests for the diagnosis of adrenal insufficiency: systematic review and meta-analysis. J Clin Endocrinol Metab. 2016 Feb;101(2):427–34. [PMID: 26649617]

Puar TH et al. Adrenal crisis: still a deadly event in the 21st century. Am J Med. 2016 Mar;129(3):339.e1–9. [PMID: 26363354]

Raff H et al. Physiological basis for the etiology, diagnosis, and treatment of adrenal disorders: Cushing's syndrome, adrenal insufficiency, and congenital adrenal hyperplasia. Compr Physiol. 2014 Apr;4(2):739–69. [PMID: 24715566]

Hyperaldosteronism

Asbach E et al. Recent developments in primary aldosteronism. Exp Clin Endocrinol Diabetes. 2016 Jun;124(6):335–41. [PMID: 27219889]

Douillard C et al. SFE/SFHTA/AFCE consensus on primary aldosteronism, part 2: first diagnostic steps. Ann Endocrinol (Paris). 2016 Jul;77(3):192–201. [PMID: 27177498]

Funder JW. Genetic disorders in primary aldosteronism—familial and somatic. J Steroid Biochem Mol Biol. 2017 Jan;165(Pt A):154–7. [PMID: 27013018]

Funder JW et al. The management of primary aldosteronism: case detection, diagnosis, and treatment: an Endocrine Society Clinical Practice Guideline. J Clin Endocrinol Metab. 2016 May;101(5):1889–916. [PMID: 26934393]

Monticone S et al. Understanding primary aldosteronism: impact of next generation sequencing and expression profiling. Mol Cell Endocrinol. 2015 Jan 5;399:311–20. [PMID: 25240470]

Reznik Y et al. SFE/SFHTA/AFCE consensus on primary aldosteronism, part 3: Confirmatory testing. Ann Endocrinol (Paris). 2016 Jul;77(3):202–7. [PMID: 27318644]

Stowasser M et al. Primary aldosteronism: changing definitions and new concepts of physiology and pathophysiology both inside and outside the kidney. Physiol Rev. 2016 Oct;96(4):1327–84. [PMID: 27535640]

Hypoaldosteronism

Sousa AG et al. Hyporeninemic hypoaldosteronism and diabetes mellitus: pathophysiology assumptions, clinical aspects and implications for management. World J Diabetes. 2016 Mar 10;7(5):101–11. [PMID: 26981183]

Wilczynski C et al. Selective hypoaldosteronism: a review. Endocr Pract. 2015 Aug;21(8):957–65. [PMID: 26121445]

Congenital Adrenal Hyperplasia

Bachelot A et al. Management of endocrine disease: congenital adrenal hyperplasia due to 21-hydroxylase deficiency: update on the management of adult patients and prenatal treatment. Eur J Endocrinol. 2017 Apr;176(4):R167–81. [PMID: 28115464]

Bulsari K et al. Clinical perspectives in congenital adrenal hyperplasia due to 11β-hydroxylase deficiency. Endocrine. 2017 Jan;55(1):19–36. [PMID: 27928728]

Falhammar H et al. Biochemical and genetic diagnosis of 21-hydroxylase deficiency. Endocrine. 2015 Nov;50(2):306–14. [PMID: 2633683]

Parsa AA et al. Steroid 21-hydroxylase deficiency in congenital adrenal hyperplasia. J Steroid Biochem Mol Biol. 2017 Jan;165(Pt A):2–11. [PMID: 27380651]

Raff H et al. Physiological basis for the etiology, diagnosis, and treatment of adrenal disorders: Cushing's syndrome, adrenal insufficiency, and congenital adrenal hyperplasia. Compr Physiol. 2014 Apr;4(2):739–69. [PMID: 24715566]

Speiser PW. Congenital adrenal hyperplasia. F1000Res. 2015 Aug 20;4(F100 Faculty Review):601. [PMID: 26339484]

Disorders of the Female Reproductive Tract

Erika B. Johnston-MacAnanny, MD,
Bansari G. Patel, MD, & Robert N. Taylor,
MD, PhD

Disorders of the female reproductive system can occur as a result of disease in one of the many reproductive organs: the ovaries, the fallopian tubes, the uterus, the cervix, the vagina, or the breast. During the reproductive years, these disorders often present as **altered menstruation**, **pelvic pain**, or **infertility**. Cancers arising in these tissues occur more often in the late reproductive or menopausal years. Unfortunately, for several reasons, they often have high mortality rates and a high incidence of metastases when diagnosed. Some organs are located deep and are relatively inaccessible to palpation (ovaries). Others have few sensory nerves (ovary, fallopian tubes) and hence remain asymptomatic. Additionally, the breasts have large amounts of adipose tissue, which can make early detection of breast cancer difficult. The one exception is the uterine cervix. Its easy access enables screening by use of the Papanicolaou smear and human papillomavirus (HPV) testing; this screening has led to a dramatically reduced mortality rate of cervical cancer.

Disorders of the female reproductive system can also occur as a result of disease in other organs whose function affects reproductive organs (eg, brain, hypothalamus, pituitary, thyroid, adrenals, kidney, liver). The presentation of these disorders is typically painless.

Conversely, disorders of the reproductive system can cause disorders in other tissues. Ovarian hormones are necessary for the maintenance and health of most tissues in women. Alterations in these hormones can lead to **osteoporosis** (loss of bone mass), atrophy and inflammation of estrogen-deprived tissues (eg, atrophic vaginitis), atherogenesis and alterations in cardiovascular compliance, and an increased risk of some forms of cancer (eg, endometrial carcinoma as a consequence of estrogen excess and progesterone deficiency). Dysfunction of the reproductive system can also contribute to unique variants of systemic disorders, such as gestational diabetes and the hypertensive syndrome of preeclampsia-eclampsia, affecting 5% of pregnancies and associated with a high risk of cardiovascular death.

CHECKPOINT

1. How do female reproductive system disorders present during the reproductive years?
2. To what might you ascribe the lack of reduction in mortality rate from ovarian cancer in contrast to cervical cancer?
3. What are some consequences of reproductive system dysfunction?

NORMAL STRUCTURE & FUNCTION OF THE FEMALE REPRODUCTIVE TRACT

ANATOMY

The reproductive pelvic organs include the vagina, cervix, uterus, fallopian tubes, and ovaries (Figure 22–1). The two **ovaries** contain thousands of **follicles**, each with an **oocyte** surrounded by a layer of **granulosa cells** and **thecal cells**. These supporting cells produce steroids and paracrine products important in follicular maturation and the coordination of events in reproduction. The **fallopian tubes**, which are open to the peritoneal space, connect the ovaries to the uterus. The **uterus** contains an internal hormone-sensitive mucosal lining, the **endometrium**. During nonpregnant cycles, menstrual bleeding occurs as the monthly culmination of endometrial growth, differentiation, and sloughing in response to changes in blood levels of estrogen and progesterone (Figure 22–2).

FIGURE 22–1 Anatomic landmarks of the uterus and adjacent organs. (Redrawn, with permission, from Chandrasoma P et al. *Concise Pathology*, 3rd ed. Originally published by Appleton & Lange. Copyright © 1998 by The McGraw-Hill Companies, Inc.)

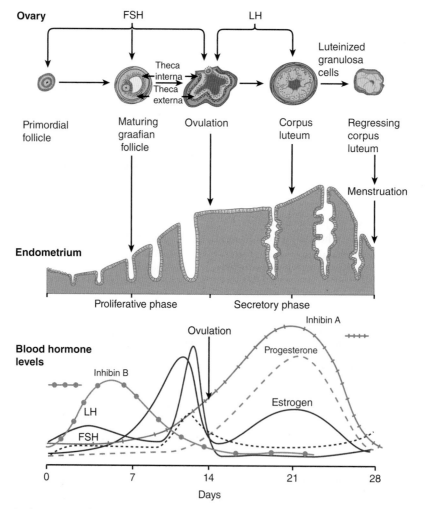

FIGURE 22–2 Changes in the ovary, endometrium, and blood hormone levels during the menstrual cycle. Anti-müllerian hormone levels stay constant during the cycle. (FSH, follicle-stimulating hormone; LH, luteinizing hormone.) (Redrawn, with permission, from Chandrasoma P et al. *Concise Pathology*, 3rd ed. Originally published by Appleton & Lange. Copyright © 1998 by The McGraw-Hill Companies, Inc.)

During pregnancy, the endometrium produces a wide variety of endocrine and paracrine products, which promote embryonic implantation (see Figure 22–1). Surrounding the endometrium is the smooth muscle layer of the uterus, the **myometrium**. Contractions of the myometrium lead to menstrual cramps or expel the fetus at parturition. The cervix is contiguous with the uterus and is the conduit for passage of menses or the fetus into the **vagina**, the muscular tube opening into the vulva.

The **breasts** (Figure 22–3) produce, store, and eject milk upon appropriate hormonal and physical stimulation.

SEXUAL DIFFERENTIATION & MATURATION OF ESTROGEN-DEPENDENT TISSUES

Embryonic Sexual Differentiation

During embryonic development, the primordial gametes originate in the endoderm of the yolk sac, allantois, and hindgut and migrate to the genital ridge by week 5 or 6 of gestation. Once at the genital ridge, they multiply and induce male or female gonads depending on the identity of the sex chromosomes.

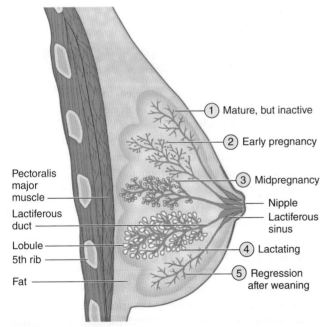

Pectoralis major muscle
Lactiferous duct
Lobule
5th rib
Fat

1. Mature, but inactive
2. Early pregnancy
3. Midpregnancy
Nipple
Lactiferous sinus
4. Lactating
5. Regression after weaning

FIGURE 22–3 Schematic drawing of the sequence of changes that occur in the alveolar secretory units and duct system of the female breast before, during, and after pregnancy and lactation: (1) Before pregnancy, the glands are inactive, with small ducts and only a few small secretory alveoli; (2) early in pregnancy, alveoli develop and begin to grow; (3) by midpregnancy, the alveoli and ducts are enlarged with dilated lumens; (4) at parturition and during lactation, the alveoli are greatly dilated and active in milk production; and (5) after weaning, the alveoli and ducts regress by apoptotic cell death. (Redrawn, with permission, from Mescher AL. *Junqueira's Basic Histology*, 14th ed. McGraw-Hill, 2016.)

Until week 8 of gestation, the sex of the embryo cannot be determined morphologically; therefore, this period is termed the **indifferent phase** of sexual development. After this time, differentiation of the internal and external genitalia occurs, determining the **phenotypic sex** of the individual, which becomes fully developed after puberty. During embryogenesis, the internal genitalia are formed from a dual genital duct system within the urogenital ridge. The first to form is the wolffian duct, followed by the müllerian duct, the development of which depends on prior wolffian duct development. After 8 weeks of gestation, the production of **anti-müllerian hormone** by Sertoli cells in the fetal testes leads to regression of the müllerian ducts, whereas production of **testosterone** by the Leydig cells leads to the persistence of the wolffian duct and the subsequent development of the prostate, epididymis, and seminal vesicles. In the absence of these secretions, female internal reproductive organs are formed from the müllerian ducts, and the wolffian structures degenerate. Similarly, male external genitalia develop in the presence of dihydrotestosterone; in the absence of this hormone, the common embryologic structures give rise to female external genitalia. Exposure to androgens can result in virilization of the external genitalia of female embryos, whereas androgen deficiency results in defective male development (Figure 22–4). In contrast to the extensive study of male differentiation, relatively little is known about ovarian development. Since Jost discovered in the 1940s that the removal of embryonic gonads from rabbits leads to a female phenotype (regardless of the chromosome constitution), the female pathway was long thought to be a passive, or "default," pathway that will be followed unless overridden by the regulatory cascade triggered by the *SRY* gene in males. However, recent research strongly suggests that both the female and male pathways actively suppress the opposing developmental program to ensure proper ovarian or testicular development and function. Mouse studies have shown that this battle of the sexes is not only important during embryonic development, but continues when fully functional differentiated gonads have formed in the adult. The main components of the female pathway are the transcription factor FOXL2, one of the earliest markers of the developing ovary, and the WNT-signaling pathway with its activating components, WNT4 and R-Spondin1 (RSPO1). Homozygous *RSPO1* null mutations have been reported to cause 46,XX testicular disorder of sex development (DSD), whereas large duplications on chromosome 1, which contain both *WNT4* and *RSPO1*, can cause 46,XY gonadal dysgenesis. Based on the mouse studies, it has been suggested that over-activation of β-catenin by WNT4 and RSPO1 is able to override the testis pathway and trigger ovarian development.

During female development, the female ovaries contain about 7 million oogonia by 24 weeks of gestation. The majority of these cells die during intrauterine life, leaving only about 1 million primary oocytes at birth. This decreases to about 400,000 by puberty. The surviving oogonia are arrested at the prophase of meiosis I. Completion of the first meiotic division does not occur until the time of ovulation, and the

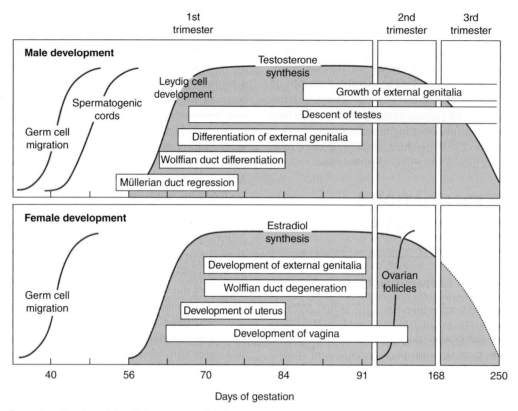

FIGURE 22–4 Timing of male and female human sexual differentiation. (Redrawn, with permission, from Kovacs WJ et al. *Textbook of Endocrine Physiology*, 6th ed. Oxford University Press, 2012. By permission of Oxford University Press, USA.)

second meiosis is completed with fertilization. Only about 400 of these oocytes mature and are released by ovulation during a woman's lifetime; the others undergo **atresia** at various stages of development.

PUBERTY

Secondary sexual characteristics develop at puberty, when maturation of the capacity for adult reproductive function occurs. The changes that occur in the brain and hypothalamus that initiate the onset of puberty involve, first, the establishment of sleep-dependent and, later, the truly pulsatile release of gonadotropin-releasing hormone (GnRH) from the hypothalamus. The hypothalamic kisspeptin/GPR54 ligand/receptor pair appears to be the key mediator of the onset of puberty.

The increase in GnRH leads to an increase in and a pulsatile pattern of luteinizing hormone (LH) and then follicle-stimulating hormone (FSH) secretion, hormones collectively termed gonadotropins. Before about age 10 years in girls, gonadotropin secretion is at low levels and does not display a pulsatile character. After this age, the pulsatile release of GnRH begins and initiates folliculogenesis, leading to cyclic changes in estrogen and progesterone production. These changes allow estrogen-dependent tissues, such as the breasts and the endometrium, to begin their maturation. The appearance of breast development is referred to as **thelarche**, and the first menstrual period is termed **menarche**.

CHECKPOINT

4. What is the difference between the chromosomal, gonadal, and phenotypic sex of an individual?
5. Approximately what percentage of the total number of oocytes present in the ovaries of a female at birth completes their maturation and is released upon ovulation over the course of her reproductive life?
6. Describe some changes that occur in the female with the onset of puberty.

THE MENSTRUAL CYCLE

Normal female reproductive function involves coordinated interactions between the brain and ovaries under the influence of other organs such as the liver (which metabolizes hormones and makes steroid-binding globulins), adrenals, and thyroid. With this coordination, cyclic changes during the course of the menstrual cycle allow the reproductive organs to perform specific functions at different points in time to optimize the chances for successful reproduction. When these mechanisms malfunction, the result may be infertility, altered menstrual bleeding, amenorrhea, or even cancer.

The menstrual cycle has three phases. The **follicular** phase typically lasts 12–14 days and culminates in the production of a mature oocyte. Initially, a cohort of follicles begins to grow,

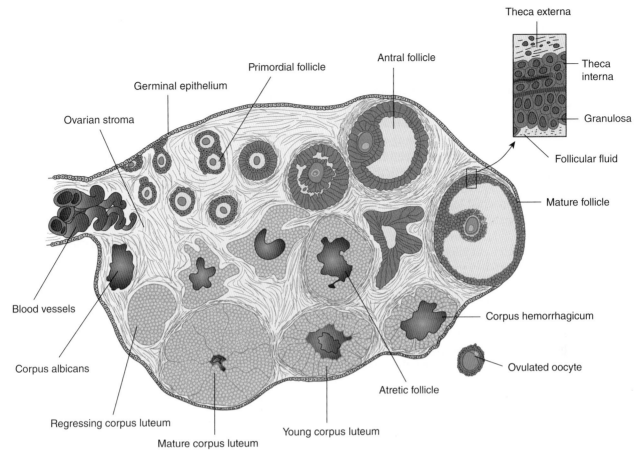

FIGURE 22–5 Diagram of the ovary, showing the sequential development of a follicle and the formation of a corpus luteum. An atretic follicle is shown in the center, and the structure of the wall of the mature follicle is detailed at the upper right. (Redrawn, with permission, from Barrett KE et al, eds. *Ganong's Review of Medical Physiology*, 25th ed. McGraw-Hill, 2016.)

but ultimately a single dominant follicle is selected, and the rest undergo a process of degeneration and apoptotic death, termed **atresia** (Figure 22–5). The follicular phase is followed by **ovulation**, in which the dominant follicle releases its mature oocyte to be transported through the uterine tubes for fertilization and subsequent implantation in a receptive uterus. The third, **luteal**, phase also averages 14 days and is characterized by luteinization of the ruptured follicle to produce the corpus luteum. The physiology of each of these phases in the menstrual cycle is best understood by considering different compartments: neuroendocrine, ovarian, and target tissues, most notably the uterus (Figure 22–6).

The neuroendocrine axis involves the brain, hypothalamus, pituitary, and ovary. Neurons within the hypothalamus synthesize the peptide **GnRH**, and its secretion is modulated by endogenous opioids and corticotropin-releasing hormone (CRH). GnRH is secreted directly into the portal circulation of the pituitary in a pulsatile fashion. This pulsatility is required for proper activation of its receptor located on the **gonadotropes**, which are cells located in the anterior pituitary. In response, the gonadotropes secrete the polypeptides **FSH** and **LH**, collectively called gonadotropins, which stimulate the ovary to produce estrogen and inhibin. Inhibin feeds back to

suppress FSH secretion but has no effect on LH. Estrogen also affects the pituitary by increasing the number of GnRH receptors and its sensitivity to GnRH stimulation. With estradiol production by the ovaries, a critical concentration is reached for a sufficient time to induce a midcycle LH surge and subsequent ovulation. After this surge, high levels of progesterone

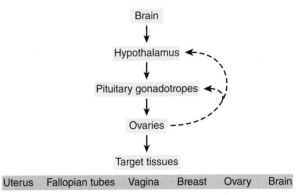

FIGURE 22–6 Female reproductive neuroendocrine feedback axis. Solid arrows indicate stimulation; dashed arrows indicate inhibition.

produced by the corpus luteum suppress gonadotropin release for the duration of the luteal phase.

Within the ovary, LH and FSH lead to the synthesis and secretion of steroid hormones and other paracrine/autocrine proteins, directing the maturation of a single oocyte for ovulation. During the early follicular phase, FSH stimulates the growth of a cohort of follicles and increases the production of inhibin and activin in granulosa cells. Activin acts in the ovary to augment the effect of FSH, increasing aromatase activity and increasing the production of FSH and LH receptors. LH stimulates the production of androgens in the thecal cells, which is augmented by inhibin. Androgens diffuse into the granulosa cells to be converted to estrogens through the enzymatic reaction of aromatization. As the follicular phase progresses, inhibin production comes under the control of LH, and the increasing amounts of inhibin lead to the further conversion of androgens to produce the high levels of estrogen needed for the LH surge.

The midcycle LH surge triggers the final steps of oocyte maturation and the resumption of meiosis within the dominant oocyte. Changes in prostaglandins and proteases allow the digestion of the follicular wall leading to oocyte extrusion and ovulation. The follicular cells remaining after ovulation develop into a structure called the **corpus luteum**, which synthesizes and releases large amounts of both estradiol and progesterone. Continued secretion from the corpus luteum requires LH (or **human chorionic gonadotropin [hCG]**, as discussed below) stimulation; in its absence, degeneration occurs.

The uterine compartment reacts to the steroids produced from the ovaries throughout the menstrual cycle. During the follicular phase, the endometrium proliferates under the influence of estrogen, creating straight glands with thin secretions and microvascular proliferation. During the luteal phase, the high levels of estradiol and progesterone promote the maturation of the endometrium, which develops tortuous glands engorged with thick secretions and proteins (see Figure 22–2). Additionally, the endometrium secretes a number of endocrine and paracrine factors (Table 22–1). These changes optimize the environment for implantation. In the absence of pregnancy, the corpus luteum cannot sustain the high levels of progesterone production, and the endometrial vasculature cannot be maintained. This leads to a sloughing of the endometrium and the onset of menstruation, which is marked by the nadir of estradiol and progesterone levels, ending the cycle (see Figure 22–2).

Contraception

Birth control pills are a pharmacologic means of preventing pregnancy by disrupting the precise timing of the hormone-directed events necessary for reproduction. Current formulations include progestins alone as well as combinations of estrogens and progestins. Most preparations of estrogen and progestin block the LH surge at midcycle, thereby preventing ovulation. However, other contraceptive actions include effects on estrogen- and progesterone-sensitive tissues, such

TABLE 22–1   Endocrine and paracrine products of the endometrium.

Lipids	Cytokines	Peptides and Others
Prostaglandins	Interleukin-1α	Prolactin
Thromboxanes	Interleukin-1β	Relaxin
Leukotrienes	Interleukin-6	Renin
	Interleukin-8	Endorphin
	Interferon-γ	Epidermal growth factor
	Colony-stimulating factor-1	IGFs
	VEGF	Fibroblast growth factor
		Platelet-derived growth factor
		Transforming growth factor β
		IGF-binding proteins
		Glycodelin
		Tumor necrosis factor
		PTHrP

IGF, insulin-like growth factor; PTHrP, parathyroid hormone–like peptide; VEGF, vascular endothelial growth factor.

Modified and reproduced, with permission, from Fritz M et al. The uterus. In: *Clinical Gynecologic Endocrinology and Infertility*, 8th ed. Lippincott Williams & Wilkins, 2011.

as inducing antifertility changes in cervical mucus and the endometrial lining that are unfavorable to sperm transport and embryonic implantation, respectively.

In order to mitigate the unpleasant side effects of nausea and bloating, as well as the dangerous side effect of thrombosis, the doses of estrogen and progestin have been decreased over the years. Non-oral formulations also have been developed, including long-term intrauterine and subdermal systems that deliver progestins. A transdermal patch allows the absorption of estrogen and progestin without "first-pass" metabolism in the liver. Transvaginal absorption is also available with a soft ring placed monthly in the vagina. Each of these formulations provides contraceptive efficacy equal to or better than oral contraceptive pills.

PHYSIOLOGY OF OVARIAN STEROIDS

Like the adrenal gland, the ovary is a steroid factory. The ovary secretes three types of steroids: **progesterone**, containing 21 carbons; **androgens**, containing 19 carbons; and **estrogens**, containing 18 carbons. Steroid synthesis occurs by conversion from cholesterol in a series of oxidative biochemical reactions catalyzed by enzymes in the mitochondria and the endoplasmic reticulum (see Chapter 21). The rate-limiting steps in steroid production involve the transport (StAR) and side chain cleavage of cholesterol within the mitochondrion by the enzyme cytochrome P450, family 11, subfamily A, polypeptide 1 (CYP11A1) to generate the basic steroid backbone, pregnenolone. This steroid is further modified in the endoplasmic reticulum to generate the various steroid hormones. Because steroids are synthesized by a cascade of enzyme reactions in various pathways, a block in one step (eg, resulting from a congenital enzyme defect or inhibition by certain drugs) can result in a lack of synthesis of downstream products and a "spillover" of precursors. Such defects are the hallmark of congenital adrenal hyperplasia (also discussed in Chapter 21).

The classical mechanism of steroid hormone action involves diffusion across the plasma membrane, binding of the steroid to receptor proteins in the cytoplasm or nucleus, and, after association with chromatin, activation of the transcription of selected genes by binding of the steroid–receptor complex to specific regions of DNA. In this way, the pattern of gene expression is changed in the various steroid-responsive tissues (ie, those that contain steroid receptors). Membrane-bound steroid receptors have also been shown to activate phosphorylation cascades typically regulated by growth factors.

CHECKPOINT

7. What are the primary target tissues for GnRH? For gonadotropins? For ovarian steroids?

8. Why is the pulsatile secretion of GnRH important?

9. What are some specialized features of GnRH action?

10. What are the specific effects of gonadotropins on the ovary?

11. How does the structure of the uterine lining differ in the midfollicular versus the midluteal stages, and for what reproduction-related events is each stage optimized?

12. What products are made by a granulosa cell in the dominant follicle over the course of its lifetime?

PREGNANCY

Prerequisites for a Successful Pregnancy

A number of changes must occur in reproductive and other organs to successfully establish and complete a pregnancy. Fertilization requires successful ovulation, capture of the mature oocyte by the fimbria of the fallopian tubes, and transport of the zygote to the uterus. Because fertilization usually occurs in the ampulla, it also requires the effective transport of viable sperm into the distal tube.

After implantation, a placenta forms consisting of two functional epithelial layers, the cytotrophoblast and the syncytiotrophoblast, as well as an adjacent maternal layer, the endometrial decidua, with its underlying mesenchymal core (Figure 22–7). The placenta allows the intimate apposition of maternal and fetal circulations for the exchange of nutrients, oxygen, and waste products. In addition, the placenta secretes a variety of important hormones, including an LH-like hormone termed

human chorionic gonadotropin (hCG). Unlike LH secretion by the gonadotrophs of the anterior pituitary, placental hCG secretion is neither pulsatile nor inhibited by the high levels of estrogen and progesterone. hCG maintains the corpus luteum for a period of 8–10 weeks until the full progesterone-producing capacity of the placenta has developed. At that point, hCG levels fall and the mature placenta produces progesterone from maternal cholesterol (Figure 22–8). Other factors produced by the placenta include a growth hormone–like protein called human chorionic somatomammotropin (hCS), also known as human placental lactogen (hPL) (Table 22–2).

During most of a pregnancy, the fetus provides the placenta with androgens, which are aromatized to make estrogens and secreted into the maternal circulation (Figure 22–9). This reflects the action of a special zone in the fetal adrenal cortex engaged in androgen production. Toward the end of pregnancy, increasing ACTH secretion by the fetal pituitary triggers the fetal adrenal to produce cortisol in addition to androgen. This switch may play a role in triggering the onset of labor by modulating the expression of progesterone receptors in the myometrium.

In addition to the changes in organs with pregnancy-specific functions, physiologic changes occur in essentially every maternal organ system. These include increased blood volume (increased by more than 40% by the middle of the third trimester), increased total body water (increased by 6–8 L), and increased cardiac output because of increased stroke volume (increased by 30%) and heart rate (increased by 15%). A striking increase in minute ventilation (increased by 50% compared with the nonpregnant state) without any change in respiratory rate is observed as a result of increased tidal volume (see Chapter 9). Dramatic increases in renal blood flow and the glomerular filtration rate (increased by 40%) are also seen. Most of these alterations are related in complex ways to the effects of hormones produced in pregnancy.

Effects of Ovarian Steroids in Pregnancy

The physiological effects of various sex steroids in pregnancy are incompletely understood. The demonstrated and proposed roles of progesterone in pregnancy include (1) promotion of implantation; (2) suppression of the maternal immune response to fetal antigens, thus preventing rejection of the allogeneic fetus; (3) increased cardiovascular compliance; (4) provision of substrate for manufacture of glucocorticoids and mineralocorticoids by the fetal adrenal; (5) maintenance of myometrial quiescence through gestation; and (6) a role in parturition. Estrogens contribute to (1) volume expansion; (2) cardiac remodeling; and (3) the preparative production of clotting factors, anticipating blood loss that commonly follows delivery.

Human Chorionic Somatomammotropin & Fuel Homeostasis in Pregnancy

Another example of fetal–placental–maternal interactions is seen in the actions of hCS (Figure 22–10). This

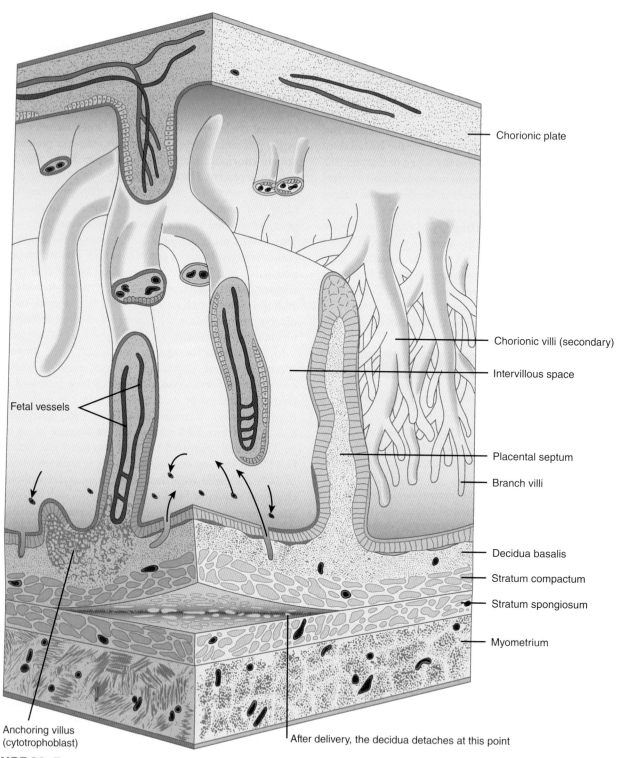

Chorionic plate

Chorionic villi (secondary)

Intervillous space

Fetal vessels

Placental septum

Branch villi

Decidua basalis

Stratum compactum

Stratum spongiosum

Myometrium

Anchoring villus
(cytotrophoblast)

After delivery, the decidua detaches at this point

FIGURE 22–7 Placental anatomy.

"counter-regulatory" hormone (ie, a hormone whose actions oppose those of insulin) appears to serve as a defense against fetal hypoglycemia. From a metabolic standpoint, pregnancy is a form of "accelerated starvation" characterized by fasting hypoglycemia, as fuel substrates produced by the mother are consumed by the growing fetus. The hCS produced by the placenta in response to hypoglycemia serves to increase lipolysis, thereby raising maternal free fatty acid levels and, ultimately, blood glucose and ketone levels. This "diabetogenic" role of hCS is a major burden on the maternal compartment and contributes to the tendency for diabetes mellitus to emerge in susceptible individuals during pregnancy. Normally, glucose is the major fuel source for the fetus. However, in the event of glucose deprivation, ketones provide a ready emergency fuel

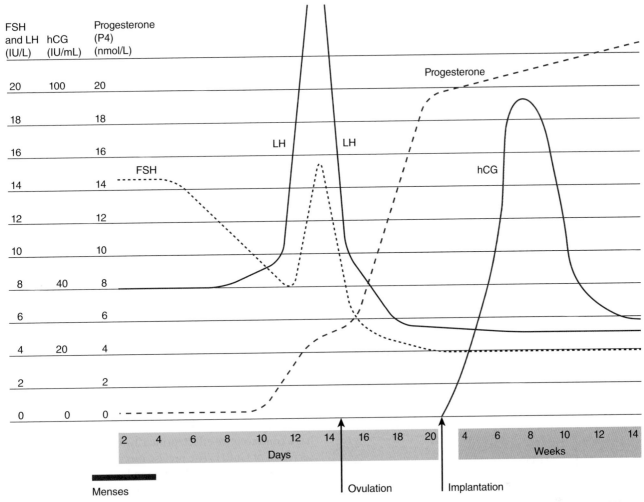

FIGURE 22–8 Hormone production during pregnancy. (FSH, follicle-stimulating hormone; hCG, human chorionic gonadotropin; LH, luteinizing hormone.) (Redrawn and modified, with permission, from Fritz M et al. Regulation of the menstrual cycle. In: *Clinical Gynecologic Endocrinology and Infertility*, 8th ed. Lippincott Williams & Wilkins, 2011.)

supply (as they do in starvation) for both the mother and, via the placenta, the fetus.

CHECKPOINT

13. How is the corpus luteum maintained until the placenta has developed adequately?

14. What are some possible roles of steroids during pregnancy?

15. Why is new-onset diabetes mellitus a common complication of pregnancy?

LACTATION

Breast Structure & Development

The rudiments for breast development are established during embryonic development. During puberty, rising estrogen levels stimulate breast growth as one of a number of female secondary sexual characteristics. Breast growth involves the proliferation and branching of lactiferous ducts, as well as the accumulation of adipose and connective tissue. In the mature breast, each terminal lactiferous duct drains clusters of tubuloalveolar secretory units lined by milk-secreting epithelial cells and is suspended in connective and adipose tissue well populated with lymphocytes. The mature female breast consists of a cluster of 15–25 lactiferous ducts, each emerging independently at the nipple (see Figure 22–3). Both the pubertal and pregnant phases of breast growth require the permissive influence of glucocorticoids, thyroxine, and insulin for full development, and their actions are potentiated by estrogen and progesterone.

Initiation & Maintenance of Milk Synthesis & Secretion

During pregnancy, prolactin, progesterone, and hCS play a dominant role in stimulating breast growth and the capacity for milk production. Actual lactation, or milk release, however, is

TABLE 22–2 Endocrine and paracrine products in pregnancy other than steroids.

Fetal Compartment	Placental Compartment	Maternal Compartment
Alpha-fetoprotein	Hypothalamic-like hormones	Decidual proteins
	CRH	Prolactin
	TRH	Fibronectin
	Somatostatin	VEGF
	Pituitary-like hormones	Relaxin
	hCG	IGFBP-1
	hCS	Interleukin-1
	GH-P	Colony-stimulating factor-1
	ACTH	Glycodelin (progesterone-associated endometrial protein)
	Growth factors	Corpus luteum proteins
	IGF-1	Relaxin
	Epidermal growth factor	Prorenin
	Platelet-derived growth factor	
	Fibroblast growth factor	
	Transforming growth factor-β	
	Inhibin/Activin	
	Cytokines	
	Interleukin-1	
	Interleukin-6	
	Colony-stimulating factor	
	Other	
	Opioids	
	Prorenin	
	Pregnancy-specific β-glycoprotein	
	Pregnancy associated plasma protein A	

ACTH, adrenocorticotropic hormone; GH-P, growth hormone (placental); hCG, human chorionic gonadotropin; hCS, human chorionic somatomammotropin; IGF-1, insulin-like growth factor-1; IGFBP-1, insulin-like growth factor–binding protein 1; VEGF, vascular endothelial growth factor.

Data from Cowan BD et al. Management of abnormal genital bleeding in girls and women. (Current concepts.) N Engl J Med. 1991;324:1710.

inhibited by the high levels of placental steroids present before birth. After delivery of the placenta, estrogen and progesterone levels fall dramatically, removing this block. The maintenance of milk secretion requires the integrated action of both anterior and posterior pituitary factors (Figure 22–11), as well as interaction between the mother and infant. Suckling stimulates afferent neural pathways that suppress dopamine levels in the hypothalamus, thereby maintaining the high levels of prolactin necessary for milk synthesis. At the same time, afferent sensory nerve fibers in the breast (as well as other stimuli such as the infant's cry) stimulate the synthesis, transport, and secretion of oxytocin from the posterior pituitary. Oxytocin promotes the contraction of mammary myoepithelial cells, thereby triggering the ejection of milk from the mammary epithelial alveoli and out the nipple.

Toward the end of pregnancy, there is an increase in the lymphocyte population in the vasculature and connective tissue of the breast. These lymphocytes secrete immunoglobulin A (IgA) into the local bloodstream, from which it is taken up by the mammary epithelial cells. By the process of transcytosis, IgA crosses the mammary epithelial cells into the luminal secretion (milk). This mechanism, coupled with the transplacental transport of maternal IgG, is responsible for conferring passive immunity on the newborn. The earliest mammary gland secretion after birth, termed colostrum, has a particularly high immunoglobulin content.

The high level of prolactin maintained during lactation also has a contraceptive effect, primarily by inhibiting the pulsatile secretion of GnRH. The precise mechanism is not known but may involve a short feedback loop by which prolactin stimulates dopamine release, which, in turn, elevates endogenous opioid release and inhibits GnRH secretion. There may also be effects of prolactin directly on the ovary that contribute to lactational anovulation and amenorrhea. However, it should be noted that the contraceptive effect of prolactin is only moderate and, therefore, of low reliability.

CHECKPOINT

16. Which hormones are involved in breast development?
17. Why is milk rarely secreted before parturition?
18. What is the probable mechanism of lactational amenorrhea?

Menopause

Menopause is the point in a woman's life when, as a result of the exhaustion of the supply of functioning ovarian follicles, menstrual cycles cease. Ten years before menopause, at approximately age 40 years, reproductive function starts to diminish. This is manifested as a decreased frequency of ovulation and alterations in menstrual patterns. During this time, in the setting of few remaining follicles, increased GnRH-stimulated LH and FSH secretion is observed. Higher levels of estradiol circulate, particularly in the follicular phase from

FIGURE 22–9 Fetal–placental–maternal cooperation in steroidogenesis. (3β-Hydroxysteroid dehydrogenase, hydroxy-Δ-5-steroid dehydrogenase, 3 β- and steroid Δ-isomerase (HSD3β); 17α-Hydroxylase, 17α-hydroxylase activity of cytochrome P450, family 17, subfamily A, polypeptide 1 (CYP17A1); LDL, low-density lipoprotein.) (Reproduced, with permission, from Fritz M et al. The endocrinology of pregnancy. In: *Clinical Gynecologic Endocrinology and Infertility*, 8th ed. Lippincott Williams & Wilkins, 2011.)

ages 35–48 years, and then estradiol levels sharply decline just prior to menopause. This transitory period of diminishing reproductive function approaching menopause is termed the **climacteric**.

During the climacteric transition, the hormonal status of women changes from a cyclic high-estrogen state to a steady-state, low-estrogen, postmenopausal state. This leads to **vasomotor symptoms** such as hot flushes ("hot flashes"), sweating, and chills. Psychologic symptoms such as irritability, tension, anxiety, and depression may also be observed. After menopause, other more gradual changes can appear. In addition to the atrophy of estrogen-dependent tissues such as the vaginal epithelium, a gradual loss in bone density leading to **osteoporosis** can occur.

A modest degree of androgen production from thecal cells of the residual ovarian stroma continues even in the absence of follicular growth. In postmenopausal women, ovarian and adrenal androgens continue to be aromatized into estrogens by the enzyme aromatase (cytochrome P450, CYP19A1) in adipose tissue and hair follicles. The significance of peripheral aromatization in relation to the severity of menopause symptoms varies in different individuals.

In the medical literature, menopause was often viewed as an "endocrinopathy," specifically as a disorder of estrogen deficiency. To treat the vasomotor symptoms and osteoporosis, hormone therapy (HT) was often prescribed. Given the interaction of estrogen with the cardiovascular system, HT had also been thought to have protective cardiovascular effects, and

several early trials had suggested its usefulness in the primary and secondary prevention of coronary heart disease. Results of large prospective studies, however, showed no benefit in cardiovascular protection with HT. The Women's Health Initiative randomized clinical trial showed that the increased risk of thromboembolic disease and invasive breast cancer associated with estrogen and progesterone replacement outweighed the benefit of fewer events of colon cancer and hip fracture. Treatment with estrogen replacement therapy without progesterone in women who had undergone hysterectomy did not show any increase in breast cancer but instead suggested possible breast cancer prevention. The other risks and benefits were similar. From these studies, it is recognized that HT should not be used for cardiovascular prevention or initiated in women older than 60 years. Use for the symptomatic relief of menopausal symptoms is still considered appropriate after counseling the patient about the global risks and benefits of treatment.

CHECKPOINT

19. What are the symptoms of menopause?
20. What is the primary source of the estrogen found in the bloodstream of postmenopausal women not on estrogen replacement therapy?
21. Compare LH and FSH levels before puberty, during the reproductive years, and after menopause.

A. hCS changes in the fasting state

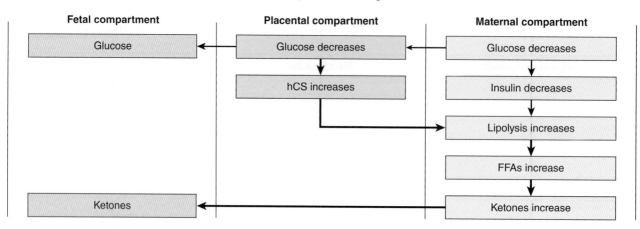

B. hCS changes in the fed state

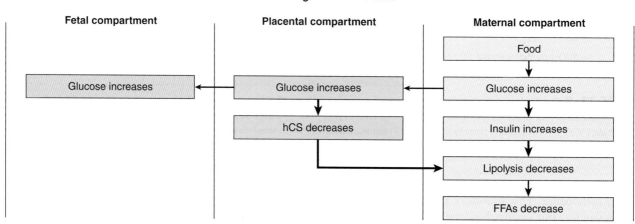

FIGURE 22–10 Fetal–placental–maternal cooperation in fuel homeostasis. (FFA, free fatty acid; hCS, human chorionic somatomammotropin.) (Reproduced, with permission, from Fritz M et al. The endocrinology of pregnancy. In: *Clinical Gynecologic Endocrinology and Infertility*, 8th ed. Lippincott Williams & Wilkins, 2011.)

OVERVIEW OF FEMALE REPRODUCTIVE TRACT DISORDERS

Many female reproductive disorders can be traced to a particular level of the neuroendocrine feedback axis and thus can be categorized as resulting from central (pituitary, hypothalamus, or other brain centers that influence the hypothalamus), ovarian, or end-organ (target tissue, eg, uterine) dysfunction.

DISORDERS OF CENTRAL HYPOTHALAMIC–PITUITARY FUNCTION

Any change in the precise rate or amplitude of GnRH secretion by the hypothalamus can result in altered pituitary responsiveness (eg, downregulation of GnRH receptors, altered gonadotropin secretion). This altered pituitary function, in turn, results in disordered ovarian function (eg, inadequate steroidogenesis with or without anovulation) and altered target tissue response (eg, endometrial atrophy and menstrual abnormalities). Many central (eg, psychic stress) and peripheral (eg, body fat content) inputs affecting pulsatile GnRH release are integrated in the hypothalamus. Thus, altered GnRH release from the hypothalamus is a common cause of amenorrhea (eg, in athletic young women).

DISORDERS OF THE OVARY

Proper ovarian function involves responsiveness to gonadotropins, the intrinsic viability of follicles, and a host of paracrine interactions within and between individual follicles. Polycystic ovary syndrome (PCOS) is an example of ovarian dysfunction resulting from a self-perpetuating cycle of altered feedback relationships (see later discussion). PCOS is manifested by anovulation, hirsutism, infertility, dyslipidemia, and either abnormal uterine bleeding or amenorrhea.

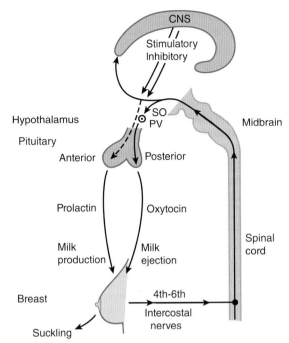

FIGURE 22–11 The role of anterior and posterior pituitary factors in milk synthesis and secretion. (CNS, central nervous system; PV, paraventricular nucleus; SO, supraoptic nucleus.) (Redrawn, with permission, from Rebar RW. The breast and physiology of lactation. In: Creasy RK et al, eds. *Maternal–Fetal Medicine: Principles and Practice*, 4th ed. Saunders, 1999.)

DISORDERS OF THE UTERUS, FALLOPIAN TUBES & VAGINA

Because normal menstrual bleeding is most directly a function of the growth state of the uterine endometrium, disorders of the uterus, including hormonal dysfunction, myomas (fibroids, benign tumors of the underlying myometrium), and cancer of the endometrium itself, often present with abnormal vaginal bleeding.

Pelvic infections can produce adhesions and scarring of the endometrium or fallopian tubes that may result in infertility. The initial presentation typically includes abdominal and pelvic (cervical and adnexal) pain. Usually, fever is also present with a concomitant elevation of the white blood cell count and a positive endocervical culture. Common infectious agents include gonorrhea, anaerobic bacteria, and *Chlamydia*. Multiple organisms are usually involved, and symptoms may be minimal or absent in as many as half of infected women. Aggressive screening programs and prompt antibiotic therapy are important in treating these infections to limit permanent damage to sensitive reproductive structures. Pelvic infections can develop into tubo-ovarian abscesses requiring surgical drainage.

DISORDERS OF PREGNANCY

The normal events of pregnancy can set the stage for a wide array of localized and systemic disorders. Abnormalities in the process of implantation, for example, appear to predispose to recurrent miscarriage and preeclampsia-eclampsia (see later). In addition, a genetic predisposition to disease that might otherwise remain latent for decades may manifest first—often transiently—during pregnancy.

A good example of the latter is the genetic predisposition to the development of diabetes mellitus. As discussed, pregnancy is a counter-regulatory state, with an elevation of multiple blood glucose–elevating hormones, especially hCS. Because of the insulin-resistant features of pregnancy, blood glucose control in diabetics who become pregnant is more difficult. Nondiabetic patients can also develop diabetes transiently during pregnancy (gestational diabetes mellitus). Gestational diabetes mellitus is common and occurs in 2–5% of all pregnancies in the United States. Many of these individuals go on to manifest type 2 diabetes mellitus later in life.

Poor control of blood glucose during pregnancy has effects on the mother, the course of the pregnancy, and the fetus. Maternal retinopathy and nephropathy may appear during the course of the pregnancy, although the long-term severity of the mother's disease is probably not altered by pregnancy. There is a higher incidence of acute diabetes complications during pregnancy, including ketoacidosis, hypoglycemia, and infections. Patients with gestational and pregestational diabetes mellitus are at greater risk for preeclampsia-eclampsia. Poor glucose control also increases the rate and risk of cesarean section with its associated anesthetic and surgical morbidity.

The effects of poor glucose control on the fetus are even more profound. Unexplained fetal deaths, spontaneous abortions, and **congenital anomalies** are increased. Just how gestational diabetes increases the risk of congenital anomalies is not well understood. Some studies have implicated altered myoinositol and prostaglandin metabolism. Other studies have demonstrated embryopathic effects of oxygen free radicals generated at elevated levels in diabetic pregnancies.

Fetal **macrosomia** (large body size) is often the result of gestational diabetes. High maternal blood glucose levels trigger increased fetal insulin secretion, resulting in a larger fetus. As the fetus becomes larger, the risk of fetopelvic disproportion increases, which contributes to traumatic vaginal deliveries and an increased frequency of cesarean section. Neonatal hypoglycemia, hypocalcemia, polycythemia, and hyperbilirubinemia may also occur.

The high levels of steroids and other products in the pregnant state can lead to a range of other serious medical complications. Pregnancy is paradoxically associated with both hemorrhage and thrombosis (Table 22–3). Both are related to the special functions of the placenta and its adaptations in the course of mammalian evolution.

Separation of the placenta from the wall of the uterus at birth poses a threat of massive, life-threatening hemorrhage given the intimate apposition of the placenta and the maternal blood supply, 10% of which is funneled to the uterus at term. As an adaptation to this risk, pregnancy is a hypercoagulable state established in part by estrogen stimulation of hepatic coagulation proteins. Physiologically, this increased tendency toward coagulation and decreased activity of the fibrinolytic system

TABLE 22–3   Factors predisposing to thrombosis in pregnancy.

Factor	Mechanism
Hormonal effects	Alterations in blood flow resulting in increased hemostasis
	Increased blood viscosity due to impaired erythrocyte deformability
	Increased production of coagulation factors I (fibrinogen), VII, VIII, IX, X, and XII and decreased antithrombin
Nonhormonal effect	Depressed fibrinolytic activity

may serve to control postpartum hemorrhage. Pathologically, these same factors pose a risk of inappropriate thrombosis. It has been calculated that the risk of thrombophlebitis is increased nearly 50 times in the first month postpartum compared with the nonpregnant state. When thrombosis does occur, therapy is complicated by the teratogenic risks associated with warfarin. Therefore, pregnant patients with thrombosis are given subcutaneous heparin therapy.

Miscarriage, Ectopic Pregnancy & Placental Disorders

At least 15% of all pregnancies terminate in spontaneous abortion as a result of genetic or environmental factors before the period when extrauterine life is possible (about 24 weeks of gestation and 750 g body weight). Inevitable abortion presents with heavy bleeding, pain, and dilation of the internal os. Threatened abortion is considered when painless uterine bleeding occurs with a closed, uneffaced cervix.

For patients presenting with vaginal bleeding and pain in the first trimester, miscarriage must be distinguished from molar and ectopic pregnancy. Ectopic pregnancy typically results from implantation of the blastocyst into the lining of the tube rather than the endometrium. Damaged or scarred fallopian tubes, from previous pelvic infections or endometriosis, impede transit of the zygote, leading to a predisposition for ectopic pregnancies. In this location, the embryo is not viable, and its growth results in rupture and potentially life-threatening hemorrhage unless it is surgically or medically eliminated. Diagnosis is made by a failure of serum β-hCG to rise appropriately in the first several weeks of pregnancy and failure to localize an intrauterine pregnancy by ultrasonography.

Third-trimester bleeding is typically associated with **placenta previa** (placental obstruction of all or part of the internal cervical os) or **placental abruption** (premature separation of a normally implanted placenta). Women who have had multiple prior pregnancies, and particularly those who have had multiple cesarean section deliveries, are at increased risk of placenta previa, which is believed to be due to scar tissue formation from previous implantations. Hypertension, smoking, and multiple pregnancies increase the risk of hemorrhage into the decidual plate and subsequent placental abruption. Hemorrhage can be massive and life-threatening.

TROPHOBLASTIC DISEASES

Complete molar pregnancies are abnormal growths resulting from trophoblastic proliferation. Rarely, they coexist with a fetus (**partial mole**). The prevalence in the United States is approximately 1 per 1500 pregnancies, but in certain areas of Asia, it is as high as 1 per 125 pregnancies. The tissue in complete moles has higher malignant potential and is purely of paternal origin, whereas that of partial moles is usually benign and typically contains an extra set of paternal chromosomes (triploidy). Most moles present with vaginal bleeding and are diagnosed during an evaluation of threatened abortion by (1) the lack of a fetus; and (2) the presence of hydropic trophoblastic tissue on ultrasound imaging. Particularly severe nausea of pregnancy, a uterus larger than expected for gestational age, and an extremely elevated hCG level are suggestive, but not diagnostic, of molar pregnancy.

The complications of hydatidiform mole include high risks of (1) **choriocarcinoma**, a malignant trophoblastic neoplasm with high potential for metastasis, especially to the lung and brain; (2) hyperthyroidism with the added risk of thyroid storm during anesthesia induction; and (3) severe hemorrhage or trophoblastic tissue pulmonary embolism during suction curettage to remove the molar products. The extremely high levels of hCG that occur with molar pregnancy and choriocarcinoma can result in a cross-activation of the thyroid-stimulating hormone (TSH) receptor and trigger hyperthyroidism in some patients. Approximately 5% of women with hydatidiform mole subsequently develop choriocarcinoma. The serum β-hCG can be used as a sensitive test to detect the continued presence of malignant tissue. The exquisite sensitivity of choriocarcinoma to chemotherapy has made it a readily curable malignancy if detected early.

DISORDERS OF THE BREAST

Intrinsic disorders of the breast are either malignant (breast cancer) or benign (eg, fibrocystic disease). Breast disease can also occur as a result of the effects of other disorders or drug therapy (eg, galactorrhea). The breast, like other estrogen- and progesterone-target tissues, displays cyclic changes throughout the menstrual cycle. Subtle imbalances in the relative levels of estrogen and progesterone may be the cause of **benign breast disease**. This term refers to abnormalities ranging from normal premenstrual breast tenderness relieved with menstruation at one extreme to so-called fibrocystic disease at the other. In fibrocystic disease, breast fibrosis and cysts are associated with mammary epithelial hyperplasia. True fibrocystic disease with epithelial cell hyperplasia is a risk factor for breast cancer in much the same way that endometrial hyperplasia resulting from unopposed estrogen action is a risk factor for endometrial cancer.

DISORDERS OF SEXUAL DEVELOPMENT (FORMERLY PSEUDOHERMAPHRODITISM)

Under certain circumstances, aberrations can occur during embryogenesis that alter the normal course of events in chromosomal, gonadal, or phenotypic sexual development. An example of such an aberration in chromosomal sex is **Turner syndrome** (45,X). Individuals with Turner syndrome are phenotypic females with primary amenorrhea, absent secondary sexual characteristics, short stature, a webbed neck, a shield chest, and bilateral streak gonads.

An example of altered gonadal sex is the syndrome of pure **gonadal dysgenesis**. Affected individuals have bilateral streak gonads and an immature female phenotype, but unlike those with Turner syndrome, they are of normal height, have no associated somatic defects, and have a normal female karyotype.

Disorders of phenotypic sex include disorders that result from exposure of female embryos to excessive maternal or exogenous androgens (eg, congenital adrenal hyperplasia) (see Chapter 21) during sexual differentiation or from defects in androgen synthesis or tissue sensitivity in the embryo (eg, androgen insensitivity).

PATHOPHYSIOLOGY OF SELECTED FEMALE REPRODUCTIVE TRACT DISORDERS

MENSTRUAL DISORDERS

Disorders of the menstrual cycle include (1) **amenorrhea** (lack of menstrual bleeding), which may be considered primary (ie, the failure of menstrual periods to begin by age 16) or secondary (ie, the lack of menstrual periods for 6 months in a previously menstruating woman); (2) **dysmenorrhea** (pain and other symptoms accompanying menstruation); or (3) **heavy menstrual bleeding** (previously known as **menorrhagia**) or **intermenstrual bleeding** (previously known as **metrorrhagia**).

Etiology

A. Amenorrhea

The cause of amenorrhea can be traced to one of four broad categories of conditions (Table 22–4):

1. Normal physiologic processes such as pregnancy and menopause.
2. Disorders of the uterus or the pathway of menstrual flow such as the destruction of the endometrium after curettage coupled with infection within the uterus (**Asherman syndrome**).
3. Disorders of the ovary such as gonadal failure resulting from a range of chromosomal, developmental, and structural abnormalities; autoimmune disorders; premature follicle loss; and poorly understood syndromes in which ovaries with follicles are resistant to gonadotropin stimulation.
4. Disorders of the hypothalamus or pituitary resulting in either a lack of or disordered GnRH secretion and, as a consequence, insufficient gonadotropin secretion to maintain ovarian steroid production. The causes of hypothalamic and pituitary dysfunction include prolactin-secreting tumors, hypothyroidism, excessive stress and exercise, and weight loss.

Within these categories, amenorrhea can have very diverse specific causes.

B. Dysmenorrhea

Dysmenorrhea is pain, typically cramping in character and lower abdominal in location, occurring in the days just before and during menstrual flow. Dysmenorrhea can occur as a primary disorder in the absence of identifiable pelvic disease, or it may be secondary to an underlying pelvic disease such as endometriosis or leiomyomas (Table 22–5).

C. Abnormal Uterine Bleeding

Uterine bleeding is abnormal if it occurs (1) prepubertally; (2) at the time of usual menses but is of longer duration than usual; (3) at the time of usual menses but is heavier than usual; (4) between menstrual periods; or (5) after menopause in the absence of pharmacologic hormone replacement therapy. Table 22–6 lists the categories of abnormal uterine bleeding and some specific causes.

Pathology & Pathogenesis

A. Amenorrhea

The pathogenesis of amenorrhea depends on the level of the neuroendocrine reproductive axis from which the disorder stems and whether it is due to a structural problem or to a functional problem of hormonal control. In a previously menstruating patient presenting with amenorrhea, it is important first to rule out pregnancy and then to assess thyroid (serum

TABLE 22–4   Causes of amenorrhea.

Category	Common Causes	Pathophysiologic Mechanisms	How to Make a Diagnosis	Intervention
Normal physiologic processes	Pregnancy	Sustained high estrogen and progesterone	Serum hCG, history	Prenatal care
	Menopause	Lack of estrogen	Clinical diagnosis	Recommendations for osteoporosis prevention
Disorders of the uterus and outflow tract	Disorders of sexual development	Excessive androgen exposure	Physical examination	Surgical treatment
	Congenital anomalies (eg, imperforate hymen)		Physical examination	Surgical treatment
	Asherman syndrome	Endometrial adhesions following vigorous curettage	Lack of response to estrogen–progestin trial; visualization of scant endometrium	Hysteroscopy, lysis of adhesions
Disorders of the ovary	Gonadal dysgenesis	Deletion of genetic material from the X chromosome	Karyotype	Remove streak gonads if Y chromosome is present in view of high risk of dysgerminoma
	Premature ovarian insufficiency	Lack of viable follicles	Check gonadotropins; ultrasound for atretic follicles	HRT for osteoporosis prevention
	Polycystic ovary syndrome	Altered intraovarian hormone relationships	Clinical diagnosis in patients with chronic anovulation and androgen excess	Decrease ovarian androgen secretion (wedge resection, oral contraceptives); increase FSH secretion
Disorders of the hypothalamus or pituitary	Stress, athletic endeavor, underweight	Altered GnRH pulses	Check serum TSH, PRL, gonadotropins	Replacement if deficient; search for tumor if excessive

FSH, follicle-stimulating hormone; GnRH, gonadotropin-releasing hormone; hCG, human chorionic gonadotropin; HRT, hormone replacement therapy; PRL, prolactin; TSH, thyroid-stimulating hormone.

TABLE 22–5   Categories of dysmenorrhea.

Category	Etiology	Distinguishing Features
Primary dysmenorrhea	Prostaglandins	Lack of organic pelvic disease
Secondary dysmenorrhea		
Endometriosis	Ectopic endometrium, including intramyometrial endometrial tissue	Finding of endometriosis lesions on laparoscopy
Pelvic inflammatory disease	Infection	Positive culture
Anatomic lesions (imperforate hymen, intrauterine adhesions, leiomyomas, polyps)	Congenital, inflammatory, or neoplastic	Findings on physical examination, ultrasound
Premenstrual syndrome (PMS)	Unknown	Association with emotional, behavioral, and other symptoms

TSH level) and pituitary (serum prolactin level) function before approaching the workup of amenorrhea.

1. **Uterine Disorders**—Damage to the underlying stem cells from which the endometrium proliferates can lead to amenorrhea. In most cases, this occurs in the setting of endometritis after **curettage** (scraping of the endometrium) either for postpartum bleeding or abnormal uterine bleeding and subsequent failure of the endometrium to regenerate. Ultrasound typically reveals a thin lining (<5 mm).

   To establish a functional endometrium, an amenorrheic patient is given either progesterone alone or the sequential combination of estrogen and progesterone. Renewed vaginal bleeding after cessation of the hormonal therapy suggests that the endometrium is intact. This response also indicates that the cause of the amenorrhea lies elsewhere (ie, is due to an endocrine defect causing a lack or insufficiency of cyclic estrogen and progesterone stimulation).

2. **Ovarian Insufficiency**—Amenorrhea resulting from ovarian insufficiency can be either primary or secondary to dysfunction higher in the neuroendocrine

TABLE 22–6   Causes of abnormal vaginal or uterine bleeding.

Childhood	
Genital lesions	**Endocrine changes**
Vaginitis	Estrogen ingestion
Foreign body	Precocious puberty
Trauma	Ovarian tumors
Tumors	
Adolescents and adults	
Abnormal uterine bleeding	**Malignant diseases**
Estrogen breakthrough	Endometrial cancer
Estrogen withdrawal	Cervical cancer
Diseases of the genital tract	Vaginal cancer
Benign conditions	**Pregnancy**
Uterine leiomyoma	Ectopic pregnancy
Cervical polyp	Threatened abortion
Endometrial polyp	Miscarriage
Genital laceration	**Other causes**
Endometrial hyperplasia	Thyroid disease
	von Willebrand disease
	Thrombocytopenia

reproductive axis. Primary (or premature) ovarian insufficiency occurs with a premature loss of follicles. This can result from genetic disorders, autoimmune disorders (lymphocytic oophoritis), metabolic problems (galactosemia), or exogenous insults such as chemotherapy, toxins, or radiation. Secondary ovarian insufficiency is caused by a lack of gonadotropin stimulation of otherwise normal ovaries, resulting in failure to produce the estrogen and progesterone needed for menstrual cycles.

a. **Primary ovarian insufficiency**—Primary ovarian insufficiency occurs when follicle atresia is accelerated in an ovary of a woman of reproductive age. It presents with symptoms and signs of menopause resulting from estrogen deficiency in patients younger than 40 years. Serum LH and FSH levels are elevated. There is a lack of estrogen production and an absence of viable follicles. In some instances, primary ovarian insufficiency is just one manifestation of an autoimmune polyglandular failure syndrome in which autoantibodies destroy a number of endocrine tissues. These patients may also have associated diabetes mellitus, hypothyroidism, or adrenal insufficiency, as discussed elsewhere (see Chapters 18, 20, and 21).

Genetic causes of primary ovarian insufficiency include abnormalities of the *FMR1* gene. An expansion of CGG trinucleotide repeats of between 55 and 200 copies is defined as the fragile X premutation and is associated with a premature depletion of ovarian function (see Chapter 2); Turner syndrome (an absence of, or abnormality in, an X chromosome [ie, 45,X]); or Turner mosaicism (ie, multiple cell lines of varying sex chromosome composition). Approximately 40% of patients who appear to have Turner syndrome prove to be mosaics. The presence of any Y chromosome in the karyotype of these individuals carries a high risk for gonadal germ cell tumors and is an indication for gonadectomy. Thus, a karyotype should be performed on any amenorrheic individual younger than 30 years with high serum FSH and LH levels.

b. **Chronic anovulation**—Other patients are found to have adequate numbers of follicles, but these fail to mature and ovulate. This condition is known as **chronic anovulation** and is manifested as amenorrhea with intermittent bleeding (caused by uncoordinated overgrowth of the endometrium in response to stimulation by estrogen alone). Left untreated, the high estrogen level places the individual at increased risk for endometrial carcinoma. Among the causes of chronic anovulation is thyroid dysfunction (Table 22–7). Both hyperthyroidism and hypothyroidism can alter ovarian function and the metabolism of androgens

TABLE 22–7   Causes and mechanisms of chronic anovulation.

Causes	Mechanisms
Thyroid disease	Altered estrogen clearance
Hyperthyroidism Hypothyroidism	Decreased androgen clearance with resulting increased peripheral aromatization to estrogen
Hyperprolactinemia	Altered gonadotropin-releasing hormone (GnRH) pulses
Obesity	Increased peripheral aromatization of androgens to estrogens
	Decreased steroid hormone–binding globulin, resulting in increased free estrogen and testosterone
	Increased insulin resistance, resulting in increased insulin secretion, which increases ovarian stromal production of androgens
Ovarian insufficiency	Genetic disorders (eg, Turner syndrome, fragile X premutation)
	Cytotoxic drugs
	Irradiation
	Autoimmune disorders

TABLE 22–8   Clinical consequences of chronic anovulation in polycystic ovary syndrome.

Infertility
Menstrual dysfunction (either amenorrhea or abnormal uterine bleeding)
Hirsutism and acne (androgen excess state)
Increased risk of endometrial cancer
Possible increased risk of breast cancer
Increased risk of hyperlipidemia
Increased risk of diabetes mellitus (insulin resistance and hyperinsulinemia)

and estrogens, resulting in a variety of menstrual disorders. Another cause of chronic anovulation is hyperprolactinemia. It has been proposed that progressively more severe hyperprolactinemia presents first as an inadequate luteal phase with recurrent abortion, then as anovulation with intermittent bleeding, and finally as amenorrhea. Table 22–8 summarizes the clinical consequences of chronic anovulation.

c. **Hormonal feedback disorders**—PCOS affects 2–5% of reproductive-age women and presents with amenorrhea and hirsutism (Table 22–9). Patients are often obese with hyperinsulinemia, insulin resistance, and dyslipidemia. In addition, they have elevated plasma androgens, together with elevated plasma estrogens that are predominantly estrone derived from the peripheral aromatization of adrenal androgens in the granulosa cell by the enzyme aromatase (cytochrome P450, CYP19A1).

The hyperinsulinemia is believed to be a key etiologic factor. Insulin results in the decreased hepatic synthesis of steroid hormone-binding globulin

TABLE 22–9   Manifestations of polycystic ovary syndrome.[1]

Hirsutism	95%
Large ovaries	95%
Infertility	75%
Amenorrhea	55%
Insulin resistance and hyperinsulinemia	50%
Obesity	40%
Dysmenorrhea	28%
Persistent anovulation	20–50%

[1]Figures are percentage of patients with syndrome manifesting each symptom or sign.

Modified, with permission, from Baulieu EE et al, eds. *Hormones: From Molecules to Disease.* Chapman & Hall, 1990.

(SHBG) and insulin-like growth factor binding protein-1 (IGFBP-1) (Figure 22–12). The decreased levels of binding proteins result in an increase in free androgens, estrogens, and IGF-1. IGF-1 and high levels of insulin stimulate the IGF-1 receptor, leading to increased thecal androgen production in response to LH, contributing to the hyperandrogenemic state. The high levels of androgens impede developing follicles and disrupt the feedback relationships that normally result in the selection of a dominant follicle for ovulation (see Figure 22–12). The resulting anovulation is associated with amenorrhea and estrogen-induced endometrial hyperplasia with breakthrough bleeding. The elevated estrogen levels also are implicated in the development of endometrial cancer. Thus, events occurring in the brain, ovary, and bloodstream of these patients work together to constitute a vicious cycle that maintains the aberrant feedback relationships.

The high levels of androgens in the bloodstream are responsible for hirsutism. Patients with elevated androgens from totally different causes (eg, Cushing disease, congenital adrenal hyperplasia) also display amenorrhea associated with polycystic ovaries, suggesting that the structural changes in the ovaries are secondary to the disordered feedback.

d. **Pituitary disorders**—Head trauma resulting in pituitary stalk transection with loss of hypothalamic–pituitary communication should be considered in patients with new-onset infertility with amenorrhea. The same is true of vascular accidents such as occurs in **Sheehan syndrome**, in which postpartum hemorrhage causes hypotension and consequent ischemic pituitary necrosis. Enlargement of the anterior pituitary during pregnancy may predispose to ischemia under conditions of hypotension. The pituitary approximately doubles in size during normal pregnancy, largely as a result of hypertrophy and hyperplasia of prolactin-secreting lactotrophs.

e. **Hypothalamic disorders**—Inputs from various central pathways impinge on the mediobasal portion of the hypothalamus, including the arcuate nucleus, from which GnRH pulses originate. Medications and illicit drugs that affect the neurotransmitters used in these pathways (opioids, dopamine, norepinephrine) can also affect GnRH secretion. This underscores the importance of a taking a detailed medication and social history in the workup of amenorrhea.

Also important is a detailed history of behavioral patterns and any recent life changes. Psychic stress (eg, that associated with moving to a different country) can lead to altered GnRH secretion and subsequent amenorrhea that lasts up to 1 year. Vigorous exercise and excessive weight loss can also lead to impaired GnRH pulsatility, accounting for the amenorrhea seen in competitive athletes and in **anorexia nervosa**.

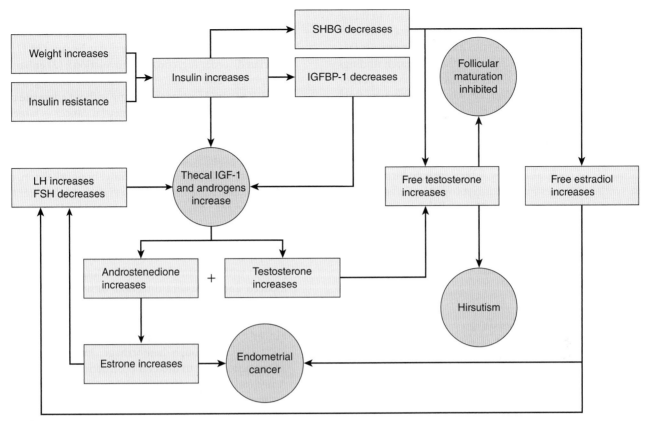

FIGURE 22–12 Pathogenesis of the various clinical manifestations of polycystic ovary syndrome. (FSH, follicle-stimulating hormone; IGF, insulin-like growth factor; IGFBP-1, insulin-like growth factor binding protein-1; LH, luteinizing hormone; SHBG, steroid hormone-binding globulin.)

(Redrawn, with permission, from Barnes HV. *Clinical Medicine: Selected Problems with Pathophysiologic Correlations.* Year Book Medical Publishers, 1988. Copyright © Elsevier.)

Thus, a wide range of factors that alter the pulsatile release of GnRH can influence female reproductive physiology. Lack of menstrual periods because of a change in one of these factors is termed **hypothalamic amenorrhea** and is a common cause of infertility. Correction of the underlying cause often leads to a return of normal cyclic ovulation.

f. **Indirect influences**—In addition to factors that work directly on the GnRH-secreting neurons, indirect influences must be considered. Primary hypothyroidism, as well as primary or secondary hyperprolactinemia, can result in altered GnRH pulse frequency and amplitude. The subsequent diminished gonadotropin secretion produces a secondary ovarian failure and amenorrhea. Examples of conditions that result in secondary hyperprolactinemia include lactation and treatment with drugs that have dopamine-blocking effects (eg, antipsychotic agents).

CHECKPOINT

25. Identify environmental and lifestyle factors that cause altered GnRH secretion and hypothalamic amenorrhea.

26. What are the consequences of untreated amenorrhea?

B. Dysmenorrhea

Primary dysmenorrhea is thought to be due to disordered prostaglandin production by the secretory endometrium. Prostaglandin F2α (PGF2α) stimulates myometrial contractions of the nonpregnant uterus, whereas prostaglandins of the E series tend to inhibit its contraction. It appears that patients with severe dysmenorrhea generally experience excessive PGF2α production rather than increased sensitivity to this prostaglandin. Unabated contractions of the myometrium result in uterine muscle ischemia, which stimulates the uterine pain fibers of the autonomic nervous system. Anxiety, fear, and stress may lower the pain threshold and thereby exaggerate the prominence of these symptoms.

Among the secondary causes of dysmenorrhea is **endometriosis**, a disorder in which extrauterine implants of ectopic endometrial tissue respond cyclically to estrogen and progesterone production (see Table 22–5). This is a common disorder, affecting 10–25% of women of reproductive age. The presenting symptoms of patients with endometriosis can range from pain and cramping during menstruation to adhesions with bowel obstruction in severe cases. Typical locations for ectopic endometrial tissue include the pelvic portion of the peritoneal cavity and the ovaries. The establishment of endometrial tissue in these locations is believed to occur by either or both of two mechanisms: (1) transport of sloughed endometrial tissue by retrograde menstruation through the fallopian tubes; or (2) metaplasia of undifferentiated celomic mesenchyme in the peritoneum, perhaps under the influence of growth factors present in retrograde menstrual efflux. Research findings support the hypothesis of a vicious cycle involving peritoneal inflammation with elevated cytokines in peritoneal fluid and the secretion of angiogenic factors that maintain ectopic endometrial tissue. A characteristic feature of endometriosis is amelioration after pregnancy and after menopause. These observations provide a therapeutic rationale for the most common modes of medical therapy, which include birth control pills; synthetic progestins (medroxyprogesterone acetate) or androgens (danazol), which block gonadotropin production; and long-acting GnRH analogs that downregulate the reproductive neuroendocrine axis. Some of these drugs may also work by downregulating cytokine production. It is unclear how endometriosis causes infertility, although inflammatory cytokines have been invoked.

C. Abnormal Uterine Bleeding

The pathogenesis of abnormal uterine bleeding depends on its cause. In an effort to standardize the nomenclature used to describe the pathogenesis of abnormal uterine bleeding, the International Federation of Gynecology and Obstetrics proposed a new classification system in 2011. This system encompasses the most common pathologies associated with abnormal uterine bleeding and includes uterine polyp, adenomyosis, leiomyoma, malignancy (and endometrial hyperplasia); coagulopathy; ovulatory dysfunction; and endometrial, iatrogenic, and not-yet-classified causes. This nomenclature system is collectively recognized by the acronym **PALM-COEIN** and is now universally accepted. The term "dysfunctional uterine bleeding," once frequently used to refer to abnormal uterine bleeding without any definable pathology, is not a part of the new classification system, and its use has, therefore, been discontinued. Similarly, the terms "heavy menstrual bleeding" and "intermenstrual bleeding" have now replaced the obsolete terms "menorrhagia" and "metrorrhagia," respectively.

1. **Structural Lesions**—Structural lesions that alter the contour of the endometrial cavity often lead to uterine bleeding. Endometrial polyps present with premenstrual or intermenstrual bleeding. Leiomyomas, however, more often cause abnormal uterine bleeding with aberrations in both timing and severity. When these benign tumors are located within the endometrial cavity or within the wall of the uterus, they can disrupt the endometrial vasculature. Very heavy prolonged or sporadic bleeding can occur.

2. **Adenomyosis**—The presence of endometrial glands in the myometrium, known as adenomyosis, is a common cause of a spectrum of menstrual abnormalities, ranging from heavy menstrual bleeding to severe dysmenorrhea.

3. **Malignancy**—Both precancerous and cancerous lesions of the uterus or cervix can produce abnormal vaginal bleeding. Endometrial hyperplasia is often the consequence of excessive estrogen production and stimulation

without progesterone exposure. It can progress to endometrial cancer with continued estrogen excess. Unopposed estrogen stimulation can occur because of (1) an ovarian disorder (eg, chronic anovulation); (2) enhanced peripheral aromatization of adrenal androgens by CYP19A1; or (3) estrogen therapy without adequate progestin supplementation. Endometrial cancer is largely a perimenopausal and postmenopausal disease; only 5% of cases occur during the reproductive years. Endometrial cancer spreads by direct involvement of the lymphatics with distant metastases to the lung, brain, skeleton, and abdominal organs. Patients with endometrial cancer typically present with abnormal vaginal bleeding. As with ovarian cancer, ascites, bowel obstruction, and associated pleural effusions occur in widespread disease.

Dysplasia of the cervix and cervical cancer can also present with abnormal vaginal bleeding. Carcinogens in tobacco and persistent infection with certain subtypes of human papillomavirus (HPV) have been shown to increase the risk of cervical cancer. If untreated, cervical cancer spreads directly to the other pelvic organs; death often occurs through hemorrhage, infection, or renal failure secondary to ureteral obstruction. Currently, the American College of Obstetricians and Gynecologists recommends that uninfected girls and young women between the ages of 9 and 26 years (and, as their potential sexual partners, boys and men between the ages of 11 and 26 years) be vaccinated against HPV to prevent cervical cancer.

4. **Systemic Conditions with Altered Coagulation**— Normal blood clotting involves both coagulation factors and platelets. Disorders affecting the production, quality, and survival of either clotting factors or platelets can cause abnormal vaginal bleeding (Table 22–10).

5. **Functional Disorders**—Endocrine disorders, as described previously, can sometimes result in altered amounts and timing of hormonal stimulation of the genital tract, at times causing a complete cessation of menses. Systemic disorders resulting in oligo-ovulation or anovulation may cause significant menstrual aberrations, including heavy and intermenstrual uterine bleeding. These aberrations are due to overgrowth and a lack of progesterone-induced stabilization of the endometrium.

6. **Endometrial Factors**—Abnormal uterine bleeding occurring in the context of cyclic menstrual bleeding (typical of ovulatory cycles) and, particularly when no other definable causes are identified, are referred to as primary disorders of the endometrium. Endometrial dysfunction may result from failure to regulate hemostasis due to an overproduction of vasodilators including prostaglandin E2 and prostacyclin.

7. **Iatrogenic Factors**—Medical interventions and devices often contribute to the pathogenesis of abnormal uterine bleeding. Hormonal interventions with progestins and intrauterine devices (IUDs) that secrete progestins, such as the levonorgestrel IUD, are a cause of abnormal

TABLE 22–10   Disorders of coagulation.

A. Disorders resulting in thrombocytopenia	B. Disorders resulting in clotting factor deficiency
Decreased platelet production	**Acquired**
Congenital bone marrow failure (eg, Fanconi anemia, Wiskott–Aldrich syndrome)	Liver diseases (cirrhosis, acute hepatic failure, liver transplantation, thrombopoietin deficiency)
Acquired bone marrow failure (eg, aplastic anemia, myelodysplasia, leukemia)	Renal failure
Exposure to chemotherapy, irradiation	Vitamin K deficiency (malabsorption syndrome, prolonged antibiotic therapy, malnutrition, prolonged biliary obstruction)
Marrow infiltration (neoplastic, infectious/granulomatous)	Hematologic disorders (acute leukemias [particularly promyelocytic], myelodysplasias, monoclonal gammopathies, essential thrombocythemia)
Nutritional (deficiency of vitamin B_{12}, folate, iron; alcohol)	Acquired antibodies against coagulation factors
Increased platelet destruction	Disseminated intravascular coagulation (sepsis, malignancies, trauma, obstetric complications, retained products of conception, malignancies, giant hemangiomas)
Immune thrombocytopenia (primary)	Drugs (antiplatelet agents, anticoagulants, antithrombins; thrombolytic, hepatotoxic, and nephrotoxic agents)
Immune thrombocytopenia (secondary), including hepatitis C virus, HIV-related, and drug-induced	Vascular
Heparin-induced thrombocytopenia	Nonpalpable purpura ("senile," solar, and factitious purpura), vitamin C deficiency, thromboembolic, purpura fulminans)
Thrombotic microangiopathy	Palpable-purpura (Henoch–Schönlein, vasculitis, dysproteinemias, amyloidosis)
Disseminated intravascular coagulation	**Inherited**
Post-transfusion purpura	Deficiencies of coagulation factors (hemophilia A [factor VIII deficiency], hemophilia B ([actor IX deficiency]; deficiencies of fibrinogen factors II, V, VII, X, XI, and XIII; von Willebrand disease)
Mechanical (aortic valvular dysfunction; extracorporeal bypass)	Fibrinolytic disorders (a_2-antiplasmin deficiency, plasminogen activator inhibitor-1 deficiency)
von Willebrand disease, type 2B	Vascular (hemorrhagic telangiectasias)
Hemophagocytosis	Connective tissue disorders (Ehlers–Danlos syndrome)
Increased platelet sequestration	
Hypersplenism (eg, related to cirrhosis, myeloproliferative disorders, lymphoma)	
Other conditions causing thrombocytopenia	
Gestational thrombocytopenia	
Bernard–Soulier syndrome, gray platelet syndrome, May–Hegglin anomaly	
Pseudothrombocytopenia	

Modified, with permission, from Papadakis MA et al, eds. *Current Medical Diagnosis & Treatment 2018*, 57th ed. McGraw-Hill, 2018; and Kaushansky K et al, eds. *Williams Hematology*, 9th ed. McGraw-Hill, 2016.

uterine bleeding (especially intermenstrual bleeding). The administration of anticoagulants, including warfarin and heparin, is another cause of iatrogenic abnormal uterine bleeding. These agents impair the coagulative function of the endometrial vasculature and can cause severe bleeding diatheses.

CHECKPOINT

27. What are effective medical therapies for endometriosis, and how do they work?
28. What factors predispose to cervical cancer?

Clinical Manifestations

A. Amenorrhea

The clinical symptoms and signs that accompany amenorrhea depend on its category (see Table 22–4). In genetic disorders, particularly disorders of ovarian development, various degrees of delayed puberty, such as lack of breast development and absence of pubic hair, may accompany amenorrhea. In outflow tract disorders (eg, imperforate hymen), pain from occult, obstructed menstruation may occur on a cyclic basis. Generally, disorders of the uterus and the hypothalamic–pituitary axis that result in amenorrhea are painless. Ovarian insufficiency resulting in amenorrhea is often preceded by symptoms referable to decreased estrogen and progesterone production. These include hot flushes and other vasomotor symptoms.

The most common complication in the nonpregnant patient with amenorrhea is infertility. Additional complications depend on the specific cause of lack of menstruation. Osteoporosis is a major potential long-term complication of inadequate estrogen production. Inadequate estrogen can also be associated with a thinning of estrogen-dependent epithelia, such as that of the vagina, resulting in atrophic vaginitis. This symptom usually responds to topical estrogen cream. In the case of inadequate progesterone production—typically associated with irregular vaginal bleeding but also seen in some cases of amenorrhea—the risk of endometrial cancer is greatly increased. Endometrial cancer is the most common cancer of the female genital tract; 34,000 new cases are identified annually in the United States. Risk factors for endometrial cancer include early menarche, late menopause, nulliparity, obesity, hypertension, and diabetes mellitus.

B. Dysmenorrhea

Dysmenorrhea may be accompanied by a variable constellation of symptoms, including sweating, weakness and fatigue, insomnia, nausea, vomiting, diarrhea, back pain, headache (including both migraine and tension headaches; see Chapter 7), dizziness, and syncope. Prostaglandin synthesis inhibitors (nonsteroidal anti-inflammatory agents) often alleviate many of these symptoms if treatment is initiated prior to menses and averts the cascade of events that occur with the production of prostaglandins.

With **premenstrual syndrome** (**PMS**), dysmenorrhea is accompanied by additional symptoms, including a sensation of bloating, weight gain, edema of the hands and feet, breast tenderness, acne, anxiety, aggression, mood irritability, food cravings, and change in libido. An initial approach should be to encourage changes in lifestyle if indicated by the history (eg, more sleep; exercise; improved diet; and less tobacco, alcohol, and caffeine). Pharmacologic therapy with selective serotonin reuptake inhibitors (SSRIs) has proven beneficial in addition to behavioral modification.

C. Abnormal Vaginal Bleeding

The symptoms and signs that accompany abnormal vaginal bleeding vary with the cause. In children, vulvovaginitis is the most frequent disorder, accompanied by a mucopurulent discharge that may become bloody with mucosal erosion. Other prominent causes, including foreign objects and tumors, can be assessed by physical examination. In adolescents and adults, anovulatory uterine bleeding is most common, but other causes must be considered. These include pregnancy (assessed by serial serum hCG determinations and ultrasound examination), trauma (by history and physical examination), cancer (by colposcopy and hysteroscopy), and systemic disorders such as a hemorrhagic diathesis (by platelet, prothrombin, and partial thromboplastin time determinations) and thyroid disease (by serum TSH and total and free thyroxine determinations). In postmenopausal women, one-fifth of vaginal bleeding cases prove to be endometrial cancer.

INFERTILITY

Infertility is defined as the absence of conception after at least 1 year of regular sexual intercourse.

Etiology

Males are found to be solely responsible for 20-30% of infertility cases (eg, inadequate sperm count) and to contribute to 50% of cases (eg, via antisperm antibodies) overall (see Chapter 23). For female infertility, about 40% of cases are due to ovulatory failure, about 40% are due to endometrial or tubal disease, about 10% are due to rarer causes (eg, thyroid disease

TABLE 22–11   Causes of female infertility.[1]

Cause	Patients with Infertility
Ovulatory dysfunction	40%
Diminished ovarian reserve	
Oligo-ovulation or amenorrhea	
Polycystic ovary syndrome (PCOS)	
Hypothalamic amenorrhea	
Other	
Tubal or pelvic pathology	40%
Endometriosis	
Scarring and adhesions (from pelvic inflammatory disease, chronic infection, tubal surgery, ectopic pregnancy, or ruptured appendix)	
Miscellaneous	10%
Thyroid disease	
Pituitary disease (hyperprolactinemia)	
Unexplained	10%

[1]In infertile couples, problems in the male account for 30% of the total.

or hyperprolactinemia), and about 10% remain unexplained after full workup (Table 22–11).

Pathology & Pathogenesis

A. Ovulatory Causes

Infertility due to ovarian dysfunction can result from disorders of the hypothalamus or pituitary, resulting in inadequate gonadotropic stimulation of the ovary; from ovarian disorders, resulting either in inadequate secretory products or failure to ovulate; and occasionally from both types of disorder occurring at the same time. Correction of the underlying cause will often restore fertility. In many cases, the administration of exogenous gonadotropins will stimulate the ovaries to produce follicular growth. The oocytes can then be released in vivo and fertilized by intercourse or by artificial insemination. Alternatively, the mature oocytes can be removed via transvaginal aspiration and subsequently fertilized using in vitro fertilization (IVF), with or without the technique of intracytoplasmic sperm injection (ICSI), in the laboratory. The resultant embryos can then be returned to the uterus transcervically. Testing the embryos via biopsy of the trophectoderm, termed preimplantation genetic screening (PGS), is being applied widely to increase IVF success rates, reduce miscarriages, and reduce multiple births as a result of fertility treatments.

One of the most common ovarian disorders, called diminished ovarian reserve, is age related and can involve both the oocytes themselves and the secretory products of the ovary.

There is an accelerated loss of follicles with the approach of menopause. With follicular depletion, FSH levels tend to rise, reflecting an inadequate production of inhibin, and anti-müllerian hormone (AMH) levels fall. This could result from an inadequate number of follicles, diminished competence of the remaining follicles, diminished steroidogenesis by the aging ovary, or some combination of these factors. Regardless of the specific reason, the net effect is a shortened follicular phase, which is associated with increased rates of infertility. Treatment with clomiphene citrate, a weak estrogen antagonist, is a means of diminishing negative feedback and increasing the endogenous gonadotropin stimulation of the ovary and restoring ovulation. Similarly, a common treatment to encourage multifollicular development in the setting of infertility is the self-administration of exogenous gonadotropins (FSH and LH) in the follicular phase of the cycle.

Other etiologies of ovulation dysfunction include conditions that alter the coordination between ovary and hypothalamus, such as PCOS and hypothalamic amenorrhea. In these scenarios, the oocytes do not undergo the appropriate development and maturation to lead to regular ovulation.

B. Tubal and Pelvic Causes

With normal follicles and reproductive neuroendocrine axis function, the major cause of infertility is an abnormality in the endometrium or fallopian tubes. Prior or ongoing pelvic infections, with adhesions or inflammation, can result in a failure of sperm or egg transport, a failure of implantation, or implantation in an inappropriate location (ectopic pregnancy).

Endometriosis, presumably occurring due to the cyclic proliferation and sloughing of ectopic endometrial tissue, results in inflammation and adhesion formation. New data suggest that endometriosis may arise from a circulating endometrial stem cell population. This condition should be suspected when infertility is associated with severe dysmenorrhea, dyspareunia, or central pelvic pain. Intermenstrual pain is another common endometriosis-related symptom. Surgical and medical therapies are efficacious in the reduction of endometriosis-associated pain. Newer oral treatments using GnRH agonists have been advocated and are promising for this population.

C. Other Causes of Female Infertility

Most of the less common causes of infertility can be grouped into those disorders that affect the production of GnRH by the hypothalamus or the hormone's effect on the pituitary (eg, thyroid disease and hyperprolactinemia).

CHECKPOINT

29. What are the most common causes of infertility in couples?
30. What feature of the history suggests a tubal or uterine cause of infertility?

PREECLAMPSIA-ECLAMPSIA

Pregnancy is associated with a host of medical complications the clinical management of which requires an understanding of both the underlying physiology of pregnancy and the pathophysiology of the particular disorder. The syndrome of preeclampsia-eclampsia, characterized by hypertension, proteinuria, and edema, is chosen for focus here for several reasons. First, preeclampsia-eclampsia is one of the most common causes of maternal death in the United States and the developed world. Second, it illustrates how pathophysiologic mechanisms in pregnancy may be far more complex—and the clinical consequences far more serious—than would have been expected from a simple consideration of each of the presenting symptoms in isolation. Third, advances have significantly altered our current thinking about the pathogenesis of this disorder.

Clinical Presentation

Hypertension can develop during pregnancy as an isolated finding (**pregnancy-induced hypertension [PIH]**) or as a component of a dangerous syndrome (**preeclampsia-eclampsia**). Treatment guidelines for PIH are different from those for essential hypertension in the nonpregnant patient: Elevated maternal blood pressure is often left untreated unless symptomatic or if severe hypertension develops. Because placental perfusion depends on a pressure difference between the maternal and fetal circulations, decreases in maternal blood pressure can lead to underperfusion of the placenta. This can result in **placental insufficiency** with fetal growth restriction and distress.

The hypertension seen in preeclampsia is associated with proteinuria and edema. This syndrome occurs in approximately 5% of pregnancies in the United States. Eclampsia, the superimposition of generalized tonic-clonic seizures on pregnancy-induced hypertension, can occur as the initial presenting sign of this syndrome or during its progression and is life-threatening. Table 22–12 summarizes the symptoms and signs of preeclampsia-eclampsia.

Etiology

Preeclampsia-eclampsia is thought to derive from faulty implantation, resulting in a systemic disorder of endothelial cell activation (see later discussion). Predisposing factors for the development of preeclampsia include first pregnancy, obesity, pre-existing diabetes or hypertension, hydatidiform mole, malnutrition, and a family history of preeclampsia.

Pathology & Pathogenesis

The placenta of a preeclamptic patient shows signs of premature aging, including apoptosis, hyaline deposition, calcification, and congestion. The maternal decidua also shows hemorrhage and necrosis with thrombosis of the spiral arteries and diffuse infarcts.

Normally, blood vessels of the uterine wall undergo striking morphologic changes at the site of implantation, facilitating

TABLE 22–12   Indicators of mild to moderate versus severe preeclampsia-eclampsia.

Site	Indicator	Mild to Moderate	Severe
Central nervous system	Symptoms and signs	Hyperreflexia	Seizures
			Blurred vision
			Scotomas
			Headache
			Clonus
			Irritability
Kidney	Proteinuria	0.3–5 g/24 h	>5 g/24 h or catheterized urine with 4+ protein
	Urinary output	>30 mL/h	<30 mL/h
Liver	AST, ALT, LD	Normal liver enzymes	Elevated liver enzymes
			Epigastric pain
			Ruptured liver
Hematologic	Platelets		<100,000/mcL
	Hemoglobin	Normal	Low, normal, or elevated
Vascular	Blood pressure	<160/110 mm Hg	>160/110 mm Hg
	Retina	Arteriolar spasm	Retinal hemorrhages
Fetal–placental unit	Growth restriction	Absent	Present
	Oligohydramnios	Absent	Present
	Fetal distress	Absent	Present

ALT, alanine aminotransferase; AST, aspartate aminotransferase; LD, lactate dehydrogenase.

Reproduced, with permission, from Papadakis MA et al, eds. *Current Medical Diagnosis & Treatment 2018*, 57th ed. McGraw-Hill, 2018.

placental perfusion. The diameters of the spiral arteries increase and the muscular and elastic components are lost. However, for unknown (perhaps immune-mediated) reasons, these early angiogenic changes of implantation do not occur—or at least not fully—in patients who will develop preeclampsia-eclampsia later in gestation. As a result, a condition of relative placental ischemia is established, with the release of lipid and protein factors that damage the maternal vascular endothelium, at first within the decidua and later systemically. Oxidative injury is believed to potentiate the effects of maternal factors (eg, obesity, diabetes, diet, genes) to cause generalized endothelial cell damage.

Endothelial activation has two important pathophysiologic consequences. First, the balance between vasodilation and vasoconstriction is altered, specifically by a diminished production of vasodilator products, such as prostacyclin and nitric oxide, and an increased production of vasoconstrictive thromboxane, endothelin, and platelet-derived growth factor. As a result, there is increased vasoconstriction of the placental bed arterioles, with hypoperfusion and ischemia of the downstream tissues and systemic hypertension. Second, the endothelial cell barrier between platelets and the collagen of basement membranes is breached, promoting thrombosis.

As a result of the latter changes, platelet aggregation, activation of the clotting cascade, and the production of vasoactive substances cause capillary leak. This results in further tissue hypoperfusion, edema formation, and proteinuria, the hallmarks of preeclampsia-eclampsia. Because these processes result in further vascular endothelial damage, a vicious circle is established.

Recent speculation has centered on the potential of serotonin to modulate vasodilation and angiogenic growth factors. New data also invoke a role for agonistic autoantibodies directed against the second extracellular loop of the angiotensin II AT1 receptor, resulting in the vasospasm associated with preeclampsia. A short angiotensin peptide (Ang 1-7) with vasodilator activity is reported to be reduced in preeclampsia.

Clinical Manifestations

Preeclampsia has a plethora of manifestations (see Table 22–12). Beyond the clinical triad of hypertension, edema, and proteinuria, patients may also experience increased deep tendon reflexes or placental abruption. Hepatic periportal congestion, hemorrhage, and necrosis can lead to elevated liver function tests and ultimately result in rupture of the hepatic capsule. Severe preeclampsia can also produce renal changes, including glomerular endothelial cell swelling, mesangial proliferation, and marked narrowing of glomerular capillary lumens. The renal cortex displays significant cortical ischemia that may progress to frank necrosis and acute kidney injury. Thrombocytopenia, disseminated intravascular coagulopathy (DIC), and cerebral vascular accidents may also occur (Table 22–13). Eclampsia, with its characteristic additional neurological features such as maternal seizures resulting from cerebral ischemia and petechial hemorrhage, can occur in this setting or can appear as the first manifestation of this disease. Preeclampsia-eclampsia also carries risks for the fetus. Placental deterioration and insufficiency can result in intrauterine growth restriction (IUGR) and fetal hypoxia. Delivery of the fetus and placenta is the only definitive cure for this syndrome, which carries a high risk of morbidity and mortality for both mother and child (see Table 22–13).

CHECKPOINT

31. What are the hallmarks of preeclampsia-eclampsia?
32. What are the risks to the fetus of untreated maternal hypertension?
33. What are some of the maternal sequelae of preeclampsia-eclampsia?

TABLE 22–13 Complications of preeclampsia-eclampsia.

Cerebral hemorrhage
Cortical blindness
Retinal detachment
HELLP syndrome (*hemolysis, elevated liver enzymes, low platelets*)
Hepatic rupture
Disseminated intravascular coagulation (DIC)
Pulmonary edema
Laryngeal edema
Acute renal cortical necrosis
Acute renal tubular necrosis
Abruptio placentae
Intrauterine fetal asphyxia and death

Data from Roberts JM et al. Pre-eclampsia: more than pregnancy-induced hypertension. Lancet. 1993;341:1447.

CASE STUDIES

Yeong Kwok, MD

(See Chapter 25, p. 786–88 for answers)

CASE 119

A 27-year-old woman comes to a gynecology appointment for the evaluation of amenorrhea. She underwent menarche at age 14 but, since menarche, has always had irregular periods, varying 1 to 3 months between menstrual periods. Her last period was about 12 months earlier. She has been sexually active with her boyfriend for the past 2 years, using condoms sporadically. She has never been pregnant and has never had any gynecologic infections, procedures, or surgeries. The physical examination shows her to be obese, with a body mass index of 35. The examination is notable for facial hair and acne.

Questions

A. What are the four broad categories of amenorrhea?
B. What is its likely cause in this patient?
C. What is the underlying pathophysiology of this condition?

CASE 120

A 24-year-old woman presents to the clinic complaining of painful menses. She states that for the last several years, she has had cramping pain in the days preceding her menses as well as during her menses. In addition, she notes bloating and weight gain in the week before her menses, with swelling of her hands and feet. She experiences irritability and severe mood swings during that time, such that she cries easily and for no reason seems to become enraged at her family or boyfriend. On a review of systems, she denies urinary symptoms, vaginal discharge, and gastrointestinal symptoms. She has no significant medical history. She has never been pregnant. She has never had a sexually transmitted infection. She is sexually active only with her long-standing boyfriend and states that they always use condoms. She takes no medications. Her physical examination is unremarkable.

Questions

A. What are some possible causes of this woman's dysmenorrhea? Which do you think is most likely? Why?
B. What is the pathophysiologic mechanism responsible for her dysmenorrhea?
C. How would you treat her symptoms?

CASE 121

A 57-year-old woman presents to her primary care doctor's office with abnormal vaginal bleeding. Her last menstrual period was 7 years before at age 50. After menopause, she had some mild hot flashes for 1–2 years but experienced no other symptoms. During the week before presentation, she "a very heavy period," with the passage of a large amount of blood and clots from her vagina. A pelvic ultrasound shows a thickened endometrium of 10 mm. An endometrial biopsy reveals endometrial cancer.

Questions

A. What is the current classification system for abnormal uterine bleeding?
B. What uterine condition can lead to endometrial carcinoma?
C. What fraction of cases of vaginal bleeding in postmenopausal women result from endometrial cancer?

CASE 122

A 28-year-old woman presents to the clinic with a complaint of infertility. She states that she and her husband have been trying to get pregnant for approximately 1 year without success. She had menarche at age 14 years. Since that time, she has had regular menses lasting 5 days, without significant dysmenorrhea or abnormal bleeding. She has never been pregnant. The medical history is notable for gonorrhea and trichomoniasis at age 18 years. In addition, she has had an abnormal Pap smear consistent with human papillomavirus at age 20 years, with normal Pap smears since that time. She takes no medications. She has been married for 2 years and is sexually active only with her husband. Before her marriage, she had approximately 25 sexual partners, mostly during her college years. Her physical examination is unremarkable.

Questions

A. What are the most common causes of female infertility?
B. What do you suspect is the cause of this patient's infertility? Why?

CASE 123

A 28-year-old woman presents to her obstetrician for her regularly scheduled prenatal examination. She is 30 weeks pregnant. She has noted some swelling of her hands and feet in the last 2 weeks that seems to be getting progressively worse, such that she is no longer able to wear her rings and can only wear open-heeled shoes. She is otherwise without complaints. She has no past medical problems. This is her first pregnancy. She has had regular prenatal care and no complications thus far. She is taking only prenatal multivitamins. Her family history is notable for maternal hypertension and diabetes. She is married and works as a schoolteacher. She denies alcohol, tobacco, and drug use. On examination she appears to be well, with a blood pressure of 152/95 mm Hg. The fundal height is consistent with gestational age. The fetal heart rate is 140 bpm. There is a 1+ lower extremity edema to the knees and trace edema of the hands. A urine dipstick reveals 3+ protein.

Questions

A. What is the likely diagnosis?

B. What are some risk factors for developing this condition?

C. How does this condition develop? How does it result in maternal hypertension, edema, and proteinuria?

D. What are the risks to the fetus if this condition is left untreated?

E. What are the maternal sequelae of leaving this condition untreated? What is the treatment?

REFERENCES

General

Committee on Practice Bulletins—Gynecology. Practice bulletin no. 128: diagnosis of abnormal uterine bleeding in reproductive-aged women. Obstet Gynecol. 2012 Jul;120(1):197–206. [PMID: 22914421]

Croft B et al. Review disorders of sex development: the evolving role of genomics in diagnosis and gene discovery. Birth Defects Res C Embryo Today. 2016 Dec;108(4):337–50. Erratum in: Birth Defects Res. 2017 Jul 3;109 (11):869–71. [PMID: 28033663]

Fritz M et al. *Clinical Gynecologic Endocrinology and Infertility*, 8th ed. Lippincott Williams & Wilkins, 2011.

Haghshenas MR et al. Efficacy of human papillomavirus L1 protein vaccines (Cervarix and Gardasil) in reducing the risk of cervical intraepithelial neoplasia: a meta-analysis. Int J Prev Med. 2017 Jun 1;8:44. [PMID: 28656100]

Hoffman BL et al, eds. *Williams Gynecology*, 3rd ed., McGraw-Hill, 2016.

Oktay K et al. Fertility preservation in women with Turner syndrome: a comprehensive review and practical guidelines. J Pediatr Adolesc Gynecol. 2016 Oct;29(5):409–16. [PMID: 26485320]

Infertility

American College of Obstetricians and Gynecologists Committee on Gynecologic Practice; Practice Committee of the American Society for Reproductive Medicine. Female age-related fertility decline. Committee Opinion No. 589. Obstet Gynecol. 2014 Mar;123(3):719–21. [PMID: 24553169]

Baskind NE et al. Hypothalamic-pituitary, ovarian and adrenal contributions to polycystic ovary syndrome. Best Pract Res Clin Obstet Gynaecol. 2016 Nov;37:80–97. [PMID: 27137106]

Broughton DE et al. Obesity and female infertility: potential mediators of obesity's impact. Fertil Steril. 2017 Apr;107(4):840–7. [PMID: 28292619]

Dumesic DA et al. Scientific statement on the diagnostic criteria, epidemiology, pathophysiology, and molecular genetics of polycystic ovary syndrome. Endocr Rev. 2015 Oct;36(5):487–525. [PMID: 26426951]

Franasiak J et al. Chapter 19: Preimplantation genetic diagnosis and genetic screening. In Falcone T et al, eds. *Clinical Reproductive Medicine and Surgery: A Practical Guide*, 3rd ed. Springer, 2017, pp. 329–45.

Garg D et al. The role of AMH [anti-Müllerian hormone] in the pathophysiology of polycystic ovarian syndrome. Reprod Biomed Online. 2016 Jul;33(1):15–28. [PMID: 27174394]

Hanson B et al. Female infertility, infertility-associated diagnoses, and comorbidities: a review. J Assist Reprod Genet. 2017 Feb;34(2):167–77. [PMID: 27817040]

Qi X et al. The role of anti-Müllerian hormone in the pathogenesis and pathophysiological characteristics of polycystic ovary syndrome. Eur J Obstet Gynecol Reprod Biol. 2016 Apr;199:82–7. [PMID: 26914398]

Traeger-Synodinos J. Pre-implantation genetic diagnosis. Best Pract Res Clin Obstet Gynaecol. 2017 Feb;39:74–88. [PMID: 27856159]

Trikudanathan S. Polycystic ovarian syndrome. Med Clin North Am. 2015 Jan;99(1):221–35. [PMID: 25456652]

Menstrual Disorders

Collins G et al. Primary ovarian insufficiency: current concepts. South Med J. 2017 Mar;110(3):147–53. [PMID: 28257537]

Molitch ME. Diagnosis and treatment of pituitary adenomas: a review. JAMA. 2017 Feb7;317(5):516–24. [PMID: 28170483]

Munro MG et al; FIGO Working Group on Menstrual Disorders. FIGO classification system (PALM-COEIN) for causes of abnormal uterine bleeding in nongravid women of reproductive age. Int J Gynaecol Obstet. 2011 Apr;113(1):3–13. [PMID: 21345435]

Taylor HS et al. Treatment of endometriosis-associated pain with Elagolix, an oral GnRH antagonist. N Engl J Med. 2017 Jul 6;377(1):28–40. [PMID: 28525302]

Pregnancy

Henderson JT et al. Preeclampsia screening: evidence report and systematic review for the U.S. Preventive Services Task Force. JAMA. 2017 Apr 25;317(16):1668–83. [PMID: 28444285]

Karumanchi SA et al. Preeclampsia and pregnancy-related hypertensive disorders. Hypertension. 2016 Feb;67(2):238–42. [PMID: 26693822]

Narayan B et al. Medical problems in pregnancy. Clin Med (Lond). 2016 Dec;16(Suppl 6):s110–s116. [PMID: 27956450]

Pauli JM et al. Preeclampsia: short-term and long-term implications. Obstet Gynecol Clin North Am. 2015 Jun;42(2):299–313. [PMID: 26002168]

Roberts JM. Pathophysiology of ischemic placental disease. Semin Perinatol. 2014 Apr;38(3):139–45. [PMID: 24836825]

Salzer L et al. Metabolic disorder of pregnancy (understanding pathophysiology of diabetes and preeclampsia). Best Pract Res Clin Obstet Gynaecol. 2015 Apr;29(3):328–38. [PMID: 25481558]

U.S. Preventive Services Task Force; Bibbins-Domingo K et al. Screening for preeclampsia: U.S. Preventive Services Task Force recommendation statement. JAMA. 2017 Apr 25;317(16):1661–7. [PMID: 28444286]

Puberty

Abitbol L et al. Evaluation of delayed puberty: what diagnostic tests should be performed in the seemingly otherwise well adolescent? Arch Dis Child. 2016 Aug;101(8):767–71. [PMID: 27190100]

Li P et al. Gonadotropin releasing hormone agonist treatment to increase final stature in children with precocious puberty: a meta-analysis. Medicine (Baltimore). 2014 Dec;93(27):e260. [PMID: 25501098]

Maïmoun L et al. Endocrine disorders in adolescent and young female athletes: impact on growth, menstrual cycles, and bone mass acquisition. J Clin Endocrinol Metab. 2014 Nov;99(11):4037–50. [PMID: 24601725]

Wei C et al. Recent advances in the understanding and management of delayed puberty. Arch Dis Child. 2016 May;101(5):481–8. [PMID: 26353794]

Disorders of the Male Reproductive Tract

Mikkel Fode, MD, PhD, Jens Sønksen, MD, PhD, & Dana A. Ohl, MD

Male reproductive tract functions include androgen homeostasis, spermatogenesis, sperm transport and storage, and normal erectile and ejaculatory function ability. The control of these functions involves the pituitary gland, central and peripheral nervous systems, and genitalia. In addition to a review of normal male reproductive anatomy and physiology, this chapter considers two common disorders of the male reproductive tract: male infertility and benign prostatic hyperplasia.

NORMAL STRUCTURE & FUNCTION OF THE MALE REPRODUCTIVE TRACT

ANATOMY & PHYSIOLOGY

The male reproductive tract is composed of the testes, genital ducts, accessory glands, and penis (Figure 23–1).

The testes are responsible for the production of testosterone and spermatozoa. Each testis is approximately 4 cm in length and 20 mL in volume. The testis is divided into lobules consisting of seminiferous tubules (inside which sperm are produced) and connective tissue (Figure 23–2). The seminiferous tubules converge to form another network of tubules called the rete testis through which spermatozoa are transported to the epididymis.

The seminiferous tubules are surrounded by a basal membrane and a specialized epithelium containing Sertoli cells that provide protection and nourishment to germ cells. At puberty, tight junctions develop between adjacent Sertoli cells, creating an impermeable lining called the blood–testis barrier. This barrier divides the seminiferous tubules into a basal compartment and an adluminal compartment, separating more advanced germ cells from the immune system. The separation is necessary because mature sperm are potentially antigenic since they are not present at the prepubertal interval when much of the immune tolerance is established. The Leydig cells in the intertubular connective tissue produce testosterone.

Both testosterone production and spermatogenesis are controlled by the hypothalamic–pituitary–gonadal axis. The hypothalamus produces gonadotropin-releasing hormone (GnRH) in a pulsatile fashion. GnRH courses through the hypothalamic–pituitary portal system to stimulate the anterior pituitary gonadotropes to secrete (also in a pulsatile fashion) the two gonadotropins: luteinizing hormone (LH) and follicle-stimulating hormone (FSH). FSH stimulates the Sertoli cells to produce paracrine growth factors and other products supporting spermatogenesis. FSH also stimulates the production of inhibin in response to active spermatogenesis and androgen-binding globulin (ABP).

Under the influence of LH, the Leydig cells produce testosterone. Concentrations of testosterone in the seminiferous tubules are 80–100 times greater than in the general circulation. Androgens act on spermatogenesis via the Sertoli cells, and high testicular levels of androgens are essential for spermatogenesis. Circulating testosterone provides negative feedback on the secretion of GnRH, LH, and FSH by acting on both the hypothalamus and the pituitary. Gonadal inhibin exerts negative feedback on FSH secretion by the pituitary.

During spermatogenesis, primitive germ cells develop into mature spermatozoa while moving from the basement membrane to the lumen of the tubules. The immature germ cells near the basement membrane are called spermatogonia and

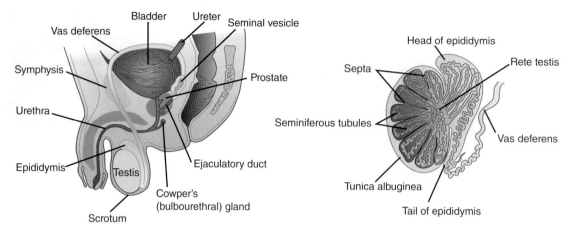

FIGURE 23–1 Anatomy of the male reproductive system (left) and the duct system of the testis (right). (Redrawn, with permission, from Barrett KE et al. *Ganong's Review of Medical Physiology*, 25th ed. McGraw-Hill, 2016.)

have the normal diploid number of 46 chromosomes. Beginning at puberty and continuing throughout life, the spermatogonia divide mitotically, maintaining the population. Some of the spermatogonia differentiate into primary spermatocytes and enter the first meiotic division. During the prophase of the first meiotic division, DNA duplication, homologous chromosome pairing, and crossing over take place in the spermatocytes as they develop a duplicated set of 46 chromosomes. The spermatocytes (now called secondary spermatocytes) then undergo the second meiotic division producing spermatids, which have a haploid number of unduplicated chromosomes. In this way, four spermatids are produced from each

spermatogonium. Spermatids then undergo a maturation process called spermiogenesis to form spermatozoa. In this process, the nuclear chromatin condenses, and the enzyme-filled acrosome cap is formed. The spermatids also elongate and develop flagella. Spermiogenesis ends with the spermatozoa being released from the germinal epithelium. The process in which the primary spermatogonia divide and develop into mature spermatozoa takes about 74 days.

After spermiogenesis, spermatozoa are released into the lumen of the seminiferous tubule and then course through the rete testis into the epididymis. During a 5-to-14-day epididymal transit, spermatozoa mature and become capable of progressive movement in a process involving changes in membrane, metabolism, and morphology. Sperm are stored in the cauda epididymis until the time of ejaculation. During ejaculation, sperm travel through the vas deferens via the inguinal canal and medially to the posterior and inferior part of the urinary bladder, where the vas deferens fuses with the duct of the seminal vesicle, forming the combined ejaculatory duct. The ejaculatory ducts enter the prostatic portion of the urethra at the verumontanum distal to the internal bladder sphincter (Figure 23–3).

During normal erection, parasympathetic fibers travel from S2–S4 through the pelvic nerve and the pelvic plexus to the cavernous nerve, where they release acetylcholine (ACh) and nitric oxide (NO). This release causes the smooth muscles of the penile corpora to relax, which in turn leads to increased blood flow and blood trapping, resulting in erection.

The ejaculatory reflex is initiated primarily by afferent input from the dorsal nerves of the penis, although cerebral erotic stimuli also play a role. The ejaculate is transported from the ampulla of the vas deferens into the posterior urethra in a process called seminal emission. This is the result of peristaltic contractions of smooth muscle cells in the epididymis, vas deferens, and accessory sex glands under sympathetic control from fibers arising from T10–T12. After seminal emission, contraction of the posterior urethra and closure of the bladder neck (preventing retrograde ejaculation into the bladder)

FIGURE 23–2 Schematic section of testis. (Redrawn, with permission, from Barrett KE et al. *Ganong's Review of Medical Physiology*, 25th ed. McGraw-Hill, 2016.)

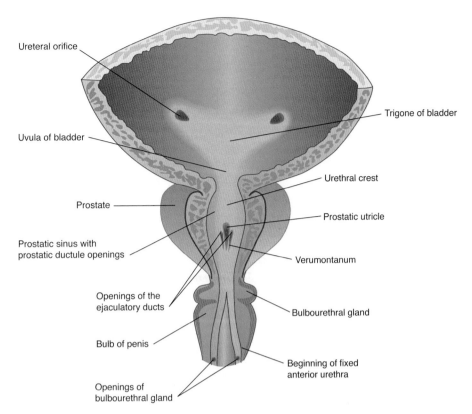

FIGURE 23–3 Anatomic relationships of the prostate. (Redrawn, with permission, from Lindner HH. *Clinical Anatomy*. Originally published by Appleton & Lange. Copyright © 1989 by The McGraw-Hill Companies, Inc.)

are initiated by sympathetic nerve fibers, while the external urethral sphincter relaxes. These events are followed by rhythmic contractions of the periurethral and pelvic floor muscles mediated by the somatic fibers from S2–S4 running through the pudendal nerve. This results in the projectile phase of ejaculation.

In the female reproductive tract, the spermatozoa must migrate through the cervical mucus and then undergo a series of functional and structural changes collectively termed capacitation. These changes are necessary for the spermatozoa's ability to fertilize the oocyte as they facilitate the acrosome reaction, during which the sperm plasma membrane fuses with the outer acrosomal membrane. This exposes the contents of the acrosome, such as acrosin and hyaluronidase, allowing oocyte penetration. Capacitation can also be induced by incubation in a suitable laboratory medium.

Sperm cells make up only 1–2% of the semen volume, with the rest coming from the accessory male sex glands. The seminal vesicles produce two-thirds of the ejaculate volume and provide fructose as an energy source, as well as seminogellin, which contributes to seminal coagulation. The prostate supplies about one-third of the ejaculate, and this includes prostate-specific antigen, a proteolytic enzyme that cleaves seminogellin, effecting liquefaction. Finally, the bulbourethral glands contribute a small amount of clear mucoid discharge, released mainly during sexual stimulation before ejaculation.

PHYSIOLOGY

Androgen Synthesis, Protein Binding & Metabolism

The testes secrete two steroid hormones essential to male reproductive function: testosterone and dihydrotestosterone. Figure 23–4 illustrates the pathways of testicular androgen biosynthesis.

Testosterone, a C_{19} steroid, is synthesized from cholesterol by the interstitial (Leydig) cells of the testes and from androstenedione secreted by the adrenal cortex. The majority of circulating testosterone is bound to sex hormone–binding globulin (SHBG) and is unavailable for biological activity.

The remainder is loosely bound to albumin and is available for target tissue action. Only about 2% is unbound in circulation. The albumin-bound and free fractions make up the "bioavailable" testosterone in circulation. SHBG is synthesized in the liver and may be increased in certain clinical conditions. The effect of increasing SHBG in the circulation is to lower the bioavailable fraction, so that while the serum total testosterone level is normal, hypogonadism occurs at the tissue level because of protein binding. The most common causes of increased SHBG are liver dysfunction, hyperestrogenemia, obesity, and aging. Figure 23–5 illustrates the normal testosterone levels throughout the lifespan. Figure 23–6 depicts the negative feedback control mechanisms for testosterone.

FIGURE 23–4 Biosynthesis and metabolism of testosterone. Heavy arrows indicate major pathways. Circled numbers represent enzymes as follows: ①cytochrome P450, family 11, subfamily A, polypeptide 1 (CYP11A1); ②hydroxy-Δ-5-steroid dehydrogenase, 3β- and steroid Δ-isomerase (HSD3β); ③17α-hydroxylase activity of cytochrome P450, family 17, subfamily A, polypeptide 1 (CYP17A1); ④17,20-lyase activity of cytochrome P450, family 17, subfamily A, polypeptide 1 (CYP17A1); ⑤hydroxysteroid (17β) dehydrogenase (HSD17β); ⑥steroid-5α-reductase, polypeptide 2 (3-oxo-5α-steroid Δ4-dehydrogenase α) (SRD5A); ⑦cytochrome P450, family 19, subfamily A, polypeptide 1 (CYP19A1). (Modified and redrawn, with permission, from Gardner DG et al. *Greenspan's Basic and Clinical Endocrinology*, 10th ed. McGraw-Hill, 2017.)

Dihydrotestosterone (DHT) is derived both from direct secretion by the testes (~20%) and from the conversion in peripheral tissues (~80%) of testosterone and other sex steroid precursors secreted by the testes and adrenals. DHT circulates in the bloodstream. The normal plasma DHT level for the adult male is 27–75 ng/dL (0.9–2.6 nmol/L) (Table 23–1).

Estradiol is produced by the aromatization of testosterone in the peripheral circulation. The aromatase enzyme is present in abundant amounts in fatty tissue. Thus, obesity can increase the conversion of testosterone, resulting in hyperestrogenemia, downregulation of the hypothalamic–pituitary–gonadal axis, and hypogonadism.

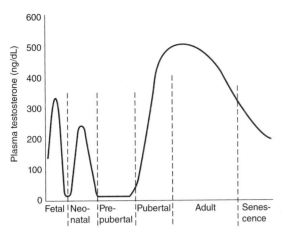

FIGURE 23–5 Plasma testosterone levels at various ages in males. (Redrawn, with permission, from Barrett KE et al. *Ganong's Review of Medical Physiology*, 25th ed. McGraw-Hill, 2016.)

TABLE 23–1 Normal plasma levels of pituitary and gonadal hormones in men.

Hormone	Conventional Units	SI Units
Testosterone, total	280–900 ng/dL	10.0–31.3 nmol/L
Testosterone, free	50–210 pg/mL	173–729 pmol/L
Dihydrotestosterone	27–75 ng/dL	0.9–2.6 nmol/L
Androstenedione	50–250 ng/dL	1.7–8.5 nmol/L
Estradiol	10–50 pg/mL	3.67–18.35 pmol/L
Estrone	15–65 pg/mL	55.5–240 pmol/L
FSH	1.0–7.0 mIU/mL	1.0–7.0 IU/L
LH	1.0–7.0 mIU/mL	1.0–7.0 IU/L
PRL	5–18 ng/mL	218–780 nmol/L

FSH, follicle-stimulating hormone; LH, luteinizing hormone; PRL, prolactin.

Data from Gardner DG et al. *Greenspan's Basic and Clinical Endocrinology*, 10th ed. McGraw-Hill, 2017.

Effects of Androgens

Circulating testosterone or DHT crosses the membrane of the target cell and enters the cytoplasm. Testosterone may be converted to the more potent DHT inside the target cell. Testosterone or DHT binds to the androgen receptor, and the complex is then transported to the cell's nucleus, where it binds to DNA and initiates mRNA synthesis. The resultant proteins synthesized account for the subsequent androgenic changes that occur (Figure 23–7).

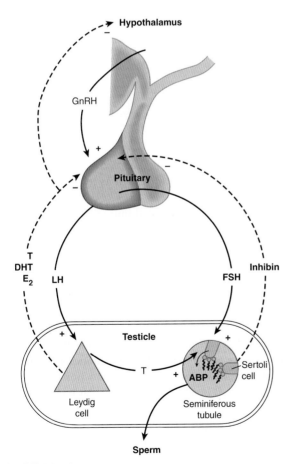

FIGURE 23–6 Endocrine control of the male reproductive system. (ABP, androgen-binding protein; DHT, dihydrotestosterone; E$_2$, estradiol; GnRH, gonadotropin-releasing hormone; T, testosterone.) (Redrawn and modified, with permission, from Gardner DG et al. *Greenspan's Basic and Clinical Endocrinology*, 10th ed. McGraw-Hill, 2017.)

FIGURE 23–7 Mechanism of androgen action. (DHT, dihydrotestosterone; R$_c$, cytoplasmic receptor, which becomes the nuclear receptor, R$_n$, in the nucleus; T, testosterone.) (Redrawn, with permission, from Gardner DG et al. *Greenspan's Basic and Clinical Endocrinology*, 10th ed. McGraw-Hill, 2017.)

TABLE 23–2   Pubertal development of male secondary sex characteristics.

External genitalia	Penis increases in length and width, scrotum becomes pigmented and rugose
Internal genitalia	Seminal vesicles enlarge and secrete
Larynx	Larynx enlarges, vocal cords increase in length and thickness, voice deepens
Hair	Beard appears; scalp hairline recedes anterolaterally; pubic hair appears with male pattern (triangle with apex up); axillary, chest, and perianal hair appears
Musculoskeletal	Shoulders broaden, skeletal muscles enlarge
Skin	Sebaceous gland secretions increase and thicken
Mental	More aggressive, active attitude appears; libido develops

Modified, with permission, from Barrett KE et al. *Ganong's Review of Medical Physiology*, 25th ed. McGraw-Hill, 2016.

In the fetus, androgens are necessary for the normal differentiation and development of the internal and external male genitalia. During puberty, androgens are needed for the normal growth of the male genital structures, including the scrotum, epididymis, vas deferens, seminal vesicles, prostate, and penis. During adolescence, androgens and estrogens cause rapid growth of skeletal muscle and bone. Androgens are also responsible for the development of the secondary sex characteristics summarized in Table 23–2. During adult life, androgens are necessary for normal male reproductive function. Specifically, androgens stimulate erythropoiesis, preserve bone structure and muscle mass, and maintain libido and erectile function.

CHECKPOINT

1. What is the purpose of seminiferous tubule tight junctions?
2. What are the roles of the two major cell populations in the testis, the Leydig cells and the Sertoli cells?
3. How is testosterone secretion regulated?
4. What are the target cells of luteinizing hormone (LH) and follicle-stimulating hormone (FSH)?
5. What are the relative concentrations of testosterone in the peripheral circulation and the testicular tissue?
6. Describe the sequence of events leading up to and during ejaculation.
7. How is estradiol created in men?
8. What are the effects of androgens?

PATHOPHYSIOLOGY OF SELECTED MALE REPRODUCTIVE TRACT DISORDERS

MALE INFERTILITY

For conception to occur, spermatogenesis must be normal and the seminal accessory glands must produce seminal fluids. The ducts for sperm transport must also be patent, and ejaculation must occur so the sperm can be delivered near the female's cervix. Next, the spermatozoa must be able to travel to the fallopian tubes, and they must undergo functional changes that allow them to fuse with the oolemma (plasma membrane of oocyte). Any defect in these mechanisms can result in infertility.

Infertility is defined as the inability of a couple to achieve pregnancy despite unprotected intercourse for a period of more than 12 months. About 15% of all couples are infertile. Males are found to be solely responsible for 20-30% of infertility cases and to contribute to 50% of cases overall. In spite of this, the evaluation of the male partner is often neglected, mainly because of the high pregnancy rates that can be achieved by assisted reproductive techniques (ARTs). This practice is unfortunate because male infertility can often be cured, sparing the female partner the extensive treatment and cost of ART. Furthermore, evidence suggests that ART procedures can be associated with increased risks for both mother and child, in part owing to an increase in multiple births.

Finally, neglecting to examine the infertile man properly risks overlooking serious conditions such as testicular cancer that may coexist with infertility.

Male infertility can be divided into pretesticular, testicular, and post-testicular forms. Table 23–3 provides a comprehensive list of etiologies; Table 23–4 lists genetic causes of male infertility; and Table 23–5 lists the causes of testicular atrophy.

A. Pretesticular Causes

The pretesticular causes of infertility originate in either the hypothalamus (GnRH) or the pituitary (LH and FSH). These endocrinopathies are most often caused by mutations in genes involved in the biosynthesis of the hormones, growth factors or receptors, and associated signal transduction pathways. The deficiencies result in a loss of intratesticular testosterone production and the cessation of spermatogenesis.

Hypogonadotropic hypogonadism is an uncommon cause of male infertility but is important to recognize because replacement therapy can be initiated. The condition is characterized either by reduced GnRH production, causing circulating levels of FSH and LH to diminish, or by rare disorders of the pituitary (with normal GnRH) that result in primary deficiencies of FSH and/or LH. These defects result in deficient androgen secretion and spermatogenesis.

TABLE 23–3 Etiology of male infertility.

Pretesticular	Testicular	Post-testicular
Hypothalamic–pituitary disorders	Varicocele	Ductular obstruction, scarring
Panhypopituitarism	Trauma	Pelvic, retroperitoneal, inguinal, or scrotal surgery (eg, retroperitoneal lymphadenectomy, herniorrhaphy, Y-V-plasty, transurethral prostate resection, vasectomy)
Gonadotropin deficiency	Testicular torsion	Genital tract infections (eg, venereal disease, prostatitis, tuberculosis)
Isolated LH deficiency (fertile eunuch)	Orchiopexy	Cystic fibrosis
Biologically inactive LH	Infection	Retrograde ejaculation (eg, diabetic autonomic neuropathy, postsurgical, medications)
Combined LH and FSH deficiency (eg, Kallmann syndrome)	Mumps orchitis	Antibodies to sperm or seminal plasma
Prader–Willi syndrome	Drugs and toxins	Developmental abnormalities
Laurence–Moon–Biedl syndrome	Medications (eg, sulfasalazine, cimetidine, nitrofurantoin, cyclophosphamide, chlorambucil, vincristine, methotrexate, procarbazine)	Penile anatomic defects (eg, hypospadias, epispadias, chordee)
Cerebellar ataxia	Ingestants (eg, alcohol, marijuana)	Congenital absence (bilateral or unilateral) of the vas deferens; bilateral ejaculatory duct obstruction; or bilateral obstructions within the epididymides—all associated with mutations in the cystic fibrosis transmembrane conductance regulator (*CFTR*) gene
Pituitary tumors (eg, prolactinoma) Systemic illness (eg, cirrhosis, uremia)	Environmental exposures (eg, pesticides, radiation, thermal exposure)	Androgen insensitivity (eg, androgen receptor deficiency, testicular feminization syndrome)
Thyroid disorders (eg, hyperthyroidism, hypothyroidism)	Chromosomal abnormalities (eg, Klinefelter syndrome [XXY seminiferous tubule dysgenesis], Y chromosome microdeletions)	Poor coital technique
Adrenal disorders (eg, adrenal insufficiency, congenital adrenal hyperplasia)	Developmental abnormalities	Sexual dysfunction, impotence
Drugs (eg, phenytoin, androgens)	Cryptorchidism	Idiopathic
	Congenital absence of vas deferens, seminal vesicles	
	Immotile cilia syndrome	
	Bilateral anorchia (vanishing testes syndrome)	
	Leydig cell aplasia	
	Noonan syndrome (male Turner syndrome)	
	Myotonic dystrophy	
	Defective androgen biosynthesis (eg, 5α-reductase deficiency)	

FSH, follicle-stimulation hormone; LH, luteinizing hormone.

Disorders resulting in abnormal GnRH synthesis and release are most often caused by mutations, small deletions, or polymorphic expansions within genes involved in the regulation of sexual development and function. Disorders of GnRH synthesis and release can also be caused by hypothalamic tumors. Disorders without a known cause are termed idiopathic hypogonadotropic hypogonadism. Men suffering from GnRH deficiencies have firm prepubertal-sized testes and a small penis.

TABLE 23–4   Chromosomal and genetic disorders causing male infertility.

Disorder	Cause of Infertility	Defect
Chromosomal		
Klinefelter syndrome	Oligoazoospermia, hyalinization of seminiferous tubules	47,XXY or 46,XY/47,XXY mosaic karyotype
XX male syndrome	SCOS	46,XX SRY translocation to short arm of X
XYY male syndrome		47,XYY karyotype
Genetic		
Disorders of GnRH secretion		
Kallmann syndrome		
GnRH receptor defects		
Prader–Willi syndrome	Decreased GnRH secretion	*KAL* gene mutation
Congenital adrenal hypoplasia	Defects in G protein coupled for GnRH	*GNRHR* gene mutation 15q11q13 mutation
Idiopathic hypogonadotropic hypogonadism	Decreased GnRH secretion	*DAX1* gene mutation Prohormone convertase-1 (*PC1*) gene mutation Kisspeptin or *GPR54* mutation
Disorders of androgen function		
Congenital adrenal hyperplasia	Excessive androgens inhibit pituitary secretion of gonadotropins	Steroidogenic enzyme mutations
Androgen insensitivity syndromes (Reifenstein syndrome, testicular feminization, Lub syndrome, Rosewater syndrome)	Androgen insensitivity	*AR* gene mutation
Kennedy syndrome		Expansion of polyglutamine tract in the AR transactivation domain
5α-reductase deficiency		5α-reductase gene mutations
Y chromosome microdeletions		
AZFa		*DBY*, *USP9Y* gene defect
Complete deletion	SCOS	
Partial deletion	Variable phenotype: oligozoospermia to SCOS	
AZFb		*RBMY1* gene defect
Complete deletion	Spermatogenic arrest	
Partial deletion	Variable phenotype: oligozoospermia to SCOS	
AZFc		*DAZ* gene defect
Complete or partial deletion	Variable phenotype: oligozoospermia to SCOS	
Yq complete deletion	Azoospermia	
Cystic fibrosis	Congenital absence of vas deferens	*CFTR* gene defect

AR, androgen receptor; AZF, azoospermia factor; GnRH, gonadotropin-releasing hormone; SCOS, Sertoli cell–only syndrome.

TABLE 23–5 Causes of testicular atrophy.

Trauma
Testicular torsion
Hypopituitarism
Cryptorchidism
Klinefelter syndrome (47,XXY)
Alcoholism and cirrhosis
Infection (eg, mumps orchitis, gonococcal epididymitis)
Malnutrition and cachexia
Radiation
Obstruction to semen outflow
Aging
Drugs (eg, estrogen therapy for prostatic cancer)

Modified, with permission, from Chandrasoma P et al. *Concise Pathology*, 3rd ed. Originally published by Appleton & Lange. Copyright © 1998 by The McGraw-Hill Companies, Inc.

Kallmann syndrome is a syndrome of defective olfaction with hypogonadotropic hypogonadism caused by failed olfactory and GnRH axonal migration during fetal development. This is caused by a mutation in the *KALIG1* gene on Xp22.3. It results in a deficiency in GnRH secretion and consequent failure of pubertal initiation along with anosmia or hyposmia. In addition, patients tend to be tall and may experience congenital deafness, asymmetry of the cranium and face, cleft palate, cerebellar dysfunction, cryptorchidism, or renal abnormalities. However, some Kallmann syndrome patients present only with isolated gonadotropin deficiency, manifesting as infertility.

Other causes of pubertal failure include mutations in the hypothalamic kisspeptin peptide or its cognate receptor, GPR54. With clinical implications for the diagnosis and treatment of infertility and related disorders, this ligand–receptor pair has proven to be one of the key mediators of pubertal onset.

Mutations of the X-linked *Dax1* gene are associated with hypogonadotropic hypogonadism and congenital adrenal hypoplasia. Dax1 is a nuclear receptor that plays a critical role in the development of the hypothalamus, pituitary, adrenal, and gonads.

GnRH receptor mutations are also associated with hypogonadotropic hypogonadism. The GnRH receptor is a G protein–coupled receptor for GnRH. Patients with GnRH mutations experience a spectrum of reproductive dysfunction from partial to complete hypogonadism.

Mutations in the *PC1* or convertase-1 gene are associated with hypogonadotropic hypogonadism in conjunction with obesity and diabetes mellitus. PC1 is essential in the cleavage of multiple propeptides to their active peptide hormone. The *PC1* gene is believed to have a role in GnRH secretion and release.

Prader–Willi syndrome is caused either by mutations or deletions of a specific locus within paternal chromosome 15 or, less commonly, by maternal uniparental disomy (two maternal copies) of this locus. Symptoms include obesity, mild or moderate mental retardation, infantile hypotonia, and hypogonadotropic hypogonadism.

Hemochromatosis is associated with treatable hypogonadotropic hypogonadism; some men with hemochromatosis develop primary testicular failure.

Biologically inactive LH or FSH can result from genetic mutations in either the hormones or their receptors. The mutations result in a spectrum of dysfunction ranging from hypogonadism to complete virilization failure.

Pituitary mass lesions are uncommon but are recognized causes of hypogonadotropic hypogonadism and male infertility. Such lesions interfere with the release of LH and FSH, either by directly compressing the portal system or by decreasing the secretion of these gonadotropins.

In **hyperprolactinemia**, the elevated serum prolactin level causes hypogonadism because it interferes with the normal pulsatile release of GnRH. Adenomas of the pituitary can cause hyperprolactinemia (owing to infundibular compression and the resultant inhibition of hypothalamic dopamine that tonically inhibits prolactin synthesis and secretion), together with headaches and visual field impairment (owing to direct compression of the optic chiasm). Selective serotonin reuptake inhibitors can also cause hyperprolactinemia.

Spermatogenesis depends on a high androgen concentration. Genetic steroidogenic enzyme deficiencies can result in combined defects in multiple steroid hormones including testosterone and/or DHT. Androgen deficiency results in a spectrum of phenotypic abnormalities ranging from incomplete virilization to completely feminized genitalia and cryptorchid testes. Alternatively, in **congenital adrenal hyperplasia**, impaired corticosteroid and androgenic steroid synthesis often results in ACTH-dependent elevations in adrenal androgens (see Chapter 21).

The X-linked androgen receptor (AR) is a nuclear steroid receptor that is classically activated upon androgen binding to facilitate the transcriptional activation of a host of target genes. **Androgen insensitivity syndromes** result from mutations in AR structure and/or function. The complete loss of AR function results in the complete feminization of 46,XY individuals. Because testosterone is converted to estradiol by peripheral aromatization, estradiol levels are usually elevated and feminization occurs in a similar fashion to that of normal XX females at the time of puberty. In less severe cases, the phenotypic spectrum ranges from simple male infertility to ambiguous genitalia and hypospadias.

Thyroid disorders may also influence fertility, although the exact mechanisms are not fully elucidated. Hypothyroidism may cause disturbances in the production and metabolism of androgens, thereby indirectly influencing fertility. It may also result in delayed ejaculation, which, in rare cases, can inhibit the occurrence of natural pregnancies. On the other hand, hyperthyroidism may result in increased oxidative stress and subsequent damage to the testicular tissue or the developing sperm cells.

Anabolic steroid abuse results in negative feedback at the level of the hypothalamus and pituitary, and LH and FSH release is reduced. This in turn disables endogenous testosterone production and spermatogenesis, because normal spermatogenesis requires both FSH and adequate intratesticular testosterone. Decreased testicular size and gynecomastia can also be seen in association with long-time anabolic steroid abuse. The extent and reversibility of these detrimental effects depend on dose and duration of use. Normal hormonal function usually returns after these agents are discontinued.

Although the topic is still controversial, emerging data suggest that **obesity** may reduce male fertility. Increasing body mass index (BMI) is correlated with decreased male fertility. The detrimental effects of increased fat mass may be mediated through a number of diverse mechanisms including obesity-related comorbidities (eg, diabetes mellitus, heart disease), sexual dysfunction, endocrine derangements, and possibly epigenetic alterations in spermatogenesis.

B. Testicular Causes

A number of conditions damage spermatogenic potential through direct effects on the testicles.

Varicoceles are considered the most common cause of subfertility in men. The term **varicocele** refers to abnormally dilated scrotal veins. A varicocele is present in about 15% of the normal male population but in approximately 40% of men presenting with infertility.

Possible pathogenic mechanisms in varicocele formation include the anatomical configuration of the left internal spermatic vein, incompetent or absent valves, and the potential for partial left renal vein compression between the aorta and the superior mesenteric artery. An acute varicocele can also be caused by retroperitoneal malignancies compressing the venous system.

Varicoceles are associated with impaired spermatogenesis by one of several mechanisms: increased scrotal temperatures, alterations in testicular blood flow, reduced testicular size, accumulation of adrenal steroid metabolites, increased oxidative stress (which may damage cell membrane integrity or cause DNA damage), and alterations in the hypothalamic–pituitary–gonadal axis, leading to decreased serum testosterone levels. The pathophysiology of the impaired spermatogenesis is likely multifactorial in many cases.

Several studies have shown decreased semen quality and increased sperm DNA damage in varicocele patients compared with normal controls. Moreover, accumulating data indicate improvement in both semen parameters and pregnancy rates with varicocele repair.

Genetic disorders are characterized as (a) abnormalities of entire chromosomes (abnormalities of the karyotype); (b) deletions of specific areas of chromosomes; or (c) specific mutations within genes. These disorders can alter spermatogenesis and impair the normal development of the genital tract, thus decreasing fertilization capacity.

Chromosomal defects are categorized as either numerical or structural. Numerical chromosome abnormalities include deletion or duplication of whole chromosomes. Structural chromosome abnormalities include deletion, inversion, or duplication of a portion of a chromosome, or translocation of part of one chromosome to another chromosome. Both autosomal and sex chromosomes may be affected. Such abnormalities occur with much greater frequency in infertile men than in the general population. About 1 in 20 infertile men has a chromosomal abnormality, and most of these cases involve a sex chromosome. These men are usually azoospermic or severely oligospermic.

Klinefelter syndrome (47,XXY) is the most common chromosomal disorder associated with infertility. Patients with Klinefelter syndrome are severely oligospermic or azoospermic. The phenotype of men with Klinefelter syndrome varies but can include increased height, female hair distribution, gynecomastia, a decreased level of intelligence, diabetes mellitus, obesity, an increased incidence of leukemia and nonseminomatous extragonadal germ cell tumors, small firm testes, and infertility. Laboratory studies show increased serum FSH, normal or increased serum estradiol, and normal or low serum testosterone (with a tendency to decrease with age). Leydig cell function is commonly impaired in men with Klinefelter syndrome. Patients with Klinefelter syndrome who are mosaics with 46,XY/47,XXY have a less severe phenotype, with a variable sperm production.

There are other less common chromosomal defects. Most patients with **mixed gonadal dysgenesis** have a mosaic karyotype of 45,X/46,XY, but others have a normal 46,XY. Affected individuals can have male, female, or ambiguous genitalia; streak gonads; or normal testes. The **XX male syndrome** (46,XX) is caused by translocation of the *SRY* sex-determination gene from the paternal Y chromosome to the paternal X of the offspring, resulting in "normal" development of testes in the XX fetus but a lack of all spermatogenic genes normally found on the Y chromosome. The **XYY male syndrome** (47,XYY) is characterized by decreased intelligence, antisocial behavior, an increased incidence of leukemia, and impairment of spermatogenesis.

Microdeletions of the Y chromosome have been shown to be of great importance in male infertility. The long arm of the Y chromosome contains genes critical for spermatogenesis (Figure 23–8). The genes most often mutated in patients with defective spermatogenesis are found in the azoospermia factor

FIGURE 23–8 Diagrammatic representation of areas responsible for male infertility on the long arm of the Y chromosome (Yq). (Redrawn, with permission, from Iammarrone E et al. Male infertility. Best Pract Res Clin Obstet Gynaecol. 2003;17:211. Copyright © Elsevier.)

(AZF) region, where three nonoverlapping intervals (AZFa, AZFb, and AZFc) exist. Y chromosome microdeletions are detected by polymerase chain reaction–based mapping of molecular markers and genes. The most frequently deleted region is AZFc (~60% of Y chromosome deletions), followed by AZFb (35%) and AZFa (5%). There can also be large deletions that span more than one region.

Microdeletions in the AZF region are responsible for azoospermia or severe oligozoospermia (sperm concentrations of less than 5 million/mL). Such AZF microdeletions are estimated to account for about 7–10% of male factor infertility. Affected men do not have other phenotypic abnormalities.

Among men with microdeletions in the AZFc region of the Y chromosome, 70% still have sufficient sperm production to allow sperm extraction via testis biopsy. If spermatozoa are obtained from patients with the Y deletion, they can be used for in vitro fertilization (IVF), but the deletion and infertility are transmitted to male offspring. Men with microdeletions in the AZFb and AZFa regions do not have sperm on testicular biopsy.

Cryptorchidism is the term used when testicular descent does not proceed normally during development, and the testis remains in the abdominal cavity or groin. The prevalence of cryptorchidism is approximately 3% in full-term newborns but only 1–2% by age 6 months. About 85% of cases of cryptorchidism are unilateral.

Failure of normal testicular descent can result in impaired spermatogenesis. Without treatment, 50–70% of unilaterally cryptorchid men will be oligospermic or azoospermic, and almost 100% of bilaterally cryptorchid men will be azoospermic.

Exposure to toxins has also been postulated to cause defects in spermatogenesis. While numerous substances and occupations have been suspected, inadequate study sample size and confounding factors make causal relationships difficult to confirm.

The different germ cell populations display unique sensitivities to different toxins. Spermatogonia are located outside the blood–testis barrier and are exposed to any toxins in the interstitial fluid. Conversely, spermatocytes and spermatids are located inside the blood–testis barrier, which offers them some protection. Toxins that injure Sertoli cells can also impair spermatogenesis, whereas injury to the Leydig cells can reduce testosterone levels. Toxins may also interfere with hormone balance by causing alterations in androgen or gonadotropin receptor binding, alterations in circulating gonadotropin levels, and alterations in the metabolism of androgens. The effects of toxins may be reversible if the agents are removed before azoospermia occurs.

Cigarette smoking has been associated with a reduction in sperm count and motility and an increase in abnormal forms. Cigarette smoking can also cause damage to sperm DNA. A meta-analysis of 21 studies examining the effects of cigarette smoking on semen quality revealed that smoking lowered sperm concentration by 13–17% in 7 studies but had no adverse spermatogenic outcome in 14 studies. Therefore, it remains controversial whether smoking actually decreases male fertility rates.

Also controversial is whether second-hand smoke from a male partner can affect female fertility. There is, however, some evidence that maternal smoking may be related to decreased sperm counts in the male offspring. Finally, the risk of developing erectile dysfunction is almost doubled for smokers compared with nonsmokers, and this can limit male fertility.

Testicular temperatures are approximately 2°C below core body temperature, and spermatogenesis depends on this cooler temperature. Factors such as clothing, lifestyle, season, and fever can cause increases in scrotal temperature. Increases in scrotal temperature reduce sperm quantity and quality.

Chemotherapy and **radiation therapy**, used in men with testicular cancer, Hodgkin disease, or leukemia, are potent **gonadotoxins**. For example, both radiation therapy and chemotherapy can cause damage to the germinal epithelium, and spermatogenesis may not recover. Therefore, it is recommended that patients bank their semen before such therapy. If the semen quality is good, specimens can be preserved in aliquots large enough for intrauterine insemination. If only a single specimen is available, the sample should be divided into smaller aliquots that can be used for IVF or intracytoplasmic sperm injection.

If patients receiving chemotherapy remain azoospermic after recovery from cancer, there is still a significant chance (41% in one study) that sperm can be obtained with testicular sperm extraction for IVF or intracytoplasmic sperm injection.

Testicular or **epididymal infections** may lead to infertility. For example, although mumps is generally a self-limited disease in children, mumps may result in orchitis in postpubertal males. Necrosis from acute swelling and increased intratesticular pressure can cause permanent testicular atrophy and infertility.

Epididymitis can lead to scarring of the tubules and obstruction of sperm flow (discussed below). In the absence of ductal obstruction, however, the role of infection in causing infertility is controversial. The potential deleterious effects of infection on male fertility include decreases in spermatogenesis, breaches in the blood–testis barrier leading to sperm autoimmunity, and seminal oxidative stresses owing to an increase in seminal fluid oxidant levels or a decrease in seminal fluid antioxidant levels. However, such effects have never been conclusively proven.

Torsion of the spermatic cord with interruption of testicular blood flow results in acute, intense testicular pain. If untreated, the absence of blood flow after 4–6 hours of torsion causes irreparable damage. Torsion may also induce sperm autoimmunity owing to a breakdown of the blood–testis barrier during the ischemic event.

Testicular trauma can lead to scrotal or testicular edema, hematoma, hematocele, hydrocele, torsion, fracture, or rupture. These may result in testicular atrophy as well as the development of antisperm antibodies. In both testicular rupture and torsion, early surgery is needed to ensure testicular salvage. The ruptured testicle can be restored in up to 90% of patients if the rupture is treated within 72 hours, but torsion of the testicle must be treated within 6 hours to obtain a similar result.

C. Post-testicular Causes

Ductal obstruction can occur anywhere along the male reproductive system, and results of semen analysis vary with the site of obstruction. Complete obstruction of the ejaculatory duct results in a low-volume, acidic, fructose-negative ejaculate. Obstruction of the vasa or epididymides results in a normal-volume, alkaline, fructose-positive ejaculate. Men with ductal obstruction as the only cause of their infertility have normal serum testosterone and FSH levels.

Obstruction is either congenital or acquired. Congenital causes include congenital atresia or stenosis of the ejaculatory ducts and utricular or müllerian and wolffian duct cysts. Acquired vasal obstruction may be caused by inguinal or pelvic surgery but is most commonly the result of a **vasectomy**. Epididymal obstruction may be caused by scrotal surgery or epididymitis. **Epididymitis** is an inflammation most commonly due to infection. In men younger than 35 years, the most common pathogens are the sexually transmitted organisms *Chlamydia trachomatis* and *Neisseria gonorrhoeae*. In young children and older men, the most common pathogen is *Escherichia coli*. Epididymitis in a child mandates exclusion of a urinary tract anomaly.

Congenital bilateral absence of the vas deferens (CBAVD) is part of the phenotypic spectrum of cystic fibrosis (CF). CF is an autosomal recessive disease, and about 1 in 25 Caucasians are heterozygous carriers. Mutations of the cystic fibrosis transmembrane conductance regulator (*CFTR*) gene cause the disease; more than 500 such mutations have been identified. CBAVD occurs in 1–2% of infertile men, making it the most common congenital abnormality of the wolffian duct system. Although most patients with classic CF carry severe mutations on both *CFTR* gene loci, patients with CBAVD can have a severe mutation in only one *CFTR* gene, coupled with a minor mutation in the other, or minor mutations on both loci. Men with CBAVD also have hypoplastic, nonfunctional seminal vesicles and ejaculatory ducts, as well as epididymal remnants frequently composed of only the caput regions, which are firm and distended. Other manifestations of CF, such as pulmonary, pancreatic, and gastrointestinal dysfunction, are usually absent.

However, spermatogenesis is not impaired in these patients, and they can undergo sperm-retrieval procedures and have their semen used in ART. To diminish the possibility of transmitting CF to the offspring, men with CBAVD and their partners should be referred to genetic counseling and screened for *CFTR* mutations before proceeding with sperm retrieval and IVF.

Men with idiopathic epididymal obstruction have also been found to have an increased incidence of CF mutations and probably simply represent a variant phenotype from the patient with classic CBAVD. These men should also undergo CF testing before epididymal sperm aspiration or reconstructive surgery. Finally, patients presenting with a unilateral absence of the vas deferens are also at risk of mutations and should undergo analysis of the *CFTR* gene.

Ejaculatory duct obstruction is an uncommon cause of male infertility, representing about 1% of cases. Most cases are bilateral because of the close proximity of the ostia of both ejaculatory ducts. The condition may be congenital or acquired. Occasionally, congenital isolated ejaculatory duct obstruction may be associated with *CFTR* mutations, and genetic screening is appropriate. Acquired cases may be due to genitourinary infections, pelvic surgery, urethral trauma, chronic prostatitis, or inspissated secretions in the ejaculatory ducts causing calculi. Utricular cysts may also obstruct the ejaculatory ducts.

Symptoms from ejaculatory duct obstruction include infertility, decreased ejaculate volume, reduced ejaculatory force, hematospermia, pain with ejaculation, and dysuria. The physical examination of patients with ejaculatory duct obstruction is usually normal. However, some may have a palpable seminal vesicle or mass on rectal examination, or prostatic or epididymal tenderness.

Clinically, ejaculatory duct obstruction must be considered in patients with azoospermia, low ejaculate volume, an absence of fructose in the ejaculate, and normal hormone profiles. Transrectal ultrasonography (TRUS) has led to the identification of patients with seminal vesicle dilation or genitourinary cysts causing reduced ejaculatory volume with oligospermia or azoospermia.

Partial obstruction of the ejaculatory duct has also been recognized. Affected patients have low-volume ejaculate and variable semen quality. Unfortunately, semen quality may worsen after attempting corrective surgery. Seminal vesicle aspiration after ejaculation may aid in diagnosing partial ejaculatory duct obstruction.

Immunologic infertility may result from a breach in the blood–testis barrier, exposing the mature spermatozoa to the immune system with the formation of **antisperm antibodies**. These antibodies may be present in the blood or in seminal fluids. Risk factors for the formation of antisperm antibodies include trauma to the testes, epididymitis, congenital absence of the vas deferens, and vasectomy. It may also be caused by the dysregulation of normal immunosuppressive activities within the male reproductive tract. Antisperm antibodies are found in 5–10% of infertile couples but are also present in 1–3% of fertile men. Antisperm antibodies react with all major regions of sperm and can impair sperm motility, sperm penetration through the cervical mucus, the acrosome reaction, and sperm–oocyte interactions and fertilization.

High levels of circulating antisperm antibodies may reduce the likelihood of a successful outcome from treatment by intercourse, intrauterine insemination, or IVF. However, if intracytoplasmic sperm injection is used in conjunction with IVF, antisperm antibodies do not have a negative effect on the outcome of the procedure.

Disorders of ejaculation are uncommon but important causes of male infertility. The disorders can be divided into premature ejaculation, anejaculation, and retrograde ejaculation.

Premature ejaculation is the inability to control ejaculation for a satisfactory length of time during intercourse. The condition has been reported to affect up to 31% of men 18–59 years of age. Premature ejaculation causes distress as a sexual dysfunction for both partners but seldom leads to infertility, as ejaculation usually occurs intravaginally.

Anejaculation describes the complete absence of seminal emission into the posterior urethra. True anejaculation is always connected with central or peripheral nervous system dysfunction or with drugs. Orgasm (climax) may or may not be achieved. **Spinal cord injury** is the most common neurological cause of anejaculation, even though many men with spinal cord injury do have reflex erections and some capability for vaginal intercourse. Congenital spinal abnormalities, such as spina bifida, and other neurological conditions that affect spinal cord function or its sympathetic outflow (multiple sclerosis, transverse myelitis, vascular spine injuries) can also impair ejaculation. These disorders resemble the spinal cord injury group in their dysfunction. Periaortic or pelvic surgery, including retroperitoneal lymph node dissection, can damage the nerves and cause ejaculatory dysfunction. Finally, men with diabetes mellitus are at risk for neuropathy, which can affect ejaculatory function. Typically, men with diabetic neuropathy develop ejaculatory dysfunction in a slowly progressive fashion, going from a decreased amount of ejaculate to retrograde ejaculation to anejaculation. As with other long-term complications of diabetes, this condition is related to poor blood sugar control. Several classes of drugs are also potentially responsible for anejaculation: α-adrenergic blockers, antipsychotics, and antidepressants. Anejaculation can also be psychogenic or idiopathic.

Retrograde ejaculation accounts for 0.3–2% of cases of male infertility. It is caused by a dysfunction in bladder neck closure that results in a total or partial absence of antegrade ejaculation. In this condition, with ejaculation, the ejaculate flows into the bladder, the path of least resistance. Because bladder neck closure is controlled by the α-adrenergic neurons of the sympathetic nervous system, the condition can be caused by the same conditions as neurogenic anejaculation: retroperitoneal lymph node dissection, diabetes mellitus, bladder neck surgery, and transurethral resection of the prostate (TURP). The condition may also be idiopathic. Drugs that may cause retrograde ejaculation include $α_1$-adrenoreceptor antagonists, antipsychotics, and antidepressants.

Retrograde ejaculation is diagnosed when, after absent or intermittent emission of ejaculate during ejaculation, sperm is found in the bladder urine, which may be cloudy. Patients usually experience a normal or slightly decreased orgasm but may note a "dry" ejaculation.

D. Idiopathic Oligospermia

Despite advances in molecular diagnostics, the pathophysiology of spermatogenic failure remains unknown in many infertile men. In such cases, the infertility is classified as idiopathic. Although, research is still needed in the area, many such cases are now believed to be caused by unknown genetic alterations or complex epigenetic modifications, such as DNA methylation and histone tail modifications. ARTs are the best treatment option for patients with idiopathic oligospermia.

Pathology

Percutaneous or open testicular biopsy specimens may show any of several lesions involving the entire testis or only a portion. The most common lesion is "**maturation arrest**," defined as failure to complete spermatogenesis beyond a particular stage. There are early- and late-arrest patterns, with cessation of development at either the primary spermatocyte or the spermatogonial stage of the spermatogenic cycle. The second most common and least severe lesion is "**hypospermatogenesis**," in which all stages of spermatogenesis are present but there is a reduction in the number of germinal epithelial cells per seminiferous tubule. Peritubular fibrosis may be present. "**Germ cell aplasia**" is a more severe lesion characterized by a complete absence of germ cells, with only Sertoli cells lining the seminiferous tubules (**Sertoli cell–only** syndrome [SCOS]). The most severe lesion (eg, in Klinefelter syndrome) involves the hyalinization, fibrosis, and sclerosis of the tubules. These findings usually indicate irreversible damage.

CHECKPOINT

9. What are the major categories of causes of male infertility? Name several specific causes in each category.

10. From the perspective of the male reproductive system, what steps must occur for conception?

11. What is the value of testing for a *CFTR* mutation or Y chromosome microdeletion?

12. What is the most common cause of obstructive azoospermia?

Clinical Manifestations

A. Symptoms and Signs

A couple should undergo an evaluation for infertility if pregnancy fails to occur within one year of regular unprotected intercourse. Evaluation should be done before one year if there are risk factors for infertility either in the male or in the female. Also, an evaluation can be initiated sooner if the couple has a good understanding of ovulation timing, and they have had more than simple, random attempts at pregnancy. The reason for initiating an examination sooner rather than later is that the longer a couple remains infertile, the less likely it is that treatment will work.

The evaluation should attempt to identify an underlying cause of the infertility in order to initiate treatment or ART or to recommend donor insemination or adoption. The evaluation should also identify any underlying pathology that requires medical attention. If the couple is to undergo ART, a genetic evaluation of the infertile man is important in order to avoid transferring possible abnormalities on to the child.

The full evaluation of the infertile man should consist of a history, physical examination, and laboratory tests, including both semen analysis and endocrine evaluation.

History—A complete general medical history and a comprehensive reproductive history are required.

With regard to reproductive history, the duration of infertility and information on coital technique, frequency, and timing are assessed. Because sperm survive in the female reproductive tract for about 2–5 days, the most effective time for intercourse is in the first 48 hours after ovulation. Pregnancy rates are highest with daily intercourse around this time. The history should ask about the use of lubricants since many of these are spermicidal. The patient is also asked about general sexual function, including erectile and ejaculatory function.

The general medical history must also include developmental history, including congenital abnormalities, childhood illnesses, and pubertal development. Treatment for delayed puberty is obviously salient.

Information on systemic medical illnesses, prior surgeries or traumas, and genitourinary infections should be noted. Respiratory problems are especially important, as there is a correlation between sinopulmonary conditions and infertility.

Past surgeries may have an impact on fertility. Any pelvic surgery can interrupt the vas deferens or cause neurogenic erectile or ejaculatory dysfunction. Retroperitoneal surgery can impair seminal emission owing to injury to the sympathetic nervous system. Hernia repair can cause an iatrogenic injury to the vas deferens.

Current and past medications should be listed. Of particular interest are alpha blockers, antidepressants, and anabolic steroids, such as testosterone and others contained in dietary supplements. Possible gonadotoxin exposure must be assessed. The patient should be asked specific questions regarding cigarette smoking, marijuana use, and excessive alcohol intake, which may all suppress spermatogenesis. The family history should include questions regarding reproduction, hypogonadism, cryptorchidism, congenital defects, and cystic fibrosis.

Physical Examination—The physical examination should include a general evaluation, but it should also focus on the secondary sex characteristics and genitalia.

Androgen status is evaluated by assessing the secondary sex characteristics, including body habitus, virilization, body hair, and gynecomastia. The penis should be examined to look for the location of the urethral meatus and penile curvature.

Examination of the genitalia is performed by palpating the testes with the patient standing. Testicular size is measured by means of calipers, orchidometer, or ultrasound. The normal adult testis is ovoid, measuring 4–5 cm in length and 2–3 cm in both transverse and anteroposterior dimensions, and has a mean volume of at least 20 mL. Small testes most likely indicate impaired spermatogenesis, since the seminiferous tubules

form over 90% of the testis. Abnormal testicular dimensions are present in about two-thirds of men with infertility. In men with severe spermatogenic defects, such as those with Klinefelter syndrome or Y chromosome microdeletions, the testicular size is that of a prepubertal male.

The examination should also identify the presence of scrotal pathology including hydroceles, spermatoceles, varicoceles, and hernias. The vas deferens and epididymis should be examined for obstruction, manifested by induration and enlargement of these structures. Physical examination may reveal an absence of the vas deferens and epididymis. In such patients, a renal ultrasound should be performed because vasal agenesis can be associated with renal anomalies.

Varicocele examination should be done in a warm room to allow for complete relaxation of the scrotal wall. The patient needs to be examined standing, at rest, and again with the Valsalva maneuver. Approximately 90% of varicoceles are left sided. Varicoceles are graded from 1 to 3. With the patient standing, a grade 3 varicocele is readily visible; a grade 2 varicocele is palpable without employing the Valsalva maneuver; and a grade 1 varicocele is palpable only with the Valsalva maneuver. The patient should also be examined in the lying position, to ensure that the dilated veins collapse. If they remain dilated after assuming a recumbent position, there is a higher likelihood of retroperitoneal pathology as the source of the varicocele, and an imaging study is indicated. Also, a large difference in spermatic cord diameter between standing and recumbent positions may be an indication that a varicocele is present.

Semen Analysis—Semen collection should be done by masturbation into a glass container, because plastic may contain spermatocidal chemicals. Standard instructions for semen collection include abstinence for 2–3 days. Longer periods of abstinence lead to decreased sperm motility, and shorter periods result in low semen volume and sperm concentration.

Semen analysis provides information on semen volume and sperm concentration, motility, and morphology. This information helps define the severity of the male factor in a couple's infertility. Semen analysis also includes an examination of the spermatozoa and the seminal fluid. In normal men, the ejaculate volume is ≥1.5 mL or more, and the normal semen pH is slightly alkaline (≥7.2). According to the latest standards of the World Health Organization, normal sperm parameters include a sperm concentration of ≥15 million sperm/mL, a progressive motility of ≥32% motile sperm, and a normal morphology of ≥44%. Sperm motility is defined as the percentage of sperm moving in 10 random high-power fields. Sperm morphology is evaluated by the Kruger criteria, which divide sperm into normal and abnormal morphology on the basis of a normal range of more than 4%. Table 23–6 provides standard semen analysis criteria.

A semen analysis can diagnose 9 out of 10 men with reduced semen quality. However, because semen quality varies over time and is often affected by exogenous factors, a single semen analysis has low specificity. Therefore, two to three tests at least one month apart are recommended.

TABLE 23–6   Semen analysis: Normal values and definitions.

Characteristic	Reference Standard
Ejaculate volume	>1.5 mL
pH	≥7.2
Sperm concentration	≥15 million/mL
Sperm count	≥39 million/mL
Sperm motility	≥40% total motility and 32% with progressive motility
Sperm morphology	≥4%[1] with normal forms

Term	Definition
Normospermia	Normal ejaculate (as defined by reference standards above)
Oligozoospermia	Sperm concentration <15 million/mL
Asthenozoospermia	<32% of spermatozoa with progressive motility
Azoospermia	No spermatozoa in ejaculate
Aspermia	No ejaculate

[1]Strict criterion.

Data from World Health Organization. Reference values of semen variables. In: *WHO Laboratory Manual for the Examination of Human Semen*, 5th ed. World Health Organization, 2010.

If sperm are completely absent on semen analysis, the specimen should be centrifuged to assess for very low sperm numbers. The finding of any sperm rules out complete ductal obstruction and the complete absence of spermatogenesis. If persistent low volume is seen, an examination of post-orgasm urine should be undertaken to exclude retrograde ejaculation.

Evidence of sperm agglutination should be noted; increased clumping is suggestive of inflammatory or immunologic processes. Testing for antisperm antibodies is indicated in such cases.

About 25% of men with sperm concentrations below 12.5 million/mL can father a child through spontaneous conception; conversely, 10% of men are infertile despite a sperm concentration of up to 25 million/mL. This indicates that some men may have dysfunctional sperm despite normal semen parameters. In other words, the normal ranges for the semen analysis provide an indication of a man's fertility, but its values are not absolute. In such men, a number of specialized tests can be used to assess the reason for infertility.

Additional tests of the ejaculate can also be important. Absent or low-volume ejaculate suggests retrograde ejaculation, lack of emission, ejaculatory duct obstruction, hypogonadism, or CBAVD. With low semen volumes (<1 mL) and azoospermia, the seminal pH and fructose content should be determined. If both are low, it suggests agenesis, decreased function, or obstruction of the seminal vesicles.

Patients with partial ejaculatory duct obstruction often present with low-volume semen, oligoasthenospermia, and poor forward progression of sperm (see the section on **post-testicular causes**).

Endocrine Evaluation—An endocrine evaluation of the hypothalamic–pituitary–testicular axis should be performed if sperm concentration is reduced. Spermatogenesis is evaluated by serum FSH and inhibin, whereas Leydig cell function is evaluated by serum LH, testosterone, sex hormone–binding globulin (SHBG), and free or bioavailable testosterone. A single measurement is usually sufficient to determine a patient's clinical endocrine status. The relative values of testosterone, LH, FSH, and prolactin can often identify the cause of the reduced semen parameters.

Men without sperm production produce very low levels of inhibin, leading to high FSH levels. Conversely, normal FSH and inhibin levels in an azoospermic man suggest normal spermatogenesis with obstruction. In men with spermatogenic arrest, normal values of FSH and inhibin can be found, especially if maturation arrest is present, since there may be enough spermatogenic progress to allow inhibin secretion. A combination of both inhibin and FSH levels has been shown to have a better diagnostic value than either one alone.

Low or nonmeasurable FSH and LH levels are found in patients with pituitary or hypothalamic hypogonadism and in patients with human chorionic gonadotropin (hCG)–producing testicular tumors. Such levels are also seen in patients with a history of anabolic steroid abuse. Notably, these synthetic substances are not measurable by standard testosterone assays.

A combined elevation of FSH and LH levels reflects a decline in both Sertoli cell and Leydig cell function caused by direct testicular damage.

Men with hypogonadotropic hypogonadism should undergo magnetic resonance imaging (MRI) of the pituitary gland and the hypothalamus to evaluate the possibility of a pituitary tumor. If the serum gonadotropin levels are low and the serum testosterone level is half the lower limit of normal, further evaluation of the remaining pituitary hormones should also be performed. This includes assessing other pituitary–end organ axes to exclude panhypopituitarism. The thyroid axis is most commonly checked by obtaining serum thyroid-stimulating hormone (TSH) and free T_4 levels. Serum prolactin should be measured to exclude a prolactin-secreting adenoma. Finally, if the hypogonadotropic hypogonadism remains unexplained, serum iron, total iron-binding capacity, and ferritin levels should be obtained to exclude hemochromatosis.

Fructose is produced in the seminal vesicles, and its absence in the semen implies obstruction of the ejaculatory ducts. This test is currently used sparingly, as more emphasis is placed on low semen volume as a screening test and **transrectal ultrasound of the prostate** as a confirmatory test. Obstruction of the ejaculatory ducts is strongly suggested by a seminal vesicle anteroposterior diameter of 1.5 cm or more on ultrasound.

Leukospermia (an excessive number of leukocytes in the semen) may adversely affect sperm movement and fertilization ability, perhaps because of an excessive generation of reactive oxygen species by the leukocytes. Also, with active prostatic infection, prostate swelling can lead to a functional obstruction of the ejaculatory ducts. The finding of leukospermia should prompt further investigations to exclude a genital tract infection.

A variety of in vitro tests have been developed to assess sperm function in an attempt to explain previously hidden male factors in couples with unexplained infertility. These couples have significantly lower IVF rates compared with those in whom simple uterine tubal problems can be identified. These tests are designed to uncover defects in sperm capacitation and motion, in binding to the zona pellucida, in acrosome reaction, and in the ability to penetrate the oocyte. The in vitro **sperm mucus-penetration test** assesses the capacity of spermatozoa to move through a column of midcycle cervical mucus and helps detect impaired motility caused by antibodies.

In the optimized **sperm mucus-penetration test**, the infertile man's sperm are placed in egg yolk buffer, cooled, and stored at cold temperature overnight, and then subjected to rapid heating in the morning and incubated with hamster oocytes that have had the zona pellucida removed enzymatically to allow penetration. Results are reported as either the percentage of ova that have been penetrated (normal is 100% of the oocytes penetrated) or as the number of sperm penetrations per ovum, termed the sperm capacitation index (normal is >5).

The **hemizona assay** assesses the fertilizing capability of sperm using the zona pellucida from a nonfertilizable, nonliving human oocyte. The zona is divided in half. One half is incubated with the infertile man's sperm, and the other half is incubated with sperm from a known fertile donor. The number of sperm binding to the zona is compared and expressed as a ratio. However, a major problem with this assay is the limited availability of human ova. The identification of zona pellucida glycoprotein 3 (ZP3) as the primary determinant of sperm–zona binding has led to an exploration of the use of recombinant human ZP3 rather than the zona itself for testing sperm–zona interactions.

High-resolution **transrectal ultrasound** can be used to evaluate the seminal vesicles for dysplasia or obstruction; the ejaculatory ducts for scarring, cysts, or calcifications; and the prostate for calcifications.

Internal spermatic venography is occasionally used to demonstrate testicular venous reflux in a man with a suspected varicocele when the physical examination is difficult or when he is suspected of a recurrence after surgical repair.

Testicular biopsy is useful in azoospermic men to distinguish intrinsic testicular abnormalities from ductal obstruction. Testicular biopsy can recover some spermatozoa for intracytoplasmic sperm injection in nearly all men with azoospermia owing to obstruction and in 40–75% of men with nonobstructive azoospermia, depending on the reason for the poor production. The best yield of operative sperm retrieval is in men with hypospermatogenesis, followed by those with germinal aplasia (owing to the presence of patchy normal sperm production). The prognosis is worst in men with maturation arrest, in whom a probable genetic "block" of advanced sperm production is a likely cause.

Figure 23–9 illustrates a suggested algorithm for evaluating and treating male infertility.

BENIGN PROSTATIC HYPERPLASIA

Benign prostatic hyperplasia is nonmalignant growth of the prostate stroma and epithelial glands that causes enlargement of the prostate gland. Growing slowly over decades, the gland can eventually reach up to 10 times the normal adult prostate size in severe cases. Benign prostatic hyperplasia is a common age-related disorder. Each year more than 500,000 men in the United States undergo transurethral resection of the prostate (TURP).

Etiology

The cause of benign prostatic hyperplasia is unknown. However, aging and hormonal factors are both clearly important. Age-related increases in prostate size are evident at autopsy, and the development of symptoms is age related. Data from autopsy studies show pathologic evidence of benign prostatic hyperplasia in less than 10% of men in their 30s, in 40% of men in their 50s, in more than 70% of men in their 60s, and in almost 90% of men in their 80s. Clinical symptoms of bladder outlet obstruction are seldom found in men younger than 40 years but are found in about one-third of men older than 65 years and in up to three-fourths of men at age 80 years. Prostatic androgen levels, particularly DHT levels, play an important role in the development of the disorder; these factors are discussed below. In addition, it has become clear that there is a strong association, supported by epidemiologic studies, between metabolic syndrome and both prostate size and development of voiding problems. Prostatic growth is more pronounced in men with components of metabolic syndrome. Furthermore, weight loss may partially alleviate symptoms. Possible pathophysiological explanations include insulin-mediated prostatic growth, low-grade inflammation in the urinary tract, and a decreased capacity of the smooth muscle to relax upon voiding.

Pathology

The normal prostate is composed of both stromal (smooth muscle) and epithelial (glandular) elements. Growth of each of these elements—alone or in combination—can result in hyperplastic nodules and ultimately the symptoms of benign prostatic hyperplasia. Pathologically, the hyperplastic gland is enlarged, with a firm, rubbery consistency. Although small nodules are often present throughout the gland, benign prostatic hyperplasia arises most commonly in the periurethral and transition zones of the gland (Figure 23–10). With advancing age, there is an increase in the overall size of the

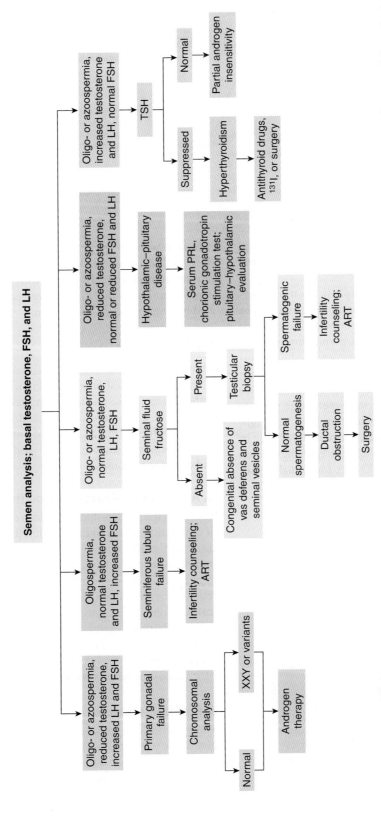

FIGURE 23–9 Approach to the diagnosis of male infertility. (ART, assisted reproductive technologies; FSH, follicle-stimulating hormone; LH, luteinizing hormone; PRL, prolactin; TSH, thyroid-stimulating hormone.) (Redrawn, with permission, from Gardner DG et al. *Greenspan's Basic and Clinical Endocrinology*, 9th ed. McGraw-Hill, 2011.)

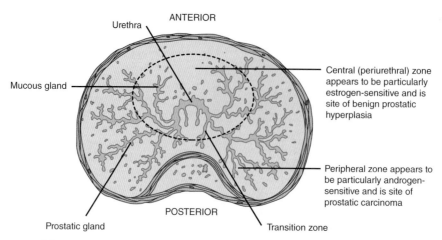

ANTERIOR

Urethra

Mucous gland

Central (periurethral) zone appears to be particularly estrogen-sensitive and is site of benign prostatic hyperplasia

Peripheral zone appears to be particularly androgen-sensitive and is site of prostatic carcinoma

POSTERIOR

Prostatic gland

Transition zone

FIGURE 23–10 Structure of the prostate. (Redrawn, with permission, from Chandrasoma P et al. *Concise Pathology*, 3rd ed. Originally published by Appleton & Lange. Copyright © 1998 by The McGraw-Hill Companies, Inc.)

transition zone, as well as an increase in the number—and later the size—of nodules. The urethra is compressed and has a slit-like appearance.

Histologically, benign prostatic hyperplasia is a true hyperplastic process with an increase in prostatic cell number. The prostatic nodules are composed of both hyperplastic glands and hyperplastic stromal muscle. Most periurethral nodules are stromal in character, but transition zone nodules most often consist of glandular tissue. The glands become larger than normal, with stromal muscle between the proliferative glands. Perhaps as much as 40% of the hyperplastic prostate is smooth muscle. The cellular proliferation leads to a tight packing of glands within a given area. There is an increase in the height of the lining epithelium, and the epithelium often shows papillary projections (Figure 23–11). Individual epithelial cells also show some hypertrophy.

FIGURE 23–11 Benign prostatic hyperplasia. (Reproduced, with permission, from Chandrasoma P et al. *Concise Pathology*, 3rd ed. Originally published by Appleton & Lange. Copyright © 1998 by The McGraw-Hill Companies, Inc.)

In men with benign prostatic hyperplasia, the bladder can show both detrusor (bladder wall) smooth muscle hypertrophy and trabeculation associated with an increase in collagen deposition. This is due to the increased bladder pressure created by urinary system obstruction.

Pathogenesis

Although the actual cause of benign prostatic hyperplasia is undefined, several factors are known to be involved in its pathogenesis. These include age-related prostatic growth, the presence of a prostatic capsule, androgenic hormones and their receptors, stromal–epithelial interactions and growth factors, prostatic smooth muscle and adrenergic receptors, and detrusor responses.

A. Age-Related Prostatic Growth

The size of the prostate does not always correlate with the degree of obstruction. The amount of periurethral and transition zone tissue may relate more to the degree of obstruction than the overall prostate size. However, the idea that the clinical symptoms of benign prostatic hyperplasia are due simply to a mass-related increase in urethral resistance is probably too simplistic. Instead, some of its symptoms may be due to obstruction-induced detrusor dysfunction and neural alterations in the bladder and prostate. This has been demonstrated in men with lower urinary tract symptoms undergoing urodynamic testing, which measures the perfusion pressure of the urethra.

B. Prostatic Capsule

The presence of a capsule around the prostate is thought to play a role in development of obstructive symptoms. Besides human males, dogs are the only animal known to develop benign prostatic hyperplasia. However, the canine prostate lacks a capsule, and dogs do not develop obstructive symptoms. In men, the capsule presumably causes the "pressure" created by the expanded periurethral–transition zone tissue that is transmitted to the urethra, leading to an increase in urethral resistance. Surgical incision of the prostatic capsule or removal of the obstructing portion of the prostate, whether by transurethral resection or by open prostatectomy, is effective in relieving symptoms.

C. Hormonal Regulation of Prostatic Growth

The development of benign prostatic hyperplasia requires testicular androgens as well as aging. There are several lines of evidence for this relationship. First, men who are castrated before puberty or who have disorders of impaired androgen production or action do not develop benign prostatic hyperplasia. Second, the prostate, unlike other androgen-dependent organs, maintains its ability to respond to androgens throughout life. Androgens are required for normal cell proliferation and differentiation in the prostate. They may also actively inhibit cell turnover and death. Finally, androgen deprivation at various levels of the hypothalamic–pituitary–testicular axis can reduce prostate size and improve obstructive symptoms (Table 23–7).

Although androgenic hormones are clearly required for the development of benign prostatic hyperplasia, testosterone is not the primary androgen that acts on the prostate. Instead, 80–90% of prostatic testosterone is converted to the more active metabolite DHT by the enzyme 5α-reductase. Two subtypes of 5α-reductase (type 1 and type 2) have been described. Both type 1 and type 2 isoenzymes are found in the skin and liver, but only the type 2 isoenzyme is found in the fetal and adult urogenital tract, including both basal epithelial cells and stromal cells in the prostate. Two 5α-reductase inhibitor drugs are used clinically: Finasteride inhibits only the type 2 isoenzyme, and dutasteride inhibits both the type 1 and 2 isoenzymes (see later). In the prostate, it appears that DHT synthesis largely depends on the type 2 enzyme and that, once it is synthesized, the DHT acts in a paracrine fashion on androgen-dependent epithelial cells. The nuclei of these cells contain large numbers of androgen receptors (Figure 23–12). DHT levels are the same in hyperplastic and normal glands. However, prostatic levels of DHT remain high with aging even though peripheral levels of testosterone decrease. These decreases in plasma androgen levels are further amplified by an age-related increase in the plasma SHBG level, resulting in relatively greater decreases in free testosterone than in total testosterone levels.

Androgen suppression leads to a reduction in prostate size and relief of symptoms of bladder outlet obstruction. True anti-androgens, which block the action of testosterone and DHT in the prostate, should be distinguished from agents that impair androgen production (see Table 23–7). GnRH agonists work by paradoxically downregulating GnRH receptors in the pituitary, producing a transient increase and subsequent long-term reduction in LH concentrations. A variety of anti-androgen treatment approaches have been used clinically,

TABLE 23–7 Mechanisms and side effects of anti-androgenic treatment for benign prostatic hyperplasia.

Agent	Mechanism	Side Effects[1]
Androgen ablation		
GnRH agonists (eg, nafarelin, leuprolide, buserelin, goserelin)	Inhibits pituitary LH secretion, decreases T and DHT. Reduces prostate volume by ≈35%	Hot flushes, loss of libido, impotence, gynecomastia
Abiraterone	Inhibitor of cytochrome P450	
True anti-androgens		
(eg, flutamide, bicalutamide)	Androgen receptor inhibition	Gynecomastia or nipple tenderness; no significant incidence of impotence
5α-Reductase inhibitors[2]		
(eg, finasteride, dutasteride)	Decreases DHT, no alteration in T or LH. Reduces prostate volume by ≈20%	3–4% incidence of impotence and decreased libido
Mixed mechanism of action		
Progestins (eg, megestrol acetate, hydroxyprogesterone caproate, medrogestone)	Inhibits pituitary LH secretion, decreases T and DHT, androgen receptor inhibition	Loss of libido, impotence, heat intolerance.
Cyproterone acetate	Androgen receptor inhibition, inhibits pituitary LH secretion, variable decreases in T and DHT	Loss of libido, impotence (variable)

DHT, dihydrotestosterone; GnRH, gonadotropin-releasing hormone; LH, luteinizing hormone; T, testosterone.

[1]Other than gastrointestinal, hematologic, and central nervous system reactions.

[2]5α-Reductase: steroid-5α-reductase, α polypeptide 2 (3-oxo-5α-steroid α4-dehydrogenase α) or SRD5A.

Modified and reproduced, with permission, from McConnell JD. Benign prostatic hyperplasia: hormonal treatment. Urol Clin North Am. 1995;22:387. Copyright © Elsevier.

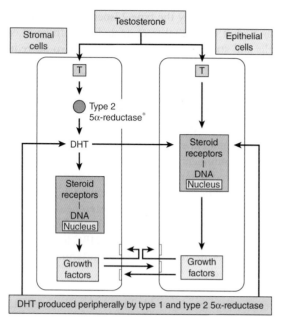

FIGURE 23–12 Mechanism of androgen action on prostatic stromal and epithelial cells. After testosterone (T) diffuses into the cell, it can interact directly with the androgen (steroid) receptors bound to the promoter region of androgen-related genes. In the stromal cell, a majority of T is converted into dihydrotestosterone (DHT), which acts in an autocrine fashion in the stromal cell and in a paracrine fashion after diffusing into nearby epithelial cells. DHT produced peripherally in the skin and liver can also diffuse into the prostate and act in an endocrine fashion. *5α-Reductase: steroid-5α-reductase, α polypeptide 2 (3-oxo-5α steroid Δ4-dehydrogenase α) or SRD5A.

including GnRH agonists (nafarelin, leuprolide, buserelin), androgen receptor inhibitors (cyproterone acetate, flutamide), progestogens, and 5α-reductase inhibitors (finasteride, dutasteride) (Figure 23–13). The complete suppression of androgen action can lead to intolerable adverse effects, such as erectile dysfunction, flushing, and loss of libido. However, the 5α-reductase inhibitors finasteride and dutasteride suppress both plasma and prostatic DHT levels by approximately 65–95%. Treatment with these agents has been shown to induce significant decreases in the size of the prostate as a whole and in the size of the periurethral zone. The 5α-reductase inhibitors must be given for at least 6–12 months to have beneficial effects and must be continued indefinitely thereafter. Both GnRH agonists and 5α-reductase inhibitors have been shown to be effective in improving symptoms and urinary flow rates in patients with benign prostatic hyperplasia, particularly in men with larger (>40 g) prostates. The 5α-reductase inhibitors are less effective than GnRH agonists in reducing the size of the prostate but cause fewer side effects. Because of the adverse side effects produced by total androgen deprivation with GnRH agonists, and because the 5α-reductase inhibitors are effective without these side effects, GnRH agonists are not used in the everyday treatment of benign prostatic hyperplasia symptoms.

Androgen receptor levels remain high with aging, thus maintaining the mechanism for androgen-dependent cell growth. Nuclear androgen receptor levels have been found to be higher in the prostatic tissue of men with benign prostatic hyperplasia than in that of normal controls. The regulation of androgen receptor expression in benign prostatic hyperplasia is now being studied at the transcriptional level.

Finally, androgens are not the only important hormones contributing to the development of benign prostatic hyperplasia. Estrogens appear to be involved in inducing the androgen receptor. Serum estrogen levels increase in men with age, absolutely or relative to testosterone levels. Age-related increases in estrogens may thus increase androgen receptor expression in the prostate, leading to increases in cell growth (or decreases in cell death). Intraprostatic levels of estrogen are increased in men with benign prostatic hyperplasia. Patients with benign prostatic hyperplasia who have larger prostatic volumes tend

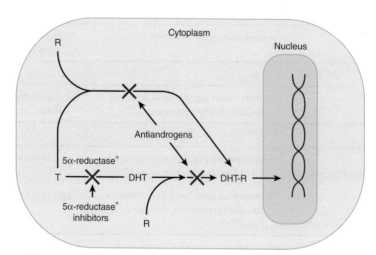

FIGURE 23–13 Site of action of anti-androgens and 5α-reductase inhibitors. X, site of blockade. *5α-Reductase: steroid-5α-reductase, α polypeptide 2 (3-oxo-5α-steroid Δ4-dehydrogenase α) or SRD5A. (Redrawn, with permission, from Oesterling JE. Endocrine therapies for symptomatic benign prostatic hyperplasia. Urology. 1994 Feb;43[2 Suppl]:7–16. Copyright © Elsevier.)

to have higher plasma levels of estradiol. Studies of prostatic specimen tissue have documented an accumulation of DHT, estradiol, and estrone that correlates with patient age. The results show a dramatic increase in the estrogen–androgen ratio with increasing age, particularly in the stroma of prostatic tissue.

Investigations have demonstrated powerful cell-specific, nontranscriptional effects of estradiol on the human prostate. Estradiol, acting in concert with SHBG, has been found to produce an eightfold increase in intracellular cAMP in hyperplastic prostatic tissue. This increase in cAMP does not occur with estrogens such as diethylstilbestrol, which do not bind to SHBG, and is not blocked by the anti-estrogen tamoxifen. Both of these findings suggest that the classic estrogen receptor is not involved. On the other hand, DHT, which blocks the binding of estradiol to SHBG, completely negates the effect of estradiol on cAMP. Finally, the SHBG–estradiol-responsive second-messenger system has been primarily localized to the prostatic stromal cells and not to the epithelial cells.

Thus, estrogens may be causally linked to the onset of benign prostatic hyperplasia and may have an important supportive role in its maintenance. Aromatase inhibitors, such as the investigational agent atamestane, can produce marked reductions in both serum levels and intraprostatic concentrations of estrogens, including estradiol and estrone. However, to date, clinical trials with aromatase inhibitors for benign prostatic hyperplasia have been disappointing.

D. Growth Factors

Evidence suggests that prostatic growth is under the direct control of specific growth factors and only indirectly modulated by androgens. According to this evidence, growth factors from both the fibroblast growth factor (FGF) family and the transforming growth factor (TGF) "superfamily" act together to regulate growth. These growth factors are polypeptides that modulate cell proliferation. The FGF family stimulates cell division and growth: Basic fibroblast growth factor (bFGF) stimulates the growth of both stroma and blood vessels (angiogenesis), and fibroblast growth factor 7 (FGF7; also known as keratinocyte growth factor [KGF]) stimulates the growth of epithelial cells. On the other hand, members of the TGF-β family inhibit cell division. $TGF-\beta_1$ primarily inhibits the growth of stroma, and $TGF-\beta_2$ primarily inhibits the growth of epithelial cells. In the normal prostate, the rate of cell death is equaled by the rate of cell production. It is hypothesized that a balance exists in the stroma between the stimulatory effects of bFGF and the inhibitory effects of $TGF-\beta_1$ and in the epithelial glands between FGF7 stimulation and $TGF-\beta_2$ inhibition. In benign prostatic hyperplasia, when an excess growth of stroma predominates, bFGF is overproduced relative to its regulator $TGF-\beta_1$; when an excess growth of epithelial glands occurs, FGF7 is overproduced relative to $TGF-\beta_2$.

Other growth factors, including epidermal growth factor and insulin-like growth factors (IGF-1 and IGF-2), are also known to stimulate prostatic tissue growth. The IGF axis has been implicated in the pathogenesis of benign prostatic hyperplasia via the paracrine action of IGFs and IGF-binding proteins (IGFBPs). It is hypothesized that DHT may increase IGF-2 activity, mainly in the periurethral region, which in turn induces the benign proliferation of both epithelial and stromal cells characteristic of benign prostatic hyperplasia. In normal prostatic stromal cells, $TGF-\beta_1$ exerts its antiproliferative effects by stimulating the production of IGFBP-3, which acts as an inhibitory factor for cell growth, either indirectly by inhibiting IGFs, or directly by interacting with cells. In cells cultured from hyperplastic prostatic tissue, prostatic stromal cells have a reduced IGFBP-3 response to $TGF-\beta_1$ and a demonstrate decreased $TGF-\beta_1$–induced growth inhibition relative to normal prostatic stromal cells. Growth factors undoubtedly also play a role in the development of bladder hypertrophy in response to outflow obstruction (see later). TGF-β is known to stimulate collagen synthesis and deposition in the bladder.

Targeting peptide growth factors offers a potential means of regulating prostatic enlargement and relieving symptoms associated with benign prostatic hyperplasia. Preliminary clinical trials of growth factor antagonists have led to significant improvements in urinary symptoms, maximal flow rates, and residual volumes.

E. Prostatic Smooth Muscle, Adrenergic Receptors & Phosphodiesterase Type 5

Prostatic smooth muscle represents a significant proportion of the gland. Urethral elasticity and the degree of bladder outlet obstruction are undoubtedly influenced by the relative content of smooth muscle within the prostate in patients with benign prostatic hyperplasia. Undoubtedly, resting and dynamic prostatic smooth muscle tone plays a major role in the pathophysiology of benign prostatic hyperplasia. Smooth muscle cells in the prostate—at the bladder neck and in the prostatic capsule—are richly populated with α-adrenergic receptors. Contraction of the prostate and bladder neck are mediated by α_1-adrenergic receptors. Stimulation of these receptors results in a dynamic increase in prostatic urethral resistance. $Alpha_1$-adrenergic receptor blockade clearly diminishes this response and has been found to improve symptoms, urinary flow rates, and residual urine volumes in patients with benign prostatic hyperplasia within 2–4 weeks after starting therapy. The selective α_1-blockers prazosin, terazosin, doxazosin, and alfuzosin have been extensively studied and found to be effective (Table 23–8). Because the bladder's smooth muscle cells do not contain a significant number of α_1 receptors, alpha-blocker therapy can selectively diminish urethral resistance without affecting detrusor smooth muscle contractility.

Studies have suggested that the α_1 receptors involved in the contraction of prostate smooth muscle appear to be α_{1a} receptors (previously called α_{1c} receptors). Clinical studies have established the efficacy of the subtype-selective α_{1a} antagonists, tamsulosin and silodosin.

Contractile protein gene expression in stromal smooth muscle cells is significantly altered after alpha blockade. This

TABLE 23–8   Alpha-receptor blockade for benign prostatic hyperplasia.

Agent	Site and Mechanism of Action	Side Effects
Alfuzosin	Postsynaptic α_{1a} blockade	Hypotension (especially postural hypotension leading to syncope)
Doxazosin	Postsynaptic α_1 blockade	
Prazosin	Postsynaptic α_1 blockade	
Terazosin	Postsynaptic α_1 blockade	
Silodosin	Postsynaptic α_{1a} blockade	
Tamsulosin	Postsynaptic α_{1a} blockade	
Tadalafil	Phosphodiesterase type 5 inhibitor	

Reproduced, with permission, from Papadakis MA et al, eds. *Current Medical Diagnosis & Treatment 2018*, 57th ed. McGraw-Hill, 2018.

suggests that alpha-blocking agents may work not only by the simple relaxation of muscle tone but also by affecting the phenotypic expression of contractile proteins in prostatic smooth muscle cells.

Alpha-blockers may also work by changing the balance between prostate cell growth and death. Some investigators hypothesize that benign prostatic hyperplasia occurs as a result of a decrease in apoptosis (programmed cell death), allowing more cells to accumulate in the prostate, hence causing its enlargement. The alpha-blockers doxazosin and terazosin have been shown to induce apoptosis in the stroma of the prostate.

Another means of relaxing smooth muscle and reducing the symptoms of benign prostatic hyperplasia may be phosphodiesterase type 5 (PDE5) inhibitors. The PDE5 enzyme has been found throughout the urinary tract, where it works to break down the intracellular smooth muscle relaxant, cyclic guanosine monophosphate (cGMP). This means that PDE5 inhibition may reduce smooth muscle tone in the prostate, urethra, and bladder, although the exact mechanism of action in relation to urinary symptoms is still to be determined. Nevertheless, trials have shown that PDE5 inhibitors can improve urinary symptoms by approximately the same magnitude as alpha-blockers and may increase urinary flow.

F. Possible Mechanisms of Bladder Outlet Obstruction

There are several ways in which benign prostatic hyperplasia might cause obstruction of the bladder neck. The prominent median lobe may simply act as a ball valve; restriction may occur from the nondistensible capsule; static obstruction may result from the enlarged prostate surrounding the prostatic urethra; and dynamic obstruction may occur from an inability to relax prostatic smooth muscle. In fact, clinical data support a role for each of these proposed factors. For example, TURP frequently relieves obstructive symptoms, as does simple surgical incision of the prostatic capsule. Medications that shrink the prostate or relax smooth muscle also relieve bladder outlet obstruction and increase urinary flow rates.

Various thermal therapies have been investigated as less invasive surgical procedures than TURP for benign prostatic hyperplasia, including transurethral microwave, high-intensity focused ultrasound, laser-delivered interstitial thermal therapies, and transurethral needle ablation (TUNA) of the prostate. These procedures use different forms of energy such as microwave, ultrasound, laser, and radiofrequency to produce the thermal injury. It is unclear whether these procedures work by anatomic shrinkage, debulking of the obstructing enlarged prostate, or physiologic alteration of voiding function. In pathologic studies of TUNA of the prostate, for example, coagulative necrosis gradually changes to retractile fibrous scar. This could cause a decrease in the volume of the treated area even without a significant decrease in prostatic volume. Alternatively, severe thermal damage to intraprostatic nerve fibers may reduce the dynamic component of the bladder outlet obstruction by denervating the receptors or sensory nerves.

G. Bladder Response to Obstruction

Many of the clinical symptoms of benign prostatic hyperplasia are related to obstruction-induced changes in bladder function rather than to outflow obstruction per se. Thus, one-third of men continue to have significant voiding problems even after surgical relief of obstruction. Obstruction-induced changes in bladder function are of two basic types. First, there are changes that lead to **detrusor overactivity** (**instability**). These are clinically manifested by frequency and urgency. These two symptoms cause much of the distress related to benign prostatic hyperplasia and are sometimes quite out of proportion to the degree of obstruction. Thus, treating the bladder overactivity may have more impact than treating the obstruction. Second, there are changes that lead to **decreased detrusor contractility**. These are clinically manifested by symptoms of decreased force of the urinary stream, hesitancy, intermittency, increased residual urine, and, in a minority of cases, **detrusor failure**.

The bladder's response to obstruction is largely adaptive (Figure 23–14). The initial response is the development of detrusor smooth muscle hypertrophy. It is hypothesized that this increase in muscle mass, though an adaptive response to increased intravesical pressure and one that maintains urinary outflow, is associated with significant intracellular and extracellular changes in smooth muscle cells that predispose to detrusor instability. In experimental animal models, unrelieved obstruction results in significant increases in detrusor extracellular matrix (collagen).

In addition to obstruction-induced changes in the smooth muscle cells and extracellular matrix of the bladder, there is increasing evidence that chronic obstruction in patients with untreated benign prostatic hyperplasia may alter neural responses as well, occasionally predisposing to detrusor failure.

Traditional therapies for symptoms associated with bladder obstruction have been directed toward relief of bladder outflow resistance (see Table 23–8). Newer treatments of detrusor instability include anticholinergic medications and the

Clinical response   **Bladder response**

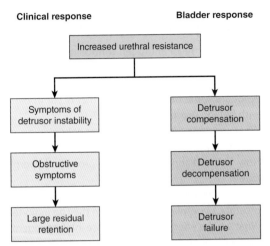

FIGURE 23–14 Schematic of the natural history of benign prostatic hyperplasia. (Redrawn, with permission, of John Wiley & Sons Ltd from McConnell JD. The pathophysiology of benign prostatic hyperplasia. J Androl. 1991 Nov-Dec;12(6):356–63. Copyright © American Society of Andrology.)

β_3 agonist, mirabegron. In the past, such drugs were avoided because of the fear that inhibiting bladder activity would lead to acute urinary retention, but that fear has not been substantiated in recent studies of men with minimal (<200 mL) residual urine after voiding.

The effects of chronic bladder obstruction are still not well understood. Future studies must examine the importance of changes in receptor density, affinity, and distribution, as well as the agonist release and degradation that occur during chronic obstruction and the ultrastructural and physiologic changes that occur with relief of obstruction.

Clinical Manifestations

A. Symptoms and Signs

Urinary outflow obstruction and bladder dysfunction are responsible for the major symptoms and signs of benign prostatic hyperplasia.

There are two types of symptoms: irritative, which are related to bladder filling, and obstructive, which are related to bladder emptying. **Irritative symptoms** occur as a consequence of bladder hypertrophy and dysfunction and include urinary frequency, nocturia, and urgency. These observations may be more related to the bladder's response to the obstruction, rather than to the direct effects of the obstruction itself. **Obstructive symptoms** result from the distortion and narrowing of the bladder neck and prostatic urethra, leading to incomplete bladder emptying. Obstructive symptoms include difficulty initiating urination, decreased force and caliber of the urinary stream, intermittency of the urinary stream, urinary hesitancy, and dribbling.

To objectively evaluate the severity and complexity of symptoms in benign prostatic hyperplasia, a symptom index has been developed by the American Urological Association. The self-administered questionnaire evaluates patient symptoms, such as bladder emptying, frequency, intermittency, urgency, and nocturia, as well as quality of life. The symptom index has been validated and found to have good test–retest reliability and to discriminate well between affected patients and controls. In clinical trials, there have been good correlations between urinary symptoms and total score, and the instrument has proved useful to describe changes in symptoms over time and after treatment.

In severe cases, prostatic enlargement may cause either acute or chronic urinary retention. **Acute urinary retention** causes painful bladder dilation, with an inability to void. Acute urinary retention is often precipitated by prostate swelling caused by the infarction of a nodule or by certain medications. **Chronic urinary retention** has both obstructive and irritative voiding symptoms. Occasionally, a patient presents with marked urinary retention, yet few if any symptoms. Complications of chronic bladder dilation include hypertrophy of the bladder wall musculature and the development of diverticula; urinary tract infection as a result of the stagnant bladder urine; hematuria, particularly with infarction of a prostatic nodule; and chronic kidney disease and azotemia from bilateral hydroureter and hydronephrosis. Bladder dilation can be treated with a permanent catheter or by teaching the patient the technique of intermittent self-catheterization to empty the bladder about every 4 hours.

Digital rectal examination may reveal either focal or diffuse prostate enlargement. However, the size of the prostate as estimated by digital rectal examination does not correlate well with either the symptoms or signs of benign prostatic hyperplasia or the need for treatment. Examination of the lower abdomen may reveal a distended bladder, consistent with urinary retention.

B. Laboratory Tests and Evaluation

Laboratory tests performed to evaluate patients with benign prostatic hyperplasia include blood urea nitrogen (BUN) and serum creatinine to exclude renal failure, and urinalysis and urine culture to exclude urinary tract infection. Elevations of BUN or serum creatinine from benign prostatic hyperplasia occur only rarely. CT scan and ultrasound are usually not performed in patients with normal findings on these simple laboratory tests. Instead, these tests are generally reserved for patients with hematuria or suspected hydronephrosis. When a CT scan or ultrasound is performed in a man with benign prostatic hyperplasia, it typically shows elevation of the bladder base by the enlarged prostate; trabeculation, thickening, and diverticula of the bladder wall; elevation of the ureters; and poor bladder emptying. Uncommonly, in a neglected patient, the CT or ultrasound shows hydronephrosis, putting the patient at risk for acute kidney failure.

The most useful technique for assessing the significance of benign prostatic hyperplasia is urodynamic evaluation with uroflowmetry and cystometry. In these tests, the patient voids and various measurements are made. In uroflowmetry, the maximal urinary flow rate is recorded. If the peak flow rate is less than 10 mL/s, the patient is considered to have significant bladder outlet obstruction. However, the patient must void at least 150 mL for the measurement to be considered reliable. Pressure–flow studies are simultaneous recordings of urinary bladder pressure and urinary flow rates, which provide information about urethral resistance. These pressure–flow studies can help determine which patients are less likely to benefit from prostatic surgery by providing information on detrusor function. Cystourethroscopy is usually reserved for patients who have hematuria that remains unexplained despite a CT or ultrasound or preoperatively for patients who require TURP. Validated symptom scores, an estimation of prostate volume, and a determination of serum prostate-specific antigen can help predict the progression of benign prostatic hyperplasia. New ultrasound techniques also hold promise.

CHECKPOINT

13. Which is the major androgen controlling prostate size?
14. What are some ways to provide relief of obstructive symptoms?
15. What are some bladder changes that occur in patients with benign prostatic hyperplasia?
16. What are some symptoms and signs of benign prostatic hyperplasia?
17. How is the diagnosis of benign prostatic hyperplasia made?
18. What is the role of α_1-adrenergic receptors in benign prostatic hyperplasia, and how can they be inhibited?
19. What are the effects of 5α-reductase inhibitor agents on men with benign prostatic hyperplasia?

CASE STUDIES

Yeong Kwok, MD

(See Chapter 25, p. 788–89 for answers)

CASE 124

A married couple presents to a primary care physician with a complaint of infertility. They have been trying to get pregnant for approximately 1 year. During that time, they have had intercourse approximately three or four times a week without birth control. There is a 3-year-old child from the woman's prior marriage. The man has never had a child to his knowledge. He denies sexual dysfunction. He had both gonorrhea and chlamydial infection in his early 20s and one episode of prostatitis for which he was treated. His medical history is otherwise unremarkable. He takes no medications. He denies tobacco and drug use and drinks only rarely. On examination, his testes are approximately 4.5 × 3 × 2.5 cm bilaterally. The epididymis is irregular to palpation bilaterally. There are no varicoceles or hernias. The vas deferens is present and without abnormality. The prostate is of normal size, with no bogginess or tenderness. The penis has no fibrosis or angulation. The urethral meatus is appropriately situated.

Questions

A. What are the categories of male infertility? Give the major causes in each category.
B. What do you suspect is the likely cause of infertility in this patient? Why?
C. Given the likely diagnosis, what would you expect to find on semen analysis? Why? What would you expect the serum testosterone, LH, and FSH to be? Why?
D. What other tests may be helpful in confirming the diagnosis?

CASE 125

A 68-year-old man presents to the physician with a complaint of urinary frequency. He states that he has noted increased urgency and frequency for approximately 1 year, but his symptoms have become progressively worse. He states that currently he seems to have to urinate "all the time" and often feels as if he has not completely emptied his bladder. He must get up to urinate three or four times each night. In addition, in the last month, he sometimes has postvoid dribbling. He denies fevers, weight loss, and bone pain. His medical history is notable only for hypertension. His medications include atenolol and aspirin. The family history is negative for malignancy.

On examination, he appears healthy. His vital signs are notable for a blood pressure of 154/92 mm Hg. The prostate is diffusely enlarged, with no focal nodule or tenderness. Benign prostatic hyperplasia is suspected.

Questions

A. How would you make the diagnosis of benign prostatic hyperplasia?

B. What factors are known to be responsible for the pathogenesis of this disorder?

C. How would you classify this patient's symptoms? What is the mechanism by which benign prostatic hyperplasia causes these symptoms?

REFERENCES

General

Barrett KE et al. *Ganong's Review of Medical Physiology*, 26th ed. McGraw-Hill, 2018.

Kumar V et al. *Robbins & Cotran Pathologic Basis of Disease*, 9th ed. Elsevier, 2014.

Melmed S et al. *Williams Textbook of Endocrinology*, 13th ed. Elsevier, 2015.

Male Infertility

Bachir BG et al. Infectious, inflammatory, and immunologic conditions resulting in male infertility. Urol Clin North Am. 2014 Feb;41(1):67–81. [PMID: 24286768].

Cooper TG et al. World Health Organization reference values for human semen characteristics. Hum Reprod Update. 2010 May-Jun;16(3):231–45. [PMID: 19934213]

Craig JR et al. Obesity, male infertility, and the sperm epigenome. Fertil Steril. 2017 Apr;107(4):848–59. [PMID: 28366411]

Davis SM et al. Testis development and fertility potential in boys with Klinefelter syndrome. Endocrinol Metab Clin North Am. 2015 Dec;44(4):843–65. [PMID: 26568497]

Esteves SC. Novel concepts in male factor infertility: clinical and laboratory perspectives. J Assist Reprod Genet. 2016 Oct;33(10):1319–35. [PMID: 27423664]

Fode M et al. Sexually transmitted disease and male infertility: a systematic review. Eur Urol Focus. 2016 Oct;2(4):383–93. [PMID: 28723470]

Fode M et al. A step-wise approach to sperm retrieval in men with neurogenic anejaculation. Nat Rev Urol. 2015 Nov;12(11):607–16. [PMID: 26481575]

Fronczak CM et al. The insults of illicit drug use on male fertility. J Androl. 2012 Jul-Aug;33(4):515–28. [PMID: 21799144]

Gunes S et al. The role of epigenetics in idiopathic male infertility. J Assist Reprod Genet. 2016 May;33(5):553–69. [PMID: 26941097]

Hotaling JM. Genetics of male infertility. Urol Clin North Am. 2014 Feb;41(1):1–17. [PMID: 24286764]

Hotaling JM et al. Male endocrine dysfunction. Urol Clin North Am. 2014 Feb;41(1):39–53. [PMID: 24286766]

Jensen CFS et al. Varicocele and male infertility. Nat Rev Urol. 2017 Sep;14(9):523–33. [PMID: 28675168]

Kathrins M et al. Diagnosis and treatment of infertility-related male hormonal dysfunction. Nat Rev Urol. 2016 Jun;13(6):309–23. [PMID: 27091665]

Mintziori G et al. Consequences of hyperthyroidism in male and female fertility: pathophysiology and current management. J Endocrinol Invest. 2016 Aug;39(8):849–53. [PMID: 26956000]

Niederberger CS. Chapter 24. Male infertility. In: Wein AJ et al, eds. *Campbell–Walsh Urology*, 11th ed. Elsevier, 2015.

Ohlander SJ et al. Testosterone and male infertility. Urol Clin North Am. 2016 May;43(2):195–202. [PMID: 27132576]

Winters BR et al. The epidemiology of male infertility. Urol Clin North Am. 2014 Feb;41(1):195–204. [PMID: 24286777].

Benign Prostatic Hyperplasia

Aaron L et al. Review of prostate anatomy and embryology and the etiology of benign prostatic hyperplasia. Urol Clin North Am. 2016 Aug;43(3):279–88. [PMID: 27476121]

Burke N et al. Systematic review and meta-analysis of transurethral resection of the prostate versus minimally invasive procedures for the treatment of benign prostatic obstruction. Urology. 2010 May;75(5):1015–22. [PMID: 19854492]

Cox L et al. Urodynamics in male LUTS: when are they necessary and how do we use them? Urol Clin North Am. 2014 Aug;41(3):399–407, viii. [PMID: 25063596]

Cunha GR et al. A historical perspective on the role of stroma in the pathogenesis of benign prostatic hyperplasia. Differentiation. 2011 Nov-Dec;82(4-5):168–72. [PMID: 21723032]

De Nunzio C et al. Benign prostatic hyperplasia in 2014: innovations in medical and surgical treatment. Nat Rev Urol. 2015 Feb;12(2):76–8. [PMID: 25558836]

Egan KB. The epidemiology of benign prostatic hyperplasia associated with lower urinary tract symptoms: prevalence and incident rates. Urol Clin North Am. 2016 Aug;43(3):289–97. [PMID: 27476122]

Gratzke C et al. EAU guidelines on the assessment of non-neurogenic male lower urinary tract symptoms including benign prostatic obstruction. Eur Urol. 2015 Jun;67(6):1099–109. [PMID: 25613154]

Thorner DA et al. Benign prostatic hyperplasia: symptoms, symptom scores, and outcome measures. Urol Clin North Am. 2009 Nov; 36(4):417–29. [PMID: 19942042]

Vignozzi L et al. Lower urinary tract symptoms, benign prostatic hyperplasia and metabolic syndrome. Nat Rev Urol. 2016 Feb;13(2):108–19. [PMID: 26754190]

Inflammatory Rheumatic Diseases

Allan C. Gelber, MD, MPH, PhD, Stuart M. Levine, MD, FACP, & Erika Darrah, PhD

The inflammatory rheumatic diseases form a group of disorders that are highly variable in their phenotypic expression. However, they have in common the presence of localized and/or systemic inflammation, which results in characteristic musculoskeletal system and internal organ damage. Among these diseases, the specific clinical and pathologic features of each disorder likely reflect the initiating and propagating stimuli that determine the specific tissues targeted and the inflammatory effector mechanisms that predominate.

Although the spectrum of inflammatory rheumatic diseases is broad, some general principles provide a framework within which to discuss the pathophysiology of all. One of the most useful constructs is a kinetic one, which focuses on disease initiation, propagation, and flares. It is useful for discussing both acute and chronic diseases. Understanding the stimuli and mechanisms responsible for each of these phases among the different rheumatic diseases permits a deeper insight into these fascinating and complex syndromes.

OVERVIEW OF INFLAMMATORY RHEUMATIC DISEASES

ACUTE DISEASES

The initiating force of acute diseases (eg, gout, immune complex vasculitis) is often clearly recognizable and can be endogenous (eg, crystal deposition) or exogenous (eg, new medication, systemic bacterial or viral infection) in origin. The disease is self-limited owing to the success of the inflammatory response in removing the offending initiating stimulus (eg, urate crystals in gout, bacterial antigen or drug in immune complex vasculitis) (Figure 24–1). Despite resolution of the acute episode, flares may occur upon re-exposure to the initiating stimulus.

CHRONIC DISEASES

The initiating force in chronic diseases (eg, systemic lupus erythematosus [SLE], rheumatoid arthritis) is often remote and no longer recognizable once the unique disease phenotype becomes fully established and the diagnosis clear. Propagation of the disease typically occurs as a result of an autoimmune response that induces a self-amplifying cycle of damage. Autoimmune diseases are characteristically driven by "self-antigens" (eg, nucleosomes [composed of DNA and histones] in SLE) and can elicit both cellular and humoral immune responses. Conditions leading to the initiation of chronic autoimmune diseases occur rarely, but once a disease is established, flares are frequent. This circumstance probably reflects the abundant capacity of the immune system to "remember" previously encountered antigens and to respond to them with greater vigor when encountered again, even at lower concentrations (see Figure 24–1).

Different tissues are affected in various diseases (eg, specific synovial joints in gout and rheumatoid arthritis; skin, joints, kidneys, serosal surfaces, nervous system, and blood cell lines in SLE).

PATHOGENESIS OF INFLAMMATION

The nature of tissue damage and joint injury is determined in part by the inflammatory and immune effector functions that predominate. In addition, the pathologic features of the chronic inflammatory disorders reflect the combination of inflammatory damage and the consequences of healing.

Acute diseases

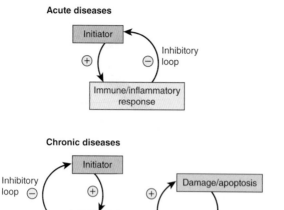

Chronic diseases

FIGURE 24–1 Kinetics of acute and chronic inflammatory rheumatic diseases.

ENDOTHELIAL ACTIVATION

The recruitment and activation of specific subsets of inflammatory and immune cells are essential determinants of the pathologic features. In this regard, the role of regional blood vessel endothelium activation by pro-inflammatory cytokines (eg, tumor necrosis factor alpha [TNFα], interleukin [IL]-1β) must be emphasized. Several cytokines induce the expression on endothelial cells of ligands for the adhesion-promoting receptors of inflammatory cells (integrins and selectins) and allow neutrophils and monocytes to adhere to the vessel wall in the inflamed area and migrate into the underlying tissues.

CYTOKINES

Distinct classes of immune effector function are activated depending on the pattern of cytokines that predominate during initiation of the inflammatory response. For example, some cytokines (eg, IL-12) produced by infected monocyte-macrophages skew the lymphocyte response toward T_H1 cells (which generate the T_H1 cytokines IL-2, interferon-γ, and TNFα) that are associated with activating macrophage killing functions and protecting against invading intracellular pathogens. In contrast, the presence of IL-4 during the initial response induces the differentiation of T_H2 lymphocytes, which generate T_H2 cytokines (eg, IL-4, IL-5, IL-6, IL-10). These cytokines have their predominant function in activating B cells and generating antibodies. A new subset of helper T cells that develop in the presence of the cytokines TGF-γ and IL-6 has recently been described. These cells are termed T_H17 cells because of their characteristic secretion of IL-17. They appear to be critically involved in recruiting granulocytes, protecting against certain types of bacteria, and generating chronic inflammation and autoimmunity.

Although significant overlap exists, specific pathologic features tend to accompany the different cytokine patterns (eg,

granulomas for T_H1 versus immune complex disease for T_H2). In addition, significant data point to an important role for type I interferons in inducing novel pathways of monocyte differentiation in patients with SLE that enhance responses to "self-antigens."

COMPLEMENT PATHWAY

The classical complement pathway is activated when antibody binds to its specific antigen. Activation of the complement cascade induces inflammatory cell recruitment and activation (with all the consequences mentioned later), other features of the acute inflammatory response (eg, increased capillary permeability), and cellular damage mediated by terminal components of the complement cascade (ie, membrane attack complex).

MYELOMONOCYTIC CELLS & IMMUNE COMPLEX FORMATION

Although myelomonocytic cells (neutrophils and macrophages) have numerous effector pathways that function to rid the host of foreign invaders, some of these effector mechanisms can damage healthy tissue if released in large amounts. These include free radical species generated during the respiratory burst, as well as a variety of secretory products contained in the granules of these inflammatory cells. Important granule contents include a variety of proteases such as cathepsins, elastase, and collagenase. These products are liberated into the extracellular medium in the inflammatory locus, where they accumulate and may have damaging effects on normal connective tissue. In addition, numerous pro-inflammatory mediators released in this environment (including TNFα, IL-1β, IL-6, prostaglandins, and leukotrienes) attract further inflammatory cells to the area and amplify the potential to generate tissue damage if the inflammatory response is not adequately quenched.

Numerous studies have emphasized the roles of the complement pathway and immunoglobulin Fc gamma receptors (FcγRs) in the activation of the myelomonocytic cell effector function that results in tissue damage. For example, Fc receptors play a critical role in generating the pathologic picture characteristic of immune complex–mediated diseases (see Immune Complex Vasculitis and Systemic Lupus Erythematosus). Clinical conditions in which this situation might arise include drug reactions, serum sickness, and infections (infective endocarditis, streptococcal skin and pharyngeal infections, and others). Under conditions such as these that lead to the liberation of significant amounts of "self-antigen" from host tissue (cell damage or death), immune complex formation, Fc receptor binding, and complement activation may result.

The consequences of immune complex formation and deposition are similar whether caused by foreign antigens or "self-antigens." Notably, immune complex–mediated renal disease and vasculitis that occur in several murine models of SLE are completely absent in the FcγR knockout mouse.

CELLULAR CYTOTOXICITY

Lymphocyte-Mediated Cytotoxicity

Cytotoxic T lymphocytes (ie, CD8+ T cells) are capable of killing target cells. When target cell destruction exceeds the capacity for renewal, impaired tissue function can result. As with other lymphocyte functions, this effector function is activated only on ligation of the T-cell receptor by a specific peptide (bound within the cleft of a major histocompatibility complex [MHC] class I molecule). On recognition of antigen on the surface of a target cell, cytotoxic T lymphocytes induce the death of those cells, using several distinct mechanisms. One prominent mechanism involves the Fas/Fas-ligand (FasL) pathway, whereby FasL present on activated lymphocytes binds to the Fas receptor on target cells and activates target cell apoptosis. The second critical mechanism involves the release of cytotoxic T-lymphocyte secretory granules. These granules contain at least two distinct classes of proteins. One, called **perforin**, allows water, salt, and proteins (including the second class of granule protein, the granzymes) to enter the target cell cytoplasm through mechanisms that still remain unclear. The **granzymes**, a family comprising several proteases, target a number of critical cellular substrates and activate the process of apoptosis within the target cell.

Antibody-Dependent Cellular Cytotoxicity

The destruction of antibody-coated target cells by natural killer cells is called antibody-dependent cellular cytotoxicity (ADCC) and occurs when the Fc receptor of a natural killer (NK) cell binds to the Fc portion of the surface-bound antibody. The cytotoxic mechanism involves the release of cytoplasmic granules containing perforin and granzymes into the cytoplasm of the antibody-coated cell (similar to cytotoxic T lymphocyte–mediated killing, described previously).

This mechanism has been implicated in autoantibody-mediated syndromes, in which the autoantigen resides at the cell surface or relocates to this site after an insult. An example of this is the photosensitive skin disease that occurs in patients with SLE who possess the Ro autoantibody. On exposure to ultraviolet light, the Ro antigen is expressed on the surface of apoptotic keratinocytes within surface blebs. Circulating Ro antibodies bind the antigen at the cell surface, with induction of FcR-mediated effector pathways.

HOST TISSUE DIFFERENTIATION

In response to inflammatory mediators (including cytokines) and T cells, cells in tissues ordinarily unrelated to the immune response can alter their form and function to support (and in some cases drive) a chronic inflammatory response. This mechanism has been described in myositis (see Inflammatory Myopathies), in which the inflammatory and autoimmune response is focused on areas of ongoing damage and regeneration.

CHECKPOINT

1. What is the hallmark of the rheumatic diseases?
2. What three kinetic features account for the specific clinical and pathologic characteristics of the different rheumatic diseases?
3. What six inflammatory effector mechanisms account for the inflammation seen in the rheumatic diseases? Give an example of a disease that illustrates each principle.

PATHOPHYSIOLOGY OF SELECTED RHEUMATIC DISEASES

GOUT

Clinical Presentation

Gout is the classic example of crystal-induced inflammation of synovial joints. It is a common condition, presenting in approximately 4% of the adult American population, and it is approximately three times more common in men than women. The deposition of monosodium urate crystals in the joint space leads to episodes of severe acute joint pain and swelling (particularly in the great toe, midfoot, ankle, and knee). These episodes tend to resolve completely and spontaneously within a week, even in the absence of therapy. If not properly treated, however, this acute, self-limited form of the disease can evolve over many years into a chronic, destructive pattern resulting in more frequent and sustained periods of pain and resultant joint deformity. Accumulations of urate crystals elsewhere in the body can lead to subcutaneous deposits called tophi ("tophus" in the singular).

Etiology

The critical initiating factor in gout is the precipitation of monosodium urate crystals in synovial joints. This occurs when body fluids become supersaturated with uric acid (generally at serum levels >7 mg/dL). Indeed, the degree of hyperuricemia correlates well with the development of gout, with annual incidence rates of about 5% for serum uric acid levels more than 9 mg/dL. Increased levels of serum uric acid result either from the underexcretion (90% of patients)

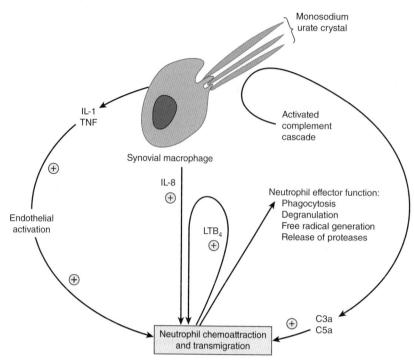

FIGURE 24–2 The mechanisms of the initiation and amplification of the acute inflammatory response in gout involve both cytokines and humoral mediators.

or overproduction (10%) of uric acid. A decreased glomerular filtration rate is the most frequent cause of decreased uric acid excretion and may be due to numerous causes (see Chapter 16), but, regardless of etiology, impaired renal function is clearly related to the occurrence of gout. Diuretic administration is also a frequent cause of decreased uric acid excretion. Overproduction defects can result from primary defects in the purine salvage pathway (eg, hypoxanthine–guanine phosphoribosyl transferase deficiency), leading to an increase in de novo purine synthesis and high flux through the purine breakdown pathway. Diseases causing increased cell turnover (eg, myeloproliferative disorders, psoriasis) and DNA degradation (eg, tumor lysis syndrome) are secondary causes of hyperuricemia.

Pathophysiology

Although the concentration of monosodium urate in joint fluid slowly equilibrates with that in the serum, crystal formation is markedly influenced by physical factors such as temperature and blood flow. The propensity for gout to involve distal joints (eg, great toes and ankles), which are cooler than more proximal body parts, probably reflects the presence of local physical conditions at these sites remote from the body core that favor crystal formation.

Monosodium urate crystals are not biologically inert. Their highly negatively charged surfaces function as efficient initiators of the acute inflammatory response. The crystals are potent activators of the classic complement pathway, generating complement cleavage products (eg, C3a, C5a) that are

strong chemoattractants for neutrophil influx (Figure 24–2). The crystals also activate the kinin system and in that way induce local vasodilation, pain, and swelling. Crystal phagocytosis by synovial macrophages activates the inflammasome (a complex of proteins that sense certain intracellular stressors and activate IL-1β maturation) and stimulates the release of pro-inflammatory cytokines (eg, IL-1β, TNFα, IL-8, PGE₂). These products increase adhesion molecule expression on local vessel endothelium to facilitate neutrophil adhesion and migration and are also potent chemoattractants for neutrophils. Neutrophils also amplify their own recruitment by releasing leukotriene LTB₄ upon urate crystal phagocytosis (see Figure 24–2).

The intense inflammatory response in gout typically resolves spontaneously and completely over the course of several days, even without therapy. This down-modulation of the inflammatory response is a typical feature of acute inflammation, whereby the inflammatory response itself successfully removes the pro-inflammatory stimulus (Table 24–1). Numerous mechanisms appear to be responsible: (1) efficient crystal phagocytosis, preventing the activation of newly recruited inflammatory cells; (2) increased heat and fluid influx, altering the local physical and chemical conditions to favor crystal solubilization; (3) coating of crystals with serum proteins, rendering the surface of the crystals less inflammatory; (4) secretion of a variety of anti-inflammatory cytokines (eg, TGF-β) by activated joint macrophages; and (5) phagocytosis of previously activated apoptotic neutrophils by macrophages in the joint, altering the balance of cytokines secreted by these macrophages in such a way that pro-inflammatory cytokine

TABLE 24–1   Mechanisms causing down-modulation of the inflammatory response in gout.

Efficient crystal phagocytosis
Increased heat and fluid influx, favoring solubilization
Coating of crystals with serum proteins, shielding their pro-inflammatory surfaces
Secretion of anti-inflammatory cytokines (eg, TGF-β) by activated joint macrophages
Apoptotic neutrophil phagocytosis, enhancing anti-inflammatory effects

secretion is inhibited while anti-inflammatory cytokine secretion is enhanced.

Thus, gout represents an excellent example of an acute inflammatory response initiated by a pro-inflammatory force. The response is acute, highly focused, and self-limited rather than self-sustaining and is associated with little tissue destruction in the acute phase. Flares of disease represent a recurrence of crystals in a pro-inflammatory form in the joints. Myelomonocytic cells and humoral factors (eg, cytokines and the complement and kinin cascades) are critical mediators of the acute syndrome.

Clinical Manifestations

A. Podagra and Episodic Oligoarticular Arthritis

Podagra—severe inflammatory arthritis at the first metatarsophalangeal joint—is the most frequent manifestation of gout. Patients typically describe waking in the middle of the night with dramatic pain, redness, swelling, and warmth of the area. Flares of gout typically produce one of the most intense forms of inflammatory arthritis. The toes and, to a lesser extent, the midfoot, ankles and knees, are the most common sites for gout flares. Gout attacks frequently occur in circumstances that increase serum uric acid levels, such as metabolic stressors leading to increased DNA or adenosine triphosphate (ATP) turnover (eg, sepsis or surgery) or dehydration. Agents that reduce prostaglandin synthesis (eg, nonsteroidal anti-inflammatory drugs), reduce neutrophil migration into the joints (eg, colchicine), or decrease the activation of myelomonocytic cells (eg, corticosteroids) reduce the duration of a gouty flare.

Gouty arthritis can be diagnosed by examining synovial fluid aspirated from an actively inflamed joint under a polarizing microscope. Monosodium urate crystals can be seen as negatively birefringent, needle-like structures that extend across the diameter of and are engulfed by polymorphonuclear neutrophils.

B. Tophi Formation

Firm, irregular, subcutaneous deposits of monosodium urate crystals may occur in patients with chronic gout and are referred to as tophi. A tophus most often forms along tendinous tissues on the extensor surfaces of joints and tendons, as well as on the outer helix of the ear. Such tophi may extrude chalky material, containing urate crystals, onto the skin surface that can be viewed for diagnostic purposes using polarized microscopy.

C. Chronic Erosive Polyarthritis

In some patients, the total body burden of uric acid increases greatly over years; deposits of monosodium urate crystals occur at multiple joint sites. This may result in a persistent but more indolent inflammatory arthritis associated with the remodeling of the thin synovial membrane into a thickened inflammatory tissue. Destructive and irreversible joint deformities resulting from bone and cartilage erosions often develop in this circumstance. Renal tubular injury and nephrolithiasis can also develop under these conditions.

Treatment

Therapy for acute gouty arthritis consists of agents that decrease inflammatory cell recruitment and activation to the involved joints. In contrast, the prevention or prophylaxis of recurrent attacks of gouty arthritis requires chronic therapy to decrease serum uric acid levels into the normal range, in which the dissolution of crystals is favored. Several agents are available that can accomplish this. These include uricosuric agents (eg, probenecid), which enhance the excretion of uric acid into the urine; allopurinol and febuxostat, which impede uric acid synthesis by inhibiting xanthine oxidase (a critical enzyme in the uric acid synthetic pathway); and pegloticase, which converts uric acid to allantoin, an inactive and soluble metabolite readily excreted by the kidneys. Conceptually, the xanthine oxidase inhibitors, allopurinol and febuxostat, are most appropriate for the treatment of uric acid overproduction (10% of patients); the uricosuric agent, probenecid, for the treatment of uric acid underexcretion (90% of patients); and pegloticase for the rare cases of refractory tophaceous gout. However, agents that decrease uric acid production can be used for hyperuricemia therapy irrespective of cause and are often more convenient in terms of dosage regimens.

CHECKPOINT

4. What physical factors other than uric acid concentration influence crystal formation in gout?
5. What are some pro-inflammatory products released by synovial macrophages upon urate crystal phagocytosis?
6. Suggest five reasons why the intense acute inflammatory response in gout typically resolves spontaneously over the course of several days even in the absence of therapy.
7. What are three metabolic conditions that can precipitate a gout flare?
8. Name three chronic sequelae of recurrent gout flares.

IMMUNE COMPLEX VASCULITIS

Clinical Presentation

Immune complex vasculitis is an acute inflammatory disease of the small blood vessels that occurs in the setting of ongoing antigen load and an established humoral (antibody) immune response. Tissues affected include the skin (leukocytoclastic vasculitic rash), joints (inflammatory arthritis of small and medium-sized joints), and kidneys (immune complex–mediated glomerulonephritis).

Etiology

Antigens are frequently derived from exogenous sources, including infections (eg, streptococcal skin infections, hepatitis B virus) and numerous drugs (especially antibiotics). An intense inflammatory response to such antigens accounts for one of the names ("hypersensitivity vasculitis") given to this disorder. The release of endogenous antigens in the setting of an autoimmune response may similarly initiate the vasculitic process (see Systemic Lupus Erythematosus).

Pathophysiology

Any antigen that elicits a humoral immune response may give rise to circulating immune complexes if the antigen remains present in abundant quantities once antibody is generated. Immune complexes are efficiently cleared in most circumstances by the reticuloendothelial system and are rarely pathogenic. Their pathogenic potential is realized when circulating immune complexes are deposited in the subendothelium, where they set in motion the complement cascade and activate myelomonocytic cells. The propensity for immune complexes to deposit is a function of the relative amounts of antigen and antibody and of the intrinsic features of the complex (ie, composition, size, solubility). The solubility of immune complexes is not a fixed property, because it is profoundly influenced by the relative concentrations of antigen and antibody, which generally change as an immune response evolves. For physicochemical reasons, soluble immune complexes formed at concentrations of slight antigen excess are not effectively cleared by the reticuloendothelial system and are of a size that allows them to gain access to and be deposited at subendothelial and extravascular sites (Figure 24–3). When antibody is present in excess, immune complexes are rapidly cleared by the reticuloendothelial system, and deposition does not occur.

Thus, if foreign antigens (eg, drugs, infectious organisms) induce an antibody response in the setting of slight antigen excess, significant numbers of immune complexes of the appropriate size are formed, and they may then be deposited in small vessels within various target organs (in the skin, joints, kidneys, or blood vessel walls) where they activate several effector pathways (eg, FcR receptor, classic complement cascade) and where they may lead to the characteristic skin rashes (eg, palpable purpura), arthritis, and glomerulonephritis that are the hallmarks of small-vessel vasculitis. As the immune response progresses and titers of specific antibody rise, or as the offending agent is removed, complexes are more effectively cleared, leading to resolution of the vasculitis.

A classic example of the altered pathogenicity of immune complexes at various antigen–antibody ratios is serum sickness. (Penicillin-induced hypersensitivity vasculitis represents a similar example.) When serum products from animals (eg, horses) are injected into humans for a therapeutic purpose (eg, as once was used for passive immunization against snake venom), the foreign serum proteins stimulate an immune response, with antibodies first appearing approximately 1 week after injection. Soon thereafter, immune complexes appear, followed by the development of fever, arthritis, rash, and glomerulonephritis, consistent with the deposition of soluble immune complexes and myelomonocytic cell activation at multiple tissue sites. As the antibody titers rise, immune complexes are no longer formed at great antigen excess but approach the zone of

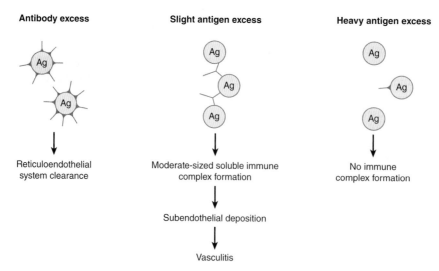

FIGURE 24–3 Immune complex formation and the impact of concentrations of antigens and antibodies.

equivalence and then the zone of antibody excess. The latter complexes are effectively cleared and thus lose their pathogenicity as the immune response evolves. Provided that antigen administration is not sustained, the inflammatory disease will resolve spontaneously as those immune complexes that were deposited early (during the soluble phase) are cleared. Such significant clinical effects of immune complexes usually occur only when the initial antigen load is great (eg, a large bacterial load or drug administration).

Clinical Manifestations of Immune Complex Vasculitis

Affected tissues are all highly enriched in small blood vessels, which are the target of injury in this syndrome.

A. Cutaneous Small-Vessel (Leukocytoclastic) Vasculitis

A common clinical presentation of immune complex–induced vasculitis in the skin is palpable purpura, which appears as red or violaceous papules. Cutaneous immune complex vasculitis seldom causes severe pain or tissue breakdown and only rarely leads to long-term injury (see Chapter 8).

B. Polyarthritis

The most common pattern of joint involvement with immune complex disease is that of a severe, rapid-onset, and self-limited symmetric polyarthritis. As the immune complexes undergo phagocytosis and are cleared, the immune response remits unless further waves of immune complexes are deposited.

C. Glomerulonephritis

Glomeruli are beds of small blood vessels in the kidneys where immune complexes are likely to be deposited. Acute immune complex glomerulonephritis causes proteinuria, hematuria, and the formation of red blood cell casts owing to a disruption of the glomerular basement membrane caused by subendothelial immune complex deposition. In cases of extensive immune complex–mediated injury, immune complex vasculitis can cause oliguria and acute kidney injury.

The most effective treatment for immune complex vasculitis is the elimination of the inciting antigen (eg, by discontinuing an offending drug). Medications that reduce the degree of activation of myelomonocytic cells (eg, corticosteroids) are also helpful.

Contrast Between Immune Complex Vasculitis, Granulomatosis with Polyangiitis (formerly Wegener Granulomatosis) & Polyarteritis Nodosa

The vasculitides are a diverse group of inflammatory syndromes characterized by the inflammatory destruction of blood vessels. However, not all forms of vasculitis are caused

TABLE 24–2 Classification of vasculitic syndromes based on vessel size.

Vessel Size	Examples	Epidemiology and Demographics
Small vessel	Immune complex–mediated; Henoch–Schönlein purpura	Common, evanescent; predominantly in children, relatively common compared with other autoimmune conditions
Medium vessel	Polyarteritis nodosa	Rare; ~5 cases per million
Large vessel	Giant cell arteritis	Only in patients older than 50 years; ~100 cases per million

by immune complex deposition. This fact is highlighted by the current classification system for the systemic vasculitides, which segregates diseases on the basis of the size of the blood vessel involved (Table 24–2), by the presence of circulating autoantibodies, and by the histologic presence or absence of immune complexes.

It is useful to contrast the clinical and pathophysiologic features of immune complex vasculitis (see prior discussion) with those of the "pauci-immune" vasculitic processes, which include granulomatosis with polyangiitis [GPA] and polyarteritis nodosa. The clinical hallmarks of GPA include the granulomatous inflammation of the upper airway (eg, sinusitis, epistaxis) and lower airway (eg, trachea, lungs), as well as a necrotizing vasculitis involving the kidneys and many other organs. Although immune complex deposition is not a prominent feature in the pathophysiology of GPA, a specific group of antibodies highly specific to this disease may play an important propagating role. These "ANCA" antibodies [*anti*-*neutrophil cytoplasmic antibodies*], directed against components situated within neutrophil cytoplasmic granules, may bind to and activate neutrophils at the interface of the plasma and vessel wall and cause them to degranulate and damage vascular walls at these sites. Recent genome-wide association studies suggest that the propensity to generate these antibodies may be genetically determined. In patients with antibodies generated against the most common ANCA antigen, proteinase 3 (PR3), associations with polymorphisms in both the PR3 locus itself and that of its major endogenous inhibitor α-1 antitrypsin (SERPINA1 locus) were noted.

In contrast, neither ANCA antibodies nor immune complex deposition plays a central role in the pathogenesis of polyarteritis nodosa, a vasculitis affecting medium-sized muscular arteries and arterioles. In this condition, the pathologic hallmark is an intense and destructive myelomonocytic cellular infiltrate in the blood vessel wall (called fibrinoid necrosis), leading to vessel occlusion, marked luminal narrowing, and obsolescence. The dominant pathologic features of this disease, therefore, are organ and tissue ischemia–mediated dysfunction related to decreased perfusion and subsequent impaired oxygen delivery from severely damaged medium-sized vessels. Common manifestations of this condition include infarction of nerve trunks (eg, mononeuritis multiplex), bowel ischemia (eg, mesenteric insufficiency causing abdominal angina), kidney ischemia (eg, renal insufficiency), and deep cutaneous ulcerations. The different vasculitic syndromes, therefore, express unique phenotypes, clinical symptoms and signs, and pathologic features reflecting their distinct underlying pathophysiologic mechanisms.

CHECKPOINT

9. In what two immunologic settings does immune complex vasculitis occur?
10. What are the three most prominent organ systems affected by immune complex vasculitis? Describe the typical manifestations in each.
11. What three physical properties determine whether immune complexes will be deposited in vessel walls?
12. What happens once subendothelial deposition has occurred?
13. Why does the pathogenicity of immune complexes generally decrease as antibody titers rise?

SYSTEMIC LUPUS ERYTHEMATOSUS

Clinical Presentation

Systemic lupus erythematosus is the prototypic systemic autoimmune rheumatic disease, characterized by chronic inflammatory injury to, and the subsequent damage of, multiple organ systems. A key feature of this disease is the unique adaptive immune response, driven by antigens contained in "self" tissues, which is apparently responsible for much of the widespread pathologic consequences of the disease. Clinically, SLE is episodic in nature, with a course characterized by flares and remissions. It is also highly variable in severity, ranging from mild to life threatening. Tissues frequently affected include the skin, joints, kidneys, blood cell lines, serosal surfaces, and brain.

Epidemiology

The prevalence of SLE is approximately 30 cases per 100,000 in the general population in the United States. It occurs about nine times more frequently in women than in men and is most prevalent in blacks. Prevalence estimates rise to approximately 1 in 250 young African American women.

Etiology

SLE is a complex disease because of an interplay between inherited susceptibilities (>20 different genetic loci are implicated) and poorly defined environmental factors. Genetic deficiencies of the proximal components of the classic complement

pathway (eg, C1q, C1r, C1s, C4), although rare in most populations, are the strongest known risk factors defined for the development of lupus. Studies have demonstrated that the classic complement pathway is required for the efficient non-inflammatory clearance of apoptotic cells by macrophages. The development of lupus in individuals with these deficiencies may relate to the impaired clearance of apoptotic cells in this setting, with pro-inflammatory consequences (see Initiation, below). The mechanisms whereby environmental factors (eg, drugs, viral infections) function to initiate or propagate SLE are not yet well understood.

Pathophysiology

It is useful to view the pathogenesis of SLE in discrete phases even though these phases are not clearly separable clinically. Indeed, it is likely that events underlying initiation occur before the onset of clinically defined disease, which requires chronic amplification of the propagation phase to become clinically apparent.

A. Initiation

The exuberant autoantibody response in lupus targets a highly specific group of "self-antigens" (Table 24–3). Although this group of autoantigens does not share common features (eg, structure, distribution, function) in healthy cells, these molecules are unified during apoptotic cell death, when they become clustered and structurally modified in apoptotic surface blebs (Figure 24–4). Indeed, studies suggest that the initiating event in lupus is a unique form of apoptotic cell death that occurs in a pro-immune context (eg, viral infection). Several environmental exposures have been persuasively associated with disease initiation in SLE. These include sunlight exposure (associated with both disease onset and flares), viral infection (Epstein–Barr virus exposure is strongly associated with SLE in children), and certain drugs. These are agents to which humans are commonly exposed, suggesting that those individuals who develop SLE have underlying abnormalities that render them particularly susceptible to disease initiation.

TABLE 24–3 Autoantigens in systemic lupus erythematosus.

Nuclear	Nucleosomes (dsDNA and histone core)
	Ribonucleoprotein complexes
	Sm
	nRNP
	Ro (60 kDa)
	La
Cytoplasmic	Ribosomal protein P
	Ro (52 kDa)
Membrane associated	Anionic phospholipids or phospholipid-binding proteins

Small blebs:
Ro (52 kDa)
Ribosomal P
Calreticulin
Fodrin
Jo-1

Apoptotic cell

Apoptotic bodies:
Nucleosomes
Ro (60 kDa)
La
Sm
U1-70 kDa
Ku/DNA-PK
Mi-2
PARP
NUMA

Entire surface membrane:
C1q
PS-protein complexes

FIGURE 24–4 Although sharing no features in healthy cells, autoantigens become unified in apoptotic cells. Here, they become clustered at the surface of the apoptotic cells, and their structure is modified.

A critical susceptibility defect for the development and propagation of SLE appears to be an impairment of the normal clearance of apoptotic cells in tissues. Thus, in normal individuals, the fate of most apoptotic cells is rapid and efficient phagocytosis by macrophages, and antigens ingested in this way are rapidly degraded. Furthermore, the phagocytosis of apoptotic cells inhibits the secretion of pro-inflammatory cytokines from macrophages and induces the secretion of several anti-inflammatory cytokines, contributing to the impaired ability of apoptotic cells to initiate a primary immune response. Last, the avid phagocytosis of apoptotic cells by normal macrophages prevents significant numbers from accessing dendritic cell populations, which are highly efficient initiators of primary immune responses. Together, these factors ensure that normal individuals do not efficiently immunize themselves with apoptotic material derived from their own tissues. In contrast, an impaired clearance of apoptotic cells is observed in a subgroup of patients with SLE. If apoptotic material is not efficiently cleared by macrophages (eg, in C1q deficiency), suprathreshold amounts of it may gain access to potent antigen-presenting cell populations. Under pro-immune conditions, it will initiate a response to molecules whose structure has been modified during delayed apoptotic cell death.

B. Propagation

Autoantibodies in lupus can cause tissue injury by a variety of mechanisms:

1. The most common pathogenic mechanism is the generation and deposition of immune complexes, in which antigen is derived from damaged and dying cells. When the concentration and size of the relevant complexes favor subendothelial deposition, these markedly pro-inflammatory complexes initiate inflammatory effector functions that result in tissue damage (see prior discussion). Of particular importance is the ability of immune complexes to ligate the Fcγ receptor, which activates myelomonocytic cell effector functions. The deposition of immune complexes in the kidneys, joints, and skin underlies several of the central clinical features of SLE.

2. Autoantibodies bind to extracellular molecules in the target organs and activate inflammatory effector functions at that site, with consequent tissue damage. Examples of this phenomenon include autoimmune hemolytic anemia and antibody-mediated thrombocytopenia, as well as the photosensitive skin disease of neonatal lupus syndrome (see Clinical Manifestations, below).

3. Autoantibodies directly induce cell death by ligating cell surface molecules or by penetrating into living cells and exerting functional effects.

It is important to note that the intracellular antigens that drive the immune response in SLE can be derived from damaged or apoptotic cells. Such damage or apoptosis occurs commonly in the course of immune effector pathways. Thus, these effector pathways can generate additional antigen, further stimulating the immune system and generating still more antigen. This auto-amplification is a central feature of the propagation phase of lupus.

Type I interferons have recently been shown to play a central role in amplification pathways in SLE, with clear evidence of increased type I interferon activity during active disease. Type I interferons induce the differentiation of monocytes into potent antigen-presenting dendritic cells. Additionally, type I interferons enhance signaling through toll-like receptors (TLRs), specifically increasing the pro-inflammatory signaling of SLE antigens containing nucleic acids through TLRs 3, 7, and 9. Additionally, type I interferons sensitize target cells to death through various inflammatory effector pathways, increasing the antigen load presented to the immune system.

C. Flares

One of the characteristic features of an immune response is the establishment of immunologic memory, so that when the organism again encounters the antigen, the immune system responds more rapidly and vigorously to lower concentrations than were required to elicit the primary response. Flares in SLE appear to reflect immunologic memory, occurring in response to rechallenge of the primed immune system with antigen. Apoptosis not only occurs during cell development and homeostasis (particularly of hematopoietic and epithelial cells), but also in many disease states. Thus, numerous stimuli (eg, ultraviolet light exposure, viral infection, endometrial and breast epithelial involution) may conceivably provoke disease flares.

Clinical Manifestations

SLE is a multisystem autoimmune disease that predominantly affects women during the childbearing years (mean age at diagnosis is 30 years). It is characterized clinically by periodicity, and the numerous exacerbations that occur over the years are termed flares. The symptoms are highly variable but tend to be stereotyped in a given individual (ie, the prominent clinical features often remain constant over years). The production of specific autoantibodies is a universal feature. Several organ systems are frequently affected. Prominent among these is the skin. Photosensitivity and a variety of SLE-specific skin rashes (including a rash over the malar region, discoid pigmentary changes to the external ear, and erythema over the dorsum of the fingers) are common. Like those with other immune complex–mediated diseases, patients with SLE may manifest a nonerosive symmetric polyarthritis. Renal disease, which takes the form of a spectrum of glomerulonephritides, is a frequent major cause of morbidity and mortality. Patients may manifest a variety of hematologic disturbances (including hemolytic anemia, thrombocytopenia, and leukopenia), inflammation of serosal surfaces (including pleuritic and pericarditic chest pain and peritonitis), as well as several neurologic syndromes (eg, seizures, organic brain syndrome).

An intriguing neonatal SLE syndrome occurs in the offspring of mothers with antibodies directed against the Ro, La, or U1-RNP proteins. In this condition, the passive transfer of maternal autoantibodies across the placenta results in disease in the fetus as a result of the antibody-associated destruction of developing tissues that transiently express these antigens. These antibodies commonly induce transient photosensitivity in the neonate, and anti-Ro (SSA) antibodies can cause permanent damage to the cardiac conduction system leading to congenital heart block.

CHECKPOINT

14. What are the antigens against which antibodies are directed in SLE?

15. How many different genetic loci are believed to confer susceptibility to SLE? Which are the strongest ones?

16. What is believed to be the relationship of apoptosis to the initiation of SLE?

17. What prevents normal individuals from being immunized to apoptotic cell debris? Why does this host defense break down in patients with SLE?

18. What are three stimuli that typically provoke SLE flares?

19. What are the most prominently affected organ systems in SLE?

SJÖGREN SYNDROME

Clinical Presentation

Sjögren syndrome is a prevalent and slowly progressive autoimmune rheumatic disorder in which the exocrine glands are the primary target tissue. Affected individuals frequently manifest an intense dryness of their eyes (xerophthalmia) and mouth (xerostomia), giving rise to the alternative name keratoconjunctivitis sicca. Histologically, an intense mononuclear inflammatory infiltrate is observed in affected lacrimal and salivary glands, respectively. Like other autoimmune rheumatic diseases, prominent polyclonal hypergammaglobulinemia and high-titer levels of characteristic autoantibodies are frequent features of the syndrome.

Epidemiology

Sjögren syndrome occurs in approximately 1–3% of the adult population. As with SLE, the prevalence is about nine times more frequent in women than men. The prototypic affected individual is a woman in the fourth or fifth decade of life. Sjögren syndrome occurs as both a primary disorder and as a secondary process in the context of another well-defined autoimmune rheumatic disorder (especially SLE and rheumatoid arthritis).

Etiology

Viruses have been implicated in the development of Sjögren syndrome, but conclusive data are lacking. Epithelial cells in salivary glands can be infected by a number of viral pathogens (including Epstein-Barr virus, cytomegalovirus [CMV], hepatitis C, HIV, and coxsackievirus). In an autoimmune mouse model, CMV infection leads to initial infection of the salivary glands, followed later by autoimmune salivary gland inflammation. Whether a similar process occurs during initiation of the human disease is not yet known.

Pathophysiology

Although the cause of Sjögren syndrome remains unclear, several pathways have been implicated in its pathogenesis. Central among these is autoimmunity to epithelial tissues, with an immune response directed against several ubiquitously expressed antigens (eg, Fodrin, Ro, and La), as well as to some antigens expressed specifically in secretory epithelial cells (eg, type 3 muscarinic acetylcholine receptors [M3Rs]). The antibodies to M3R are believed to prevent the stimulated secretion of saliva and tears and may be important generators of the hyposecretion that characterizes the disease. In addition, exocrine tissues are also infiltrated with activated cytotoxic lymphocytes, which induce the death of duct and acinar epithelium, with a progressive loss of functioning salivary tissue. The enrichment of HLA-DR3 in patients with Sjögren syndrome may reflect the enhanced ability of these molecules to present peptides contained within the pathogenic autoantigens.

Clinical Manifestations

The most prominent presenting symptoms in Sjögren syndrome are ocular and oral dryness. Intense xerophthalmia (ocular dryness) may express itself as eye irritation, with a foreign body sensation or with pain. Such impairment in tear production heightens the risk of corneal ulcer and perforation.

Impaired saliva production, at rest and with stimulation when eating, contributes to the prominent symptom of xerostomia (dry mouth). Affected persons often report difficulty in swallowing dry foods or in speaking at length without access to a beverage. An altered sensation of taste or a sensation of oral burning may occur. Characteristically, individuals affected by Sjögren syndrome are susceptible to new-onset and severe dental caries at the gum line in mid-adult life.

This reflects the loss of the essential antibacterial functions of saliva, with a consequent excessive concentration of bacteria at dental surfaces.

Other epithelial surfaces may be similarly affected by diminished secretions and contribute to dryness. For example, patients may complain of skin and vaginal dryness. Dryness in the respiratory tract may give rise to hoarseness and recurrent bronchitis. Moreover, it is noteworthy that when immune activation is severe, patients experience systemic symptoms, including fatigue, arthralgia, myalgia, and low-grade fever. Other potentially affected organ systems include the kidneys, lungs, joints, and liver (resulting in interstitial nephritis, interstitial pneumonitis, nonerosive polyarthritis, and intrahepatic bile duct inflammation). As many as half of affected individuals experience autoimmune thyroid disease. Those patients with particularly severe disease are at increased risk of cutaneous vasculitis (including palpable purpura and skin ulceration) and lymphoproliferative disorders (eg, mucosa-associated lymphoid tissue [MALT] lymphoma).

Treatment

Current therapy is aimed primarily at symptomatic improvement. Available agents include artificial tears, which serve as topical lubricants to aid with eye dryness. Maintaining oral hydration, with access to a regular supply of beverages, is encouraged. Use of sugar-free gum and lozenges may stimulate salivary flow. More recently, new cholinergic agonists have come to market aimed at improving oral hydration by stimulating increased salivary production, via muscarinic receptors, in affected submandibular salivary glands. Effective anti-inflammatory and immunosuppressive treatment for Sjögren syndrome has not yet been found, indicating that the components of the critical amplification loops have not yet been discovered. For those affected by severe disease sequelae (including systemic vasculitis and mononeuritis multiplex), the administration of systemic immunosuppression is necessary.

CHECKPOINT

20. What are the key targets of the inflammatory process that define the classic phenotypic features of Sjögren syndrome? Which immune effector cells infiltrate these tissues?

21. What antigens are specifically targeted by autoantibodies in Sjögren syndrome?

INFLAMMATORY MYOPATHIES

Clinical Presentation

The inflammatory myopathies are characterized by the gradual development of progressive motor weakness affecting the arms, legs, and trunk in association with characteristic histologic evidence of muscle inflammation. While such inflammation predominantly involves striated muscle, it is important to recognize that smooth muscle and even cardiac muscle may similarly, though less commonly, be affected. Often, the afflicted patient experiences increasing difficulty when rising from a seated position, getting out of bed, or ascending a flight of stairs. It may become increasingly difficult to reach up and lift dishes from an upper shelf or even to brush one's hair.

At the most severe end of the disease spectrum, affected persons may develop profound impairment in swallowing solid foods and in full lung expansion, arising from the pathologic involvement of visceral muscle affecting the esophageal and diaphragmatic muscle tissues, respectively. These disease manifestations may result in the nasal regurgitation of swallowed liquids and in profound respiratory compromise with hypoventilation. There is also a predilection for extramuscular involvement to occur, including of the lung parenchyma (interstitial pulmonary fibrosis) and peripheral joints (inflammatory polyarthritis), and in those with dermatomyositis, mild, moderate, or even severe inflammation of the integument. At the same time, diplopia (double vision resulting from a paretic ocular muscle) is distinctly uncommon in patients with inflammatory myopathies.

Epidemiology

The inflammatory myopathies are relatively rare disorders. Two main types have traditionally been defined (polymyositis and dermatomyositis), although recent insights into the pathogenesis of these conditions suggests that "pure" polymyositis may be rarer than originally thought. A third type, referred to as immune-mediated necrotizing myopathy has now been recognized. Polymyositis has been estimated to occur with an annual incidence of approximately 5 cases per million. Women are affected twice as often as men. Interestingly, dermatomyositis has a bimodal distribution in terms of age at onset; the first peak occurs in childhood, and the second peak occurs in mid- and late adult life. As noted, polymyositis may rarely occur as a primary disorder, however, the polymyositis phenotype may also occur in the context of another well-defined autoimmune rheumatic disorder, such as SLE, from which it is otherwise clinically and histologically indistinguishable.

Etiology

Autoantibodies are present in approximately 60% of all patients with an inflammatory myosis. Several of these antibodies are closely linked to distinct clinical phenotypes, and their presence may provide insight into both the diagnosis and prognosis of the disease in question. Examples include anti-Jo-1 antibodies (which target histidyl *t*RNA synthetase), which are found in approximately 20% of all patients with myositis and in approximately 70% of patients with a myositis/interstitial lung disease overlap syndrome, and several antibodies associated with unique subphenotypes in dermatomyositis: (a) anti-Mi-2 antibodies that target a DNA binding protein; (b) anti-NXP2 antibodies, associated with calcinosis; (c) anti-MDA5 antibodies, associated with rapid progression to lung disease, together with a unique form of cutaneous ulceration; and (d) anti-TIF1γ antibodies, associated with an increased risk of malignancy and severe skin disease. Since both nuclear and cytoplasmic antigens are targeted for an immune response in these diseases, both antinuclear antibodies (ANA) and anticytoplasmic antibodies can be found. Notably, Jo-1-positive myositis is the prototypic antisynthetase disorder.

Recent studies suggest that one source of these autoantigens is the regenerating muscle cell itself, which expresses higher levels of myositis autoantigens than its normal counterpart. Some tumor cells also express these same antigens at high levels. An intriguing pathophysiologic hypothesis is that the immune response that targets similar antigens in both tumor and inflamed muscle cells might be responsible for the link between inflammatory myositis and malignancy.

Pathophysiology

The inflammatory myopathies share several similar pathologic features but also possess distinct ones. These include patchy involvement, the presence of inflammatory infiltrates, and areas of muscle damage and regeneration. However, careful interpretation of biopsy specimens is critical since (1) several of these changes (especially damage/regeneration) can be seen in the muscle of patients with noninflammatory "mimics" such as the muscular dystrophies; and (2) inflammatory infiltrates are only rarely seen in the necrotizing myopathies. In polymyositis, inflammation is located around individual muscle fibers ("perimyocyte"), and the infiltrate is T cell (CD8+ > CD4+) and macrophage predominant. It has been suggested that the inflammation seen in polymyositis is driven by autoantigens expressed in the muscle environment, given the restricted T-cell repertoire in both circulating and muscle-infiltrating lymphocytes. Pro-inflammatory cytokines may induce a striking upregulation of MHC class I molecules seen on affected muscle cells but not on adjacent normal myocytes. This MHC class I upregulation may lead to muscle damage through antigen-specific interactions with infiltrating CD8+ T cells, or through indirect mechanisms by triggering a cell-damaging unfolded protein response ("UPR" or "ER stress") in the muscle itself. Further damage occurs when infiltrating T cells degranulate and release perforin and proteolytic granzymes at specific sites of contact within the affected muscle.

In dermatomyositis, the pathology looks quite different, although the outcome—profound muscle weakness—is the same. The major pathologic hallmarks of this condition include atrophy at the periphery of muscle bundles ("perifascicular atrophy"), and a predominantly B-cell and CD4+ T-cell infiltrate localized to the perifascicular and perivascular space surrounding capillaries (which are reduced in number). Activation of the complement cascade is seen as well. Major involvement of the capillaries has led many experts to suggest that the primary disorder in dermatomyositis is a small-vessel vasculitis, with myositis occurring later as a result of tissue ischemia and repair. The characteristic skin and nailfold capillary changes seen in patients with dermatomyositis lend support to this notion. Recent evidence has implicated the type 1 interferon pathway in the pathogenesis of dermatomyositis. The localized expression and induction of IFN-inducible proteins occurs at the site of muscle injury in dermatomyositis patients, and gene-expression profiling has shown an increased expression of associated transcripts in dermatomyositis muscle. Furthermore, changes characteristic of IFN expression have been noted in affected muscle capillary walls, suggesting a localized expression at these sites.

A specific antibody association has been described in up to 40% of patients with one form of necrotizing myopathy. In a subset of patients given a statin medication to treat their high cholesterol level, antibodies to the cellular target of the statin itself, anti-HMG CoA-reductase, have been demonstrated. These patients have a severe form of necrotizing myopathy that may persist even after the statin medication is withdrawn.

Clinical Manifestations

The inflammatory myopathies characteristically begin over a number of weeks to a few months. The hallmark symptom is weakness. This characteristically involves the upper and lower extremities and is predominantly proximal rather than distal in location. While muscle pain or myalgia may be present, weakness is the predominant symptom. Routine daily activities that one might otherwise take for granted can become quite a chore, or even an impossible ordeal, to perform. An example is standing up from a chair or toilet seat. In addition, the cutaneous features of dermatomyositis can be quite debilitating and include a painful, burning sensation of the affected skin, as well as skin cracking and even breakdown with open ulceration.

There are four characteristic criteria for the diagnosis of polymyositis: (1) weakness; (2) elevated laboratory parameters of muscle tissue (eg, creatine phosphokinase or aldolase); (3) an irritable electromyogram upon electrodiagnostic evaluation (producing sharp waves and spontaneous discharges); and (4) an inflammatory infiltrate upon histologic evaluation. In patients with dermatomyositis, a fifth criterion is a characteristic skin rash. Erythematous and/or violaceous discoloration may occur around the outside of the eye, or in a V-neck distribution on the trunk. These prototypic skin changes are termed the periorbital heliotrope and the shawl sign, respectively. Erythematous scaly eruptions may also occur over the extensor surface of the metacarpophalangeal (MCP) and proximal interphalangeal (PIP) joints and are termed the Gottron sign. Extensive sheets of muscle and soft tissue calcification may occur in children with dermatomyositis. Though recent efforts to modify the original diagnostic criteria, by integrating newer imaging modalities including magnetic resonance imaging or using newer autoantibodies with specificities for the inflammatory myopathies, have been proposed, the original criteria remain the foundation for these two muscle disorders.

An important additional clinical feature of the inflammatory myopathies has been the finding of an association with cancer in multiple demographic groups and among diverse populations. In adult patients, the new diagnosis of an inflammatory myopathy frequently heralds the co-occurrence or subsequent development within 1–5 years of a malignancy. The veracity of this observation has been confirmed in several population-based studies that link the diagnoses of dermatomyositis and polymyositis with cancer in cancer registries. A diagnosis of dermatomyositis carries a twofold greater risk of incident malignancy, particularly cancers of the stomach, lung, breast, colon, and ovary.

Treatment

Corticosteroids are the first-line therapy for the inflammatory myopathies and are often required in high doses, for an extended period of time, to bring the marked inflammation in affected muscle tissues under control and to restore the patient's full functional capacity. Therefore, a careful review of the clinical and histologic evidence supporting the diagnosis of an inflammatory myopathy is indicated in order to be confident that the potential drug-associated toxicity to which the patient will be exposed is warranted. In addition, the clinician also must recognize that a subset of treatment-refractory patients with presumed polymyositis may in fact be cases of a toxic myopathy (ie, related to the use of colchicine or a statin) or be attributable to a different myopathy (eg, inclusion body myositis). Second-line immunosuppressive agents integrated into treatment algorithms for the inflammatory myopathies include methotrexate, mycophenolate mofetil, intravenous immunoglobulin, and rituximab.

CHECKPOINT

22. Which parts of the body can become weak, and which types of muscle cell are targeted by the immune system in the various clinical forms of the inflammatory myopathies?

23. What is the antigen target and the most prominent visceral manifestation of the prototypic antisynthetase syndrome?

24. Which type of myelomonocytic cell is typically present in the inflammatory infiltrate characteristic of polymyositis, and where in the muscle tissue is it observed? How about in dermatomyositis?

RHEUMATOID ARTHRITIS

Clinical Presentation

Rheumatoid arthritis (RA) is a chronic systemic inflammatory disease characterized by the persistent symmetric inflammation of multiple peripheral joints. It is one of the most common inflammatory rheumatic diseases and is characterized by the development of a chronic inflammatory proliferation of the synovial linings of diarthrodial joints, which leads to aggressive cartilage destruction and progressive bony erosions. Untreated, RA often leads to progressive joint destruction, disability, and premature death.

Epidemiology

The prevalence of RA in the United States is approximately 1% in the general population; similar prevalence rates have been observed worldwide. The disorder occurs approximately three times more frequently in women than in men and has its peak onset in the fifth to sixth decade of life.

Etiology

RA is a systemic autoimmune disease in which the abnormal activation of B cells, T cells, and innate immune effectors causes damage to the patient's own ("self") tissues. While the majority of inflammatory activity in RA occurs in the joint synovium, other tissue such as the lungs, skin, and blood vessels can be affected. Although the cause of RA is unknown, a complex set of genetic and environmental factors appears to contribute to disease susceptibility. Because the incidence of RA has been observed to be similar in many cultures and geographic regions across the globe, it is assumed that the environmental exposures that provoke RA must be widely distributed. Early RA is closely mimicked by transient inflammatory arthritis precipitated by several microbial pathogens. However, although a role for infection in the development of RA has long been postulated, it has not yet been satisfactorily proven. Specific MHC class II alleles (eg, HLA-DR4) have been strongly linked to disease susceptibility and severity in RA (see Genetic Factors).

Pathophysiology

Much of the pathologic damage that characterizes RA is centered around the synovial linings of joints. Normal synovium is composed of a thin cellular lining (one to three cell layers thick) and an underlying interstitium, which contains blood vessels but few cells. The synovium normally provides nutrients and lubrication to adjacent articular cartilage. RA synovium, in contrast, is markedly abnormal, with a greatly expanded lining layer (8–10 cells thick) composed of activated cells; a highly inflammatory interstitium replete with B cells, T cells, and macrophages; and vascular changes, including thrombosis and neovascularization. At sites where synovium and articular cartilage are contiguous, RA synovial tissue (called pannus) invades and destroys adjacent cartilage and bone. A major role for osteoclasts (multinucleated cells that mediate bone resorption) in disease pathogenesis is also suggested by the frequently observed erosive bone disease in RA patients. Studies have shown that pro-inflammatory factors present in the RA joint can amplify osteoclast formation and activity.

Although the causes of RA remain unclear, several important components of pathogenesis have been elucidated. Specific genetic and environmental factors have been identified that predispose to the development of RA, as have dysregulated pathways that drive ongoing inflammation. As discussed previously (see Systemic Lupus Erythematosus), it is useful to separate the initiating and propagating phases of the disease and to recognize that the established RA phenotype reflects a self-sustaining and amplified inflammatory state.

A. Initiation

1. Genetic Factors—A clear role for genetic factors is demonstrated by studies showing a 15–35% concordance rate among identical twins. The most striking of these genetic factors defined to date is a specific subset of MHC class II alleles whose presence appears to predominantly determine disease development and severity (patients homozygous for disease-associated alleles have the most severe disease). These MHC molecules function as antigen-presenting scaffolds, which present peptides to CD4 T cells. Disease-associated alleles (eg, HLA-DR4, HLA-DR1, others) share a consensus QKRAA motif in the peptide-binding groove and are therefore termed the "shared-epitope" alleles. It has been postulated that these alleles present critical antigens to autoreactive T cells, which play a role in initiating and driving disease progression. Among these, self-peptides, in which arginine residues have been post-translationally modified to the nonclassical amino acid citrulline, have been shown to bind preferentially to the groove of shared-epitope alleles. Recent high-throughput genome-wide genetic association studies have identified several additional genetic risk factors associated with the development of RA. These genes (ie, *PADI4*, *PTPN22*, *CTLA4*, *STAT4*, others) are involved in generating and propagating inflammatory responses and possibly also producing autoantibodies.

2. Environmental Factors—Cigarette smoking and infection are the two environmental factors that have been most strongly implicated in RA pathogenesis. Growing evidence suggests that immune responses to the "self-antigens" targeted in RA may begin outside the joints, at sites directly exposed to a variety of environmental insults. At mucosal surfaces such as the periodontium and lung, environmental factors may interact with genetic-risk alleles to induce autoimmune disease. Although numerous bacterial and viral pathogens have been investigated as perhaps having a role in the initiation of RA, scrutiny has failed to identify a clear causal role for any specific infectious cause. It is conceivable that any one of several different infectious agents might be able to induce changes that culminate in the initiation of joint disease in susceptible individuals.

3. Autoantibodies—Immune recognition of a specific set of "self-antigens" appears to be an important factor in generating the RA phenotype. A hallmark feature of the disease is the development of antigen-driven autoantibodies, including IgG rheumatoid factors (antibodies that recognize the Fc portion of other IgG molecules) and anti-citrullinated protein antibodies (ACPAs). Highly specific for RA, ACPAs are detected by the anti-cyclic citrullinated peptide (anti-CCP) antibody test. Importantly, both rheumatoid factor and ACPAs can be present in the serum of patients years before disease onset, making them valuable diagnostic markers.

B. Propagation

1. Citrullination—Once disease is established, autoantigens and components of the immune system interact to amplify the disease process. In established disease, ACPAs appear to be a marker of a more destructive and aggressive RA phenotype. Citrullinated proteins may therefore play important roles in both the development and propagation of RA, but the reasons these modified proteins are targeted in RA are unknown. Potential explanations include an increase in the expression or activity of the peptidyl arginine deiminase (PAD) enzymes in RA target tissues. The PAD family of enzymes mediate the conversion of arginine to citrulline, generating the citrullinated protein targets of ACPAs. These citrullinated peptides also bind preferentially to the disease-associated shared-epitope alleles and are recognized by autoreactive T cells. Among the five PAD enzyme family members, PAD2 and PAD4 are the most strongly implicated in RA pathogenesis. Notably, polymorphisms in both genes (*PADI2* and *PADI4*) have been linked to RA development; both enzymes are increased in the RA joint; and both enzymes have been shown to generate citrullinated autoantigens. Autoantibodies to the PAD4 enzyme itself are also found in a subset of patients with RA and are associated with severe joint damage. This suggests that ongoing PAD activity and the continual production of citrullinated autoantigens may be important contributors to disease propagation in patients with RA.

2. Cytokines—Enhanced pro-inflammatory cytokine production is a dominant feature of RA with the production of T_H1 (eg, IFNγ, TNFα), T_H17 (eg, IL-17, IL-23), and innate (eg, IL-1β, IL-6, granulocyte–macrophage colony-stimulating factor [GM-CSF]) cell cytokines. Although the cytokine profile in RA synovium is highly complex, with numerous cytokines being expressed simultaneously, studies have persuasively demonstrated that the inhibition of even a single key cytokine can have dramatic therapeutic benefit. In particular, TNFα is an important upstream mediator in the propagation of the RA inflammatory process. Thus, when pathways downstream of TNFα are inhibited with soluble TNFα receptors or monoclonal antibodies to TNFα, a rapid and markedly beneficial effect on the inflammatory synovitis and overall state of well-being is noted in many patients (see Treatment). Interestingly, it is clinically appreciated that the effects of anti-TNFα treatment are limited to the duration of therapy, and symptoms and signs of inflammation often return rapidly upon therapy discontinuation. This points to ongoing pro-inflammatory cytokine secretion as an important driver of disease propagation in RA.

Clinical Manifestations

RA is most typically a persistent, progressive disease presenting in women in the middle years of life. Fatigue and joint inflammation, characterized by pain, swelling, warmth, and morning stiffness, are hallmarks of the disease. Almost invariably, multiple small and large synovial joints are affected on both the right and left sides of the body in a symmetric distribution. Involvement of the small joints of the hands, wrists, and feet, as well as the larger peripheral joints, including the hips, knees, shoulders, and elbows, is typical. Involved joints are demineralized, and joint cartilage and juxta-articular bone are eroded by the synovial inflammation, inducing joint deformities. Although the lower spine is spared, cervical involvement can occur, potentially leading to spinal instability. In highly active cases, extra-articular manifestations can occur. These include lung nodules, interstitial lung disease, subcutaneous "rheumatoid" nodules (typically present over extensor surfaces), ocular inflammation (including scleritis), and small- to medium-sized arteritis.

Treatment

Prompt and aggressive treatment to control inflammation in RA can slow or even arrest progressive joint erosion. A number of immunomodulatory medications have shown benefit in treating RA. The primary pathway through which methotrexate—the drug most commonly used as single-agent therapy for RA—acts to diminish joint inflammation is still debated. One hypothesis suggests that methotrexate induces an increased local release of adenosine, a short-acting anti-inflammatory mediator.

RA is one of the first conditions in which biologic modifiers of defined pathogenic pathways have been used successfully to treat disease. TNFα inhibitors were the first to be developed and act by sequestering the cytokine and blocking its disease-promoting functions. This can be achieved either by administering a recombinant, soluble form of the TNFα receptor (etanercept) or monoclonal antibodies to TNFα (eg, infliximab, adalimumab). Similar therapeutic strategies have been adopted for blocking the inflammatory effects of IL-1β (eg, with anakinra) and IL-6 (eg, with tocilizumab) and are being developed for other RA-associated cytokines. Although these agents have a high likelihood of achieving benefit in patients with RA, their use is still limited by their high cost and potential risks of drug-associated toxicity (including susceptibility to infections and malignancies, and induction of other autoimmune syndromes). Furthermore, although they are among the most potent agents yet described for the control of RA, there remain patients who fail to experience disease remission when treated with only a single agent. As a general principle of therapy in RA, it appears that using multiple agents with (presumably) different and complementary mechanisms of action can lead to additional benefit. The recent success of small-molecule inhibitors that block cytokine signaling pathways (eg, janus kinase inhibitors) offers a new strategy for simultaneously blocking the pro-inflammatory effects of

multiple cytokines. T cells, B cells, and antigen-presenting cells (APCs), as well as the interactions among these cells, play important roles in the propagation phase of RA. It is therefore not surprising that additional biological agents have also shown efficacy in the treatment of RA, including, but not limited to, agents that inhibit B cells (eg, rituximab) and that induce the co-stimulation of T cells by APCs (eg, CTLA4-Ig).

CHECKPOINT

25. What is the shared epitope, and how is it thought to contribute to RA pathogenesis?
26. Which two environmental factors have been implicated as having a role in the initiation of RA?
27. What are the common autoantibodies present in patients with RA, and which antigens do they target?
28. Describe five features of the inflammatory arthritis observed in patients with RA.
29. Select four RA therapeutic agents with distinct mechanisms of action, and describe how they reduce inflammation.

SPONDYLOARTHROPATHY

Clinical Presentation

The spondyloarthropathies are a group of inflammatory rheumatic diseases that characteristically present with inflammatory low back pain and an asymmetric oligoarthritis of the peripheral joints. These disorders—ankylosing spondylitis, reactive arthritis, inflammatory bowel disease–associated arthritis, and psoriatic arthritis—are more common among men and usually commence in young adult life.

Etiology

Extensive research over many decades has linked the MHC class I molecule HLA-B27 (B27) with susceptibility to the spondyloarthropathies. There is both compelling population-based and animal model data to support this association. The large majority (>90% of Caucasian patients with ankylosing spondylitis) are positive for the HLA-B27 allele. Though its frequency is lower among African Americans with ankylosing spondylitis, about half of whom harbor the B27 gene, the frequency of HLA-B27 in both racial groups greatly exceeds that of the general population. Notably, the background frequency of HLA-B27 is 8% among Caucasian and 4% among African American populations, underscoring the strength of its association with ankylosing spondylitis.

In addition, in a well-established rodent model, rats that are both genetically engineered to possess the human B27 gene and raised in an environment with exposure to anaerobic bacteria develop inflammation of the skin and articular and gastrointestinal tissues at 10 weeks of life. By reproducing the human phenotype in an animal model, it reinforces the role of exposure to foreign organisms among genetically susceptible hosts in disease development. In contrast, similar rodents possessing mutant B27, or those possessing human B27 but raised under germ-free conditions, do not develop a spondyloarthropathy.

Pathophysiology

In terms of laboratory profile, persons affected by a spondyloarthropathy are seronegative for the rheumatoid factor but are usually positive for the cell-surface major histocompatibility surface marker HLA-B27. Anemia may be observed as a consequence of inflammation and as an acute-phase reactant response.

Although B27 has been linked to the spondyloarthropathies for decades, how it interfaces with the immune system to facilitate disease initiation and propagation remains unclear. One hypothesis is that "self" or foreign (microbial) antigens, bound to the HLA-B27 binding groove, may be recognized by the T-cell receptors of autoreactive CD8+ T cells, inciting an inflammatory response. An alternative hypothesis is that a misfolding of the B27 molecule within the cell results in endoplasmic reticulum stress that triggers an unfolded protein response and an upregulation of IL-23 cytokine levels. Yet a third hypothesis is that B27 free heavy chains, when expressed at the cell surface, are recognized by cells bearing killer immunoglobulin-like receptors and trigger an inflammatory response.

The cytokine milieu is also an important component of spondyloarthropathy-associated inflammation. An emerging and prominent role for IL-17 and IL-23 has come to light in the pathogenesis of the spondyloarthropathies, particularly ankylosing spondylitis and psoriatic arthritis. Elevated levels of IL-12 have been detected as well. Genome-wide association studies have demonstrated a linkage between the IL-23 receptor and single nucleotide polymorphisms of the IL-12 receptor in ankylosing spondylitis. Further, an intergenic region between these two loci modulates enhancer activity and heightened levels of T_H1 cell differentiation. In addition, T_H17 cells have been detected in the circulation, spinal facet joints, and synovium of patients with high disease activity. These activated cytokines and effector cells also play a role in bone resorption and remodeling.

Clinical Manifestations

Among all spondyloarthropathy disorders, **inflammatory low back pain** is common, as is **asymmetric oligoarthritis**, often involving lower, rather than upper, extremity joints. Not only may axial and peripheral synovial joints become stiff, painful, or swollen, but there is a predilection for **enthesitis**, or inflammation at the anatomic site where the tendon or ligament inserts itself into bone. A notable extra-articular feature common to these disorders is **inflammation of the eye**, particularly anterior uveitis or iridocyclitis, producing a red, painful, photophobic eye.

A. Ankylosing Spondylitis

The hallmark of ankylosing spondylitis is inflammatory low back pain. Affected patients characteristically report achiness, stiffness, or pain in the midline lower back. Such back discomfort characteristically has its onset at the start of the day, upon awakening from sleep, and improves over the next few hours coincident with ambulation and activity. Systemic features of ankylosing spondylitis include a predilection for the ocular (acute anterior uveitis), pulmonary (apical lung bullae, interstitial fibrosis), and cardiac (aortic regurgitation, atrioventricular conduction block) organ systems.

B. Reactive Arthritis

There is a well-established temporal and causal relationship between the onset of an intense asymmetric oligoarthritis and an antecedent gastrointestinal or genitourinary tract infection. Affected patients characteristically experience a painful, stiff, swollen knee followed by pain and swelling of a wrist or ankle on the opposite side of the body. The classic triad of uveitis, urethritis, and arthritis can be remembered by using the mnemonic that affected patients "cannot see, pee, or climb a tree!" *Chlamydia trachomatis* is a common organism that infects the genitourinary tract, inducing a urethritis, and thereafter predisposing to this so-called "reactive arthritis." Enteric gram-negative bacteria, including *Shigella flexneri*, *Yersinia enterocolitica*, and *Campylobacter jejuni*, may first cause inflammation of the gastrointestinal tract and later a post-dysentery reactive arthritis.

C. Inflammatory Bowel Disease–Associated Arthritis

Both Crohn's disease and ulcerative colitis may provoke recurrent episodes of abdominal pain, associated with diarrhea, bloody stools, fever, weight loss, and malaise. Among affected young adults, 1 in 4 develop an associated inflammatory arthritis, particularly of lower extremity joints. Patients may also experience inflammation of the lumbar spine and/or pelvic joints, giving rise to radiographic evidence of vertebral body enthesophytes (also called syndesmophytes) and/or sacroiliitis. Furthermore, the level of disease activity in affected peripheral joints closely parallels disease activity within the gastrointestinal tract, as assessed clinically, endoscopically, and histologically. In contrast, radiographic evidence of disease propagation in the axial skeleton (ie, spondylitis, sacroiliitis) may proceed and progress independent of bowel disease activity.

D. Psoriatic Arthritis

An estimated 1% of the U.S. adult population harbors cutaneous evidence of psoriasis, characterized by well-demarcated erythematous scaly plaques, some of whom develop a related arthritis. In fact, there are several distinct subsets of psoriatic arthritis, including (a) an asymmetric oligoarthritis affecting lower extremity joints; (b) a symmetric polyarthritis affecting upper and lower extremity joints; (c) monoarticular involvement of a distal interphalangeal joint alone; (d) a destructive finger joint arthritis that produces "telescoping," a shortening of the digit as a consequence of aggressive bone destruction and resorption (arthritis mutilans); and (e) axial skeleton involvement (spondylitis, sacroiliitis).

Treatment

For decades, the first-line approach to the management of spinal stiffness and peripheral joint arthritis for those with an active spondyloarthropathy disorder was non-steroidal anti-inflammatory agents. Next, and in similar fashion to the treatment of RA, both methotrexate and sulfasalazine became, in the 1980s and 1990s, frequent second-line drugs used to control the pain and stiffness of these conditions. Then, as with RA, over the next 20 years came insights from the laboratory of the crucial roles of cytokines, particularly TNFα, in disease propagation. These investigative insights furnished a biologic basis for a new therapeutic modality by identifying specific cytokines to antagonize. Thereafter, the U.S. Food and Drug Administration (FDA) approved the use of TNFα inhibitors for patients with ankylosing spondylitis, psoriatic arthritis, and spondyloarthritis in active inflammatory bowel disease (both moderate to severe Crohn's disease and ulcerative colitis).

The FDA then approved the use of secukinumab, an inhibitor of IL-17A, for the treatment of ankylosing spondylitis and psoriatic arthritis. In addition, ustekinumab, yet another novel monoclonal antibody that targets IL-12 and IL-23, has similarly been approved by the FDA for the same indications. The therapeutic benefit of these cytokine antagonists demonstrated in randomized clinical trials further underscores their role in mediating disease activity in the spondyloarthropathy disorders.

More recently, apremilast, a phosphodiesterase-4 inhibitor that raises intracellular cyclic adenosine monophosphate (cAMP) levels, has demonstrated therapeutic benefit in patients with psoriatic arthritis. Each of these novel biologic agents seemingly alters the balance between and pro- and anti-inflammatory mediators to achieve clinical benefit.

CHECKPOINT

30. Which disorders constitute the spectrum of the spondyloarthropathies?
31. Which gene confers susceptibility to developing a spondyloarthropathy, most evident in ankylosing spondylitis?
32. Which cytokines have been found at heightened levels in the spondyloarthropathies? How have they been targeted in clinical practice to ameliorate disease activity?

CASE STUDIES

Yeong Kwok, MD

(See Chapter 25, p. 789–91 for answers)

CASE 126

A 58-year-old man with a long history of treated essential hypertension and mild renal insufficiency presents to the urgent care clinic complaining of pain in the right knee. His primary care provider saw him one week ago and added a thiazide diuretic to improve his blood pressure control. He had been feeling well until the night before the clinic visit, when he noted some redness and slight swelling of his knee. He went to sleep and was awakened early by significant swelling and pain. He was able to walk only with assistance. He has no history of knee trauma.

The physical examination confirmed the presence of a swollen right knee, which was erythematous and warm. Joint aspiration recovered copious dark yellow, cloudy synovial fluid. A microscopic analysis demonstrated 30,000 leukocytes/μL, a negative Gram stain, and many needle-like, negatively birefringent crystals consistent with acute gout.

Questions

A. What factors may have precipitated this gout flare?
B. Describe the inflammatory pathways involved in acute gout.
C. What agents should the urgent care physician consider in treating this gout flare? What are their mechanisms of action?

CASE 127

A 24-year-old man presents with a worsening rash. One week ago, he had been at an urgent care center with a sore throat and was diagnosed with "strep throat." He was prescribed penicillin and had been getting better. The day before presentation, he noted the development of a pink rash on his trunk, and on the day of his evaluation, it had spread to his arms and legs. On examination, the patient has a symmetric maculopapular rash covering his extremities and trunk. Some of the lesions on his legs are palpable.

Questions

A. What is the likely cause of this patient's rash?
B. What is the underlying pathophysiology in this case?
C. Which other organs can this disorder affect, and why?

CASE 128

A 22-year-old African American woman with a family history of SLE reports intermittent knee arthralgias. She denies any facial rash, photosensitivity, chest pain, and shortness of breath. She is convinced she has lupus and requests confirmatory blood tests.

Questions

A. What additional history may be helpful in supporting the diagnosis of lupus as the cause of this patient's arthralgias?
B. Why is it essential to elicit a medication history when considering this diagnosis?
C. Describe three possible mechanisms of autoantibody-induced tissue injury in SLE.
D. Describe the natural history of the disease. Which stimuli have been implicated in the exacerbations that punctuate its course?

CASE 129

A 45-year-old woman comes to the clinic complaining of progressive worsening of dry eyes and mouth over the past year. At first, she thought it may have been a worsening of her allergies, but her eyes feel irritated all the time, as if she has sand in them. She gets mild relief with over-the-counter eye drops. Her mouth has also felt dry, and she has found it difficult to eat certain foods, such as bread and crackers, and to carry on prolonged conversations owing to her tongue sticking to the roof of her mouth. She recently saw her dentist and was found to have two cavities, the first since childhood. The physical exam is notable for mild injection of her conjunctiva but is otherwise normal.

Questions

A. What is this patient's likely diagnosis, and what are the two most common presenting symptoms of this condition?
B. What are potential complications of this syndrome in severe disease?

CASE 130

A 55-year-old woman comes to your office with a progressive feeling of weakness. She had been in good health until about six weeks ago when she began having trouble getting up from a low chair. This symptom has become more pronounced over time, and she has also noted difficulty climbing stairs and brushing her hair. Her shoulders and thighs are mildly achy but not painful. She is well appearing with normal vital signs and an essentially normal physical examination, with the exception of mild shoulder and thigh muscle tenderness. She does not have a rash. Laboratory tests are notable for a creatine phosphokinase level of 840 IU/L (normal female: 26–180 IU/L) and an aldolase value of 32 IU/L (normal: 1.0–7.0 IU/L). Her electromyogram shows her muscles producing sharp waves and spontaneous discharges. She is diagnosed with polymyositis.

Questions

A. What are the pathologic similarities and differences between polymyositis and dermatomyositis?
B. What are the four characteristic criteria for the diagnosis of polymyositis?
C. What condition(s) is this patient at risk for during the next few years?

CASE 131

A 47-year-old woman presents to the clinic with a four-week history of fatigue, bilateral hand pain and stiffness, and hand and wrist joint swelling. About a month before presentation, she noticed that her hands were stiffer in the morning but thought that it was due to too much typing. However, the stiffness has worsened, and she now needs about an hour each morning to "loosen up" her hands. As the day goes on, the stiffness improves, although it does not go away entirely. She has also noticed that her knuckles and wrists are swollen and feel somewhat warm. The physical examination reveals warm, erythematous wrists and metacarpal joints bilaterally. Hand x-ray films show periarticular demineralization and erosions, and blood test results are significant for a mild anemia, elevated sedimentation rate, and a positive rheumatoid factor. The patient is diagnosed with rheumatoid arthritis.

Questions

A. What is the basic pathogenic process in rheumatoid arthritis?
B. Describe the interplay between genetic and environmental factors that leads to the pathogenic process.
C. How are novel treatments being used to treat this condition?

CASE 132

A 23-year-old man comes into the doctor's office for increasing back pain. He states that over the past 3 months, he has had gradually worsening pain in the middle of his lower back. The pain is at its worst first thing in the morning and gradually improves as the day goes on. He has also been more tired than usual and has had some intermittent low-grade fevers. He has experienced no radiation of the pain into his legs, no weakness or sensory changes in the legs, and no changes in bowel or bladder function. He denies injury and new activities. He has not had any diarrhea, dysuria, skin rash, or other joint pain. Two years ago, he had an episode of unexplained painful, red right eye, which was treated with eye drops. He has tested positive for HLA-B27.

Questions

A. What is the likely diagnosis?
B. What are the possible roles of HLA-B27 in this condition? What other factors may be involved?
C. What potential treatments could be offered to this patient?

REFERENCES

General

Fox C et al. Evolving spectrum of HIV-associated rheumatic syndromes. Best Pract Res Clin Rheumatol. 2015 Apr;29(2):244–58. [PMID: 26362742]

Shaw AT et al. Mediators of inflammation and bone remodeling in rheumatic disease. Semin Cell Dev Biol. 2016 Jan;49:2–10. [PMID: 26481971]

Gout

Dalbeth N et al. Gout. Lancet. 2016 Oct 22;388(10055):2039–52 [PMID: 27112094]

Juraschek SP et al. Gout, urate-lowering therapy and uric acid levels among adults in the United States. Arthritis Care Res (Hoboken). 2015 Apr;67(4):588–92. [PMID: 25201123]

Neogi T. Gout. Ann Intern Med. 2016 Jul 5;165(1):ITC1–ITC16. [PMID: 27380294]

Neogi T et al. 2015 Gout Classification Criteria: an American College of Rheumatology/European League Against Rheumatism collaborative initiative. Arthritis Rheumatol. 2015 Oct;67(10):2557–68. Erratum in: Arthritis Rheumatol. 2016 Feb;68(2):515. [PMID: 26352873]

Newberry SJ et al. Diagnosis of gout: a systematic review in support of an American College of Physicians Clinical Practice Guideline. Ann Intern Med. 2017 Jan 3;166(1):27–36. [PMID: 27802505]

Vasculitis

Buttgereit F et al. Polymyalgia rheumatica and giant cell arteritis: a systematic review. JAMA. 2016 Jun 14;315(22):2442–58. [PMID: 27299619]

Cacoub P et al. Cryoglobulinemia vasculitis. Am J Med. 2015 Sep;128(9):950–5. [PMID: 25837517]

Cheadle C et al. Transcription of proteinase 3 and related myelopoiesis genes in peripheral blood mononuclear cells of patients with active Wegener's granulomatosis. Arthritis Rheum. 2010 Jun;62(6):1744–54. [PMID: 20155833]

Dejaco C et al. The spectrum of giant cell arteritis and polymyalgia rheumatica: revisiting the concept of the disease. Rheumatology (Oxford). 2017 Apr 1;56(4):506–15. [PMID: 27481272]

Lyons PA et al. Genetically distinct subsets within ANCA-associated vasculitis. N Engl J Med. 2012 Jul 19;367(3):214–23. [PMID: 22808956]

Yates M et al. ANCA-associated vasculitis. Clin Med (Lond). 2017 Feb;17(1):60–4. [PMID: 28148583]

Systemic Lupus Erythematosus

Arriens C et al. Systemic lupus erythematosus biomarkers: the challenging quest. Rheumatology (Oxford). 2017 Apr 1;56(Suppl 1): i32–i45. [PMID: 28013203]

Caielli S et al. Oxidized mitochondrial nucleoids released by neutrophils drive type I interferon production in human lupus. J Exp Med. 2016 May;213(5):697–713. [PMID: 27091841]

Thong B et al. Systemic lupus erythematosus diagnosis and management. Rheumatology (Oxford). 2017 Apr 1;56(Suppl 1):i3–i13. [PMID: 28013206]

Zharkova O et al. Pathways leading to an immunological disease: systemic lupus erythematosus. Rheumatology (Oxford). 2017 Apr 1;56(Suppl 1):i55–i66. [PMID: 28375453]

Sjögren Syndrome

Al Kindi MA et al. Secreted autoantibody repertoires in Sjögren's syndrome and systemic lupus erythematosus: a proteomic approach. Autoimmun Rev. 2016 Apr;15(4):405–10. [PMID: 26804757]

Hall JC et al. Molecular subsetting of interferon pathways in Sjogren's syndrome. Arthritis Rheumatol. 2015 Sep;67(9):2437–46. [PMID: 25988820]]

Ramos-Casals M et al; EULAR Sjögren Syndrome Task Force. Characterization of systemic disease in primary Sjögren's syndrome: EULAR-SS Task Force recommendations for articular, cutaneous, pulmonary and renal involvements. Rheumatology (Oxford). 2015 Dec;54(12):2230–8. [PMID: 26231345]

Sada PR et al. Biologic treatment in Sjögren's syndrome. Rheumatology (Oxford). 2015 Feb;54(2):219–30. [PMID: 25342375]

Shiboski CH; International Sjögren's Syndrome Criteria Working Group. 2016 American College of Rheumatology/European League Against Rheumatism classification criteria for primary Sjögren's syndrome: a consensus and data-driven methodology involving three international patient cohorts. Arthritis Rheumatol. 2017 Jan;69(1):35–45. [PMID: 27785888]

Singh AG et al. Rate, risk factors and causes of mortality in patients with Sjögren's syndrome: a systematic review and meta-analysis of cohort studies. Rheumatology (Oxford). 2016 Mar;55(3):450–60. [PMID: 26412810]

Thompson N et al. Exploring BAFF: its expression, receptors and contribution to the immunopathogenesis of Sjögren's syndrome. Rheumatology (Oxford). 2016 Sep;55(9):1548–55. [PMID: 26790457]

Inflammatory Myopathy

Basharat P et al. Immune-mediated necrotizing myopathy: update on diagnosis and management. Curr Rheumatol Rep. 2015 Dec;17(12):72. [PMID: 26515574]

Cavazzana I et al. The clinical and histological spectrum of idiopathic inflammatory myopathies. Clin Rev Allergy Immunol. 2017 Feb;52(1):88–98. [PMID: 26514357]

Chhibber S et al. Clinical evaluation and management of inflammatory myopathies. Semin Neurol. 2015 Aug;35(4):347–59. [PMID: 26502759]

Findlay AR et al. An overview of polymyositis and dermatomyositis. Muscle Nerve. 2015 May;51(5):638–56. [PMID: 25641317]

Lahouti AH et al. Polymyositis and dermatomyositis: novel insights into the pathogenesis and potential therapeutic targets. Discov Med. 2015 Jun;19(107):463–70. [PMID: 26175404]

Mammen AL. Statin-associated autoimmune myopathy. N Engl J Med. 2016 Feb 18;374(7):664–9. [PMID: 26886523]

Meyer A et al. Incidence and prevalence of inflammatory myopathies: a systematic review. Rheumatology (Oxford). 2015 Jan;54(1):50–63. [PMID: 25065005]

Satoh M et al. A comprehensive overview on myositis-specific antibodies: new and old biomarkers in idiopathic inflammatory myopathy. Clin Rev Allergy Immunol. 2017 Feb;52(1):1–19. [PMID: 26424665]

Tieu J et al. Idiopathic inflammatory myositis. Best Pract Res Clin Rheumatol. 2016 Feb;30(1):149–68. [PMID: 27421222]

Rheumatoid Arthritis

Chen XM et al. Role of micro RNAs in the pathogenesis of rheumatoid arthritis: novel perspectives based on review of the literature. Medicine (Baltimore). 2015 Aug;94(31):e1326. [PMID: 26252320]

Darrah E et al. Peptidylarginine deiminase 2, 3 and 4 have distinct specificities against cellular substrates: novel insights into autoantigen selection in rheumatoid arthritis. Ann Rheum Dis. 2012 Jan;71(1):92–8. [PMID: 21859690]

Darrah E et al. Proteolysis by granzyme B enhances presentation of autoantigenic peptidylarginine deiminase 4 epitopes in rheumatoid arthritis. J Proteome Res. 2017 Jan 6;16(1):355–65. [PMID: 27700100]

Her M et al. Alterations in immune function with biologic therapies for autoimmune disease. J Allergy Clin Immunol. 2016 Jan;137(1):19–27. [PMID: 26768759]

Mikuls TR et al. Autoimmunity of the lung and oral mucosa in a multisystem inflammatory disease: the spark that lights the fire in rheumatoid arthritis? J Allergy Clin Immunol. 2016 Jan;137(1):28–34. [PMID: 26768760]

Smolen JS et al. Rheumatoid arthritis. Lancet. 2016 Oct 22;388(10055):2023–38. Erratum in: Lancet. 2016 Oct 22;388(10055):1984. [PMID: 27156434]

Spondyloarthropathy

Roberts AR et al. An ankylosing spondylitis-associated genetic variant in the IL23R-IL12RB2 intergenic region modulates enhancer activity and is associated with increased Th1-cell differentiation. Ann Rheum Dis. 2016 Dec;75(12):2150–6. [PMID: 26916345]

Schmitt SK. Reactive arthritis. Infect Dis Clin North Am. 2017 Jun;31(2):265–77. [PMID: 28292540]

Taurog JD et al. Ankylosing spondylitis and axial spondyloarthritis. N Engl J Med. 2016 Jun 30;374(26):2563–74. [PMID: 27355535]

Case Study Answers

Yeong S. Kwok, MD

CASE 1

A. The four types of osteogenesis imperfecta are type I (mild), type II (perinatal, lethal), type III (progressive, deforming), and type IV (deforming with normal scleras). All forms of osteogenesis imperfecta are characterized by an increased susceptibility to fractures ("brittle bones"), but there is considerable phenotypic heterogeneity, even within individual subtypes. Approximately 60% of the cases of type I and type IV osteogenesis imperfecta represent new mutations; in the remainder, the history and examination of other family members reveal findings consistent with autosomal dominant inheritance. Type III is also transmitted as an autosomal dominant trait, although type III can occasionally be transmitted in an autosomal recessive manner. Type II, the most severe form, generally occurs as a result of a sporadic dominant mutation.

B. Type II osteogenesis imperfecta presents at birth (or even in utero) with multiple fractures and bony deformities, resulting in death in infancy and, therefore, is unlikely to be seen in a child 4 year of age. Type III presents at birth or in early infancy with multiple fractures—often prenatal—and progressive bony deformities. The absence of prenatal fractures and early deformities in this patient's history is most suggestive of type I or type IV osteogenesis imperfecta. These individuals generally present in early childhood with one or a few fractures of long bones in response to minimal or no trauma, as seen in this case. Type I and type IV osteogenesis imperfecta are differentiated by their clinical severity and scleral hue. Type I tends to be less severe, with 10–20 fractures during childhood plus short stature but few or no deformities. These patients tend to have blue scleras. Patients with type IV osteogenesis imperfecta tend to have more fractures, resulting in significant short stature and mild to moderate deformities. Their scleras are normal or slightly gray.

C. In patients with type I osteogenesis imperfecta, the fracture incidence decreases after puberty, and the main features in adult life are mild short stature, conductive hearing loss, and occasionally dentinogenesis imperfecta (defective dentin formation in tooth development).

D. Advances in the last two decades demonstrate two genetically different groups: the "classical" group, in which more than 90% of cases are caused by a pathogenic variant (previously, "mutation") of the *COL1A1* or *COL1A2* genes, which encode the subunits of type I collagen, proα1(I) and proα2(I), respectively, and a newer group, caused by loss-of-function variants in proteins required for the proper folding, processing, and secretion of collagen. The fundamental defect in most individuals with type I osteogenesis imperfecta is a reduced synthesis of type I collagen resulting from loss-of-function variants in *COL1A1*. Several potential molecular defects are responsible for *COL1A1* variants in type I osteogenesis imperfecta, including alterations in a regulatory region leading to reduced transcription, splicing abnormalities leading to reduced steady-state levels of RNA, and the deletion of the entire *COL1A1* gene. However, in many cases, the underlying defect is a single base pair change that creates a premature stop codon (also known as a **nonsense mutation**) in an internal exon. In a process referred to as nonsense-mediated decay, partially synthesized mRNA precursors that carry the nonsense codon are recognized and degraded by the cell. Each of these variants gives rise to greatly reduced (partial loss-of-function) or no (complete loss-of-function) mRNA. Because the normal *COL1A1* allele continues to produce mRNA at a normal rate (ie, there is no dosage compensation), heterozygosity for a complete loss-of-function variant results in a 50% reduction in the total rate of proα1(I) mRNA synthesis, whereas heterozygosity for a partial loss-of-function variant results in a less severe reduction. A reduced concentration of pro1(I) chains limits the production of type I procollagen, leading to both a reduced amount of structurally normal type I collagen and an excess of unassembled proα2(I) chains, which are degraded inside the cell. This ultimately results in fragile bones.

CASE 2

A. The primary metabolic defect in phenylketonuria (PKU) is the inability to hydroxylate phenylalanine, an essential step in the conversion of phenylalanine to tyrosine and the synthesis of protein. This condition is most commonly due to a defect in phenylalanine hydroxylase, the responsible enzyme, or less commonly, to a defect in the metabolism of tetrahydrobiopterin (BH_4), an essential co-factor in the hydroxylation of phenylalanine. This leads to the accumulation of phenylalanine and its metabolites.

B. The accumulation of phenylalanine and its metabolites, especially phenylpyruvate, directly reduces energy production and protein synthesis and affects neurotransmitter homeostasis in the developing brain, since many neurotransmitters are derived from amino acids. Elevated levels of phenylalanine also inhibit amino acid transport across the blood–brain barrier, causing an amino acid deficit in the cerebrospinal fluid. All these effects combine to cause intellectual disability, developmental delay, and seizures. Affected individuals also suffer from eczema, the mechanism of which is not well understood, and have hypopigmentation owing to an inhibition of melanocytes from the excess phenylalanine. Most, if not all, of the above consequences of PKU can be prevented by strict dietary management to ensure that excessive serum phenylalanine concentrations do not occur.

C. PKU is inherited as an autosomal recessive trait. The reproductive fitness of affected untreated individuals is poor, meaning that they are unlikely to produce offspring. Theories have been proposed about why the trait has persisted at a relatively high rate in the population. It is known that the rate of spontaneous PKU mutation is low. Two potential explanations for the high rate of the defective gene are the founder effect and heterozygote advantage. The founder effect occurs when a population founded by a small number of ancestors has by chance a high frequency of a deleterious gene. Heterozygote advantage refers to the fact that certain genes may actually confer a benefit in the heterozygote state even though the homozygote state is disadvantageous. This is the case for the genetic defect in sickle cell disease, in which heterozygote carriers have a relative resistance to malaria.

CASE 3

A. Fragile X–associated mental retardation is a syndrome caused by a genetic mutation of the X chromosome. The mutation leads to a failure of the region between bands Xq27 and Xq28 to condense at metaphase, thereby increasing the "fragility" of the region. The mutation appears as an amplification of a $(CGG)_n$ repeat within the untranslated region of a gene named *FMR1*. The *FMR1* gene encodes an RNA-binding protein named FMR1. However, in affected individuals, amplification of the gene results in methylation of an area known as the CpG island, located at Xq27.3. This methylation prevents expression of the FMR1 protein.

The FMR1 protein is normally expressed in the brain and testes. This protein resembles a group of proteins named heterogeneous nuclear RNA-binding proteins (hnRNPs) that function in the processing or transport of nuclear mRNA precursors. It is believed that the FMR1 protein plays a general role in the cellular metabolism of nuclear RNA but only in the tissues in which it is primarily expressed (ie, the central nervous system [CNS] and testes). This would explain in part the symptoms of mental retardation and enlarged testes. It is not known why the absence of *FMR1* expression leads to joint laxity and hyperextensibility and facial abnormalities.

B. Fragile X–associated mental retardation is an X-linked disease. Given that a male child inherits his X chromosome from his mother, she is clearly the carrier of the mutation.

The boy's mother and grandparents do not demonstrate the phenotype of fragile X–associated mental retardation because of the processes of premutation and parental imprinting. As mentioned, the mutation in fragile X is associated with the amplification of a segment of DNA containing the sequence $(CGG)_n$. This segment is highly variable in length. In individuals who are neither carriers nor affected, the number of repeats is generally less than 50. In transmitting males and unaffected carrier females, the number of repeats is usually between 70 and 100. Alleles with 55 or more repeats are unstable and often exhibit expansion after maternal transmission; these individuals are generally considered to carry the premutation. They are unaffected phenotypically, but the regions are unstable, and when transmitted from generation to generation, the regions tend to undergo amplification into a full mutation. Although premutation carriers do not develop a typical FMR syndrome, recent studies indicate that female premutation carriers exhibit a 20% incidence of premature ovarian failure, whereas male premutation carriers are at increased risk for a tremor–ataxia syndrome. In both cases, the mechanism is likely explained by somatic expansion of the premutation. Full mutations, observed in all affected individuals, always have more than 200 amplifications.

The most important determinant of whether a premutation allele is subject to amplification is the sex of the parent who transmits the premutation allele. A premutation allele transmitted by a female expands to a full mutation with a likelihood proportionate to the length of the premutation. In contrast, a premutation allele transmitted by a male rarely expands to a full mutation regardless of the length of the premutation. This process is called parental imprinting. Thus, it is likely that the boy's mother and grandfather are carriers of a premutation allele and are, therefore, unaffected and that this gene amplified to a full mutation on transmission to the boy.

C. The chance that her unborn child will be affected depends on its gender. If it is a boy, the chance that it will be affected is approximately 80%, whereas if it is a girl, the chance is only 32%.

CASE 4

A. Leber hereditary optic neuropathy (LHON) arises from a pathogenic variant (previously, "mutation") in mitochondrial

DNA (mtDNA). The mtDNA encodes protein components of the electron transport chain involved in the generation of adenosine triphosphate (ATP). Mutations in the mtDNA can result in the inability to generate ATP. This defect especially affects tissues with intensive ATP use such as skeletal muscle and the central nervous system. It is not understood why the defect in LHON is largely confined to the optic nerve and retina. Other mitochondrial disorders do affect skeletal muscle, most notably mitochondrial encephalomyopathy with ragged red fibers (MERRF).

B. LHON is inherited through mtDNA pathogenic variants. All the mtDNA in our bodies comes exclusively from the egg. The sperm makes no contribution of mtDNA. Therefore, LHON is inherited only from the mother. In addition, a typical cell carries 10–100 separate mtDNA molecules, only a fraction of which carry the pathogenic variant. This is known as **heteroplasmy**. Within any one affected woman, the level of abnormal DNA in different eggs may vary from 50% to 90%. Thus, some offspring may be severely affected, whereas others may not show any signs. Furthermore, within any given offspring, the level of abnormal mtDNA will vary from tissue to tissue and from cell to cell.

C. LHON affects males 4 to 5 times more often than females. This difference is thought to be due to a factor on the X chromosome that modifies the severity of a mitochondrial pathogenic variant. Even though mtDNA encodes essential components of the electron transport chain, there are copies for most mitochondrial components also encoded on the nuclear genome.

CASE 5

A. Down syndrome occurs approximately once in every 700 live births. Common features include developmental delay, growth restriction, congenital heart disease (in 50%), immunodeficiency, and characteristic major and minor facial and dysmorphic phenotypic features, including upslanting palpebral fissures (82%), epicanthal folds (59%), brushfield spots on the iris, brachycephaly (75%), excess skin on the back of the neck (81%), folded or dysplastic ears (50%), a flat nasal bridge (68%), a protruding tongue, hyperextensible joints (75%), a wide gap between the first and second toes, short and broad toes, a short and incurved fifth finger, and transverse palmar creases (53%).

B. There are two major genetic abnormalities associated with Down syndrome. The most common abnormality occurs in children born to parents with normal karyotypes. It is caused by the nondisjunction of chromosome 21 during meiotic segregation, resulting in one extra chromosome 21 (trisomy 21), with 47 chromosomes on karyotyping. Alternatively, Down syndrome can be caused by DNA rearrangement resulting in the fusion of chromosome 21 to another acrocentric chromosome via its centromere. This abnormal chromosome is called a robertsonian translocation chromosome. Unlike those with

trisomy 21, these individuals have 46 chromosomes on karyotyping. This type of translocation can sometimes be inherited from a carrier parent.

Both these genetic abnormalities result in a 50% increase in gene dosage for nearly all genes on chromosome 21. In other words, the amount of protein produced by all or nearly all genes on chromosome 21 is approximately 150% of normal in Down syndrome. The genes that have been shown to contribute to the Down syndrome phenotype include the gene that encodes the amyloid protein found in the senile plaques of Alzheimer disease and the one that encodes the cytoplasmic form of superoxide dismutase, which plays an important role in free radical metabolism.

C. It is not known why advanced maternal age is associated with an increased risk of Down syndrome as a result of trisomy 21. One theory suggests that biochemical abnormalities affect the ability of paired chromosomes to disjoin and that these abnormalities accumulate over time. Because germ cell development is completed in females before birth, these biochemical abnormalities are able to accumulate within the egg cells as the mother ages, thereby increasing the risk of nondisjunction. Another hypothesis is that structural, hormonal, and immunologic changes occur in the uterus as the woman ages, producing an environment less able to reject a developmentally abnormal embryo. Therefore, an older uterus would be more likely to support a trisomy 21 conceptus to term. Alternatively, it is possible that a combination of these and other genetic factors may contribute to the relationship between advanced maternal age and an increased incidence of Down syndrome.

CASE 6

A. Babies born with Down syndrome may exhibit developmental delay, growth restriction, congenital heart disease (in 50%), and immunodeficiency, as well as characteristic major and minor facial and dysmorphic phenotypic features, including upslanting palpebral fissures, epicanthal folds, Brushfield spots on the iris, brachycephaly, excess skin on back of the neck, folded or dysplastic ears, a flat nasal bridge, a protruding tongue, hyperextensible joints, a wide gap between the first and second toes, short and broad toes, a short and incurved fifth finger, and transverse palmar creases.

B. For a female carrier of a balanced robertsonian translocation, 45,XX,+t(14q;21q), the chance of having a child with Down syndrome is 10%. Unlike with Down syndrome as a result of trisomy 21 (47,XX+21 or 47,XY+21), this risk not affected by maternal age.

C. Down syndrome illustrates the principle of gene dosage, which states that the amount of a gene product produced per cell is proportionate to the number of copies of that gene present. In other words, the amount of protein produced by all or nearly all genes that lie on chromosome 21 is 150% of normal in trisomy 21 cells. There may be a critical region of chromosome 21, which, when present in triplicate, is both necessary and sufficient to produce the phenotypic features of Down syndrome.

CASE 7

A. The cross-linking of surface-bound IgE by antigen activates tissue mast cells and basophils, inducing the immediate release of preformed mediators and the synthesis of newly generated mediators. Mast cells and basophils also have the ability to synthesize and release pro-inflammatory cytokines, which are growth and regulatory factors that interact in complex networks. The interaction of mediators with various target organs and airway cells can induce a **biphasic allergic response**: an early phase mediated chiefly by the release of histamine and other stored mediators (tryptase, chymase, heparin, chondroitin sulfate, and tumor necrosis factor [TNF]), whereas late-phase events are induced after the generation of arachidonic acid metabolites (leukotrienes and prostaglandins), platelet-activating factor, and de novo cytokine synthesis.

Histologically, the early response is characterized by vascular permeability, vasodilatation, tissue edema, and a mild cellular infiltrate of mostly granulocytes. The late-phase response is characterized clinically by erythema, induration, heat, burning, and itching and microscopically by significant influx of mainly eosinophils and mononuclear cells. Changes consistent with airway remodeling and tissue hyper-reactivity may also occur.

B. Patients with allergic rhinitis develop chronic or episodic paroxysmal sneezing; nasal, ocular, or palatal pruritus; and watery rhinorrhea triggered by exposure to a specific allergen. Patients may demonstrate signs of chronic pruritus of the upper airway, including a horizontal nasal crease from frequent nose rubbing ("allergic salute") and palatal "clicking" from rubbing the itching palate with the tongue. Symptoms of nasal obstruction may become chronic as a result of persistent late-phase allergic mechanisms. Nasal mucous membranes may appear pale blue and boggy. Children frequently show signs of obligate mouth breathing, including long facies, narrow maxillae, flattened malar eminences, a marked overbite, and high-arched palates (so-called adenoid facies).

C. Serous otitis media and sinusitis are major comorbidities in patients with allergic rhinitis. Both conditions occur secondary to the obstructed nasal passages and sinus ostia in patients with chronic allergic or nonallergic rhinitis. Complications of chronic rhinitis should be considered in patients with protracted rhinitis unresponsive to therapy, refractory asthma, or persistent bronchitis. Serous otitis results from an auditory tube obstruction by mucosal edema and hypersecretion. Children with serous otitis media can present with conductive hearing loss, delayed speech, and recurrent otitis media associated with chronic nasal obstruction.

Sinusitis may be acute, subacute, or chronic depending on the duration of symptoms. The obstruction of osteomeatal drainage in patients with chronic rhinitis predisposes to bacterial infection in the sinus cavities. Patients manifest symptoms of persistent nasal discharge, cough, sinus discomfort, and nasal obstruction. Examination may reveal chronic otitis media, infraorbital edema, inflamed nasal mucosa, and purulent nasal discharge. Radiographic diagnosis by sinus x-ray film or computed tomographic (CT) scan reveals sinus opacification, membrane thickening, or the presence of an air–fluid level.

CASE 8

A. The most likely cause of this child's recurrent infections is severe combined immunodeficiency disease (SCID). These patients experience a complete or near-complete failure of development of both the cellular and humoral components of the immune system. Placental transfer of maternal immunoglobulin is insufficient to protect these children from infection, and for that reason they present at a very early age with severe infections.

B. SCID is a heterogeneous group of genetic and cellular disorders characterized by a failure in the cellular maturation of lymphoid stem cells, resulting in reduced numbers and function of both B and T lymphocytes and hypogammaglobulinemia. The genetic and cellular defects can occur at many different levels, starting with surface membrane receptors, but also including deficiencies in signal transduction or metabolic biochemical pathways. Although the different molecular defects may cause clinically indistinguishable phenotypes, the identification of specific mutations has allowed for improved genetic counseling, prenatal diagnosis, and carrier detection.

The most common genetic defect is an X-linked form of SCID (XSCID) in which the maturation defect is mainly in the T-lymphocyte lineage and is due to a point mutation in the γ chain of the IL-2 receptor. This defective γ chain is shared by the receptors for IL-4, IL-7, IL-9, and IL-15, leading to dysfunction in all these cytokine receptors. Defective signaling through the IL-7 receptor appears to block the normal maturation of T lymphocytes. Circulating B-cell numbers may be preserved, but defective IL-2 responses inhibit the proliferation of T, B, and NK cells, explaining the combined immune defects seen in XSCID patients.

Several other forms of SCID have also been identified. A defect in the α chain of the IL-7 receptor can lead to an autosomal recessive form of SCID through mechanisms similar to XSCID but with intact NK cells.

About 20% of SCID cases are caused by a deficiency of adenosine deaminase (ADA), an enzyme in the purine salvage pathway responsible for adenosine metabolism. Absence of the ADA enzyme results in an accumulation of toxic adenosine metabolites within the cells. These metabolites inhibit normal lymphocyte proliferation and lead to extreme cytopenia of both B and T lymphocytes. The combined immunologic deficiency and clinical presentation of this disorder, known as SCID-ADA, are identical to those of the other forms of SCID. Skeletal abnormalities and neurologic abnormalities may be associated with this disease.

An alternative autosomal recessive form of SCID is a deficiency of ZAP-70, a tyrosine kinase important in normal T-lymphocyte function. Deficiency of this tyrosine kinase results in the total absence of CD8 T lymphocytes and functionally defective CD4 T lymphocytes, but normal B-lymphocyte and NK activity. Mutations of the CD3δ, CD3γ, and CD3ε subunits may lead to the partially arrested development of TCR expression and a severe T-cell deficiency.

Deficiencies of both p56^{kk} and Janus kinase 3 (Jak3) can also lead to SCID through defective signal transduction; p56^{kk} is a T-cell receptor–associated tyrosine kinase essential for T-cell differentiation, activation, and proliferation. Jak3 is a cytokine receptor–associated signaling molecule. Finally, patients have been identified with defects in enzymes participating in VDJ recombination. (VDJ recombination is the process by which T cells and B cells in their early stages of development randomly assemble different gene segments—known as variable [V], diversity [D], and joining [J] genes—to generate a highly diverse repertoire of antibodies [immunoglobulins] found on B cells and antigen receptors found on T cells, respectively, that collectively can recognize many different types of antigen molecules.) Recombination-activating genes (RAG-1 and RAG-2) initiate the recombination of antigen-binding receptor genes, immunoglobulins, and T-cell receptors. The defect leads to both quantitative and qualitative (functional) deficiencies in T and B lymphocytes.

C. Without treatment, most patients with SCID die within the first 1–2 years.

CASE 9

A. This child has X-linked agammaglobulinemia, formerly called Bruton agammaglobulinemia. The history of multiple infections occurring after the age of 6 months, the family history of a maternal uncle with lethal infection, the severe current infection with *Streptococcus pneumoniae*, and the absence of circulating B lymphocytes are characteristic of this disorder.

B. The main defect is a mutation in the *BTK* (Bruton tyrosine kinase) gene, located on the X chromosome. This gene's product is a B cell–specific signaling protein necessary for normal B-cell maturation. The mutation affects the catalytic domain of the protein, halting B-cell maturation. This, in turn, leads to an absence or greatly reduced levels of the immunoglobulins IgA, IgG, and IgM. Their absence or reduction is a particular problem for fighting infections from encapsulated bacteria because these bacteria require antibody binding for efficient opsonization. Therefore, patients are particularly susceptible to infections with bacteria such as *Haemophilus influenzae* and *S pneumoniae*. Because they cannot mount an antibody response, they also develop very little immunity to these infections and are thus susceptible to repeated infections with the same organism.

C. The affected child is relatively protected by circulating maternal antibodies until 4–6 months of age. The child's immune system is otherwise unaffected, but as the levels of maternal antibodies decrease, the child becomes increasingly susceptible to infection, particularly from encapsulated bacteria.

CASE 10

A. Individuals with common variable immunodeficiency (CVI) commonly develop recurrent sinopulmonary infections such as sinusitis, otitis media, bronchitis, and pneumonia. Common pathogens are encapsulated bacteria such as *S pneumoniae*, *H influenzae*, and *Moraxella catarrhalis*. Bronchiectasis may develop as a result of these recurrent infections. Patients may also develop gastrointestinal (GI) malabsorption from bacterial overgrowth or from chronic *Giardia* infection in the small bowel.

B. CVI is a heterogeneous disorder in which the primary immunologic abnormality is a marked reduction in antibody production, with normal or reduced numbers of circulating B cells. This is most commonly caused by a defect in the terminal differentiation of B lymphocytes in response to T lymphocyte–dependent and T lymphocyte–independent stimuli. However, defects in B-lymphocyte development have been shown to occur at any stage of the maturation pathway.

In many patients, the defect is intrinsic to the B-lymphocyte population. Approximately 15% of patients with CVI demonstrate defective B-cell surface expression of the transmembrane activator and calcium modulator and cyclophilin ligand interactor (TACI), a member of the TNF receptor family. Lacking a functional TACI, the affected B cells do not respond to B cell–activating factors, resulting in deficient immunoglobulin production. Another defect that may lead to CVI involves the deficient expression of the B-cell surface marker, CD19. When complexed with CD21 and CD81, CD19 facilitates cellular activation through B-cell receptors. B-cell development is not affected, but humoral function is deficient. A variety of T-cell abnormalities may also lead to immune defects with subsequent impairment of B-cell differentiation. A mutation of the inducible T-cell costimulator gene, expressed by activated T cells and responsible for B-cell activation and antibody production, may be the molecular defect in some cases of CVI. T-lymphocyte dysfunction can be manifested as increased suppressor T-lymphocyte activity, decreased cytokine production, defective synthesis of B-lymphocyte growth factors, defective cytokine gene expression in T cells, decreased T-cell mitogenesis, and deficient lymphokine-activated killer cell function.

C. Individuals with CVI are at increased risk of autoimmune disorders and malignancies. The autoimmune disorders most commonly seen in association with CVI include immune thrombocytopenic purpura, hemolytic anemia, and symmetric seronegative arthritis. The malignancies associated with CVI include lymphomas, gastric carcinoma, and skin cancers.

D. Treatment is mainly symptomatic along with the replacement of immune globulin with monthly IVIG infusions.

CASE 11

A. Chronic granulomatous disease is typically inherited as an X-linked condition. It is characterized by impaired granulocyte function. The boy's mother is likely to be a carrier of the defective gene. Her male children have a 50% chance of inheriting it.

B. Defects in the gene coding for nicotinamide adenine dinucleotide phosphate (NADPH) oxidase inhibit oxidative metabolism and severely compromise the killing activity of neutrophils. NADPH oxidase is normally assembled from two membrane and two cytosolic components after phagocytic cell activation; its assembly leads to the catalytic conversion of molecular oxygen into superoxide. Oxidative burst and intracellular killing rely on the production of superoxide, which is later converted to hydrogen peroxide and sodium hypochlorite (bleach). Although microbial killing is deficient in patients with chronic granulomatous disease, other neutrophil functions such as chemotaxis, phagocytosis, and degranulation remain intact.

C. Catalase-negative bacteria are effectively killed because microbes produce small amounts of peroxide, concentrated in phagosomes, leading to microbial death. Catalase-positive organisms scavenge these relatively small amounts of peroxide and are not killed without neutrophil oxidative metabolism. Since *Staphylococcus aureus* and *Serratia marcescens* produce catalase, they are not killed by the defective neutrophils.

CASE 12

A. Pneumocystis pneumonia is commonly seen in AIDS. An HIV-1 antibody test should be obtained whenever a diagnosis of *Pneumocystis jirovecii* is suspected.

B. AIDS is the consequence of infection with HIV-1, a retrovirus that infects multiple cell lines, including lymphocytes, monocytes, macrophages, and dendritic cells. With HIV infection, there is an absolute reduction of CD4 T lymphocytes, an accompanying deficit in CD4 T-lymphocyte function, and an associated increase in CD8 cytotoxic T lymphocytes (CTLs). In addition to the cell-mediated immune defects, B-lymphocyte function is altered such that many infected individuals have marked hypergammaglobulinemia but impaired specific antibody responses. The resultant immunosuppression predisposes patients to the constellation of opportunistic infections and malignancies that characterizes AIDS.

The loss of CD4 cells seen in HIV infection is the result of multiple mechanisms, including (1) the direct HIV-mediated destruction of CD4 T lymphocytes during viral replication; (2) depletion by the fusion and formation of multinucleated giant cells; (3) the toxicity of viral proteins to CD4 T lymphocytes and precursors; (4) the loss of T lymphocyte costimulatory factors such as CD28; and (5) the induction of apoptosis of uninfected T cells.

C. The clinical manifestations of HIV infection and AIDS are the direct consequence of progressive and severe immunosuppression and can be correlated with the degree of CD4 T lymphocyte destruction. HIV infection may present as an acute, self-limited febrile syndrome. This is often followed by a long, clinically silent period, sometimes associated with generalized lymphadenopathy. The time course of disease progression varies, but the median time before the appearance of clinical disease is about 10 years in untreated individuals. Approximately 10% of those infected manifest rapid progression to AIDS within 5 years of infection. A minority of individuals who demonstrate long-term disease nonprogression are termed "elite controllers." Genetic factors, host cytotoxic immune responses, viral load, and virulence all appear to have an impact on susceptibility to infection and the rate of disease progression. Although not curative, modern antiretroviral therapies (ART) can suppress viral replication and restore immune function, leading to clinical recovery and markedly extended life expectancy.

As the CD4 count declines, the incidence of infection increases. At CD4 counts between 200/μL and 500/μL, patients are at an increased risk for bacterial infections, including pneumonia and sinusitis. The risk of *Mycobacterium tuberculosis* reactivation is 5–10% per year in HIV-infected patients compared with a lifetime risk of 10% in those without HIV. As CD4 counts continue to drop—generally below 200/μL—patients are at high risk for other opportunistic infections such as *Pneumocystis jirovecii* pneumonia, candidiasis, toxoplasmosis, cryptococcal meningitis, cytomegalovirus (CMV) retinitis, and *Mycobacterium avium* complex infection. HIV-infected individuals are also at increased risk for certain malignancies, including Kaposi sarcoma, non-Hodgkin lymphoma, primary CNS lymphoma, invasive cervical carcinoma, and anal squamous cell carcinoma. Other manifestations of AIDS include AIDS dementia complex, peripheral neuropathy, monoarticular and polyarticular arthritides, unexplained fevers, and weight loss. Since patients are living longer owing to treatment with potent ART, cardiovascular complications are becoming more prominent. ART has been associated with dyslipidemia and metabolic abnormalities including insulin resistance. HIV infection may be atherogenic as well, through effects on lipids and pro-inflammatory mechanisms.

CASE 13

A. This patient's presentation is characteristic of untreated infective endocarditis, an infection of the cardiac valves. The most common predisposing factor is the presence of structurally abnormal cardiac valves related to rheumatic heart disease, congenital heart disease, a prosthetic valve, or prior endocarditis. Injection drug use is also an important risk factor for this disease. The patient's history of significant illness as a child after a sore throat suggests the possibility of rheumatic heart disease.

B. The most common infectious agents causing native valve endocarditis are gram-positive bacteria, including viridans group streptococci, *S aureus*, and enterococci. Given the history of recent dental work, the most likely pathogen in this patient is viridans group streptococci, which are normal mouth flora that can become transiently blood-borne after dental work.

C. The painful papules found on the pads of this man's fingers and toes are Osler nodes. They are thought to be caused by the deposition of immune complexes in the skin. The painless hemorrhagic macules (Janeway lesions) and splinter hemorrhages are thought to result from the microembolization of the cardiac vegetations.

D. In addition to the symptoms described in this man (fever, chills, night sweats, malaise, Roth spots, Janeway lesions, splinter hemorrhages, and Osler nodes), patients with infective endocarditis can develop multisystemic complaints, including headaches, back pain, focal neurologic symptoms, shortness of breath, pulmonary edema, chest pain, cough, decreased urine output, hematuria, flank pain, abdominal pain, among others. These symptoms and signs reflect (1) hemodynamic changes from valvular damage; (2) end-organ damage by septic emboli (right-sided endocarditis causes emboli to the lungs; left-sided endocarditis causes emboli to the brain, spleen, kidney, GI tract, and extremities); (3) immune complex deposition causing acute glomerulonephritis; and (4) persistent bacteremia and distal seeding of infection, resulting in abscess formation.

Death is usually caused by hemodynamic collapse after the rupture of the aortic or mitral valves or by septic emboli to the CNS, resulting in brain abscesses or mycotic aneurysms with a resultant intracranial hemorrhage. Risk factors for a fatal outcome include left-sided cardiac involvement, bacterial causes other than viridans group streptococci, medical comorbidities, complications from endocarditis (heart failure, valve ring abscess, or embolic disease), and, for those with large vegetations and significant valvular destruction, delayed valvular surgery.

E. Endothelial damage from turbulent blood flow (valvular disease) or microabrasions (injection drug use) promotes the deposition of fibrin, platelets, and adhesion proteins, forming sterile vegetations. When bacteremia occurs, such as after dental work, microorganisms can be deposited on these sterile thrombi. Once infected, the lesions continue to grow through further deposition of platelets and fibrin. These infected vegetations act as a sanctuary from host defense mechanisms such as phagocytosis and complement-mediated lysis. They also act as mechanical barriers to antibiotic penetration. It is for this reason that the prolonged administration of bactericidal antibiotics and possible operative intervention are required for cure.

CASE 14

A. The most likely diagnosis in this patient is meningitis. The acuity and severity of presentation are most consistent with a pyogenic bacterial cause, although viral, mycobacterial, and fungal causes should be considered as well. In adults, the most likely bacterial pathogens are *Neisseria meningitidis* and *S pneumoniae*. In infants younger than 3 months, the most

common pathogens are those to which the infant is exposed in the maternal genitourinary canal, including *E coli* and other gram-negative bacilli, group B and other streptococci, and *Listeria monocytogenes*. Between the ages of 3 months and 15 years, *N meningitidis* and *S pneumoniae* are the most common pathogens.

B. Most cases of bacterial meningitis begin with colonization of the host's nasopharynx. This is followed by local invasion of the mucosal epithelium and subsequent bacteremia. Cerebral endothelial cell injury follows and results in increased blood–brain barrier permeability, facilitating meningeal invasion. The resultant inflammatory response in the subarachnoid space causes cerebral edema, vasculitis, and infarction, ultimately leading to decreased cerebrospinal fluid flow, hydrocephalus, worsening cerebral edema, increased intracranial pressure, and decreased cerebral blood flow.

The bacterial pathogens responsible for meningitis possess several characteristics that facilitate the steps just listed. Nasal colonization is facilitated by pili on the bacterial surface of *N meningitidis* that assist in mucosal attachment. *N meningitidis*, *H influenzae*, and *S pneumoniae* also produce IgA proteases that cleave IgA, the antibody commonly responsible for inhibiting the adherence of pathogens to the mucosal surface. By cleaving the antibody, the bacteria are able to evade this important host defense mechanism. In addition, *N meningitidis*, *H influenzae*, and *S pneumoniae* are often encapsulated, which can assist in nasopharyngeal colonization as well as systemic invasion. The capsule inhibits neutrophil phagocytosis and resists classic complement-mediated bactericidal activity, enhancing bacterial survival and replication.

It remains unclear how bacterial pathogens gain access to the CNS. It is thought that cells of the choroid plexus may contain receptors for them, facilitating movement into the subarachnoid space. Once the bacterial pathogen is in the subarachnoid space, host defense mechanisms are inadequate to control the infection. Subcapsular surface components of the bacteria, such as the cell wall and lipopolysaccharide, induce a marked inflammatory response mediated by IL-1, IL-6, matrix metalloproteinases, and TNF. Despite the induction of a marked inflammatory response and leukocytosis, there is a relative lack of opsonization and bactericidal activity such that the bacteria are poorly cleared from the cerebrospinal fluid. The host inflammatory response, with cytokine and proteolytic enzyme release, leads to a loss of membrane integrity, with resultant cellular swelling and cerebral edema, contributing to many of the pathophysiologic consequences of this disease.

C. Cerebral edema may be vasogenic, cytotoxic, or interstitial in origin. Vasogenic cerebral edema is principally caused by the increase in the blood–brain barrier permeability that occurs when the bacteria invade the cerebrospinal fluid. Cytotoxic cerebral edema results from swelling of the cellular elements of the brain. This occurs because of toxic factors released by the bacteria and neutrophils. Interstitial edema is due to the obstruction of cerebrospinal fluid flow.

D. Any patient suspected of having bacterial meningitis should have emergent lumbar puncture with Gram stain and cerebrospinal fluid culture. If there is concern about a focal neurologic problem—such as may occur with abscess—CT or MRI of the brain may be performed before lumbar puncture.

Antibiotics should be started immediately, without waiting for imaging study or lumbar puncture if a delay is anticipated in these procedures. Corticosteroids should also be given if pneumococcal meningitis is suspected. The importance of the immune response in triggering cerebral edema has led researchers to study the role of adjuvant anti-inflammatory medications for bacterial meningitis. A meta-analysis of studies of concurrent glucocorticoid and first-dose antibiotic administration has shown a slight decrease in the risk of sensorineural hearing loss and in mortality among adults with pneumococcal meningitis.

CASE 15

A. The patient has a moderately severe infection and an underlying diagnosis of COPD, requiring hospitalization but not ICU admission. The most likely pathogens are *S pneumoniae*, *H influenzae*, and *M catarrhalis*. Other potential pathogens include *Mycoplasma pneumoniae*, *Chlamydophila pneumoniae*, *Legionella pneumophila*, and respiratory viruses. Tuberculosis and fungi should also be considered, although these are less likely in this patient with such an acute presentation. Anaerobes are also unlikely without a history of substance abuse or recent depressed mental status. If this patient required ICU admission, the atypical pathogens, *M pneumoniae* and *C pneumoniae*, are much less likely, and *S aureus* and *Pseudomonas aeruginosa* should be added to the differential diagnosis, particularly if the patient had been recently hospitalized.

B. Pulmonary pathogens reach the lungs by one of three routes: (1) direct inhalation of infectious droplets into the lower airways; (2) aspiration of oropharyngeal content; or (3) hematogenous spread.

C. Normal pulmonary antimicrobial defense mechanisms include the following: (1) aerodynamic filtration by subjecting incoming air to turbulence in the nasal passages and then abrupt changes in the direction of the airstream as it moves through the pharynx and tracheobronchial tree; (2) the cough reflex to remove aspirated material, excess secretions, and foreign bodies; (3) the mucociliary transport system, moving the mucous layer upward to the larynx; (4) phagocytic cells, including alveolar macrophages and polymorphonuclear neutrophils (PMNs), as well as humoral and cellular immune responses, which help to eliminate the pathogens; and (5) pulmonary secretions containing surfactant, lysozyme, and iron-binding proteins, which further aid in bacterial killing.

D. Common host risk factors include the following: (1) an immunocompromised state, resulting in immune dysfunction and increased risk of infection; (2) chronic lung disease, resulting in decreased mucociliary clearance; (3) alcoholism or

other reduction of the level of consciousness, which increases the risk of aspiration; (4) injection drug abuse, which increases the risk of hematogenous spread of pathogens; (5) environmental or animal exposure, resulting in inhalation of specific pathogens; (6) residence in an institution, with its associated risk of microaspirations, and exposure via instrumentation (catheters and intubation); and (7) recent influenza infection, leading to disruption of respiratory epithelium, ciliary dysfunction, and inhibition of PMNs. This patient has a history of chronic lung disease, increasing his risk of pneumonia, and he is immunocompromised by the use of corticosteroids for his COPD.

CASE 16

A. There are many primary modes of pathogen transmission causing infectious diarrhea. Pathogens such as *Vibrio cholerae* are water-borne and transmitted via a contaminated water supply. Several pathogens, including *S aureus* and *Bacillus cereus*, are transmitted by contaminated food. Some pathogens, such as *Shigella* and *Rotavirus*, are transmitted by person-to-person spread and are, therefore, commonly seen in institutional settings such as child care centers. Finally, *Clostridium difficile* infection can result from overgrowth after antibiotic administration.

B. The description of this patient's diarrhea as profuse and watery suggests a small bowel site of infection. The small bowel is the site of significant electrolyte and fluid transportation. Disruption of this process leads to the production of profuse watery diarrhea, as seen in this patient.

C. The most likely cause of diarrhea in this patient, who has recently returned from Mexico, is enterotoxigenic *E coli* (ETEC), which is the most common cause of traveler's diarrhea. Diarrhea results from the production of two enterotoxins that "poison" the cells of the small intestine, causing watery diarrhea. ETEC produces both a heat-labile and a heat-stable enterotoxin. The heat-labile enterotoxin activates adenylyl cyclase and the formation of cAMP, which stimulates water and electrolyte secretion by intestinal endothelial cells. The heat-stable toxin produced by ETEC results in guanylyl cyclase activation, also causing watery diarrhea.

CASE 17

A. The factors that contribute to hospital-related sepsis are invasive monitoring devices, indwelling catheters, extensive surgical procedures, and increased numbers of immunocompromised patients.

B. Sepsis generally starts with a localized infection. Bacteria may then invade the bloodstream directly (leading to bacteremia and positive blood cultures) or may proliferate locally and release toxins into the bloodstream. Gram-negative bacteria contain an endotoxin, the lipid A component of the lipopolysaccharide–phospholipid–protein complex present in the outer cell membrane. Endotoxin activates the coagulation cascade, the complement system, and the kinin system, as well as the release of several host mediators such as cytokines, platelet-activating factor, endorphins, endothelium-derived relaxing factor, arachidonic acid metabolites, myocardial depressant factors, nitric oxide, and others. As sepsis persists, host immunosuppression plays a critical role. Specific stimuli such as the organism, inoculum, and site of infection stimulate CD4 T cells to secrete cytokines with either inflammatory (type 1 helper T cell) or anti-inflammatory (type 2 helper T cell) properties (Figure 4–11). Patients who die of sepsis experience a significant loss of cells essential for the adaptive immune response (B lymphocytes, CD4 T cells, dendritic cells). Apoptosis is thought to play a key role in the decrease in these cell lines and downregulates the surviving immune cells.

C. A hyperdynamic circulatory state, described as distributive shock to emphasize the maldistribution of blood flow to various tissues, is the common hemodynamic finding in sepsis. The release of vasoactive substances (including nitric oxide) results in a loss of the normal mechanisms of vascular autoregulation, producing imbalances in blood flow, with regional shunting and the relative hypoperfusion of some organs. Myocardial depression also occurs, with reductions in both the left and right ventricular ejection fractions and increases in end-diastolic and end-systolic volumes. This myocardial depression has been attributed to the direct toxic effects of nitric oxide, TNF, and IL-1. Refractory hypotension can ensue, resulting in end-organ hypoperfusion and injury.

D. Organ failure results from a combination of decreased perfusion and microvascular injury induced by local and systemic inflammatory responses to infection. The maldistribution of blood flow is accentuated by impaired erythrocyte deformability, with microvascular obstruction. The aggregation of neutrophils and platelets may also reduce blood flow. The demargination of neutrophils from the vascular endothelium results in a further release of inflammatory mediators and the subsequent migration of neutrophils into tissues. Components of the complement system are activated, attracting more neutrophils and releasing locally active substances such as prostaglandins and leukotrienes. The net result of all these changes is microvascular collapse and, ultimately, organ failure.

E. The outcome in sepsis depends on the number of organs that fail, with a mortality rate of 70% in patients who develop failure of three or more organ systems.

CASE 18

A. Carcinoid tumors arise from neuroendocrine tissue, specifically the enterochromaffin cells. These cells migrate during embryogenesis to the submucosal layer of the intestines and the pulmonary bronchi. Therefore, carcinoid tumors are most commonly found in the intestines and lungs.

B. Since carcinoid tumors are derived from neuroendocrine tissue, they can secrete many peptides that have systemic effects. This secretion is due to the inappropriate activation of the latent synthetic ability that all neuroendocrine cells possess. Many of the peptides, such as serotonin, can cause vasodilation, resulting in flushing. They can also cause wheezing, diarrhea, excessive salivation, and fibrosis of the heart valves and other tissues.

C. Serotonin production is characteristic of gut carcinoid tumors. Serotonin is metabolized to 5-HIAA. Therefore, finding high levels of 5-HIAA in a 24-hour urine collection in a patient with flushing or other symptoms is highly suggestive of the diagnosis. Bronchial carcinoids rarely produce 5-HIAA and, therefore, rarely present with carcinoid syndrome; instead, they often produce ectopic ACTH, resulting in Cushing syndrome.

CASE 19

A. Adenomas are thought to be related to colorectal carcinoma by means of stepwise genetic alterations (or hits), with adenomas representing a precancerous lesion that may ultimately progress to cancer. It is believed that stepwise genetic alterations, including both oncogene activation and tumor suppressor gene inactivation, result in phenotypic changes that progress to neoplasia.

B. Two principal lines of evidence support the model of stepwise genetic alterations in colon cancer: (1) Familial colon cancer syndromes are known to result from germline mutations, implicating a genomic cause. Familial adenomatous polyposis is the result of a mutation in the APC gene, whereas hereditary nonpolyposis colorectal carcinoma is associated with mutations in the DNA repair genes hMSH2 and hMLH1. (2) Several factors linked to an increased risk of colon cancer are known to be carcinogenic. Substances derived from bacterial colonic flora, foods, and endogenous metabolites are known to be mutagenic. Levels of these substances can be decreased by following a low-fat, high-fiber diet. Epidemiologic studies suggest that such a change in diet might reduce the risk of colon cancer.

C. The earliest molecular defect in the pathogenesis of colon cancer is the acquisition of somatic mutations in the APC gene in the normal colonic mucosa. This defect causes abnormal β-catenin regulation, which leads to abnormal cell proliferation and the initial steps of tumor formation. Subsequent defects in the TGF-β signaling pathway inactivate this important growth inhibitory pathway and lead to further tumor mucosal proliferation and the development of small adenomas. Mutational activation of the K-ras gene leads to the constitutive activation of an important proliferative signaling pathway and is common at these stages. It further increases the proliferative potential of the adenomatous tumor cells. The deletion or loss of expression of the DCC gene is common in the progression to invasive colon cancers. The DCC protein is a transmembrane protein of the immunoglobulin superfamily and may be a receptor for certain extracellular molecules that guide cell growth or apoptosis. Mutational *p53* inactivation is also a commonly observed step in the development of invasive colon cancer, seen in late adenomas and early invasive cancers, and leads to the loss of an important cell cycle checkpoint and the inability to activate the p53-dependent apoptotic pathways. In parallel to these sequential abnormalities in the regulation of cell proliferation, colon cancers also acquire defects in mechanisms that protect genomic stability. These generally involve mutations in mismatch repair genes that prevent chromosomal instability, including *MSH2*, *MLH1*, *PMS1*, and *PMS2*. Germline mutations in these genes cause hereditary nonpolyposis colorectal cancer (HNPCC) syndrome. Nonhereditary colon cancers develop genomic instability through defects in the chromosomal instability (CIN) genes. Defects in these genes lead to the gain or loss of large segments or entire chromosomes during replication, leading to aneuploidy.

D. Early in the progression of dysplasia, disrupted architecture results in the formation of fragile new blood vessels and the destruction of existing blood vessels. These changes often occur before invasion of the basement membrane and, therefore, before progression to true cancer formation. These friable vessels can cause microscopic bleeding. This can be screened for by fecal occult blood tests, an important tool in the early detection of precancerous and cancerous colonic lesions.

CASE 20

A. Linkage analysis has identified genetic markers known to confer a high risk of developing breast cancer. Two such genes in particular have been found: *BRCA1* and *BRCA2*. Both are involved in DNA repair. Inherited mutations of *BRCA1* or *BRCA2* are associated with a lifetime risk in women of developing breast cancer of up to 70%. Mutations in these genes are also associated with a high incidence of ovarian cancer in females and an increased incidences of prostate cancer, melanoma, and breast cancer in males.

B. There are two major subtypes of breast cancer. Ductal carcinomas, the majority, arise from the collecting ducts in the breast glandular tissue. Lobular carcinomas arise from the terminal lobules of the glands.

C. While it is still contained by the basement membrane, the tumor is called carcinoma in situ. Invasive carcinoma occurs when tumor cells breach the basement membrane. Both ductal and lobular carcinomas may be either in situ or invasive. By definition, an in situ tumor does not carry a risk of spreading to the lymph nodes or of creating distant metastases. Finding an in situ tumor increases the affected individual's risk of developing a subsequent breast cancer, in either breast and of either subtype. Therefore, carcinoma in situ is a marker of heightened susceptibility to developing invasive breast cancer.

D. There are specific therapies that target receptors present in breast cancer. The amount of estrogen exposure is correlated with breast cancer risk. Antiestrogen therapy has long been used with success in patients with estrogen receptor–positive breast cancer, although half of patients diagnosed with breast cancer are estrogen receptor negative. More recently, antibodies that target the HER2 receptor, a tyrosine kinase growth factor receptor, are used in tumors with an overexpression of the HER2 receptor.

CASE 21

A. Testicular cancer arises from germinal elements within the testes. Germ cells give rise to spermatozoa and thus can theoretically retain the ability to differentiate into any cell type. The pluripotent nature of these cells is witnessed in the production of mature teratomas. These benign tumors often contain mature elements of all three germ cell layers, including hair and teeth.

B. During early embryogenesis, the germline epithelium migrates along the midline of the embryo. This migration is followed by the formation of the urogenital ridge and ultimately the aggregation of germline cells to form the testes and ovaries. The pattern of migration of the germline epithelium predicts the location of extragonadal testicular neoplasms. These neoplasms are found in the midline axis of the lower cranium, mediastinum, and retroperitoneum.

C. One can monitor the serum concentrations of proteins expressed during embryonic or trophoblastic development to monitor tumor progression and response to therapy. These proteins include alpha-fetoprotein and human chorionic gonadotropin.

CASE 22

A. Sarcomas arise from mesenchymal tissue. These include myocytes, adipocytes, osteoblasts, chondrocytes, fibroblasts, endothelial cells, and synovial cells.

B. Many sarcomas are more common in younger people. This is thought to be because the cells of origin, such as chondrocytes or osteoblasts, divide more rapidly in childhood and adolescence than in adulthood.

C. Because osteosarcomas arise from osteoblasts, they retain their ability to produce a bone matrix of calcium and phosphorus within the tumor.

CASE 23

A. The theory that chronic immune stimulation or modulation may play an early role in the formation of lymphoma is supported by several observations. Iatrogenic immunosuppression, as seen in this patient and in other transplant patients, can increase the risk of B-cell lymphoma, possibly associated with Epstein–Barr virus infection. An increased risk of lymphoma is also seen in other immunosuppressed patients, such as those with AIDS or other autoimmune diseases. Chronic immune stimulation such as chronic gastritis from *Helicobacter pylori* may give rise to gastric mucosa-associated tissue (MALT) lymphomas.

B. This patient has been diagnosed with a follicular cleaved cell lymphoma, a well-differentiated or low-grade lymphoma. Low-grade lymphomas retain the morphology and patterns of gene expression of mature lymphocytes, including cell surface markers such as immunoglobulin in the case of B lymphocytes. Their clinical course is generally more favorable, being characterized by a slow growth rate. Paradoxically, however, these lymphomas tend to present at a more advanced stage, as in this case.

C. Follicular lymphomas arise from lymphoblasts of the B-cell lineage. Common chromosomal abnormalities include translocations of chromosome 14, including t(14;18), t(11;14), and t(14;19). The t(14;18) translocation results in a fusion gene known as IgH;*bcl-2*, which juxtaposes the immunoglobulin heavy chain enhancer on chromosome 14 in front of the *bcl-2* gene on chromosome 18. This results in the enhanced expression of an inner mitochondrial protein encoded by *bcl-2*, which has been found to inhibit the natural process of cell death, or apoptosis. Apoptosis is required to remove certain lymphoid clones whose function is not needed. Inhibition of this process probably contributes to the proliferation of lymphoma cells.

D. This patient's symptoms of fever and weight loss are known as B symptoms. They are thought to be mediated by a variety of cytokines produced by lymphoma cells, or they may occur as a reaction of normal immune cells to the lymphoma. Two commonly implicated cytokines are IL-1 and TNF.

CASE 24

A. Like all neoplasms, leukemias are classified by their cell of origin. The first branch point is whether the malignant cell is of myeloid or lymphoid lineage, resulting in either a myeloid or lymphocytic leukemia. All types can be acute, presenting with more than 20% blasts on bone marrow biopsy, or chronic, presenting in a more indolent fashion, usually with a slowly progressive course of many years. Lymphocytic leukemias are further divided into T-cell or B-cell leukemias depending on the type of lymphoid cell of origin. The type can be distinguished by the cluster of differentiation (CD) antigens found on the surface of the tumor cells. Myeloid leukemias are also divided into subtypes depending on the type of myeloid cell from which the leukemia arises. AML types M1–M3 arise from myeloblasts. Types M4 and M5 arise from monocytes. Type M6 arises from erythrocyte precursors called normoblasts. Type M7 arises from platelet precursors called megakaryoblasts.

B. Acute leukemias typically present with pancytopenia, a decrease in the count of all normal blood cells, including the

normal white cells (the leukemic cells accounting for almost all the high total WBCs), red blood cells, and platelets. This is caused by the crowding out of normal precursors in the bone marrow by the abnormally dividing blast cells, and by the inhibition of normal hematopoiesis owing to the secretion of cytokines and inhibitory substances. The patient's presenting symptoms are directly related to the blood abnormalities. The fatigue and pallor are due to the anemia (lack of red blood cells) and the resulting reduced oxygen-carrying capacity. The petechiae and bleeding are from the lack of platelets, inhibiting the ability of the blood to clot. Patients with leukemia are susceptible to serious infections owing to the lack of normal WBCs. Finally, the markedly elevated number of leukemic cells can clog small blood vessels and result in strokes, retinal vein occlusion, and pulmonary infarction.

C. Chromosomal deletions, duplications, and translocations have been identified in leukemias. One such genetic abnormality is the so-called Philadelphia chromosome, a balanced translocation of chromosomes 9 and 22, that is commonly found in chronic myelogenous leukemia (CML). This translocation results in a fusion gene, *bcr-abl*, that encodes a kinase that phosphorylates key proteins involved in cell growth. Targeted therapies that inhibit the enzymatic function of the bcr-abl kinase by competing with the ATP-binding site induce remissions in most patients in chronic phases of CML.

CASE 25

A. The patient's confusion and decreased level of consciousness likely result from his high serum calcium level (hypercalcemia). Hypercalcemia of this magnitude can result in altered sensorium, coma, and even death.

B. Hypercalcemia can occur in many types of malignancies. It has several causes, including the secretion of a parathyroid hormone–like peptide as a result of the activation of the parathyroid hormone–related protein (PTHrP) gene, as well as the elaboration of locally acting cytokines that increase bone uptake in areas of tumor infiltration.

C. Hyponatremia caused by the syndrome of inappropriate antidiuretic hormone (SIADH) can also occur as a paraneoplastic phenomenon, occurring most often in patients with small cell lung cancer. The result of ectopic ADH production is a retention of free water and consequent hyponatremia. Severe hyponatremia can result in altered sensorium, coma, and death.

CASE 26

A. The most likely cause of anemia in this patient is iron deficiency. Iron deficiency anemia is the most common form of anemia. In developed nations, it is primarily the result of iron loss, almost always through blood loss. In men and in postmenopausal women, blood is most commonly lost from the GI tract, as in this case. In premenopausal women, menstrual blood loss is the major cause of iron deficiency.

In this man, there are no symptoms of significant bleeding from the gut as would be manifested by gross blood (hematochezia) or metabolized blood in the stool (melena, usually described as black-colored stool), and he has no GI complaints. This makes some of the benign GI disorders such as peptic ulcer, arteriovenous malformations, and angiodysplasias less likely. He has no symptoms of inflammatory bowel disease such as diarrhea or abdominal pain. Concern is thus aroused about a possible malignancy, particularly colon cancer.

When no source of bleeding is uncovered, insufficient dietary intake (eg, strict vegetarian diets) and GI malabsorption should be considered as a possible cause of iron deficiency anemia. Such malabsorption occurs in patients with celiac disease, *H pylori* infection, partial gastrectomy, or gastric bypass surgery. Other mechanisms of iron deficiency anemia include intravascular hemolysis (paroxysmal nocturnal hemoglobinuria or cardiac valvular disease) and iron depletion in response to erythropoietin treatment.

B. Blood loss results in anemia via a reduction in heme synthesis. With a loss of blood comes a loss of iron, the central ion in the oxygen-carrying molecule, heme. In iron deficiency, the final step in heme synthesis, during which ferrous iron is inserted into protoporphyrin IX, is interrupted, resulting in inadequate heme synthesis. Globin biosynthesis is inhibited by heme deficiency through a heme-regulated translational inhibitor (HRI). Elevated HRI activity (a result of heme deficiency) inhibits a key transcription initiation factor for heme synthesis, eIF2. Thus, there are both less heme and fewer globin chains available in each red cell precursor. This directly causes anemia, a decrease in the hemoglobin concentration of the blood.

C. In this symptomatic man, the peripheral blood smear is likely to be significantly abnormal. As the hemoglobin concentration of individual red blood cells falls, the cells take on the classic picture of microcytic (small), hypochromic (pale) erythrocytes. There is also apt to be anisocytosis (variation in size) and poikilocytosis (variation in shape), with target cells. The target cells occur because of the relative excess of red cell membrane compared with the amount of hemoglobin within the cell, leading to a "bunching up" of the membrane in the center.

D. Laboratory tests may be ordered to confirm the diagnosis. The most commonly ordered test is serum ferritin, which, if low, is diagnostic of iron deficiency. Results may be misleading, however, in acute or chronic inflammation and severe illness. Because ferritin is an acute-phase reactant, it can rise in these conditions, resulting in a normal ferritin level. Serum iron and transferrin levels can also be misleading because these levels can fall not only in anemia but also in many other illnesses. Typically in iron deficiency, however, serum iron levels are low, whereas total iron-binding capacity (TIBC) is elevated. The ratio of serum iron to TIBC is less than 20% in uncomplicated iron deficiency. Serum (soluble) transferrin receptor (TfR), released by erythroid precursors, is elevated

in iron deficiency. A high ratio of TfR to ferritin may predict iron deficiency when ferritin is not diagnostically low. Though helpful, this test has seen limited use in clinical practice.

Occasionally when blood tests are misleading, a bone marrow biopsy is performed to examine for iron stores. Iron is normally stored as ferritin in the macrophages of the bone marrow and is stained blue by Prussian blue stain. A decrease in the amount of iron stores on bone marrow biopsy is diagnostic of iron deficiency. More commonly, however, the response to an empiric trial of iron supplementation is used to determine the presence of iron deficiency in complicated cases.

E. Fatigue, weakness, and shortness of breath are the direct results of decreased oxygen-carrying capacity, which leads to decreased oxygen delivery to metabolically active tissues, causing this patient's symptoms. He is pale because there is less oxygenated hemoglobin per unit of blood, and oxygenated hemoglobin is red, giving color to the skin. Pallor also results from a compensatory mechanism whereby superficial blood vessels constrict, diverting blood to more vital structures.

CASE 27

A. The probable cause of this woman's anemia is vitamin B_{12} (cobalamin) deficiency, which is characterized by anemia, glossitis, and neurologic impairment. Vitamin B_{12} deficiency results in anemia via effects on DNA synthesis. Cobalamin is a crucial cofactor in the synthesis of deoxythymidine from deoxyuridine. Cobalamin accepts a methyl group from methyltetrahydrofolate, leading to the formation of methylcobalamin and reduced tetrahydrofolate. Methylcobalamin is required for the production of the amino acid methionine from homocysteine. Reduced tetrahydrofolate is required as the single-carbon donor in purine synthesis. Thus, cobalamin deficiency depletes tetrahydrofolate stores, lowering purine production and impairing DNA synthesis. Impaired DNA synthesis results in a decreased production of red blood cells. It also causes megaloblastic changes in the blood cells in the bone marrow. These cells are subsequently destroyed in large numbers by intramedullary hemolysis. Both processes result in anemia.

B. The peripheral blood smear varies depending on the duration of cobalamin deficiency. In this patient, because she is profoundly symptomatic, we would expect a full-blown megaloblastic anemia. The peripheral smear would show significant anisocytosis and poikilocytosis of the red cells and hypersegmentation of the neutrophils. In severe cases, morphologic changes in peripheral blood cells may be difficult to differentiate from those seen in leukemia.

Other laboratory tests that may be ordered include a lactate dehydrogenase (LDH) level and indirect bilirubin determination. Both should be elevated in cobalamin deficiency, reflecting the intramedullary hemolysis that occurs in vitamin B_{12} deficiency. Serum vitamin B_{12} would be expected to be low. Yet there remain high rates of both false-positive and false-negative tests owing to the fact that only 20% of total measured serum B_{12} is bound to the cellular delivery protein, transcobalamin; the rest is bound to haptocorrin, which is not available for cells to use. Antibodies to intrinsic factor are usually detectable. Concurrent elevations of serum methylmalonic acid and serum homocysteine are highly predictive of B_{12} deficiency.

The various causes of megaloblastic anemia can often be differentiated by a Schilling test. This test measures the oral absorption of radioactively labeled vitamin B_{12} with and without added intrinsic factor, thereby directly evaluating the mechanism of the vitamin deficiency. It must be performed after cobalamin stores have been replenished.

C. Pernicious anemia is caused by autoimmune destruction of the gastric parietal cells, which are responsible for the production of stomach acid and intrinsic factor. Autoimmune destruction of these cells leads to achlorhydria (loss of stomach acid), which is required for the release of cobalamin from foodstuffs. The production of intrinsic factor decreases. Intrinsic factor is required for the effective absorption of cobalamin by the terminal ileum. Together, these mechanisms result in vitamin B_{12} deficiency.

There is strong evidence that parietal cell destruction is autoimmune in nature. Pathologically, patients with pernicious anemia demonstrate gastric mucosal atrophy with infiltrating lymphocytes, predominantly antibody-producing B cells. Furthermore, more than 90% of patients with this disease demonstrate antibodies to parietal cell membrane proteins, primarily to the proton pump. More than half of patients also have antibodies to intrinsic factor or to the intrinsic factor–cobalamin complex. These patients are also at increased risk for other autoimmune diseases.

D. The patient's tachycardia is probably a reflection of profound anemia. Unlike many other causes of anemia, pernicious anemia often leads to very severe decreases in the hemoglobin concentration. This results in a marked decrease in the oxygen-carrying capacity of the blood. The only way to increase oxygenation to metabolically active tissues is to increase cardiac output. This is accomplished by raising the heart rate. Over time, the stresses this puts on the heart can result in high-output heart failure.

The neurologic manifestations—paresthesias and impaired proprioception—seen in this patient are caused by demyelination of the peripheral nerves and posterolateral spinal columns, respectively. The lack of methionine caused by vitamin B_{12} deficiency appears to be at least partly responsible for this demyelination, but the exact mechanism is unknown. Demyelination eventually results in neuronal cell death. Therefore, neurologic symptoms may not be improved by treating the vitamin B_{12} deficiency.

CASE 28

A. Classic, childhood-onset, cyclic neutropenia results from mutations in the gene for a single enzyme: neutrophil elastase.

Most cases reflect an autosomal dominant inheritance; however, sporadic adult cases also occur, and these are also associated with neutrophil elastase mutations.

Studies of neutrophil kinetics in affected patients reveal that the gene defect results in the abnormal production—rather than abnormal disposition—of neutrophils. In cyclic neutropenia, it is hypothesized that the mutant neutrophil elastase may have an overly inhibitory effect, causing prolonged trough periods and inadequate storage pools to maintain a normal peripheral neutrophil count. This production defect affects other cell lines as well, resulting in cyclic depletion of all storage pools. Because the development of neutrophils from the progenitor stage to maturity takes 2 weeks and the life span is only 12 days, depletion of the neutrophil cell line becomes clinically apparent. The other cell lines have longer life spans, and although they too undergo cyclic decreases in production, these decreases do not become clinically apparent.

The exact cause of the relationship between the cyclic waves of maturation and the neutrophil elastase mutation is not known. Because multiple cell lines are seen to cycle, it is believed that neutrophil elastase mutations accelerate the process of apoptosis in early progenitor cells unless they are "rescued" by granulocyte colony-stimulating factor (G-CSF). Some evidence suggests that neutrophil elastase can antagonize G-CSF action, but the relationship of mutated neutrophil elastase to G-CSF action in cyclic neutropenia is not well understood.

Clinically, administering pharmacologic doses of G-CSF (filgrastim) to affected individuals has three interesting effects that partially overcome the condition. First, although cycling continues, mean neutrophil counts increase at each point in the cycle, such that patients are rarely neutropenic. Second, cycling periodicity decreases immediately from 21 days to 14 days. Third, other cell line fluctuations change in parallel; their cycle periodicity also decreases to 14 days, suggesting that an early progenitor cell is indeed at the center of this illness. However, the fact that cycling does not disappear demonstrates that there are other abnormalities yet to be discovered. It also suggests that there may be an inherent cycling of all stem cells in normal individuals, which is modulated by multiple cytokines in the marrow.

B. The periodic neutropenia with spontaneous remission seen in this patient is characteristic of cyclic neutropenia. In this disease, patients develop a drop in neutrophil count approximately every 3 weeks (19–22 days), with nadirs (low neutrophil counts) lasting 3–5 days. Patients are generally well during periods when the neutrophil cell count is normal and become symptomatic as the count drops below 250/μL. Neutrophils are responsible for a significant portion of the immune system's response to both bacterial and fungal infections. Thus, the primary clinical manifestation of cyclic neutropenia is recurrent infection. Each nadir is usually characterized by symptoms of fever and malaise. Cervical lymphadenopathy and oral ulcers, as seen in this patient, are also common. Life-threatening bacterial and fungal infections are uncommon but can occur, particularly as a result of infection from endogenous gut flora. More commonly, however, patients develop skin infections and chronic gingivitis.

C. The peripheral blood smear should be normal except for a paucity of neutrophils. The neutrophils present would be normal in appearance. The bone marrow, however, would be expected to show increased numbers of myeloid precursors such as promyelocytes and myelocytes. Mature neutrophils would be rare. If marrow examination were repeated in 2 weeks—after neutrophil counts have improved—the results would be normal.

CASE 29

A. The most likely diagnosis in this patient is drug-associated immune thrombocytopenia. Many drugs—but most commonly heparin—have been associated with this phenomenon. There is a 10-fold increased risk for heparin-induced thrombocytopenia (HIT) in patients receiving unfractionated heparin (UFH) compared with those receiving low-molecular-weight heparin (LMWH). Cardiac or orthopedic surgery patients have a higher risk of clinical HIT (1–5%) than medical or obstetric patients (0.1–1%) when receiving UFH. Women have twice the risk for HIT as men.

B. Heparin leads to thrombocytopenia via two distinct mechanisms, both involving antibodies. It appears that heparin can bind to a platelet-produced protein, platelet factor 4 (PF4), which is released by platelets in response to activation. The heparin–PF4 complex acts as an antigenic stimulus, provoking the production of IgG. IgG can then bind to the complex, forming IgG–heparin–PF4. The new complex can bind to platelets via the Fc receptor of the IgG molecule or via the PF4 receptor. This binding can lead to two distinct phenomena. The first is platelet destruction by the spleen. Antibody adherence to the platelets changes their shape, causing the spleen to recognize them as abnormal and destroy them. This leads to simple thrombocytopenia, with few sequelae.

The second phenomenon is platelet activation, which can lead to more significant sequelae. After the formation of an IgG–heparin–PF4 complex, both IgG and PF4 can bind to platelets. The platelets can become cross-linked, leading to platelet aggregation. This decreases the number of circulating platelets, leading to thrombocytopenia. However, it may also lead to the formation of a thrombus, or "white clot."

C. Even though the platelet count in drug-associated immune thrombocytopenia may be very low, significant bleeding is unusual. Most commonly, the primary manifestation is easy bruising, and, at platelet counts fewer than 5000/μL, petechiae may be seen on the skin or mucous membranes. When actual bleeding does occur, it is generally mucosal in origin, such as nosebleed, gingival bleeding, or GI blood loss.

As noted, when thrombocytopenia is due to heparin, paradoxical clotting may occur instead of bleeding. Thrombus formation often occurs at the site of previous vascular injury

or abnormality and can present as either arterial or venous thrombosis.

CASE 30

A. The Virchow triad consists of three possible contributors to the formation of a clot: (1) decreased blood flow; (2) blood vessel injury or inflammation; and (3) changes in the intrinsic properties of the blood. This patient has no history of immobility or other cause of decreased blood flow. She does, however, have a history of blood vessel injury (ie, deep vein thrombosis). Despite the absence of symptoms of a lower extremity thrombus, this is still the most likely site of origin of the pulmonary embolus. Finally, the recurrence now of thrombus formation along with the family history of clots is suggestive of a change in the intrinsic properties of the blood, as seen in the inherited hypercoagulable states.

B. The most common hypercoagulable states include activated protein C resistance (factor V Leiden), protein C deficiency, protein S deficiency, antithrombin III deficiency, and hyperprothrombinemia (prothrombin gene mutation). Except for hyperprothrombinemia, each of these results in clot formation because of a lack of adequate anticoagulation rather than an overproduction of procoagulant activity; hyperprothrombinemia is caused by excess thrombin generation.

The most common site of the problem in the coagulation cascade is at factor Va, which is required for the formation of the prothrombinase complex with factor Xa, which leads to the thrombin burst and fibrin generation during hemostasis. Protein C is the major inhibitor of factor Va. It acts by cleaving factor V into an inactive form, thereby slowing the activation of factor X. The negative effect of protein C is enhanced by protein S. A quantitative or qualitative reduction in either of these two proteins thus results in the unregulated procoagulant action of factor Xa.

Activated protein C resistance is the most common inherited hypercoagulable state. It results from a mutation in the factor V gene. This mutation alters the three-dimensional conformation of the cleavage site within factor Va, where protein C usually binds. Protein C is then unable to bind to factor Va and is, therefore, unable to inactivate it. Coagulation is not inhibited.

Antithrombin inhibits the coagulation cascade at an alternative site. It inhibits the serine proteases: factors II, IX, X, XI, and XII. Antithrombin deficiency results in an inability to inactivate these factors, allowing the coagulation cascade to proceed unrestrained at multiple coagulation steps.

Hyperprothrombinemia is the second most common hereditary hypercoagulable state and the only one so far recognized as being due to the overproduction of procoagulant factors. It is caused by a mutation of the prothrombin gene that leads to elevated prothrombin levels. The increased risk of thrombosis is thought to be due to excess thrombin generation when the Xa–Va–Ca^{2+}–PL complex is activated.

C. This patient may be evaluated by various laboratory tests for the presence of an inherited hypercoagulable state.

A quantitative evaluation of the relative amounts of protein C, protein S, and antithrombin can be performed. Qualitative tests that assess the ability of these proteins to inhibit the coagulation cascade can be measured via clotting assays. The presence of the specific mutation in factor V Leiden can be assessed via polymerase chain reaction testing.

CASE 31

A. The patient has cerebellar ataxia, likely from long-term alcohol abuse. The causes of ataxia are varied. Ataxia may result from vascular insults to the cerebellum, toxic insults (including alcohol), infections, autoimmune disorders, vitamin deficiency (eg, thiamine, vitamin E), and degenerative disorders (inherited or sporadic).

B. The clinical features of cerebellar ataxia include (1) ataxic gait, which results in a widened base, staggering, falls, and, if severe, wheelchair confinement; (2) truncal ataxia, which can result in the inability of patients to sit unsupported by their arms; (3) dysmetria, which refers to an impaired ability to perform accurate movements during ballistic movements owing to a faulty estimation of distance; (4) limb ataxia, which results in difficulty with coordinated tasks; (5) vertigo with nausea and vomiting resulting from damage to the vestibulocerebellum; (6) static and kinetic tremor, also called intention tremor; (7) cerebellar dysarthria, also termed scanning speech, resulting in slurred speech and, in severe cases, unintelligible speech; (8) the eye movement abnormalities of nystagmus and ocular dysmetria.

C. One might suspect an inherited form of cerebellar ataxia. Mutations in more than 450 genes are associated with cerebellar ataxia, some inherited dominantly and some recessively. The largest group of dominantly inherited ataxias result from glutamine-encoding CAG repeats in various disease genes. These include spinocerebellar ataxia (SCA) types 1, 2, 3, 6, 7, and 17. The pathogenesis of the dominant polyglutamine ataxias is thought to be a gain-of-function mutation causing an expanded number of glutamine repeats in the respective disease proteins. Although the putative roles of these different proteins are diverse, the clinical features of the polyglutamine SCAs are remarkably similar, and it is difficult clinically to distinguish one type of SCA from another. The mechanism by which polyglutamine expansion leads to ataxia remains unknown.

CASE 32

A. The most common form of motor neuron disease in adults is amyotrophic lateral sclerosis (ALS), in which mixed upper and lower motor neuron deficits are found in limb and bulbar muscles. In 80% of patients, the initial symptoms are due to limb muscle weakness. Complaints are often bilateral but asymmetric. The involvement of bulbar muscles causes difficulty swallowing, chewing, speaking, breathing, and coughing.

Neurologic examination reveals a mixture of upper and lower motor neuron signs. There is usually no involvement of the extraocular muscles or sphincters. The disease is progressive and generally fatal within 3–5 years, with death usually resulting from pulmonary infection and respiratory failure.

B. In ALS, there is a selective degeneration of motor neurons in the primary motor cortex and the anterolateral horns of the spinal cord. Many affected neurons show cytoskeletal disease with accumulations of intermediate filaments in the cell body and axons. There is only a subtle glial cell response and little evidence of inflammation.

C. There are several theories concerning the molecular pathogenesis of ALS. Glutamate is the most abundant excitatory neurotransmitter in the CNS and functions to generate an excitatory postsynaptic potential and raise the concentration of free intracellular Ca^{2+} in the cytosol of the postsynaptic neuron. This Ca^{2+} signal activates calcium-sensitive enzymes and is quickly terminated by the removal of glutamate from the synapse and by mechanisms for calcium sequestration and extrusion in the postsynaptic cell. In 60% of patients with sporadic ALS, there is a large decrease in glutamate transport activity in the motor cortex and spinal cord, but not in other regions of the CNS. This has been associated with a loss of the astrocytic glutamate transporter protein excitatory amino acid transporter 2 (EAAT2), perhaps resulting from a defect in the splicing of its messenger RNA. In cultured spinal cord slices, the pharmacologic inhibition of glutamate transport induces motor neuron degeneration.

About 10% of ALS cases are familial, and 20% of these familial cases are due to missense mutations in the cytosolic copper–zinc superoxide dismutase (*SOD1*) gene on the long arm of chromosome 21. *SOD1* catalyzes the formation of hydrogen peroxide from superoxide anion. Hydrogen peroxide is then detoxified by catalase or glutathione peroxidase to form water. Not all mutations reduce *SOD1* activity, and the disorder is typically inherited as an autosomal dominant trait, suggesting that familial ALS results from a gain of function, rather than a loss of function, of the SOD1 gene product. One hypothesis suggests that the mutant enzyme has an altered substrate specificity catalyzing the reduction of hydrogen peroxide to yield hydroxyl radicals and using peroxynitrite to produce the nitration of tyrosine residues in proteins.

A role for neurofilament dysfunction in ALS is supported by the finding that neurofilamentous inclusions in cell bodies and proximal axons are an early feature of ALS pathology. In addition, mutations in the heavy chain neurofilament subunit (NF-H) have been detected in some patients with sporadic ALS, suggesting that NF-H variants may be a risk factor for ALS.

The exciting discovery of the protein called transactive response DNA-binding protein 43 (TDP 43) may offer new clues to the etiology of this disorder. This newly discovered protein is the major component of the ubiquitinated, tau-negative inclusions that are the pathological hallmark of sporadic and familial ALS and frontotemporal dementia (FTD). It is also found in some cases of Alzheimer disease and Parkinson disease. Mutations in this gene, located on chromosome 1, co-segregate with disease in familial forms of ALS and FTD and are not found in *SOD1* familial ALS. FTD and ALS overlap in approximately 15–25% of cases, and these disorders are starting to be referred to as "TDP-43 proteinopathies." Several other genes and gene regions have been identified to cause both FTD and ALS, including *TARDBP* on chromosome 1p36.2, *MAPT* on chromosome 7q21, and *DCTN1* on chromosome 2p13.

The major genetic cause of ALS and/or FTD was recently discovered. Two independent groups identified hexanucleotide repeats in an intron of C9ORF72 on chromosome 9 in 34% of familial ALS cases, 6% of sporadic ALS cases, 26% of familial FTD cases, and 5% of sporadic FTD cases. The protein is of unknown function. These mutations likely induce a gain-of-function mutation similar to other noncoding repeat-expansion disorders. This discovery of another disorder caused by nucleotide repeats provides an additional rationale for the development of one or more new drugs focused on decreasing the expression of these toxic repeats.

CASE 33

A. This patient has parkinsonism. The resting tremor (which improves with activity), "cog-wheeling" rigidity, and difficulty with gait (especially with initiating walking and changing direction) are all characteristic of parkinsonism. While there are many causes of parkinsonism, including toxins, head trauma, drugs, encephalitis, and other degenerative diseases, the most common cause is Parkinson disease, an idiopathic degenerative neurological disorder.

B. Parkinson disease results from the selective degeneration of the monoamine-containing neurons in the basal ganglia and brainstem, particularly the pigmented dopaminergic neurons of the substantia nigra. This region is involved in regulating movement, particularly initiating and stopping actions. In addition to the degeneration of the dopaminergic neurons, scattered neurons elsewhere contain eosinophilic cytoplasmic inclusion bodies called Lewy bodies.

C. Through studies of familial cases of Parkinson disease and cases of parkinsonism produced by toxins, some of the molecular processes involved have been discovered. One cause of parkinsonism is 1-methyl-4-phenyl-1,2,3,6-tetrahydropyridine (MPTP), a neurotoxin once a contaminant in illicit opioid drugs. It causes parkinsonism by being metabolized to *N*-methyl-4-phenylpyridinium (MPP+), which is taken up through dopamine uptake sites on dopamine nerve terminals and concentrated in mitochondria. This leads to disturbed mitochondrial function and ultimately to cell death.

In familial cases of Parkinson disease, several mutations have been identified involving genes encoding several proteins: parkin, alpha-synuclein, DJ-1, ubiquitin, and PTEN-induced kinase. Mutations in the glucocerebrosidase (GCase) enzyme account for 3% of sporadic Parkinson disease cases and 25% of

juvenile-onset Parkinson disease cases. This enzyme is involved in lysosomal processing. The enzyme activity is reduced by 58% in the substantia nigra of patients with heterozygous familial Parkinson disease (it is reduced by 33% in the substantia nigra in those with sporadic [non-genetic] disease). The inhibition of this enzyme leads to an accumulation of α-synuclein, which in turn leads to the further inhibition of the enzyme. These mutations are being studied to find clues about the molecular mechanisms involved in the pathogenesis of Parkinson disease.

CASE 34

A. The most likely diagnosis in this patient is myasthenia gravis, a disease characterized by fluctuating fatigue and weakness in muscles with small motor units, particularly the ocular muscles. Myasthenia gravis is an autoimmune disorder resulting in a simplification of the postsynaptic region of the neuromuscular end plate.

Patients with this disease have lymphocytic infiltration at the end plate plus antibody and complement deposition along the postsynaptic membrane. Circulating antibodies to the receptor are present in 90% of patients, blocking acetylcholine binding and activation. The antibodies can cross-link the receptor molecules, leading to receptor internalization and degradation. They also activate the complement-mediated destruction of the postsynaptic region, resulting in the simplification of the end plate.

Many patients who lack antibodies to the acetylcholine receptor instead have autoantibodies against the muscle-specific receptor tyrosine kinase, which is an important mediator of acetylcholine receptor clustering at the end plate. These antibodies inhibit receptor clustering in muscle cell cultures. Thus, patients with myasthenia gravis have an impaired ability to respond to acetylcholine released from the presynaptic membrane.

Referred to as double-sero-negative patients, some myasthenia gravis patients have no antibodies for either acetylcholine receptor antibodies or MuSK. Recently, a new antibody has been found in 50% of these patients. Antibodies to lipoprotein-related protein 4 (LRP4), which is the agrin-binding receptor of the MuSK complex, disrupt agrin-induced acetylcholine receptor clustering, causing the disease symptoms. The clinical presentation of these patients is similar to that of patients with acetylcholine receptor myasthenia gravis without thymoma.

B. Muscles with small motor units are the muscles most affected in myasthenia gravis. The ocular muscles are most frequently affected; oropharyngeal muscles, flexors and extensors of the neck and proximal limbs, and erector spinae muscles are the next most commonly involved. In severe cases and without treatment, the disease can progress to involve all muscles, including the diaphragm and intercostal muscles, resulting in respiratory failure.

C. Normally, the number of quanta of acetylcholine released from the nerve terminal decreases with repetitive stimuli.

There are usually no clinical consequences of this decrease because a sufficient number of acetylcholine receptor channels are opened despite the reduced amount of neurotransmitter. In myasthenia gravis, however, there is a deficiency in the number of acetylcholine receptors. Therefore, as the number of quanta released decreases, there is a decremental decline in neurotransmission at the neuromuscular junction. This is manifested clinically as muscle fatigue with sustained or repeated activity.

D. Myasthenia gravis is associated both with a family history of autoimmune disease and with the presence of coexisting autoimmune diseases. Hyperthyroidism, rheumatoid arthritis, systemic lupus erythematosus, and polymyositis are all seen with increased frequency in these patients. These patients also have a high incidence of thymic disease; most demonstrate thymic hyperplasia, and 10–15% have thymomas.

E. There are two basic strategies for treating this disease: decreasing the immune-mediated destruction of the acetylcholine receptors and increasing the amount of acetylcholine available at the neuromuscular junction. As noted previously, many patients with myasthenia gravis demonstrate disease of the thymus gland. The thymus is thought to play a role in the pathogenesis of myasthenia gravis by supplying helper T cells sensitized to thymic nicotinic receptors. Removing the thymus of patients with generalized myasthenia gravis can improve symptoms and even induce remission. Plasmapheresis, corticosteroids, and immunosuppressant drugs can all be used to reduce the levels of antibody to acetylcholine receptors, thereby suppressing disease. Increasing the amount of acetylcholine available at the neuromuscular junction is accomplished by the use of cholinesterase inhibitors. Cholinesterase is responsible for the breakdown of acetylcholine at the neuromuscular junction. By inhibiting the breakdown of acetylcholine, cholinesterase inhibitors can compensate for the normal decline in released neurotransmitter during repeated stimulation and thus decrease symptoms.

CASE 35

A. The characteristic pathologic finding in Alzheimer disease (AD) is the presence of neuritic plaques, made of a dense amyloid core surrounded by dystrophic neuritis, reactive astrocytes, and microglia. There are also neurofibrillary tangles, synaptic loss, and neuronal loss. Interestingly, the severity of disease does not correlate with plaque number.

B. In neurologic disorders, the location of the lesion predicts what function will be affected. In AD, the neuritic plaques are most prominent in the hippocampus, entorhinal cortex, association cortex, and basal forebrain. These are areas involved in memory and higher-order cortical functions such as judgment and insight. This explains why memory loss, poor judgment, and denial are such common presenting symptoms. In contrast, the motor and sensory cortexes are not prominently affected, and thus a loss of motor and

sensory function does not present until much later in the course of the disease.

C. The major protein in neuritic plaques is amyloid beta-peptide. This is a protein derived from beta-amyloid precursor protein (APP), which is encoded by a gene on chromosome 21. Increased APP production results in increased amyloid beta-peptide, which is known to be toxic to cultured neurons. Individuals who produce excess APP, such as people with trisomy 21 or those with inherited mutations of the APP gene, develop early-onset AD.

D. Currently, there is no role for genetic testing in AD. Only about 10% of cases of AD are familial, and in these cases, several different mutations have been identified. It has also been recognized that individuals with subtype 4 of apolipoprotein E are at an increased risk of developing AD. However, 15% of the population carries this subtype, and most cases of AD develop in people who do not carry this subtype. Even among carriers, many never develop AD. Therefore, testing for it is not recommended.

CASE 36

A. Generalized tonic-clonic seizures are characterized by a sudden loss of consciousness followed rapidly by tonic muscle contractions, causing limb extension and back arching. This phase lasts approximately 10–30 seconds and is followed by a clonic phase of limb jerking. The jerking builds in frequency, peaking after 15–30 seconds, and then it gradually slows over another 15–30 seconds. The patient may remain unconscious for several minutes after the seizure. The seizure is generally followed by a period of confusion lasting minutes to hours.

B. Recurrent seizures are in many cases idiopathic, particularly in children. Seizures may also be due to brain injury from trauma, stroke, mass lesion, or infection. Finally, one must consider metabolic causes such as hypoglycemia, electrolyte abnormalities, and alcohol withdrawal. The cause of this patient's seizure is unknown because of the lack of an available history. However, because he has focal neurologic findings, with decreased movement on his left side, one must suspect an underlying brain lesion in the right cerebral hemisphere.

C. Seizures occur when neurons are activated synchronously. The kind of seizure depends on the location of the abnormal activity and the pattern of spread to different parts of the brain. The formation of a seizure focus in the brain may result from a disruption of normal inhibitory circuits. This disruption may occur because of alterations in ion channels or from injury to inhibitory neurons and synapses. Alternatively, a seizure focus may be formed when groups of neurons become synchronized by the reorganization of neural networks following a brain injury. After the formation of a seizure focus, local discharge may then spread. This spread occurs by a combination of mechanisms. After the synchronous depolarization of abnormally excitable neurons—known as the paroxysmal depolarizing shift—extracellular potassium accumulates, depolarizing nearby neurons. The increased depolarization frequency then leads to an increased calcium influx into nerve terminals. This increases the neurotransmitter release at excitatory synapses by a process known as post-tetanic potentiation, whereby normally quiescent, voltage-gated, N-methyl-D-aspartate (NMDA) receptor–gated excitatory synaptic neurotransmission is increased and inhibitory synaptic neurotransmission is decreased. The net effect of these changes is the recruitment of neighboring neurons into a synchronous discharge, causing a seizure.

CASE 37

A. The diagnosis in this patient is stroke, characterized by the sudden onset of focal neurologic deficits that persist for at least 24 hours owing to an abnormality of the cerebral circulation. The focal symptoms and signs that result from stroke correlate with the area of the brain supplied by the affected blood vessel. In this case, the patient has weakness and sensory loss on the right side. These symptoms suggest involvement of the left middle cerebral artery or at least its associated vascular territory. The vascular territory supplied by the middle cerebral artery includes the lateral frontal, parietal, lateral occipital, and anterior and superior temporal cortex and adjacent white matter, as well as the caudate, putamen, and internal capsule.

B. Risk factors for stroke include age, male sex, hypertension, hypercholesterolemia, diabetes, smoking, heavy alcohol consumption, and oral contraceptive use.

C. Stroke is classified as either ischemic or hemorrhagic in origin. Ischemic stroke may result from the thrombotic or embolic occlusion of the vessel. Hemorrhagic stroke may result from intraparenchymal hemorrhage, subarachnoid hemorrhage, subdural hemorrhage, epidural hemorrhage, or hemorrhage within an ischemic infarction. Given the CT scan result, it is likely that this man has sustained an ischemic, rather than a hemorrhagic, stroke. Hemorrhagic and ischemic strokes can be difficult to differentiate on clinical grounds, but the former often produce a less predictable pattern of neurologic deficits. This is because the neurologic deficits in hemorrhagic stroke depend both on the location of the bleed and on factors that affect brain function at a distance from the hemorrhage, including increased intracranial pressure, edema, the compression of neighboring brain tissue, and rupture of blood into the ventricles or subarachnoid space.

D. The most likely underlying cause of stroke in this patient is atherosclerosis. Atherosclerosis arises from vascular endothelial cell injury, often caused by chronic hypertension or hypercholesterolemia, both present in this man. Endothelial injury stimulates the attachment of circulating monocytes and lymphocytes that migrate into the vessel wall and stimulate the proliferation of smooth muscle cells and fibroblasts. This results in plaque formation. Damaged endothelium also serves as a nidus of platelet aggregation that further stimulates the proliferation of smooth muscle and fibroblasts. The plaques formed may enlarge and occlude the vessel, leading to thrombotic stroke, or they may rupture, releasing emboli and causing embolic stroke.

CASE 38

A. The lesions described are characteristic of psoriasis vulgaris. Psoriasis is both a genetic and an environmental disorder. A genetic origin is supported by several lines of evidence. There is a high rate of concordance for psoriasis in monozygotic twins and an increased incidence of psoriasis in the relatives of affected individuals. Furthermore, the overexpression of gene products of class I alleles of the major histocompatibility complex (MHC) is seen in patients with psoriasis. However, psoriasis is unlikely to be completely genetic in nature. Individuals with a genetic predisposition to the disorder appear to require environmental triggers, at least in some cases, such as trauma, cold weather, infections, stress, and drugs.

B. In psoriasis, there is a shortening of the usual duration of the keratinocyte cell cycle and a doubling of the proliferative cell population. This excessive epidermatopoiesis results in skin thickening and plaque formation. In addition to skin thickening, cell cycle truncation leads to an accumulation of cells within the cornified layer with retained nuclei. This pattern is known as parakeratosis and results in neutrophil migration into the cornified layer. Together, these form the silvery scale characteristic of psoriasis. Finally, psoriasis induces endothelial cell proliferation, resulting in the pronounced dilation, tortuosity, and increased permeability of the capillaries in the superficial dermis and causing erythema.

C. A large number of immunologic abnormalities that involve both innate and adaptive immunity have been documented in psoriatic skin. Antigenic stimuli are thought to activate the innate immune response, leading to the production of cytokines, such as interferon, TNF, IL-23, and IL-12, by macrophages, dendritic cells, and neutrophils. This leads to the attraction, activation, and differentiation of T cells. These T cells, most importantly T_H1 and T_H17 cells, produce cytokines that lead to epidermal hyperplasia, the recruitment of inflammatory cells, and ultimately a positive feedback loop that perpetuates the pathologic process.

CASE 39

A. The lesions described are characteristic of the "pruritic polygonal purple papules" of lichen planus. Although the triggers of lichen planus are often obscure, several drugs have been implicated. Antimalarial agents (eg, chloroquine) and therapeutic gold are the drugs most closely linked to this phenomenon. It is believed that these agents and other unknown triggers result in a cell-mediated autoimmune reaction leading to damage of the basal keratinocytes of the epidermis.

B. As mentioned, the triggers leading to lichen planus formation are often idiopathic. However, it appears that some form of antigenic stimulation leads to the infiltration and activation of CD4 T lymphocytes. These stimulated CD4 cells elaborate cytokines, leading to the recruitment of cytotoxic T lymphocytes. Cell-mediated cytotoxicity, cytokines, interferon-γ, and TNF combine to injure keratinocytes and contribute to cell vacuolization and necrosis. Injured, enucleated keratinocytes coalesce to form colloid bodies. Melanocytes are destroyed as "innocent bystanders," and melanin is phagocytosed by macrophages.

C. The appearance of the lichen planus papules is a direct reflection of the underlying histopathologic features. The dense array of lymphocytes in the superficial dermis yields the elevated, flat-topped appearance of the papule. Minute whitish streaks, known as Wickham striae, result from chronic inflammation and hyperkeratosis of the cornified layer of the epidermis. The purple hue of the lesions is caused by the macrophage phagocytosis of the released melanin to form melanocytes. Although the melanin is brown-black, the melanophages are embedded in a colloid matrix. This causes an extensive scattering of light by an effect known as the Tyndall effect, resulting in an interpretation of the lesion as dusky or violaceous by the human eye.

CASE 40

A. The lesions described are characteristic of erythema multiforme. The lack of mucosal involvement suggests erythema multiforme minor.

B. Erythema multiforme is similar to lichen planus in that both are interface dermatitides, and both are caused by some inciting agent that results in lymphocyte migration to the epidermis and papillary dermis. Cytotoxic T cells then combine with elaborated cytokines, interferon-γ, and TNF to kill keratinocytes, resulting in enucleation, vacuolization, and coalescence to form colloid bodies.

Unlike lichen planus, with its dense dermal inflammatory infiltrate, the dermal infiltrate of lymphocytes in erythema multiforme is sparse. Thus, the vacuolated keratinocytes widely distributed in the epidermal basal layer are more conspicuous.

C. Many cases of erythema multiforme minor are triggered by herpes simplex virus (HSV), as seen in this patient. The evidence to support this association derives from both clinical and molecular data. Clinically, it has long been documented that erythema multiforme is often preceded by herpes simplex infection. Furthermore, antiherpetic agents such as acyclovir can suppress the development of erythema multiforme in some individuals. Molecular studies have confirmed the presence of herpes simplex DNA within skin from erythema multiforme lesions. HSV DNA is also present in the peripheral blood lymphocytes and lesional skin after resolution of the rash but is not found in nonlesional skin. Other known causes

include *Mycoplasma* infection, contact dermatitis, drugs, and radiation.

D. The target-like lesions seen in erythema multiforme reflect zonal differences in the inflammatory response and its deleterious effects. At the periphery of the lesion, inflammation and vacuolization are sparse, resulting in the erythematous halo. The dusky bull's eye in the center, on the other hand, is an area of dense epidermal vacuolization and necrosis.

CASE 41

A. The term "bullous" reflects the blisters (or bullae) that are characteristic of this condition. The term "pemphigoid" reflects the clinical similarity of bullous pemphigoid to pemphigus vulgaris, another more serious blistering skin disease characterized by intraepidermal, rather than subepidermal, vesiculation.

B. Microscopically, bullous pemphigoid lesions show a subepidermal cleft containing lymphocytes, eosinophils, neutrophils, and eosinophilic material, representing extravasated macromolecules such as fibrin. An inflammatory infiltrate of eosinophils, neutrophils, and lymphocytes is also present in the dermis beneath the cleft.

C. Direct immunofluorescence microscopy demonstrates IgG and C3 bound in a linear distribution along the epidermal–dermal junction. These autoantibodies are bound to a 230-kDa protein within the lamina lucida, known as the bullous pemphigoid antigen. This antigen has been localized to the hemidesmosomal complex of the epidermal basal cell. Its role has not been established.

D. Blister formation is believed to begin with the binding of IgG to the bullous pemphigoid antigen, activating the complement cascade. Complement fragments then induce mast cell degranulation and attract neutrophils and eosinophils. The granulocytes and mast cells release multiple enzymes, resulting in enzymatic digestion of the epidermal–dermal junction and separation of the layers. It is also possible that the bullous pemphigoid antigen plays a vital structural role that is compromised when the autoantibodies bind, leading to cleavage of the epidermal–dermal junction.

CASE 42

A. Palpable purpura over the distal lower extremities or other dependent areas—recurring over a period of months—and histologic study revealing fibrinoid necrosis are most consistent with leukocytoclastic vasculitis. Common precipitants include infections and medications. Bacterial, mycobacterial, and viral infections can all trigger leukocytoclastic vasculitis; *Streptococcus* and *Staphylococcus* are the most common infectious precipitants. *S pneumoniae* is the most common cause of pneumonia in this age group and may have been the precipitant in this man. Hepatitis C is also associated with leukocytoclastic vasculitis. Many drugs have been associated with this disorder, including antibiotics, thiazides, and nonsteroidal anti-inflammatory drugs (NSAIDs). Of the antibiotics, penicillins, such as the amoxicillin given to this man, are the most common offenders.

B. Eliciting factors such as microbial antigens or medications trigger the formation of immune complexes, consisting of antibodies bound to the exogenous antigen. For reasons not yet clear, these complexes are preferentially deposited in the small cutaneous vessels (venules). After becoming trapped in the tissue of the venules, the immune complexes activate the complement cascade, and the localized production of chemotactic fragments and vasoactive molecules ensues. This attracts neutrophils, which release enzymes, resulting in destruction of the immune complexes, neutrophils, and vessels. Ultimately, erythrocytes and fibrin are able to exude through the vessel wall and enter the surrounding dermis, resulting in the classic finding of palpable purpura.

C. Leukocytoclastic vasculitis lesions are raised and papular because lesional skin is altered and expanded by an intense vasocentric infiltrate containing numerous neutrophils. The lesions are purpuric or erythematous because of the extravasated red blood cells that accumulate in the dermis.

D. Leukocytoclastic vasculitis may also involve small vessels in other parts of the body, including the joint capsules, soft tissues, kidneys, liver, and GI tract. The most common systemic symptoms are arthralgias, myalgias, and abdominal pain. It would be important to inquire about these symptoms and order laboratory tests to assess liver or renal involvement.

CASE 43

A. The diagnosis is likely to be *Rhus* dermatitis ("poison ivy," "poison oak," and "poison sumac"), a form of allergic contact dermatitis. The history of hiking in a heavily wooded area 2 days before onset of the rash is a helpful clue. However, the finding on physical examination of blisters arranged in straight lines helps make the diagnosis. Straight lines and angles suggest an exogenous cause for a skin eruption. In this case, poison ivy leaves traced a line across the skin as the patient walked through the brush, and she developed an allergic contact dermatitis in the pattern of the exposure to its sticky, long-lasting oil (known as urushiol).

B. A common misconception regarding *Rhus* dermatitis is that blister fluid from broken blisters (or even touching the blistered area) causes the eruption to spread. In fact, once the eruption has developed, the urushiol allergen has been irreversibly bound to other proteins or has been so degraded that it cannot be transferred to other sites. In this case, the patient developed large blisters or bullae in response to the contactant at the original sites of contact, the legs. This means that she had a severe reaction to the allergen. Intense inflammation such as this can result in the autosensitization phenomenon,

which in this case explains the development of ill-defined erythematous plaques with small papules and vesicles within the plaques seen on this patient's arms and trunk. Alternatively, inadvertent contact with contaminated clothes or other surfaces (eg, a pet's fur) can induce new areas of dermatitis. The *Rhus* allergen is tremendously stable and can persist on unwashed clothing and remain capable of inducing allergic contact dermatitis for up to 1 year.

C. If the allergen exposure is transient, the first exposure to a *Rhus* antigen often does not result in a reaction at the exposure site. However, a contingent of "armed-and-ready" memory T cells is now policing the skin, waiting for the allergen to reappear, and the individual is said to be sensitized. When the person is exposed to the urushiol antigen again, the elicitation phase begins. Langerhans cells process antigen and migrate to lymph nodes, but presentation and T-cell proliferation also occur at the site of contact with the allergen. Nonspecific T cells in the vicinity are recruited and stimulated by the inflammatory cytokines released by the specifically reactive T cells, and an amplification loop ensues, eventuating in clinically recognizable dermatitis. This complex series of events takes time to develop, resulting in the 24- to 48-hour delay between re-exposure and rash eruption.

CASE 44

A. The probable diagnosis is erythema nodosum (EN), given the tender, ill-defined nodules. The anterior lower legs are the most common locations for such (node-like) lesions to develop. This patient probably has subclinical streptococcal pharyngitis. The fact that the patient herself had symptoms of pharyngitis, which were alleviated with antibiotics, is helpful. However, because the antibiotics course was much shorter than required (2 days vs. the standard 10), she must be suspected of having a partially treated (subclinical) infection. Until the infection is adequately treated, the patient will continue to manifest EN as a hypersensitivity response. Once the infection has been eradicated, the skin lesions should subside within several weeks. Persistent EN despite adequate antibiotic treatment of the pharyngitis should prompt a thorough search for an alternative cause.

B. Common causes of EN besides streptococcal pharyngitis include many different medications (including sulfa drugs), estrogen-containing oral contraceptives, pregnancy, and inflammatory bowel disease. There are numerous other possible causes.

C. Erythema nodosum is thought to represent a systemic, delayed-type hypersensitivity reaction that localizes to the subcutis for unknown reasons.

D. In erythema nodosum, the inflammatory response consists of lymphocytes, histiocytes, neutrophils, and eosinophils scattered throughout the septal compartment of the subcutis with frequent multinucleated histiocytes. The septa are thickened and may become fibrotic, depending on the density of the infiltrate and the duration of the reaction. Even though the infiltrate is largely confined to subcutaneous septa, there is commonly an element of fat necrosis at the edges of the subcutaneous lobules in erythema nodosum. Microscopically, evidence of fat necrosis may be seen in the form of an infiltrate of "foamy" (lipid-laden) macrophages at the periphery of subcutaneous lobules or in the form of small stellate clefts within multinucleate macrophages, indicating an element of lipomembranous fat necrosis.

CASE 45

A. The likely diagnosis is sarcoidosis. Because sarcoidosis is a diagnosis of exclusion, a thorough workup for specific causes is warranted. A skin biopsy should demonstrate changes typical of sarcoidosis (non-caseating granulomata), with negative histochemical stains for mycobacterial and fungal organisms. Additionally, a tissue culture of affected skin should be negative. A chest x-ray film is helpful to rule out tuberculosis and to search for hilar adenopathy. Bone films may demonstrate characteristic findings as well.

B. This patient has sarcoidal papules around the edges of the nostrils, a finding known as lupus pernio or nasal rim sarcoidosis. This finding indicates that the patient is at high risk for significant involvement of the tracheobronchial tree or lung parenchyma. The complaint of chronic cough should also suggest lung involvement. Regardless of symptoms and dermatologic presentation, the possibility of pulmonary involvement should always be investigated in all cases of sarcoidosis because it is quite common and sometimes asymptomatic.

C. Sarcoidosis is a nodular dermatitis with histiocytic granulomas situated within the dermis. There are few lymphocytes present in and around the granulomas. Multinucleated histiocytes are frequently present.

D. Sarcoidosis is seen clinically as an elevation (papule, plaque, or nodule) caused by the expansion of the dermis by the infiltrate. There is no scale overlying the lesions because the epidermis is not affected.

CASE 46

A. Contrary to popular perception, acne is not caused by dirt clogging the pores. In fact, "blackheads" (open comedones) are black because of the oxidation of the keratinaceous debris within the dilated follicles, not because of "dirt." However, some exogenous substances such as oily cosmetics or petrolatum-based hair care products may promote comedone formation and thus exacerbate acne. Cleansing does not affect any of the four steps essential to the development of acne, because all steps occur within the follicles. Cleansing merely removes surface debris and oil. The patient should be advised to use a gentle soap or nonsoap cleanser designed for the face and to avoid scrubbing the skin with rough cloths, towels, or scrubbing pads, which is not helpful in ameliorating acne and

may cause secondary irritation, making topical treatments less tolerable. She should also be advised to use nongreasy cosmetics, usually those labeled as "noncomedogenic," as well as hair care products without petrolatum.

B. Keratinocytes fail to slough from the follicles as they should. As a result, the follicle becomes plugged (a comedo). The buildup of sebum behind the plug expands the follicle. *Propionibacterium acnes* overgrowth in the follicle breaks down sebum. Bacterial factors and sebum breakdown products attract neutrophils to the follicle, thus forming a pustule. Follicular rupture induces an intense inflammatory response in the dermis seen clinically as an inflammatory papule or pustule. Scarring may be the end result.

C. Follicular plugging may be corrected with retinoids (vitamin A analogues) either topically or, if the condition is severe enough, orally. Retinoids promote the proper desquamation of keratinocytes. Bacteria are controlled with topical or oral antibiotics. Some common topical antibiotic agents include benzoyl peroxide and clindamycin. Oral antibiotics such as erythromycin or tetracycline are frequently used in addition to topical antibiotics. These agents are not merely antibacterial but are known to have anti-inflammatory properties independent of their antibacterial action. Last, sebum production may be decreased through the use of retinoids, again topically or orally, although oral therapy is much more effective for this purpose, or with antiandrogen medications such as spironolactone and oral contraceptives.

CASE 47

A. Urticaria affects approximately 15–25% of the population, including people of all ages. In some patients, a specific cause can be identified, such as sunlight, water, medication, pressure, vibration, heat, cold, exercise, or emotional stress. In other patients, no specific trigger can be pinpointed. This patient's urticaria is likely exercise induced.

B. Urticaria is the result of mast cell degranulation resulting in a release of histamine and other pro-inflammatory cytokines such as prostaglandins, leukotrienes, and platelet activating factor. While the type I hypersensitivity reaction mediated by IgE is the classic cause for mast cell degranulation, there are in fact many other mediators of mast cell degranulation, including complement activation, physical stimuli (such as exercise or cold temperatures), viral infections, and autoantibodies. The release of histamine causes capillary vasodilation in the superficial dermis with the subsequent extravasation of protein-rich fluid into the superficial aspects of the skin and the development of the urticarial papules and/or plaques. The lesions resolve when the fluid gets resorbed.

C. Urticaria is associated with angioedema in approximately 50% of affected patients, whereas about 40% of patients have urticaria alone, and 10% have angioedema alone. Angioedema is due to the same process (mast cell degranulation) as urticaria, although it involves the deep dermis and subcutaneous tissue. Angioedema typically manifests as diffuse swelling, rather than as discrete papules or plaques, owing to the deeper location of the changes. Angioedema lesions present as diffuse swelling, most often of mucous membranes and/or the hands and feet. They can persist for up to 3 days. If the respiratory tract is involved, the swelling can be life-threatening.

CASE 48

A. The fundamental abnormality in asthma is an increased reactivity of the airways to stimuli. Asthma can be induced by many provocative agents (triggers). These can be broadly categorized as (1) physiologic or pharmacologic mediators of asthmatic airway responses; (2) allergens that can induce airway inflammation and reactivity in sensitized individuals; and (3) exogenous physicochemical agents or stimuli that produce airway hyper-reactivity. This patient's history (seasonal predilection) is most consistent with allergen-induced asthma. The worsening symptoms in the last few months may be due to an allergic reaction to the roommate's cat.

B. The earliest events in asthma are the activation of local inflammatory cells, primarily mast cells and eosinophils, by the provocative agents described previously. This can occur by specific IgE-dependent mechanisms or indirectly by chemical irritant exposure or osmotic stimuli. Acute-acting mediators, including leukotrienes, prostaglandins, and histamine, induce smooth muscle contraction, mucus hypersecretion, and vasodilation with endothelial leakage and local edema formation. Epithelial cells also participate, releasing leukotrienes, prostaglandins, and inflammatory cytokines. Additional inflammatory cells, including neutrophils and eosinophils, are recruited to the airway mucosa. In addition, the cell cytokines released promote the growth of mast cells and eosinophils, the influx and proliferation of T cells, and the differentiation of B lymphocytes into IgE- and IgA-producing plasma cells. Ultimately, this ongoing inflammation results in injury to epithelial cells, denudation of the airway, and greater exposure of afferent sensory nerves, and subsequently to smooth muscle hyper-responsiveness, chronic inflammation, submucosal gland hypersecretion, and increased mucus volume. In addition to the classic paradigm of allergic asthma described above, there are also nonallergic asthma and asthma in the obese patient, entities that have a different, but incompletely understood, pathogenesis.

C. Wheezing is caused by a combination of smooth muscle contraction and mucus hypersecretion and retention, resulting in airway caliber reduction and prolonged turbulent airflow. The sensations of shortness of breath and chest tightness are also the result of a number of concerted changes. These include the detection by spindle cell stretch receptors of the greater muscular effort required to overcome the increased airway resistance, as well as the detection of thoracic distention resulting from chest hyperinflation, decreased lung compliance, and increased work of breathing. These are sensed by the chest wall nerves and manifested as chest tightness and shortness of breath. As the obstruction worsens, hypoxemia and CO_2 retention occur, further stimulating respiratory drive through peripheral and central chemoreceptors. This stimulus in the setting of respiratory muscle fatigue produces progressive dyspnea.

D. This patient's symptoms are relatively mild, occurring only intermittently. In between exacerbations, her pulmonary function tests may be normal. During an attack, all indices of expiratory airflow may be reduced, including FEV_1, FEV_1/FVC, and peak expiratory flow rate. FVC may also be reduced as a result of premature airway closure. Total lung capacity, functional residual capacity, and residual volume may be increased as a consequence of airflow obstruction and incomplete emptying of lung units. DLCO may be increased because of increased lung and capillary blood volume.

CASE 49

A. Chronic obstructive pulmonary disease (COPD) is defined by the presence of persistent respiratory symptoms and airflow limitation caused by airway and alveolar abnormalities resulting from exposure to noxious particles or gases. COPD is often described as two distinct processes, chronic bronchitis and emphysema, both of which can lead to the development of fixed airway obstruction. Any given individual may have components of both processes present.

Chronic bronchitis is defined by a clinical history of productive cough for 3 months of the year for 2 consecutive years. Both dyspnea and airway obstruction, often with an element of reversibility, are intermittently to continuously present. Chronic bronchitis predominantly impacts the airways. Inflammation of the larger airways leads to mucosal thickening and mucus hypersecretion, which contributes to the productive cough. Extension of the inflammatory changes into smaller bronchioles produces airflow obstruction.

Pulmonary emphysema is a condition marked by an irreversible enlargement of the airspaces distal to the terminal bronchioles, accompanied by the destruction of their walls, most often without obvious fibrosis. In contrast to chronic bronchitis, the primary pathologic defect in emphysema is not in the airways but rather in the respiratory unit walls, where the loss of elastic tissue results in a loss of the recoil tension necessary to support distal airways during expiration. Progressive dyspnea and nonreversible obstruction accompany the airspace destruction without mucus hypersecretion or productive cough. Furthermore, the loss of alveolar surface area and the accompanying capillary bed for gas exchange contribute to progressive hypoxia and dyspnea.

B. The chronic productive cough and thick sputum production present in this patient are characteristic of chronic bronchitis. Cigarette smoking remains the principal cause of disease in up to 90% of patients with chronic bronchitis and emphysema. Beyond tobacco exposure, population-based studies suggest that chronic dust (including silica and cotton) or chemical fume exposure is a significant contributing risk factor for COPD. In the developing world, indoor exposure to smoke from burning biofuels is a major cause of COPD. The most important identified genetic risk factor for the evolution of COPD is a deficiency of the α_1-protease (α_1-antitrypsin) inhibitor. Reduced circulating and tissue levels can lead to the early onset of severe emphysema, but not chronic bronchitis.

C. Diffuse airway obstruction is demonstrated on pulmonary function testing as a global reduction in expiratory flows and volumes. FEV_1, FVC, and the FEV_1/FVC ($FEV_1\%$) ratio are all reduced. The expiratory flow–volume curve shows substantial flow limitation. Some patients may respond to bronchodilators. Lung volume measurement reveals an increase in the RV and FRC, reflecting air trapped in the lung as a result of diffuse airway obstruction and early airway closure at higher lung volumes. This is characterized by a flattened diaphragm on chest x-ray. DLCO is typically normal, reflecting a preserved alveolar capillary bed.

D. Ventilation/perfusion mismatching is common in chronic bronchitis. The A–a ΔPO_2 is increased, and hypoxemia is common mainly because of significant areas of low ratios (physiologic shunt); hypoxemia at rest tends to be more profound than in emphysema. Mismatch is also present in emphysema, but patients with emphysema typically adapt to high ratios by increasing their minute ventilation. They may maintain nearly normal PO_2 and PCO_2 levels despite advanced disease. However, with greater disease severity and further loss of capillary perfusion, the DLCO falls, leading to exercise-related and, ultimately, resting arterial hemoglobin desaturation. In both conditions, increasing PCO_2 (hypercapnia) and respiratory acidosis, with compensatory metabolic alkalosis, are seen in severe disease.

CASE 50

A. The pathophysiology of interstitial pulmonary fibrosis (IPF) and its histopathologic correlate, usual interstitial pneumonia (UIP), is an active area of research. Mounting evidence implicates repetitive microinjury to the alveolar epithelium followed by aberrant wound repair as the predominant mechanism of disease pathogenesis. Defects (both genetic and acquired) in type II alveolar epithelial cells increase the susceptibility of these cells to injury and apoptosis and also interfere with their regenerative capacity. It is currently unknown what environmental challenges are responsible for the repetitive microinjury to the susceptible type II alveolar epithelial cell (hence the idiopathic designation). It is likely that multiple different insults contribute.

Following epithelial injury, fibroblasts accumulate in the lung interstitium and typically differentiate into myofibroblasts. Myofibroblasts are highly contractile and contribute to tissue destruction. They are also responsible for the synthesis and deposition of extracellular matrix proteins such as fibronectin and collagen. The (myo)fibroblasts in IPF persist longer than usual and lead to the progressive nature of the disease. Current evidence suggests that the damaged type II alveolar epithelial cells secrete profibrogenic mediators, including transforming growth factor–β (TGF-β), connective tissue growth factor, and platelet-derived growth factor, leading to the (myo)fibroblast activation. Disruption of the epithelium also leads to plasma leak, TGF-β activation, clotting cascade activation, and thrombin generation, which can activate fibroblasts through the cleavage of protease-activated receptors. In turn, the fibrogenic mediators, in conjunction with the development of a stiff, cross-linked, collagen-rich extracellular matrix, drive myofibroblast differentiation and apoptosis resistance.

B. An intermittent, irritating, nonproductive cough and a slowly progressive dyspnea are often the first symptoms of IPF. The cough may be refractory to antitussive therapy. The mechanism is likely multifactorial, with fibrotic damage to terminal respiratory units causing bronchial and bronchiolar distortion, leading to alterations in both the stimulatory and inhibitory nerve fibers involved in cough reflexes.

Multiple factors contribute to dyspnea in patients with IPF. Fibrosis of the lung parenchyma decreases lung compliance; in combination with alterations in surfactant turnover, the distending pressure required to inflate the lungs increases, as does the work of breathing. Increased stimuli from C fibers in fibrotic alveolar walls or stretch receptors in the chest wall may sense the increased force necessary to inflate less compliant lungs.

Tachypnea results from increased lung sensory receptor stimuli and the attempt to maintain a normal alveolar minute ventilation (and hence normal $PaCO_2$) as lung volumes decrease. A rapid, shallow breathing pattern also reduces ventilatory work in the face of increased lung elastic recoil. The diminished capillary bed and thickened alveolar–capillary membrane contribute to hypoxemia with exercise. In advanced disease, altered gas exchange with severe mismatching can produce hypoxemia at rest.

The diffuse inspiratory crackles reflect the successive opening on inspiration of respiratory units that are collapsed owing to fibrosis and loss of normal surfactant. The cause of digital clubbing is unknown.

C. Characteristic chest radiograph findings include reduced lung volumes with increased reticular opacities that are prominent in the lung periphery and cause a loss of definition of the vascular structures, hemidiaphragms, and cardiac border. Fibrosis surrounding expanded small airspaces is seen as honeycombing. With pulmonary hypertension, central pulmonary arteries may be enlarged. Pulmonary fibrosis produces a restrictive pattern on pulmonary function tests. This is manifested as reductions in TLC, FEV_1, and FVC, with preservation of or increases in FEV_1/FVC and expiratory flow rates. DLCO decreases progressively as fibrosis continues and lung capillaries are obliterated.

CASE 51

A. The four factors that account for almost all cases of pulmonary edema are (1) an increase in the hydrostatic pressure gradient (cardiogenic pulmonary edema); (2) an increase in vascular endothelial cell and/or alveolar epithelial cell permeability (noncardiogenic pulmonary edema); (3) a decrease in the oncotic pressure gradient (usually owing to a low plasma protein content); and (4) impaired lymphatic drainage either from physical lymphatic obstruction or from lymphatic obliteration, which can occur in the setting of radiation treatment. This patient's history of prior myocardial infarction, long-standing history of hypertension, and possible recent ischemia make it likely that he has cardiogenic pulmonary edema.

B. Cardiogenic or hydrostatic pulmonary edema classically results from elevated pulmonary venous and left atrial pressures owing to left ventricular systolic or diastolic failure, mitral stenosis, or mitral regurgitation. This is primarily a mechanical process resulting in an ultrafiltrate of plasma. Edema fluid in this setting has a relatively low protein content, generally less than 60% of a patient's plasma protein content. In normal individuals, pulmonary capillary pressure (ie, pulmonary capillary wedge pressure) must exceed approximately 20 mm Hg before the fluid leaving the vascular space exceeds the rate of resorption, leading to the accumulation of interstitial (Figure 9–25) and ultimately alveolar fluid that we describe as pulmonary edema.

CASE 52

A. Thromboemboli that cause pulmonary embolism almost never originate in the pulmonary circulation; they arrive there by dislodging from their site of origin and traveling through the venous circulation. More than 95% of pulmonary thromboemboli arise from the deep veins of the lower extremity: the popliteal, femoral, and iliac veins. The findings of right lower extremity warmth, erythema, and swelling in this patient support the view that this is very likely the site of origin of the thromboembolism. It is important to note, however, that the absence of such lower extremity findings does not exclude the diagnosis of thrombus from the lower extremity, because findings are insensitive.

B. This patient has multiple risk factors for pulmonary embolism, and he was at high risk for such an event. He is older than 40 years, was anesthetized for more than 30 minutes for his total knee replacement, and underwent orthopedic surgery (risk imposed by immobilization). His risk for calf vein thrombosis is as high as 84%, and the risk of fatal pulmonary embolism is approximately 5%. All such patients should receive prophylactic anticoagulant therapy postoperatively.

C. All patients with pulmonary emboli have some degree of mechanical obstruction of the pulmonary circulation. The severity of the mechanical obstruction depends on the clot burden, on the neurohumoral reflexes stimulated by the thrombus, and on the presence or absence of pre-existing cardiopulmonary disease. As the degree of obstruction of pulmonary circulation increases, pulmonary artery pressures rise, ultimately leading to right ventricular strain. In severe pulmonary embolism, occlusion of the pulmonary outflow tract may occur, severely reducing cardiac output and causing cardiovascular collapse and death.

D. The immediate effect of a pulmonary embolism is the generation of increased "dead space" ventilation (ie, regions of the lung with preserved $\dot{V}$ but absent $\dot{Q}$). This increase in dead space impairs the elimination of carbon dioxide with minimal effect on oxygenation. However, in the setting of thromboembolism, patients typically compensate for the increase in dead space ventilation by increasing their total minute ventilation. In fact, patients classically overcompensate for the increase in dead space and exhibit a respiratory alkalosis on their arterial blood gas analysis.

CASE 53

A. Acute respiratory distress syndrome (ARDS) is the archetypal example of increased-permeability edema. While the underlying pathophysiology is complex, the fundamental mechanism is an inflammation-mediated disruption of the alveolar capillary barrier. Through loss of endothelial and epithelial barrier integrity, the normal homeostatic mechanisms of fluid balance are disrupted, and protein-rich fluid accumulates in the alveolar space. This loss of integrity may result from direct injury to the alveolar epithelium following the local activation of inflammation by inhaled toxins or pulmonary infection. Or it may occur after injury to the pulmonary capillary endothelium following the systemic activation of inflammation by circulating toxins, as, for example, in sepsis or pancreatitis. Whether the injury occurs directly or indirectly, the insult activates the innate immune response through resident immune cells such as the alveolar macrophage. These cells recognize both exogenous factors, such as those derived from microorganisms, and endogenous factors, elaborated by local or distant cellular injury, through "pattern recognition" receptors (eg, toll-like receptors). Receptor activation stimulates pro-inflammatory responses. Through the release of cytokines and chemokines such as IL-1B, TNFα, IL-6, and IL-8, circulating inflammatory cells including neutrophils and monocytes are recruited to the lung and undergo activation, which further potentiates the pro-inflammatory signal. The propagation of this inflammatory cascade results in direct and indirect tissue injury through the release of a variety of factors, including other cytokines and chemokines, proteases, eicosanoids, and reactive oxygen species. Loss of the barrier integrity as a result of injury to both the alveolar epithelium and capillary endothelium ultimately leads to the leakage of protein-rich fluid into the alveolar spaces throughout the lung. There, the edema fluid inactivates surfactant, increasing surface tension with resultant alveolar instability and atelectasis. Increased surface tension also decreases the interstitial hydrostatic pressure, further favoring fluid movement into the alveolus. The loss of surfactant activity and the filling of airspaces cause the significant physiologic derangements that characterize ARDS, including decreases in both lung compliance and lung volume, resulting in severe hypoxemia (secondary to low $\dot{V}/\dot{Q}$ and shunt).

B. ARDS is the final common pathway of a number of different serious medical conditions, all of which lead to increased pulmonary capillary leak. The range of clinical presentations includes all the diagnoses in the adult ICU, including sepsis, pneumonia, pancreatitis, aspiration of gastric contents, shock, lung contusion, nonthoracic trauma, toxic inhalation, near-drowning, and multiple blood transfusions. About one-third of ARDS patients initially have sepsis syndrome.

C. The severe hypoxia found in ARDS is due to several factors. Damage to endothelial and epithelial cells causes increased vascular permeability and reduced surfactant production and activity. These abnormalities lead to interstitial and alveolar pulmonary edema, alveolar collapse, a significant increase in surface forces, markedly reduced pulmonary compliance, and hypoxemia. As the process worsens, there may be a further fall in compliance and disruption of pulmonary capillaries, leading to areas of true shunting and refractory hypoxemia. The combination of increased work of breathing and progressive hypoxemia usually requires mechanical ventilation. The underlying process is heterogeneous, with normal-appearing lung adjacent to atelectatic or consolidated lung. Therefore, ventilating patients at typical tidal volumes may overdistend normal alveoli, reduce blood flow to areas of adequate ventilation, and precipitate further lung injury ("volu-trauma"). Hypoxemia can be profound in ARDS, typically followed days later by hypercapnia owing to increasing dead space ventilation.

CASE 54

A. The atrioventricular (AV) node normally forms the only electrical connection between the atria and the ventricles. However, an accessory AV connection is found in approximately 1 in 1000 persons. This accessory pathway is usually composed of normal atrial or ventricular tissue. Because part of the ventricle is "pre-excited" over the accessory pathway, rather than via the AV node, the surface ECG shows a short PR interval and a relatively wide QRS with a slurred upstroke, termed a **delta wave**.

B. Because the atria and ventricles are linked by two parallel connections, re-entrant tachycardias are readily initiated. For example, a premature atrial contraction could be blocked in the accessory pathway but still conduct to the ventricles via the AV node. If enough time has elapsed that the accessory pathway has recovered excitability, the cardiac impulse can travel in retrograde fashion to the atria over the accessory pathway and initiate a re-entrant tachycardia.

C. First, an increased automaticity resulting from more rapid phase 4 depolarizations can cause rapid heart rate. Second,

if repolarization is delayed (longer plateau period), spontaneous depolarizations (caused by the reactivation of sodium or calcium channels) can sometimes occur in phase 3 or phase 4 of the action potential. These depolarizations are called "triggered activity" because they depend on the existence of a preceding action potential. If these depolarizations reach threshold, tachycardia can occur in certain pathologic conditions.

CASE 55

A. Heart failure can be caused by (1) inappropriate workloads placed on the heart, such as volume overload or pressure overload; (2) restricted filling of the heart; (3) myocyte loss; or (4) decreased myocyte contractility. Each of these causes has several possible underlying mechanisms. This patient has myocyte loss and decreased myocyte contractility from the myocardial infarction, the most common cause of myocyte loss in developed countries. She may also have restricted filling owing to impaired myocyte relaxation if she has ongoing ischemia.

B. In **systolic dysfunction**, the isovolumic systolic pressure curve of the pressure–volume relationship is shifted downward. This reduces the stroke volume of the heart with a concomitant decrease in cardiac output. To maintain cardiac output, the heart can respond with three compensatory mechanisms: First, an increased return of blood to the heart (preload) can lead to increased sarcomere contraction (Frank–Starling relationship). Second, an increased release of catecholamines can increase cardiac output by both increasing the heart rate and shifting the systolic isovolumetric curve to the left. Finally, cardiac muscle can hypertrophy and ventricular volume can increase, shifting the diastolic curve to the right. Although each of these compensatory mechanisms can temporarily maintain cardiac output, each is limited in its ability to do so, and if the underlying cause of systolic dysfunction remains untreated, the heart ultimately fails.

In **diastolic dysfunction**, the position of the systolic isovolumic curve remains unchanged (myocyte contractility is preserved). However, the diastolic pressure–volume curve is shifted to the left, with an accompanying increase in left ventricular end-diastolic pressure and symptoms of heart failure (Figure 10–17). Diastolic dysfunction can be present in any disease that causes decreased relaxation, decreased elastic recoil, or increased stiffness of the ventricle. Hypertension, which often leads to compensatory increases in left ventricular wall thickness, can cause diastolic dysfunction by changing all three parameters. A lack of sufficient blood delivered to myocytes (ischemia) can also cause diastolic dysfunction by decreasing relaxation. If ischemia is severe, as in myocardial infarction, irreversible damage to the myocytes can occur, with the replacement of contractile cells by fibrosis, which will lead to systolic dysfunction. In most patients, a combination of systolic and diastolic dysfunction is responsible for the symptoms of heart failure.

C. Shortness of breath is likely due to the rise in pulmonary capillary pressure relative to plasma oncotic pressure, which causes fluid to move into the interstitial spaces of the lung (pulmonary edema). Interstitial edema probably stimulates juxtacapillary J receptors, which in turn causes reflex shallow, rapid breathing. Replacement of air in the lungs by blood or interstitial fluid can cause a reduction of vital capacity, restrictive physiology, and air trapping as a result of the closure of small airways. The work of breathing increases as the patient tries to distend stiff lungs, which can lead to respiratory muscle fatigue and the sensation of dyspnea. Alterations in the distribution of ventilation and perfusion result in relative ventilation/perfusion mismatch, with a consequent widening of the alveolar–arterial O_2 gradient, hypoxemia, and increased dead space.

The sudden onset of severe respiratory distress at night—paroxysmal nocturnal dyspnea—probably occurs because of the reduced adrenergic support of ventricular function that occurs with sleep, the increase in blood return as described previously, and the normal nocturnal depression of the respiratory center.

Shortness of breath occurs in the recumbent position (orthopnea) because of reduced blood pooling in the extremities and abdomen, and because the patient is operating on the steep portion of the diastolic pressure–volume curve, any increase in blood return leads to marked elevations in ventricular pressures. Patients usually learn to minimize orthopnea by sleeping with the upper body propped up by two or more pillows.

CASE 56

A. The three most common causes of aortic stenosis are congenital abnormalities (unicuspid, bicuspid, or fused leaflets), rheumatic heart disease, and degenerative valve disease resulting from calcium deposition. The most likely cause in this patient is rheumatic heart disease. Congenital aortic stenosis generally presents before age 30 years, whereas degenerative aortic stenosis is the most common cause in persons older than 70 years. Furthermore, this patient has a history of recurrent streptococcal sore throat, suggesting the possibility of rheumatic heart disease.

B. Syncope in aortic stenosis is usually due to decreased cerebral perfusion from the fixed obstruction, but it may also occur because of transient atrial arrhythmias with the loss of effective atrial contribution to ventricular filling. Arrhythmias arising from ventricular tissue are also more common in patients with aortic stenosis and can result in syncope.

C. Angina can be caused by a number of different mechanisms. Approximately half of all patients have comorbid significant coronary artery disease, which can lead to angina. Even without coronary artery disease, aortic stenosis causes compensatory ventricular hypertrophy. Ventricular hypertrophy causes an increase in oxygen demand as well as the compression of the

vessels traversing the cardiac muscle, resulting in decreased oxygen supply. The result is relative ischemia of the myocytes. Finally, in the case of calcified aortic valves, calcium emboli can cause coronary artery obstruction, although this is rare.

D. Carotid upstroke is decreased (pulsus parvus) and late (pulsus tardus) because of the fixed obstruction to flow. Left ventricular hypertrophy causes the apical impulse to be displaced laterally and become sustained. The increased dependence on atrial contraction is responsible for the prominent S_4. Flow through the restricted aortic orifice results in the midsystolic murmur, whereas regurgitant flow causes the diastolic murmur.

E. Once symptoms occur in aortic stenosis, the prognosis is poor without treatment. Life expectancy is 2 years if aortic stenosis causes angina and 3 years if aortic stenosis causes syncope.

CASE 57

A. The fundamental problem in aortic regurgitation is volume overload of the left ventricle during diastole. In aortic regurgitation, blood enters the left ventricle from both the pulmonary veins and the aorta (through the leaky aortic valve). The left ventricular stroke volume can increase dramatically, although the effective stroke volume may be minimally changed since much of the increase in stroke volume leaks back into the left ventricle. If the regurgitation develops slowly, the heart responds to the increased diastolic volume with sarcomere elongation (dilation) and wall thickening (hypertrophy). This can result in an enlarged heart that is displaced to the left. All these changes are characteristic of slowly progressive aortic regurgitation. However, if the condition develops quickly, over a few days, such as during aortic valve destruction as a result of infective endocarditis, these compensatory mechanisms do not have a chance to develop.

B. In aortic regurgitation, the pulse pressure is widened both because of an increase in systolic pressure and a falling diastolic pressure. The systolic pressure increases owing to the increased stroke volume. The diastolic pressure decreases owing to the regurgitant flow back into the left ventricle and the increased compliance of the great vessels. This large difference between systolic and diastolic pressures is readily felt in the peripheral pulse as a sudden rise, then drop, in pressure. There are many physical signs resulting from this phenomenon, including the so-called water-hammer pulse (Corrigan pulse), head bobbing (de Musset sign), uvula pulsation (Müller sign), and arterial nailbed pulsations (Quincke pulse).

C. The high-pitched diastolic murmur at the left lower sternal border is from the regurgitant flow through the leaky aortic valve. The diastolic rumbling at the apex, also known as the Austin Flint murmur, is from the regurgitant flow impinging on the anterior leaflet of the mitral valve, causing a functional mitral stenosis. The systolic murmur at the left upper sternal border is from the increased stroke volume flowing across the aortic valve during systole.

D. Early in aortic regurgitation, there is no heart failure because the left ventricle adapts to the increased volume by enlarging and thickening. However, at some point the compensatory mechanisms fail, and the end-diastolic pressure in the left ventricle rises. This rise in end-diastolic pressure is transmitted through the pulmonary veins to the lungs, where it results in pulmonary edema owing to increases in hydrostatic pressure. This buildup of fluid in the alveoli causes impaired oxygenation, leading to shortness of breath. In milder cases, the shortness of breath may become evident only when there is increased demand; in severe cases, it may manifest at rest. For example, increased demand can occur during exertion. It may also occur during sleep, when the supine position allows the interstitial fluid from dependent tissues to re-enter the circulation, causing an increased intravascular volume.

CASE 58

A. The likely diagnosis in this patient is mitral stenosis. The history of a long illness following a sore throat in childhood is suggestive of acute rheumatic fever, the most common cause of mitral stenosis. The diastolic murmur results from impaired blood flow across the narrowed mitral valve. The irregularly irregular rhythm is due to atrial fibrillation, and the shortness of breath and rales are due to the heart failure of advanced mitral stenosis.

B. The normal mitral valve area is 5–6 cm². When it becomes narrowed to less than 1 cm², the flow of blood from the left atrium to the left ventricle is compromised enough to result in elevated left atrial pressure and volume. These elevations cause the left atrium to dilate, disrupting the orderly initiation of each heartbeat. Chaotic electrical activity replaces the usual control of the heart rhythm by the sinoatrial node, and atrial fibrillation ensues. The elevated left atrial pressure is also transmitted to the pulmonary veins and capillaries, resulting in heart failure, pulmonary edema, and hemoptysis from the leakage of engorged pulmonary veins.

C. The blood in the dilated left atrium is relatively static, and clots form there in approximately 20% of patients with mitral stenosis. If these thrombi enter the left ventricle, they can be pumped out to the systemic circulation causing a sudden arterial blockage, such as a stroke.

CASE 59

A. The patient's decompensation was likely triggered by the development of acute mitral regurgitation. The leaflets of the mitral valve are tethered by chordae tendineae, which are in turn attached to the ventricular wall by papillary muscles. The papillary muscles derive their blood supply from the left circumflex coronary artery and can become ischemic and even rupture if the blood supply is interrupted. When this happens, the leaflet is no longer tethered, and the valve no longer closes with systole, resulting in the sudden development of acute mitral regurgitation.

B. In mitral regurgitation, blood regurgitates into the left atrium from the left ventricle during systole. This leads to both volume and pressure overload of the left atrium, which in turn is transmitted to the pulmonary vasculature. It can also lead to dilation of the atrium and disruption of the heart's electrical system, causing arrhythmias such as atrial fibrillation. The increased pulmonary pressures can lead to heart failure. Also, in contrast to mitral stenosis, there is also an element of volume overload on the left ventricle, as the regurgitant blood from the left atrium flows back into the left ventricle during diastole.

C. If mitral regurgitation develops more slowly, the heart has a chance to adapt to the increased volume. The left ventricle, in particular, can dilate and hypertrophy in response to the increased stroke volume (though usually not to the extent that this left ventricular dilation and hypertrophy happen in aortic regurgitation). As a result, the apical impulse becomes displaced to the left.

CASE 60

A. The most likely diagnosis in this patient is coronary artery disease, specifically angina pectoris. Because the symptoms are exertional only and have been stable for several months, this patient would be classified as having stable angina. If the pain occurred at rest, with less and less activity, or more frequently or for a longer duration despite similar activity levels, he would be classified as having unstable angina.

B. By far the most common cause of coronary artery disease is atherosclerosis of the large epicardial arteries, and this is the most likely cause in this patient. A less common cause is coronary artery vasospasm, found more commonly in Japanese individuals. Vasospastic angina is most often nonexertional. Rare causes include emboli and congenital abnormalities.

C. This patient has several cardiac risk factors, including male gender, a family history of coronary artery disease, hyperlipidemia, smoking, and hypertension.

D. The mechanism by which atherosclerotic plaques form remains unclear and is the subject of much debate. It appears that atherosclerosis starts early in life, when the endothelial linings of the blood vessels are exposed to shear stress. The injury that results causes the endothelial cells to release vascular cell adhesion molecules to which monocytes become attached and enter the subendothelium, where they engulf oxidized low-density lipoprotein (LDL), forming foam cells. The injured endothelium, in combination with the foam cells, forms the fatty streak characteristic of atherosclerosis. Oxidized LDL causes the release of cytokines and the inhibition of NO. Vascular smooth muscle moves from the media to the intima, where it proliferates, laying down collagen and matrix and taking up oxidized LDL to form more foam cells. T cells also accumulate in the growing plaque. T cells, smooth muscle cells, and endothelial cells produce various cytokines and growth factors responsible for further cell migration and proliferation. Ultimately, the thickened and distorted artery wall takes up calcium, creating a brittle plaque.

E. Chest pain is due to myocardial ischemia, which occurs when cardiac oxygen demand exceeds supply. In the case of stable angina, the fixed narrowing of one or more coronary arteries by atherosclerotic plaque occurs. When the patient exercises, cardiac oxygen demand increases. However, because of the decreased diameter of the coronary arteries, insufficient blood flow, and, therefore, insufficient oxygen, is supplied to the heart. Chest pain has been attributed to this ischemia; however, it has been shown that up to 80% of all ischemic episodes are asymptomatic. When present, chest pain is thought to be triggered by adenosine release, stimulating the sympathetic afferent fibers that innervate the atrium and ventricle. These fibers then traverse the sympathetic ganglia and five upper thoracic dorsal roots of the spinal cord. These fibers converge with fibers from other structures in the spinal cord, which accounts for the frequent sensation of pain in the chest wall, back, and arm.

CASE 61

A. The probable diagnosis in this patient is pericarditis.

B. The most common cause of pericarditis is infection. Although bacteria, protozoa, and fungi can all cause pericarditis, viruses are the most common offender, in particular the coxsackieviruses. Coxsackievirus infection is the most likely cause in this patient given his young age, absence of underlying diseases, and viral prodrome. Pericarditis also occurs after injury (eg, myocardial infarction, thoracotomy, chest trauma, radiation therapy). Less common causes include collagen-vascular diseases (lupus erythematosus, scleroderma, rheumatoid arthritis), neoplasms, and renal failure.

C. The chest pain is probably due to pericardial inflammation. The pleuritic nature of the chest pain may be due to inflammation of the adjacent pleura.

D. The sound heard on cardiac examination is characteristic of a pericardial friction rub, which is pathognomonic for pericarditis. It is believed to be caused by friction between the visceral and parietal pericardial surfaces. The three components are attributable to the rapid movements of the cardiac chambers. The systolic component is related to ventricular contraction and is the one most commonly heard. There are two diastolic components: one in early diastole resulting from rapid ventricular filling and one late in diastole caused by atrial contraction. The two diastolic components frequently merge, so a two-component rub is most often heard.

E. One complication of pericarditis is pericardial effusion. The sudden onset of pericardial effusion may lead to tamponade.

This sudden addition of fluid increases pericardial pressure to the level of right atrial and ventricular pressures, causing chamber collapse and inadequate filling. Physical findings consistent with tamponade include elevated jugular venous pressure, hypotension, paradoxical pulse, and muffled heart sounds.

A second complication of pericarditis is fibrosis resulting in constrictive pericarditis. In constrictive pericarditis, early diastolic filling is normal, but the filling is suddenly stopped by the nonelastic fibrotic pericardium. This cessation of filling is probably responsible for the diastolic knock classically heard in this disease. In addition, because of the limited flow into the heart, systemic and, therefore, jugular venous pressures are elevated. The Kussmaul sign may also be present (ie, inappropriate increase in jugular venous pressure with inspiration). Finally, elevated systemic venous pressures can lead to fluid accumulation in the liver and intraperitoneal space, resulting in hepatomegaly and ascites.

CASE 62

A. The three classic signs of pericardial tamponade are called the Beck triad, after the surgeon who described them in 1935: (1) hypotension; (2) elevated jugular venous pressure; and (3) muffled heart sounds. In addition, the patient may have a decrease in systemic pressure with inspiration (paradoxic pulse).

B. The pericardium is normally filled with a small amount of fluid (30–50 mL), with an intrapericardial pressure that is usually about the same as the intrapleural pressure. With the sudden addition of fluid, the pericardial pressure can increase, at times to the level of the right atrial and right ventricular pressures. The transmural distending pressure of the ventricle decreases and the chamber collapses, preventing appropriate filling of the heart from systemic venous return. The four chambers of the heart occupy a relatively fixed volume in the pericardial sac, and hemodynamic evaluation reveals equilibration of ventricular and pulmonary artery diastolic pressures with right atrial and left atrial pressures, all at approximately intrapericardial pressure.

C. The arterial systolic blood pressure normally drops 10–12 mm Hg with inspiration. A marked inspiratory decrease in systolic blood pressure (>20 mm Hg) is an important physical finding in the diagnosis of cardiac tamponade but can also be seen in severe pulmonary disease and, less commonly, in constrictive pericarditis. A marked inspiratory decline in left ventricular stroke volume occurs because of a decreased left ventricular end-diastolic volume. With inspiration, increased blood return augments the filling of the right ventricle, which causes the interventricular septum to bow to the left and reduce the left ventricular end-diastolic volume (reverse Bernheim effect). Also during inspiration, flow into the left atrium from the pulmonary veins is reduced, further reducing left ventricular preload.

CASE 63

A. This patient likely has angina pectoris and intermittent claudication owing to underlying atherosclerosis.

B. The initial event in atherosclerosis is the infiltration of low-density lipoproteins (LDLs) into the subendothelial region. The endothelium is subject to shear stress, the tendency to be pulled along or deformed by flowing blood. This is most marked at points where the arteries branch, and this is where the lipids accumulate to the greatest degree. The LDLs are oxidized or altered in other ways and activate various components of the innate immune system, including macrophages, natural antibodies, and innate effector proteins such as C-reactive protein and complement. The oxidized LDL is taken up into macrophages, forming foam cells. The foam cells form fatty streaks. Vascular smooth muscle cells in the vicinity of foam cells are stimulated and move from the media to the intima, where they proliferate, lay down collagen and other matrix molecules, and contribute to the bulk of the lesion. Smooth muscle cells also take up oxidized LDL and become foam cells. Lipids accumulate both intracellularly and extracellularly. The intercellular "soup" in the plaques contains a variety of cell-damaging substances, including ozone. In addition, the "loading" of macrophages with cholesterol can be lipotoxic to the endoplasmic reticulum, resulting in macrophage apoptosis and plaque necrosis. Cholesterol crystals associated with necrotized macrophages further stimulate inflammation and lead to the recruitment of neutrophils. As the atherosclerotic lesions age, T cells of the immune system and monocytes are attracted to them, creating a vicious cycle of necrosis and inflammation. As plaques mature, a fibrous cap forms over them. The plaques with defective or broken caps are most prone to rupture. The lesions alone may distort vessels to the point that they are occluded, but it is usually the rupture or ulceration of plaques that triggers thrombosis, blocking blood flow.

C. This patient is postmenopausal and a smoker, has high blood pressure, and is diabetic. Estrogen increases cholesterol removal by the liver, and the progression of atherosclerosis is less rapid in premenopausal women than in men. On the other hand, large estrogen doses increase the incidence of blood clots, and even small doses produce a slight increase in clotting. In addition, in several studies, estrogen treatment of postmenopausal women failed to prevent second heart attacks. The reason for the discrepancies between the epidemiologic and experimental data is currently unsettled. The deleterious effects of smoking include endothelial damage caused by carbon monoxide–induced hypoxia. Other factors may also be involved. Thus, stopping smoking is a major way to slow the progression of atherosclerosis. Because of the increased shear stress imposed on the endothelium by an elevated blood pressure, hypertension is another important modifiable risk factor for atherosclerosis. Lowering blood pressure has its greatest effect in reducing the incidence of stroke, but there are beneficial effects on ischemic heart disease as well. In diabetics, there are both microvascular and macrovascular complications.

The latter are primarily related to atherosclerosis. There is a twofold increase in the incidence of myocardial infarction in diabetics compared with nondiabetics; severe circulatory deficiency in the legs with gangrene is relatively common; they experience more thrombotic strokes; and chronic kidney disease is a serious problem.

CASE 64

A. Hypertension is generally defined as a blood pressure greater than 140/90 mm Hg on three consecutive doctor's office visits, and prehypertension as blood pressures of 120–139/80–89 mm Hg. Although this patient would certainly be considered to have high blood pressure on this visit, he would not yet be diagnosed with hypertension.

B. In long-standing severe hypertension, one may note hypertensive retinopathy, including narrowed arterioles or even retinal hemorrhages and exudates. Cardiac enlargement resulting from hypertrophy may be noted as a displaced and prominent point of maximal impulse on cardiac palpation. An S_4 may be heard on cardiac auscultation.

C. Complications of hypertension include accelerated atherosclerosis resulting in ischemic heart disease, thrombotic strokes, cerebral hemorrhages, and renal failure. In severe hypertension, encephalopathy may occur.

D. By far the most common cause of hypertension is essential hypertension, and that is probably the cause in this patient. Because the patient is black, salt sensitivity may be a contributory factor. Other relatively common causes are diffuse renal disease, medications, renal arterial disease, and neurologic disorders. Less commonly, coarctation of the aorta, mineralocorticoid excess, glucocorticoid excess, and catecholamine excess can cause hypertension.

CASE 65

A. The four major pathophysiologic types of shock are hypovolemic, distributive, cardiogenic, and obstructive. Given the patient's age, history of severe trauma, and physical findings, the most likely type in this case is hypovolemic shock.

B. In hypovolemic shock, decreased blood volume leads to inadequate tissue perfusion. This results in increased anaerobic glycolysis and the production of lactic acid. Lactic acidosis depresses the myocardium, decreases peripheral vascular responsiveness to catecholamines, and may cause coma. Decreased mean arterial blood pressure decreases arterial baroreceptor firing, resulting in increased vasomotor discharge. This causes generalized vasoconstriction. Vasoconstriction in the skin causes coolness and pallor.

C. There are five causes of hypovolemic shock: hemorrhage, trauma, surgery, burns, and fluid loss resulting from vomiting or diarrhea. This patient was in a motor vehicle accident, resulting in traumatic shock. This was caused by blood loss into the abdomen, as suggested by the physical examination.

CASE 66

A. Other historical features to be elicited include chest pain (12%), flushing (14%), excessive sweating (50%), fainting (40%), and GI symptoms such as nausea or vomiting (19%), abdominal pain (14%), and diarrhea (6%). In addition, a medical history or family history of genetic diseases increasing the risk of pheochromocytoma should be elicited, as should a family history of pheochromocytoma independent of other genetic syndromes. Approximately 20–30% of pheochromocytomas are familial. Most familial cases are caused by one of four syndromes: neurofibromatosis type 1, von Hippel–Lindau syndrome, multiple endocrine neoplasia type 2 (MEN-2), and hereditary paraganglioma syndrome. Germline mutations in *RET*, *VHL*, *SDHx*, and others account for about 30–40% of cases of isolated pheochromocytomas and paragangliomas.

B. Pheochromocytoma is usually diagnosed by demonstrating abnormally high concentrations of catecholamines or their breakdown products in the urine or plasma. Increases in plasma metanephrine and normetanephrine concentrations are greater and more consistent than increases in plasma catecholamines. The administration of clonidine, 0.3 mg orally, can also be used to differentiate patients with pheochromocytoma from those with essential hypertension. Clonidine normally suppresses sympathetic nervous system activity and substantially lowers plasma norepinephrine levels, reducing blood pressure. However, in patients with pheochromocytoma, clonidine has little or no effect on blood pressure or plasma catecholamine level because these tumors behave autonomously.

C. As a tumor of adrenal medullary tissue, a pheochromocytoma produces symptoms of catecholamine excess. Anxiety, headache, and palpitations are direct effects of catecholamine discharge; weight loss is secondary to one of the metabolic effects of excessive circulating catecholamines. These include an increase in basal metabolic rate and an increase in glycolysis and glycogenolysis, leading to hyperglycemia and glycosuria.

CASE 67

A. This patient likely has achalasia, a condition in which the lower esophageal sphincter fails to relax properly. Under normal circumstances, the lower esophageal sphincter is a 3–4 cm ring of smooth muscle that is contracted, under stimulation by vagal cholinergic inputs. When a swallow is initiated, vagal inhibitory fibers allow the sphincter to relax so that the bolus of food can pass into the stomach. In achalasia, there is a degeneration of the myenteric plexus and a loss of the inhibitory neurons that allow this relaxation. Therefore, the sphincter remains tightly closed. The neural dysfunction can also extend further up the esophagus as well, and effective esophageal peristalsis is also often lost.

B. Injecting botulinum toxin into the lower esophageal sphincter of patients with achalasia diminishes the excitatory pathways responsible for the tonic contraction of the sphincter and allows its partial relaxation.

C. The tight closure of the lower esophageal sphincter in achalasia can result in a dilation of the lower portion of the esophagus and the storage of up to 1 L of material there. This material can become infected and be aspirated into the lungs. It can also cause esophageal mucosal ulceration and even perforation or rupture.

CASE 68

A. This patient appears to suffer from reflux esophagitis. Normally, the tonically contracted lower esophageal sphincter provides an effective barrier to acid reflux from the stomach back into the esophagus. This is reinforced by secondary esophageal peristaltic waves in response to transient lower esophageal sphincter relaxation. The effectiveness of that barrier can be altered by the loss of lower esophageal sphincter tone, an increased frequency in transient relaxations, the loss of secondary peristalsis after a transient relaxation, increased stomach volume or pressure, or increased acid production, all of which can make the more likely reflux of acidic stomach contents sufficient to cause pain or erosion. Recurrent reflux can damage the mucosa, resulting in inflammation, hence the term "reflux esophagitis." Recurrent reflux itself predisposes to further reflux because the scarring that occurs with healing of the inflamed epithelium renders the lower esophageal sphincter progressively less competent as a barrier.

B. Many factors such as her food choices (eg, chocolate), medications such as benzodiazepines, and smoking decrease lower esophageal sphincter tone, resulting in the reflux of acid-rich gastric contents into the esophageal lumen. This process is exacerbated at night when she lies down to sleep.

C. The most common complication is the development of stricture in the distal esophagus. Progressive obstruction, initially to solid food and later to liquid, presents as dysphagia. Other complications of recurrent reflux include hemorrhage or perforation; hoarseness, coughing, or wheezing; and pneumonia as a result of aspirating gastric contents into the lungs, particularly during sleep. Epidemiologic studies suggest that cigarette smoking and alcohol abuse associated with recurrent reflux result in a change in the esophageal epithelium from squamous to columnar histology, termed Barrett esophagus. In 2–5% of cases, Barrett esophagus leads to the development of esophageal adenocarcinoma.

CASE 69

A. Excessive acid secretion or diminished mucosal defenses predispose to the development of acid–peptic disease, specifically gastric ulcer. Most gastric ulcers are believed to be related to impaired mucosal defenses, because the acid and pepsin secretory capacity of some affected patients is normal or even below normal. Motility defects have been proposed to contribute to development of gastric ulcer in at least three ways: (1) by a tendency of duodenal contents to reflux back through an incompetent pyloric sphincter (bile acids in the duodenal reflux material act as an irritant and may be an important contributor to a diminished mucosal barrier against acid and pepsin); (2) by delayed emptying of gastric contents, including reflux material, into the duodenum; and (3) by delayed gastric emptying and hence food retention, resulting in increased gastrin secretion and gastric acid production. It is unknown whether these motility defects are a cause or a consequence of gastric ulcer formation. Mucosal ischemia may also play a role in the development of a gastric ulcer (see answer B). Subsets of gastric ulcer patients with each of these defects have been identified. Thus, the risk factors (NSAID ingestion, smoking, psychologic stress, *H pylori* infection) that have been associated with gastric ulcer probably act by diminishing one or more mucosal defense mechanisms.

B. Prostaglandins are known to increase mucosal blood flow, as well as bicarbonate and mucus secretion, and to stimulate mucosal cell repair and renewal. Thus, their deficiency, resulting from NSAID ingestion or other insults, may predispose to gastritis and gastric ulcer, as might diminished bicarbonate or mucus secretion owing to other causes.

C. *H pylori* can cause acid–peptic disease by multiple mechanisms, including altered signal transduction, resulting in increased inflammation, increased acid secretion, and diminished mucosal defenses. It may also affect apoptosis in the GI tract. Despite the high rate of association of inflammation with *H pylori* infection, the important role of other factors is indicated by the fact that only about 15% of *H pylori*–infected individuals ever develop a clinically significant ulcer. These other factors (both genetic and environmental, such as cigarette smoking) must account for the individual variations and are pathophysiologically important. Nevertheless, the role of *H pylori* is of particular clinical importance because, of patients who do develop acid–peptic disease, most have *H pylori* infection. Furthermore, treatment that does not eradicate *H pylori* is associated with the rapid recurrence of acid–peptic disease in most patients. Recent studies have also associated different strains of *H pylori* with different forms and degrees of acid–peptic disease and implicated *H pylori* infection in the development of GI tract cancers. Cornerstones of therapy for this patient include discontinuing ibuprofen, initiating proton pump inhibitors to decrease acid production, and initiating antibiotics to treat the *H pylori* infection.

CASE 70

A. Normal gastric emptying is influenced in part by the intrinsic enteric nervous system and its autonomic control. These systems are compromised by long-standing diabetes mellitus and its associated autonomic neuropathy.

It is likely that this patient's elevated fingerstick glucose is due to poor adherence to the medical regimen. This is supported by 6 months of worsening peripheral neuropathy. The newly diagnosed gastroparesis may, however, complicate attempts at improved glucose control.

B. The cause of his diarrhea may be multifactorial. Poorly coordinated pyloric contractions may result in entry into the duodenum of too large a bolus of chyme, which is ineffectively handled by the small intestine. Malabsorption results, leading to diarrhea. This malabsorption also predisposes to bacterial overgrowth, which may further exacerbate his diarrhea.

CASE 71

A. Many factors are involved in gallstone formation, but they can be divided into factors affecting bile composition and factors affecting gallbladder motility. Factors affecting the lithogenicity of bile include the cholesterol content; the presence of nucleating factors, prostaglandins, and estrogen; the rate of bile formation; and the rate of water and electrolyte absorption. Gallbladder motility also plays a major factor. Usually, bile does not stay in the gallbladder long enough to form a gallstone, but it may happen if stasis occurs.

B. In premenopausal women, high levels of serum estrogens promote gallstone formation in two ways: Estrogens both increase the cholesterol concentration of bile and decrease gallbladder motility. Bile stasis and the elevation of its cholesterol concentration enable gallstone formation.

C. A gallstone may become lodged in the cystic duct, obstructing gallbladder emptying. This can lead to the inflammation (cholecystitis) and infection of the static contents (empyema) of the gallbladder. If untreated, such inflammation and infection can lead to necrosis of the gallbladder and sepsis. If a gallstone becomes lodged in the common bile duct, it can cause obstructive jaundice with an elevation in serum bilirubin levels. If it lodges farther along the common bile duct and blocks the pancreatic duct near the sphincter of Oddi, it can cause acute pancreatitis, perhaps because the digestive enzymes of the pancreas are trapped in the pancreatic duct and cause inflammation in the pancreas.

CASE 72

A. Lactose intolerance is the most common problem of carbohydrate digestion. It results mainly from the reduction of intestinal brush border lactase activity in adults. Lactase is normally expressed at high levels in the jejunum of neonatal and infant humans. In many parts of the world, lactase levels are gradually reduced after weaning. However, lactase levels do not decrease significantly in populations in which milk products are an important part of the adult diet. Lactase activity is rate-limiting for lactose digestion in most adults throughout other regions of the world.

B. Carbohydrates, which are mainly present in the diet as polysaccharides and disaccharides, must be digested to monosaccharides for absorption. If lactase is deficient, nondigested lactose is not absorbed. The nonabsorbed lactose retains water in the lumen to maintain the osmolality of chyme equivalent to that of plasma. This fluid retention causes abdominal pain (cramps), nausea, and diarrhea. Bacterial fermentation of lactose in the distal small intestine and colon further exacerbates these symptoms.

CASE 73

A. Crohn disease is a regional enteritis that primarily affects the distal ileum and colon but may affect the GI tract from mouth to anus as evidenced by the significant oral aphthous ulcers seen in this patient.

B. The pathogenesis of Crohn disease remains unclear. Many factors have been speculated to contribute to the development of Crohn disease, including microorganisms (bacteria and viruses), dietary factors, genetic factors, defective immune responses, and psychosocial factors. The association of Crohn disease with other known hereditary disorders, such as cystic fibrosis and ankylosing spondylitis, is indirect evidence of a genetic component. The normal gut is able to modulate frank inflammatory responses to its constant bombardment with dietary and microbial antigens in the lumen. This modulation may be defective in Crohn disease, resulting in uncontrolled inflammation.

There has been considerable recent interest in the role of cytokines, such as interleukins and TNF, in Crohn disease. Cytokine profiles of the T_H1 category have been implicated in Crohn disease. Mice lacking IL-10 have a T_H1 cytokine profile and develop a Crohn disease–like inflammation of the intestine. Monoclonal antibodies to TNF reduce inflammation in affected animals and humans.

C. Acute and chronic inflammation causes a relapsing and remitting clinical course. Complications such as small bowel obstruction can occur as a result of active inflammation or, more commonly, from chronic fibrotic stricturing. Fistulization, abscesses, perianal disease, carcinoma, and malabsorption are other known complications of Crohn disease.

D. Extraintestinal manifestations include migratory arthritis; inflammatory disorders of the skin, eye, and mucous membranes; gallstones from the malabsorption of bile salts from the terminal ileum; and nephrolithiasis from increased oxalate absorption. Amyloidosis is a serious complication of Crohn disease, as is thromboembolic disease.

CASE 74

A. The patient likely has ulcerative colitis. This condition is characterized by multiple episodes of bloody diarrhea lasting several weeks in the absence of intestinal infection and by continuous colitis that extends from the rectum to the sigmoid.

B. Ulcerative colitis also responds to therapy that uses monoclonal antibodies against the inflammatory cytokine tumor necrosis factor α (TNFα). This monoclonal antibody therapy is now commonly used to treat patients with moderate to severe disease since its benefit-to-risk profile is better than that of glucocorticoids. Moreover, this class of corticosteroid-sparing agent can be used long term to maintain clinical remission. Newer and developing therapies for inflammatory bowel disease include those that target cytokines (interleukin-23), inflammatory signaling kinases (Janus kinase [JAK]), and cell trafficking (integrins and adhesions molecules).

C. Patients with ulcerative colitis are at an increased risk of colonic adenocarcinoma that increases with the duration of the disease. Therefore, these patients need more frequent colonoscopic screening for colon cancer. Chronic disease can also damage the muscularis propria, resulting in a thin-walled, dilated, poorly motile area of the colon that is susceptible to rupture (toxic megacolon).

CASE 75

A. Diverticular disease (diverticulosis) commonly affects older patients and is caused by the herniation of mucosa and submucosa through the muscularis layer of the colon. There are both structural and functional abnormalities that contribute to its development. The structural integrity of the muscularis layer may be compromised by abnormal connective tissue. The functional abnormality may involve the development of a pressure gradient between the colonic lumen and the peritoneal space, which results from the vigorous wall contractions needed to propel stool through the colon. Higher pressures are created to compensate for poor dietary fiber intake affecting normal stool bulk. Epidemiologic data support this assertion because the incidence of diverticular disease has increased with our society's reliance on fiber-poor foods and consequent constipation.

B. Opioids for abdominal pain control should be avoided because they directly raise intraluminal pressure and may increase the risk of perforation.

C. There are two important complications of diverticulosis. Diverticular bleeding from intramural arteries that rupture into the diverticula is a common cause of lower GI tract bleeding in the elderly. Diverticulitis, as seen in this patient, is due to a focal area of inflammation in the wall of a diverticulum in response to irritation from retained fecal material. Fever, abdominal pain, and diarrhea or constipation are typically present. The local infection may progress to an abscess with or without perforation, requiring surgical intervention.

CASE 76

A. This patient likely has irritable bowel syndrome, as she has the three classic symptoms: crampy abdominal pain, alternating constipation and diarrhea, and bloating. She also has normal laboratory and colonoscopy results. The onset of irritable bowel syndrome after a bout of gastroenteritis is common.

B. Irritable bowel syndrome is a complex and not well understood condition. Affected patients have decreased intestinal motility along with increased intestinal pain sensitivity, also known as visceral hyperalgesia. Both of these can result from alterations in the intrinsic and extrinsic nervous systems of the intestine. Microbial dysbiosis (imbalance) is another important potential etiology. One hypothesis is that intestinal inflammation from an infection or other insult results in these intestinal nervous system changes, which in turn lead to altered intestinal motility, secretion, and sensation.

CASE 77

A. Acute hepatitis is an inflammatory process causing liver cell death, which can be initiated by viral infection or, in this case, by toxic exposure. Prescription and nonprescription drugs are common inciters of acute hepatic injury and can be divided into predictable, dose-related toxicity (eg, acetaminophen) and unpredictable, idiosyncratic reactions such as occurs with isoniazid. Isoniazid is an infrequent but important cause of acute hepatitis and, in susceptible individuals, may be due to a genetic predisposition to certain pathways of drug metabolism that create toxic intermediates. Synergistic reactions between drugs have also been implicated in acute liver failure. Normal hepatic function recovery typically follows prompt discontinuation of the offending agent.

B. Histologic findings in acute hepatitis include focal liver cell degeneration and necrosis, portal inflammation with mononuclear cell infiltration, bile duct prominence, and cholestasis. Less commonly, acute hepatitis may result in bridging hepatic necrosis. Normal lobular architecture is largely restored in the recovery phase. Rarely, in massive hepatic necrosis (<1% of patients), the liver becomes small, shrunken, and soft.

C. Jaundiced skin and icteric sclera on physical examination suggest hyperbilirubinemia from intrahepatic cholestasis caused by the acute hepatic injury. As a result, conjugated bilirubin is inadequately excreted into the bile, explaining the appearance of clay-colored stools. Conjugated bilirubin is also extruded from hepatocytes into the bloodstream, and its water-soluble metabolites are excreted by the kidneys, darkening the urine. These changes in stool and urine often precede clinically evident jaundice. Yellowing of the skin reflects the accumulation of water-insoluble bilirubin metabolites and is usually not appreciated on examination until the serum bilirubin rises above 2.5 mg/dL.

CASE 78

A. This patient has chronic hepatitis B infection. The absence of recurrent acute episodes and extrahepatic involvement suggests chronic persistent infection. Further histologic, serologic,

and autoimmune markers are helpful to determine more precisely whether hepatitis B infection is a chronic persistent or chronic active infection.

B. Approximately 5% of patients acutely infected with hepatitis B will mount an immune response that fails to clear the liver of virus, resulting in a chronic carrier state. Two-thirds of these patients will develop chronic persistent infection characterized by a relatively benign course and rare progression to cirrhosis. One-third will develop chronic active disease marked by histologic changes such as piecemeal necrosis, portal inflammation, distorted lobular architecture, and fibrosis. Chronic active hepatitis patients are at greater risk of progression to cirrhosis and, independently of this risk, are predisposed to hepatocellular carcinoma.

C. Hepatitis D superinfection increases the likelihood of chronic active hepatitis beyond that which usually follows isolated hepatitis B infection. Coinfection is associated with a high incidence of fulminant hepatic failure.

D. Immune-mediated damage is supported by liver biopsy results demonstrating inflammation with lymphocytic infiltration. Viral DNA integrates itself into the genome of the infected cell, and viral antigens are expressed on the surface associated with class I HLA determinants, resulting in lymphocytic cytotoxicity. The degree of injury is largely related to viral replication and the host's immune response.

CASE 79

A. Ethanol has both direct and indirect toxic effects on the liver. Its direct liver injury effects may result from the increased fluidity of biologic membranes and the resulting disruption of cellular functions. Its indirect effects may result from the oxidation of ethanol to acetaldehyde and then to acetate, leading to the promotion of fatty acid synthesis. Acetaldehyde can also be a direct toxin to hepatocytes. In addition, ethanol can alter the pattern of gene expression, resulting in an increased sensitivity to other toxins. Oxidative stress in the liver leading to hepatocyte damage and immune response can propagate further injury. Other molecular mechanisms triggered by ethanol and implicated in the development of alcoholic liver disease include (1) the induction of oxidative stress with resultant mitochondrial damage; (2) the activation of programmed hepatocyte necrosis; (3) the development of pericentral hypoxia; (4) disruption of the gut microbiome; and (5) alteration of the intestinal epithelium resulting in increased permeability and the influx of lipopolysaccharides into the liver, which can, in turn, cause systemic inflammation and trigger apoptotic pathways.

B. Portal hypertension is in part responsible for many of the complications of cirrhosis, including clinically apparent ascites, a sign of liver disease associated with poor long-term survival. Although no single hypothesis can explain its pathogenesis, portal hypertension and inappropriate renal sodium retention are important elements of any theory. Portal hypertension changes the hepatocellular architecture, resulting in increased intrahepatic vascular resistance. This elevates the sinusoidal pressures transmitted to the portal vein and other vascular beds. Splenomegaly and portal-to-systemic shunting result. Vasodilators such as nitric oxide are shunted away from the liver and not cleared from the circulation, resulting in peripheral arteriolar vasodilation. Decreased renal artery perfusion from this vasodilation is perceived as an intravascular volume deficit by the kidney, encouraging sodium and water resorption. By overwhelming oncotic pressure, increased hydrostatic pressure from fluid retention in the portal vein results in ascites formation. Exceeding lymphatic drainage capacity, ascites accumulates in the peritoneum.

C. Splenomegaly and hypersplenism are direct consequences of elevated portal venous pressure. Thrombocytopenia and hemolytic anemia occur as a result of both sequestration of these formed elements by the spleen and the depressive effect of alcohol on the bone marrow. The frequent bruising and elevated prothrombin time in this patient highlight the coagulopathy seen in cirrhosis and chronic liver disease. As a result of inadequate bile excretion, there is an impaired absorption of the fat-soluble vitamin K, a vitamin necessary for the activation of specific clotting factors. In addition, the inadequate hepatic synthesis of other clotting factors causes a coagulopathy.

CASE 80

A. Biliary tract disease is a common cause of acute pancreatitis. It is hypothesized that the inciting event is an obstruction of the common bile and main pancreatic ducts by a gallstone lodged in the ampulla of Vater. Parenchymal injury may be caused by the local reflux of bile or duodenal contents. It has also been proposed that inflammation is caused by bacterial toxins or free bile acids transported from the gallbladder to the pancreas through the lymphatics.

B. Although choledocholithiasis appears to be the most likely cause of this patient's acute pancreatitis, other causes should be considered; for example, alcohol use, infection (viral, bacterial, parasitic), concomitant drugs, recent surgeries, comorbid rheumatologic disease, autoimmune pancreatitis, and hereditary pancreatitis. Laboratory studies such as a serum calcium and lipid panel, including triglycerides, would be helpful in ruling out important metabolic causes of pancreatitis. Of note, however, the cause of the pancreatitis remains unclear despite workup in approximately 15–25% of cases. To help guide prognosis, the Ranson criteria require an assessment of the white blood cell count, serum glucose, LDH, and AST.

C. Acute respiratory distress syndrome (ARDS) may be caused, in part, by activated pancreatic enzymes such as circulating phospholipases, which are released systemically and interfere with the normal function of pulmonary surfactant. In addition, the systemic release of both the CC and CXC

families of cytokines and endotoxin, beginning shortly after pain onset and peaking 36–48 hours later, corresponds temporally with the profound clinical decline observed. In particular, substance P, neurokinin-1, and platelet activating factor (PAF) are involved in the pro-inflammatory responses seen in pancreatitis-associated acute lung injury. Elevated serum levels of IL-6 have been associated with the severity of lung injury in acute pancreatitis, an effect mediated by NFκB activation in pancreatic acinar cells. IL-6 and other inflammatory signaling pathways may prove to be appropriate therapeutic targets in severe acute pancreatitis, although to date no therapeutic agents have been found effective in clinical trials.

CASE 81

A. Alcoholism is the most common cause of chronic pancreatitis, accounting for 70–80% of cases. The risk is directly related to the duration and amount of alcohol consumed, but in fact, only 5–10% of heavy drinkers develop the disease. Recent epidemiologic evidence identifies cigarette smoking as a strong independent risk factor for the development of chronic pancreatitis. Moreover, tobacco exposure appears to have a dose-dependent relationship with its incidence. The number of daily cigarettes smoked as well as the duration of tobacco smoke exposure appear to be important risk factors. Last, the combination of significant alcohol use and cigarette smoking augments the risk of chronic pancreatitis.

B. It is thought that ethanol causes the secretion of insoluble pancreatic proteins that calcify and occlude the pancreatic duct. This results in the progressive fibrosis and subsequent destruction of glandular tissue. In addition, deficiencies of dietary antioxidants such as zinc and selenium may lead to the buildup of toxic free radicals. Unlike other forms of chronic pancreatitis, alcohol-related chronic disease may evolve from multiple episodes of severe acute pancreatitis.

C. Proton pump inhibitors may be helpful adjuvant therapy along with pancreatic enzyme replacement by decreasing postprandial gastric acid secretion, commonly seen in patients with severe pancreatic insufficiency.

CASE 82

A. Because pancreatic lipase is essential for fat digestion, its absence leads to steatorrhea (the occurrence of greasy, bulky, light-colored stools). On the other hand, although pancreatic amylase and trypsin are important for carbohydrate and protein digestion, other enzymes in gastric and intestinal juice can usually compensate for their loss. Thus, patients with pancreatic insufficiency seldom present with maldigestion of carbohydrate and protein (nitrogen loss).

B. In severe cases of fat malabsorption, deficiencies of the fat-soluble vitamins (vitamins A, D, E, and K) may occur and require parenteral supplementation. Diarrhea results from the cathartic action of hydroxylated fatty acids. These fatty acids inhibit the absorption of sodium and water by the colon. Hypocalcemia, hypophosphatemia, tetany, osteomalacia, osteopenia (low bone mineral density), and osteoporosis can occur both from deficiency of the fat-soluble vitamin D and from the binding of dietary calcium to unabsorbed fatty acids, forming insoluble calcium–fat complexes (soaps) in the gut. These soaps also prevent the normal binding of dietary oxalate to calcium. Dietary oxalate remains in solution and is absorbed from the colon, causing hyperoxaluria and predisposing to nephrolithiasis. About 40% of patients with pancreatic insufficiency demonstrate malabsorption of vitamin B_{12} (cobalamin), although clinical manifestations of vitamin B_{12} deficiency (anemia, subacute combined degeneration of the spinal cord, and dementia) are rare. The malabsorption of vitamin B_{12} appears to result from reduced degradation by pancreatic proteases of the normal complexes of vitamin B_{12} and its binding protein (R protein), resulting in less free vitamin B_{12} to bind to intrinsic factor in the small intestine. Finally, long-standing malabsorption leads to protein catabolism and consequent weight loss, muscle wasting, fatigue, and edema. At times, weight loss occurs in patients with chronic pancreatitis because eating exacerbates their abdominal pain or because narcotics used to control pain cause anorexia.

CASE 83

A. A palpable gallbladder in the right upper quadrant is referred to as the Courvoisier law. A palpable gallbladder makes gallstones of the common bile duct less likely than carcinoma of the pancreas because gallstones typically result in inflammation and subsequent scarring, resulting in a shrunken, not distended, gallbladder.

B. Adenocarcinomas of the pancreas may present with anemia, migratory thromboembolic disease, or disseminated intravascular coagulation. The coagulopathies may be related to thromboplastins released within the mucinous secretions of the adenocarcinoma.

C. Clinical prognostic factors include tumor size, site, clinical stage, lymph node metastasis, type of surgery, anemia requiring blood transfusion, performance status, and adjuvant radiation therapy. The poor overall prognosis (5-year survival of <5%, and only 15–20% of patients undergoing curative tumor resections living >5 years) can be attributed primarily to the advanced stage of the disease by the time it presents clinically, the rapid rate of local tumor expansion, and the early systemic dissemination.

CASE 84

A. The clinical summary and the elevated creatine kinase suggest rhabdomyolysis-induced acute tubular necrosis (ATN). Crush injuries release myoglobin into the bloodstream that precipitates in the renal tubules, causing intrarenal toxicity and subsequent failure. With this underlying defect, antibiotic therapy may exacerbate the situation or may induce a separate inflammatory interstitial nephritis. The absence of documented hypotension makes ischemia-mediated ATN less likely. Thus, the patient has an intrarenal cause of acute kidney injury.

B. Besides the likely intrarenal mechanism of disease, she may also have a prerenal cause as a result of dehydration from being trapped or from poor oral intake. To distinguish between these two possibilities, one can calculate the fractional excretion of sodium. The fractional excretion of sodium, FE_{Na+}, derived from measuring the urine and plasma sodium and creatinine, reflects the ability of the kidney to generate a concentrated urine. This function is essentially lost in the setting of acute tubular necrosis, and the patient's urine osmolarity is probably less than 350 mOsm/L. More commonly in the setting of myoglobinuria-induced ATN, her FE_{Na+} would be greater than 2%; however, the FE_{Na+} has been noted to be less than 1% in some cases of rhabdomyolysis.

C. Mainstays of treatment involve maintaining a vigorous alkaline diuresis to prevent myoglobin precipitation in the tubules and adjusting renally cleared antibiotics to prevent further nephrotoxicity.

CASE 85

A. This patient probably suffers from osteoporosis, accelerated by her underlying renal failure. The pathogenesis of bone disease is multifactorial. Calcium is poorly absorbed from the gut because of decreased renally generated vitamin $1,25\text{-}(OH)_2D_3$ levels. Hypocalcemia results and is further exacerbated by high serum phosphate levels from impaired phosphate excretion by the kidney. Low serum calcium and hyperphosphatemia trigger PTH secretion, which depletes bone calcium and contributes to osteomalacia and osteoporosis. Also implicated are the diminished responsiveness of bone to vitamin D_3 and chronic metabolic acidosis.

B. Easy fatigability is often attributable to a worsening normochromic, normocytic anemia seen in chronic kidney disease. This occurs primarily because of impaired erythropoietin synthesis by the kidney and thus decreased erythropoiesis. To improve symptoms, exogenous erythropoietin is started to raise the hematocrit of 25–28%, typically seen in chronic kidney disease patients.

C. A pericardial friction rub suggests uremia-related pericarditis. This is thought to occur from uremic toxins that irritate and inflame the pericardium. The absence of this finding, lack of asterixis, and clear mentation suggest that despite underlying chronic kidney disease, the patient does not exhibit evidence of uremia at this time.

CASE 86

A. Poststreptococcal glomerulonephritis results from a skin infection with a nephritogenic strain of group A (β-hemolytic) streptococci such as type 12. The abrupt onset of hematuria ("cola-colored" urine), edema, and variable degrees of hypertension most commonly occur 7–14 days after streptococcal pharyngitis or impetigo and can occur sporadically or in clusters. Significant glomerular damage can lead to rapid progression to oliguria and acute kidney injury.

B. Bacterial infections can cause glomerular damage through the deposition of antibody–antigen complexes. However, vasculitis does not occur in the setting of all infections. Rather, the subendothelial deposition of immune complexes is required to damage highly vascularized nephrons by fixing complement (this explains the serum levels measured) and by activating myelomonocytic cells. Deposition of these complexes can occur only in the presence of excess antigens to make the complexes soluble, permitting them access to the subendothelial space and enabling them to cause injury.

C. This disorder is usually self-limited; 95% of individuals recover normal renal function within 2 months after onset. As antibody titers rise, immune complex formation decreases, and soluble complexes are eventually cleared provided that antigen administration is not sustained. Treating underlying infectious substrates may hasten the resolution of the glomerulonephritis.

CASE 87

A. Patients with nephrotic syndrome have hypoalbuminemia and profoundly decreased plasma oncotic pressures because of the loss of serum proteins in the urine. This leads to intravascular volume depletion and the activation of the renin–angiotensin–aldosterone system and the sympathetic nervous system. Vasopressin secretion is also increased. Such patients also have altered renal responses to atrial natriuretic peptide. Despite signs of volume overload such as edema or anasarca, patients may develop signs of intravascular volume depletion, including syncope, shock, and acute kidney injury.

B. Minimal change disease, as the name suggests, is associated with few or no changes apparent on light microscopy, as opposed to other subtypes of glomerulonephritis associated with varying degrees of segmental sclerosis or basement membrane thickening. Immunofluorescence staining is generally unremarkable, whereas membranous glomerulonephritis is characterized by IgG and C3 deposited uniformly along capillary loops. However, the pathologic changes are most evident on electron microscopy, which reveals the obliteration of epithelial foot processes and slit diaphragm disruption. Minimal change disease is typically seen in children, but when found in adults it can be idiopathic or can follow an upper respiratory tract infection, can be associated with tumors such as Hodgkin disease, or can be related to hypersensitivity reactions.

C. Hypercoagulability is a clinically significant manifestation of nephrotic syndrome and is caused by renal losses of proteins C and S and antithrombin, as well as elevated serum

fibrinogen and lipid levels. Immobilization from a prolonged hospital stay puts this patient at additional risk for deep venous thrombosis.

CASE 88

A. This patient is presenting with his first episode of renal stone disease. At least 75% of stones are calcium containing and reflect idiopathic hypercalciuria. Hyperparathyroidism and hyperuricosuria are other important causes of calcium stones. Other types of stone are uric acid stones, cysteine stones, and struvite stones. If the patient is able to collect a passed stone, an analysis of its composition would be helpful in diagnosing the subtype and tailoring treatment.

B. After effective pain control is achieved, the patient may return home, and the need for adequate hydration with at least 2 L/day should be reinforced. Hydration may dilute unknown substances that predispose to stone formation and minimize the likelihood of Ca^{2+} precipitation in the nephron. High-protein diets in known stone formers are inadvisable since they predispose to recurrent calcium nephrolithiasis. This results from a transient increase in calcium resorption from bone and increased filtration through the nephron in response to a protein load that stimulates the GFR. A high-sodium diet should be avoided because Na^+ predisposes to Ca^{2+} excretion and increases the saturation of monosodium urate, which acts as a nidus for calcium oxalate stone formation. Dietary calcium restriction is not recommended because it can actually increase oxalate absorption and thus may not decrease urinary calcium excretion. Finally, citrate supplementation may be considered because of the ability of citrate to chelate calcium in solution, forming soluble complexes as opposed to calcium oxalate or phosphate.

C. Fragments of renal pelvis stones that break off and travel down the ureter produce the pain syndrome known as renal colic. In the setting of acute obstruction, distention at the level of the renal pelvis, ureter, or renal capsule can produce pain that can become quite intense.

CASE 89

A. Primary hyperparathyroidism accounts for most cases of hypercalcemia in the outpatient setting. Given the chronic nature of this woman's symptoms and the history of recurrent renal stones, this is the most likely diagnosis. However, particularly in older individuals, hypercalcemia of malignancy is another important cause to consider. Medications, particularly lithium and the thiazide diuretics, also cause hypercalcemia. Other causes include familial hypocalciuric hypercalcemia, thyrotoxicosis, granulomatous diseases, milk–alkali syndrome, and adrenal insufficiency.

B. In primary hyperparathyroidism there is an excessive secretion of PTH in relation to the serum calcium. This is due both to an increase in parathyroid cell mass and to a reduced sensitivity to serum calcium levels, resulting in a qualitative regulatory defect in serum PTH secretion.

The *PRAD1* gene, which produces D1 cyclin, has been implicated in the pathogenesis of primary hyperparathyroidism. Cyclins are cell cycle–regulatory proteins. *PRAD1* and the gene encoding PTH are both located on the long arm of chromosome 11. An inversion event occurs leading to the juxtaposition of the 5′-regulatory domain of the PTH gene upstream to the *PRAD1* gene. This leads to an abnormally regulated transcription of the *PRAD1* gene in a parathyroid-specific manner. The overproduction of the *PRAD1* gene product, D1 cyclin, increases cell proliferation.

The *MEN1* gene, also on chromosome 11, has been implicated in both MEN-1 kindreds and in up to 25% of people with nonfamilial benign primary hyperparathyroidism. *MEN1* appears to be a tumor suppressor gene. The hyperparathyroidism in MEN-2a and MEN-2b appears to be caused by mutations in the RET protein.

C. The diagnosis of primary hyperparathyroidism is confirmed by at least two simultaneous measurements of serum calcium and intact PTH. An elevated or normal PTH in the setting of hypercalcemia confirms the diagnosis.

CASE 90

A. The likely diagnosis in this patient is familial hypocalciuric hypercalcemia (FHH). The diagnosis is suggested by the findings of an elevated serum calcium level with normal levels of intact parathyroid hormone (PTH) and 1,25-OH vitamin D. It is possible that the patient also has mild primary hyperparathyroidism, but the low urinary calcium excretion strongly suggests FHH rather than hyperparathyroidism.

B. This condition results from a defect in the CaSR, a member of the G protein receptor family. CaSR is highly expressed in the kidney and parathyroid glands. In the kidney, CaSR detects the serum calcium concentration and adjusts the urinary calcium excretion accordingly. In the parathyroid glands, CaSR regulates the secretion of PTH. If CaSR is defective, it misreads the serum calcium concentration as inappropriately low and causes the kidneys to retain calcium and the parathyroid glands to secrete excess PTH. Fortunately, in FHH, the elevation in serum calcium tends to be mild, and most patients are clinically asymptomatic. A rare, severe form that manifests in infancy is called neonatal severe primary hyperparathyroidism. Although this is a genetic disorder with an autosomal dominant mode of inheritance, there is no genetic testing available for the condition because the various responsible mutations are dispersed over the large gene encoding the calcium receptor.

CASE 91

A. Hypercalcemia is most commonly seen in solid tumors, primarily squamous cell carcinomas, renal cell carcinoma, and breast carcinoma. It also occurs frequently in plasma cell myeloma. It occurs less commonly in lymphomas and leukemias. Given this patient's long-standing smoking history and abnormal lung examination, the most likely diagnosis is squamous cell carcinoma of the lung.

B. Serum PTH should be undetectable, and PTHrP should be elevated. This is due to the fact that 70–80% of malignancy-induced hypercalcemia is caused by tumor PTHrP secretion. In particular, this is true of squamous cell carcinoma–induced hypercalcemia.

C. PTHrP is homologous with PTH at its amino terminal and is recognized by the type 1 PTH receptor. Therefore, it has effects on bone and kidney similar to those of PTH, including increasing bone resorption, increasing phosphate excretion, and decreasing renal calcium excretion.

CASE 92

A. The parathyroid glands lie in close proximity to the thyroid gland and are, therefore, at risk of trauma, devascularization, or removal during thyroid surgery. Damage to the parathyroid glands results in decreased PTH release, with a resultant inability to maintain normal serum calcium concentrations. Because PTH is required to stimulate the renal production of 1,25-$(OH)_2D$, levels of 1,25-$(OH)_2D$ are low in patients with hypoparathyroidism. This leads to reduced intestinal calcium absorption. In the absence of adequate PTH and 1,25-$(OH)_2D$, the mobilization of calcium from bone is abnormal. Furthermore, because less PTH is available to act in the distal nephron, urinary calcium excretion may be high. A combination of these mechanisms is responsible for the hypocalcemia seen in hypoparathyroidism.

There may be a prolonged latent period before symptomatic hypocalcemia develops. Hypoparathyroidism may vary in severity. In this case, it is likely that the patient has decreased parathyroid reserve only. The increased stress on her parathyroid glands because of her pregnancy has probably precipitated her symptomatic hypocalcemia.

B. The Chvostek sign is elicited by tapping on the facial nerve anterior to the ear. Twitching of the ipsilateral facial muscles is a positive test. A positive Trousseau sign is demonstrated by inflating the sphygmomanometer above the systolic blood pressure for 3 min. Painful carpal muscle contractions and spasms signify a positive test. Both signs indicate latent tetany secondary to hypocalcemia.

C. Serum phosphate is often but not invariably elevated in hypoparathyroidism. Hyperphosphatemia occurs because the proximal tubular effect of PTH to promote phosphate excretion is lost. Due to the decrease in its release, the serum PTH will be low.

CASE 93

A. Medullary carcinoma of the thyroid is a C-cell neoplasm. Because C cells are neuroendocrine cells, they have the capacity to release several hormones. The secretion of serotonin, prostaglandins, or calcitonin probably causes the watery (secretory) diarrhea this patient has. Flushing is generally caused by the tumor producing either substance P or calcitonin gene–related peptide, both of which are vasodilators.

B. The diagnosis would be made most efficiently by fine-needle aspiration of the thyroid nodules. They should demonstrate the characteristic C-cell lesion with positive immunostaining for calcitonin. A serum calcitonin level would also be beneficial, because it is typically elevated in medullary carcinoma and correlates with extent of tumor burden. Calcitonin levels may be monitored during treatment to assess response.

C. As noted, serum calcitonin levels are a useful means of assessing tumor burden and for monitoring disease progression during and after treatment. Serum carcinoembryonic antigen (CEA) is also frequently elevated in patients with medullary carcinoma and is present at all stages of the disease. Rapid increases in CEA predict a worse clinical course.

All patients with medullary carcinoma of the thyroid should be tested for the *RET* oncogene. Although this patient denies a family history of MEN, she is young (<40 years) and has bilateral tumors, both of which are concerning for hereditary forms of medullary carcinoma and the MEN syndromes. More than 95% of patients with MEN-2 harbor *RET* mutations. Even sporadic cases of medullary carcinoma should be tested for *RET* mutations, because new mutations in the *RET* gene are frequently present, and family members can then be screened for these mutations.

If MEN-2 syndrome is detected in this patient, she should be tested for pheochromocytoma, as well as for hyperparathyroidism, before undergoing thyroid surgery. This can be done by testing plasma fractionated metanephrines together with serum calcium and PTH; additional biochemical testing or imaging would be undertaken as indicated.

CASE 94

A. Genetics are very important in determining peak bone mass and loss. However, a number of hormonal and environmental factors can reduce the genetically determined peak bone mass or hasten the loss of bone mineral and thus present important risk factors for osteoporosis. The most important etiologic factor in osteoporosis is a deficiency of gonadal sex steroids, either estrogen in the case of postmenopausal women or testosterone in hypogonadal men. Another important cause is excess cortisol, either in the form of exogenous corticosteroid use or endogenous excess in Cushing syndrome. Other medications such as heparin, thyroid hormone, and anticonvulsants can also cause osteoporosis. Immobilization, alcohol abuse, and smoking are additional important risk factors. Adequate dietary calcium and vitamin D intake and weight-bearing exercise are vital because they are necessary to build peak bone mass and minimize loss. Many other disorders affecting the GI, hematologic, and connective tissue systems can contribute to the development of osteoporosis (Table 17–10).

B. This patient likely has a combination of postmenopausal and age-related osteoporosis. Postmenopausal osteoporosis is caused by accelerated bone resorption. Although bone formation is also increased, it is insufficient to fully counteract bone resorption, and net bone loss occurs. The cellular basis for the activation of bone resorption in postmenopausal osteoporosis is somewhat unclear. Osteoclasts have estrogen receptors, and this may account at least in part for their activation during estrogen deficiency. There is also evidence that osteoclast-stimulating cytokines, such as IL-6, are released from other bone cells after menopause.

The pathogenesis of age-related or senile osteoporosis is even less clear. Again, there is an uncoupling of bone resorption and bone formation, such that bone formation does not keep pace with resorption. A deficiency of dietary calcium and $1,25\text{-}(OH)_2D$ is one important pathogenic factor. As people age, intestinal calcium absorption is decreased while renal calcium loss is preserved, resulting in an increased need for dietary calcium. This occurs at a time when most people reduce their calcium intake, often related to lactose intolerance.

In addition, some older individuals may be deficient in vitamin D, further impairing their ability to absorb calcium. Particularly in northern climates, where sunlight exposure is reduced in the winter months, borderline low levels of $1,25\text{-}(OH)_2D$ and mild secondary hyperparathyroidism are evident by the end of winter.

Secondary hyperparathyroidism may also occur in older people due to changes in multiple organ systems that occur with aging, including decreased renal function. As renal function decreases, so may renal production of $1,25\text{-}(OH)_2D$, thereby increasing PTH secretion. Reduced $1,25\text{-}(OH)_2D$ secretion also results in decreased calcium absorption, exacerbating the intrinsic inability of the aging intestine to absorb calcium. Because the responsiveness of the parathyroid gland to calcium seems to be reduced in aging, the hyperparathyroidism seen in aging seems to be the result of the combined effects of aging on the kidney, intestine, and parathyroid gland.

C. There are three major risk factors for fractures in osteoporosis: decreased bone density, poor bone quality, and falls. For every standard deviation below the mean bone density for age, there is a 2- to 3-fold increased risk of fracture. The microarchitecture of bone also determines its mechanical strength and its ability to withstand stress. Finally, fractures rarely occur unless people fall or otherwise sustain trauma. Muscle weakness, impaired vision, impaired balance, sedative use, and environmental factors (eg, stairs, carpeting) are all important risk factors for falls and, therefore, fractures.

D. The 6-month mortality rate for hip fracture is approximately 20%, much of it resulting from the complications of immobilizing a frail person in a hospital bed. These complications include pulmonary embolus and pneumonia. About half of elderly people with a hip fracture will never walk freely again.

E. Treatments for reduced bone mass include calcium and vitamin D supplementation, estrogen replacement therapy with hormone replacement therapy or raloxifene, antiresorptive agents such as the bisphosphonates, calcitonin, denosumab (a monoclonal antibody to RANK ligand), and PTH. In contrast to the bone resorption caused by continuous PTH elevations such as occur in hyperparathyroidism, a single daily injection of PTH stimulates bone formation and, to a lesser extent, bone resorption, resulting in net gains in bone density and decreased fracture risk.

CASE 95

A. Osteomalacia can result from vitamin D deficiency, phosphate deficiency, hypophosphatasia, and several toxic substances (fluoride, aluminum, and phosphate-binding agents) with effects on bone. Vitamin D deficiency is the likely cause in this patient. She is bed-bound, living in a basement apartment without adequate sunlight exposure. She is a strict vegetarian, even refraining from ingesting dairy products, so she has limited to no exposure to dietary vitamin D supplementation. Finally, the x-ray evidence of pseudofracture of the pubic rami is strongly indicative of vitamin D–deficient osteomalacia.

B. Vitamin D deficiency produces osteomalacia in two stages. Initially, decreased vitamin D leads to decreased intestinal calcium absorption and secondary hyperparathyroidism. Serum calcium is maintained at the expense of increased renal phosphate excretion and hypophosphatemia. Ultimately, however, hypocalcemia ensues. Poor delivery of calcium and phosphate to bone results in impaired matrix mineralization. Osteoid or unmineralized matrix, therefore, accumulates at the bone-forming surfaces.

C. If bone undergoes biopsy for quantitative histomorphometry, osteoid seams and a reduction in the mineralization rate are found.

CASE 96

A. Type 1 diabetes mellitus (DM) is an autoimmune disease caused by the selective destruction of pancreatic β cells by T lymphocytes targeting ill-defined β-cell antigens. An asymptomatic stage of β-cell autoantibody positivity, which peaks in incidence at 1–2 years of age, is followed by at least 1–2 years of dysglycemia (abnormal OGTT and hemoglobin A_{1C} and loss of first-phase insulin release) attributable to gradual T cell–mediated dysfunction and/or destruction of the islets (Figure 18–7). The clinical onset of symptoms, and thus diagnosis, occurs only after sufficient β-cell mass (more than 70%) has been lost to cause extreme insulinopenia.

B. At least 50% of the genetic susceptibility in type 1 DM has been linked to the genes of the major histocompatibility complex (MHC) that encode class II human leukocyte antigen (HLA) molecules expressed on the surface of specific antigen-presenting cells such as macrophages. While 95% of individuals with type 1 DM have either DR3-DQ2 or DR4-DQ8 haplotypes, they share this genotype with 40% of the general population. In addition, only 6% of children with high-risk HLA types will develop diabetes. Also, only 15% of newly diagnosed patients with type 1 diabetes have a positive family history, and there is only a 30% concordance rate in identical twins. Therefore, environmental factors also play a large role in the pathogenesis. Evidence suggests that viral infections, such as congenital exposure to rubella, may precipitate disease, particularly in genetically susceptible individuals. It is hypothesized that an immune response to foreign antigens could incite β-cell destruction if these foreign antigens have some homology with islet cell antigens (molecular mimicry). For example, coxsackievirus infections are also associated with the onset of type 1 DM, and one particular coxsackie viral protein shares homology with the islet cell antigen glutamic acid decarboxylase (GAD). Vitamin D deficiency also correlates with a greater risk of type 1 DM, which may partially explain the increased incidence of type 1 DM at higher latitudes where populations have less exposure to sunlight.

C. Patients with type 1 DM are always insulinopenic due to the destruction of pancreatic β cells. A profound loss of insulin activity leads not only to increased serum glucose levels because of increased hepatic glucose output and decreased glucose uptake by insulin-sensitive tissues, but also to ketogenesis. In the absence of insulin, lipolysis is stimulated, providing fatty acids that are preferentially converted to ketone bodies in the liver by unopposed glucagon action. Most patients with type 2 DM have enough insulin to prevent the initiation of such ketone production in the liver.

CASE 97

A. Ketoacidosis is caused by a severe lack of insulin, seen most commonly in patients with type 1 DM, and it may be the initial presentation of this disorder. However, in this patient with a long-standing history of type 2 DM, resultant insulin resistance, and true insulinopenia, ketosis was precipitated by acute infection. In this case, severe cellulitis induced counter-regulatory hormone production, which inhibits insulin's action. Thus, in the effective absence of insulin, lipolysis generates fatty acids that are preferentially converted to ketone bodies by the liver, resulting in ketoacidosis.

B. Altered mental status in diabetic ketoacidosis, as in hyperosmolar coma, most closely correlates with the degree of hyperosmolality induced by hyperglycemia and the associated osmotic diuresis. Profound intracellular dehydration is seen in the brain as fluid shifts in response to elevated plasma osmolality. The effective osmolality in this patient is calculated as follows: $2(132 + 3.7) + (488 \div 18) = 298.5$. Coma occurs when the effective plasma osmolality reaches 340 mOsm/L. Although alterations in mental status can occur as plasma osmolality rises above the upper limit of normal (295 mOsm/L), patients usually do not exhibit anything more than mild to moderate drowsiness at the level of osmolarity seen in this patient. Therefore, other possible causes of altered mental status should be considered, including stroke, infection, and drugs.

C. This patient exhibits Kussmaul breathing (hyperpnea that effectively drops the PCO_2 to partially compensate for the underlying metabolic acidosis). This respiratory pattern is commonly seen with a blood pH less than 7.20. In addition, the fruity odor detected on his breath is due to the keto acid acetone produced in this disorder.

D. Mainstays of treatment for diabetic ketoacidosis include concomitant insulin therapy along with free water and electrolyte replacement. The osmotic diuresis results in significant free water loss and total body potassium depletion. However, the serum potassium appears normal because of the shift of K^+ out of cells and into the extracellular space—induced by acidosis, hyperglycemia, and insulinopenia. Correction of the acidosis and hyperglycemia with insulin therapy shifts potassium back into cells. Unless carefully monitored and replete, serum K^+ levels can drop dangerously low, leading to potentially fatal cardiac arrhythmias. Phosphate depletion can also be seen, but replacement is considered only in severe cases because of the risks of intravenous phosphate repletion.

CASE 98

A. The Whipple triad sets forth the diagnostic criteria for hypoglycemia: (1) symptoms and signs of hypoglycemia; (2) an associated low plasma glucose level; and (3) an improvement in symptoms with the administration of glucose. This patient's self-diagnosis of hypoglycemic attacks meets these criteria.

B. The patient's age and the fasting hypoglycemia are suggestive of insulinoma, an insulin-secreting tumor of the B cells of the islets of Langerhans. Normally during exercise, insulin levels decline, allowing for significant glycogen uptake in the periphery. In addition, glucagon-stimulated hepatic glucose output increases to maintain adequate serum glucose levels, and counter-regulatory hormones mobilize fatty acids for ketogenesis and fatty acid oxidation by muscle. However, during exercise, an elevated insulin level secreted by an insulinoma suppresses the glucagon-mediated glucose output while insulin-induced peripheral glucose uptake continues. Thus, the patient becomes hypoglycemic, and his symptoms recur.

C. Hypoglycemia in the setting of an elevated serum insulin level essentially rules out examples of non–insulin-mediated causes of hypoglycemia such as Addison disease, sepsis, and severe hepatic injury. The differential diagnosis of insulin-mediated hypoglycemia includes surreptitious insulin injection, oral hypoglycemic use (stimulating endogenous insulin production), and the presence of insulin antibodies. In this patient, a C peptide measurement was elevated, suggesting that this was not due to surreptitious injections or antibodies. A greater challenge is to distinguish insulinoma from oral hypoglycemic use, both of which show an elevated C peptide

and, therefore, require the direct measurement of serum levels of oral hypoglycemic agents to confirm the latter diagnosis.

CASE 99

A. Necrolytic migratory erythema is typically a late manifestation of glucagonoma and may be the result of hypoaminoacidemia stemming from the excessive glucagon-mediated hepatic uptake of amino acids. This nutritional deficiency, rather than a direct effect of glucagon itself, is linked to the dermatologic manifestations.

B. Diabetes or glucose intolerance is usually mild, seen in response to the hyperstimulation of hepatic glucose output by supranormal glucagon levels. Subsequently, serum insulin is increased, which prevents lipolysis and an associated ketotic state.

C. Glucagonomas are usually malignant, and weight loss and liver metastasis are present in 50–90% of patients at the time of diagnosis. Surgical resection is rarely pursued. Once diagnosed, the median survival is typically less than 3 years.

CASE 100

A. Somatostatinomas are very rare tumors, typically associated with a triad of findings including diabetes, steatorrhea, and cholelithiasis. The latter finding is thought to be due to somatostatin-induced gallbladder hypomotility.

B. Because somatostatin suppresses both insulin and glucagon secretion, the resulting hyperglycemic state is mild and not accompanied by glucagon-mediated hepatic ketogenesis.

CASE 101

A. Body weight is controlled by a complex interaction of hormones that act on the hypothalamus to maintain body weight over the short and long term. A key mechanism by which short-term food intake and satiety are regulated is communication via the "gut–brain axis." The gut–brain crosstalk uses two main routes of communication: neural components (ie, afferent vagal fibers) and hormonal components (cholecystokinin [CCK], glucagon-like peptide-1 [GLP-1], and ghrelin). In contrast to the short-term control of body weight, long-term regulation is largely influenced by the degree of obesity. Fat cells secrete hormones including leptin in proportion to the amount of triglyceride they have stored. Leptin decreases appetite and increases metabolism through effects in the CNS.

B. Body mass index (BMI) is the most commonly used index of overweight and obesity. The BMI is calculated as the patient's body weight (in kilograms) divided by height (in meters squared). The normal range is defined as a BMI of 18.5–25; overweight is defined as a BMI of 25.1–30; and obesity is defined as a BMI of more than 30.

C. Obesity increases the risk of developing many medical conditions. Obesity increases insulin resistance and can lead to the development of type 2 diabetes. Obese people have increased vascular tone and sodium retention, leading to hypertension. These two risk factors, as well as decreases in high-density lipoprotein cholesterol and increases in low-density lipoprotein cholesterol, in obese persons can lead to coronary artery disease or stroke. The excess soft tissue in the head and neck can lead to obstructive sleep apnea. Increases in serum estrogen and cholesterol levels in obese individuals can lead to gallstones. The excess wear and tear on joints can lead to osteoarthritis. Uric acid levels can be elevated and lead to gout. Also, obese individuals have an increased risk of several cancers.

CASE 102

A. The likely diagnosis is pituitary adenoma.

B. The pituitary adenoma probably developed from a single cell with altered growth control and feedback regulation. At least four different syndromes caused by defined genetic mutations are known to significantly raise the incidence of pituitary tumor formation: multiple endocrine neoplasia type 1 (MEN-1), Carney complex (CNC), McCune–Albright syndrome, and *AIP* (aryl hydrocarbon receptor–interacting protein)-related predisposition to pituitary adenoma. In this patient, a multistep process of genetic alterations and local cell reactions likely led to the formation of the adenoma. Several known and proposed factors have been shown to be contribute to the transformation of pituitary cells (eg, GNAS1, PTTG).

C. Both this patient's bitemporal hemianopia and her headaches are symptoms of the mass effect of the pituitary adenoma. The bitemporal hemianopia occurs because the crossing fibers of the optic tract, which lie directly above the pituitary gland and innervate the part of the retina responsible for temporal vision, are compressed by the tumor. Her headaches are caused by stretching of the dura by the tumor.

D. Irregular menses and galactorrhea are symptoms of prolactin excess. Galactorrhea occurs because of the direct effect of prolactin, and irregular menses are due to the indirect effect of prolactin suppressing gonadal function.

CASE 103

A. This patient probably suffers from amenorrhea resulting from hypopituitarism. Her history of pituitary radiation is strongly suggestive of this cause. Radiation therapy frequently results in progressive destruction of the pituitary gland. This results in LH and FSH deficiency, causing menstrual irregularity and ultimately amenorrhea.

B. The patient's history of fatigue and weight gain, in conjunction with the physical examination findings of dry, brittle hair and a delayed relaxation phase in her deep tendon reflexes,

suggests the diagnosis of hypothyroidism. Again, given her history of pituitary radiation, TSH deficiency is the probable cause.

C. One should be concerned about the diagnosis of panhypopituitarism in this patient. In addition to LH, FSH, and TSH deficiency, she may also have deficiencies of ACTH and vasopressin. Because mineralocorticoid secretion is only partially controlled by ACTH, sufficient glucocorticoid may be present even in the absence of ACTH. Adrenal insufficiency may go unnoticed until another unrelated medical emergency occurs and the patient is unable to mount a normal protective stress response. Vasopressin deficiency may go unnoticed as long as the patient is able to maintain adequate fluid intake to compensate for the inability to concentrate urine.

CASE 104

A. Both central and nephrogenic diabetes insipidus result in the same symptoms: polyuria, polydipsia, hypotonic urine, and hypernatremia. The history of lithium use, however, is suggestive of nephrogenic diabetes insipidus. To confirm the diagnosis, one must assess responsiveness to injected vasopressin. In central diabetes insipidus, vasopressin causes a dramatic decrease in urine volume and an increase in urine osmolarity. This occurs because the basic defect in central diabetes insipidus is a lack of vasopressin. In nephrogenic diabetes insipidus, injected vasopressin has little or no effect because the kidneys are unable to respond to the circulating vasopressin.

B. Vasopressin receptors in the kidney appear to be sensitive to lithium and other salts, preventing vasopressin binding and therefore disabling the kidney's ability to retain water.

C. Polyuria in nephrogenic diabetes insipidus results from the inability to conserve water in the distal nephron because of a lack of vasopressin-dependent water channels. These channels are normally inserted into the apical plasma membrane in response to vasopressin stimulation, resulting in water conservation. In nephrogenic diabetes insipidus, the kidneys are resistant to circulating vasopressin and unable to respond to it. Thirst results from the hypertonicity brought on by the inability to concentrate the urine.

D. If the patient is unable to maintain sufficient water intake for any reason, dehydration and hypernatremia result. This can lead to progressive obtundation, myoclonus, seizures, and ultimately coma.

CASE 105

A. The syndrome of inappropriate ADH (vasopressin) secretion (SIADH) is caused by a variety of vasopressin-secreting tumors, CNS disorders, pulmonary disorders, and drugs. Small cell bronchial carcinoma is an important cause of SIADH and is present in this patient. His lung examination and fever suggest the possibility of pneumonia, another cause of SIADH. Although this patient is not currently undergoing therapy for lung cancer, several chemotherapeutic agents can cause SIADH, including vincristine and vinblastine, and it would be important to determine whether the patient was given either of these drugs during his therapy.

B. SIADH is due to a secretion of vasopressin in excess of what is appropriate for hyperosmolarity or intravascular volume depletion. The pathophysiologic mechanisms behind most cases of SIADH are poorly understood. However, in this patient, the most likely cause is small cell lung cancer, which is probably secreting vasopressin.

C. The patient's neurologic symptoms are the result of osmotic fluid shifts causing brain edema and elevated intracranial pressures. These are the result of hyponatremia.

D. Hyponatremia resulting from SIADH is treated with simple water restriction. Treatment of the underlying disease can help as well.

CASE 106

A. Other historical features to be elicited include heat intolerance, excessive sweating, nervousness, irritability, emotional lability, restlessness, poor concentration, muscle weakness, palpitations, and increased frequency of bowel movements.

B. The examiner should evaluate the eyes for stare, lid lag, proptosis, and abnormal eye movements; the heart for irregular rhythm, flow murmur, and heart failure; the breasts for gynecomastia; the nails for onycholysis; the pretibial area for dermopathy; and the deep tendon reflexes for a rapid relaxation phase.

C. The free thyroxine (free T_4) level should be high; the TSH level should be low. Rarely, hyperthyroidism is caused by secondary or tertiary hyperthyroidism as a result of excessive TSH or TRH production, respectively. In these cases, TSH would be elevated.

D. Possible causes of this patient's condition include thyroid hormone overproduction (in Graves disease, toxic multinodular goiter, and autonomous hyperfunctioning follicular adenoma), thyroid gland destruction with the release of stored hormone (in thyroiditis), or the ingestion of excessive exogenous thyroid hormone.

E. Graves disease is the most common cause of hyperthyroidism. In Graves disease, TSH receptor autoantibodies, TSH-R [stim] Ab, also known as thyroid-stimulating antibodies (TSIs), are present in the circulation. These are autoantibodies of the IgG class, directed against TSH receptors on the follicular cell membrane. When they bind to the cell membrane TSH receptors, they stimulate the thyroid follicular cells to produce excessive amounts of T_4 and T_3, causing hyperthyroidism. The precipitating cause of this antibody production is unknown, but an immune response against a viral antigen that shares homology with TSH-R may be responsible. Another theory of the pathogenesis of Graves disease is a defect of suppressor T

lymphocytes, which allows helper T lymphocytes to stimulate B lymphocytes to secrete antibodies directed against follicular cell membrane antigens, including the TSH receptor.

F. Tachycardia is thought to be related to the direct effects of excess thyroid hormone on the cardiac conducting system. The pathogenesis of thyroid dermopathy may involve lymphocyte cytokine stimulation of fibroblasts. Thyroid dermopathy is associated with a very high serum titer of TSH-R [stim] Ab. Weight loss results from an increase in the basal metabolic rate. Autoantibodies have been identified that stimulate the growth of thyroid epithelial cells and produce the goiter of Graves disease. The muscle weakness is related to increased protein catabolism and muscle wasting, decreased muscle efficiency, and changes in myosin.

CASE 107

A. Other features to be elicited in the history include cold intolerance, mental slowing, forgetfulness, lethargy, muscle weakness or cramps, and hair loss. The examiner should also evaluate the body temperature, the musculature for weakness, the face and skin for puffiness and carotenemia, the extremities for edema, and the deep tendon reflexes for sluggishness and a slowed ("hung-up") relaxation phase.

B. Weight gain is related to a decrease in the basal metabolic rate. Constipation is caused by decreased GI motility. Menorrhagia results from anovulatory menstrual cycles. Thyroid atrophy and fibrosis may result from lymphocytic infiltration and the destruction of thyroid follicles, the destruction of the thyroid by surgery or radiation, or atrophy as a result of diminished TSH secretion. The skin changes of hypothyroidism are the result of an accumulation of polysaccharides in the dermis.

The quiet heart sounds may be related to the development of pericardial effusion or of cardiomyopathy caused by the deposition of mucopolysaccharides in the interstitium between myocardial fibers.

C. Serum TSH is the most sensitive test for detecting hypothyroidism. TSH is elevated in almost all cases of hypothyroidism, with the rare exceptions of pituitary and hypothalamic disease. Free thyroxine levels should be low.

D. In the adult, hypothyroidism may result from Hashimoto (autoimmune) thyroiditis, lymphocytic thyroiditis, thyroid ablation (via surgery or radiation), hypopituitarism or hypothalamic disease, or drugs. The most likely cause of this patient's hypothyroidism is Hashimoto thyroiditis, both because it is the most common cause and because of the atrophic thyroid gland on examination.

E. Other autoimmune disorders, including endocrine disorders such as diabetes mellitus and hypoadrenalism, and nonendocrine disorders such as pernicious anemia, systemic lupus erythematosus, and myasthenia gravis are all seen with increased frequency in patients with Hashimoto thyroiditis.

CASE 108

A. The physician should ask about causes of goiter such as an increased intake of foods containing goitrogens (eg, rutabaga, cabbage, turnip, cassava), a diminished intake of foods containing iodine (eg, fish), and the use of medications associated with goiter (eg, propylthiouracil, methimazole, nitroprusside, sulfonylureas, lithium). Symptoms of thyroid encroachment on surrounding structures such as respiratory or swallowing difficulties should be elicited. Because of this patient's fatigue and depression, the physician should also probe for other symptoms of hypothyroidism.

B. The most common cause of goiter in developing nations is dietary iodine deficiency. Because this patient is 40 years of age and recently emigrated from Afghanistan, iodine deficiency would be the most likely cause. A diet low in iodine (<10 μg/d) hinders the synthesis of thyroid hormone, resulting in decreased thyroid hormone secretions and an elevated TSH level. The elevation in serum TSH level results in diffuse thyroid hyperplasia. If TSH stimulation is prolonged, the diffuse hyperplasia is followed by focal hyperplasia with necrosis, hemorrhage, and nodule formation.

C. The serum TSH should be determined to exclude hypothyroidism.

CASE 109

A. Primarily on the basis of the history consistent with hyperthyroidism and the presence of a single thyroid nodule palpable on examination, this patient most likely has hyperthyroidism resulting from an autonomous hyperfunctioning follicular adenoma.

B. A serum TSH should be ordered and possibly a free thyroxine index. The free thyroxine index will be elevated and the serum TSH suppressed if the patient is truly hyperthyroid.

C. A radioactive iodine scan could be performed to confirm the diagnosis. Radioactive iodine uptake will be elevated in the region of the nodule and suppressed elsewhere. The thyroid scan will show a "hot" nodule.

D. A biopsy of the nodule will show normal follicles of varying size. An excisional biopsy will show compression of surrounding normal thyroid and areas of hemorrhage, fibrosis, and calcification or cystic degeneration. Biopsy is important to rule out the diagnosis of thyroid cancer, although given the patient's symptoms of hyperthyroidism, this is less likely.

CASE 110

A. Although this patient has an elevated total T_4 level, she has no symptoms or signs of hyperthyroidism. An elevated total T_4 level in clinically euthyroid individuals may be idiopathic or may be due to pregnancy, acute or chronic hepatitis, acute intermittent porphyria, estrogen-producing tumors, or hereditary disorders. Drugs that may cause elevated total T_4 levels are estrogens (including oral contraceptives), methadone, heroin, perphenazine, and clofibrate.

B. The resin uptake of T_4 or T_3 (RT_4U or RT_3U) should be determined and the free thyroxine index calculated. The serum TSH level should be normal if the patient is euthyroid.

C. Elevated TBG levels in pregnancy lead to an increased binding of free T_4. When the free T_4 level falls, the pituitary secretes more TSH. This, in turn, leads to increased T_4 production by the gland and equilibration at a new level at which the total T_4 level is elevated but the free T_4 level is again normal.

D. A syndrome of familial euthyroid hyperthyroxinemia is most likely. These inherited syndromes may be caused by several mechanisms, including the abnormal binding of T_4 (but not T_3) to albumin, an increased serum level of transthyretin, an altered affinity of transthyretin for T_4, or pituitary and peripheral resistance to thyroid hormone.

CASE 111

A. In the presence of circulating thyroid (anti-TPO) autoantibodies, approximately 5% of individuals with subclinical hypothyroidism progress to overt hypothyroidism each year, compared with 2% per year or less among those without thyroid autoantibodies.

B. Subclinical hypothyroidism is associated with an increased risk of atherosclerotic heart disease and heart failure, particularly in individuals whose TSH levels are greater than 10 mU/L. Other studies suggest the risk of cardiovascular complications may be limited to younger individuals (those younger than 55 years). Some, but not all, studies suggest subtle neurocognitive abnormalities, particularly related to executive functions.

C. Unfortunately, there have not yet been any large randomized trials of the treatment of subclinical hypothyroidism with clinical endpoints such as heart disease or heart failure. Some individuals report improved exercise tolerance and an improved sense of well-being when given sufficient thyroxine to normalize serum TSH, but there is insufficient evidence to recommend the routine treatment of individuals with persistent subclinical hypothyroidism that does not progress to overt hypothyroidism. A large multicenter placebo-controlled trial in Europe (TRUST) has been designed to address this issue, and published results have revealed that levothyroxine provided no symptomatic benefits for elderly patients with subclinical hypothyroidism.

CASE 112

A. Prospective studies have demonstrated subtle abnormalities of cardiac contractility in individuals with subclinical hyperthyroidism, and one prospective study found that individuals older than 65 years with TSH levels of less than 0.1 mU/L had a threefold greater risk of developing atrial fibrillation than those with normal TSH levels. In postmenopausal women, subclinical hyperthyroidism may also be associated with bone loss and fracture. In a prospective study of women older than 65 years, the risks of hip and spine fracture were two to three times higher among those with TSH levels less than 0.1 mU/L (mostly from over-replacement with thyroid hormone) compared with those with normal TSH levels.

B. Autonomous thyroid nodules and early Graves disease are believed to account for the majority of cases.

C. On one hand, the desire to avoid atrial fibrillation and serious fractures, mentioned above, may drive the clinician to recommend treatment. However, the natural history of subclinical hyperthyroidism is not well known. One study of postmenopausal women with endogenous subclinical hyperthyroidism found that more than 50% had normal TSH levels after 1 year of follow-up, arguing for observation and laboratory test monitoring, at least for a limited time.

CASE 113

A. Additional features of Cushing syndrome include hirsutism (82%), muscular weakness (58%) and muscular atrophy (70%), back pain (58%), acne (40%), psychological symptoms (40%), edema (18%), headache (14%), polyuria and polydipsia (10%), and hyperpigmentation (6%).

B. The exact cause of hypertension in hypercortisolism remains unclear. It may be related to salt and water retention from the mineralocorticoid effects of the excess glucocorticoid, the increased secretion of angiotensinogen or deoxycorticosterone, or a direct effect of glucocorticoids on blood vessels.

The cause of the obesity and redistribution of body fat seen in Cushing syndrome is also somewhat unclear. It may be explained by the increase in appetite or by the lipogenic effects of hyperinsulinemia caused by cortisol excess. The striae result from increased subcutaneous fat deposition, which stretches the thin skin and ruptures the subdermal tissues. These striae are depressed below the skin surface because of the loss of underlying connective tissue.

C. Major causes of Cushing syndrome include Cushing disease (ACTH-secreting pituitary adenoma), ectopic ACTH syndrome, a functioning adrenocortical adenoma or carcinoma, and long-term high-dose exogenous glucocorticoid intake (iatrogenic Cushing syndrome).

In Cushing disease and in ectopic ACTH syndrome, the production of both ACTH and cortisol is excessive. Adrenocortical adenomas or carcinomas are characterized by the autonomous secretion of cortisol and the suppression of pituitary ACTH. The most likely cause in this patient, a 38-year-old woman with a gradual onset of symptoms, is Cushing disease (ACTH-secreting pituitary adenoma).

D. Current recommendations involve a stepwise approach to diagnostic evaluation. The first step is to demonstrate pathologic hypercortisolemia and confirm the diagnosis of Cushing syndrome. The measurement of free cortisol in a 24-hour urine specimen collected on an outpatient basis demonstrates an excessive excretion of cortisol (24-hour urinary free cortisol levels >150 μg/24 h) and is the most sensitive and specific screening test for Cushing syndrome. Urinary free cortisol values are rarely normal in Cushing syndrome. Performance of an overnight 1 mg dexamethasone suppression test will demonstrate a lack of the normal suppression by exogenous corticosteroid (dexamethasone) of adrenal cortisol production. The overnight dexamethasone suppression test is accomplished by prescribing 1 mg of dexamethasone at 11:00 PM and then obtaining a plasma cortisol level the following morning at 8:00 AM. In normal individuals, the dexamethasone suppresses the early-morning surge in cortisol, resulting in plasma cortisol levels of less than 5 μg/dL (0.14 μmol/L); in Cushing syndrome, cortisol secretion is not suppressed to as great a degree, and values are more than 10 μg/dL (0.28 μmol/ L). If the overnight dexamethasone suppression test result is normal, the diagnosis is very unlikely; if the 24-hour urine free cortisol level is also normal, Cushing syndrome is excluded. If both test results are abnormal, hypercortisolism is present, and the diagnosis of Cushing syndrome can be considered established, provided that conditions causing false-positive results (pseudo-Cushing syndrome) are excluded (acute or chronic illness, obesity, high-estrogen states, drugs, alcoholism, and depression). The CRH test is a useful adjunct in patients with borderline elevated urinary cortisol levels resulting from a probable pseudo-Cushing state. In patients with equivocal or borderline results, a 2-day low-dose dexamethasone suppression test is often performed (0.5 mg every 6 hours for eight doses). Normal responses to this test exclude the diagnosis of Cushing syndrome. Normal responses are an 8:00 AM plasma cortisol less than 5 μg/dL (138 nmol/L); a 24-hour urinary free cortisol less than 10 μg/24 h (<28 μmol/24 h); and a 24-hour urinary 17-hydroxycorticosteroid level less than 2.5 mg/24 h (6.9 μmol/24 h) or 1 mg/g creatinine (0.3 mmol/mol creatinine).

The second step is to distinguish ACTH-independent disease from ACTH-dependent disease (Figure 21–14) with assay of the plasma ACTH level. The high-dose dexamethasone suppression test is useful for differentiating pituitary from ectopic ACTH secretion.

The final step for patients with ACTH-dependent disease is to determine the anatomic localization of the ACTH source by MRI or thin-section CT (pituitary, adrenal, lung, or other) or, if equivocal, by inferior petrosal sinus sampling (IPSS) or cavernous sinus sampling (CSS).

CASE 114

A. An incidentally found adrenal mass is often referred to as an adrenal incidentaloma. The mass could be an adrenal adenoma or a non-adenoma, which could be a malignancy (primary adrenocortical carcinoma, pheochromocytoma, or a metastatic cancer from a different source), infiltrating process, hemorrhage, or cyst. The evaluation of an adrenal mass requires both a functional and an anatomic workup. The functional evaluation is to determine whether the mass is producing excess adrenal hormone by performing a dexamethasone suppression test (or 24-hour urine free cortisol) to exclude hypercortisolism, by measuring the plasma or urinary metanephrines to exclude pheochromocytoma, and by measuring the serum potassium and aldosterone-to-renin ratio to exclude hyperaldosteronism.

B. Anatomically, the lesion needs to be evaluated to determine level of concern for malignancy. Lesions like the one in this patient that are small (<3 cm), homogeneous, and low in signal intensity (<10 HU) are likely benign, lipid-rich adenomas. Lesions that are large (>6 cm), heterogeneous, and not low in signal intensity can be malignant. Lesions that are functional and those that do not fulfill the criteria for benignity are usually removed. Recommended monitoring for patients with a mass that is not definitively benign consists of one surveillance CT scan 6–12 months later to ensure that it is not enlarging, which would suggest malignancy. Clinical and/or hormonal re-evaluation can be repeated periodically if the patient develops symptoms consistent with a hyperfunctional adrenal tumor since nonfunctioning adenomas may (rarely) develop hormone overproduction at a later time.

CASE 115

A. Other symptoms of chronic adrenal insufficiency include anorexia, nausea, vomiting, hypoglycemia, and personality changes. The examiner should also look for orthostatic changes in blood pressure and pulse, hyperpigmentation of the mucous membranes and other areas, vitiligo, and loss of axillary and pubic hair.

B. The serum sodium is typically low and the serum potassium high. In Addison disease, the deficiency of cortisol is associated with a deficiency of aldosterone, resulting in an unregulated renal loss of sodium and a retention of potassium. Additional blood chemistry findings suggesting Addison disease include mild acidosis, azotemia, and hypoglycemia.

C. The diagnosis of hypoadrenocorticism can be established by performing an ACTH stimulation test. In Addison disease, there is a low 8:00 AM plasma cortisol and virtually no increase in plasma cortisol 30 minutes and 60 minutes after administering 250 μg of synthetic ACTH (cosyntropin) intravenously or intramuscularly. At a specificity of 95%, the sensitivity of the 250 μg cosyntropin stimulation test is 97% for primary adrenal insufficiency.

D. Hypotension, including recumbent hypotension, occurs in about 90% of patients with Addison disease and may cause orthostatic symptoms and syncope. These symptoms are related to the volume contraction resulting from unregulated renal sodium losses.

Cortisol deficiency commonly results in loss of appetite and in GI disturbances, including nausea and vomiting. Weight loss is common and, in chronic cases, may be profound (≥15 kg).

In primary adrenal insufficiency, the persistently low or absent plasma cortisol level results in a marked hypersecretion of ACTH by the pituitary. ACTH has intrinsic melanocyte-stimulating hormone activity, causing a variety of pigmentary changes in the skin, including generalized hyperpigmentation.

CASE 116

A. The major consequences of chronic aldosterone excess are sodium retention and potassium and hydrogen ion wasting by the kidney. Aldosterone binds to a mineralocorticoid receptor in the cytosol. The steroid–receptor complex then moves into the nucleus of the target cell and increases DNA transcription, mRNA induction, and protein synthesis stimulation by ribosomes. The aldosterone-stimulated proteins have two effects: a rapid effect, to increase the activity of epithelial sodium channels (ENaCs) by increasing the insertion of ENaCs into the cell membrane from a cytosolic pool, and a slower effect to increase the synthesis of ENaCs. One of the genes activated by aldosterone is the gene for serum- and glucocorticoid-regulated kinase (sgk), a serine-threonine protein kinase. The *sgk* gene product increases ENaC activity (Figure 21–10). Aldosterone also increases the mRNA for the three subunits that compose the ENaCs. Aldosterone also binds directly to distinct membrane receptors with a high affinity for aldosterone and, by a rapid, nongenomic action, increases the activity of membrane Na^+–K^+ exchangers to increase intracellular Na^+. In the distal renal tubules and collecting ducts, aldosterone acts to promote the exchange of Na^+ for K^+ and H^+, causing Na^+ retention, K^+ diuresis, and increased urine acidity. Elsewhere, it acts to increase the reabsorption of Na^+ from the colonic fluid, saliva, and sweat. Increased sodium is associated with fluid retention, blunting the hypernatremia. The net effect in primary aldosteronism is the mild hypernatremia, hypokalemia, and acidosis seen in this patient.

Hypertension results from the underlying sodium retention and subsequent expansion of plasma volume. The prolonged potassium diuresis produces symptoms of potassium depletion, including muscle weakness, muscle cramps, nocturia (frequent nighttime urination), and lassitude. A blunting of baroreceptor function, manifested by postural falls in blood pressure without reflex tachycardia, may develop.

B. Prolonged potassium depletion damages the kidney (hypokalemic nephropathy), causing a resistance to antidiuretic hormone (vasopressin). Patients may be unable to concentrate urine (nephrogenic diabetes insipidus), resulting in symptoms of thirst and polyuria and the finding of a low urine specific gravity (<1.010). Urinary electrolytes show an inappropriately large amount of potassium in the urine.

C. The diagnosis of primary aldosteronism is already suggested by finding hypokalemia in an untreated patient with hypertension. Currently, the best screening test for primary aldosteronism involves determining the plasma aldosterone concentration (normal: 1–16 ng/dL) and plasma renin activity (normal: 1–2.5 ng/mL/h) and calculating the plasma aldosterone–renin ratio (normal: <25). Patients with aldosterone–renin ratios of 30 or more require further evaluation.

Subsequent workup entails measuring the 24-hour urinary aldosterone excretion and the plasma aldosterone level with the patient on a diet containing more than 120 mEq of Na^+ per day. The urinary aldosterone excretion exceeds 14 µg/d, and the plasma aldosterone is usually more than 90 pg/mL in primary aldosteronism. High-resolution CT or MRI of the adrenal glands can also help to differentiate between **adrenal adenoma** and bilateral **adrenal hyperplasia**. The gold standard for diagnosis is bilateral adrenal venous sampling, which is more sensitive and specific than imaging, to identify a unilateral cause, namely an adrenal adenoma causing the primary aldosteronism.

CASE 117

A. This patient probably has hyporeninemic hypoaldosteronism (type IV renal tubular acidosis), a disorder characterized by hyperkalemia and acidosis in association with (usually mild) chronic kidney disease. The syndrome is thought to be due to an impairment of renin production by the juxtaglomerular apparatus, associated with underlying renal disease. Chronic kidney disease is usually not severe enough by itself to account for the hyperkalemia. The impaired secretion of both potassium and hydrogen ion in the renal tubule causes the observed hyperkalemia and metabolic acidosis.

B. Other causes of hypoaldosteronism include (1) bilateral adrenalectomy; (2) acute or chronic adrenocortical insufficiency; (3) the ingestion of exogenous mineralocorticoids (fludrocortisone) or inhibitors of the 11β-hydroxysteroid dehydrogenase type 2 enzyme (licorice), leading to sodium retention, volume expansion, and the suppression of renin production; (4) long-standing hypopituitarism, resulting in atrophy of the zona glomerulosa; (5) congenital adrenal hypoplasia, caused by one or more enzymatic abnormalities in mineralocorticoid biosynthesis; and (6) pseudohypoaldosteronism, in which there is renal tubular resistance to mineralocorticoid hormones, presumably because of a deficiency of mineralocorticoid hormone receptors.

C. Plasma and urinary aldosterone levels and plasma renin activity are consistently low and unresponsive to stimulation by ACTH administration, upright posture, dietary sodium restriction, and furosemide administration.

CASE 118

A. Congenital adrenal hyperplasia is a relatively common disease, occurring in 1 in 5000 to 1 in 15,000 births. By far, the most frequent cause of congenital adrenal hyperplasia is 21β-hydroxylase deficiency. During the newborn period, there are two classic presentations of congenital adrenal hyperplasia resulting from classic 21β-hydroxylase deficiency: salt wasting and non–salt wasting (also called "simple virilizing"). Neonates with the salt-wasting form have severe cortisol and aldosterone deficiencies and, if undiagnosed and untreated, will develop potentially lethal adrenal crisis and salt wasting at 2–3 weeks of age. Since this is a serious condition that is relatively common with a known treatment, it is sensible to screen newborns for this condition.

B. More than 90% of cases are due to a deficiency of the enzyme steroid 21β-hydroxylase. The 21β-hydroxylase enzyme (cytochrome P450c21) is encoded by the gene *CYP21A2*. More than 50 different *CYP21A2* mutations have been reported, perhaps accounting for a wide range of congenital adrenal hyperplasia phenotypes. The 15 most common mutations, which constitute 90–95% of alleles, derive from the intergenic recombination of DNA sequences between the *CYP21A2* gene and a neighboring pseudogene (an inactive gene that is transcribed but not translated). These intergenic *CYP21A2* mutations are caused by the conversion of a portion of the active *CYP21A2* gene sequence into a pseudogene sequence, resulting in a less active or inactive gene (gene conversion).

C. Impaired *CYP21A2* or *CYP11B1* activity causes deficient production of both cortisol and aldosterone. The low serum cortisol stimulates ACTH production; adrenal hyperplasia occurs, and precursor steroids—in particular 17-hydroxyprogesterone—accumulate. The accumulated precursors cannot enter the cortisol synthesis pathway and thus spill over into the androgen synthesis pathway, forming androstenedione and DHEA/DHEAS. Prenatal exposure to excessive androgens results in masculinization of the female fetus, leading to ambiguous genitalia at birth. Newborn males have normal genitalia.

CASE 119

A. The causes of amenorrhea may be classified into four broad categories: (1) normal physiologic processes, such as pregnancy and menopause; (2) disorders of the uterus or the pathway of menstrual flow, such as the destruction of the endometrium coupled with an intrauterine infection after curettage (Asherman syndrome); (3) disorders of the ovary, such as gonadal failure resulting from a range of chromosomal, developmental, and structural abnormalities; autoimmune disorders; premature follicle loss; and poorly understood syndromes in which ovarian follicles are resistant to gonadotropin stimulation; and (4) disorders of the hypothalamus or pituitary, resulting in either a lack of or disordered GnRH secretion and, as a consequence, insufficient ovarian steroid production. Causes of hypothalamic or pituitary dysfunction include prolactin-secreting tumors, hypothyroidism, excessive stress and exercise, and weight loss.

B. This patient likely has polycystic ovary syndrome (PCOS), evidenced by her obesity, amenorrhea, and hirsutism. But pregnancy must be ruled out since she has been sexually active with questionable birth control measures.

C. Patients with PCOS are often obese with hyperinsulinemia, insulin resistance, and dyslipidemia. In addition, they have elevated plasma androgen levels, together with elevated plasma estrogen levels. The predominant estrogen is estrone derived from the peripheral aromatization of adrenal androgens in the granulosa cell (by the enzyme aromatase [cytochrome P450, CYP19A1]).

Hyperinsulinemia is believed to be a key etiologic factor in PCOS. Insulin results in the decreased hepatic synthesis of steroid hormone-binding globulin (SHBG) and insulin-like growth factor binding protein-1 (IGFBP-1) (Figure 22–12). The decreased levels of these binding proteins result in an increase in free androgens, estrogens, and IGF-1. The high levels of insulin and IGF-1 stimulate the IGF-1 receptor, leading to increased thecal androgen production in response to LH, contributing to the hyperandrogenemia. The high androgen levels impede developing follicles and disrupt the feedback relationships that normally result in the selection of a dominant follicle for ovulation. The resulting anovulation is associated with amenorrhea and estrogen-induced endometrial hyperplasia with consequent breakthrough bleeding. The elevated estrogen levels are also implicated in the development of endometrial cancer. Thus, events occurring in the brain, ovary, and bloodstream of patients with PCOS work together to create a vicious cycle that maintains the aberrant feedback relationships.

CASE 120

A. Dysmenorrhea may be a primary disorder in which no identifiable pelvic disease is present, or it may be secondary to an underlying pelvic disease. Among the most common causes are endometriosis, leiomyomas, chronic pelvic infections, and adhesions from prior infections or ectopic pregnancies. Finally, dysmenorrhea may occur as a part of premenstrual syndrome, in which it is associated with other symptoms, including bloating, weight gain, edema, irritability, mood swings, and acne. This patient's constellation of symptoms in combination with her lack of prior medical problems and normal physical examination make premenstrual syndrome the most likely diagnosis.

B. Dysmenorrhea in premenstrual syndrome and in primary dysmenorrhea is due to disordered or excessive prostaglandin production by the secretory endometrium of the uterus. Patients with dysmenorrhea have an excessive production of prostaglandin $F_{2\alpha}$, which stimulates myometrial contractions of the uterus. Excessive contractions of the myometrium cause ischemia of the uterine muscle, thereby stimulating uterine pain fibers. Anxiety, fear, and stress may lower the pain threshold and thereby exaggerate the prominence of these symptoms from one patient to another and over time in a given patient.

C. The first step in treating patients with premenstrual syndrome is to encourage lifestyle changes such as more sleep,

exercise, improved diet, and discontinuation or decreased use of tobacco, alcohol, and caffeine. Pharmacologic therapy with selective serotonin reuptake inhibitors (SSRIs) has proven beneficial in addition to behavioral modification. Additionally, pain may be treated with monthly pharmacotherapy with prostaglandin synthesis inhibitors such as NSAIDs.

CASE 121

A. In an effort to standardize the nomenclature used to describe the causes of abnormal uterine bleeding, the International Federation of Gynecology and Obstetrics proposed a new classification system in 2011. This system encompasses the most common pathologies associated with abnormal uterine bleeding. It includes uterine **P**olyp, **A**denomyosis, **L**eiomyoma, **M**alignancy (and endometrial hyperplasia); **C**oagulopathy; **O**vulatory dysfunction; and **E**ndometrial, **I**atrogenic, and **N**ot yet classified causes. This now universally accepted nomenclature system is perhaps easily remembered by the acronym **PALM-COEIN**.

B. Unopposed estrogen exposure without progesterone in the perimenopausal or postmenopausal period can lead to endometrial hyperplasia. With continued estrogen excess, this endometrial hyperplasia can progress to endometrial cancer. Unopposed estrogen stimulation can occur because of (1) ovarian disorders (eg, chronic anovulation); (2) the enhanced peripheral aromatization of adrenal androgens by CYP19A1; or (3) estrogen therapy without adequate progestin supplementation.

C. In postmenopausal women, one-fifth of cases of vaginal bleeding prove to be endometrial cancer.

CASE 122

A. About 15% of couples are infertile. It is estimated that infertility is due to female factors about 30% of the time and that about 30% of cases are due to a combination of female and male factors. (About 30% of cases are due to male factors alone, and about 10% of cases are unexplained.) Forty percent of cases of female infertility are due to ovulatory failure, as occurs in hypothalamic, pituitary, and ovarian disorders. Another 40% of cases are due to endometrial or tubal disease, as occurs with pelvic infections and endometriosis. Ten percent are due to less common causes, such as those that affect the production of GnRH by the hypothalamus or the hormone's effect on the pituitary (thyroid disease, hyperprolactinemia) and those that affect ovarian feedback (hypergonadism, polycystic ovary disease). The final 10% of cases are of unknown cause.

B. The most likely cause of this patient's infertility is endometrial and tubal scarring as a result of her prior sexually transmitted infections. Infections such as gonorrhea and the often-asymptomatic chlamydial infections can cause scarring and adhesions. This scarring may impede sperm or egg transport and implantation. Her history of regular menses and her normal examination argue against the other causes of female infertility (other than idiopathic). Finally, it is possible that the infertility results from her husband (male factor infertility) and not the patient herself.

CASE 123

A. The most likely diagnosis is preeclampsia-eclampsia. Although preeclampsia can be difficult to differentiate from essential hypertension developing during pregnancy, the fact that the patient's hypertension developed after week 20 and was associated with edema and proteinuria strongly suggests a diagnosis of preeclampsia.

B. Predisposing factors for the development of preeclampsia include first pregnancy, multiple previous pregnancies, pre-existing diabetes mellitus or hypertension, hydatidiform mole, malnutrition, and a family history of preeclampsia.

C. For unclear (perhaps immune-mediated) reasons, changes that normally occur in the blood vessels of the uterine wall early in implantation do not occur in patients with preeclampsia-eclampsia. A condition of relative placental ischemia is established. Undetermined factors are released that cause damage to the vascular endothelium. This damage occurs first within the placenta and later throughout the body. Endothelial damage alters the balance between vasodilation and vasoconstriction, with increased vasoconstriction of small blood vessels and resultant hypoperfusion and ischemia of downstream tissues and systemic hypertension. The endothelial cell barrier between platelets and the collagen of basement membranes is breached. As a result of these changes, platelet aggregation increases, the clotting cascade is activated, and vasoactive substances are produced, causing capillary leak. Further tissue hypoperfusion, edema formation, and proteinuria result. These processes all cause further endothelial damage, thus establishing a vicious circle. Interesting recent speculation has centered on the potential of serotonin to modulate vasodilation or vasoconstriction, respectively, via the 5-HT_1 or 5-HT_2 serotonin receptors. New data also invoke a role for agonistic autoantibodies directed against the second extracellular loop of the angiotensin II AT1 receptor, resulting in the vasospasm associated with preeclampsia.

D. The risks to the fetus of preeclampsia-eclampsia are the consequence of placental deterioration and insufficiency and include intrauterine growth retardation and hypoxia.

E. Patients can develop multiple complications as a result of preeclampsia-eclampsia, including malignant hypertension, hepatic damage (periportal necrosis, congestion, and hemorrhage can lead to elevated liver function tests and ultimately rupture of the hepatic capsule), renal changes (glomerular endothelial cell swelling, mesangial proliferation, a marked narrowing of the glomerular capillary lumens, and cortical ischemia that may progress to frank necrosis and acute kidney injury), thrombocytopenia, disseminated intravascular coagulopathy, and cerebrovascular accidents. Eclampsia, or maternal seizures resulting from cerebral ischemia and petechial hemorrhage, can occur in this setting or can appear as the first manifestation of disease. Delivery of the fetus is the only definitive cure for this syndrome, which carries a high mortality rate for mother and child.

CASE 124

A. It is estimated that infertility is due to male factors in about 30% of cases and due to a combination of male and female factors in another 30%. Overall, of the cases due to male factors, approximately 50% are potentially treatable. Identifiable causes of male infertility are classified into three major categories: (1) pretesticular causes; (2) testicular causes; and (3) post-testicular causes. Pretesticular causes are generally hormonal in nature and include hypothalamic–pituitary disorders, thyroid disorders, adrenal disorders, and drugs that can affect hormonal secretion or action. Testicular causes may be chromosomal (Klinefelter syndrome) or developmental (cryptorchidism) or may result from varicocele, trauma, infection (mumps), or drugs and toxins. Post-testicular causes include ductal obstruction and scarring, retrograde ejaculation, antibodies to sperm or seminal plasma, developmental abnormalities (penile anatomic defects), androgen insensitivity, poor coital technique, and sexual dysfunction. Despite evaluation, many cases of male infertility are idiopathic in nature, without a currently identifiable cause.

B. Considering the history of sexually transmitted infections and the physical examination findings of epididymal irregularity, the most likely diagnosis is bilateral obstruction to sperm outflow.

C. Semen analysis should reveal oligospermia (<15 million sperm/mL semen) or, more likely, azoospermia (the absence of sperm). These abnormalities would be expected because the epididymal abnormalities on examination suggest bilateral obstruction to the outflow of sperm. LH, FSH, and testosterone should all be normal because no defects are present in the hypothalamic–pituitary axis or in the testes themselves.

D. Testing for fructose in the seminal fluid was once performed because fructose is produced in the seminal vesicles, and its absence in the semen implies an obstruction of the ejaculatory ducts. This test is currently used sparingly, with more emphasis placed on low semen volume as a screening test and transrectal ultrasound of the prostate as a confirmatory test. Obstruction of the ejaculatory ducts is strongly suggested by a seminal vesicle anteroposterior diameter of more than 1.5 cm on ultrasound. Testicular biopsy may also be helpful in distinguishing intrinsic testicular pathology from ductal obstruction.

CASE 125

A. The diagnosis of benign prostatic hyperplasia is suspected based on the history and physical examination. A symptom index questionnaire may be administered to the patient to objectively evaluate the severity and complexity of symptoms. Digital rectal examination reveals the prostatic enlargement. Prostatic enlargement may be focal or diffuse, and the degree of enlargement does not necessarily correlate with the degree of symptoms. Blood urea nitrogen and serum creatinine are measured to exclude renal failure, and urinalysis is performed to rule out infection. In most patients, this is enough to make the diagnosis of benign prostatic hyperplasia. A urodynamic evaluation with uroflowmetry and cystometry may be undertaken to assess the significance of the disorder. These pressure–flow studies can help determine which patients are less likely to benefit from prostatic surgery by providing information on detrusor function. Renal ultrasonography or intravenous urography may be performed on patients with hematuria or suspected hydronephrosis. Ultrasonography of the prostate with possible biopsy may be necessary to exclude prostate cancer as the cause of symptoms.

B. Although the actual cause of benign prostatic hyperplasia is unclear, several factors have been identified as contributing factors. These include age-related growth of the prostate, the presence of a prostatic capsule, androgenic hormones and their receptors (especially dihydrotestosterone), stromal–epithelial interactions and growth factors (FGF, TGF), and detrusor responses.

C. This patient has both irritative symptoms and obstructive symptoms. His irritative symptoms include urinary frequency, nocturia, and urgency. These occur as the result of bladder hypertrophy and dysfunction. His obstructive symptoms include incomplete emptying and postvoid dribbling. These are caused by distortion and narrowing of the bladder neck and prostatic urethra, leading to incomplete bladder emptying.

CASE 126

A. Gout flares are typically precipitated by a combination of metabolic and physical stressors in the setting of either urate underexcretion, seen in the vast majority of cases, or urate overproduction. The mild renal insufficiency may be associated with a decreased glomerular filtration rate and thus poor urate excretion. The recent addition of a diuretic further exacerbated this underlying impairment.

B. Multiple inflammatory pathways are invoked by the negatively charged urate crystals. For example, they activate the classic complement pathway whose cleavage products serve as effective neutrophil chemoattractants. The kinin system is stimulated by crystals as well, contributing to the inflammatory signs seen on examination, such as tenderness and erythema from local vasodilation. In addition, macrophages phagocytose urate crystals, initiating the release of proinflammatory cytokines (eg, IL-1, TNF1β, TNFα, IL-8, PGE2), which activate the vascular endothelium, encouraging neutrophil adhesion and migration. Neutrophils are able to simulate their own recruitment by releasing leukotriene B4 in response to urate crystal phagocytosis.

C. Therapy for an acute gouty attack should target the proinflammatory mediators described previously. NSAIDs such as ibuprofen reduce prostaglandin synthesis; colchicine impairs the migration of neutrophils into the joints; and corticosteroids deactivate myelomonocytic cells responsible for crystal phagocytosis and subsequent cytokine release. Because gouty flares are typically self-limited events, treatment is offered to alleviate symptoms and reduce the duration of the flare. On the other hand, probenecid (which is a uricosuric agent, inhibiting renal tubular urate resorption), allopurinol and febuxostat (which are xanthine oxidase inhibitors, interfering with the conversion of hypoxanthine and xanthine to uric acid), and pegloticase, (which converts uric acid to allantoin, an inactive and soluble metabolite readily excreted by the kidneys) are typically reserved for the prevention of future attacks.

CASE 127

A. This patient likely has an immune complex vasculitis. When it manifests itself in the skin, it is also called cutaneous small vessel or leukocytoclastic vasculitis.

B. Immune complexes are generated by the combination of an antigen and an antibody. In this case, the antigen is the penicillin that the person has been taking regularly for a week. The penicillin stimulated an antibody response, leading to antibody production against, and then binding to, the penicillin. The antigen–antibody complexes are soluble and are deposited in the subendothelial space; in this case, in the small vessels of the skin. There, they trigger an inflammatory response, which causes a rash. If the supply of new antigen is cut off (eg, by stopping the medication), the immune complexes are cleared by the immune system, and the process resolves.

C. The same process can also affect the joints and the kidneys, both areas rich in small blood vessels. The specific organ(s) affected depend on the solubility of the specific antigen–antibody complex.

CASE 128

A. This patient's suspicion that her arthralgias may be explained by lupus is supported by a high prevalence of systemic lupus erythematosus (SLE) among African American women—approximately 1 in 250—as well as her family history of this disorder. The symptoms are highly variable but tend to be stereotyped in a given individual (ie, the prominent clinical features often remain constant over years). Since SLE can affect many organs, it is important to do a thorough review of systems. Skin symptoms such as photosensitivity and a variety of SLE-specific skin rashes (including a rash over the malar region, discoid pigmentary changes to the external ear, and erythema over the dorsum of fingers) are common. Like those with other immune complex–mediated diseases, patients with SLE may manifest a nonerosive symmetric polyarthritis. Renal disease, which takes the form of a spectrum of glomerulonephritides, can present with hematuria or symptoms of renal failure. Patients may manifest a variety of hematologic disturbances (including hemolytic anemia, thrombocytopenia, and leukopenia), inflammation of serosal surfaces (including pleuritis, pericarditis, and peritonitis), as well as several neurologic syndromes (eg, seizures, organic brain syndrome).

B. Several environmental exposures have been definitively associated with disease initiation in SLE. These include sunlight exposure (associated with both disease onset and flares), viral infection (Epstein–Barr virus exposure is strongly associated with SLE in children), and certain drugs. These are agents to which humans are commonly exposed, suggesting that individuals who develop SLE have underlying abnormalities that render them particularly susceptible to disease initiation.

C. These mechanisms include (1) subendothelial deposition of immune complexes, in which antigens are derived from damaged or dying cells; (2) autoantibody binding to extracellular molecules in the target organs (eg, skin, joints, kidneys, blood elements), which activates inflammatory effector functions and induces damage at that site; and (3) the induction of cell death by autoantibodies.

D. The natural history of SLE is characterized by a relapsing, remitting course. Flares reflect immunologic memory, sparked by rechallenge of a primed immune system with antigen. Numerous stimuli such as viral infections, ultraviolet light exposure, and endometrial and breast epithelial involution may induce apoptosis, which resupplies immune-inciting antigens. Despite this course, 10-year survival rates commonly exceed 85%.

CASE 129

A. This patient has Sjögren syndrome, which occurs in approximately 1–3% of the adult population. Sjögren syndrome is approximately 9 times more prevalent in women than in men. Affected individuals frequently manifest intense dryness of the eyes (xerophthalmia) and mouth (xerostomia), giving rise to the alternative name keratoconjunctivitis sicca.

B. Dryness in the respiratory tract may give rise to hoarseness and recurrent bronchitis. Moreover, when immune activation is severe, patients experience systemic symptoms, including fatigue, arthralgia, myalgia, and low-grade fever. Other potentially affected organ systems include the kidneys, lungs, joints, and liver (resulting in interstitial nephritis, interstitial pneumonitis, nonerosive polyarthritis, and intrahepatic bile duct inflammation, respectively). As many as half of affected individuals experience autoimmune thyroid disease. Those patients with particularly severe disease are at increased risk for cutaneous vasculitis (including palpable purpura and skin ulceration) and lymphoproliferative disorders (eg, mucosa-associated lymphoid tissue [MALT] lymphoma).

CASE 130

A. The inflammatory myopathies, polymyositis and dermatomyositis, share several similar pathologic features but possess distinctive ones as well. These include patchy involvement, the presence of inflammatory infiltrates, and areas of muscle damage and regeneration. In polymyositis, inflammation is located around individual muscle fibers ("perimyocyte"), and the infiltrate is T cell (CD8+ > CD4+) and macrophage predominant. It has been suggested that the inflammation seen in polymyositis is driven by autoantigens expressed in the muscle environment, given the restricted T-cell repertoire in both circulating and muscle-infiltrating lymphocytes.

In dermatomyositis, the pathology looks quite different, although the outcome—profound muscle weakness—is the same. The major pathologic hallmarks of this condition include atrophy at the periphery of muscle bundles ("perifascicular atrophy") and a predominantly B-cell and CD4+ T-cell infiltrate localized to the perifascicular and perivascular space surrounding capillaries (which are reduced in number). Activation of the complement cascade is seen as well. Major involvement of the capillaries has led many experts to suggest that the primary disorder in dermatomyositis is a small-vessel vasculitis, with myositis occurring later as a result of tissue ischemia and repair. The characteristic skin and nail-fold capillary changes seen in patients with dermatomyositis lend support to this notion.

B. There are four characteristic criteria for the diagnosis of polymyositis: (1) weakness; (2) elevated laboratory parameters of muscle tissue (eg, creatine phosphokinase or aldolase); (3) an irritable electromyogram upon electrodiagnostic evaluation (producing sharp waves and spontaneous discharges); and (4) an inflammatory infiltrate upon histologic evaluation.

C. In adult patients, the new diagnosis of an inflammatory myopathy frequently heralds the co-occurrence or subsequent development (within 1–5 years) of a malignancy. The veracity of this observation has been confirmed in several population-based studies that link the diagnoses of dermatomyositis and polymyositis with various types of cancer in cancer registries. A diagnosis of dermatomyositis carries a twofold greater risk of incident malignancy, particularly cancers of the stomach, lung, breast, colon, and ovary.

CASE 131

A. The pathophysiology of rheumatoid arthritis is centered around the synovial linings of joints. The normal synovium is 1–3 cell layers thick. In rheumatoid arthritis, the synovium is markedly thickened and contains inflammatory cells in the interstitium, including T cells, B cells, and macrophages. This inflammatory tissue can invade adjacent bone and cartilage, accounting for the bony erosions and joint destruction.

B. Rheumatoid arthritis is thought to arise when an environmental factor (such as an infection) triggers an autoimmune response to antigens present in the synovium and elsewhere in the body. However, the specifics have not been identified. No definite infectious agents have been identified as causal agents in rheumatoid arthritis. The autoimmune mechanisms involved in triggering and maintaining the rheumatoid inflammatory response have also not been definitively identified, although TNF plays a central role. Genetic factors have been found, arising from the observation that identical twins have a 15–35% concordance rate of developing rheumatoid arthritis. A specific subset of MHC class II alleles has been found that determine disease development and severity.

C. For many years, the mainstay of treatment for rheumatoid arthritis involved nonspecific immunosuppressant agents. More recently, biologic modifiers of defined pathogenic pathways have been used successfully to treat disease. TNFα inhibitors were the first to be developed, and they function by sequestering TNFα so that it cannot maintain the inflammatory response. They are either soluble TNFα receptors or monoclonal antibodies that bind the free TNFα and clear it from the body. Similar therapeutic strategies have been used to block the inflammatory effects of IL-1β and IL-6, and new agents are being developed for still other RA-associated cytokines.

CASE 132

A. This patient likely has ankylosing spondylitis. This diagnosis is suggested by the age of presentation (he is in his 20s), early-morning stiffness, fatigue, low-grade fevers, previous episode of inflammatory eye disease (likely anterior uveitis), and his HLA-B27 positivity.

B. Although HLA-B27 has been linked to the spondyloarthropathies for decades, how it interfaces with the immune system to facilitate disease initiation and propagation remains unclear. One hypothesis is that "self" or foreign (microbial) antigens, bound to the HLA-B27 binding groove, may be recognized by the T-cell receptors of autoreactive CD8+ T cells, inciting an inflammatory response. An alternative hypothesis is that a misfolding of the B27 molecule within the cell results in endoplasmic reticulum stress that triggers an unfolded protein response and an upregulation of IL-23 cytokine levels. A third hypothesis is that, when expressed at the cell surface, B27 free heavy chains are recognized by cells bearing killer immunoglobulin-like receptors and trigger an inflammatory response.

The cytokine milieu is also an important component of the inflammation associated with this spondyloarthropathy. An emerging and prominent role for IL-17 and IL-23 has come to light in the pathogenesis of the spondyloarthropathies, particularly ankylosing spondylitis and psoriatic arthritis. Elevated levels of IL-12 have been detected as well. Genome-wide association studies have demonstrated a linkage between the IL-23 receptor and single nucleotide polymorphisms of the IL-12 receptor in ankylosing spondylitis. Further, an intergenic region between these two loci modulates enhancer activity and heightened levels of T_H1 cell differentiation. In addition, in patients with high disease activity, T_H17 cells have been detected in the circulation, spinal facet joints, and synovium. These activated cytokines and effector cells also play a role in bone resorption and remodeling.

C. Older, established agents used in the treatment of ankylosing spondylitis are anti-inflammatory drugs, including nonsteroidal anti-inflammatory agents, methotrexate, and sulfasalazine. Newer, more targeted agents that have more recently been approved by the FDA for the treatment of ankylosing spondylitis (and other spondyloarthropathies) include TNFα inhibitors (eg, etanercept, adalimumab), an IL-17A inhibitor (secukinumab), and a novel monoclonal antibody that targets IL-12 and IL-23 (ustekinumab).

Index